D1220918

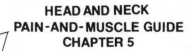

PART 1

HEAD AND NECK
PAIN-AND-MUSCLE GUIDE
CHAPTER 5

PART 2

UPPER BACK,
SHOULDER AND ARM
PAIN-AND-MUSCLE GUIDE
CHAPTER 18

PART 3

ELBOW TO FINGER
PAIN-AND-MUSCLE GUIDE
CHAPTER 33

PART 4

TORSO
PAIN-AND-MUSCLE GUIDE
CHAPTER 41

Pictorial index. The muscles that are likely to refer pain to an illustrated region of the body are listed in the Pain-and-muscle Guide to the corresponding Part of the *Manual*. A Guide is found at the beginning of each Part, which is marked by red thumb tabs.

VOLUME 1

Myofascial Pain and Dysfunction

The Trigger Point Manual

THE UPPER EXTREMITIES

This is the first of two planned volumes, and contains information relating to the "upper half" of the body. The proposed volume 2 will deal with the "lower half" of the body.

VOLUME 1

Myofascial Pain and Dysfunction

The Trigger Point Manual

THE UPPER EXTREMITIES

JANET G. TRAVELL, M.D.

Emeritus Clinical Professor of Medicine
The George Washington University School of Medicine
Washington, D.C.

DAVID G. SIMONS, M.D.

Clinical Professor
Department of Physical Medicine and Rehabilitation
University of California, Irvine

Clinical Chief
Electromyography and Electrodiagnosis Section
Rehabilitation Medicine Service
Veterans Administration Medical Center
Long Beach, California

Illustrations by Barbara D. Cummings

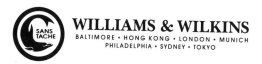

WILLIAMS & WILKINS
BALTIMORE • HONG KONG • LONDON • MUNICH
PHILADELPHIA • SYDNEY • TOKYO

Copyright ©, 1983
Williams & Wilkins
428 E. Preston Street
Baltimore, Md 21202, U.S.A.

All rights reserved. This book is protected by copyright. No part of this book may be reproduced in any form or by any means, including photocopying, or utilized by any information storage and retrieval system without written permission from the copyright owner. However, this book may be reproduced royalty free for United States Governmental purposes.

Accurate indications, adverse reactions, and dosage schedules for drugs are provided in this book, but it is possible that they may change. The reader is urged to review the package information data of the manufacturers of the medications mentioned.

Made in the United States of America

Library of Congress Cataloging in Publication Data

Travell, Janet, 1901–
  Myofascial pain and dysfunction, Volume 1.
  Includes index.
   1. Myalgia—Handbooks, manuals, etc. 2. Muscles—Diseases—Handbooks, manuals, etc. 3. Fasciae (Anatomy)—Diseases—Handbooks, manuals, etc. I. Simons, David G. II. Title. III. Title: Trigger point manual. [DNLM: 1. Myofascial Pain Syndromes. 2. Muscles. WE 500 T779m]
RC925.5.T7 1982   616.7′4   82-8555
ISBN 0-683-08366-X   AACR2

94 95 96 97
20

TO
Suzanne Hanson Poole
and
Ute M. Simons

whose enthusiastic support made this work possible.

Foreword

Rene Cailliet

At last a text is presented about the pain and dysfunction of myofascial tissues, a condition that confronts the medical practitioner daily, but remains poorly understood and frequently overlooked by the medical profession. Yet, patients continue to present themselves with symptoms that are attributable to myofascial trigger-point pathophysiology. These patients often fail to receive proper evaluation and, therefore, appropriate treatment.

"Trigger points" have been inadvertently discovered by patients, their spouses, therapists, nonmedical practitioners; yet, many of their physicians who have examined them, have attributed their condition to various etiologies, and treated them with ineffectual methods. Failure to achieve success has resulted in the assumption that patients in their noncompliance are the cause of failure, rather than therapeutic misguidance.

For decades, Janet Travell has labored to document the scientific basis of myofascial pain and dysfunction. Her clinical reports have been ridiculed and ignored by some, but believed and confirmed by many. Unfortunately, until this text, it has been mandatory to observe her and be directly involved in a presentation of her concepts and techniques, as numerous as they have been, by this indefatigable missionary. Too few have been privileged to observe and learn her techniques.

David Simons became an avid exponent of the Travell concepts, and performed a yeoman task in surveying the international literature and in supplying much needed neurophysiological verification in the clinic and in the laboratory. He, too, has been tireless in his efforts to train staff and residents under his tutelage in the techniques and documentation of myofascial pain.

Together, they have compiled a documentary which will be a classic for years to come. The format of their text is ideal in that it clarifies terminology, and clearly and scientifically identifies the anatomical basis of pain and dysfunction.

The medical education of today, and even the continuing medical education efforts currently employed, do not sufficiently instruct the clinician in functional anatomy, surface anatomy, kinesiology, and the techniques of evaluating this musculoskeletal aspect of the human body. Trauma is too simply considered to be the evidence of external contact, but is not documented as postural stress, occupational unphysiologic postures, or faulty mechanical activities of everyday living. Yet, these are important in the full evaluation and management of myofascial pain syndromes.

Examination of the patient today is also so dependent upon machines and equipment that the use of touch, palpation and manual examination of joints, muscles and ligaments remains a lost art. This art is resurrected in this text by Travell and Simons.

The text is, therefore, structured to depict the clinical aspects of the pain based always on the anatomical attachments and innervation of the involved neuromuscular unit. This is extremely well done and, per se, would be a classic text of kinesiology. Symptoms and signs are very clearly depicted, as is the examination of the patient. Treatment follows in a logical sequence based on the anatomical diagnosis and verification of the patterns of referred pain. Corrective measures are undertaken by the patient, which helps to insure relieving the pain and overcoming the dysfunction, and also to prevent recurrence.

The speciality of Physical Medicine and Rehabilitation, in fact, all medical orthopaedics and therapeutic neurology, will benefit from the clarification of this previously neglected modality and from this neurophysiological concept of musculoskeletal pain. The authors are sincerely thanked for their contribution and for their precise, readable, understandable, and applicable dissertation on this common human affliction.

Rene Cailliet, M.D.
Formerly, Professor and Chairman
Department of Rehabilitative Medicine
University of Southern California
School of Medicine
Los Angeles, California
Director,
Department of Rehabilitation Medicine
Santa Monica Hospital,
Santa Monica, California

Foreword

Parker E. Mahan

One of the most difficult and controversial diagnoses the practicing dentist must make is that of the temporomandibular joint dysfunction syndrome (TMJ) or myofascial pain dysfunction syndrome (MPD). Controversy still abounds in our literature and at professional meetings even though almost all involved therapists agree that head and neck muscles are affected in the syndromes. The champions of each concept of etiology tend to ignore or belittle the conflicting concepts as though there can be only one cause of TMJ-MPD problems.

The many factors that seem to be related to muscle pain with local spot tenderness in a tense band of muscle fibers are poorly understood by our profession. The role of referred pain from muscle trigger points in facial pain syndromes is often not considered when a diagnosis is made. Such factors as nutritional deficiencies, endocrine imbalances, chronic infection, allergy, psychological stress, nerve entrapment, congenital skeletal abnormalities and trauma to muscles are often overlooked when these unfortunate patients are examined and treated.

In many parts of our country the dentist cannot find health therapists in any field who are experienced at diagnosing and treating these muscle problems. Other therapists must be partners in the treatment of patients with etiological factors extending beyond the head and neck, and it becomes the responsibility of the knowledgeable dentist to motivate and educate his fellow health team members to study these diagnostic and treatment procedures.

The stretch and spray and anesthetic injection and other stretch treatment procedures used to relieve trigger point pain are similar to injection and manipulation procedures routinely practiced by the dentist. With his knowledge of muscle, blood vessel and nerve anatomy of the head and neck, the dentist can quickly become an expert at these treatment procedures.

This book deals with the examination, diagnosis and treatment of each head and neck muscle individually. It presents the basic concepts of muscle function and referred pain patterns that the therapist must know in order to manage these problems. The book reviews the various theories of TMJ-MPD syndromes and integrates the concept of muscle trigger point pain into each of these theories in a very logical way.

Drs. Travell and Simons are to be commended for their creative and detailed presentation of an important and often overlooked concept of muscle pain etiology and its treatment. The book is not only informative for the clinician but makes many heuristic points and will serve to stimulate further research into the many questions it identifies.

Parker E. Mahan, D.D.S., Ph.D.
Professor and Chairman
Department of Basic Dental Sciences
University of Florida
Gainesville, Florida

Preface

Myofascial trigger points are a frequently overlooked and misunderstood source of the distressingly ubiquitous musculoskeletal aches and pains of mankind. This manual, for the first time in the English language, assembles in one place the information necessary for the student and the practitioner to recognize and treat myofascial pain syndromes; appropriate therapy requires a correct diagnosis. This first volume presents the introductory general information on this subject and descriptions of the individual single-muscle syndromes for the upper half of the body.

In some patients, the myofascial pain is referred from trigger points in only one muscle. These single-muscle syndromes are easily managed. More often, the pain represents a composite pattern referred from several muscles; the practitioner must become a sleuth and recognize the component parts. Much of the detective work lies in tracking down not only what specific stress or stresses initiated the patient's trigger points, but also what *other* factors are perpetuating them. Chapter 4 of this manual presents, for the first time, a detailed consideration of the many perpetuating factors that may cause recurrence of pain after initial relief by specific myofascial therapy. The identification of these factors requires skillful medical detective work in areas that are often neglected or dismissed as unimportant.

This manual describes individually the component parts of the myofascial jigsaw puzzle. The reader must piece them together to fit the clinical picture of each patient, while remembering that no two persons are alike.

A handy index of muscle chapters, alphabetically arranged, is located inside the front cover.

Since the pain referred from most myofascial trigger points appears at some distance from the trigger point, the practitioner needs a guide to tell which muscles most commonly refer pain to a particular area of the body. The chapters in each of four parts of this volume concern those muscles that refer pain chiefly to one large region of the body. The pictorial index on the front fly leaf illustrates the four regions covered. Red thumb tabs separately identify each part, which begins with a pain-and-muscle guide. The guide illustrates the areas within that region and lists the muscles that are most likely to refer pain to each of those areas. For convenience, the pain-and-muscle guide also lists the number of the chapter that deals with each muscle.

Every muscle chapter is uniformly arranged with fourteen headings and begins with HIGHLIGHTS, a summary section that introduces the key points of the chapter. The sections of introductory Chapter 3, Apropos Of All Muscles, have the same fourteen numbered headings as does each muscle chapter. Thus, each section of Chapter 3 serves as a general introduction to the corresponding section for every muscle. It presents information applicable to all muscles. *Some of this information that is critical to the management of a patient's myofascial pain syndrome is not repeated in the muscle chapters.*

In recognition of the widespread interest of the dental profession in myofascial pain syndromes, Chapter 5 includes an extensive introduction to the masticatory muscles and their relationship to temporomandibular joint dysfunction. The individual masticatory muscles are discussed in Chapters 8 through 12.

This manual is the product of a remarkably close collaboration between the coauthors that evolved over nearly 2 decades. They brought together two very different backgrounds that were compatible and complementary. They learned to resolve their many differences of opinion by determining *what* was correct, not *who* was correct.

Dr. Travell describes in detail her introduction to myofascial trigger points in her autobiography, *Office Hours: Day and Night*. Although she was brought up on the unitary concept of disease that all of the patient's symptoms should be explained by one diagnosis, she soon learned that life is not like that. The man who has both heart disease and pulmonary tuberculosis may suddenly die of cancer of the lung. Patient complaints that originate in the musculoskeletal system usually have multiple causes responsible for the total picture.

Early in her medical career, Dr. Travell served simultaneously on a pulmonary, cardiology, and general medical service. On all the services, the major complaint she encountered among the patients was pain. The patient might be dying of a serious illness, but when asked, "How are you?" would answer, "Well, ok, except I have this terrible pain in my shoulder. I can't sleep. I can't lie on that side." When asked the cause of the pain, the resident on the pulmonary service would say that it was reflex from the lung. On the cardiology service, in another hospital, patients had the same complaint of shoulder pain, but the resident explained the pain as reflex from the heart, of course. In the general medical clinic, a secretary who spent all day typing and pulling heavy file drawers would describe precisely the same pain complaint; but its origin was said to be "psychosomatic." In none of these patients did the doctors find objective evidence of disease to account for the patient's pain, but the skeletal muscles had not been examined. When Dr. Travell examined these patients, all three groups had isolated tender spots in muscles which, when compressed, reproduced the patient's pain in the shoulder, arm or chest. The common ailment was an unrecognized myofascial trigger point syndrome.

Fortunately, these observations were made in an environment rich in experimental expertise. She regularly taught pharmacology to medical students whom, to answer their question, she inspired to perform the appropriate experiments for themselves in the laboratory. The inquisitive students and faculty at the Cornell University Medical College helped Dr. Travell formulate her investigation of the nature of trigger points and how they function.

She herself was inspired by the interchange of ideas and the criticism of leaders in basic and clinical research at the New York Hospital, Cornell Medical College Center. Foremost among these were Drs. Harry Gold, McKeen Cattell, Vincent du Vigneaud, Ephraim Shorr, Harold G. Wolff, Eugene F. Dubois, and the renowned neurologist, Frank Fremont-Smith, Director of the Josiah Macy Foundation. During the many years of their association, she was especially indebted to her cardiologist collaborator, Seymour H. Rinzler.

The successful care rendered Senator Kennedy 5 years prior to his election as President led Dr. Travell to the position of White House Physician under Presidents John F. Kennedy and Lyndon B. Johnson. Except for that one short detour, she has never strayed from her primary focus on the diagnosis and management of myofascial pain syndromes due to trigger points.

Dr. Simons and Dr. Travell met when she lectured at the School of Aerospace Medicine at Brooks Air Force Base in San Antonio, Texas, just a few years before he completed his military career as a United States Air Force Flight Surgeon pioneering aerospace medical research. The early years, between 1947 and 1951, were spent under the inspired guidance of James P. Henry, M.D. developing, for the first time, instrumentation techniques to monitor the physiological responses of animals while weightless in suborbital rocket flights.

Later, stationed at Holloman Air Force Base, he explored the stress factors and radiation hazards of a space-like environment using high altitude balloon flights. This culminated in his Man High flight to the edge of space (pre-Sputnik). It set a world altitude record in 1957 for manned balloon flight.

Before completing his Air Force career, Dr. Simons directed another laboratory that pioneered the development of personalized telemetry (including the electroencephalogram) to measure the physiological responses of crew members to stresses during flight. He was exploring computer analyses of the relations among reflex responses in multiple physiological measures.

After retiring from the Air Force in 1965, Dr. Simons became chief of the Physiometrics Research Laboratory at the Houston Veterans Administration Hospital. He also was responsible for monitoring and stimulating research in physical medicine and rehabilitation for the Central Office of the Veterans Administration. This responsibility took him frequently to Washington, D.C. where Dr. Travell lived. About once a month, he visited her to discuss the nature of trigger points. She, in turn, went to his laboratory in Houston, several times where they recorded experiments.

Deciding, in 1970, that he would now focus on the clinical and pathophysiological characteristics of myofascial pain syndromes, Dr. Simons trained as a resident in physical medicine and rehabilitation in Dr. Justus Lehmann's program, Seattle, Washington.

Following his appointment to the Rehabilitation Medicine Service at the Veterans Administration Hospital at Long Beach in 1974, he immediately established a close working relationship with Dr. Travell through her frequent visits to lecture on the West Coast. A research and training fund given by friends, Suzanne Hanson Poole and her mother, Adelyn Hanson, for training materials handed out to the University of California, Irvine, residents at the Long Beach Veterans Administration Hospital and also for Dr. Travell's repeated trips that were required for the initial stages of writing this manual. The fourth essential member joined the team when Barbara D. Cummings began making illustrations for this book in September 1977.

The authors recognize great indebtedness to their respective physician fathers for the aura of mystery and excitement that they cast over the practice of medicine. They owe an especially deep debt of gratitude to Michael D. Reynolds, M.D., and June S. Rothberg, Ph.D., for their dedicated meticulous review of the entire manuscript and express appreciation to Rene Cailliet, M.D., for his critical review of selected muscle chapters. The authors are grateful to A. J. Nielsen, R.P.T., for his endless enthusiasm and willing participation as the subject in pictures from which many of the drawings were made. They thank Richard Marlink, M.D., who, when still a medical student, helped greatly to organize the early chapters. W. R. (Paul) Patterson, M.D. provided inspirational discussions and shared his clinical expertise with us, and Earle Davis, M.D. kindly extended privileges for the anatomical dissection of cadavers.

The undersigned wish to mention the secretaries who labored over the text: Donna Murray, Topaz Emery, Terry Hacker, Ann Starbuck, Barbara Zastrow and Celine Humphrey. Members of Medical Media at the Veterans Administration Medical Center, Messrs. John Newby, Robert Walker and Walter Thill, and Mrs. Phyllis Kirkbride, helpfully provided us with needed photographic services. The librarians who retrieved the numerous references deserve a special word of appreciation: Ute M. Simons, Ann Gupta, Karen Vogel and Betty Connolly.

Dr. Simons especially thanks his residents at the Long Beach Veterans Administration Hospital for their penetrating and stimulating questions. He also expresses deep appreciation to William A. Spencer, M.D. for essential support at a critical time, and to Ralph Bodfish, M.D. and to Herbert Kent, M.D. for their encouragement and administrative support. We are grateful for Mrs. Adelyn Hanson's support.

Special gratitude is expressed for the considerable effort expended by the dentists who reviewed the chapters dealing with the masticatory muscles: Drs. Samuel H. Adams, II, John Ingle, Parker E. Mahan, Douglas H. Morgan, Yale S. Palchick, Eric Paul Shaber, William A. Solberg and Wayne Thompson.

Helpful advice and assistance with a number of preliminary drawings was provided by Richard Oden. We reserve until last the expression of our deepest respect and gratitude to the artist, Barbara D. Cummings, for seemingly inexhaustible patience with us and unending concern for the accuracy of the smallest details. She never failed to generate an ingenious solution to the most vexing of problems, and always with a smile!

Janet G. Travell, M.D.
David G. Simons, M.D.

Contents

PART 1

PART 2

PART 3

PART 4

PART 3

PART 4

PART 1

PART 2

PART 3

PART 4

CHAPTER 1
Glossary

The glossary comes first: to make sure that the reader knows what a term means as it is used in this manual, and to help the reader become acquainted with unfamiliar terms. The glossary is in front to encourage frequent reference to it, whenever it is needed. Comments concerning a definition are added in italics.

Abduction: Movement away from the midline. For **fingers**, it is movement away from the midline of the middle digit. For the **thumb**, it is movement perpendicular to, and away from, the plane of the palm. For the **hand**, at the wrist, it is radial deviation of the hand, which is away from the midline of the body in the anatomical position of the hand. For the **arm**, at the shoulder, abduction raises the elbow away from the body sideways until the elbow is overhead. For the **scapula**, it is rotation to make the glenoid fossa face upward, as the scapula glides across the chest wall away from the midline.

Active Range of Motion: The extent of movement (usually expressed in degrees) of an anatomical part at a joint when the movement is produced only by voluntary effort of that part of the body being tested.

Active Myofascial Trigger Point: A focus of hyperirritability in a muscle or its fascia that is symptomatic with respect to pain; it refers a pattern of pain at rest and/or on motion that is specific for the muscle. An active trigger point is always tender, prevents full lengthening of the muscle, weakens the muscle, usually refers pain on direct compression, mediates a local twitch response of muscle fibers when adequately stimulated, and often produces specific referred autonomic phenomena, generally in its pain reference zone. *To be distinguished from a latent myofascial trigger point.*

Acute: Of recent onset (hours or days).

Adduction: Movement toward the midline. For **fingers**, it is movement toward the midline of the middle digit. For the **thumb**, it is movement perpendicular to, and toward, the plane of the palm. For the **hand**, it is ulnar deviation at the wrist. For the **arm**, at the shoulder, it is movement of the elbow to the flank in the frontal plane from the abducted position of the arm. For the **scapula**, it is rotation to make the glenoid fossa face downward, as the scapula glides across the chest wall toward the midline.

Agonists: Muscles, or portions of muscles, so attached anatomically that when they contract, they develop forces that reinforce each other.

Antagonists: Muscles, or portions of muscles, so attached anatomically that when they contract, they develop forces that oppose each other.

Associated Myofascial Trigger Point: A focus of hyperirritability in a muscle or its fascia that develops in response to compensatory overload, shortened range, or referred phenomena caused by trigger-point activity in another muscle. *Satellite and secondary trigger points are types of associated myofascial trigger points.*

Bruxism: Grinding or gnashing of the teeth when not masticating or swallowing.[2]

Centric Occlusion: The position of jaw closure with full tooth contact (maximum intercuspation). *It is defined more formally as:* the centered contact position of the occlusal surfaces of the mandibular teeth against the occlusal surfaces of the maxillary teeth.[1]

Centric Relation: The most retruded position of the mandible from which it can make lateral excursions.[1]

1

Chronic: Long-standing (weeks, months or years), but NOT necessarily incurable. *Symptoms may be mild or severe.*

Composite Pain Pattern: Total referred pain pattern of two or more closely adjacent muscles. *No distinction is made among the pain patterns of the individual muscles.*

Contracture: Sustained intrinsic activation of the contractile mechanism of the muscle fibers. With contracture, muscle shortening occurs in the absence of motor unit action potentials. *This physiological definition, as used in this manual, must be differentiated from the clinical definition, which is shortening due to fibrosis. Contracture also must be distinguished from spasm.*

EMG: Electromyographic.

Essential Pain Zone (Area): The region of referred pain (indicated by solid red areas in pain pattern figures) that is constantly present in nearly every patient when the trigger point is active. *To be distinguished from a spillover referred pain zone.*

Fibrositis: *A term with multiple meanings. Some authors use it to identify myofascial trigger points. Other authors use the term very differently (see Chapter 2). We avoid using the term because of its ambiguity.*

Flat Palpation: Examination by finger pressure that proceeds across the muscle fibers at a right angle to their length, while compressing them against a firm underlying structure, such as bone. *It is used to detect taut bands and trigger points. To be distinguished from pincer and snapping palpation.*

Horizontal Extension: Movement of the arm backward toward the back of the chest, starting at 90° of abduction at the shoulder.

Horizontal Flexion: Movement of the arm toward the front of the chest, starting at 90° of abduction at the shoulder.

Incisal Path: The path of a point in the groove between the lower central incisor teeth in relation to the saggital plane as the jaws are opened and closed.

Interfering Occlusal Contact: An initial contact of teeth that stops or deviates the arc of closure of the mandible between centric relation and centric occlusion.[1, 4]

Involved Muscle: A muscle that has developed one or more active or latent trigger points.

Ischemic Compression: (also Acupressure, Myotherapy, Shiatzu, "Thumb" Therapy): Application of progressively stronger, painful pressure on a trigger point for the purpose of eliminating the point's tenderness. *This action blanches the compressed tissues, which usually become hyperemic (flushed) on release of the pressure.*

Jump Sign: A general pain response of the patient, who winces, may cry out, and may withdraw in response to pressure applied on a trigger point. *At one time, we erroneously used this term to describe the local twitch response of muscle fibers to trigger-point stimulation.*

Latent Myofascial Trigger Point: A focus of hyperirritability in muscle or its fascia that is clinically quiescent with respect to spontaneous pain; it is painful only when palpated. *A latent trigger point may have all the other clinical characteristics of an active trigger point, from which it is to be distinguished.*

Local Twitch Response: Transient contraction of the group of muscle fibers (usually a palpable band) that contains a trigger point. The contraction of the fibers is in response to stimulation (usually by snapping palpation or needling) of the same, or sometimes of a nearby trigger point. *The local twitch response has erroneously been called a jump sign.*

MCP: Metacarpophalangeal (joint).

Muscular Rheumatism (Muskel Rheumatismus): Muscular pain and tenderness attributed to "rheumatic" causes (especially exposure to cold), as distinguished from articular rheumatism. *Often used as synonymous with myofascial trigger points.*

Myalgia: Pain in a muscle or muscles.[2] It is used in two ways, to signify: (1) diffusely aching muscles due to systemic disease, such as a virus infection; and (2) the spot tenderness of a muscle or muscles as in myofascial trigger points. *The reader must distinguish which use an author has in mind.*

Myofascial Pain-dysfunction Syndrome: A term widely used by the dental profession to identify facial (craniomandibular) pain with a significant myofascial component. The syndrome is characterized by preauricular pain; muscle tenderness; joint clicking or popping, which is often unilateral; and limitation or distortion of jaw movement.

Myofascial Pain Syndrome: Synonymous with Myofascial Syndrome and with Myofasciitis.

Myofascial Syndrome: Pain and/or autonomic phenomena referred from active myofascial trigger points with associated dysfunction. The specific muscle or muscle group that causes the symptoms should be identified.

Myofascial Trigger Point: A hyperirritable spot, usually within a taut band of skeletal muscle or in the muscle's fascia, that is painful on compression and that can give rise to characteristic referred pain, tenderness, and autonomic phenomena. A myofascial trigger point is to be distinguished from cutaneous, ligamentous, periosteal and nonmuscular fascial trigger points. Types include active, latent, primary, associated, satellite and secondary.

Myofasciitis: Pain, tenderness, other referred phenomena, and the dysfunction attributed to myofascial trigger points.

Myogelosis: Circumscribed firmness and tenderness to palpation in a muscle or muscles. The name is derived from the concept that the regions of circumscribed firmness were due to localized gelling of muscle proteins. Focal tenderness and palpable taut muscle fibers are also characteristic of myofascial trigger points. Most patients diagnosed as having myogelosis also would be diagnosed as having myofascial trigger points.

Myotatic Unit: A group of agonist and antagonist muscles, which function together as a unit because they share common spinal-reflex responses. The agonist muscles may act in series, or in parallel.

Occlusal Disharmony: Occlusal contacts that interfere with centric occlusion of the teeth or with functional mandibular excursions from centric occlusion.[4, 6] Includes interceptive and deflective occlusal contacts.

Occlusal Interference: Premature occlusal contact that prevents full (balanced and stable) centric occlusion of the teeth. Synonymous with occlusal disharmony.

Palpable Band (Taut Band, or Nodule): The group of taut muscle fibers that is associated with a myofascial trigger point and is identifiable by tactile examination of the muscle. Contraction of the fibers in this band produces the local twitch response.

Passive Range of Motion: The extent of movement (usually tested in a given plane) of an anatomical part at a joint when movement is produced by an outside force without voluntary assistance or resistance by the subject. The subject must relax the muscles crossing the joint.

Pincer Palpation: Examination of a part by holding it in a pincer grasp between the thumb and fingers. Groups of muscle fibers are rolled between the tips of the digits to detect taut bands of fibers, to identify tender points in the muscle, and to elicit local twitch responses. To be distinguished from flat and snapping palpation.

Primary Myofascial Trigger Point: A hyperirritable spot within a taut skeletal muscle band that was activated by acute or chronic overload (mechanical strain) of the muscle in which it occurs, and was not activated as a result of trigger-point activity in another muscle of the body. To be distinguished from secondary and satellite trigger points.

Reactive Cramp: Synonymous with shortening activation.

Reference Zone: see **Zone of Reference**

Referred Autonomic Phenomena: Vasoconstriction (blanching), coldness, sweating, pilomotor response, ptosis, and/or hypersecretion that is caused by activity of a trigger point in a region separate from the trigger point. The phenomena usually appear in the same area to which that trigger point refers pain.

Referred (Trigger-Point) Pain: Pain that arises in a trigger point, but is felt at a distance, often entirely remote from its source. The pattern of referred pain is reproducibly related to its site of origin. The distribution of referred trigger-point pain rarely coincides with the entire distribution of a peripheral nerve or dermatomal segment.

Referred (Trigger-Point) Phenomena: Sensory and motor phenomena, such as, pain, tenderness, increased motor unit activity (spasm), vasoconstriction, vasodilatation, and hypersecretion caused by a trigger point, which usually occur at a distance from the trigger point.

Rest Position (Myocentric Relation): The relation of the mandible to the maxilla when the muscles of the jaws are at their most relaxed length, placing the condyles in their most unstrained position.[1, 3, 5]

Satellite Myofascial Trigger Point: A focus of hyperirritability in a muscle or its fascia that became active because the muscle was located within the zone of reference of another trigger point. To be distinguished from a secondary trigger point.

Screening Palpation: Digital examination of a muscle to determine the absence, or presence, of palpable bands and tender trigger points using flat and/or pincer palpation.

Secondary Myofascial Trigger Point: A hyperirritable spot in a muscle or its fascia that became active because its muscle was overloaded as a synergist substituting for, or as an antagonist countering the tautness of, the muscle that contained the primary trigger point. To be distinguished from a satellite trigger point.

Shortening Activation: Activation of latent myofascial trigger points by unaccustomed shortening of a muscle during stretch therapy of its antagonist. The activated latent trigger points increase antagonist muscle tension and can cause severe referred pain.

Snapping Palpation: A fingertip is placed against the tense band of muscle at right angles to the direction of the band and suddenly presses down while drawing the finger back so as to roll the underlying fibers under the finger. The motion is similar to that used to pluck a guitar string, except that contact with the surface is maintained. To most effectively elicit a local twitch response, the band is palpated and snapped at the trigger point, with the muscle at a neutral length or slightly longer. To be distinguished from flat and pincer palpation.

Spasm: Increased tension with or without shortening of a muscle due to non-voluntary motor nerve activity. Spasm cannot be stopped by voluntary relaxation. To be distinguished from contracture.

Spillover Pain Zone (Area): The region where some, but not all, patients experience referred pain beyond the essential pain zone, due to greater hyperirritability of a trigger point. The spillover zone is indicated by red stippling in the pain-pattern figures. To be distinguished from an essential referred pain zone.

Synergistic Muscles: Muscles that reinforce each other when they contract.

Thoracic Outlet: The triangular aperture bounded anteriorly by the scalenus anterior muscle, posteriorly by the scalenus medius muscle, and below by the first rib.

TMJ: Temporomandibular joint.

TP: Trigger point.

TPs: Trigger points.

Trigger Point (Trigger Zone, Trigger Spot, Trigger Area): A focus of hyperirritability in a tissue that, when compressed, is locally tender and, if sufficiently hypersensitive, gives rise to referred pain and tenderness, and sometimes to referred autonomic phenomena and distortion of proprioception. Types include myofascial, cutaneous, fascial, ligamentous and periosteal trigger points.

Zone of Reference: The specific region of the body at a distance from a trigger point, where the phenomena (sensory, motor, autonomic) that it causes are observed.

References

1. Adisman IK, et al.: Glossary of prosthodontic terms. J Prosthet Dent 38:70–109, 1977 (pp. 75).
2. Agnew LRC, et al.: Dorland's Illustrated Medical Dictionary, Ed. 24. W.B. Saunders, Philadelphia, 1965.
3. Jankelson B: Neuromuscular aspects of occlusion. Dent Clin North Am 23:157–168, 1979.
4. Mahan PE: Personal communication, 1981.
5. Morgan DH: Personal communication, 1981.
6. Shaber EP: Personal communication, 1981.

CHAPTER 2
Background and Principles

HIGHLIGHTS: The first section, **BACKGROUND**, reviews some of the literature on myofascial trigger points (TPs), which includes a multitude of related terms. Some are nearly synonymous, while others have accrued a confusing diversity of additional meanings. The most distinctive **CLINICAL CHARACTERISTICS OF MYOFASCIAL TRIGGER POINTS** include a typical pattern of pain referred from the TP and, on examination, local spot tenderness (the TP) in a palpably tense band of muscle fibers within a muscle that is shortened and weak. The TP also may respond to rapid changes of pressure with the pathognomonic local twitch response. The **DIFFERENTIAL DIAGNOSIS** must distinguish other sources of similar pain. The **MECHANISMS OF TRIGGER POINTS** remain controversial. Electromyographic, clinical, and experimental evidence all suggest that a myofascial TP, which begins with muscular strain, becomes the site of sensitized nerves, increased metabolism and reduced circulation. This initial neuromuscular dysfunction phase, if untreated, may progress to a dystrophic phase that causes demonstrable histological changes in the muscle.

A. BACKGROUND

Importance

Voluntary (skeletal) muscle is the largest single organ of the human body and accounts for 40% or more of body weight.[13, 95, 152] The number of muscles counted in the body depends on the degree of subdivision that is considered a muscle, and on the number of variable muscles that are included. Bardeen[13] quoted the *Basle Nomina Anatomica* as recognizing 347 paired, and 2 unpaired muscles for a total of 696 muscles. Not counting heads, bellies and other parts of muscles, the *Nomina Anatomica* reported by the International Anatomical Nomenclature Committee under the Berne Convention,[121] list 200 paired muscles, or a total of 400 muscles. Any one of these muscles can develop myofascial trigger points (TPs) that refer pain and other distressing symptoms, usually to a remote location.

Yet the muscles receive little attention in modern medical school teaching and medical textbooks. This manual describes a neglected, major cause of pain and dysfunction in the largest organ of the body.

The contractile muscle tissues are extremely subject to the wear and tear of daily activities, but it is the bones, joints, bursae and nerves on which physicians usually concentrate their attention.

Prevalence. Myofascial TPs are extremely common and become a distressing part of nearly everyone's life at one time or another. *Latent* TPs, which may cause some stiffness and restricted range of motion, are far more common than *active* TPs.

Among 200 unselected, asymptomatic young adults, Sola et al.[241] found focal tenderness representing latent TPs in the shoulder-girdle muscles of 54% of the female, and 45% of the male subjects. Referred pain was demonstrated in 5% of these subjects. No comparable study of the prevalence of latent TPs in symptom-free groups of other ages has been reported.

In a population of hospitalized and ambulatory Physical Medicine and Rehabilitation Service patients, with the fibrositis syndrome (TPs), the greatest number were between 31 and 50 years of age.[139] These data agree with our clinical impression that individuals in their mature years of

5

maximum activity are most likely to suffer from the pain syndromes of active myofascial TPs. With advancing age and reduced activity, the stiffness and restricted range of motion of latent TPs become more prominent than pain.

The importance of myofascial TPs has been described in the literature on acupuncture,[101, 167] anesthesiology,[26, 34] dentistry,[20, 145, 265] general practice,[76, 190] orthopaedics,[8, 15, 54] pediatrics,[16] physical therapy,[186, 187] rehabilitation medicine,[38, 139, 209, 269, 290, 298] and rheumatology.[202, 256]

Severity. The severity of symptoms from myofascial TPs ranges from painless restriction of motion due to latent TPs, so common in the aged, to agonizing incapacitating pain caused by very active TPs. The potential severity of this common malady is illustrated by one housewife who, while bending over cooking, activated a quadratus lumborum TP that felled her to the floor and caused pain so severe that she was unable to reach up and turn the stove off to prevent a pot from burning through its bottom.

Patients who have had other kinds of severe pain, such as that due to a heart attack, broken bones, or renal colic, say that the myofascial pain from TPs can be just as severe. Despite their painfulness, myofascial TPs are not directly life threatening, but their painfulness can, and often does, devastate the quality of life.

Cost. Unrecognized myofascial headache, shoulder pain and low back pain that have become chronic are major causes of industrial lost time and compensation applications. Bonica[28] pointed out that disabling chronic pain costs the American people billions of dollars annually. Low back pain alone cost the people of California $200 million. Analgesics to relieve chronic pain are costly and a significant cause of nephropathy.[81] The considerable portion of chronic pain due to myofascial TPs can be relieved by their diagnosis and appropriate treatment.

How many more people are there, who do carry on, yet bear the misery of nagging TP pain that would respond, if diagnosed and treated for what it is? When the myofascial nature of pain is unrecognized, such as the mimicking of cardiac pain by TPs in the pectoral muscles, the symptoms are likely to be diagnosed as neurotic,[32]

adding frustration and self-doubt to the patient's misery. Active myofascial TPs are largely responsible for that scourge of mankind, musculoskeletal pain. The total cost is enormous.

Historical Review

Why should so common and serious a problem be so neglected by modern medicine? A look at the past literature helps to answer this question.

The large and confusing literature on muscle pain syndromes includes many terms used to describe only a part of the myofascial trigger point picture, and often includes other conditions as well. Many authors have contributed different pieces to this jigsaw puzzle, but few have presented a complete picture. Two key pieces of the picture that remain controversial are the pathophysiological nature of the TP itself, and what it is that makes palpable bands palpable. Simons[227] reviewed and summarized the literature on muscle pain syndromes, selecting only 85 references from a much larger field. Recently, Reynolds[203] reviewed the subject more extensively, selecting over 100 representative references. The literature was already extensive early in this century; in 1920, Port cited 78 references.[196]

Clinical interest in pain of muscular origin has ebbed and flowed through the years as new names and new concepts of its cause have come and gone. In 1843, Froriep[71] used the term "Muskelschwiele," or muscle callouses, to identify occasionally tender spots in muscle that felt like a tendinous cord, or a wide band, and were related to serious rheumatic pain complaints. The name and idea of serous exudation were conceptually combined by subsequent authors with an 1852 paper of Virchow[280] attributing such changes to muscular rheumatism or rheumatic fever. By 1898 Strauss[253] concluded that anatomical studies had failed to substantiate a "callus" of deposited connective tissue to account for the hard cords palpable in painful muscles. Meanwhile, the work of Helleday[110] in Sweden focused clinicians' attention on tender points and nodules in muscles.

A similar wave of interest was evolving in the English-language literature. A 1904 paper on lumbago by Gowers[92] introduced the term fibrositis as a more specific name than muscular rheumatism because he attributed the local tenderness and regions of palpable hardness in the muscle to inflammation of fibrous tissue. He assumed that sciatica was due to fibrositis and described fibrositis of the arm (frozen shoulder), of the back, and of other locations. Stockman,[249] in the same year, attributed similar symptoms to connective tissue hyperplasia, which he illustrated histologically. In 1915, Llewellyn and Jones[151] sanctified this union of Gower's term and Stockman's tissue changes by publishing a book, *Fibrositis*, that entrenched the term in the language and confused its definition. It included, as fibrositis, unmistakable descriptions of rheumatoid arthritis and gout, as well as myofascial pain syndromes. However, inflammatory pathology of connective tissue was not substantiated as the cause of most cases of fibrositis in subsequent biopsy studies.[1, 46, 235, 278] This led to the concept of "fibrositis" as a wastebasket term, useful to describe pain of non-organic origin.[285] Fibrositis remains a term in search of redefinition and continues to welcome diagnoses by default.

In Germany, studies by a medical officer during World War I initiated a new cycle. In 1919, Schade[219] reported the persistence of tender hardenings in muscles during deep anesthesia and after death until rigor mortis. This finding discredited a nerve-activated, muscular contraction mechanism as the cause of the palpable bands. Schade[219a] later postulated an increase in the viscosity of muscle colloid and proposed the term "Myogelose," translated as "myogelosis." In the same year, an orthopaedic surgeon in Munich, F. Lange, and G. Eversbusch[143] described tender points associated with regions of palpable hardness in muscles, which he termed "Muskelhärten," translated as "muscle hardenings" or "indurations." His student, M. Lange,[144] later equated these muscle hardenings to Schade's myogeloses and described the hardened part of the muscle as having the consistency of muscle in rigor mortis. He used fingers, knuckles, or a blunt wood probe to apply forceful massage (Gelotripsie), which was therapeutically effective. His 1931 book[144] presented the history and experimental basis of the concept of myogelosis. The book described

many pain syndromes associated with specific tender muscles, illustrated the location of hardenings in many muscles, and included 41 patient examples.

Two German studies that will be described later reported 24 biopsies in 1951,[79] and 77 biopsies in 1960.[173] Both studies found characteristic non-specific changes by light microscopy.

Before 1938, only a few authors recognized that, characteristically, pain was referred to a distance from the tender spot (myofascial TP) in the muscle.[51, 110, 249] Either the close relationship was overlooked, or the distant pain was attributed to an associated "neuralgia."[279]

Kellgren,[125] in 1938, reported that many of his patients experienced referred pain in areas remote from the tender points in the muscle that were causing the pain. He explored what tissues, including individual muscles, referred pain to a distance in the body. Working with Sir Thomas Lewis,[150a] and often using himself as a subject, he established the scientific credibility of referred pain arising in skeletal muscles.[124] He injected 0.1–1.3 ml of 6% hypertonic saline into many major muscles. Pain often appeared in remote portions of the same limb or, at times, several spinal segments away from the site of injection. Since the complexity of the spinal cord and the extensive sensory interconnections between segments were not known at that time,[131] Kellgren and his peers assumed that the referred pain was transmitted by the peripheral nerves of the same segment as that stimulated, but recognized that the pain also must have a "common path" in the central nervous system when several spinal segments were included.

The course of the history of muscle pain syndromes took a new tack when three authors blossomed independently on three continents immediately after Kellgren's work. Successive papers of each author increasingly identified a patient's pain with a specific muscle rather than a group of muscles. Each reported pain syndromes of muscles throughout the body in a large number of patients. One of the three, Gutstein, was born in Poland and first published in German.[103] He moved to Great Britain where he published in English as Gutstein-Good,[107] and then as Good.[83] He referred to the tender TP areas as "myalgic spots" and described the referred pain patterns of muscles. He also called attention to the patient's pain reaction, which was later termed the "jump sign."[139] In the 12 or more papers that he wrote between 1938[103] and 1957,[87] he repeatedly held that the process responsible for "myalgic spots" was a local constriction of blood vessels due to overactivity of the sympathetic fibers supplying the vessels.

Throughout his series of nearly a dozen papers on "fibrositis" between 1941[127] and 1963,[129] the Australian, Michael Kelly, was impressed by both the palpable hardness of the "nodule" associated with the tender point in the muscle and by the distant referral of pain from the afflicted muscle. He gradually evolved the concept that "fibrositis" was a functional, neurological disturbance originating at the myalgic lesion, which was due to a local rheumatic process. He envisioned little or no local pathology, but rather that a central nervous system reflex disturbance caused the referred pain.

In her initial 1942 paper on this subject, Travell and her coauthors[273] emphasized the pain referred from the tender TP and expressed the opinion that any fibroblastic proliferation was secondary to a functional disorder; pathologic changes occurred only if the condition existed for a long time. In 1976,[268] she summarized her concept, which had evolved through a series of at least 38 papers on TPs: the self-sustaining characteristic of TPs depended on a feedback mechanism between the TP and the central nervous system.

Others among the first in this country to describe referred pain from tender points in muscle included Hunter,[114] who, in 1933, reported pain referred from tender spots in the muscles of the abdomen (myalgia of the abdominal wall) and Edeiken and Wolferth,[61] whose 1936 paper noted that pressure on trigger zones over the left scapula caused pain to radiate into the left shoulder and arm. In 1937 and 1941, Hans Kraus[140, 141] promoted vapocoolant spray as a treatment for TPs, and later,[142] in 1970, authored a book which emphasized the importance of exercise in the treatment of patients with back pain due to TPs. Reichart[201] in 1938 described areas of referred pain from numerous muscles; Cyriax[53]

identified several muscles of the head and neck that were responsible for headache, and Gorrell[89] in 1939 reported that precordial pain suggestive of myocardial infarction originated from chest wall muscles.

A new explanation for the palpable hardness within "fibrositic" muscles was advanced by Brendstrup and his colleagues in 1957.[33]

In 1973, both Awad[11] in this country and Fassbender and Wegner[65] in Germany reported ultramicroscopic findings in biopsies of muscles that showed evidence of myofascial TPs. The German report was rewritten in English as a chapter in a book.[64] Both papers reported abnormalities of the contractile elements in muscle. Their findings will be discussed in more detail in the section on Mechanisms.

More recently, the Russian authors, Popelianskii et al.,[195] briefly summarized the history of muscle pain syndromes over the past hundred years, including not only the Western papers cited above, but a large group of Russian papers which have not been cited in the Western literature. These authors describe a two-stage process causing myofascial TPs: an initial neuromuscular dysfunctional stage, and a subsequent dystrophic pathological stage.

For a more detailed history than can be given in this summary, the reader is referred to Simons[227] and Reynolds.[203]

Confusion of Terms

A major block to a general understanding of myofascial pain disorders has been the profusion of terms with parallel meanings, overlapping meanings, and some with multiple meanings. Consider, for example, the writings of three productive authors, Good, Kelly and Travell. In his initial 1938 paper, Good (writing as Gutstein)[103] used the terms "muscular rheumatism" and "non-articular rheumatism" to describe "myalgic spots." In the text of his 1940 paper,[107] he used "idiopathic myalgia" and in 1943,[84] he added the term "muscular sciatica," all to describe essentially the same condition in the gluteal musculature, but only the last was confined to this area. A few years later he added "myalgia," "rheumatic myalgia," and "fibrositis,"[85] and then returned to "non-articular rheumatism."[86] Readers of Good's series of papers might have wondered at the time whether he was talking about many different conditions, or using different terms to describe one disorder in different locations. In perspective, it was clearly the latter. In addition to the other terms, he consistently referred to myalgia[82] (with modifying adjectives) from 1940 to 1951 and then changed to "rheumatic myopathy."

Kelly used the term "fibrositis"[127] throughout his publications. Kelly's readers, at least, could be certain that he was talking about the same disorder from paper to paper, but could well have failed to recognize its close relation to the work of Good and of Travell.

In her initial paper, Travell[273] referred to trigger points, to "idiopathic myalgia," and later to "myalgia."[261] Since then, all her papers refer to "trigger points", or "trigger areas," with the addition of the adjective "myofascial" in 1952.[268, 274] Her readers could be sure that she was referring to the same condition from paper to paper, but could easily have missed its close connection with the work of Good and Kelly. And so it has gone, year-after-year, author-after-author.

There are several reasons why authors keep introducing new names for myofascial pain syndromes.

1. Many physicians are unfamiliar with myofascial pain disorders. Upon discovering a group of patients with a myofascial pain syndrome, and being unaware of the previous papers and many different names, the authors describe it de novo and add another name to the list.[63]

2. An author may be unaware that myofascial pain disorders comprise a large family of single-muscle and muscle-group syndromes. Numerous authors have invented regional anatomical names (e.g. tennis elbow, scapulocostal syndrome[171]) without realizing that the local pain was but another instance of the family of syndromes.

3. Frustrated with the ambiguity of the term "fibrositis," other authors define new modifications of the term, like interstitial myofibrositis[11] to make it more specific. The lack of agreement as to the pathophysiology of TPs contributes to this process.

4. The necessity to make the diagnosis entirely by history and physical examination without help from the laboratory or radiographs encourages an author to select a name that emphasizes those clinical aspects that are most characteristic of that syndrome. Each author approaches the subject with a different emphasis.

The following incomplete list samples the resulting nosological confusion: myitis chronica,[110] rheumatic myositis,[295] pressure point,[51] chronic rheumatism,[249] nerve point,[52] nodular fibromyositis,[258] myogelosis,[219] muscle hardenings or indurations,[143] myofascitis,[6, 239] myofibrositis,[181] myositis,[97] fibropathic syndromes,[185] hypersensitive areas,[241] myodysneuria,[106] interstitial myofibrositis,[11] and chest wall syndrome.[63]

Usually Synonymous Terms

The literature is less misleading if the following terms that have been consistently used as synonymous with myofascial TPs are distinguished from those that are obscured by multiple meanings.

Muskelschwiele. In 1843, Froriep[71] used this term to describe the palpable hardness found in the muscles of patients suffering from "rheumatism." It was common in the German literature for more than half a century.[180, 253]

Muscular Rheumatism.[3, 64, 103, 251] This term has been in common use in English, and also in the German language as "Muskelrheumatismus"[143, 144, 219, 221] in the late 19th and throughout this century. These terms are associated with palpable tender areas in the muscle and with clinical pain complaints that are relieved by local treatment of the tender spot in the muscle. In the last 50 years, the term usually has been restricted to the condition that we define as myofascial TPs;[48] however, its use in the 19th century was often too imprecise to equate it with TPs.

Myalgia. This name, when combined with another word, usually refers to a myofascial TP problem. Gutstein[103] used "myalgic spots" extensively; others[114, 232] referred to "myalgia of (a part of the body)." Lundervold[156] studied "occupational myalgia." Good[107] employed "idiopathic myalgia," "traumatic myalgia," and "rheumatic myalgia."[85] Authors using "myalgia" terms usually have eliminated the diagnosis of myositis in their patients by the circumscribed nature of the tender areas in the muscles and their response to local treatment. Some reports of *treatment failures*, especially in the older literature, may represent use of "myalgia" to describe true myositis. When used to describe myofascial TPs, the term "myalgia" identifies the *focal* tenderness characteristic of TPs.

Myogelosis.[122] This English term was derived from the corresponding German, "Myogelose,"[79, 144, 201, 219, 296] which was coined on the theory that the palpable hardness in muscle was caused by gelling of muscle proteins. The term, *Muskelhärten*, (muscle hardenings, or indurations) frequently is used as synonymous with Myogelosen to identify the same clinical finding.[79, 140, 144, 213] Both terms refer to myofascial TPs with rare exceptions.

Interstitial Myofibrositis. This terminology was introduced by Awad in 1973,[11] based on pathological findings, with an ingenious theory of the pathophysiology causing myofascial TPs.

Myofascial (Pain) Syndrome. As early as 1940,[245] "myofascial" was used to describe the identification and treatment of trigger areas in muscles of the low back and by 1948,[205] in the pectoral muscles. In 1950, Gorrell[90] used "musculofascial pain," and in 1952 "myofascial" was adopted by the senior author.[274] She observed that during an infraspinatus muscle biopsy, stroking or pinching either the superficial fascia or the contractile tissue of the muscle evoked the referred pain pattern from that muscle.[267] In the next few years, the term was adopted by other authors.[27, 154, 241] It was quickly picked up by the dental profession.[145, 265] It is now widely employed by physicians.[16, 34, 59, 72, 99, 111, 215] The expressions, "myofasical pain," and "myofascial syndrome," have the advantages that they clearly situate the illness in the muscle or its fascia, and that they have been used consistently to identify TP phenomena, with rare application to other conditions.

Myofasciitis (or Myofascitis). This word was introduced in 1927 by Albee[6] and then adopted by others.[9, 76, 239, 246] It is useful as a diagnostic term that identifies the myofascial pain syndrome due to TPs, and is generally acceptable to carriers of medical insurance, whereas "myofascial pain" or "myofascial TPs" is not always recognized by them as a diagnosis.

Trigger Points (Trigger Areas, Trigger Zones). Prior to Kellgren's[124, 125] demonstration that stimulation of areas within a muscle projected pain to distant regions, only a few authors clearly recognized this phenomenon.[51, 110] Most of those who did erroneously attributed the distant pain to pressure on a nerve.[92, 110, 249, 253, 279] Some, however, clearly described the pain radiation to distant parts of the body as reflex in nature, and not due to direct nerve stimulation.[50, 201, 246] The expression "trigger zone" to describe the site from which pain was referred was introduced in 1936 by Edeikin and Wolferth.[61] Travell and co-workers[273] used the term "trigger point" in 1942. Her complete bibliography to 1967 is available in the appendix of her autobiography.[267] "The Myofascial Genesis of Pain",[274] which pictured most of the clinically common patterns of pain referred from individual muscles, was published in 1952 and continues to be extensively reproduced in textbooks and scientific papers. It has contributed greatly toward establishing the TP concept. A number of articles and chapters have summarized the concept of myofascial TPs.[23, 27, 47, 142, 203, 227, 255, 268]

Myofascial Pain-Dysfunction Syndrome. In 1954, Schwartz[222] reported that inactivation of TPs by procaine injection was often an important part of the management of pain in the temporomandibular joint (TMJ) region. This treatment was based on his use of the myofascial pain patterns of masticatory muscles published in 1952.[274] This disorder came to be known as the TMJ pain-dysfunction syndrome and use of the term was reinforced a few years later by Freese,[70] by Shore's textbook,[224] and by electromyographic studies.[198, 226] In 1969, Laskin[145] emphasized the psychophysiological nature of the syndrome and proposed "myofascial pain-dysfunction syndrome," instead of TMJ pain-dysfunction syndrome. The new term has been widely accepted in the dental literature, while some authors still use the earlier term.[40, 192, 289] This common syndrome[243] was reviewed recently[174] and has been included in many textbooks of dentistry.[7, 19, 74, 119, 179] The myofascial pain-dysfunction syndrome is discussed more fully in Chapter 5.

Sometimes Synonymous Terms

The following terms are sometimes used as synonymous with "myofascial TPs," and at other times have different meanings. When reading the literature, one must understand in *which sense* the author is using each.

Fibrositis. Of all the labels applied to muscle pain syndromes, fibrositis causes the most confusion, because it has been used with such a broad range of overlapping and conflicting definitions. Quoting Waylonis, "Fibrositis means many things to many people."[282]

Gowers introduced "fibrositis" in 1904[92] as a term for muscular rheumatism, citing examples in the neck, shoulder, and lumbosacral regions. His description of muscular rheumatism could represent myofascial pain due to TPs. He attributed the palpable hardness of the muscles to "inflammation of the fibrous tissues of the muscles." Independently, in the same year, Stockman[249] presented pathological evidence that the nodules (palpable bands) in "chronic rheumatism" were patches of inflammatory hyperplasia in the connective tissue of skin, muscle, subcutaneous fat, fascia or periosteum. Stockman[250] later applied Gowers' "fibrositis" to his pathological findings in a 1911 paper. The marriage of these ideas was sanctified at a 1913 meeting of the Royal Society of Medicine. The issue of the union was the book, *Fibrositis*, by Llewellyn and Jones in 1915[151]; it entrenched the term in the English language. This book classified all rheumatic diseases, including gout and rheumatoid arthritis, as some form of fibrositis. The early use of Stockman's largely, if not completely, irrelevant pathologic findings as the cause of fibrositis confounded the usefulness of this term from the beginning.

By 1945, numerous authors[1, 46, 182, 235] were unable to correlate the pathology described by Stockman with the palpable hardenings (nodules) observed clinically. In 1947 Valentine,[278] and a few years later Neufeld,[185] compiled frustrated reviews. Unable to find any consistent pathological or neurophysiological basis for fibrositis, and for the pain symptoms ascribed to it, these authors proposed complex classifications that incorporated numerous other conditions under this diagnosis.

Over the years, "fibrositis" has accrued at least five distinguishable meanings.

1. Early authors generally used this term as synonymous with "muscular rheumatism" and with what we call myofascial TPs.[14, 36, 80, 85, 89, 127, 128, 173]

2. Authors[93, 94, 109, 123, 176] have equated fibrositis, or non-articular rheumatism, with psychogenic rheumatism. Failing to identify the signs and symptoms of myofascial TPs, and lacking laboratory or X-ray evidence of a disease process that would account for the patient's pain, physicians attributed the patient's pain primarily to psychological stress. The use of Macnab's definition,[159] "low back pain of undetermined origin associated with tender nodules attributed to no specific pathological process," encourages its use as a "wastebasket" diagnosis.

Weinberger,[285] the internist, seems convinced that the only rational basis for the pain described by these patients is psychological. Recently, however, Bennett[21] expressed a growing dissatisfaction with the exclusively psychogenic definition of fibrositis.

3. The current chapter on fibrositis in a prestigious rheumatology text[237] lists four criteria for the diagnosis of the condition:

1. Widespread *aching* of more than 3 month's duration,
2. Local tenderness at 12 of 14 specific sites,
3. Skin roll tenderness over the upper scapular region,
4. Disturbed sleep, with morning fatigue and stiffness.

These criteria bear only a distant relation to what most previous authors described as fibrositis and little relation to myofascial TPs. Moldofsky et al.[178] found an associated sleep disturbance that contributed to these patients' pain symptoms. Most of these patients would be likely to have specific myofascial pain syndromes that would respond to myofascial therapy.

4. Panniculosis or panniculitis, a circumscribed subcutaneous tenderness and induration seen over the back of the shoulder and pelvic girdles, has been considered a form of fibrosis.[48, 151, 155, 252]

5. Because "fibrositis" was introduced as a description of a pathological process of connective tissues in various structures, it has been applied to disorders of connective tissue in structures that include tendinitis, bursitis, capsulitis, and tenosynovitis.[92, 151, 184] Circumscribed deposits of fibrous tissue (nodules) in the non-muscular connective tissues investing thin-walled blood vessels, periosteum, and perineurium represented forms of fibrositis to

Stockman.[251] It also has been equated, in the lumbar and gluteal regions, with painful herniated nodules of fat (episacroiliac lipomas).[49]

The term "fibrositis" has been compartmentalized by added modifiers that included myo-fibrositis,[151] fibromyalgia,[111] muscular fibrositis,[92] abdominal fibrositis,[105] brachial, lumbosacral, and intercostal fibrositis,[92] fibrositic spots,[105] fibrositis syndrome,[139, 178, 236] and interstitial myofibrositis.[11]

In our opinion, fibrositis has become a hopelessly ambiguous diagnosis because of its multiple incompatible meanings and, thus, is best avoided.

Valleix Points. In 1841, Valleix[279] described tender points which he believed were located along nerves. He attributed the pain that was projected to a distance by palpation on one of these points to normal irritability of compressed nerve fibers. His authoritative focus of attention on nerves rather than on muscles distracted the attention of his many followers from the referred nature of the pain and from its muscular source. This may help to account for the paucity of French literature on the subject of myofascial TPs.

Non-articular Rheumatism. Generally, "non-articular rheumatism" has served as a generic term denoting a diversity of conditions.[208] Following the American Rheumatological Association definition of 1962, Hench[111] included fibrositis, carpal tunnel syndrome due to median nerve entrapment at the wrist, fibrofatty nodules along the iliac crest, and other conditions. It is occasionally also used to mean specifically myofascial TPs.[64]

Anatomical Pain Terms. Many patients are given an anatomical diagnosis of temporal headache, tennis elbow (Chapter 36), subdeltoid bursitis, bicipital tendinitis, brachial neuralgia, or osteoarthritis of the spine when, actually, myofascial TPs cause the patient's pain. Additional terms include tension headache,[53, 85, 266, 283, 292] scapulocostal syndrome,[171, 172, 190] pleurisy,[89] pleurodynia,[92, 151] lumbago,[36, 92, 151] and sciatica.[36, 62, 84, 127, 132] Myofascial TP pain may mimic that of radiculopathy.[202] Myofascial TPs refer both pain and tenderness in patterns resembling these disorders, and the physician mistakenly focuses on the site of the pain rather than on its remote source. These individual pain syndromes are considered in the chapter on the muscle from which each pain arises.

Shoulder pain commonly associated with hemiplegia has been attributed to subluxation of the shoulder, often when subluxation is not apparent. Even **with** subluxation, the pain may be due primarily to active myofascial TPs in the shoulder-girdle musculature, especially in the infraspinatus and subscapularis muscles, which generally respond well to myofascial TP therapy.

Pain Terms. Understanding exactly what "pain" the patient feels is difficult and fraught with misunderstanding. Until recently, the purely subjective experiences of pain and distorted sensation have not been clearly defined in a standard "pain" vocabulary. Many times, what the patient means by a descriptive pain term is not what the examiner understands it to mean.

An important step toward standardization of pain terms was taken when the subcommittee on taxonomy of the International Association for the Study of Pain recommended definitions, with extensive notes on usage.[55, 254] This manual uses those definitions, which aid communication among professionals, but does not solve the problem of understanding what patients mean by the words they use to describe their pain and its location. This requires skillful inquiry by the examiner.

B. CLINICAL CHARACTERISTICS OF MYOFASCIAL TRIGGER POINTS

A myofascial TP is a hyperirritable locus within a taut band of skeletal muscle, located in the muscular tissue and/or its associated fascia. The spot is painful on compression and can evoke characteristic referred pain and autonomic phenomena. A myofascial TP is to be distinguished from a TP in other tissues, such as skin, ligament, and periosteum.

We classify myofascial TPs as either active or latent. An active TP causes the patient pain. A latent TP is clinically silent with respect to pain, but may cause restriction of movement and weakness of the affected muscle. A latent TP may persist for years after apparent recovery from injury; it predisposes to acute attacks of pain, since minor overstretching, overuse, or chilling of the muscle may suffice to reactivate it. Both latent and active TPs cause dysfunction; only active TPs cause pain.

The clinical characteristics listed in this section provide an operational definition of myofascial TPs. The characteristics are grouped in the order in which one is likely to encounter them during the evaluation of a patient. The methods of examining for these characteristics are covered in the next chapter.

Normal muscles do not contain TPs. Normal muscles have no taut bands of muscle fibers, are not tender to firm palpation, exhibit no local twitch responses, and do not refer pain in response to applied pressure.

Individuals of either sex and of any age can develop trigger points; sedentary, middle-aged women apparently are very vulnerable. Except in later years, women seem somewhat more likely than men to develop myofascial pain syndromes. Among 200 asymptomatic 17- to 35-year-old subjects, 54% of the women and 45% of the men had latent trigger points in the shoulder-girdle muscles. However, of the 100 subjects in each group, practically equal numbers, 13 female and 12 male subjects, experienced referred pain in response to pressure on the TPs.[241] Similarly, a group of 739 college students were studied for evidence of masticatory apparatus dysfunction. A significantly greater number of female than male students had headaches and were aware of temporomandibular joint sounds, indicative of the myofascial pain-dysfunction syndrome associated with TPs (Chapter 5). Other questions relating to masticatory pain and dysfunction were answered without evidence of sex distinction. Twice as many women as men had tenderness of the lateral pterygoid muscle.[243] However, 194 persons, who comprised a random sampling of 70-year-old male and female residents of a town in Sweden, showed no appreciable sex difference in the frequency of pain and dysfunction of the masticatory system.[4]

Apparently, women are more likely than men to seek medical aid for pain of myofascial origin. Among 91 patients who were referred to a Physical Medicine and Rehabilitation Service and who were diagnosed as suffering from "fibrositis syndrome,"[139] 69 were women and 22 were men. The dental literature generally reports more female than male patients with the myofascial pain-dysfunction syndrome; three recent studies found that 79%–84% of these pain patients were women.[37, 45, 223]

Infants have been observed with point tenderness of the rectus abdominis muscle and colic, both of which were relieved by sweeping a stream of vapocoolant over the muscle, which helps to inactivate myofascial TPs. When children were examined for them, myofascial TPs were found to be a common source of musculoskeletal pain in childhood.[17] It is our impression that the likelihood of developing pain-producing *active* TPs increases with age into the most active, middle years. As activity becomes less strenuous in later years, individuals tend to exhibit chiefly the stiffness and restricted motion of *latent* TPs.

Sola[238] found that laborers, who exercise their muscles heavily every day, are less likely to develop active TPs than are sedentary workers who tend to indulge in occasional orgies of vigorous physical activity. Our experience has been similar.

Active TPs are most likely in postural muscles of the neck, shoulder and pelvic girdles, and the masticatory muscles. The upper trapezius, scalene, sternocleidomastoid, levator scapulae and quadratus lumborum muscles are very commonly involved.

Symptoms

1. *Myofascial pain is referred from trigger points in specific patterns characteristic of each muscle.* The spontaneous pain is rarely located at the TP responsible for it. Just as pulling the trigger of a gun affects a remote target, so activation of the TP projects pain to a distant reference zone.

The referred pain of myofascial TPs usually is dull and aching, often deep, with intensity varying from low-grade discomfort to severe and incapacitating torture. It may occur at rest, or only on motion.

The referred pain can usually be elicited, or increased in intensity, by digital pressure on the TP, or by penetrating the TP precisely with a needle. The more hypersensitive the TP, the more intense and constant is the referred pain, and the more extensive is its distribution. In the myofascial TP syndromes, pain is rarely completely symmetrical on both sides of the body.

The patient usually presents with complaints due to the most recently activated TP. When this TP has been successfully eliminated, the pain pattern may shift to that of an earlier TP which also must be inactivated. If the initial TP is inactivated first, the patient may recover without further treatment.

Pain referred from myofascial TPs does not follow a simple segmental pattern. Neither does it follow familiar neurological patterns, nor the known patterns for referred pain of visceral origin. Myofascial pain frequently, but not always, occurs within the same dermatome,[96] myotome,[130] or sclerotome[120] as that of the TP, but does not include the entire segment. It often includes parts of additional segments. (A dermatome is the area of skin supplied by the afferent nerve fibers of a single posterior spinal root; a myotome is the group of muscles, and a sclerotome is the area of bone so innervated.[5])

Although Kellgren[124] concluded that the pain referred from a skeletal muscle usually followed spinal segmental patterns that were not dermatomal, he noted many exceptions when pain extended over several segments. Travell presented many examples of grossly non-segmental referred pain patterns,[262, 271, 274] as does this manual.

The severity and extent of the referred pain pattern depends on the degree of irritability of the trigger point, not on the size of the muscle. Myofascial TPs in small, obscure or variable muscles can be as troublesome to the patient as TPs in large familiar muscles.

2. *Trigger points are activated directly by acute overload, overwork fatigue, direct trauma, and by chilling (Fig 2.1).* Patients implicate an acute traumatic cause when they relate the onset of their myofascial pain to a specific event or movement (acute overload) that often had occurred months or years before. Primary myofascial TPs also develop in muscles subject to excessive repetitive or sustained contractions (overload fatigue).

3. *Trigger points are activated indirectly by other trigger points, visceral disease, arthritic joints, and by emotional distress (Fig. 2.1).* Satellite TPs are prone to develop in muscles that lie within the pain reference zone of other myofascial TPs, or within the zone of pain referred from a diseased viscus, such as the pain of myocardial infarction, peptic ulcer, cholelithiasis, or renal colic.

Secondary TPs are likely to develop in an adjacent or synergistic muscle that is chronically overloaded by "protective" spasm maintained to reduce strain on the first muscle that is hypersensitive, shortened and weakened due to primary TPs.

4. *Active myofascial TPs vary in irritability from hour-to-hour and from day-to-day.* The stress threshold required to produce myofascial pain is highly variable, compared with the reproducible activity threshold of some other muscular pains, such as effort angina and intermittent claudication, that are due to arterial insufficiency.

5. *Trigger-point irritability may be increased from a latent to an active level by many factors.* The amount of stress needed to activate a latent trigger point and thus cause a clinical pain syndrome depends on the degree of conditioning of the muscle; the greater the exercise tolerance of the muscle, the lower the susceptibility of its TPs to activation. Irritability of TPs also is influenced by the number and severity of perpetuating factors (see Chapter 4).

Specific situations likely to activate latent TPs include: leaving a muscle in the shortened position for a period of time, as when sleeping; chilling of the muscle (not just by drafts), especially when it is fatigued or suffering postexercise stiffness; and during or following a viral illness.

Sudden, unaccustomed shortening of a muscle that harbors a latent TP is likely to activate that TP: this occurs in the shortening reactivation of an antagonist muscle following release of its shortenend agonist by stretch-and-spray therapy (Section 12, next chapter).

6. *The signs and symptoms of myofascial trigger point activity long outlast the precipitating event.* When injured, most tissues heal, but muscles "learn"; they "learn" to avoid pain. Active TPs develop habits of guarding that limit movement of that muscle. Chronic muscular pain, stiffness, and dysfunction result.

With adequate rest, and in the absence

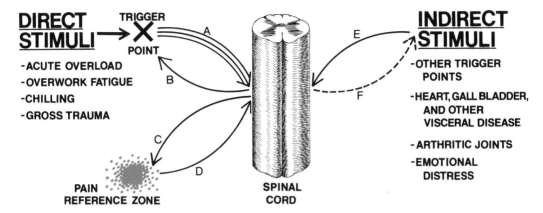

Figure 2.1.   The apparent relation of the trigger point (**X**) to factors that clinically can activate it and to its pain reference zone. The *triple arrows* (A) from the trigger point to the spinal cord represent the multiplicity of effects originating at the trigger point. The arrow returning to the trigger point (B) completes a feedback loop that is evidenced by the self-sustaining nature of many trigger points. The *long arrow* (C) to the pain reference zone represents the appearance of referred pain in neurologically distant sites that may be several segments removed from the trigger point. *Arrow D* indicates the influence on the trigger point of the vapocoolant-stretch procedure applied to the reference zone. *Arrow E* signifies the activating effect of indirect stimuli on the trigger point; *dashed arrow F* denotes effects of TPs on visceral function (After Travell,[268] Fig. 1).

of perpetuating factors, an active TP may revert spontaneously to a latent state. Pain symptoms disappear, but occasional reactivation of the TP accounts for the typical history of recurrent episodes of the same pain over a period of years.

Persistent TP activity that is resistant to adequate treatment suggests progression from a neuromuscular dysfunctional to a dystrophic phase.

7. *Phenomena other than pain are often caused by myofascial trigger points.* **Autonomic concomitants** in the pain reference zone caused by TP activity include localized vasoconstriction,[270] sweating, lacrimation, coryza, salivation, and pilomotor activity. Proprioceptive disturbances caused by TPs include imbalance, dizziness, tinnitus, and distorted perception of the weight of objects lifted in the hands.

Motoneurons serving muscles within the pain reference zone act as if their stimulation threshold is reduced (increased excitability).[270] A clinical example is given at the end of Section 4 of Chapter 38.

Several phenomena indicate disturbance of **motor coordination** by active TPs. A depressed ankle tendon jerk may be restored following inactivation of TPs in the soleus muscle. The buckling knee syndrome caused by a TP in the vastus me-

dialis seems to result from a profound inhibition of quadriceps function, occurring in lieu of pain. Patients with temporomandibular joint dysfunction and pain exhibited discoordination in the electromyographic (EMG) records of their masticatory muscles.[199] Pain induced by muscle ischemia caused serious disruption of handwriting, whereas equivalent ischemia without pain caused no appreciable disturbance.[75]

The **remote dysfunction** projected by TPs may influence muscles at a considerable distance. Inactivation of TPs that cause painful movement and restricted range of lower extremity muscles also has repeatedly resulted in a 30%–40% increase in the interincisal opening between the jaws when the restriction was caused by TPs in masticatory muscles.

Pain produced by pressure of the body on TPs during recumbency frequently **disrupts sleep**. Vice versa, Moldofsky[177] has shown that a primary sleep disturbance may, in some subjects, contribute to the pain and stiffness associated with TPs.

8. *Myofascial trigger points cause stiffness and weakness of the involved muscle.* Myofascial stiffness of the muscle is most marked after a period of inactivity, especially after a night's sleep, or after sitting in one position for an extended period.

Muscle strength becomes unreliable, e.g. things drop unexpectedly from the patient's grasp. Weakness of the involved muscle is evident when a maximum-contraction effort produces less than normal strength. Weakness apparently is due to a central inhibition that has developed to protect the muscle from a painful degree of contraction. The patient then substitutes other muscles for the weak one, often unknowingly, e.g. carrying objects with the non-dominant, stronger arm. The weakness occurs without atrophy of the affected muscle.

Findings on Examination

1. *When active TPs are present, passive or active stretching of the affected muscle increases pain.* This response was demonstrated in a series of patients by Macdonald.[157]

On stretching the muscle, at approximately the length at which pain begins, EMG activity (protective spasm) of the muscle also appears. This further increases the tension on the muscle fibers and greatly increases the painfulness of further stretch. The spasm blocks further lengthening of the muscle, unless therapeutic steps are taken to inhibit this response.

2. *The stretch range of motion is restricted.* The increased tension of the taut bands will not permit the muscle to extend to its full range. Forced attempts to do so are exquisitely painful.

3. *Pain is increased when the affected muscle is strongly contracted against fixed resistance.*[157] This effect of TPs is most marked when the muscle is placed in a shortened position prior to the contraction effort.

4. *The maximum contractile force of an affected muscle is weakened.* The weakness can usually be demonstrated by testing for strength, and is not associated with atrophy of the muscle, or with pain, unless the patient is exhorted to extreme effort.

5. *Deep tenderness and dysesthesia are commonly referred by active myofascial TPs to the zone of referred pain.* These sensory changes found in a region where the patient complains of pain are doubly misleading to the unwary.

6. *Disturbances of non-sensory function are sometimes induced in the pain refer-* *ence zone of a myofascial TP.* The referred autonomic disturbances[262] include increased vasomotor activity (pallor during stimulation of the myofascial TP, rebound hyperemia following its inactivation), lacrimation and coryza (Section 1, Chapter 7), increased sudomotor activity, and pilomotor activation (gooseflesh). Electromyographic increase in motor unit activity of muscles within the pain reference zone also occurs.[270]

7. *Muscle in the immediate vicinity of a trigger point feels tense to palpation.* These palpable hardenings have been described as "fibrositic nodules,"[151] "myogeloses,"[144] "ropiness,[139] and "tense," or "palpable bands," as we call them. Remarkably, the tenseness of the muscle fibers associated with a TP often disappears immediately following effective treatment of the TP.

8. *The trigger point is found in a palpable band as a sharply circumscribed spot of exquisite tenderness.* There is clearly a point of maximum tenderness; there is less sensitivity when digital pressure is applied a few millimeters to either side of the point.

9. *Digital pressure applied on an active trigger point usually elicits a "jump sign."* The local TP pain, which is out of proportion to the pressure applied, can be so intense that it causes the patient to "give a jump"[104] and cry out. This total response is called the "jump sign."[135, 139]

10. *Snapping palpation of the TP frequently evokes a local twitch response.* Clinically, this response, which is fully described in Section 9 of Chapter 3, is most easily elicited from active TPs in superficial muscles. The response also can be elicited from some latent TPs. It is more easily demonstrated in some muscles, such as the sternocleidomastoid, pectoralis major, deltoid, latissimus dorsi, third finger extensor, brachioradialis, vastus medialis, and gluteus maximus, than in others. Electromyographic studies showed motor unit responses only in a limited group of muscle fibers during a twitch response: these responding fibers were located where one felt the palpable band.[57, 228]

11. *Moderate, sustained pressure on a sufficiently irritable trigger point causes or intensifies pain in the reference zone of that TP.* If a TP is sufficiently active to cause pain at rest, firm pressure applied to

it usually induces referred pain, which follows the specific pattern of that TP. The referred pain pattern caused by a TP also is evoked when a needle penetrates the TP, as during injection. However, if the TP is spontaneously causing severe referred pain because it is already maximally activated, additional pressure cannot increase the pain.

12. *The skin of some patients evinces dermographia*[73, 139] *or panniculosis in the area overlying active TPs.* These phenomena are most easily observed in the skin of the back in the upper thoracic and lumbosacral areas. Panniculosis is identified by a positive skin rolling test,[161] (see Section 8, next chapter). They are not frequent concomitants of TPs in other areas.

Laboratory Findings

1. *Routine laboratory tests show no abnormalities or significant changes attributable to myofascial trigger points, per se.* The erythrocyte sedimentation rate, SMA 6 and 12, blood count and serum muscle enzymes are all normal. Abnormal serum LDH isoenzyme findings are noted below. However, many perpetuating factors are manifested by laboratory findings, as reviewed in Chapter 4. Radiographs, including films made with soft-tissue technique and computerized tomograms, have not revealed any features that are associated with myofascial TPs. With more advanced imaging techniques, this situation may change.

2. *Electromyographic examination of involved muscles at rest reveals no diagnostic abnormality.* The clinical experience of the junior author agrees with the findings of Kraft et al.[139] that the tense muscle fibers associated with myofascial TPs show no resting EMG activity. Awad[11] and Arroyo[10] reported increased numbers of polyphasic potentials in muscles afflicted with TPs. However, the number of polyphasic potentials was not quantitated and compared with control values for uninvolved muscles in the same patients. Occasionally during EMG examination, the needle will accidentally encounter a TP and thus produce a local twitch response, which is clearly palpable and visible through the skin overlying the muscle, along with a jump sign of the patient. The associated EMG activity looks like normal insertion potentials.

3. *Spontaneous motor unit activity in a muscle with trigger points can develop secondarily.* Spontaneous motor unit activity may occur when that muscle lies within the pain reference zone of a TP in *another* muscle.[270] A muscle also may develop protective spasm to relieve tension caused by TPs in an adjacent (parallel) muscle of the same myotatic unit.[268] A muscle that contains active TPs often shows EMG activity "at rest" when it is stretched to, or beyond, the point of pain.

4. *One study*[115] *reported normal serum enzyme concentrations, but a shift in the distribution of LDH-isoenzymes.* In patients with interstitial myofibrositis (myofascial TPs), the serum isoenzyme concentrations decreased in the LD_1 and LD_2 fractions and increased in the LD_3, LD_4 and LD_5 fractions. The concentrations found in biopsy specimens of involved muscles showed a nearly reversed picture. The LD_1 and LD_2 fractions were increased, and the LD_3 and LD_4 fractions were decreased. The LD_5 concentration remained normal.[115] To our knowledge, this finding has not been tested by another investigator.

5. *Thermograms of skin overlying active TPs have recently been reported to show areas of increased skin temperature, 5–10 cm in diameter.*[67] On the other hand, earlier authors reported diminished skin temperature in the vicinity of chronic muscular nodules.[136, 212]

6. *A small region of increased skin conductance (reduced skin resistance) may be observed over a trigger area.* Sola and Williams[242] observed a dramatic low-resistance deflection of the ohmmeter needle when the exploring electrode on the skin crossed over the trigger point. No controlled study is known that independently mapped myofascial trigger points and low resistance points on the skin to see how many false positives were encountered and how many TPs were overlooked. Therefore, the reliability of this procedure for locating TPs is unknown.

Perpetuating Factors

The mere passage of time often fails to bring about recovery from a myofascial pain syndrome.

In many patients, recovery depends on

the identification and elimination of one or more perpetuating factors, as reviewed in Chapter 4. These factors make the muscle more likely to develop TPs initially and to increase the irritability of existing TPs, so that the muscle's response to treatment is neither complete nor permanent.

Response to Local Therapy

One of the important clinical characteristics of TPs is their response to therapy.

1. *Frequently, the response to specific myofascial trigger point therapy is* **immediate** *disappearance of spot tenderness, referred pain, and the local twitch response, with release of the muscle's restricted motion.* The tension of the palpable band is less likely to disappear immediately when the myofascial syndrome has been present for a long time (months or years); several treatments may be required. Incomplete restoration of the normal *full* length of the muscle usually means incomplete relief of pain referred from its TPs.

2. *Hot packs applied to the muscle for a few minutes immediately following therapy, such as stretch and spray or local injection, usually provide an additional increment in the range of motion.* This application also helps significantly to reduce muscle soreness following specific myofascial therapy.

3. *Relief is more likely to be lasting when the patient moves all of the treated muscles through several cycles of their full range of motion at the end of a therapy session.* This teaches the muscles that their full range of active motion is again available and encourages the patient to use this full range in the course of daily activities. If the patient continues to guard and restrict movement of the muscle following treatment, the TP activity and pain are likely to recur.

Common Misconceptions

1. *That the pain from myofascial trigger points is solely psychogenic in origin.* Failure to recognize the signs and symptoms of myofascial TPs, and the presence of normal laboratory and radiologic findings, lead many physicians to conclude erroneously that there is no organic basis for the patient's complaints and that the symptoms, therefore, must be psychogenic.

2. *That myofascial syndromes are self-limiting and will cure themselves.* At best, an active TP spontaneously recedes to become a latent TP, awaiting some trivial stress to be reactivated. It also may persist indefinitely as a source of referred pain, until inactivated by treatment.

3. *That myofascial pain is not severe and need not be taken seriously.* A swimmer may drown from a muscle cramp produced by a myofascial TP. Myofascial pain has driven some patients to suicide. Because so many people are afflicted, this disorder exacts a frightful toll on human well-being and productivity. Myofascial back pain is a major, unrecognized source of industrial disability.

4. *That relief of pain by treatment of skeletal muscles for myofascial TPs rules out serious visceral disease.* Brief application of vapocoolant spray or infiltration of local anesthetic into the somatic pain reference zone of a viscus can temporarily relieve the pain of myocardial infarction, angina, and acute abdominal disease[288] (Chapters 42 and 49).

C. DIFFERENTIAL DIAGNOSIS

The differential diagnosis of specific myofascial pain syndromes is considered under individual muscle chapters. This section lists the criteria for identifying myofascial TPs, reviews other kinds of TPs, and notes other causes of painful muscles.

Myofascial Trigger Points

To diagnose an active myofascial TP, one looks for:

1. A history of sudden onset during or shortly following acute overload stress, or a history of gradual onset with chronic overload of the affected muscle;
2. Characteristic patterns of pain that are referred from myofascial TPs, patterns that are specific to individual muscles;
3. Weakness and restriction in the stretch range of motion of the affected muscle;
4. A taut, palpable band in the affected muscle;
5. Exquisite, focal tenderness to digital pressure (the TP), in the band of taut muscle fibers;
6. A local twitch response elicited through snapping palpation or needling of the tender spot (TP);

7. The reproduction of the patient's pain complaint by pressure on, or needling of, the tender spot (TP);
8. The elimination of symptoms by therapy directed specifically to the affected muscles.

Finding a site of local tenderness (Number 5) is essential to the diagnosis, but nonspecific. Numbers 6 and 7, a local twitch response and pain reproduction, when present, are *specific and strongly diagnostic* of a myofascial TP. The more of the remaining findings that are present, the more certain is the diagnosis, which may be recorded as myofasciitis of specific muscles for administrative or insurance purposes.

Non-myofascial Trigger Points

Skin and Scar Trigger Points. Sinclair[233] reported that, in 8 of 30 healthy young adults, sharply circumscribed TP areas were located while exploring the body by pinching the **skin** between the finger and thumb. He studied 18 TPs intensively in 4 of these subjects and performed a skin biopsy. Generally, a sharp, stinging, moderately severe pain was referred either locally or remotely to the skin from a cutaneous TP. The area of referred pain also showed modulation of sensation (referred deep tenderness or referred dysesthesia) by stimulation of the TP. Some reference zones were within the same segmental distribution, but others had no segmental relation to their skin TPs.

Trommer and Gellman[276] reported seven patients in whom skin TPs referred pain or numbness to other skin areas that were often nearby, sometimes remote. The skin TPs were found by pricking the skin with a needle, exploring for a sensitive spot that reproduced the patient's symptoms. In every case, the symptoms were relieved by repeated *intracutaneous* injections, but only if they were made precisely at the TP.

These studies do not suggest a constancy in the referred pain patterns of cutaneous TPs like that observed for myofascial TPs. Also, there was no indication in these reports, nor in our observations, that the reference zones of skin TPs bear any relation to the reference zones of TPs in underlying muscles.

In our experience, TPs that refer burning, prickling, or lightning-like jabs of pain are likely to be found in cutaneous scars. Such scar TPs may be inactivated by precise intracutaneous injection with 0.5% procaine solution, or by repeated application of the topical anesthetic, dimethisoquin hydrochloride ointment (Quotane)*. In refractory cases, the addition of a soluble steroid to the local anesthetic solution used for injection of the scar TP may be effective. Bourne[30] injected the scar TPs with triamcinolone acetonide and lidocaine (Xylocaine)†. The senior author similarly has used dexamethasone sodium phosphate (Decadron)§ with 0.5% procaine, injecting a few tenths of a milliliter at any one location.

Fascial and Ligamentous Trigger Points. In addition to occurring in the fascia and tendons of muscles, TPs also may be found in joint capsules and ligaments.

Kellgren[124] demonstrated experimentally that fascial epimysium of the gluteus medius muscle referred pain several centimeters distally when injected with 0.1 ml of 6% saline solution, and that the tendon of the tibialis anterior, similarly injected, referred pain to the medial aspect of the ankle and instep.

Travell[262] reported that an acute sprain of the ankle was accompanied by four TPs in the joint capsule, each of which referred pain to the ankle and foot. Myofascial TPs resulting from acute sprains of the knee, ankle, wrist and metacarpophalangeal joint of the thumb caused referred pain, which was at first elicited and then permanently relieved by injection of each TP with physiologic saline.[261, 272] Leriche[149] identified ligamentous TPs following fracture or sprain; the TPs responded completely to 5 or 6 injections of a local anesthetic. Gorrell[91] reviewed the anatomy of the ankle ligaments and described a technique for the identification and injection of ligamentous TPs at this joint.

Kraus[142] briefly reviewed the literature on ligamentous TPs and noted that they

---

* Dimethisoquin hydrochloride ointment is sold over-the-counter as Quotane by Menley and James Laboratories, Division of Smith Kline & French Laboratories, 1500 Spring Garden St., PA 19101.
† Xylocaine, Astra Pharmaceutical Products, 7 Neponset St., Worcester, MA 01606.
§ Decadron, Merck, Sharp & Dohme, West Point, PA 19486.

are easily localized for injection, which often gives immediate pain relief and a postinjection soreness lasting up to 10 days. Hackett[108] illustrated patterns of pain referred from the iliolumbar, sacroiliac, sacrospinal, and sacrotuberous ligaments; he recommended injection of a sclerosing agent, which was not widely used because it caused too many complications. Dittrich[58] found TPs in the aponeurosis of the latissimus dorsi muscle where it joins the lumbodorsal fascia; the TPs referred pain to the shoulder region. Weiser[287] described point tenderness at the insertion of the semimembranosus muscle in 98 patients who complained of spontaneous pain at the medial aspect of the knee. The pain was reproduced by local pressure or tension at that insertion site. Symptoms were relieved by injecting 2% lidocaine (Xylocaine†) with triamcinolone into the tender spot.

Recently, de Valera and Raftery[56] reported trigger areas in three pelvic ligaments, the sacroiliac, sacrospinous and sacrotuberous, which, when strained, become tender to palpation, refer pain, and respond to injection with a local anesthetic.

Periosteal Trigger Points. Kellgren[126] firmly established that the periosteum also can refer pain in response to injection of hypertonic saline, just as the muscles do. Among 160 experiments designed to determine the nature of referred pain originating from deep tissues, Inman and Saunders[120] reported that noxious stimulation of the periosteum by scratching it with a needle, by injecting it with 6% salt solution, or by applying a measured pressure elicited severe referred pain that sometimes radiated for considerable distances. Tenderness was referred to the muscles and bony prominences within the pain reference zone, as also happens with myofascial TPs. Repeated stimulation of the same periosteal or ligamentous attachments consistently referred pain in the same direction, but the extent of radiation varied with the intensity of the stimulus. Unfortunately, the authors did not report the distribution of these specific periosteal referred pain patterns. Autonomic reactions, such as sweating, blanching, and nausea were frequently observed in the subjects.

Clinically, the periosteum can be a potent source of referred pain.[98] Relief of this referred pain may be obtained by injecting periosteal TPs, analogous to the relief obtained by injecting myofascial or cutaneous TPs.[146]

Acupuncture and Trigger Points. The relationship between TPs and acupuncture points is frequently questioned. Superficially, they seem to have much in common. Melzack et al.[167] compared the congruence of the TP locations reported by three authors with the location of acupuncture points *related to pain*, as published by an acupuncturist. By allowing a difference of 3 cm, they found an overall correspondence of 71%. One would expect the ancient Chinese physicians who determined acupuncture points *for pain* to have discovered and included a number of the more common myofascial TP locations.

Unlike the classical acupuncture points, we do not think of the published TP sites as immutable locations, but as a guide for where to start looking. Every muscle can develop TPs; many muscles have multiple TP locations. Only the most common TP locations are shown in the published illustrations; individual muscles may have TPs in other locations. The TP sites in a given muscle vary from person to person; no two people are *exactly* alike.

Gunn[100] identified four types of acupuncture points based on the nerve arrangement penetrated by the needle. Two of the types identified nervous system structures in muscle, the motor point and Golgi tendon organs. Experiments to establish which nerves mediate nociceptive (painful) stimuli from muscle have implicated neither motor fibers nor Group IB (Golgi tendon organ) fibers, but rather, nerve fibers belonging to Groups III and IV.[170]

One experimentally well demonstrated mechanism for pain relief by acupuncture is the modulation of endorphin levels.[164] Myofascial pain is relieved primarily by inactivating the source of pain, the TP. Acupuncture apparently alleviates the awareness of pain; inactivating a TP eliminates the cause of the pain.

Acupuncturists claim effects other than pain relief by treatment of many acupuncture points; we observe no corresponding effects by inactivating myofascial TPs, only relief of pain and of the specific nonpain referred phenomena characteristic of myofascial TPs. We see no relation between non-pain acupuncture points and myofascial TPs. Acupuncture points and trigger points are derived from vastly different concepts. The fact that a number of pain points overlap does not change that basic difference. The two terms should not be used interchangeably.

Motor Points and Trigger Points. The question often arises, "What is the difference between TPs and motor points?" In 1857, Von Ziemssen demonstrated by dissection that the motor point corresponds to the entrance of the motor nerve into the muscle. Current electrodiagnostic texts agree that the motor point is found by exploring the skin for the spot where electrical stimulation with the least current produces a perceptible twitch of the muscle.[43, 88, 148] A motor point is located by *electrical stimulation*, not by palpation. Myofascial TPs are sometimes found near motor points, often not.

The functionally significant structure with regard to the innervation of muscle fibers is the myoneural junction (endplate zone), not the entry of the motor nerve into the muscle. Endplates normally lie at the midpoint of muscle fibers.[42] Some TPs are closely associated with myoneural junctions, others not. The motor point is not a reliable indicator of the endplate zone. In a few muscles, such as the gastrocnemius and peroneus longus, the motor point excites the nerve proximal to the endplates. Two muscles, the sartorius and gracilis, have scattered endplates.[42]

The terms "motor point" and "TP" have been used interchangeably.[101, 102] The motor point concerns the innervation of the whole muscle; a TP concerns a part of the muscle that includes its palpable band and the local twitch response. Motor points are located close to mid-muscle with very few exceptions. Myofascial TPs can be located anywhere throughout the length of a muscle, as seen in this manual. Although the term "motor point" has been presented as interchangeable with "trigger point,"[101, 102] motor points are not TPs, so it would be less confusing to the reader if the two concepts were clearly distinguished.

Musculoskeletal Diseases

Three major categories of musculoskeletal disease must be distinguished from the syndromes of myofascial TPs: myopathies, arthritides, and focal inflammation of musculoskeletal structures, such as tendinitis and bursitis.

Myopathies. Genetic myopathies generally are marked by painless weakness of proximal muscles; pain, if present, is usually a minor complaint. With myofascial TPs, pain is usually the chief complaint.

Polymyositis and dermatomyositis are not rare. The **polymyositis** form begins as a *painless* weakness of the proximal limb muscles, except in about 15% of cases. The exceptions have aching pain in the buttocks, joints and calves; pain often indicates the occurrence of arthritis as a manifestation of polymyositis, or the combination of polymyositis with another connective tissue disease. There is little, if any, evidence of a systemic infection. Muscle enzyme levels, such as creatine phosphokinase (CPK) and LDH, are increased in myositis, but are normal in myofascial TP syndromes, unless increased by necrosis following intramuscular injection of a long-acting local anesthetic (Section 13 of Chapter 3). **Dermatomyositis** resembles polymyositis, but with skin changes that may include erythema, a maculopapular eruption and scaling eczematoid dermatitis. A lilac color in the skin over the bridge of the nose, cheeks, forehead and around the fingernails helps, when it is present, to identify dermatomyositis.[277]

Myositis due to infection is considered for the masticatory muscles in Chapter 5. Polymyalgia rheumatica and giant cell arteritis are discussed in Section 8 of Chapter 9.

Spasticity and postexercise stiffness or soreness are reviewed in Chapter 5. Postexercise soreness occurs from 1–3 days after the exercise and, although the muscles contain exquisitely tender spots, these do not refer pain as do TPs. Postexercise tenderness is distributed in the muscle as if it were caused by sensitization with a different noxious agent, or by the sensitization of a different neural structure than that responsible for TP phenomena.

Arthritis. Pain referred from myofascial TPs to joints can closely mimic the pain of osteoarthritis, rheumatoid arthritis, gout and psoriatic arthritis. The distinctive signs of TPs are found in the involved muscles, the local signs of arthritis are found in the joints. The fact that myofascial TPs frequently refer pain *and tender-*

ness to joints is a potent source of misdiagnosis.[202]

The diagnosis of **osteoarthritis** rests primarily on local joint pain and tenderness with crepitation and bony degenerations that are substantiated by characteristic radiological changes of erosion of articular cartilage and osteoblastic reaction.[24, 160, 162] However, spurs, lipping, and joint space narrowing are not specific to osteoarthritis and, in many patients, are *not* associated with pain. One sees many patients with these structural changes who become pain free when their myofascial TPs are inactivated. All too many myofascial pain sufferers have been led to believe that their pain is due to a "degenerated spine," or "arthritis," and they erroneously conclude that the only treatment left is analgesics.

Since **rheumatoid arthritis** is a systemic disease, the American Rheumatism Association recommends that 7 of 11 criteria be met to establish this diagnosis for epidemiologic studies.[207] Among these criteria are morning stiffness, joint pain, joint swelling, symmetrical joint swelling, subcutaneous nodules, typical radiological changes, presence of rheumatoid factor, a poor mucin precipitate from synovial fluid, and characteristic histologic changes. The disease begins as a synovial inflammation with hypertrophy that progresses to characteristic radiological changes in the joints.[160, 207]

An absolute diagnosis of **gouty arthritis** is made by finding urate crystals in samples of synovial fluid, or in tissues surrounding the affected joint.[294] Most often, the diagnosis is made by the typical clinical picture of acute monarthritis of a lower limb. An elevated serum uric acid accompanying arthritis is suggestive of gout, but does not establish a diagnosis. Pseudogout mimics gout and results from the deposition of calcium pyrophosphate dihydrate crystals instead of sodium urate crystals.

The identification of **psoriatic arthritis** is made by the presence of an inflammatory arthritis in a patient with the skin or nail lesions of psoriasis, and the absence of rheumatoid factor and of rheumatoid nodules.[77, 163]

Tendinitis and Bursitis. Because myofascial TPs refer pain *and tenderness* to regions where tendons and bursae are located, these TP symptoms are commonly misdiagnosed as tendinitis or bursitis, which show local signs of inflammation. Although injection of the painful and tender reference zone with steroids and local anesthetics may be helpful, similar attention to the responsible TPs is generally more effective. Subdeltoid bursitis and rotator cuff tear are discussed in Section 8 of Chapter 21. The frozen shoulder is considered in Section 8 of Chapter 26. Tenosynovitis of the hand is covered in Section 8 of Chapter 34 and tennis elbow in Section 8 of Chapter 36.

Neurological Diseases

In general, neurological disease is identified by motor and sensory deficits in the distribution of the afflicted nerve and may be chiefly either motor or sensory. Motor signs are atrophy, weakness, diminished or absent reflexes, and acute and/or chronic neuropathic findings by electrodiagnostic examination.

Sensory changes due to neurological disease are described as numbness, tingling, burning, pins and needles, and other distortions of sensation. The pain referred by myofascial TPs, on the other hand, generally is deep and aching, but occasionally is felt as lightning-like jabs of pain. A few patients with TPs complain of loss of sensation (numbness) rather than pain, and rarely of throbbing, a sensation which usually is of vascular origin. Sensory neuropathy is tested by sensory nerve conduction studies.

The presence of **trigeminal neuralgia** (tic douloureux)[60, 225, 284] is identified by paroxysmal pain usually limited to the distribution of one division of the trigeminal nerve. The pain is sudden, sharply lancinating in quality, and lasts a matter of seconds. It may be precipitated by activity or stimuli in the region of the mouth.[78] The dystonic paroxysm, grimace, or tic of trigeminal neuralgia distinguishes it from a myofascial pain syndrome.[269]

Similarly, **glossopharyngeal neuralgia**[225] is a paroxysmal neuralgia of the glossopharyngeal nerve comparable to that of the trigeminal nerve.[31] **Sphenopalatine neuralgia**[225] is relieved by anesthetizing the sphenopalatine ganglion.[214] This neuralgia also may be associated with cluster headache that responds to the same treatment.[78]

Ménière's disease, trigeminal neuralgia, other cranial neurological lesions, and spasmodic torticollis are discussed in Section 8 of Chapter 7. Thoracic outlet entrapment, the costoclavicular syndrome, the hyperabduction syndrome, and cervical ribs are reviewed in Section 6 of Chapter 20. The cubital syndrome is considered under Section 8 of Chapter 32. Cervical radiculopathy is discussed in Section 8 of Chapter 16 and in Chapter 22, and lumbar radiculopathy in Section 8 of Chapter 48.

Visceral Disease

Active myofascial TPs in abdominal wall muscles can disturb visceral function, apparently through autonomic pathways; these visceral disorders constitute somatovisceral effects. *Vice versa*, visceral disease causes a viscerosomatic effect when it refers pain to skeletal muscles and activates satellite TPs in them. Chest somatovisceral and viscerosomatic effects are reviewed in Section 6 of Chapter 42; corresponding abdominal effects are discussed in Section 6 of Chapter 49.

Patients with pain due to ischemic heart disease usually show electrocardiographic abnormality on stress testing, if not at rest. Relief of pain by the application of vapocoolant does *not* rule out serious cardiac disease. See also Section 8 of Chapter 42. The key to distinguishing the pseudo-appendictis of active rectus abdominis TPs from underlying visceral disease is palpation of either the abdominal wall itself, or of the abdominal contents, as described in Section 8 of Chapter 49.

Infections and Infestations

Infectious myalgias that might be confused with myofascial TP pain are of viral, bacterial, or protozoan nature. Generally, the presence of symptoms other than pain indicates a non-myofascial cause of the pain. However, after recovery from the infectious illness, myofascial TPs that were activated within the painful regions may persist and require extinction for complete relief.[48]

Viral diseases. True myalgia, as distinguished from use of this term to describe TP tenderness, exhibits diffuse muscle tenderness that is a sign of viremia, rather than the spot tenderness of myofascial TPs. Viral disease also produces other symptoms of systemic illness, particularly fever.

Many viral diseases typically cause acute muscular pain and soreness in the head and neck regions, usually with fever. The list includes **Colorado tick fever, arbovirus encephalitis, Omsk hemorrhagic fever,**[216] **influenza A,**[133] **psittacosis,**[134] **Rocky Mountain spotted fever,**[293] and the prodromal phase of **smallpox**[204] and **vesicular stomatitis virus** infections.[217] Other systemic viral infections cause myalgia elsewhere in the body than the head and neck. These include the **phlebotomus fever form of arbovirus,**[216] **pleurodynia** (Devil's grip),[150] and acute **spinal paralytic poliomyelitis.**[286]

The presence of **oral herpes simplex** greatly aggravates myofascial TP syndromes, especially in the muscles of the head, neck and shoulder girdles.

Degenerative changes of a nonspecific type have been occasionally demonstrated histologically in the painful muscles of patients with viral diseases.[2]

Bacterial Diseases. Myalgia, and activation of TPs, can occur with many febrile bacterial infections, such as bacterial endocarditis. Local myalgia associated with acute **suppurative myositis,** due to staphylococci or streptococci, occurs almost always in obviously sick individuals.[2] **Streptococcal myositis** causes marked local edema, pain and crepitation.[200] **Poststreptococcal arthralgia** produces symptoms of tendinalgia or myalgia, without joint tenderness. While passive motion at the joint is painless, isometric tension of its muscles is painful.[66] **Clostridial myositis** is marked by sudden, severe local pain which develops hours-to-weeks after a penetrating wound. Edematous swelling and loss of pulses help to identify **gas gangrene.**[113] Infection with a spirochete causes **leptospirosis** (Weil's disease), which causes severe muscle aching and diffuse sensitivity to palpation; the muscles of the thighs and lumbar area are mainly involved. This myalgia, and a high spiking fever with recurrent chills and headache, typically lasts 4–9 days.[218]

Infestations. **Trichinosis** is a chronic infestation of the skeletal musculature by the larvae of the worm-like trichina, causing generalized muscle pain and tenderness, and often severe weakness.[2] The myalgia of **filariasis** is associated with lymphadenitis, progressing to lymphangitis.[193] **Malaria** characteristically produces headache and muscular pain associated with recurrent chills and fever.[194]

Neoplasm

When, after effective treatment, the patient's myofascial TP pain recurs promptly because of perpetuating factors, the local tenderness of the TPs and their other signs of hyperirritability also recur. However, when the patient's pain continues, even though the TP tenderness and signs of hyperirritability have been eliminated, one must immediately look for other, less common sources of pain, including neoplasm.

Psychogenic Pain and Pain Behavior

One occasionally sees a patient whose pain is primarily psychogenic due to conversion hysteria,[284] or is largely fabricated for conscious secondary gain. Muscle tenderness suggestive of myofascial TPs was found more frequently among psychiatric patients than among control subjects.[39] Much more frequently, patient coping behavior,[69] lack of understanding of the symptoms, lifestyle and anxieties enhance pain caused by organic disease and by myofascial TPs; the increased pain, in turn, aggravates the psychological problems.[248] Each of these components must be identified and treated individually, usually simultaneously.

Patients with predominantly hysterical or secondary gain symptoms generally fail to express emotional distress commensurate with their pain, and they *behave* as if threatened by increased function, although their *words* say they want increased function, *if* it is pain-free. A careful history with full attention to psychological overtones identifies these components and helps to establish their relative importance.

D. MECHANISMS OF TRIGGER POINTS

This section first summarizes clinical and experimental observations that need explanation relevant to TPs, then describes pathophysiological mechanisms that are germane to TP phenomena and, finally, presents an hypothesis as to the nature of TPs that relates the mechanisms

to the observed clinical and physiological facts.

Observations in Need of Explanation

Trigger Point Tenderness. Authors describing myofascial TPs consistently have reported a spot in the muscle that is hypersensitive to pressure (the TP).

Referred Pain. Of critical importance, myofascial TPs consistently refer pain to a distance in patterns that are characteristic of each muscle.

Kellgren[124] studied many of the major muscles of the body and in 1938 reported that each referred pain to a distance from the site of stimulation when the muscle belly was injected with 0.1–0.3 ml of 6% hypertonic saline. He also reported[125] that pressure on a tender spot in a muscle of certain patients with "fibrositis" reproduced the patient's pain. He used the pain patterns found by injection, in reverse, to locate which muscle had the tender spot (TP) that was causing the patient's pain complaint. The tender spot was often remote from the pain. Injection of that spot with procaine relieved the patient's related pain. Within a few years, Travell,[273] Good[82] and Kelly[127] reported extensive clinical experience that paralleled Kellgren's observations. In 1967, Hockaday and Whitty[112] confirmed Kellgren's principle findings. Active TPs sometimes referred cutaneous paresthesias and numbness instead of deep pain.[240]

We[230] found that as a single injection of a larger quantity, 5–10 ml, of a stronger saline solution, 8.5%, diffused through the latissimus dorsi muscle, it induced a sequence of referred pain patterns that overlapped in time and location. This suggested that many sites within a muscle are potentially able to refer pain, and that adjacent sites are likely to evoke different, but overlapping, pain patterns. Referred pain produced by digital pressure on an active TP may take 10 or 15 sec to appear, similar to the delay in the onset of referred pain in these saline experiments and to the delay in nociceptor response after the injection of bradykinin in experiments with cats.[297]

The referral of pain to distant sites by sensory nerves from muscle has been demonstrated experimentally in man. Ochoa and Torebjörk[189] found that intraneural stimulation of a sensory nerve fascicle from a human muscle not infrequently produced a characteristic dull pain. The pain was felt deeply, not only in a broad region of the muscle,[189] but also in distant portions of the body,[260] analogous to the referred pain patterns reported in this manual.

Myofascial referred pain did not follow dermatomal,[26] myotomal[130] or scleroto-mal[120] patterns of innervation.[240, 271]

Figure 2.1 summarizes schematically our interpretation of several clinical characteristics of myofascial TPs. The TP initiates referred pain that may be felt locally around the TP, may project to other locations within the region innervated by the same spinal segment, or may be felt in regions innervated by other spinal segments.

Referred Tenderness. Usually, an area where the patient has been experiencing referred pain also is tender to palpation. This referred tenderness disappears as soon as the TP is inactivated. Both referred tenderness and spontaneous referred pain from an active deltoid TP were greatly ameliorated by a stellate ganglion block.[73]

Non-pain Referred Phenomena. Myofascial TPs may refer vascular, secretory, and pilomotor autonomic changes. They also may produce skeletal motor, visual, vestibular, and space-perceptual disturbances.

Clinically, **vasomotor** autonomic effects are common, if one looks for them. Painful stimulation either of a TP or of an adjacent non-TP area in the upper trapezius muscle produced a transient reduction in the amplitude of temporal artery pulsations on the same and contralateral sides, during pain. However, only reduction in the TP irritability by sustained digital pressure or by precise needling and procaine injection produced a rebound increase in temporal pulse amplitude and only homolaterally, in the pain reference zone of the TP.[262] Activity of shoulder girdle TPs produced skin temperature changes.[240] Active sternocleidomastoid TPs (sternal division) produced a discharge of tears and reddening of the conjunctiva.[266]

The senior author obtained a thermogram of the face of a man with chronic tension headache. The thermogram showed an area of cooling over the right forehead where the patient was experienc-

ing mild pain referred from TPs in the clavicular division of the sternocleidomastoid muscle. Compression of this muscle at the TP caused pallor and a reduction of skin temperature of 3.8 C (7 F) in the frontal reference zone as referred head pain was intensified by the pressure on the TP.[275]

The **secretory** autonomic changes observed clinically include: coryza and lacrimation,[266] localized sweating produced on the forehead,[266] and other variations in the sweat pattern.[240] Pressure on hypersensitive TPs may cause sweat to break out in the reference zone.[262] Unilateral sweating of the forehead was observed to disappear promptly after inactivation of TPs in the sternocleidomastoid muscle.[264]

Sola and Williams[242] reported a marked decrease in skin resistance (depolarization of dermal and sweat gland membranes) as an electrode probe passed over the TP. In another study, discrete areas of low skin resistance correlated well with deep and superficial tenderness, existing musculoskeletal strain, and resting EMG activity of the paraspinal muscles. The muscle beneath some areas of reduced skin resistance had tender spots characteristic of TPs.[138] New areas of low skin resistance could be induced by postural and myofascial insults.[137] In summary, spots of decreased skin resistance are often found over TPs, but are not specific to them.

Referred **pilomotor** activity (gooseflesh) appears spontaneously and can be induced by pressure applied to active TPs that are sometimes found in specific locations.[262] Stimulation of an active trapezius TP No. 7 (Section 1 in Chapter 6) characteristically produces this response.

The influence of myofascial TPs on **skeletal muscle activity** is clinically demonstrated by the induction of satellite TPs, and increased motor unit activity of muscles in the pain reference zone.[35, 270]

Cobb et al.,[41] demonstrated that stimulation of a wrist extensor by injection of 6% saline solution, or by injection of the same solution into the periosteum of the L_1 spinous process, produced motor unit activity roughly proportional to the pain in six of seven subjects. The location of each monitoring electrode was directly over the site of injection, which would have been within the pain reference zone in the forearm, if the extensor carpi radialis longus muscle was injected.

Disturbance of **vestibular function and space perception** may originate in TPs in the clavicular division of the sternocleidomastoid muscle (Chapter 7). They can cause imbalance and disorientation of the body in space,[240] and postural dizziness.[264] Some of these patients can not gauge distances and find themselves unexpectedly bumping into one side of a doorway[262]; they veer toward the side of the most active TPs. This proprioceptive disturbance is less severe in degree, but similar in kind, to the severe disorientation, imbalance and motor incoordination observed in monkeys and baboons when their C_1, C_2 and C_3 dorsal spinal nerve roots were bilaterally anesthetized.[44]

The **visual disturbances** caused by sternocleidomastoid TPs include blurring of vision and intermittent double vision, without pupillary changes.[262]

TP activity thus modulates many central nervous system functions in addition to sensation, as indicated in Figure 2.1 by the triple arrow.

Taut Bands. These regions within the muscle substance that have increased resistance to palpation and are associated with TPs have been described as fibrositic "nodules,"[151] "ropiness" of the muscle,[139] and also as intermediate spindle-like forms.[213] In our experience, the ropiness is most apparent when the muscle is palpated by moving the fingertip across the direction of the muscle fibers repeatedly at different positions along the length of the muscle, as described and illustrated in Section 9 of Chapter 3. Examined in this way, few TPs seem nodular. The TP is the spot along any one band where local tenderness reaches its maximum. The muscle fibers of the taut band, which extend through the TP zone, show no EMG activity at rest.[35, 139, 257] Taut bands have been observed to persist after death, until obscured by rigor mortis.[219]

Although the muscle feels tense and resists stretching, the absence of EMG activity means that the muscle is *not* in spasm; it must be shortened for other reasons. Any proposed mechanism must account for the fact that this tense band, which can persist after death, frequently releases within seconds or minutes after specific TP therapy.

Nodularity. When the same taut band described above is approached by an entirely different, deep-stroking massage technique (stripping), one feels a lump or nodule at the TP. After lubricating the skin over the muscle, the thumbs of both hands, or fingers, are placed across the muscle fibers at one end of the muscle and pressed firmly into the tissue as they slide along the length of the muscle toward the TP. This produces a milking action that pushes tissue fluids ahead of the digits, leaving a white blanched region immediately behind them. One can see the erythema of cutaneous venous congestion preceding the fingers and very likely the same is occurring in the muscle beneath. Movement is recommended in the direction of venous flow. As the digits approach the region of the TP, they encounter a fullness suggestive of a lump or nodule, regardless of the direction from which the TP is approached. Since deep massage of the tender spot in the muscle was generally the treatment of choice for "muscular rheumatism" (myofascial TPs) long before the turn of this century,[110] and for "fibrositis" afterward,[291] this technique may have contributed significantly to the popularity of terms like fibrositic *nodule.* With sufficient repetitions of massage, this nodularity disappears and the thumbs can slide the length of the muscle without encountering the obstruction; the local TP tenderness and referred phenomena also disappear with it.

In summary, cross-fiber palpation reveals a taut band that includes the TP, whereas, deep palpation along the length of the same muscle fibers gives the impression of a nodule at the TP.

Local Twitch Responses and Electromyographic Activity. The local twitch response (LTR) of the fibers in the palpable band associated with a TP is produced by snapping palpation of the TP. The LTR is seen and/or felt as a contraction of the fibers in the taut band and lasts as long as 1 sec. EMG monitoring of the muscle fibers in the band reveals a sustained burst of electrical activity that has the same configuration as motor unit action potentials.[57] In one experiment on a TP in the third finger extensor, the LTR was primarily a local response and not a central nervous system reflex. The response persisted despite complete motor and sensory nerve anesthesia, which was produced by sustained pressure from a cuff around the limb.[228] The adequate stimulus to produce an LTR was sudden change of pressure on the TP. Electrical stimulation of a TP by 0.05-ms square waves at 1 pulse/sec produced referred pain, but no LTR.[228]

The moment an EMG needle electrode was inserted accurately into a TP, the needle registered a high frequency, repetitive discharge with action potential spikes of high amplitude and short duration. No discharge was recorded from the rest of the muscle, which was at rest. The potentials recorded from a TP by a coaxial needle ranged in frequency between 10 and 90/sec, with amplitude greater than 1 mV and duration 3-4 ms.[264, 267] Popelianskii[195] reported that intrusion of the electrode directly into the affected area of muscle is accompanied by volley-like activity in a muscle at rest. Arroyo[10] observed that the insertion of the needle electrode into a "fibrositic nodule" produced a continuous and prolonged burst of electrical activity similar to that of a normal voluntary muscular contraction of moderate degree. At the same time, surrounding fibers of the same muscle were inactive. This electrical insertional activity of the TP was not abolished by voluntary contraction of the antagonist muscle, but was abolished by injecting the area with procaine, and was attenuated by injecting diazepam intramuscularly into a nearby muscle. This effect could reflect either the reduction of internuncial spinal cord activity by that drug or a local action that reduced the irritability of the TP.[10]

The LTR apparently depends on local hyperirritability of motor nerves and, possibly, of sensory nerve fibers. Direct propagation of action potentials originating in the muscle fibers themselves has not been eliminated.

Self Perpetuation. A TP may persist for decades, restricting range of motion, and recurrently becoming active enough to cause attacks of referred pain without involving other muscles. Nevertheless, one treatment session may inactivate such a TP permanently.

The fact that TP activity is self-sustaining over long periods of time is illustrated schematically by its feedback loop (arrows marked A and B in Figure 2.1). Some of this self-sustaining feedback may be within the muscle itself and may not involve the spinal cord.

Responsiveness to Treatment. Many different techniques can be used to inactivate TPs.

In the **stretch-and-spray** procedure for the inactivation of myofascial TPs, passive stretch is the essential component. Correct vapocoolant spray technique facilitates stretching the muscle to its full length. Excessive spraying that cools the muscle tends to aggravate, rather than inactivate TPs.

Release of muscle tension by stretch and spray is demonstrated by increased range of motion. The procedure can release the muscular compression of an artery caused by taut myofascial bands. The arm was held in abduction with just enough external rotation so that pressure from taut bands in the involved pectoralis minor muscle occluded the radial pulse. While holding the arm fixed in the same position, vapocooling the skin over the stretched pectoralis minor muscle immediately released pressure on the artery and allowed return of the radial pulse.

For inactivating TPs in traumatized connective tissue, as in an ankle sprain, the vapocoolant is the chief agent. Here, stretch is less important.

Ischemic compression, which is firm digital pressure applied to the TP, deep stroking massage (stripping), kneading massage and vibratory massage, can be effective. Each of the first three cause blanching (ischemia) with hypoxia, followed by a reactive hyperemia.

Puncture of TPs is effective whether done by dry needling, by injection with saline, or with a local anesthetic. Dry needling requires the greatest precision, or most repetitions. Long-acting anesthetics require the least precise placement of the injection, but cause muscle necrosis.[22]

A sustained application of **ultrasound** at low intensity inactivates TPs.[188] The heating effect of ultrasound reaches deep into muscular tissue and may have some additional non-thermal effects due to agitation of the molecules by the high frequency sound waves.[147]

Histological Studies. Although authors have repeatedly alluded to negative biopsy findings,[227] only four such biopsies were reported by two authors with enough detail for the reader to know that the biopsy was taken of a muscle with point tenderness characteristic of TPs and to know what stain was used.[219, 221]

The first extensive biopsy study with complete details was reported in 1951 by Glogowski and Wallraff,[79] who described 24 biopsies that were taken from back and neck muscles and were examined by light microscopy. They found only one specimen with sufficient connective tissue proliferation to account for the palpable hardening for which the biopsy site was selected. The remaining specimens consistently showed marked non-specific changes also seen in the next study.

Miehlke et al.[173] stained paraffin sections of nearly 3 times as many biopsies with hematoxylin and eosin and, in addition, cut frozen sections prepared with histochemical and fat stains. They divided their specimens into four groups: (1) biopsies obtained from non-specific, inconstant tender areas (non-TP control specimens); (2) biopsies taken where there was spot muscle tenderness, but no associated pain complaint (latent TPs); (3) samples selected for mild to moderately severe muscular rheumatism (active myofascial TPs); and (4) specimens excised from areas of muscle causing severe clinical symptoms (vigorously active myofascial TPs).

The biopsies of the **first** group showed normal muscle.[173]

In the **second** group, biopsies of latent TPs that were processed routinely were normal, but fat-stained frozen sections showed "fat dusting," an accumulation of fine fat droplets.

The **third** group of biopsies also showed occasional "fat dusting," but, in addition, evinced mild non-specific dystrophic changes.[2] The fibers were variable in width, variable in their intensity of staining, and contained increased numbers of nuclei inside and outside the muscle fibers. The nuclei inside muscle fibers were often central, sometimes in chains. Striations remained intact.

The biopsies of the **fourth** group evinced more severe dystrophic pathology[2] that always included interstitial abnormalities, with or without marked fiber degeneration. Additional findings included contracture knots (club-like distensions of contracted myofibrils beside a section of empty sarcolemmal tube),[220] loss of cross

striations, and extreme variability in the intensity of staining of muscle fibers. Between the fibers were dense accumulations of nuclei, especially near blood vessels. Endomysial and perimysial clusters of nuclei appeared, sometimes separately and sometimes together. In severe cases, fat and connective tissue replaced muscle fibers.[173] Comparable observations were reported by others in man.[1, 11, 79] Similar degenerative dystrophic changes were also reported in the muscles of rabbits made deficient in Vitamin E.[158]

In 1957, Brendstrup et al.[33] biopsied palpable "fibrositis areas" in paraspinal muscles of 12 patients, along with the normal contralateral muscle. Sections were stained with toluidine blue. Some of the muscles showed interstitial infiltration of a metachromatically staining mucopolysaccharide. The authors thought it might account for the localized turgor felt in the muscle, since it was present in 75% of the "fibrositis" muscles and only 25% of control muscle biopsies. Awad[11] later reported finding the same substance in 8 of 10 biopsies of tender nodular areas in muscles.

Two ultramicroscopic studies of muscle fibers in the region of TPs are reported. Awad[11] noted giant (double length) sarcomeres extending beyond the Z lines of neighboring myofibrils. Some fibers showed intracellular lipid droplets, and mast cells were seen to be discharging granules. Blood platelets occurred in large clusters.

Fassbender[64, 65] reported a four-stage process of degeneration of the contractile apparatus in biopsies from regions of "focal muscular rheumatism" (TPs). In the first stage, mitochondria were swollen and myofilaments appeared moth-eaten in the region of the I bands where actin filaments attach to the Z line, which marks the end of a sarcomere. In the second stage, myofilament destruction also included the A bands (myosin filaments), but the Z bands remained intact. In the third stage,[64] disrupted sarcomere remnants were recognizable, but lay scattered and, in the last stage, complete destruction of the contractile substance left only a fine granular residue within the sarcolemma. Accumulations of collagen appeared in areas of necrosis. These observations correspond closely to the ultrastructural changes seen after ischemia of dog muscle,[247] and were similar to the interruption of myofibrils, lipid and glycogen accumulation, and enlarged and distorted mitochondria seen in the muscles of alcoholic volunteers after 1 month of alcohol ingestion.[210]

The Trigger Point Zone. When a needle thermocouple was first inserted into a TP, the temperature was higher than that of the surrounding tissue, but after 15–60 sec, the temperature fell to the level of the surrounding tissue, as the TP activity faded.[263] This means that the TP is a region of increased metabolism and/or decreased circulation. Below a critical level, the poorer the circulation in that region, the more slowly would heat being generated by the TP be carried away and the greater would be its temperature compared with the surrounding resting muscle.

Popelianskii, *et al.*[195] measured the rate at which radioactive [131]NaI was eliminated from tissue in the clinically affected area. They reported a distinct prolongation of the resorption rate of the isotope, which they interpreted as due to impaired local circulation.

Studies of the TP zone by needle EMG were noted in the section on "Local Twitch Response and Electromyographic Activity," above.

Neuromuscular Physiology

This section summarizes current concepts of pain perception, referred pain and muscle contraction.

Pain Perception. To understand the mechanisms that can be responsible for myofascial pain phenomena, one must know the fundamentals of how the body processes sensory information.

The perception of pain can originate exogenously by stimulation of a sensory end organ or of a free nerve ending. Pain may arise endogenously as central pain, or it may be displaced (referred pain). Sensory input from one location may be misinterpreted by the cortex as pain arising elsewhere.

The transmission through the central nervous system of sensations that are perceived as pain is an extremely complex process. They are intertwined with non-pain sensations. The pain "signal" on its way from muscle or skin to the cortex is transformed at least four times on at least four levels. Modulation of the signal (adjustment of its strength up or down) can occur: (1) at the receptor that converts the stimulus into nerve impulses; (2) at the spinal cord level; (3) in the network of relay stations between the spinal cord and the sensory cortex (e.g. the thalamus); and (4) in the sensory cortex itself.

The **sensory receptors and their nerves** have been studied mainly for the skin. Free nerve endings are here included as one type of sensory receptor. Some attention has recently been devoted to sensory afferents from muscle. In the skin, noxious stimuli are mediated by Group III (myelinated A_δ) and Group IV (unmyelinated C) nerve fibers. The approximately 10-times faster conduction velocity of the former is closely associated with epicritic sensation that more sharply localizes and discriminates the kind of stimulus applied to the skin.[117] Many of these A_δ fibers respond to innocuous mechanical and thermal stimuli, producing sensations other than pain; the response range of some extend to noxious (tissue damaging and therefore painful) stimuli. About one-quarter of these fibers respond only to stimuli that are potentially or frankly damaging to tissue.[29] The slower, unmyelinated C fibers are associated with the protopathic pathway that propagates delayed, less clearly localized, aching pain.[117] Nearly half of these C fibers originate as mechanoreceptors that respond to innocuous stimulation of hairy skin. The rest are either mechanical or thermal nociceptors, or combined mechanical and thermal (polymodal) nociceptors. No subgroup responds only to chemical stimuli.[117]

The activity of skin receptors is variously influenced by sensitizing noxious substances. Sensitization of the nerve ending by prior stimulation, or by exposure to certain agents such as histamine, prostaglandin, bradykinin or serotonin, causes a marked increase in the response of some nerves to the same intensity of stimulus.[191] Thus, the response to a stimulus can depend strongly on the state of sensitization of the receptors being stimulated. Such sensitization helps to explain the tenderness associated with inflammation and very likely contributes to the hyperirritability of TPs.

Although skeletal muscle is richly supplied with proprioceptive sense organs (e.g. muscle spindles and Golgi tendon organs), there is no indication that their input reaches consciousness. Unlike skin, muscle is apparently all but devoid of mechanoreceptors and thermoreceptors, but is richly supplied with Group III and Group IV fibers, *both* of which, in man, mediate the protopathic type of poorly localized aching pain.[260] The muscle nociceptors with unmyelinated axons respond to a wide variety of noxious stimuli, and can give a sustained response.[116]

More than one-half of the afferent nerve fibers from muscle are either A_δ or C fibers.[297] A large group of the A_δ fibers are ergoceptors (metaboceptors) that respond to chemical and/or other changes caused by muscular work.[170] The C fiber nociceptors in cat gastrocnemius and soleus muscles responded to bradykinin, serotonin, histamine and potassium chloride, evincing equivalent responses at respective doses of 1:30:66:4000, when each agent was injected intra-arterially.[68] In a similar study, prostaglandin E_2 and serotonin potentiated muscle afferent responses to bradykinin.[297] Great variation exists among individual muscle receptors in their responsiveness to noxious chemical and mechanical stimuli.[170]

In man, intraneural stimulation of single afferent fibers from skeletal muscle produced discrete sensations of dull pain and tension perceived as coming from the muscle, but not sharp pain or itch.[260] Both A_δ and C fiber responses were observed.[189] Stimulation of many, but less than half, of these skeletal muscle afferent fibers, unlike skin fibers, caused pain felt in other areas of the body (referred pain), in addition to pain felt in the muscle itself.[259, 260]

The dorsal horn of the **spinal cord** acts like a computer that processes the incoming sensory signals, rearranging and modulating them before sending them on to the next higher level. The process that determines which signals are emphasized and which are ignored is subject to many influences. The dorsal horn is an incredibly complex, yet precisely organized, 6-laminae structure that was described by Rexed (in Ref. 117). As dorsal rootlets penetrate the cord, the large myelinated fibers collect to form a medial bundle, whereas most of the small myelinated and unmyelinated fibers form a lateral group of fibers. Most of these incoming small fibers, which carry the pain signals, either bifurcate or bend to traverse one or two segments in the tract of Lissauer before sending collaterals to the underlying substantia gelatinosa. Intrinsic fibers, which interconnect as many as five or six spinal segments *via* the tract of Lissauer, comprise about 25% of the tract.[131] Thus, the potential for sensory input from one segment to influence the sensory signals transmitted by another segment is large. Melzack's[165] explanation of the Gate theory[168] helps one to understand, in part, how sensation is modulated at the spinal level. The recognition of descending serotonergic and noradrenergic spinal pathways that strongly inhibit pain at the spinal level is a major advance of recent years.[118]

Nociceptive impulses ascend in the spinal cord primarily *via* either the phylogenetically more recent neospinothalamic tract, which is associated with epicritic sensation, or the slower conducting, older paleospinothalamic pathway, associated with protopathic sensation. The latter pathway provokes the powerful unpleasant affective and aversive responses of avoidance and inactivity. It accounts for much of the suffering associated with pain.[29]

At the **subcortical level**, a number of structures associated with the action of morphine strongly modulate pain. When these structures are electrically stimulated or exposed to appropriate neuromodulators, they profoundly inhibit pain. The neuromodulators are called enkephalins; a molecular fragment, endorphin, has demonstrated pain relief more than 48 times the potency of morphine on a molar basis.[118] Several studies have shown that acupuncture analgesia depends on release of these neuromodulators. Melzack[166] proposes that hyperstimulation analgesia provides relief from chronic pain by "closing the spinal gate" through a central biasing mechanism, possibly located in the reticular formation of the brain stem, or by the disruption of reverberatory neural circuits responsible for the memory of pain.

At the **cortical level**, we intuitively and reflexly avoid pain. Sudden pain is interpreted as tissue-threatening injury; sustained pain is interpreted as indicating the need for rest to permit recuperation from injury.[281] When neither interpretation applies, but pain persists, the patient is confronted with chronic pain, as often happens with neglected myofascial TPs. The suffering associated with pain is enormously influenced at the cortical level by the meaning ascribed to it. The powerful effect of meaning on the perception of pain is eloquently demonstrated by religious rites that involve serious tissue damage without anesthesia, but also without evidence of pain or suffering.[165] Acute pain that diminishes in the course of the natural healing process is generally manageable psychologically. However, recurrent or persistent pain due to an unrecognized or untreatable cause threatens future function and well-being, which often leads to frustration, depression and progressive disability.[248]

When patients mistakenly believe that they must "live with" TP pain because they think it is due to arthritis or a pinched nerve that is inoperable, they restrict activity in order to avoid pain. Such patients must learn that the pain comes from muscles, not from nerve damage, and not from permanent arthritic changes in the bones. Most important, they must know it is responsive to treatment. This gives the pain a new *meaning*. When these patients realize the twin facts that their pain is myofascial and is treatable, their lives take on new meaning and they are started on the road to recovery of function.

Referred Pain. Referred pain from any source, TP or visceral, is prohibitively difficult to study in animals and, at this time, the exact mechanisms responsible for it are far from resolved. Hypotheses to account for it include peripheral branching of axons, convergence-projection, convergence-facilitation, reflex constriction of the vasa nervorum, and autonomic nociceptive feedback.

The **peripheral branching of axons**[234] would permit the response to a stimulus in one branch to be interpreted as coming from the other branch of the axon. This would require individual sensory neurons to have both visceral and somatic branches. To account thus for the pain referred from myofascial TPs, one branch would have to extend to the TP zone of a muscle and the other branch to the referred pain zone for that muscle. Extensive branching of many sensory nerves in this manner has not been reported.

The **convergence-projection** mechanism[211] is the one generally cited and can occur when cutaneous afferents and visceral (or skeletal muscle) afferents converge on the same spinal neuron. Such convergence has been demonstrated on spinal neurons of the spinothalamic tract in primates.[175] In this model, it is assumed that the sensory cortex has become accustomed to interpreting nociceptor responses of such neurons as coming from the cutaneous structures. The cortex thus misinterprets a strong visceral (or muscular) input as arising from the corresponding skin site. It is argued that, if this mechanism is exclusively responsible for referred visceral pain, anesthetizing the painful skin region should have no effect on the perception of the pain.[234]

The **convergence-facilitation** theory[211] proposes that the normal background activity of sensory afferents in the reference zone is facilitated sufficiently by abnormal visceral afferent activity to be registered as pain. Good[85] reviewed Mackenzie's introduction of this mechanism in 1921 as an "irritable focus" in the spinal cord. Should this be the mechanism responsible for referred pain, it is argued that local anesthesia of the somatic reference zone eliminates the pain for the duration of the block. In fact, local anesthetic block of the region of referred pain often provides relief that long outlasts the duration of the anesthesia, indicating that this mechanism plus another factor, such as suppression of a reverberating feedback in the central nervous system, is present.[166, 288] Considering the strong preponderance of inhibitory synapses in the dorsal horn,[131] this effect of convergence is as likely to be caused by disinhibition as by facilitation.

Roberts[206] proposed that a visceral disturbance might cause **reflex constriction of the vasa nervorum**. If these vessels nourished sensory nerves supplying the reference zone, their ischemia might cause pain to be felt in that area.

Theoretically, **autonomic nociceptive feedback** could occur if autonomic nerves reflexly released nociceptive substances in the referred pain zone.[197, 297] This mechanism would be self-sustaining if the resultant pain stimulated more such autonomic activity.[297]

Muscle Contraction. A striated muscle is an assembly of fascicles, each of which is a bundle of muscle fibers (Fig. 2.2). Each muscle fiber (a muscle cell), encloses approximately 2000 myofibrils. The basic contractile unit of skeletal muscle is the sarcomere. Sarcomeres are arranged serially to form a myofibril (Fig. 2.2). Adjacent sarcomeres are connected by the Z line (or band). Each sarcomere contains a large array of actin and myosin filaments that interact to produce the contractile force (Fig. 2.2).

The myosin heads, which are a form of adenosine triphosphatase (ATPase), interact with actin to exert contractile force. These contacts are seen through the electron microscope as cross bridges between the actin and myosin filaments. Ionized calcium triggers the interaction and adenosine triphosphate (ATP) provides the energy. The ATP releases a myosin head from the actin after one power "stroke" and immediately "recocks" it for another cycle. Many such power "strokes" are needed for the random rowing motion required of many myosin heads to accomplish one smooth twitch contraction.

In the presence of both free calcium and ATP, the actin and myosin continue to interact, expending energy and exerting force to shorten the sarcomere.[183] This interaction of actin and myosin, that produces tension and consumes energy, cannot happen if the sarcomeres are lengthened (the muscle stretched) so far that no overlap remains between actin and myosin. This has started to happen in the lowest drawing of Figure 2.2, where the actin filaments are beyond the reach of half of the myosin heads (cross bridges).

The calcium is normally sequestered in the tubular network of sarcoplasmic reticulum that surrounds each myofibril. Calcium is released from the sarcoplasmic reticulum on the arrival *via* "T" tubules of an action potential that had propagated along the surface of the muscle fiber from the myoneural junction. Normally, the free calcium is quickly recovered by the sarcoplasmic reticulum after it has been released. This return of the calcium terminates one twitch contraction of the muscle fiber.

Possible Explanations of Trigger Point Phenomena

Many observations and reports support the proposal of Popelianskii[195] that the myofascial TP process begins as a neuromuscular dysfunction, but can evolve into a histologically demonstrable dystrophic phase. The findings of Miehlke et al.,[173] which was the only extensive study that related the clinical symptoms to the biopsy findings, supported an initial dysfunctional phase that, with increased severity, developed into a dystrophic phase.

Some basic features of the neuromuscular dysfunction that characterize a TP are found below under the headings hyperirritability, increased metabolism/decreased circulation, and the palpable band. Following a discussion of dystrophic changes, the structure of the TP itself is considered, and finally, this section is summarized.

Hyperirritability. One aspect of neuromuscular dysfunction is sensory and/or motor hyperirritability at the TP as evidenced by: local tenderness to palpation; spontaneous referred pain, referred tenderness and referred autonomic phenomena; local twitch responses; and TP responses to needle penetration. The report of reduction in the threshold of the quadriceps muscles for spontaneous EMG activity[35] in response to pressure on a nearby TP illustrates its modulation of the responsiveness of neurons supplying the motor units in the region of that TP. The local twitch response depends upon hyperirritability of local motor and/or sensory nerves unless the action potentials of the response originate directly in the muscle fibers, which is considered unlikely.

These observations of hyperirritability may be accounted for if muscle afferent nerve endings have been sensitized. Substances that could act as sensitizing agents include serotonin, histamine, kinins and prostaglandins. When Awad[11] examined biopsies of TP areas under the electron microscope, he found a large number of platelets, which release serotonin, and degranulating mast cells, which release histamine.

The increased sensitivity of TPs to pressure could be mediated by sensitized mechanoreceptors or nociceptors, more

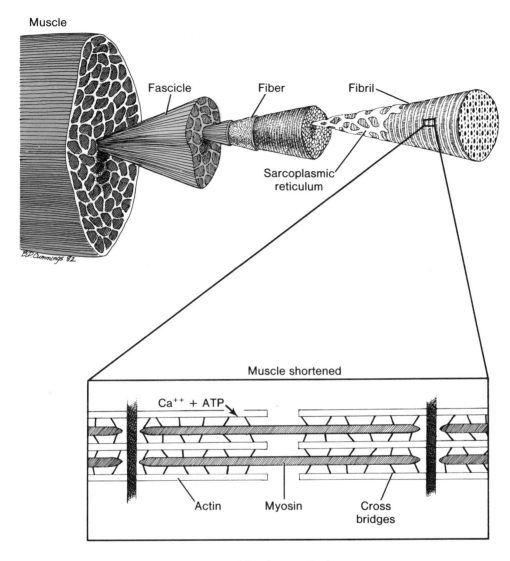

Muscle

Fascicle

Fiber

Fibril

Sarcoplasmic reticulum

Muscle shortened

Ca^{++} + ATP

Actin

Myosin

Cross bridges

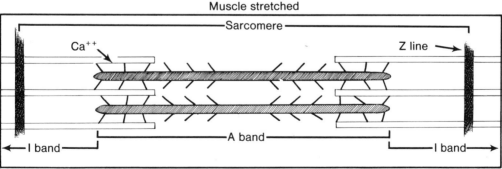

Muscle stretched

Sarcomere

Ca^{++}

Z line

A band

I band

I band

Figure 2.2.   Structure and contractile mechanism of normal skeletal muscle. The muscle is a bundle of fascicles (*light red*), each of which consists of striated muscle cells or fibers. One fiber contains on the order of 1000 myofibrils. *Insets*: adenosine triphosphate (*ATP*) and free calcium (*Ca^{++}*) activate the myosin heads (*cross bridges*) to tug on the actin filaments. This pulls the *Z lines* together and shortens the *sarcomere*, which is the contractile unit of the muscle. The portions of the actin filaments in two sarcomeres that are adjacent to a *Z line* and are free of myosin filaments form an *I band*.

likely Group III than Group IV fibers based on the rapidity and sharpness of the pain response. The afferent (sensory) fibers that run from a TP to the spinal cord and that are responsible for mediating referred pain, autonomic phenomena, and the modulation of motor neuron responsiveness need not be nociceptor fibers. Since, clinically, each of these phenomena may appear separately and since afferent nerves from muscle show a remarkable individuality of function,[68, 260] it would not be surprising if functionally different kinds of nerves represented each type of neural irritability. All afferent TP input to the CNS need not be carried by one kind of nerve. The probability of this multiple TP input to the spinal cord is identified in Figure 2.1 by the *triple arrow.*

If the referred pain is mediated by the projection-facilitation mechanism, afferent input from the TP would augment the effect on spinal cells of the normal sensory background activity from the reference zone, raising it to the pain level when transmitted cephalad. The *arrow* from the pain reference zone to the cord in Figure 2.1 represents this kind of reference zone input.

If the referred pain is mediated by projection-convergence, afferent fibers from the TP and from the referred pain zone must converge on a common spinothalamic tract neuron or on a cranial nerve central neuron. In this case, the cortex is thought to misinterpret TP activity as noxious stimulation of the reference zone afferent fibers.

The effectiveness of dry needling in terminating the hyperirritability of TPs may be due to mechanical disruption of the sensory nerve endings mediating the TP activity. Injection of any fluid, saline or anesthetic, may effectively wash out the sensitizing substances. Massage and pressure therapies that alternate ischemia and hyperemia may have a similar purgative action.

Increased Metabolism/Reduced Circulation. Diverse sources suggest that the TP is a region of increased metabolic demand and/or limited circulation, which are dysfunctions that would cause minimal histological changes. The increased temperature observed at the TP[263] could be due to **increased metabolic demand** and/or re-

duced circulation. An impressive number of important and common perpetuating factors (Chapter 4) concern **impairment of energy metabolism,** which reduces the ability of the muscle fibers to meet an increased demand. Among these factors are inadequacy of vitamins essential to energy metabolism, inadequate thyroid hormone function, anemia, and hypoglycemia.

The fine fat deposits observed in the second group of biopsies by Miehlke *et al.*[173] strongly suggest an early disturbance of fat metabolism. The abnormal mitochondria seen in the ultramicroscopic study reported by Fassbender[64] reinforce this evidence of metabolic stress.

Evidence for **impaired circulation** is based on clinical observations, biopsy studies, and temperature studies. Numerous authors have theorized, based on clinical experience, that the TP represents a region of local ischemia.[79, 144, 173, 221, 273] Fassbender[64] came to the same conclusion, based on the changes in endothelial cells of capillaries and connective tissue foci of proliferated cellular elements in his histologic studies. A radioisotope study produced evidence of slowing of perfusion in the region of the muscular lesion.[195] The feeling of fluid obstruction at the TP during stripping massage, a phenomenon that resolves with continued moving pressure, is consistent with impaired venous flow in the region of the TP.

When a needle thermocouple is first inserted into a TP, the temperature is higher than that of the surrounding tissue but, after 15–60 sec, the temperature falls to the level of the surrounding tissue, as the TP activity fades.[263] This means that the TP is a region of increased metabolism and/or decreased circulation. Below a critical level, the poorer the circulation in that region, the more slowly would heat being generated by the TP be carried away and the higher would be its temperature compared with the surrounding resting muscle.

Sympathetic mediated vasoconstriction is the most likely central feedback mechanism to maintain restricted circulation. The fact that stimulation of muscle nociceptors strongly activates γ-motor efferents to the muscle spindles[169] may contribute indirectly.

The Palpable Band. Historically, a number of explanations for the palpable hardness of the muscle containing TPs have proven inadequate. They include a deposit of fibrous tissue, a local edema or infiltrate, myogelosis (gelling of muscle colloids), and muscle spasm. Physiological contracture of muscle fibers seems the most promising explanation.

A **connective tissue deposit** as the basis for the palpable hardness in these tender muscles was assumed by authors subsequent to Froriep[71] because of his term "muscle callous," by the Scandinavians under the name "myitis," and in the histological report of Stockman in 1904.[249] Subsequent extensive biopsy studies[79, 173] eliminated this basis for explaining the texture of palpable bands.

Both **serous exudates**[1, 151] and **mucopolysaccharide deposits**[11, 33] are reported as commonly present. However, it is difficult to see how they would remain sufficiently well circumscribed and of sufficient volume to account for the palpable bands by themselves. Their presence is consistent with the inflammatory response produced by substances like histamine and prostaglandins that sensitize sensory nerves.

The concept of **myogelosis**, the gelling of muscle colloids, predates the sliding filament theory. The extensive biopsy studies designed specifically to identify this colloid[79, 173] concluded that no colloidal mass was present in the muscle that would account for the palpable hardenings associated with the tender areas in the muscle.

The early and persistent use of muscle **spasm** to account for the palpable bands and for the shortening of the muscle[18, 65, 79, 153, 173, 225, 273] is understandable because, on examination, the muscle feels as if it were in spasm. However, this explanation is untenable, primarily because motor unit activity, which is an essential component of muscle spasm, is often absent.[139] Also, central nervous system motor unit control is not known to contract certain groups of fibers in the form of bands, while the rest of the muscle remains relaxed. Normally, interdigitated muscle fibers of overlapping motor units take turns carrying the load. The situation appears more confusing when the muscle containing taut bands does develop spasm in response to an attempt to extend the muscle to its full range of motion. However, this spasm involves contraction of the muscle as a whole and not just a band of fibers in the muscle.

Contracture (contraction without action potentials) of the muscle fibers in the band would make it feel hardened and tense compared with surrounding fibers in the muscle.[231] Normally, the contractile activity of a muscle fiber is controlled by the rapid release and reabsorption of calcium stored in the sac-like sarcoplasmic reticulum. Release of calcium from this repository initiates contractile activity, return of calcium terminates contractile activity. The release of calcium is normally triggered by a brief propagated action potential. However, if the trauma activating the TP had damaged the sarcoplasmic reticulum and spilled its calcium, the sarcomeres exposed to the calcium for an extended period would sustain contractile activity as long as their ATP energy supply lasted. This contractile activity would persist despite the absence of action potentials, as long as calcium and ATP were present. The uncontrolled contractile activity of this portion of the muscle would cause equally uncontrolled local metabolism. The sustained contractile force could in turn produce the tension and hardness of the fibers that comprise the palpable band. The stimulus for reflex vasoconstriction of that region would be the need to control the runaway local metabolism.

This metabolism will terminate, and the contractile force stop if the muscle is stretched, and the sarcomeres elongated enough to separate the myosin heads from the reactive portion of the actin filaments. This could help to explain why stretching is so consistently helpful when dealing with myofascial TPs.

Dystrophic Changes. The development of the dystrophic pathologic changes identified by many authors,[11, 33, 79, 173] would account for the relatively poor response to specific myofascial therapy in some patients, and the absence of dystrophic changes, for the immediate response in others. Myofascial TPs biopsied before the development of the dystrophic phase would be expected to show few, if any, histological changes. The TPs of some patients, clinically, progress rapidly to a condition consistent with such dystrophic changes, whereas other patients may suffer from a single-muscle TP syndrome for 30 years or more that responds immediately and completely to simple stretch-and-spray therapy. Progression to the dystrophic phase apparently depends on more than time alone. Perpetuating factors may account for much of this difference in the rate of progression.

Trigger Point Structure. There is little evidence that a TP is an abnormal state of one of the sensory structures unique to muscle. Although TPs usually occur in a particular portion or portions of each muscle, they do not appear to have a fixed relation to any of the distinctive anatomical features of muscle. **Myoneural junctions** are normally placed centrally along muscle fibers,[42] where they must be located for the muscle to be mechanically efficient; TPs are sometimes close, sometimes far from mid-muscle. **Muscle spindles**[12] occur in the general vicinity of myoneural junctions, rarely toward the ends of a muscle, where TPs do occur. Muscle spindles have not been reported in biopsies of TPs, although they may have been seen and not considered important. They were not seen in biopsies of dog muscles selected for TP characteristics, where muscle spindles were specifically sought.[229] **Golgi tendon organs** and **paciniform corpuscles** are located at musculotendinous junctions[25, 244]; TPs only occasionally are located there.

On the other hand, the **free nerve endings** that occur on Groups II, III, and IV fibers from muscle are widely distributed in connective tissue between muscle fibers, in musculotendinous junction areas, and in blood vessel adventitia; free nerve endings are not restricted to any specific region of cat muscles.[244] It is likely that sensitized Group III and/or Group IV free nerve endings are responsible for the hyperirritability of a TP. The discharge of action potentials reported when penetrating the trigger area with a needle,[10, 195, 264, 267] is consistent with the TP being the site of sensitized nerves.

Using the patient's jump response and the local twitch response of the muscle as criteria of having encountered a TP, clinical experience with injecting them shows that directing a probing movement of the needle a few millimeters ($\frac{1}{16}$ in) to one side or the other determines whether the needle encounters or misses the TP. Therefore, the diameter of one TP is on the order of a few millimeters ($\frac{1}{16}$–$\frac{1}{8}$ in). However a cluster of five or six TPs can give the impression that the TP zone is a centimeter ($\frac{3}{8}$ in) or so in diameter. Experimental study of the local twitch response substantiated this observation.[57]

When one injects a TP, the needle frequently encounters a region of muscle in the immediate vicinity of the TP that is resistant like hard rubber, suggesting strongly contracted muscle fibers, organized exudate, or fibrosis. At other times, the needle encounters a firm encapsulated structure on the order of 1 or 2 mm ($\frac{1}{16}$ in) in diameter. It feels like well organized connective tissue. The nature of this structure remains to be demonstrated histologically in conjunction with TPs.

Summary. This summary proposes one way that known neuromuscular mechanisms can be fitted together to partially account for myofascial TPs. Further studies are needed to fill the gaps.

An acute muscle strain may overload the contractile elements in one region of the muscle causing tissue damage that includes tearing of the sarcoplasmic reticulum and release of its stored calcium, with loss of the ability of that portion of the muscle to remove the calcium ions. The chronic stress of the resultant sustained contraction, or excessive fatigue during repeated contractions, may cause a vulnerable region of the muscle to become disproportionately strained, repeating this same process.

The combined presence of the normal ATP energy supply and the excess calcium will initiate and maintain a sustained contracture of the fibers exposed to the calcium. This produces a region of uncontrolled metabolism within the muscle, to which the body could respond with severe local vasoconstriction. This could be a local response or a TP-mediated reflex response *via* the central nervous system and sympathetic nervous system fibers (Fig. 2.2). There is now a region of increased metabolism with decreased circulation and the muscle fibers passing through that region are strongly shortened independent of propagated action potentials. This group of taut fibers may be what is palpated as a band in the muscle.

At this point, the picture becomes less clear. The tautness of the bands, when examined clinically, suggests that at least half the total fiber length is contracted. The mechanism by which this contracture of the sarcomeres might propagate along each fiber is not clear. Another problem is the rate at which the excess calcium would diffuse through the tissues and lose its effectiveness, probably within hours, certainly within days.

A second mechanism may take over. Nearly total depletion of ATP could lead to conditions similar to others that are known to cause muscle contracture with electrical silence, as in McArdle's disease, carnatine deficiency and rigor mortis. Without ATP, the myosin heads do not release from the actin filaments and the sarcomeres become rigid at that length. For this mechanism to be responsible for a sustained contracture of the palpable band, it would help if a central region of this ATP-deficit contracture were surrounded by a region of runaway metabolism to insure that the ATP was not replenished.

Nerve-sensitizing substances, such as histamine, serotonin, kinins and prostaglandins may be released in the TP zone by several mechanisms. With the tissue injury that initiated the TP, some blood would extravasate, which Awad[11] observed to include a large number of platelets that are a source of serotonin. This is not only a sensitizing agent, but also causes local ischemia as pointed out by Awad. He also observed degranulating mast cells, which release histamine.[11] Also, the initial phase of increased metabolism with reduced circulation would create a local accumulation of metabolic products that may result in the release of additional sensitizing substances, such as prostaglandins. More research is needed.

The reported dystrophic changes,[173] which are not unlike the changes induced experimentally by muscle ischemia,[247] may result from the severe metabolic stress of a prolonged regional ischemia of critical intensity in the face of inexorable energy demands.

References

1. Abel O Jr., Siebert WJ, Earp R: Fibrositis. *J Mo Med Assoc* 36:435–437, 1939.
2. Adams RD: *Diseases of Muscle: A Study in Pathology.* Ed. 3. Harper & Row, Hagerstown, 1975 (pp. 280–291, 316, 317).
3. Adler I: Muscular rheumatism. *Med Rec* 57:529–535, 1900.
4. Agerberg G, Österberg T: Maximal mandibular movements and symptoms of mandibular dysfunction in 70-year-old men and women. *Swed Dent J* 67:147–163, 1974.
5. Agnew LRC, Aviado DM, Brody JI, et al.: *Dorland's Illustrated Medical Dictionary*, Ed. 24. W.B. Saunders, Philadelphia, 1965.
6. Albee FH: Myofascitis. A pathological explanation of many apparently dissimilar conditions. *Am J Surg* 3:523–533, 1927.
7. Alling CC, III, Mahan PE: *Facial Pain.* Ed. 2. Lea & Febiger, Philadelphia, 1977.
8. Arat A: *Neck Sprains as Muscle Injury, Tension Headache and Related Conditions*, Ed. 2. Guynes Printing Company, El Paso, Texas, 1973 (pp. 134, 136).
9. Aronson PR, Murray DG, Fitzsimons RM: Myofascitis: A frequently overlooked cause of pain in cervical root distribution. *NC Med J* 32:463–465, 1971.
10. Arroyo P: Electromyography in the evaluation of reflex muscle spasm. *J Fla Med Assoc* 53:29–31, 1966.
11. Awad EA: Interstitial myofibrositis: hypothesis of the mechanism. *Arch Phys Med* 54:440–453, 1973.
12. Banker BQ, Girvin JP: The ultrastructural features of the mammalian muscle spindle. *J Neuropathol Exp Neurol* 30:155–195, 1971.
13. Bardeen CR: The musculature, Sect. 5. In *Morris's Human Anatomy*, edited by C.M. Jackson, Ed. 6. Blakiston's Son & Co., Philadelphia, 1921 (p. 355).
14. Bateman JE: *The Shoulder and Neck.* W.B. Saunders, Philadelphia, 1972 (pp. 179–183).
15. *Ibid.* (p. 182).
16. Bates T: Myofascial pain, Chapter 14. In *Ambulatory Pediatrics II*, edited by M. Green and R.J. Haggerty. W.B. Saunders, Philadelphia, 1977 (pp. 147, 148).
17. Bates T, Grunwaldt E: Myofascial pain in childhood. *J Pediatr* 53:198–209, 1958.
18. Bayer H: Die rheumatische Muskelhärte—ein Eigenreflextetanus. *Klin Wochenschr* 27:122–126, 1949.
19. Bell WE: *Orofacial Pains—Differential Diagnosis*, Ed. 2. Year Book Medical Publishers, Chicago, 1979.
20. Bell WH: Nonsurgical management of the pain-dysfunction syndrome. *J Am Dent Assoc* 79:161–170, 1969.
21. Bennett RM: Fibrositis: misnomer for a common rheumatic disorder. *West J Med* 134:405–413, 1981.
22. Benoit PW: Reversible skeletal muscle damage after administration of local anesthetic with and without epinephrine. *J Oral Surg* 36:198–201, 1978.
23. Berges PU: Myofascial pain syndromes. *Postgrad Med* 53:161–168, 1973.
24. Berrett A: Radiographic evaluation of the temporomandibular joint: Part II, Chapter 9. In *Clinical Management of Head, Neck and TMJ Pain and Dysfunction*, edited by H. Gelb, W.B. Saun-

ders, Philadelphia, 1977 (pp. 244–251).

25. Bistevins R, Awad EA: Structure and ultrastructure of mechanoreceptors at the human musculotendinous junction. *Arch Phys Med Rehabil* 62:74–83, 1981.

26. Bonica JJ: Myofascial syndromes with trigger mechanism. In *The Management of Pain*, edited by J.J. Bonica, Lea & Febiger. Philadelphia, 1953 (pp. 1150–1151).

27. Bonica JJ: Management of myofascial pain syndromes in general practice. *JAMA* 164:732–738, 1957.

28. Bonica JJ: Preface. In *Advances in Neurology*, edited by J.J. Bonica, Vol. 4. Raven Press, New York, 1974 (p. vii).

29. Bonica JJ: Neurophysiologic and pathologic aspects of acute and chronic pain. *Arch Surg* 112:750–761, 1977.

30. Bourne IHJ: Treatment of painful conditions of the abdominal wall with local injection. *Practitioner* 224:921–925, 1980.

31. Brain WR, Walton JN: *Brain's Diseases of the Nervous System*, Ed. 7. Oxford University Press, London, 1969 (p. 189).

32. Bratolyubova TN, Vinogradov VF, Panteleeva TS: Cardiac-pain symptomatology of noncoronary genesis. *Klin Med (Musk.)* 56:93–97, 1978.

33. Brendstrup P, Jespersen K, Asboe-Hansen G: Morphological and chemical connective tissue changes in fibrositic muscles. *Ann Rheum Dis* 16:438–440, 1957.

34. Brown BR: Diagnosis and therapy of common myofascial syndromes. *JAMA* 239:646–648, 1978.

35. Brucini M, Duranti R, Galletti R, Pantaleo T, Zucchi PL: Pain thresholds and electromyographic features of periarticular muscles in patients with osteoarthritis of the knee. *Pain* 10:57–66, 1981.

36. Buckley CW: Fibrositis, lumbago and sciatica. *Practitioner* 134:129–146, 1935.

37. Butler JH, Folke LEA, Bandt CL: A descriptive survey of signs and symptoms associated with the myofascial pain-dysfunction syndrome. *J Am Dent Assoc* 90:635–639, 1975.

38. Cailliet, R: *Soft Tissue Pain and Disability*. F.A. Davis. Philadelphia, 1977 (pp. 32–35).

39. Cheney FD: Muscle tenderness in 100 consecutive psychiatric patients. *Dis Nerv Syst* 30:478–481, 1969.

40. Clark GT, Beemsterboer PL, Solberg WK, *et al.*: Nocturnal electromyographic evaluation of myofascial pain dysfunction in patients undergoing occlusal splint therapy. *J Am Dent Assoc* 99:607–611, 1979.

41. Cobb CR, deVries HA, Urban RT, *et al.*: Electrical activity in muscle pain. *Am J Phys Med* 54:80–87, 1975.

42. Cöers C, Woolf AL: *The Innervation of Muscle*. Blackwell Scientific Publications, Oxford, 1959 (pp. 3–5).

43. Cohen HL, Brumlik J: *Manual of Electroneuromyography*, Ed. 2. Harper & Row, Hagerstown, 1976 (p. 74).

44. Cohen LA: Role of eye and neck proprioceptive mechanism in body orientation and motor coordination. *J Neurophysiol* 24:1–11, 1961.

45. Cohen SR: Follow-up evaluation of 105 patients with myofascial pain-dysfunction syndrome. *J Am Dent Assoc* 97:825–828, 1978.

46. Collins DH: Fibrositis and infection. *Ann Rheum Dis* 2:114–126, 1940.

47. Cooper AL: Trigger-point injection: its place in physical medicine. *Arch Phys Med* 42:704–709, 1961.

48. Copeman WSC: Non-articular rheumatism. *Br J Clin Pract* 19:667–674, 1965.

49. Copeman WSC, Ackerman WL: Edema or herniations of fat lobules as a cause of lumbar and gluteal "fibrositis." *Arch Intern Med* 79:22–35, 1947.

50. Cornelius: Die Druck- oder Schmerzpunkte als Entstehungsurache der sogenannten funktionellen Nervenerkrankungen, ihre Entstehung und Behandlung. *Wien Med Wochenschr* 54:114–120, 1904.

51. Cornelius A: Die nervösen Magen-Darmbeschwerden, zumal der Schwangeren, und die Druckpunkttheorie. *Klin-ther Wochenschr* 10:977–981, 1006–1010, 1903.

52. Cornelius A: Nervepunkte, ihre Entstehung, Bedeutung und Behandlung mittels Nervemassage. Thieme, Leipzig 1909.

53. Cyriax J: Rheumatic headache. *Br Med J* 2:1367–1368, 1938.

54. D'ambrosia RD: *Musculoskeletal Disorders: Regional Examination and Differential Diagnosis*. J.B. Lippincott, Philadelphia, 1977 (p. 332).

55. de Jong RH: Defining pain terms. *JAMA* 244:143, 1980.

56. de Valera E, Raftery H: Lower abdominal and pelvic pain in women. In *Advances in Pain Research and Therapy*, edited by J.J. Bonica, D. Albe-Fessard, Vol. 1. Raven Press, New York, 1976 (pp. 935–936).

57. Dexter JR, Simons DG: Local twitch response in human muscle evoked by palpation and needle penetration or a trigger point. *Arch Phys Med Rehabil* 62:521, 1981.

58. Dittrich RJ: Low back pain—referred pain from deep somatic structure of the back. *J-Lancet* 73:63–68, 1963.

59. Dorigo B, Bartoli V, Grisillo D, *et al.*: Fibrositic myofascial pain in intermittent claudication. Effect of anesthetic block of trigger points on exercise tolerance. *Pain* 6:183–190, 1979.

60. Drinnan AJ: Differential diagnosis of orofacial pain. *Dent Clin North Am* 22:73–87, 1978.

61. Edeiken J, Wolferth CC: Persistent pain in the shoulder region following myocardial infarction. *Amer J Med Sci* 191:201–210, 1936.

62. Elliott FA: Tender muscles in sciatica. *Lancet* 1:47–49, 1944.

63. Epstein SE, Gerber LH, Borer JS: Chest wall syndrome—a common cause of unexplained cardiac pain. *JAMA* 241:2793–2797, 1979.

64. Fassbender HG: *Pathology of Rheumatic Diseases*. Springer-Verlag, New York, 1975. (Chapter 13, pp. 303–314).

65. Fassbender HG, Wegner K: Morphologie und Pathogenese des Weichteilrheumatismus. *Z Rheumaforsch* 32:355–374, 1973.

66. Feinstein AR: Rheumatic fever, Chapter 238. In *Harrison's Principles of Internal Medicine*, edited by M.M. Wintrobe, G.W. Thorn, R.D.

Adams, et al., Ed. 7. McGraw-Hill, New York, 1974 (p. 1173).

67. Fischer AA: Thermography and pain. Arch Phys Med Rehabil 62:542, 1981.

68. Fock S, Mense S: Excitatory effects of 5-hydroxytryptamine, histamine and potassium ions on muscular group IV afferent units: a comparison with bradykinin. Brain Res 105:459–469, 1976.

69. Fordyce WE: Behavioral Methods for Chronic Pain and Illness. C.V. Mosby, Saint Louis, 1976.

70. Freese AS: Myofascial trigger mechanisms and temporomandibular joint disturbances in head and neck pain. NY State J Med 59:2554–2558, 1959.

71. Froriep R: Ein Beitrag zur Pathologie und Therapie des Rheumatismus. Weimar, 1843.

72. Frost FA, Jessen B, Siggaard-Andersen J: A control, double-blind comparison of mepivacaine injection versus saline injection for myofascial pain. Lancet 1:8167–8168, 1980.

73. Galletti R, Procacci P: The role of the sympathetic system in the control of pain and of some associated phenomena. Acta Neurovegetativa 28:495–500, 1966.

74. Gelb H: Clinical Management of Head, Neck, and TMJ Pain and Dysfunction. W.B. Saunders, Philadelphia, 1977.

75. Gellhorn E, Thompson L: Muscle pain, tendon reflexes, and muscular coordination in man. Proc Soc Exp Biol Med 56:209–212, 1944.

76. Gillette HE: Office management of musculoskeletal pain. Texas State J Med 62:47–53, 1966.

77. Gilliland BC, Mannik M: Reiter's syndrome, psoriatic arthritis, and arthritis associated with gastrointestinal diseases, Chapter 358. In Harrison's Principles of Internal Medicine, edited by M.M. Wintrobe, G.W. Thorn, R.D. Adams, et al., Ed. 7. McGraw-Hill, New York, 1974 (p. 2000).

78. Gilroy J, Meyer JS: Medical Neurology. Macmillan, London, 1969 (pp. 80–81, 280–288, 547–549, 612–615).

79. Glogowski G, Wallraff J: Ein beitrag zur Klinik und Histologie der Muskelhärten (Myogelosen). Z Orthop 80:237–268, 1951.

80. Glyn JH: Rheumatic pains: some concepts and hypotheses. Proc R Soc Med 64:354–360, 1971.

81. Goldberg M, Murray TG: Analgesic-associated nephropathy. N Engl J Med 299:716–717, 1978.

82. Good M: Five hundred cases of myalgia in the British army. Ann Rheum Dis 3:118–138, 1942.

83. Good MG: Rheumatic myalgias. Practitioner 146:167–174, 1941.

84. Good MG: Muscular sciatica. Clin J 72:66–71, 1943.

85. Good MG: The role of skeletal muscles in the pathogenesis of diseases. Acta Med Scand 138:285–292, 1950.

86. Good MG: Objective diagnosis and curability of nonarticular rheumatism. Br J Phys Med 14:1–7, 1951.

87. Good MG: Die primäre Rolle der Muskulatur in der Pathogenese der rheumatischen Krankheit und die therapeutische Lösung des Rheumaproblems. Medizinische (Stuttgart) 13:450–454, 1957.

88. Goodgold J, Eberstein A: Electrodiagnosis of Neuromuscular Diseases, Ed. 2. Williams & Wilkins, Baltimore, 1977 (p. 3).

89. Gorrell RL: Local anesthetics in precordial pain. Clin Med Surg 46:441–442, 1939.

90. Gorrell RL: Musculofascial pain. JAMA 142:557–561, 1950.

91. Gorrell RL: Troublesome ankle disorders and what to do about them. Consultant 16:64–69, 1976.

92. Gowers WR: Lumbago: its lessons and analogues. Br Med J 1:117–121, 1904.

93. Graham W: The fibrositis syndrome. Bull Rheum Dis 3:33–34, 1953.

94. Graham W: Fibrositis and non-articular rheumatism. Phys Ther Rev 35:128–133, 1955.

95. Gray H: Anatomy of the Human Body, edited by C.M. Goss, American Ed. 29. Lea & Febiger, Philadelphia, 1973 (p. 371).

96. Ibid. (Figs. 12–29, 12–30, 12–45, 12–62).

97. Greene JA: The syndrome of psoas myositis and fibrositis; its manifestations and its significance in the differential diagnosis of lower abdominal pain. Ann Intern Med 23:30–34, 1945.

98. Gross D: Therapeutische Lokalanästhesie. Hippokrates Verlag, Stuttgart, 1972 (p. 142).

99. Grosshandler S, Burney R: The myofascial syndrome. NC Med J 40:562–565, 1979.

100. Gunn CC: Type IV acupuncture points. Am J Acupunt 5:51–52, 1977.

101. Gunn CC, Milbrandt WE: Utilizing trigger points. Osteopathic Phys 44:29–52, 1977.

102. Gunn CC, Milbrandt WE: Shoulder pain, cervical spondylosis and acupuncture. Am J Acupuncture 5:121–128, 1977.

103. Gutstein M: Diagnosis and treatment of muscular rheumatism. Br J Phys Med 1:302–321, 1938.

104. Gutstein M: Common rheumatism and physiotherapy. Br J Phys Med 3:46–50, 1940.

105. Gutstein RR: The role of abdominal fibrositis in functional indigestion. Miss Valley Med J 66:114–124, 1944.

106. Gutstein RR: A review of myodysneuria (fibrositis). Am Practit 6:570–577, 1955.

107. Gutstein-Good M: Idiopathic myalgia simulating visceral and other diseases. Lancet 2:326–328, 1940.

108. Hackett GS: Ligament and Tendon Relaxation Treated by Prolotherapy, Ed. 3. Charles C Thomas, Springfield, Ill., 1958 (pp. 27–36).

109. Halliday JL: The obsession of fibrositis. Br Med J 1:164, 1942.

110. Helleday U: Om myitis chronica (rheumatica). Ett bidrag till dess diagnostik och behandling. Nord Med Ark 8:Art. 8, 1876.

111. Hench PK: Nonarticular rheumatism. Chapter 28, In Rheumatic Diseases, Diagnosis and Management, edited by W.A. Katz. Lippincott, Philadelphia, 1977.

112. Hockaday JM, Whitty CWM: Patterns of referred pain in the normal subject. Brain 90:481–496, 1967.

113. Hook EW: Other Clostridial infections, Chapter 154. In Harrison's Principles of Internal Medicine, edited by M.M. Wintrobe, G.W. Thorn, R.D. Adams, et al., Ed. 7. McGraw-Hill, New York, 1974 (p. 853).

114. Hunter C: Myalgia of the abdominal wall. Can

Med Assoc J 28:157–161, 1933.

115. Ibrahim GA, Awad EA, Kottke FJ: Interstitial myofibrositis: serum and muscle enzymes and lactate dehydrogenase-isoenzymes. *Arch Phys Med Rehabil* 55:23–28, 1974.

116. Iggo A: Pain receptors. In *Recent Advances on Pain*, edited by J.J. Bonica, P. Procacci, C. A. Pagni. Charles C Thomas, Springfield, Ill., 1974 (pp. 24–25).

117. Ignelzi RJ, Atkinson JH: Pain and its modulation: Part 1—afferent mechanisms. *Neurosurgery* 6:577–583, 1980.

118. Ignelzi RJ, Atkinson JH: Pain and its modulation: Part 2—efferent mechanisms. *Neurosurgery* 6:584–590, 1980.

119. Ingle JI, Beveridge EE: *Endodontics*, Ed. 2. Lea & Febiger, Philadelphia, 1976.

120. Inman VT, Saunders JB, deCM: Referred pain from skeletal structures. *J Nerv Ment Dis* 99:660–667, 1944.

121. International Anatomical Nomenclature Committee: *Nomina Anatomica*. Excerpta Medica Foundation, Amsterdam, 1966 (pp. 38–43).

122. Jordan HH: Myogeloses: the significance of pathologic conditions of the musculature in disorders of posture and locomotion. *Arch Phys Ther* 23:36–54, 1942.

123. Kaplan H: Psychogenic Rheumatism. *Ariz Med* 32:280–281, 1975.

124. Kellgren JH: Observations on referred pain arising from muscle. *Clin Sci* 3:175–190, 1938.

125. Kellgren JH: A preliminary account of referred pains arising from muscle. *Br Med J* 1:325–327, 1938.

126. Kellgren JH: Deep pain sensibility. *Lancet* 1:943–949, 1949.

127. Kelly M: The treatment of fibrositis and allied disorders by local anesthesia. *Med J Aust* 1:294–298, 1941.

128. Kelly M: The nature of fibrositis: 1. the myalgic lesion and its secondary effects: a reflex theory. *Ann Rheum Dis* 5:1–7, 1945.

129. Kelly M: The relief of facial pain by procaine (novocain) injections. *J Am Geriatr Soc* 11:586–596, 1963.

130. Kendall HO, Kendall FP, Wadsworth GE: *Muscles, Testing and Function*, Ed. 2. Williams & Wilkins, Baltimore, 1971.

131. Kerr FW: Neuroanatomical substrates of nociception in the spinal cord. *Pain* 1:325–356, 1975.

132. King JS, Lagger R: Sciatica viewed as a referred pain syndrome. *Surg Neurol* 5:46–50, 1976.

133. Knight V: Influenza, Chapter 188. In *Harrison's Principles of Internal Medicine*, edited by M.M. Wintrobe, G.W. Thorn, R.D. Adams, et al., Ed. 7. McGraw-Hill, New York, 1974 (p. 939).

134. Knight V: Psittacosis, Chapter 189. In *Harrison's Principles of Internal Medicine*, edited by M.M. Wintrobe, G.W. Thorn, R.D. Adams, et al., Ed. 7. McGraw-Hill, New York, 1974 (p. 941).

135. Koenig WC, Powers JJ, Johnson EW: Does allergy play a role in fibrositis? *Arch Phys Med Rehabil* 58:80–83, 1977.

136. Kohlrausch W: Die sportbehindernden Wirkungen muskulärer Erkrankungen. *Med Klin* 32:1420–1423, 1936.

137. Korr IM: Sustained sympathicotonia as a factor in disease. In *The Neurobiologic Mechanisms in Manipulative Therapy*, edited by I.M. Korr. Plenum Press, New York, 1977 (pp. 229–268).

138. Korr IM, Goldstein MJ: Dermatomal autonomic activity in relation to segmental motor reflex threshold. *Fed Proc* 7:67, 1948.

139. Kraft GH, Johnson EW, LaBan MM: The fibrositis syndrome. *Arch Phys Med Rehabil* 49:155–162, 1968.

140. Kraus H: Behandlung akuter Muskelhärten. *Wien Klin Wochenschr* 50:1356–1357, 1937.

141. Kraus H: The use of surface anesthesia for the treatment of painful motion. *JAMA* 116:2582–2587, 1941.

142. Kraus H: *Clinical Treatment of Back and Neck Pain*. McGraw-Hill, New York, 1970 (pp. 95, 107).

143. Lange F, Eversbusch G: Die Bedeutung der Muskelhärten für die allgemeine Praxis. *Münch Med Wochenschr* 68:418–420, 1921.

144. Lange M: *Die Muskelhärten (Myogelosen)*. J.F. Lehmann's Verlag, München, 1931.

145. Laskin DM: Etiology of the pain-dysfunction syndrome. *J Am Dent Assoc* 79:147–153, 1969.

146. Lawrence RM: Osteopuncture: theory and practice. Presented at the annual meeting of the North American Academy of Manipulative Medicine, 1977.

147. Lehmann JF, De Lateur BJ: Heat and cold in the treatment of arthritis, Chapter 14. In *Arthritis and Physical Medicine*, edited by S. Licht. Williams & Wilkins, Baltimore, 1969 (pp. 344–346).

148. Lenman JAR, Ritchie AE: *Clinical Electromyography*, Ed. 2. J.B. Lippincott, Philadelphia, 1977 (pp. 86, 87).

149. Leriche R: Des effetes de l'anesthésie a la novocaine des ligaments et des insertions tendineuses peri-articulaires dans certaines maladies articulaires et dans vices de position fonctionnels des articulations. *Gazette des Hopitaux* 103:1294, 1930.

150. Lerner AM: Enteric viruses: Coxsackie viruses, ECHO viruses, reoviruses, Chapter 190. In *Harrison's Principles of Internal Medicine*, edited by M.M. Wintrobe, G.W. Thorn, R.D. Adams, et al., Ed. 7. McGraw-Hill, New York 1974 (p. 946).

150a. Lewis T, Kellgren JH: Observations relating to referred pain, visceromotor reflexes and other associated phenomena. *Clin Sci* 1:47–71, 1939.

151. Llewellyn LJ, Jones AB: *Fibrositis*. Rebman, New York, 1915.

152. Lockhart RD, Hamilton GF, Fyfe FW: *Anatomy of the Human Body*, Ed. 2. J.B. Lippincott, Philadelphia, 1969 (p. 144).

153. Long C, II: Myofascial pain syndromes: Part 1—general characteristics and treatment. *Henry Ford Hosp Med Bull* 3:189–192, 1955.

154. Long C, II: Myofascial Pain Syndromes: Part II—Syndromes of the head, neck and shoulder girdle. *Henry Ford Hosp Med Bull* 4:22–28, 1956 (Section II).

155. Luff AP: The various forms of fibrositis and their treatment. *Br Med J* 1:756–760, 1913.

156. Lundervold AJS: Electromyographic investigations of position and manner of working in typewriting. *Acta Physiol Scand* 24:(Suppl 84), 1951.

157. Macdonald AJR: Abnormally tender muscle regions and associated painful movements. *Pain* 8:197–205, 1980.

158. Mackenzie CG: Experimental muscular dystrophy. In *A Symposium on Nutrition*, edited by R.M. Herriott. The Johns Hopkins Press, Baltimore, 1953.
159. Macnab I: *Backache*. Williams & Wilkins, Baltimore, 1977 (p. 82).
160. Mahan PE: The temporomandibular joint in function and pathofunction, Chapter 2. In *Temporomandibular Joint Problems*, edited by W. K. Solberg and G.T. Clark. Quintessence Publishing, Chicago, 1980 (pp. 33–47).
161. Maigne R: Low back pain of thoracolumbar origin. *Arch Phys Med Rehabil* 61:389–395, 1980.
162. Mannik M, Gilliland BC: Degenerative joint disease, Chapter 361. In *Harrison's Principles of Internal Medicine*, edited by M.M. Wintrobe, G.W. Thorn, R.D. Adams, et al., Ed. 7. McGraw-Hill, New York, 1974 (pp. 2005–2008).
163. Marbach JJ: Arthritis of the temporomandibular joints. *Am Fam Physician* 19:131–139, 1979.
164. Mayer DJ, Price DD, Barber J, et al.: Acupuncture analgesia: evidence for activation of a pain inhibitory system as a mechanism of action. In *Advances in Pain Research and Therapy*, edited by J.J. Bonica, D. Albe-Fessard, Vol. 1. Raven Press, New York, 1976 (pp. 751–754).
165. Melzack R: *The Puzzle of Pain*. Basic Books, New York, 1973 (pp. 22–24, 153–179).
166. Melzack R: Relation of myofascial trigger points to acupuncture and mechanisms of pain. *Arch Phys Med Rehabil* 62:114–117, 1981.
167. Melzack R, Stillwell DM, Fox EJ: Trigger points and acupuncture points for pain: correlations and implications. *Pain* 3:3–23, 1977.
168. Melzack R, Wall PD: Pain mechanisms: a new theory. *Science* 150:971–979, 1965.
169. Mense S: Personal communication, 1981.
170. Mense S, Schmidt RF: Muscle pain: which receptors are responsible for the transmission of noxious stimuli? In *Physiological Aspects of Clinical Neurology*, edited by F.C. Rose. Blackwell Scientific Publications, Oxford, 1977.
171. Michele AA: Scapulocostal syndrome—its mechanism and diagnosis. *NY State J Med* 55:2485–2493, 1955.
172. Michele AA, Davies JJ, Krueger FJ, et al.: Scapulocostal syndrome (fatigue-postural paradox). *NY State J Med* 50:1353–1356, 1950.
173. Miehlke K, Schulze G, Eger W: Klinische und experimentelle Untersuchungen zum Fibrositissyndrom. *Z Rheumaforsch* 19:310–330, 1960.
174. Mikhail M, Rosen H: History and etiology of myofascial pain-dysfunction syndrome. *J Prosthet Dent* 44:438–444, 1980.
175. Milne RJ, Foreman RD, Giesler, GJ, Jr., Willis WD: Convergence of cutaneous and pelvic visceral nociceptive inputs onto primate spinothalamic neurons. *Pain* 11:163–183, 1981.
176. Moldofsky H: 'Psychogenic rheumatism' or the 'fibrositis syndrome', Chapter 10. In *Modern Trends in Psychosomatic Medicine*, edited by O. Hill, Vol 3. Butterworth, Boston, 1976 (pp. 187–195).
177. Moldofsky H, Scarisbrick P: Induction of neurasthenic musculoskeletal pain syndrome by selective sleep stage deprivation. *Psychosom Med* 38:35–44, 1976.
178. Moldofsky H, Scarisbrick P, England R, et al.: Musculoskeletal symptoms and non-REM sleep disturbance in patients with "fibrositis syndrome" and healthy subjects. *Psychosom Med* 37:341–351, 1975.
179. Morgan DH, House LR, Hall WP, Vamvas SJ: *Diseases of the Temporomandibular Apparatus: A Multidisciplinary Approach*; Ed. 2, C.V. Mosby, Saint Louis, 1982.
180. Müller A: Der Untersuchungsbefund am rheumatisch erkrankten Muskel. *Z Klin Med* 74:34–73, 1912.
181. Murray GR: Myofibrositis as a simulator of other maladies. *Lancet* 1:113–116, 1929.
182. Mylechreest WH: An investigation into the aetiology and pathology of fibrositis of the back. *Ann Rheum Dis* 4:77–79, 1945.
183. Needham DM: Biochemistry of muscle, Chapter 8. In *The Structure and Function of Muscle*, edited by G.H. Bourne, Ed. 2, Vol. 3. Academic Press, New York, 1973 (p. 377).
184. Neligan AR: The diagnosis and treatment of fibrositis and neuritis. *Practitioner* 143:263–274, 1939.
185. Neufeld I: Pathogenetic concepts of "fibrositis." *Arch Phys Med* 33:363–369, 1952.
186. Nielsen AJ: Spray and stretch for myofascial pain. *Phys Ther* 58:567–569, 1978.
187. Nielsen AJ: Case study: myofascial pain of the posterior shoulder relieved by spray and stretch. *J Orthop Sports Phys Ther* 3:21–26, 1981.
188. Nielsen AJ: Personal communication, 1981.
189. Ochoa JL, Torebjörk HE: Pain from skin and muscle. *Pain Supplement* 1:887, 1981.
190. Pace JB: Commonly overlooked pain syndromes responsive to simple therapy. *Postgrad Med* 58:107–113, 1975.
191. Perl ER: Sensitization of nociceptors and its relation to sensation. In *Advances in Pain Research and Therapy*, edited by J.J. Bonica, D. Albe-Fessard, Vol. 1. Raven Press, New York, 1976 (pp. 17–28).
192. Piecuch J, Tideman H, DeKoomen H: Short-face syndrome: treatment of myofascial pain dysfunction by maxillary disimpaction. *Oral Surg* 49:112–116, 1980.
193. Plorde JJ: Filariasis, Chapter 219. In *Harrison's Principles of Internal Medicine*, edited by M.M. Wintrobe, G.W. Thorn, R.D. Adams, et al., Ed. 7. McGraw-Hill, New York, 1974 (p. 1046).
194. Plorde JJ: Malaria, Chapter 210. In *Harrison's Principles of Internal Medicine*, edited by M.M. Wintrobe, G.W. Thorn, R.D. Adams, et al., Ed. 7. McGraw-Hill, New York, 1974 (p. 1021).
195. Popelianskii Ia Iu, Zaslavskii ES, Veselovskii VP: [Medicosocial significance, etiology, pathogenesis, and diagnosis of nonarticular disease of soft tissues of the limbs and back.] (Russian) *Vopr Revm* 3:38–43, 1976.
196. Port K: Eine für den Orthopäden wichtige Gruppe des chronischen Rheumatismus (Knötchenrheumatismus). *Arch Orthop Unfallchir* 17:465–506, 1920.
197. Procacci P, Zoppi M: Pathophysiology and clinical aspects of visceral and referred pain. *Pain Suppl* 1:6, 1981.
198. Ramfjord SP: Dysfunctional temporomandibular joint and muscle pain. *J Prosthet Dent* 11:353–374, 1961.

199. Ramfjord SP: Temporomandibular joint dysfunction; dysfunctional temporomandibular joint and muscle pain. *J Prosthet Dent* 11:353–374, 1961.

200. Rammelkamp CH, Jr.: Hemolytic streptococcal infections, Chapter 130. In *Harrison's Principles of Internal Medicine*, edited by M.M. Wintrobe, G.W. Thorn, R.D. Adams, *et al.*, Ed. 7. McGraw-Hill, New York, 1974 (p. 783).

201. Reichart A: Reflexschmerzen auf Grund von Myogelosen. *Dtsch Med Wochenschr* 64:823–824, 1938.

202. Reynolds MD: Myofascial trigger point syndromes in the practice of rheumatology. *Arch Phys Med Rehabil* 62:111–114, 1981 (Table 2).

203. Reynolds MD: The development of the concept of fibrositis. *J Hist Med Allied Sci*, (In Press), 1983.

204. Ribble JC: Smallpox, vaccinia, and cowpox, Chapter 198. In *Harrison's Principles of Internal Medicine*, edited by M.M. Wintrobe, G.W. Thorn, R.D. Adams *et. al.*, Ed. 7. McGraw-Hill, New York, 1974.

205. Rinzler SH, Travell J: Therapy directed at the somatic component of cardiac pain. *Am Heart J* 35:248–268, 1948.

206. Roberts JT: The effect of occlusive arterial diseases of extremities on the blood supply of nerves; experimental and clinical studies on the role of the vasa nervorum. *Am Heart J* 35:369–392, 1948.

207. Rodnan GP, *et al.*: *Primer on the Rheumatic Diseases*, Ed. 7. The Arthritis Foundation, New York, 1973 (pp. 25–38, 137).

208. Ronn HH: A follow-up study of the use of Benoral tablets in non-articular rheumatism. *J Int Med Res* 5:48–52, 1977.

209. Rubin D: Myofascial trigger point syndromes: an approach to management. *Arch Phys Med Rehabil* 62:107–110, 1981.

210. Rubin E: Alcoholic myopathy in heart and skeletal muscle. *N Engl J Med* 301:28–33, 1979.

211. Ruch TC: Pathophysiology of pain, Chapter 16. In *Physiology and Biophysics*, edited by T.C. Ruch and H.D. Patton, Ed. 19. W.B. Saunders, Philadelphia, 1965 (pp. 357, 358).

212. Ruhmann W: Muskelrheuma und Tastmassage. 2. Muskelrheumatische Disposition. *Med Klin* 27:1242–1245, 1279–1283, 1931.

213. Ruhmann W: Über das Wesen der rheumatischen Muskelhärte. *Dtsch Arch Klin Med* 173:625–645, 1932.

214. Ruskin AP: Sphenopalatine (nasal) ganglion: remote effects including "psychosomatic" symptoms, rage reaction, pain, and spasm. *Arch Phys Med Rehabil* 60:353–359, 1979.

215. Rutkowski B, Brzoza R: Zespoly bolowe miesniowo-powieziowe (Painful musculofascial syndromes). *Anest Reanim Inten Terap* 12:201–206, 1980.

216. Sanford JP: Arbovirus and *Arenavirus* infections, Chapter 207. In *Harrison's Principles of Internal Medicine*, edited by M.M. Wintrobe, G.W. Thorn, R.D. Adams, *et al.*, Ed. 7. McGraw-Hill, New York, 1974 (pp. 991, 994, 999, 1006).

217. Sanford JP: Other viral fevers, Chapter 208. In *Harrison's Principles of Internal Medicine*, edited by M.M. Wintrobe, G.W. Thorn, R.D. Adams *et al.*, Ed. 7. McGraw-Hill, New York, 1974 (p. 1013).

218. Sanford JP: Leptospirosis, Chapter 161. In *Harrison's Principles of Internal Medicine*, edited by M.M. Wintrobe, G.W. Thorn, R.D. Adams, *et al.*, Ed. 7. McGraw-Hill, New York, 1974 (p. 869).

219. Schade H: Beiträge zur Umgrenzung und Klärung einer Lehre von der Erkältung. *Z Gesamte Exp Med* 7:275–374, 1919.

219a. Schade H: Untersuchungen in der Erkältungstrage: III. Uber den Rheumatismus, insbesondere den Muskelrheumatismus (Myogelose). *Müench Med Wochenschr* 68:95–99, 1921.

220. Schmalbruch H: Contracture knots in normal and diseased muscle fibres. *Brain* 96:637–640, 1973.

221. Schmidt A: Zur Pathologie und Therapie des Muskelrheumatismus (Myalgie). *Münch Med Wochenschr* 63:593–595, 1916.

222. Schwartz LL: Temporomandibular joint pain—treatment with intramuscular infiltration of tetracaine hydrochloride: a preliminary report. *NY State Dent J* 20:219–223, 1954.

223. Sharav Y, Tzukert A, Refaeli B: Muscle pain index in relation to pain, dysfunction, and dizziness associated with the myofascial pain-dysfunction syndrome. *Oral Surg* 46:742–747, 1978.

224. Shore NA: *Occlusal Equilibration and Temporomandibular Joint Dysfunction*. J.B. Lippincott, Philadelphia, 1959.

225. Shore NA: *Temporomandibular Joint Dysfunction and Occlusal Equilibration*, Ed. 2. J.B. Lippincott, Philadelphia, 1976 (pp. 193–205, 237–249).

226. Shpuntoff H: Biofeedback electromyography and inhibition release in myofascial pain dysfunction cases. *NY J Dent* 47:304–309, 1977.

227. Simons DG: Muscle Pain Syndromes—Parts I and II. *Am J Phys Med* 54:289–311, 1975, and 55:15–42, 1976.

228. Simons DG, Dexter J: Unpublished data, 1982.

229. Simons DG, Stolov WC: Microscopic features and transient contraction of palpable bands in canine muscle. *Am J Phys Med* 55:65–88, 1976.

230. Simons DG, Travell J, Stark J: Unreported observations, 1978.

231. Simons DG, Travell JG: Myofascial trigger points, a possible explanation. *Pain* 10:106–109, 1981.

232. Sinaki M, Merritt JL, Stillwell GK: Tension myalgia of the pelvic floor. *Mayo Clin Proc* 52:717–722, 1977.

233. Sinclair DC: The remote reference of pain aroused in the skin. *Brain* 72:364–372, 1949.

234. Sinclair DC, Weddell G, Feindel WH: Referred pain and associated phenomena. *Brain* 71:184–211, 1948.

235. Slocumb CH: Fibrositis. *Clinics* 2:169–178, 1943.

236. Smythe HA: Non-articular rheumatism and the fibrositis syndrome. In *Arthritis and Allied Conditions*, edited by J.L. Hollander, D.J. McCarty, Ed. 8. Lea & Febiger, Philadelphia, 1972 (pp. 874–884).

237. Smythe HA: Fibrositis and other diffuse musculoskeletal syndromes, Chapter 32. In *Textbook of Rheumatology*, edited by W.N. Kelley, E.D. Harris, Jr., S. Ruddy, *et al.*, Vol. 1. W.B. Saunders, Philadelphia, 1981 (pp. 485–493).

238. Sola AE: Personal communication, 1981.
239. Sola AE, Kuitert JH: Quadratus lumborum myofasciitis. Northwest Med 53:1003–1005, 1954.
240. Sola AE, Kuitert JH: Myofascial trigger point pain in the neck and shoulder girdle. Northwest Med 54:980–984, 1955.
241. Sola AE, Rodenberger ML, Gettys BB: Incidence of hypersensitive areas in posterior shoulder muscles. Am J Phys Med 34:585–590, 1955.
242. Sola AE, Williams RL: Myofascial pain syndromes. Neurol 6:91–95, 1956.
243. Solberg WK, Woo MW, Houston JB: Prevalence of mandibular dysfunction in young adults. J Am Dent Assoc 98:25–34, 1979.
244. Stacey MJ: Free nerve endings in skeletal muscle of the cat. J Anat 105:231–254, 1969.
245. Steindler A: The interpretation of sciatic radiation and the syndrome of low-back pain. J Bone Joint Surg 22:28–34, 1940.
246. Steindler A, Luck JV: Differential diagnosis of pain low in the back. JAMA 110:106–113, 1938.
247. Stenger RJ, Spiro D, Scully RE, Shannon JM: Ultrastructural and physiologic alterations in ischemic skeletal muscle. Amer J Pathol 40:1–20, 1962.
248. Sternbach RA: Pain Patients. Academic Press, New York, 1974.
249. Stockman R: The causes, pathology and treatment of chronic rheumatism. Edinburgh Med J 15:107–116, 223–235, 1904.
250. Stockman R: The clinical symptoms and treatment of chronic subcutaneous fibrosis. Br Med J 1:352–355, 1911.
251. Stockman R: Chronic rheumatism, chronic muscular rheumatism, fibrositis, Chapter 2. In Rheumatism and Arthritis, edited by R. Stockman. W. Green & Son, Edinburgh, 1920 (pp. 41–56).
252. Stockman R: Panniculitis. In Rheumatism and Arthritis, edited by R. Stockman, W. Green & Son. Edinburgh, 1920 (pp. 57–64).
253. Strauss H: Über die sogenannte "rheumatische Muskelschwiele." Klin Wochenschr 35:89–91, 121–123, 1898.
254. Subcommittee on Taxonomy: Pain terms: a list with definitions and notes on usage. Pain 6:249–252, 1979.
255. Swezey RL: Arthritis: Rational Therapy and Rehabilitation. W.B. Saunders, Philadelphia, 1978 (pp. 144, 145).
256. Swezey RL, Spiegel TM: Evaluation and treatment of local musculoskeletal disorders in elderly patients. Geriatrics 34:56–75, 1979.
257. Taverner D: Muscle spasm as a cause of somatic pain. Ann Rheum Dis 13:331–335, 1954.
258. Telling WH: "Nodular" fibromyositis, an everyday affection, and its identity with so-called muscular rheumatism. Lancet 1:154–158, 1911.
259. Torebjörk HE: Personal Communication, 1981.
260. Torebjörk HE, Ochoa JL: Specific sensations evoked by activity in single identified sensory units in man. Acta Physiol Scand 110:445–447, 1980.
261. Travell J: Basis for the multiple uses of local block of somatic trigger areas (procaine infiltration and ethyl chloride spray). Miss Valley Med J 71:13–22, 1949.
262. Travell J: Pain mechanisms in connective tissue. In Connective Tissues, Transactions of the Sec-
ond Conference, 1951, edited by C. Ragan. Josiah Macy, Jr. Foundation, New York, 1952 (pp. 96–102, 105–109, 111).
263. Travell J: Introductory Comments. In Connective Tissues. Transactions of the Fifth Conference, 1954, edited by C. Ragan. Josiah Macy, Jr. Foundation, New York, 1954 (pp. 12–22).
264. Travell J: Symposium on mechanism and management of pain syndromes. Proc Rudolf Virchow Med Soc 16:128–136, 1957.
265. Travell J: Temporomandibular joint pain referred from muscles of the head and neck. J Prosthet Dent 10:745–763, 1960.
266. Travell J: Mechanical headache. Headache 7:23–29, 1967.
267. Travell J: Office Hours: Day and Night. The World Publishing Company, New York, 1968 (pp. 257, 274).
268. Travell J: Myofascial trigger points: clinical view. In Advances in Pain Research and Therapy, edited by J.J. Bonica and D. Albe-Fessard, Vol. 1. Raven Press, New York, 1976 (pp. 919–926).
269. Travell J: Identification of myofascial trigger point syndromes: a case of atypical facial neuralgia. Arch Phys Med Rehabil 62:100–106, 1981.
270. Travell J, Berry C, Bigelow N: Effects of referred somatic pain on structures in the reference zone. Fed Proc 3:49, 1944.
271. Travell J, Bigelow NH: Referred somatic pain does not follow a simple "segmental" pattern. Fed Proc 5:106, 1946.
272. Travell J, Bobb AL: Mechanism of relief of pain in sprains by local injection techniques. Fed Proc 6:378, 1947.
273. Travell J, Rinzler S, Herman M: Pain and disability of the shoulder and arm: treatment by intramuscular infiltration with procaine hydrochloride. JAMA 120:417–422, 1942.
274. Travell J, Rinzler SH: The myofascial genesis of pain. Postgrad Med 11:425–434, 1952.
275. Travell JG: Unreported data, 1979.
276. Trommer PR, Gellman MB: Trigger point syndrome. Rheumatism 8:67–72, 1952.
277. Tyler FH, Adams RD: Acute and subacute myopathic paralysis, Chapter 345. In Harrison's Principles of Internal Medicine, edited by M.M. Wintrobe, G.W. Thorn, R.D. Adams, et al., Ed. 7. McGraw-Hill, New York, 1974 (pp. 1921–1923).
278. Valentine M: Aetiology of fibrositis: a review. Ann Rheum Dis. 6:241–250, 1947.
279. Valleix FLI: Traité des névralgies ou affections douloureuses des nerfs. J.B. Baillière, Paris, 1841 (pp. 266–594).
280. Virchow R: Ueber parenchymatöse Entzündung. Arch Path Anat 4:261–279, 1852 (pp. 269, 270).
281. Wall PD: On the relation of injury to pain. Pain 6:253–264, 1979.
282. Waylonis GW: Long-term follow-up on patients with fibrositis treated with acupuncture. Ohio State Med J 73:299–302, 1977.
283. Webber TD: Diagnosis and modification of headache and shoulder-arm-hand syndrome. JAOA 72:697–710, 1973.
284. Weinberg LA: The etiology, diagnosis and treatment of TMJ dysfunction-pain syndrome. Part I: etiology. J Prosthet Dent 42:654–664, 1979.
285. Weinberger LM: Traumatic fibromyositis: a crit-

ical review of an enigmatic concept. *West J Med* 127:99–103, 1977.

286. Weinstein L: Poliomyelitis, Chapter 192. In *Harrison's Principles of Internal Medicine*, edited by M.M. Wintrobe, G.W. Thorn, R.D. Adams, *et al*, Ed. 7. McGraw-Hill, New York, 1974.

287. Weiser HI: Semimembranosus insertion syndrome: a treatable and frequent cause of persistent knee pain. *Arch Phys Med Rehabil* 60:317–319, 1979.

288. Weiss S, Davis D: The significance of the afferent impulses from the skin in the mechanism of visceral pain, skin infiltration as a useful therapeutic measure. *Am J Med Sci* 176:517–536, 1928.

289. Wepman BJ: Biofeedback in the treatment of chronic myofascial pain dysfunction. *Psychosomatics* 21:157–162, 1980.

290. Wiechers D, Hines M, Wongsam P, *et al.*: Hocuspocus point. *Arch Phys Med Rehabil* 61:482, 1980.

291. Wilson TS: Manipulative treatment of subacute and chronic fibrositis. *Br Med J* 1:298–302, 1936.

292. Winter SP: Reffered pain in fibrositis. *Med Rec* 157:34–37, 1944.

293. Woodward TE: Rocky mountain spotted fever, Chapter 176. In *Harrison's Principles of Internal Medicine*, edited by M.M. Wintrobe, G.W. Thorn, R.D. Adams, *et al.*, Ed. 7. McGraw-Hill, New York, 1974 (p. 913).

294. Wyngaarden JB: Gout and other disorders of uric acid metabolism, Chapter 100. In *Harrison's Principles of Internal Medicine*, edited by M.M. Wintrobe, G.W. Thorn, R.D. Adams, *et al.*, Ed. 7. McGraw-Hill, New York, 1974 (pp. 612–614).

295. Yawger NS: Chronic "rheumatic" myositis (Muskelschwielen), with cases showing some common errors in diagnosis. *Lancet* 2:292–293, 1909.

296. Zacharias VJ, Bellmann H: Die Anwendung von Myocuran bei Myogelosen—insbesondere bei degenerativen Wirbelsäulenerkrankungen. *Z Aerztl Fortbild* 64:999–1005, 1970.

297. Zimmermann M, Albe-Fessard DG, Cervero F, *et al.*: Recurrent persistent pain: mechanisms and models, group report. In *Pain and Society*, edited by H.W. Kosterlitz and L.Y. Terenius. Verlag Chemie Gmbh, Weinheim, 1980 (pp. 367–382).

298. Zohn DA, Mennell J McM: *Musculoskeletal Pain: Diagnosis and Physical Treatment*. Little, Brown, Boston, 1976 (pp. 190–194).

CHAPTER 3
Apropos Of All Muscles

HIGHLIGHTS: Considerations that apply generally to all the muscles are consolidated in this chapter. Knowledge of the **REFERRED PAIN** pattern that is characteristic of each muscle is often the most valuable single source of information to identify the muscular origin of pain. The *precise* location of all of the patient's pain is drawn on a body form to aid in diagnosis and for future reference. A clear understanding of a muscle's **ANATOMICAL ATTACHMENTS** establishes its chief action(s), functional relation to other muscles, and its location for examination, stretch and injection. The **ACTIONS** of a muscle reveal what movements and stress situations are likely to activate and perpetuate trigger points (TPs) in it. The **MYOTATIC UNIT** identifies which other muscles are functionally closely related and, therefore, also likely to develop TPs because of interacting mechanical stresses. When the onset was sudden, **SYMPTOMS** of myofascial pain and dysfunction often began after a clearly remembered movement or event at a specific time and place. In other cases, excessively prolonged or repetitive efforts insidiously activated TPs in abused muscles. The muscles strained by the stress were likely to develop the most active TPs. The stressful movement or conditions responsible for **ACTIVATION OF TRIGGER POINTS** in a particular muscle must be identified and eliminated to prevent the same stresses from reactivating and perpetuating the TPs following treatment. **PATIENT EXAMINATION** begins with observation of the patient's posture, movements, and body structure and symmetry. It progresses to screening movements that quickly identify which muscle groups have a reduced stretch range of motion due to pain, and may include tests that elicit pain when the muscle is contracted in the shortened position. These responses are characteristic of muscles with ac-

tive TPs. **TRIGGER POINT EXAMINATION** of a muscle requires first a knowledge of the location and direction of its fibers in relation to those of neighboring muscles. Objective confirmation of a TP requires special examination techniques to locate the spot tenderness and the taut band by palpation, to elicit a local twitch response by mechanical stimulation of the TP, to evoke its referred pain pattern and, perhaps, to reproduce the patient's pain. A working knowledge of the muscle's anatomy is essential. Nerve **ENTRAPMENTS** may occur because of pressure by the palpable bands of taut muscle fibers that are associated with myofascial TPs, when the nerve passes through the muscle between taut bands, or when it is compressed between such a band and bone. The neurological symptoms and signs of neurapraxia that result are easily misinterpreted if this mechanism of entrapment is not recognized. **ASSOCIATED TRIGGER POINTS** develop as satellite or as secondary TPs from primary TPs in other muscles. The **STRETCH-AND-SPRAY** technique is simple in principle, but requires practice to skillfully combine passive stretching of the involved muscle fibers with coordinated application of the vapocoolant spray. **INJECTION AND STRETCH** require accurate localization of the TP, confirmation of precise placement of the needle based on local pain and local twitch responses, and enough pressure to insure hemostasis. After injection, first passive, then active motion should be performed to stretch the muscles and reestablish normal functional range of motion. The adequacy of **CORRECTIVE ACTIONS**, including both a stretch exercise program at home and the elimination of perpetuating factors (Chapter 4), usually determines the duration of relief experienced after treatment of the involved muscles.

1. REFERRED PAIN

The patient's pattern of referred pain is usually the key to the diagnosis of a myofascial pain syndrome. This section explains how to draw and interpret distribution of the patient's pain.

Surprisingly, the patient is rarely aware of trigger points (TPs) in the muscle that are causing myofascial pain; pain evoked by lying on an infraspinatus TP at night is perceived in the shoulder, not at the guilty TP in the muscle overlying the scapula. The myofascial TP pain patterns presented throughout this manual were described by patients as situated deep (subcutaneous and muscular) and intensely aching in character, unless stated otherwise in our description.

The patterns of pain referred from TPs in a muscle are reproducible and predictable. Knowledge of these patterns is used to locate the muscles most likely to be causing the spontaneous pain, much as one suspects disease of a viscus by its specific pattern of referred pain. The diagnostic value of the patient's pain patterns depends strongly on the accuracy and detail with which this distribution is mapped at every visit.

We know of no general rule for guessing the referred pain pattern of a muscle. Pain is more likely to be projected distally than proximally in the limbs, and it is often referred to a joint moved by that muscle. However, there are many exceptions. Some muscles, like the deltoid, refer pain only locally; others, like the scaleni, refer pain extensively. The pain pattern of each muscle must be learned individually.

For individual muscles, the *solid red area* in each drawing of referred pain depicts the essential pain zone, which is present in nearly every patient when the identified TP is active. Spillover pain zones, which may or may not be present, appear as *red stippling*. A black (or white) × identifies the usual location of the TP, or TPs, in that muscle; this is intended only as a general guide. The actual location for the individual patient must be determined by physical examination, as described in Section 9 of this chapter.

Drawing the Pain Pattern

A precise pictorial representation of the patient's pain is critical for an accurate diagnosis of myofascial pain; verbal descriptions are often imprecise and misleading; a blank body form is used routinely to record the patient's pain. Figures 3.1, 3.2, and 3.3 are forms useful for this purpose.

Communication concerning pain sensations is difficult, at best. When patients say, "My shoulder hurts," some will indicate pain in front of, or behind, the shoulder; one reaches back to the scapula; another grabs the entire shoulder indicating pain deep in the joint; and yet another rubs the upper arm. The *patient* delineates the pain on his or her body using one finger, while the *practitioner* draws it on the blank form. The patient may then examine the drawing for *accuracy* and *completeness*. This procedure enhances the precision of the record, and improves communication. The locations of *all* the patient's recent pains and the dates of their first appearance are noted for future reference. Other authors also strongly endorse the use of pain drawings.[12, 81, 85] Precise delineation of the patient's pain areas is required to match them with the known pain patterns of individual muscles.

To represent the distribution of the patient's pain, one can follow the conventions in this volume. The area that hurts most severely, and/or most frequently, is drawn in solid red. Regions that are sometimes painful, or are less painful, are stippled; the lighter the stippling the less painful the area. Red is reserved for aching pain; another color such as green, or check marks, are used for numbness and tingling. A black (or white) × locates the TP area. After treatment, black diagonal lines record the areas that were stretched and sprayed. A circled × locates a TP injected with procaine. Marginal notes tell the date of onset and associated event, unusual depth of the pain (if superficial or deep in the bones and joints), and any unusual quality. The dates of onset permit reconstruction of the evolution of a series of pain patterns. When mapping back pain, it is important to record the direction of the pain, as indicated by the patient's finger movement, up and down, or across the back.

Sometimes a patient will state, "I hurt all over." When asked if the nose hurts, the answer is almost always, "No." Nor do patients complain of referred pain in the

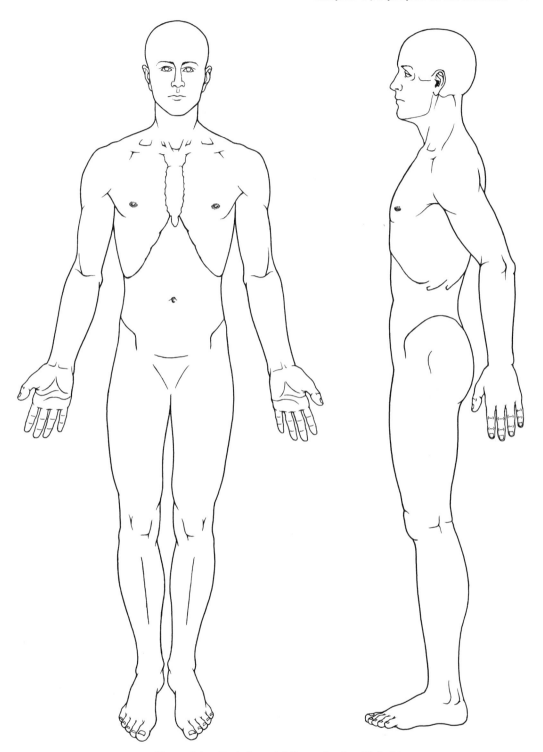

Figure 3.1.   Body form: full figure, front and left side.

fingernails. With this start, the patient begins to realize that discriminating answers are possible. Details are important, such as which side of the limb hurts, and whether the pain skips or concentrates in a joint. It does injustice to the patient and to the diagnosis to accept vague generalizations at face value.

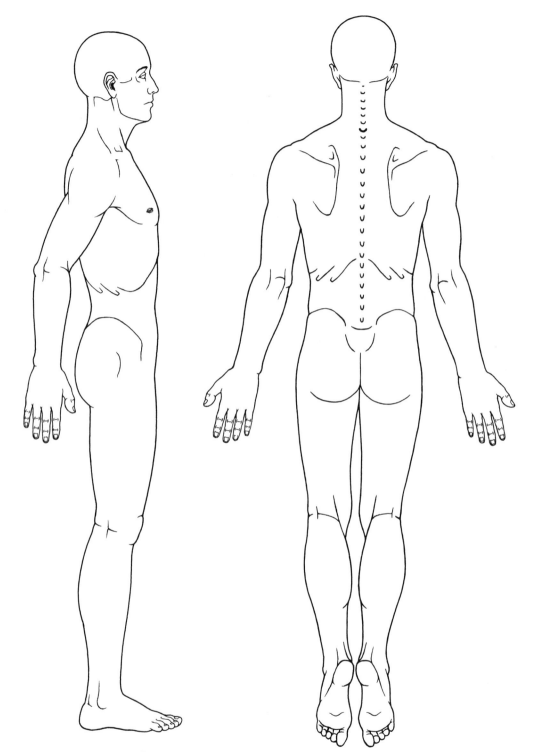

Figure 3.2. Body form: full figure, back and right side.

Interpretation of Initial Pain Patterns

Is the drawing a simple, one-muscle, myofascial TP pain pattern? Is it a com-posite of several such patterns that are superimposed, or is the distribution foreign to these pain patterns and, therefore, of non-myofascial origin? To answer these

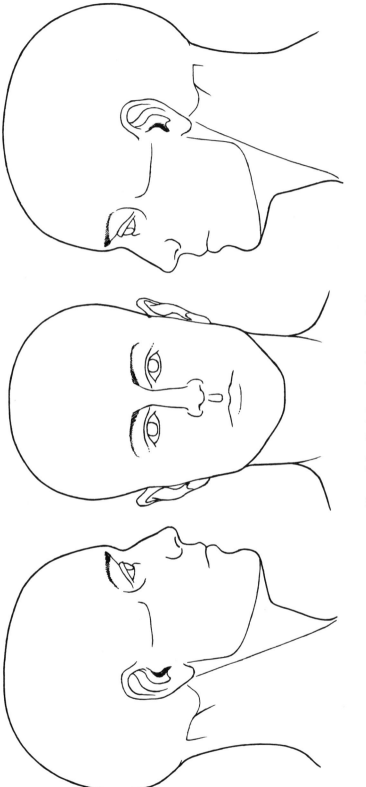

Figure 3.3.   Body form: head, front and sides.

questions one needs to be familiar with the individual myofascial referred pain patterns, and to know that myofascial pain is rarely symmetrical, and that it rarely assumes a glove-and-stocking distribution, or a pattern of hemialgia.[137] The extent of a muscle's referred pain pattern enlarges as the irritability (activity) of the TP increases.

A referred pain pattern may be composite in two ways. A total pattern may comprise overlapping patterns from different muscles, so that the extent of the pattern exceeds that of one muscle. On the other hand, if several muscles all refer pain to the same area (e.g. the shoulder), the area may be little larger, but will be more painful and hyperesthetic than if it were produced by a single muscle. Inactivation of only one of the contributing TPs may produce little amelioration of the patient's pain; inactivation of all of them achieves complete relief.

No two patients' problems are exactly alike. A few patients exhibit marked variations in the expected pain pattern, usually due to genetic variation, like anomalous muscles. Rarely are such variations hysterical symptoms.

The history should indicate whether the pain pattern has been stable, or whether it has evolved over months or years. If the pattern is stable, the pain is likely to resolve promptly with specific myofascial therapy. The progressive involvement of many muscles almost always means that perpetuating factors (Chapter 4) must be eliminated before pain relief can endure.

Interpretation of Follow-up Pain Patterns

If the patient returns pain free and the prior TP sites are no longer tender, the treatment rendered was successful.

However, if the patient returns claiming "no improvement," an accurate record of the previous pain pattern becomes critical. The earlier record is compared with a new drawing of the patient's pain. If the patient has the same degree of tenderness in the same TPs and the same pain pattern as before treatment, one asks how long pain relief lasted following treatment. If pain relief was complete for some hours or days, one can assure the patient that a muscular cause of the pain has been established, and it can be relieved, at least tem-

porarily. However, repeated treatment without first resolving the perpetuating factors that are making the TPs so hyperirritable, usually has only temporary success. The primary effort should then focus on identifying and eliminating the perpetuating factors.

On the other hand, if careful comparison of today's "no improvement" pain pattern with the patterns of the patient's previous visit shows a distinct change, and if the muscles previously treated no longer contain tender TPs, this represents satisfactory progress. Comparison of the new drawing with the initial chart of the prior pain patterns usually shows that the "new" pain is the reappearance of an old pattern. One set of TPs has been inactivated, but the absence of their pain has unmasked the referred pain pattern of the next most active TPs. Often, the patient is not aware of the shift in pain location until reminded by comparing the old and new pictorial records. Without the accurately recorded pain patterns for comparison, the person treating the patient also would be unaware of the progress made.

Occasionally, the pattern may be novel to that patient; a TP has been activated for the first time and must be managed as any acute myofascial syndrome.

2. ANATOMICAL ATTACHMENTS

By knowing exactly where a muscle attaches, one can deduce the major actions of the muscle, where to find it for palpation, and the direction of its fibers. The anatomical drawings of each muscle in this volume present the muscle alone with its bony attachments. The bones to which the muscle attaches are stippled more darkly than other bones. When necessary, additional drawings of regional anatomy show the muscle's relation to other muscles and structures. Anatomy textbooks were scoured for the needed views of muscles. When questions remained, dissections were studied in the anatomy laboratory.

Terminolgy

The names of the muscles come from *Nomina Anatomica*.[8] English usage follows the American edition of Gray's *Anatomy of the Human Body*.[56] In this manual, the words "origin" and "insertion" are avoided except in instances where the relation is unambiguous, as with finger attachments. Not uncommonly, the functions of the nominal origin and insertion become reversed, particularly during movement when muscles are likely to be strained and TPs activated; use of "attachment" helps one to keep an open mind and to think of muscle functions in realistic terms, permitting interpretation of the specific stress situation described by the patient. To stretch a muscle therapeutically, it matters not which end is fixed and which end is moved.

Unless stated otherwise, descriptions of attachments refer to the person in the upright position, standing straight, face forward, and the arms and forearms at the side with the hands supinated (Fig. 3.1). Therefore, *above* is equivalent to cephalad or proximal, and *below* is equivalent to caudad or distal.

Fiber Arrangement

A description of the fiber arrangement in muscles is commonly overlooked in anatomy texts, in the hiatus between gross and microscopic anatomy. It is rarely described adequately, except in a few older texts, such as Bardeen[7] and Eisler.[42] All the fibers of any one muscle are of nearly equal length, but usually with staggered attachments at the ends; muscle fibers usually attach to aponeuroses or to bone in a parallelogram arrangement. In long muscles with short fibers, such as the gastrocnemius, the aponeuroses overlap each other, or an aponeurosis at one end of the fibers overlaps a bony attachment at the other end.[22, 28] Individual muscle fibers may be placed so diagonally, as in the soleus, that the fiber length is barely one-half the length of the whole muscle.

In 1851, Weber[147] studied the structure of muscle and its relation to function by measuring the weight and mean fiber length of each muscle in the body. Table 3.1 extracts data for a number of the larger muscles (with correction of a few mathematical errors). The cross-sectional area of each muscle was calculated by the formula $S = P/pL$ where $S =$ the cross-sectional area, in cm^2; $P =$ the weight of the whole muscle, in grams; $p =$ the specific gravity of muscle, 1.0583 gm/cm^3; and $L =$ the mean length of the fibers in that muscle, in centimeters. This kind of measurement may vary greatly from person to person depending on body build, occupation, the degree and kind of physical activity, *etc.* Subsequent studies[22, 143] have reported results comparable to those of Weber.

Assuming similar fiber diameters among

Table 3.1
A Few of the Strongest Muscles Arranged in Their Order of Calculated Cross-sectional Area, Derived from Weber.[147]

Muscle	Cross-sectional Area	Mean Fiber Length	Total Muscle Weight
	cm^2	cm	gm
External intercostal	79	1.5	126
Multifidus	68	2.9	210
Internal intercostal	47	1.5	77
Longissimus thoracis	32	7.2	223
Deltoid	32	9.0	305
Triceps brachii, short head	26	5.8	161
Subscapularis	25	6.2	164
Infraspinatus and teres minor	17	7.4	132
Biceps femoris, long head	16	9.7	168
Triceps brachii, long head	16	7.7	131
Internal abdominal oblique	14	7.0	107
Serratus anterior	13	13.7	186
Cucularis (trapezius)	13	10.9	146
Brachialis	13	8.4	117
Pectoralis major, sternal	12	14.7	187
External abdominal oblique	10	10.9	115
Flexor digitorium profundus	10	6.7	68

muscles, the cross-sectional area is nearly proportional to the relative strength of each muscle, since this area also is proportional to the number of myofibrils contracting in parallel. This concept has been applied to the selection of muscles for transfer of tendon attachment.[22]

Supplemental References

As a convenience to those interested in different anatomical views or in a more detailed understanding of a muscle, additional illustrations are listed at the end of Section 2 of each muscle chapter, under **Supplemental References**.

3. INNERVATION

The spinal and peripheral nerves that usually supply each muscle are identified in this section. There is much individual variation; rarely do anatomists agree completely on the segmental innervation of a muscle.

4. ACTIONS

Understanding the actions of muscles is valuable diagnostically and therapeutically. Diagnostically, an accurate description of the precise movement made by the patient at the time that the TP was activated, together with a knowledge of which muscles are used to produce that movement, helps to determine which ones were likely to have been strained at the time. The strained muscles are then examined to see if they harbor active TPs.

Therapeutically, a knowledge of the movements and activities that employ the muscles being treated is needed to explain to the patient proper body mechanics. The patient must understand precisely what movements and activities should be avoided to prevent further muscular overload and perpetuation of the TPs.

In this manual, actions of muscles are described as the movement *of* a part *at* a joint; for example, the brachioradialis muscle flexes the forearm at the elbow. Terms describing directions of movement are defined in Chapter 1.

Four sources of information were used to summarize the actions of a muscle: (1) the actions listed in anatomy texts based on the attachments of the muscle; (2) the movements produced by stimulating the muscle electrically; (3) electromyographic studies that reported which movements or efforts generated motor action potentials in that muscle; and (4) the movements reported by patients, when the stresses produced TPs in that muscle.

5. MYOTATIC UNIT

The myotatic unit is emphasized because the presence of an active TP in one muscle of the myotatic unit greatly increases the likelihood that other muscles of the unit also will develop TPs. Dysfunction (weakness and shortening) of the affected muscle tends to overload other muscles of that myotatic unit. When inactivating TPs in a muscle, one must be concerned about TPs that may have developed secondarily in other muscles that work closely with it.

The physiological definition of a myotatic unit includes the synergists, which help the prime mover (agonist), and the antagonists,[107] which oppose the agonist, because these muscles are linked by interacting reflex pathways.[77, 151] The definition is sometimes extended in this manual to include muscles that do not necessarily share common reflexes, but which have one of two other close functional relationships with the agonist. One relationship is that of muscles that extend the line of pull of the affected muscle during total body movements; for example, the external abdominal oblique extends the line of pull of the serratus anterior muscle. The other involves stabilizing muscles;[107] the upper trapezius and levator scapulae muscles help control the scapula during forceful lifting movements of the upper extremity, on that side.

6. SYMPTOMS

With a thorough knowledge of individual myofascial pain syndromes and of TP referred pain patterns, one can often, with a careful history, not only establish the diagnosis of myofascial pain, but specifically identify which muscles are causing the pain. The chapters that follow note specific features of individual muscle syndromes. This section describes the features common to most myofascial pain syndromes that help to distinguish them from other painful conditions.

The myofascial pain may begin acutely with an obvious cause of muscular strain, or may begin insidiously due to obscure chronic muscular overload. In either case, symptoms may continue for months or years, if the myofascial TP source of the pain is not recognized and treated. This often, but not always, leads to the syndrome of chronic pain, which tends to become a way of life[119] and may require treatment of the pain behavior,[43] as well as the TP origin of pain. This manual concentrates on the latter.

While taking the history, the patient's comfort should be insured by demonstrating the principles of good body mechanics. A footrest is provided when the patient's legs are too short for the feet to rest firmly on the floor; additional armrest height is supplied when the elbows do not reach the armrests of the chair; a butt-lift is placed under the small hemipelvis when the patient's body is tilted because of this asymmetry; a small pillow in the lumbar hollow maintains the normal lumbar curve of the spine when the head and shoulders are hunched forward. Patients are amazed to discover the immediate relief that can be obtained by relieving the muscular strain due to these mechanical perpetuating factors. It helps the patient appreciate the strong impact that these factors have on his or her pain. A towel or scarf is provided to protect the patient's shoulders when a chilling draft causes direct cooling of the muscles. If the hands and feet are cold, a dry heating pad is placed on the abdomen to warm the core of the body and send more blood into the limbs (reflex heat). Contrary to the patient's previous experience, with the needed postural and environmental corrections he or she may now be able to sit for ½–¾ hr through the intensive interview, as comfortable at the end as at the start.

Patients who have suffered myofascial pain for months or years are likely also to have developed secondary depression and sleep disturbances, and to have restricted their activity and exercise. The ensuing restriction of body movement and the increased psychic tension aggravate their TPs, causing a vicious cycle. *All* contributory factors should be identified and managed medically.

Pain

Myofascial pain may start abruptly or gradually. With **abrupt onset**, the patient remembers clearly the first date of the pain and can usually describe in precise detail the exact event or movement, e.g. quickly getting out of bed in the morning. Pain of **gradual onset** is usually due to chronic overload of muscles; myofascial pain also may develop during or after a period of viral infection, visceral disease, or psychogenic stress.

Regardless of the mode of onset, pain referred from myofascial TPs is **characterized** as steady, deep, and aching, rarely as burning. It is to be distinguished from the prickling pain and numbness associated with paresthesias and dysesthesias of peripheral nerve entrapment or of nerve root irritation. However, two skin muscles, the platysma and palmaris longus, refer a needle-like prickling sensation superficially. Throbbing pain is more likely to be due to vascular disease or dysfunction. Occasionally, a myofascial TP initiates sharp, lancinating, or lightning-like stabs of pain.

When TPs in several muscles refer pain to one target area, such as the shoulder, or to a naturally sensitive area like the nipple, the zone of referred tenderness may become intolerant of the lightest touch and exquisitely sensitive to pressure.

Myofascial TP pain is characteristically **augmented**:

1. By strenuous use of the muscle, especially in the shortened position. Defining precisely the movement that increases the pain provides a major clue to the muscle that harbors the responsible TPs.
2. By passively stretching the muscle. However, active stretch by voluntary contraction of the antagonist does not ordinarily cause pain; the muscles quickly learn to limit this movement. The patient is aware of restricted range of motion and "weakness", but rarely thinks of the affected muscle as painful.
3. During pressure on the TP.
4. By placing the involved muscle in a shortened position for a prolonged period. Pain and stiffness are often at their worst when the patient gets out of bed in the morning, or when getting up from a chair after sitting immobile for a while.
5. By sustained or repeated contraction of the involved muscle.
6. During cold, damp weather, viral infections and periods of marked nervous tension.
7. By exposure to a cold draft, especially when the muscle is fatigued.

8. By cold packs continuously applied on the TP area. However, cold packs may afford some relief when applied to the pain reference zone. Also, relief by cold may indicate that the pain is of neuritic rather than of myofascial origin.

Myofascial TP pain is **decreased**:

1. By a *short* period of rest.
2. By slow, steady passive stretching of the involved muscles, particularly when the patient is seated under a hot shower or in a hot bath.
3. When moist heat is applied over the TP. The pain is decreased much less when the heat is applied over the reference zone.
4. By *short* periods of light activity with movement (not by isometric contraction).
5. By specific myofascial therapy (Sections 12, 13, and 13A in this chapter).

The development of a new pain during treatment must be diagnosed on its own merits and may, or may not be myofascial in origin.

Limited Range of Motion

This is rarely the chief complaint, but one that is readily elicited when investigated. Limitation of motion and increased stiffness are worse on arising in the morning and recur after periods of overactivity or immobility during the day. This painful stiffness is apparently due to the abnormal tension of the palpable bands.

Weakness

Frequently, patients are aware of weakness of certain movements, as when pouring milk from a carton, turning a doorknob, or carrying groceries in one arm. This yields clues as to which muscles are involved. The muscle learns to limit the force of its contraction below the TP pain threshold.

Other Non-pain Symptoms

Patients report excessive lacrimation, nasal secretion, pilomotor activity and occasionally changes in their sweat patterns. An involved extremity may feel cold as compared with the opposite one, due to reflex vasoconstriction. The examiner should be alert for symptoms of postural dizziness, spatial disorientation, and disturbed weight perception. All of these phenomena can be caused by myofascial TPs; some are specific to particular muscles, others are not.

Depression

A major, well-recognized cause of depression is chronic pain. Depression also may lower the pain threshold, intensify pain, and impair the response to specific myofascial therapy.

Depression must be recognized. If untreated, or undertreated, it blocks recovery from myofascial syndromes. It is diagnosed by a variety of clinical clues. Physiologic clues are insomnia, anorexia and weight loss, impotence or decreased libido, or blurred vision. Mental-outlook symptoms include a sad mood, thoughts of suicide or death, and delusions of guilt. Other clinical changes are inability to concentrate, poor memory, indecisiveness, mumbled speech, and a negative reaction to suggestion. Socially, the patient exhibits a desire to be alone, disinterest in favorite activities, a drop in job performance, and neglect of personal appearance and hygiene.

Folic acid or pyridoxine deficiency and low thyroid function are potent contributors to depression, and may, in addition, increase neuromuscular irritability and TP pain. An analysis of the problem should include, "What kind of patient has this pain?," not just, "What TP involvement does this patient have?"

With developing depression, the patient describes increasingly restricted movements and activity as their way to avoid pain. After a few weeks, most patients have discontinued their previous exercise program, and the unstretched muscles become increasingly deconditioned. This potentiates their tendency to develop TPs and makes them less responsive to treatment.

Sleep Disturbances

A careful history identifies the seriousness and nature of sleep disturbance. Depressed patients tend to fall asleep readily, but awaken in the night and have trouble sleeping again. They arise in the morning feeling more tired than when they went to bed. Some patients are awakened by their myofascial pain, others by noises. Each is dealt with by eliminating the cause.

Prognosis

Acute myofascial pain due to TPs caused by a clearly identifiable strain of one muscle is, as a rule, easily relieved. If the patient's pain has increased as the range of motion decreased, the therapeutic results are still likely to be good. If the pain has decreased as the range of motion also decreased, which may indicate increasing fibrosis, achieving relief of pain and return of function becomes more challenging.

Patients who have had a stable pattern of referred TP pain for months or longer, without extension to other muscles, are likely to respond well to treatment. When the pain has spread and is gaining momentum with successively more muscles becoming involved, multiple perpetuating factors must be eliminated before specific myofascial therapy will give sustained relief.

7. ACTIVATION OF TRIGGER POINTS

The acute events and then the chronic stresses that tend to activate TPs are considered here.

Sudden Onset

When asked, "Do you remember the day your pain started?," most patients will respond either with a clear affirmative or an unsure negative. If affirmative, the details of posture and movement at the onset permit estimation of the degree of stress that was imposed on various muscles. Sometimes, the pain was felt at the moment of stress; at other times, the patient remembers feeling "something happening" or hearing "a snap" at the moment of stress, but the pain developed gradually several hours later, reaching a maximum in 12–24 hr. Either is considered an acute single-stress onset.

The mechanical stresses that tend to activate myofascial TPs acutely include a wrenching movement, automobile accidents, falls, fractures (including chip fractures), joint sprains, dislocations, or a direct blow on the muscle.[129] Acute onset also may be associated with an episode of excessive or unusual exercise, such as packing when moving.[129] Most of the time, myofascial TPs due to such one-time gross trauma are easily inactivated as soon as the associated injury has healed; however, the TPs may persist for years if untreated.

Intramuscular injection of medicinal substances given inadvertently at the site of a latent TP may activate it.[127, 130] The patient feels a local pain before the solution is injected when the needle tip presses against or penetrates a TP. If the injection is delayed for a few seconds, this pain can be distinguished from a second intense referred pain caused by activation of the TP when a locally irritant medication is injected. It is wise to palpate for a nontender area to insert the needle and to relocate the needle before injection, if its insertion encounters TP tenderness. This activation of a latent TP can be avoided by adding procaine to make its concentration 0.5%. The procaine also minimizes postinjection soreness.

Latent TPs may be activated incidental to stretch-and-spray therapy. While one group of muscles is being passively stretched, their antagonists are shortening much more than usual. Fortunately, if latent TPs in the antagonists are painfully activated in this way, they can be inactivated quickly by also stretching and spraying them.

During injection of an especially active TP, the intense referred pain may activate latent TPs in muscles in the reference zone. For instance, injection of scalene muscles has activated TPs in the brachialis muscle, which entrapped the radial nerve and caused paresthesia and tingling of the thumb. Similarly, severe pain referred to a somatic area due to an acute visceral lesion, such as myocardial infarction or appendicitis, is likely to activate TPs in the painful region of the chest wall or abdomen.[129] Painful ischemia in a lower extremity, as in intermittent claudication due to atherosclerosis, can activate TPs in the painful calf muscle.[129]

Latent TPs in a fatigued muscle, especially in the calf or neck and shoulders, may be activated by direct cooling of the overlying skin, as by a cold draft from airconditioning or an open car window.

Gradual Onset

Locating the cause of active TPs that developed gradually due to chronic overload can be difficult, but it is important because the chronic strain, if continued, reactivates and perpetuates the TPs. Typical causes of sustained postural overload are poor work habits, such as a typist lifting the shoulders to reach an elevated keyboard, a slouched posture, or tolerating a sticking doorknob or desk drawer. If the source of strain is not obvious, the patient must help to identify it. The patient is instructed in the kind of movements that load the involved muscle, and then watches for daily activities that use that motion. The patient also notes any movement or activity that increases the referred pain, and then avoids it, or learns how to perform the activity (if essential) without overloading the muscles. Minutes spent tracking down precisely what activated the TPs can prevent recurrences and save hours of retreatment time.

Synergistic muscles that are in sustained contraction to protectively splint an involved muscle are, themselves, likely to develop secondary TPs.

A muscle that is immobilized in the shortened position for prolonged periods tends to develop active TPs.[129] This was demonstrated by the increased likelihood that patients with acute coronary thrombosis would develop a painful or frozen shoulder syndrome due to myofascial TPs when they were kept flat on their backs in bed without regular, gentle, active motion of the upper extremities.[134]

Nerve compression, such as the radiculopathy caused by a ruptured intevertebral disc, favors the development of TPs in the muscles supplied by the compressed nerve root (postdisc syndrome).[129]

The "nervous tension" associated with acute emotional stress or psychological tension produces sustained muscular activity that can induce TPs.[73, 129] Muscle pain syndromes are commonly seen in patients with any of a number of viral diseases, including acute upper respiratory tract infections.[39]

8. PATIENT EXAMINATION

This section considers the examination for myofascial TPs, which should be performed in conjunction with a general medical examination that pays special attention to neurological functions. The examination of a muscle specifically for TPs is

covered in the following Section 9. The examiner must remember that no two patients are alike. How many words can one make with 26 letters of the alphabet? How many more combinations can patients develop with 500 muscles and many perpetuating factors? The different hereditary backgrounds of patients are comparable to different languages. No two individuals have the same thumb print, not even identical twins. The challenge is to solve the riddle of how the principles of myofascial TPs apply to each patient's unique expression of them.

Patient Mobility and Posture

The patient's spontaneous posture and movements are observed while he or she walks, sits or removes articles of clothing. People with painfully active TPs tend to move slowly and protectively. They avoid, or explore gingerly, movements that might stretch the affected muscles. Some key observations: Does the patient use arms and hands bilaterally in their full range of motion? Does the body, rather than the head, turn when the patient looks around? In the sitting position, is the spine crooked and one shoulder lower than the other? Is the face symmetrical? Does the patient perform spontaneous stretching movements for relief; if so, what muscles are being stretched?

Some people have inherently poor muscular coordination; they move jerkily and quickly, just as others are tone deaf or color blind. These are the most difficult patients to treat because they keep misusing and abusing their muscles. On the other hand, the muscles of highly coordinated athletes quickly learn to inhibit movement and thus develop weakness to avoid pain. However, with treatment, these patients quickly reestablish normal function that their discriminating muscles remember well.

Neuromuscular Functions

Weakness and Restriction of Movement. A muscle containing *active* TPs is functionally shortened and somewhat weakened. Attempts to passively extend the muscle to its fully stretched length cause pain at less than normal range. Actively contracting the muscle in the shortened position also causes pain, but there is little, if any restriction of movement in that direction. Any movement, especially a quick maneuver, that markedly increases tension in the muscle, either stretching or contracting it, causes pain.

Weakness is detected by testing for muscle strength. Sudden premature cessation of effort by the patient during testing may be due to painful loading of distant stabilizing muscles, to painful loading of the muscle being tested, or to a sudden release of effort just short of painful loading that has been "learned" by the muscle being tested. The absence or presence and location of pain usually distinguish these causes of weakness due to TPs. Inactivation of the responsible TPs restores normal strength.

The painful restriction of the passive stretch range of motion can be quickly detected by screening tests. Range of motion in the shortened position shows little or no restriction, but additional contraction effort in this position is likely to be painful. This characteristic painfulness to passive stretch in one direction and to active contraction in the other was reported specifically for 10 muscles by Macdonald.[79] When screening the head and neck muscles for normal range, the seated patient should be able to place the chin firmly on the chest, to look straight up at the ceiling, to rotate the head at least 90° so that the chin points to the acromion, and to place the ear tightly against the shoulder without shrugging. When screening shoulder-girdle muscles with the Mouth-Wrap-around Test (Fig. 22.3), the hand should cover at least half of the mouth with the arm *behind* the head. When performing the Hand-to-shoulder-blade Test, the fingertips normally reach to the spine of the scapula on the non-dominant side (Fig. 22.4). Reach with the dominant hand is usually 1 or 2 cm less than with the non-dominant hand. The Mouth Wrap-around Test is restricted the most by subscapularis TPs. The Hand-to-shoulder-blade Test is restricted the most by infraspinatus and anterior deltoid TPs. Supination and pronation of the hand at the forearm are also tested because restriction can overload the shoulder muscles as they attempt to compensate.

An example of the effect of contracting a muscle in the shortened position is the Scalene-cramp Test (Fig. 20.4). The pain on contracting an affected muscle shifts to weakness as the muscle learns to avoid contractions that are forceful enough to cause pain. Several muscles are likely to show weakness and shortening because they lie in the reference zone of pain from another muscle. This is demonstrated by limited stretch of the finger extensors in the Finger-flexion Test (Fig. 20.6); this impairment of extensor digitorum communis function may develop because the muscle lies within the referred pain zone of scalene TPs. Similarly, upper trapezius TPs may cause mild to moderate impairment of opening of the jaws by restricting the stretch range of the temporalis muscle, as demonstrated by a positive Three-knuckle Test (Fig. 8.3).

The stiffness and relatively painless, but progressive, restriction of movement that characterize decrepitude of advancing age are often due primarily to latent TPs, which impair muscle function, but do not spontaneously refer pain. The muscles have learned to restrict motion to the painless range. These latent TPs respond as well to specific myofascial therapy as do active TPs, relieving this decrepitude.

Distorted Weight Perception. Testing for the disturbance of weight appreciation caused by sternocleidomastoid TPs is described in Section 8, Chapter 7. Loss of fine coordination among the muscles of mastication due to active TPs in those muscles is described in Chapter 5.

Weak Deep-tendon Reflexes. Myofascial TPs in a muscle can reduce the briskness of the deep-tendon reflex response elicited by tapping the tendon of that muscle. A weak or even absent ankle jerk due to active TPs in the soleus muscles demonstrates this, since, within minutes following inactivation of the TPs, the previously weak ankle jerk equals that of the normal side.

Cutaneous Signs

Dermographia has been strongly identified with the fibrositis syndrome (myofascial TPs) by a few authors.[69] We find that dermographia in the skin overlying muscles with active myofascial TPs occurs most often, but not invariably, when the muscles are located over the back of the torso, and less frequently with muscles in the limbs. Regular use of an antihistamine may be indicated.

Panniculosis. Despite the early use of the term panniculitis[5, 82] and the subsequent interchangeable use of panniculosis and panniculitis to characterize *diffuse* subcutaneous induration,[21] panniculitis is now described in a current rheumatology text[95] as a nodular condition of the skin that is associated with erythema nodosum and with the termination of steroid therapy. This description of panniculitis does not fit the condition we identify here as panniculosis. In panniculosis, one finds a broad, flat thickening of the subcutaneous tissue with an increased consistency that feels coarsely granular.[21] It is not associated with inflammation. Panniculosis is usually identified by hypersensitivity of the skin and the resistance of the subcutaneous tissue to "skin rolling," which is sometimes called "Rolfing," after Ida Rolf.

Skin rolling is accomplished by picking up a fold of skin and subcutaneous tissue between the fingers and the thumb, and moving the hand across the surface by rolling the fold forward, as clearly described and illustrated.[80] The peculiar, mottled, dimpled appearance of the skin in panniculosis indicates a loss of normal elasticity of the subcutaneous tissue, apparently due to turgor and congestion.[82] This "peau de orange," or orange peel effect, and the persistent indentations of the "matchstick test," but without evidence of pitting edema, has been beautifully illustrated for the skin of the back under the term trophedema.[58] However, Dorland's defines trophedema as "a disease marked by permanent edema of the feet or legs," which is not what the authors described.

Boos[21] observed that panniculosis is associated occasionally with the symptoms of "Muskelrheumatismus" (muscular rheumatism), "Muskelhartspann" (muscular firm tension) and "Myogelosen" (myogelosis), because topographically they are distributed similarly. However, they can be distinguished; the "Gewebsverhärtungen" (tissue hardenings) and "Druckpunkte" (pressure sensitive points) can be distinguished by the fact that they are located in deeper tissue layers. Boos[21] noted that freely mobile cutaneous tissue excludes panniculosis. McKeag[82] considered panniculosis a form of fibrositis. We find panniculosis in a distribution and with a frequency similar to those of dermographia (above), but not necessarily in the same patients.

Panniculosis should be distinguished from adiposa dolorosa[21] and from fat herniations.[35, 82]

It is not known why some patients with myofascial TPs show dermographia and panniculosis, and others do not. These conditions may be different forms of mild autoimmunity. Skin rolling may be therapeutic for panniculosis when done in a series of treatments.

Compression Test

When a patient presents with myofascial pain felt only during movement (not at rest), manually compressing the muscle responsible for that movement while it is being performed prevents the referred pain. Squeezing a roll of the skin overlying the involved muscle between the thumb and fingers also is often effective in blocking the referral of pain.

This Compression Test can be used to demonstrate to the patient the myofascial TP cause of the remote pain without imposing much additional pain. When patients have already heard numerous explanations for their pain from many doctors, they are naturally incredulous of this unfamiliar concept of myofascial TPs. First augmenting the patient's pain by pressure on the TP, and then relieving it by the Compression Test, helps to convince the patient that the pain has a definite muscular source, which can respond to treatment.

An example of use of the Compression Test is relief of pain in the throat during swallowing due to TPs in the sternocleidomastoid muscle; the technique is described in Section 8, Chapter 7. Section 8, Chapter 34, describes compression for TPs in the hand extensors, which cause pain during handgrip. Pain in the shoulder, when the arm is abducted at the shoulder with the thumb up, can be relieved by compressing the skin over the anterior deltoid muscle if the pain originates in a TP in that muscle. Painful abduction of the arm caused by a TP in the upper trapezius just above the scapula is relieved by firm pressure on that muscle with the palm of the hand in the midscapular line during abduction.[67]

9. TRIGGER POINT EXAMINATION

Screening tests and referred pain patterns suggest which muscles to suspect for active TPs; palpation for TPs is required to confirm which muscles are responsible for the myofascial pain.

This section deals with how to examine a muscle for TPs. If there is doubt as to where a muscle is located on the body, the anatomy drawing in the chapter on that muscle is informative. To confirm its location, the examiner has the patient perform a movement that contracts the muscle as the examiner resists the movement with one hand and feels for the contracting muscle with the other.

The optimal stretch on a muscle for palpating taut bands and TPs is just short of pain. Optimal tension for eliciting local twitch responses (LTRs) and for making the responses most visible is obtained by stretching a little less than for palpating taut bands.

While examining the muscles, the patient must be comfortable and warm. The muscle *must* be relaxed; otherwise, the distinction between tense bands and adjacent slack muscle fibers is lost.

Before the examiner attempts to palpate a muscle for TPs, the examining digits must have the fingernails trimmed short. Otherwise, the skin pain caused by long fingernails may be misinterpreted as TP tenderness.

Palpating TPs can severely exacerbate their referred pain activity for a day or two. For this reason, it is critically important to examine a muscle for TPs *only* if the examiner then applies specific myofascial therapy to the involved muscles, such as stretch and spray followed by hot moist packs. When the examiner neglects this caveat, myofascial pain patients come to dread a physical examination that includes palpating the muscles. The rule is: palpate only those muscles for TPs that can be treated during the same visit.

Taut Band and its Trigger Point

Several authors have recognized how critical are the details of the palpation technique for locating TPs.[104, 122] To palpate a taut band, the muscle is stretched until the fibers of the taut band are under tension and the uninvolved fibers remain slack (Fig. 3.4A). The stretch should be on the verge of causing pain, but should evoke only local discomfort and no referred pain. Optimal tension is usually about two-thirds of the muscle's normal stretch range of motion.

A palpable band feels like a taut cord of tense muscle fibers among the normally slackened fibers. The palpable group of muscle fibers were described as "matted together" by Wilson.[152] The examiner palpates along the taut band to locate the spot of maximum tenderness (the TP) and then maintains the pressure firmly on that spot to elicit its referred pain pattern. Flat palpation is used when the muscle can be pressed against underlying bone. Pincer palpation is used when opposite sides of the muscle are accessible so that the belly of the muscle can be grasped between digits (e.g. the sternocleidomastoid, latissimus dorsi, biceps brachii, and most of the pectoralis major).

In this manual, **flat palpation** refers to a moving fingertip that employs the mobility of the subcutaneous tissue to slide the patient's skin across the muscle fibers. This movement permits detection of changes in the underlying structures (Fig. 3.5). The skin is pushed to one side of the area to be palpated (Fig. 3.5A) and the finger slid across the fibers to be examined (Fig. 3.5B), allowing the skin to bunch on the other side (Fig. 3.5C). Any ropy structure (taut band) within the muscle is felt as it is rolled under the finger. A taut band feels like a cord 1–4 mm in diameter. Transverse snapping palpation of a taut band can be mentally compared to what plucking a violin string imbedded in the muscle would feel like. In a muscle that has many TPs, five or six such bands, or cords, may lie in such close proximity to one another that they seem to merge. If one tips the finger up on end to use the osseous spade-like end of the terminal phalanx, the individual bands in the group may be distinguishable.

When examining the abdomen, "fingertip" pressure locates spot tenderness in the abdominal wall, while "flat-hand" pressure elicits tenderness of underlying viscera.[122] Static pressure with the flat finger detects little more than underlying tenderness.

The technique of **pincer palpation** is performed by grasping the belly of the muscle between thumb and fingers (Fig. 3.6A) and squeezing the fibers between

Taut (palpable) bands in muscle

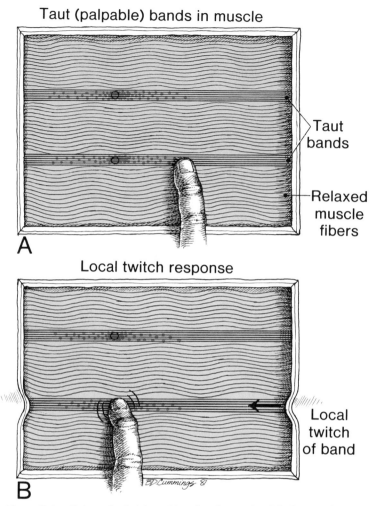

Figure 3.4. Schematic drawing of taut bands, myofascial trigger points (*dark red spots*), and a local twitch response seen in longitudinal view of the muscle (*light red*). *A*, palpation of a taut band (*straight lines*) among normally slack, relaxed muscle fibers (*wavy lines*). The density of *red stippling* corresponds to the degree of tenderness of the taut band to pressure. The trigger point is the most tender spot in the band. *B*, rolling the band quickly under the fingertip (snapping palpation) at the trigger point often produces a local twitch response that is most clearly seen toward the end of the muscle, close to its attachment.

them with a back and forth rolling motion to locate taut bands (Fig. 3.6B).

When a band is identified, it is explored along its length to locate the spot of maximum tenderness in response to minimum pressure; that is the TP.

For those who have difficulty in recognizing TPs by palpation, a dermohmeter, or similar device to measure skin conductance or skin resistance, can be used to explore the skin surface for points of high conductance (low skin resistance), which frequently, but not exclusively, overlie active TPs.

Local Twitch Response

In 1955, the senior author[129, 130] and Weeks and Travell[148] reported a localized twitch of part of the muscle when the TP was rolled under the fingers. The twitch could be vigorous enough to cause a perceptible jerk of the body part. She also observed this twitch response when a needle was inserted into a trigger area.[127]

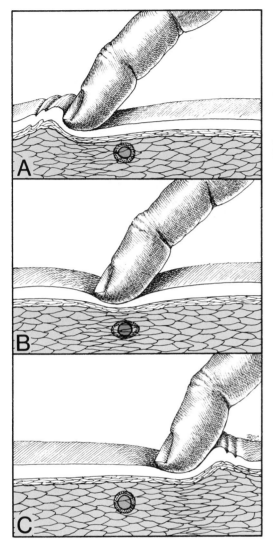

3.4*B*). It may be seen as a twitch or dimpling of the skin near the attachment of the fibers at the end of the muscle, or felt through the skin with the examining hand.

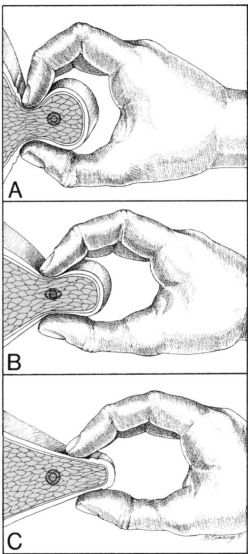

Figure 3.5. Cross-sectional schematic drawing showing flat palpation of a taut band (*black ring*) and its trigger point (*red spot*). Flat palpation is used for muscles (*light red*) that are accessible only from one direction, such as the infraspinatus. *A*, skin pushed to one side to begin palpation. *B*, fingertip slid across muscle fibers to feel the cord-like texture of the taut band rolling beneath it. *C*, skin pushed to other side at completion of snapping palpation.

Figure 3.6. Cross-sectional schematic drawing showing pincer palpation of a taut band (*black ring*) at a trigger point (*red spot*). Pincer palpation is used for muscles (*light red*) that can be picked up between the digits, such as the sternocleidomastoid, pectoralis major and latissimus dorsi. *A*, muscle fibers surrounded by the thumb and fingers in a pincer grip. *B*, hardness of the taut band felt clearly as it is rolled between the digits. The change in the angle of the distal phalanges produces a rocking motion that improves discrimination of fine detail. *C*, edge of the taut band sharply defined, as it escapes from between the fingertips, often with a local twitch response.

The EMG characteristics of local twitch responses (LTRs) were reported in 1976 by Simons,[113] but the phenomenon was then misnamed the "jump sign," which refers to a different phenomenon, as discussed below.

The LTR is a transient contraction of essentially those muscle fibers in the tense band that is associated with a TP (Fig.

The response is elicited by a sudden change of pressure on the TP, usually produced by transverse snapping palpation or needle contact with the TP.[41, 113] The closer to the TP that the taut band is stimulated by snapping, the more vigorous is the LTR. The muscle must be placed in a neutral position, neither fully lengthened nor fully shortened. This objective sign, unique to myofascial TPs, is most useful for identifying TPs clinically.

The LTR is readily elicited and perceived in the muscles that permit pincer palpation. Other superficially placed muscles, such as the deltoid, gluteus maximus, vastus medialis, and the finger and wrist extensors, are likely to exhibit strong LTRs in response to flat palpation. The LTR may not be evident in deep muscles, like the subscapularis or multifidi.

Most muscles exhibit a vigorous LTR only if they harbor active TPs, but the middle finger extensor, in many individuals, contains a latent TP that responds with a strong LTR. This LTR extends the middle finger, which makes it obvious. The relaxed arm is rested on a table or armrest of a chair with the wrist hanging over the edge. The tender spot is located in a palpable band of the middle finger extensor about 2 cm distal to the lateral epicondyle (Fig. 35.1A). With the forearm and hand to be tested fully relaxed, the TP is rolled under the fingertip with rapid, strongly applied, snapping palpation (Fig. 35.4), and the extensor response of the middle finger is observed.[113, 114]

The LTR has been studied electromyographically. It lasted from 12–76 ms in response to needle stimulation. The LTR of the middle finger extensor is clearly not a deep tendon reflex because it persisted after total motor and sensory anesthesia of the radial nerve at mid-arm.[114]

The LTR is a major diagnostic criterion of a TP in a taut band. Whether the examiner finds the band and elicits the LTR, or not, depends largely on the palpation technique. Snapping palpation requires a knack that must be mastered.

Jump Sign

Sufficient pressure on an active TP almost always elicits a jump of the patient, or jump sign. The amount of digital pressure required is one indication of the irritability of the TP. Good[51] noted, in 1949, that pressure on a myalgic spot elicits an agonizing pain accompanied by an involuntary reflex-like movement (jerk) of the body, often including a grimace. Kraft et al.[69] later dubbed this response the "jump sign," because digital pressure on the tender area produced a flinching and recoil totally disproportionate to the amount of pressure exerted. They considered it a diagnostic criterion of the fibrositis syndrome (myofascial TPs). The region of the muscle that exhibits such severe tenderness is remarkably small. This exquisite sensitivity to pressure is invaluable for locating TPs in deep-lying muscles, such as the gluteus minimus. The clear response to a slight change in the direction of the pressure exerted by the palpating finger permits one to accurately inject the TP by aiming the needle toward the maximum tenderness. The location of this jump-sign tenderness is highly reproducible for a given TP.

Induction of Referred Pain

Exploratory palpation for an active TP can elicit simultaneously a LTR, a jump sign and the referred pain pattern of that TP, as the patient might exclaim "Ouch! What did you touch? That was the pain down my arm!" Sustained firm pressure on an active TP is likely to evoke its referred pain as well as local pain at the TP.[127] Further description of the pain is found in Section 1 of this chapter. On the other hand, rapid, snapping palpation is likely to elicit an LTR with local pain, often without evoking referred pain.

If the TP is active enough to cause rest pain, digital pressure usually reproduces the patient's pain pattern; if the TP causes pain only during motion, referred pain is less likely to be elicited by pressure. The exacerbation of pain produced by examination of active TPs often does not subside for a period ranging from hours to days, unless the muscle is treated.

In eliciting referred pain, pressure on the TP first causes some local pain. The referred pain may then appear immediately, or take as long as 10 sec to develop. (Interestingly, the referred pain produced by injection of hypertonic saline also has a 5–10 sec delay before the projected pain is experienced.) Local pain appears instantly with pressure; if the pressure is too great, severe local pain may overwhelm the referred pain sensation. When the TP is so active that it already is producing maximal referred pain, pressure on the TP cannot induce additional referred pain, only local pain.

10. ENTRAPMENTS

When a nerve passes through a muscle between taut bands, or when a nerve lies between taut TP bands and bone, the unrelenting pressure exerted on the nerve can produce neurapraxia, which is loss of nerve conduction, but only in the region of compression. Table 3.2 lists the nerves observed to have been entrapped by a muscle in this manner. Occasionally, there is EMG evidence of a minor degree of neurotmesis (axonal loss) in addition to neurapraxia.

The patient with one of these entrapments is likely to have two kinds of symptoms: aching pain referred from TPs in the involved muscle, and the nerve compression effects of numbness and tingling, hypoesthesia and sometimes hyperesthesia. Patients with nerve entrapment prefer cold packs on the painful region; patients with myofascial pain usually find their symptoms aggravated by continuous cold, and relieved by heat on the TPs.

The signs and symptoms of partial neurapraxia may sometimes be relieved within minutes after inactivation of the responsible myofascial TPs, which immediately relaxes the taut bands. Effects of severe compression may require days or weeks for full recovery.

Table 3.2
Nerve Entrapments by Myofascial Taut Bands in Muscles.

Nerves	Muscles	Chapter
Supraorbital	Frontalis	14
Greater occipital	Semispinalis capitis	16
Brachial plexus, lower trunk	Scaleni	20
Sensory radial	Brachialis	31
Radial	Triceps brachii	32
Deep radial	Supinator	36
Ulnar	Flexor carpi ulnaris	38
Digital	Interossei	40
Brachial plexus	Pectoralis minor	43
Posterior primary rami	Paraspinal muscles	48

11. ASSOCIATED TRIGGER POINTS

This section in each muscle chapter identifies the other muscles of the myotatic unit that are likely to develop secondary TPs. Also, satellite TPs may develop in the pain reference zone of the primary muscle. These vulnerable muscles should be screened for TPs.

12. STRETCH AND SPRAY

Hans Kraus[93] described how he discovered that spraying ethyl chloride on the skin relieves musculoskeletal pain. Kraus was looking for a substitute for alcohol-soaked towels exposed to live steam that were then used in Germany by wrestlers as a treatment for painful sprains.[93] Kraus[71] recommends ethyl chloride spray initially, and then depends heavily on active range of motion and exercise for eventual recovery. The senior author became aware of his freezing spray technique through his 1941 paper on "surface anesthesia."[70] Her first use of it was on a young girl who had sprained her middle finger knuckle. As the spray was momentarily applied over the joint, the girl was startled and jerked her hand away. Then, mystified, she said "That feels better; put some right here." A second brief pass of vapocoolant over the other side of the joint completely relieved her pain and restored the full range of motion.[134] Obviously, refrigeration anesthesia with frosting of the skin was not an essential mechanism.

Soon Rinzler and Travell,[110] and then Travell,[126, 134] succeeded in relieving pain due to acute coronary thrombosis by applying the spray to the skin over the area of pain referred from the heart. This effectiveness of vapocoolant spray in relieving the pain of myocardial ischemia was demonstrated experimentally.[109]

In our experience, stretch and spray is the "workhorse" of myofascial therapy. Generally, it inactivates myofascial TPs more quickly, and with less patient discomfort, than local injection or ischemic compression. A single-muscle syndrome of recent onset frequently responds with full return of pain-free function when two or three sweeps of spray are applied while the muscle is being passively stretched.[124] On the other hand, when many muscles in one region of the body, such as the shoulder, are involved and the TPs are interacting strongly with one another, stretch and spray is a practical means of covering many muscles over a large territory to make significant progress toward pain relief. The stretch-and-spray technique does not require precise localization of the TP in the taut band, only identification of where in the muscle the taut bands are located, to insure that those fibers are stretched. However, considerable skill is required to coordinate the course of the spray so that it covers those fibers that are being placed on maximum tension by passive stretch.

In this manual, we use the expression "stretch and spray," not "spray and stretch," because we consider stretch the essential component, while the spray facilitates stretch. Gentle persistent stretch without spray is more likely to inactivate TPs than is spray without stretch. However, best results are obtained by spraying first, then stretching and spraying.

Stretch is the **ACTION**,

Spray is DISTRACTION.

Recently activated, acute, single-muscle TP syndromes may respond to passive stretch and hot packs without vapocooling. More chronic TPs usually require both stretch and spray.

Obvious inadequacies of body structure that perpetuate TPs should be corrected before proceeding with intensive TP therapy. When the patient has a vitamin insufficiency (B vitamins or ascorbic acid), TP injection may cause increased local muscle soreness for several days afterward, and may exacerbate, rather than relieve, the pain referred from active TPs remaining in the muscles injected. Stretch and spray is less likely to cause a similar reaction.

Myofascial TPs in the muscles of young children and babies are especially responsive to stretch-and-spray therapy.[10]

Stretch and spray is especially useful immediately after TP injection, while the local anesthesia produced by procaine remains, to inactivate any residual TPs.

Much of the shoulder pain in hemiplegic patients arises in TPs caused by strain on muscles that remain partially functional.

These functioning fibers are easily overloaded. During the first few weeks following a stroke, much temporary relief can be obtained by stretch and spray of both agonists and antagonists in the shoulder region, applied twice daily.[76] After 4–8 weeks, as the degree of paralysis and spasticity stabilizes, the relief of TP pain becomes more lasting. Such relief of pain encourages the patient to strive for function, and influences the results of rehabilitation by improving the patient's efforts to use marginally functional muscles.[35]

Immediately following major trauma, such as fracture, dislocation or whiplash injury, cold packs should be applied to the muscles to reduce tissue swelling. Stretch and spray, with heat, should be deferred until 3–5 days later as the local reaction to trauma subsides. However, the anti-inflammatory effect of the vapocoolant spray alone, without mobilization by stretch, when applied at once, may be extremely helpful in sprains, or any form of tissue damage, including burns.

As pain diminishes and stiffness with restricted motion becomes the chief complaint, the muscles tend to be less responsive to stretch-and-spray therapy, and TP injection becomes more necessary. This is evident in a "frozen shoulder" syndrome as the shoulder becomes less painful, but more limited in range of motion.[112]

Myofascial pain patients with hyperuricemia may not respond well to stretch and spray; pain recurs quickly. The response is better to injection of TPs. This may be explained by the deposition of uric acid crystals in an acid environment at the TP.

When a former patient, who has had perpetuating factors corrected, develops an acute reactivation of TPs, one may wish to wait 72 hr for the attack to subside spontaneously, while the patient avoids strain to the involved muscle, applies hot packs to the TP area, and gently stretches the muscle passively, using the body weight as the external force. The key is gentle mobility without load throughout this period. If, at the end of the 72 hr, the pain has not subsided and movement is still restricted, specific myofascial treatment is indicated.

Recovery of full function involves more than TP inactivation by stretch and spray. The muscle has learned dysfunction that restricts both its range and strength; it must relearn normal function. This requires adequate preparation for therapy, measurements of range of motion, a proper sequence of treatments, remeasurement, and post-treatment follow-up.

Patient Preparation

Patients intuitively avoid movements or activities that cause pain. Since the stretch necessary to inactivate TPs is mildly to moderately painful, the treatment contradicts intuition. Patients must understand clearly the muscular origin of their pain and that treatment requires some pain on stretching. Reproduction of the referred pain by pressure on a TP helps the patient to truly understand why treatment is directed to that muscle and not primarily to the region where pain is felt.

The portions of the skin to be sprayed should be bare. Unless it is heavily greased or thickly matted, spray penetrates the hair; but wigs and toupees must be removed.

Conservation of body heat is critical for a favorable muscular response. If the patient is chilly and the feet are cold, a dry heating pad applied to the abdomen raises the core temperature and causes reflex vasodilatation in the limbs. This is important in cold climates, chilly rooms, and whenever a patient feels cool. A blanket should cover the portion of the patient not exposed for treatment.

Before applying a specific myofascial therapy like stretch and spray, the patient should be asked if he or she has eaten recently to detect potential hypoglycemia. A banana, glass of milk, cheese, flavored "drinking" gelatin in orange juice, or a cup of instant soup may prevent a painfully adverse reaction to therapy soon afterward. Hypoglycemia aggravates TPs.

Pretreatment Measurement

Unless the patient has been given a specific frame of reference with which to judge the range of motion, he or she is likely to be unaware of the improvement gained by therapy; to the patient, a movement feels as if it "goes as far as it can go" both at restricted and at the full range of motion. During initial testing, the patient learns how to measure the exact range by answering specific questions. "How wide does your mouth open; two or three knuckles?" "How far around can you see behind you?" "Can your fingertips cover your mouth?" or "Can you reach your back pants pocket?" A mirror helps patients to see and remember what they were able to do. The measurement is retested following treatment so that the patient can judge the differences.

Stretch and Spray Sequence

Figure 3.7 demonstrates the sequence of steps in the stretch-and-spray technique, as applied to the trapezius muscle. First, the patient must be positioned *comfortably* and well supported to permit voluntary relaxation. One end of the muscle must be *anchored* so that pressure can be applied at the other end to *passively stretch* it. With the patient in the position for stretch, the first sweep of spray is applied *before* any stretch pressure is applied. A jet stream (not a diffuse mist) of *vapocoolant spray* is applied in parallel sweeps in one direction only, first over the *entire length of the muscle*, in the direction of the referred pain, and then over the *referred pain pattern*. The stretch-and-spray steps can be *repeated* until full muscle length is achieved, but any given area of skin should be covered only two or three times before rewarming. Immediate application of a moist *hot pack* rewarms the skin and helps to further relax the muscle. After the skin has rewarmed, stretch and spray can be repeated. Several cycles of *full active range of motion* complete one stretch-and-spray treatment of that muscle.

Relaxation

The involved muscle cannot be effectively stretched if it is not fully relaxed, and full relaxation requires a comfortable, warm, well-supported patient. All the limbs must be positioned comfortably when the patient is in the recumbent position. In the seated position, the patient's pelvis and shoulder-girdle axis must be leveled by adding a butt lift to compensate for any discrepancy in the size of the two halves of the pelvis. The patient is given a lumbar pad to correct a stooped posture (see Section 14 in Chapter 42). Sliding the buttocks forward slightly on the chair seat permits the patient to relax by leaning back and feeling more stable. If the oper-

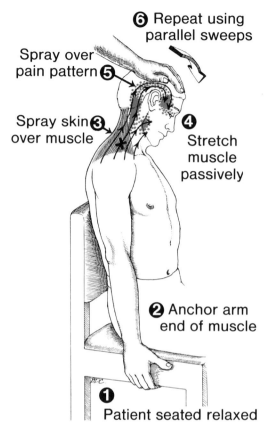

❻ Repeat using parallel sweeps

Spray over pain pattern **❺**

Spray skin **❸** over muscle

❹ Stretch muscle passively

❷ Anchor arm end of muscle

❶

Patient seated relaxed

Figure 3.7. Sequence of steps when stretching and spraying any muscle for myofascial trigger points, as applied to the upper trapezius. *1*, patient supported in a comfortable *relaxed* position. *2*, one end of the muscle (*light red*) anchored. *3*, skin sprayed with repeated parallel sweeps of the vapocoolant over the length of the muscle in the direction of pain pattern (*dark red dots*). All of the muscle is covered. *4*, immediately after the first sweep of spray, pressure is applied to stretch the muscle and is continued as spray is applied. *5*, sweeps of the spray continued to cover the referred pain pattern of that muscle. *6*, steps 3, 4 and 5 repeated only 2 or 3 times, or less if the passive range of motion becomes maximum. Hot pack and then several cycles of full *active* range of motion follow. See Figure 3.8 for details of the spray technique.

ator is extending the head, the patient is asked to lean the head back against the operator, who supports it so that the neck muscles can relax.

If a patient is tensely holding the breath, a remark like, "Don't forget to breathe," helps to release the tension. As demonstrated by Basmajian,[9] relaxation is not a passive process, but an active one that requires learning how to turn off motor unit activity.

For most patients, the trick is to divert attention from themselves and to have them concentrate on the *support*. They must feel the armrests of the chair supporting their forearms, or think about the wrinkles in the sheet on which they are lying. For those who find this difficult, deep breathing with the *abdomen* is encouraged; then stretch and spray is applied to the muscle as they slowly exhale. For most patients, abdominal breathing is much more relaxing than chest breathing.

Stabilization

To effectively stretch a muscle, one end must be anchored so that the operator can exert tension on it from the other end. Usually, the patient's body weight serves as the anchor, but at times the patient must fix one end of a muscle by holding onto something secure, e.g. the chair seat when stretching the scalene or upper trapezius muscles.

Passive Stretch

The stretch aspect of the stretch-and-spray technique has been described before.[128, 135, 136, 154] It may help to allay the patient's apprehension by calling it "instant traction."[134] To fully inactivate TPs by passive stretch, the muscle must be extended to its full normal length. However, stretching by itself usually causes pain and reflex spasm of the muscle, obstructing further movement. Patient relaxation and vapocoolant spray help to block these responses, thus permitting gradual stretch to the full range of motion, which terminates the abnormal muscle tension.

During unhurried, rhythmic, intermittent application of vapocoolant, the affected muscle is passively stretched *slowly*, with steady, gradually increasing force. The jet stream covers the length of the muscle once before the external force is applied. The stretch is then held at a point of tolerable discomfort that does not induce a stretch-reflex spasm or guarding contraction of the muscles. This requires an intensely concentrated effort on the part of the patient to relax and should be verbally reinforced frequently by the operator. As the muscle "gives up" and releases its tension, the operator *smoothly* takes up the slack to reestablish a new stretch position that maintains the same level of tension. Jerking the muscle or sudden movements by the patient must be avoided during and after stretch. Reaching the full normal length of the muscle is essential for complete inactivation of its TPs and relief of their referred pain; achieving the final few degrees of movement is critical.

Sometimes, the spray effect persists and permits the operator to maintain stretch for a few seconds, adding a small gain. Other patients react badly; the muscle begins to hurt, and tightens.

A difficult skill to be learned is "tuning in" to the tenseness of the patient's muscles and to detect immediately any muscle shortening due to voluntary contraction or to reflexes secondary to pain. If this occurs, the operator releases some stretch pressure immediately, since further stretch is impossible until the muscle relaxes. The operator asks the patient to speak up *immediately* if the tension becomes unbearable and warns the patient not to be stoical.

After completing full stretch, the return must be smooth and gradual, and the patient must not overload the muscle by suddenly lifting the member by himself.

Cooperative patients who have good neuromuscluar coordination can be taught to apply the passive stretch themselves for some muscles, while the operator applies the spray. These patients can precisely adjust the optimal amount of stretch while they are learning this self-stretch procedure for use at home. Apprehensive patients are reassured by gaining control of the stretch tension, and thus relax better.

Asking the patient to *gently* help stretch the muscle by contracting its antagonists can reap the advantage of reciprocal inhibition to reduce reflex spasm and improve relaxation. However, if the patient tries too hard and cocontracts the involved muscle, it defeats the purpose of the effort.

If the muscle seems "stuck," short of full range of motion, instead of repeating exactly the same stretch-and-spray procedure, modifications may be tried: (1) sweep the spray over functionally parallel or neighboring muscles that also may be shortened by latent TPs and could be "hanging up" the muscle being stretched; (2) place a hot pack on the muscle for a few minutes; (3) have the patient perform several cycles of the full active range of motion for that muscle and then resume stretch and spray, if indicated; and (4) try the Lewit[75] stretch technique described under Section 13A of this chapter. Effective stretch and spray of a cranky muscle is the art of adjusting the "cookbook" style to the individuality of the patient; coax the muscle a little, let the patient move it, spray again, apply a hot pack, try ischemic compression, massage it, try self-stretch, *etc.*

Vapocoolant Spray Technique

Detailed descriptions of the vapocoolant stretch-and-spray technique have been published.[46, 90, 124, 128, 135, 136, 154]

Which Vapocoolant? Both ethyl chloride and Fluori-Methane* sprays are commercially available. Ethyl chloride is too cold as usually applied, is a rapidly acting general anesthetic, flammable and explosive. It has been responsible for accidental anesthetic death and is potentially explosive when 4–15% of the vapor is mixed with air.[93] If ethyl chloride spray is used, precautions must be observed. Fire hazards must be eliminated, and the patient must not inhale the heavy vapor.[124, 135] Travell[134] assisted in the development of a safe alternative, Fluori-Methane, which is a mixture of two fluorocarbons, 85% trichloromonofluoromethane and 15% dichlorodifluoromethane.

Both volatile liquids exert pressure in a bottle at room temperature, which forces a stream of the room-temperature liquid out of the inverted bottle. The liquid immediately begins to evaporate, which cools the stream by the time it impacts the skin, where it continues to evaporate and removes heat from the tissues. Fluori-Methane is non-flammable, chemically stable, non-toxic, non-explosive and does not irritate the skin. It can freeze the skin when a stream is directed on one area for 6 sec or longer; this should be avoided.[149]

The spring cap, which seals the nozzle of the bottle, permits on-off application with no intermediate control. The bottle must be held inverted so that the fluid will flow from it; otherwise only vapor comes out. The "calibrated" nozzles are variable in bore. When an unusually fine-bore noz-

---

* Trade Name sources are listed under Suppliers at the end of the Chapter.

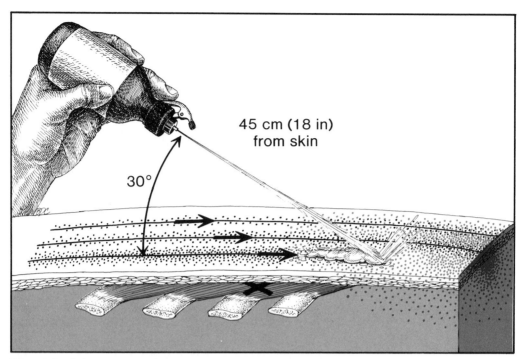

45 cm (18 in)
from skin

30°

Figure 3.8. Schematic drawing showing how the jet stream of vapocoolant is applied. Unidirectional sweeps cover, first, parallel lines of skin over those muscle fibers that are stretched the tightest, then over the rest of the muscle and its pain pattern. The lines of spray follow the direction of the muscle fibers (*solid red*), progressing toward the referred pain zones (*red stippling*). The spray bottle is held at an acute angle approximately 45 cm (18 in) from the skin, as the spray sweeps over the skin at a rate of about 10 cm (4 in)/ sec.

zle produces a thin stream, that bottle is marked "FINE" and set aside to be used on patients who exhibit unusual cold sensitivity.

After receiving adequate instruction, patients may be given the Fluori-Methane spray for home use. **Under no circumstances** do we recommend ethyl chloride spray for patient use. All of the articles by the senior author that refer to ethyl chloride (because they were written before Fluori-Methane became available) should be reinterpreted to substitute Fluori-Methane for ethyl chloride.

Urticaria owing to cold allergy has not been observed in response to spraying with Fluori-Methane for myofascial therapy, and was observed only once with ethyl chloride.[135]

Toxicity. Freon, a trademarked name for this family of fluorocarbons, was medically evaluated when it was still widely used as the propellant for aerosol hairsprays.[44] When inhaled, it had no effect on pulmonary function tests and, unlike the hairspray ingredient itself, did not compromise tracheal mucociliary transport.[44]

The major component of Fluori-Methane, trichlorofluoromethane (Freon-11), when similarly used as the propellant for pressurized aerosols of adrenergic bronchodilator drugs, was absorbed from the lungs and appeared briefly in the blood. Even with such massive inhalation doses, the concentration in the blood was not considered likely to sensitize the heart to adrenergic compounds.[102] However, under conditions of hypoxia, it may be toxic. Patients sprayed with Fluori-Methane for TPs inhale a much smaller dose and lower concentration than during the exposure in these experiments.

As a general anesthetic, ethyl chloride has a dangerously narrow margin of safety.

Technique. The closer the bottle is held to the skin, the warmer is the stream of vapocoolant on impact. One can demonstrate this easily on oneself by the length of time required to produce frosting of the skin, or how cold the stream feels, when the bottle is held at various distances from the skin.

For treatment, the jet stream of vapo-

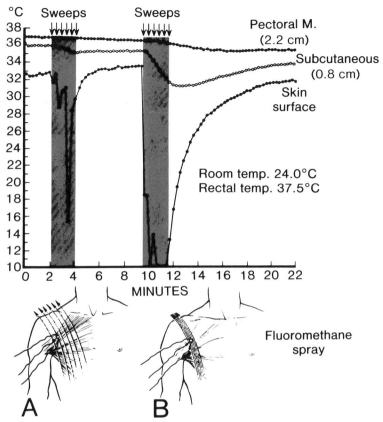

Figure 3.9. Skin surface, subcutaneous and muscle temperature effects produced by the correct (A) and incorrect (B) use of Fluori-Methane vapocoolant spray. Temperatures were recorded by a tier of three thermal sensors in needles from: (1) pectoral muscle (*upper line*) at a depth of 2.2 cm, (2) subcutaneous tissue (*middle curve*) at a depth of 0.8 cm, and (3) skin surface (*bottom curve*). The jet of vapocoolant was applied in one direction in six even sweeps at 10 cm/ sec for a total of 2 min (*shading*). A, (*bottom left*) sweeps covered adjacent parallel skin areas, and only one sweep traversed the tier of sensors. B, (*bottom right*) all six sweeps traversed the same path directly over the sensors. When a given skin area was covered only once (A), the fall in muscle temperature was negligible, 0.2 C; when the tier was covered six times (B), the muscle temperature dropped more, 1.5 C, starting during the application and continuing to drop as the overlying skin rewarmed.

coolant is directed at an acute angle to the skin (approximately 30°), not perpendicularly, and is swept over the skin parallel to the affected muscle fibers. The parallel sweeps move in one direction only, covering the entire length of the muscle, travelling toward the area of referred pain, and finally covering all of the pain reference zone. The bottle is held about 45 cm (18 in) from the skin (Fig. 3.8). Slow, even sweeps that progress over the skin at about 10 cm (4 in)/sec are spaced to provide a slight overlap of the paths of wet spray. Repetition that covers the muscle with two or three superimposed sweeps is usually

maximum; the skin must then be rewarmed. Six sweeps over the same skin area, without rewarming, are too many because that many can cool the underlying muscles (Fig. 3.9).

Frosting of the skin can cause ulceration; refrigeration anesthesia is neither necessary nor desirable.[93] Properly applied, the vapocoolant causes a rapidly changing gradient of skin temperature and an impact that produces tactile stimulation. These stimuli transmit a continuing barrage of impulses to the spinal cord.

It is best to use additional sweeps and cover a slightly larger area than necessary, being careful to include skin overlying all of the muscle. No therapeutic harm is done with some additional coverage. Full coverage also may release latent TPs in other parts of the same muscle or in adjacent muscles, where they can be limiting the range of motion.

Many patients are startled by the cold spray if they are not warned that it is coming. The impact of the spray on the operator's hand, and then on the patient's hand, should be demonstrated before starting treatment. When vapocooling the face, the eye on that side should be covered. It is startling, but not damaging, if Fluori-Methane spray accidentally hits the conjunctiva, or the eardrum.

The patient should tell the operator if he or she wants an area of skin covered that was missed by the spray. Vapocooling such an overlooked region usually further releases muscle tension. It is remarkable how precisely the skin that needs to be sprayed overlies the muscle fibers on maximum stretch. A path that is a few centimeters to one side fails to afford the release of tension that an accurately centered jet stream provides. It also is remarkable how the muscle tension sometimes melts away as the stream of spray is extended over the most distant portion of the referred pain pattern.

The direction of spraying was initially determined by subjective testing on patients by the senior author, who noted the direction of spraying that the patients preferred and that gave the maximum relief of tension and pain.

When the spray is applied for the first time over very irritable TPs, the skin may be hypersensitive to the cold, even unbearably so. However, after several passes of the spray, this extreme sensitivity usually abates. The initial distress can be alleviated by using a bottle saved for its fine-bore nozzle, by holding the bottle closer to the skin so that the spray has cooled very little before impact, and by wafting the jet stream across the skin more rapidly.

No cases are known of skin irritation or allergic reaction to Fluori-Methane spray. A white trace left behind on the skin is sebum dissolved from its pores. When patients use the spray often, the sebum can be replaced with cold cream or lanolin.

Patients generally learn quickly to self-spray their masticatory and calf muscles. However, it requires unusually skillful selective relaxation to effectively stretch and spray by oneself the shoulder-girdle, arm and neck muscles. Self treatment is useful during the transition period, while the perpetuating factors are still being identified and resolved, and for patients who seem unavoidably prone to reactivation of TPs and need to inactivate their TPs promptly themselves.

Substitute Stimuli. A variety of distracting sensory stimuli can be applied to the skin over the muscle while it is being stretched, but generally, none of these substitutes are quite as effective as vapocoolant spray. Nearly as effective is hot running water, especially if the person sits and relaxes under a hot shower, thus avoiding antigravity tension (see Fig. 16.10). Ice molded in a paper drinking cup, or an ice cube wrapped in plastic, can be stroked over *dry* skin, simulating the parallel sweeps of spray.[27, 154] The prolonged skin wetness caused by bare ice produces generalized cooling instead of a spot of rapid temperature change. Skin rolling, as used to diagnose and treat panniculosis, helps to relieve underlying muscle tension. One can use the neurologist's pinwheel, designed for testing pinprick sensation, by running it over the same paths that one would run the spray, and call it the "stretch-and-prickle" technique.

Other Uses. Ethyl chloride spray was initially used for **joint sprains**;[93] Fluori-Methane is equally effective. The sooner the vapocoolant is applied after the sprain, the more fully it relieves pain and disability. Vigorous stretching is avoided in the presence of torn tissues, but the full range of motion at the joint should be reestablished within a reasonable period.

The vapocoolant spray is effective for relieving the pain of **thermal burns**, and it also reduces their secondary hyperalgesia and erythema, as demonstrated in experimental studies.[127, 138] Burns that were sprayed until pain-free did not blister, compared with untreated control burns that did. The spray is applied to the painful area as soon as possible after the burn until it stops hurting, which usually takes several seconds. The spray is reapplied immediately if pain recurs. The number of repetitions required depends on the severity of the burn. On minor first degree burns, one application may be sufficient to completely eliminate pain.

Vapocoolant spray applied to the painful regions in acute myocardial infarction can be remarkably effective in relieving the pain without changing the course of the cardiac pathology.[109, 126] A few applications can fully replace morphine or comparable analgesics.

Vapocoolant spray partly relieves the pain of *ischemic* **calf cramps**.[93] It relieved or delayed pain during experimental ischemic contraction of forearm muscles.[139]

It relieves the pain of **bee stings**,[93] and is reported as helpful in controlling the pain of *postherpetic neuralgia*.[121]

Some **veterinarians** and animal trainers use vapocoolant spray to relieve what resembles myofascial TPs, including spot tenderness, in the muscles of horses[93] and dogs. The authors have found stretch and spray to be effective in relieving muscular pain behavior, such as limping, in these animals when examination revealed taut bands and TP-like tenderness in an appropriate muscle.

Heat

Dry heat applied to myofascial TPs is not as effective as wet heat. Many patients and athletes depend on hot tub baths or showers for maintenance of the health of their muscles and the prevention of post-exercise stiffness.

Post-treatment muscle soreness is markedly reduced by applying a hot pack for a few minutes immediately after stretch and spray. This rewarms the skin for retreatment of the same area, if needed, and promotes further reduction of muscle tension. The patient must be kept warm, and covered as much as possible; bare skin radiates a lot of heat.

In this manual, when a hot pack is mentioned, it is assumed to be moist, such as an Hydrocollator Steam Pack or comparable hot pack. A convenient alternative for home use is a *wetproof* electric heating pad covered with dampened flannel. A piece of plastic that covers the exposed side of the pad and is tucked in around its edges protects sheets, clothing and hair

from getting wet. Patients who use such electric heating pads at home must be warned not to fall asleep with the switch on high, lest they burn themselves. A hand-pumped spray bottle of water is a convenient device with which to dampen the cover of the wetproof heating pad. A thin wet towel wrapped around an old-fashioned hot water bag has been used effectively in place of a hot pad or pack.

Active Range and Remeasurement

The retraining of the muscle to full normal function is combined with a post-treatment measurement of movement for comparison with the range before treatment. The patient moves the member through three cycles of *full* range of motion, with a pause and rest between each cycle, and then the test position is held to evaluate the result of treatment. This establishes in the patient's mind the effectiveness of the myofascial therapy and fixes a specific goal for the stretch exercise program at home.

Post-treatment Instructions

Especially when trunk and lower extremity muscles are involved, the patient benefits by soaking in a hot bath at home as soon as possible after the stretch-and-spray treatment. The patient should NOT travel, go sightseeing, to the theatre, or shopping, immediately after treatment, but should allow the muscles to rest and recover normal function. The patient should know this when making an appointment, so that appropriate plans can be made. Strenuous swimming should be avoided but, in a warm pool, unstrained stretching and range-of-motion activities that cause no pain are desirable. Thus, "lazy" stretching with the body supported by the water is excellent. Specific stretching exercises for the patient to do at home are essential. They maintain, and help to extend the range of motion achieved by treatment.

Mechanisms Involved

When stretch and spray inactivates myofascial TPs, the abnormal muscle tension is released, the TP becomes non-tender, and it no longer refers pain and autonomic effects. A physiological mechanism by which the stretch could help to inactivate TPs is discussed in Chapter 2. The spray facilitates the stretching by inhibiting pain and spinal stretch reflexes. The precise mechanisms by which the vapocoolant spray exerts these effects have not been established by direct experiments. Physiological principles that help one to understand these effects include spinal inhibition, descending inhibition, and TP inhibition.

Vapocooling must exert its influence indirectly *via* skin afferent nerves, rather than by direct cooling of the muscle, because cooling barely penetrates to the subcutaneous tissues with the technique used[134, 135] (Fig. 3.8). An indirect cutaneous mechanism of cold analgesia was demonstrated by the fact that ice massage of the web between the thumb and index finger was as effective as either transcutaneous electrical stimulation or acupuncture for the relief of dental pain.[87]

Patients understand the purpose of stretch and spray when they are told that the operator is "blocking TP activity" by the procedure, and that the spray "jams the spinal switchboard" so that the muscle sensation becomes disconnected (the communication lines are all busy).

A controlled study of the effect of Fluori-Methane spray on the range of passive hip flexion in normal subjects found that the application of vapocoolant increased the range of motion.[60] Since no mention was made of screening these patients for palpable bands and latent TPs in the muscles being stretched, it is possible that the increase in range was obtained by eliminating latent TPs that were restricting the normal range.

Spinal Inhibition. Attempts to forcibly stretch a muscle that contains an active TP are blocked by pain and reflex spasm, which prevent further stretch. Figure 3.10 shows schematically how skin stimulation by vapocooling could block those responses and facilitate muscle stretching. In effect, the spray reduces the excitability of the motor neurons that supply the muscle, making the muscle less likely to contract voluntarily or reflexly.

As the stream of vapocoolant strikes the skin, it induces a sudden change in several sensory modalities. The stream of cold spray always stimulates cold and touch sensations, and sometimes pain, as reported by a few patients. The vapocoolant causes an absense of sensation if the temperature of the sensory nerves in the skin drops to 10 C (50 F). The spray technique recommended in this manual minimizes the adaptation of tactile sensors to repeated stimuli, by not stimulating them again until they have had adequate time to

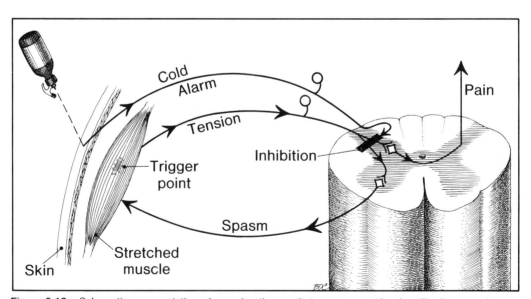

Figure 3.10. Schematic representation of neural pathways that can account for the effectiveness of vapocoolant applied to skin overlying an active myofascial trigger point (*dark red*). The sudden cold and touch stimuli of the spray inhibit the pain and reflex spasm that would otherwise prevent passive stretching of the muscle. The *black bar* in the dorsal horn of the spinal cord represents this inhibition.

rewarm. A new group of receptors are being stimulated sequentially as the spray moves along the parallel lines of skin.[29, 127] This continuing barrage of alarming stimuli from new sites on the skin is the kind of "novel" stimulus responsible for the orientation reflex of the central nervous system that initiates a preemptive "all stations alert."[116] This alert response can strongly inhibit other reflex responses.[116]

An experiment with ischemic contraction demonstrated the ability of vapocoolant spray to modulate myogenic pain.[139] The patient's endurance to deep pain caused by muscular contractions of the forearm muscles during ischemia, produced by a blood pressure cuff on the arm, was measured with and without the application of vapocoolant over those muscles. Pre-spraying the forearm before the test always increased endurance as much as two-fold. Spraying the arm on reaching the limit of pain tolerance relieved pain so that additional ischemic contractions could be performed. The pain relief could not have been due to reflex changes in the circulation of blood in the muscle.[139]

The close reflex relationship between skin sensation and function of the underlying muscle was demonstrated by studies of human withdrawal reflexes to noxious skin stimuli on both the trunk and lower extremity. Electromyographic recordings of a gentle, sustained voluntary contraction of multiple muscles throughout the region measured increases and decreases in the EMG activity induced by shock stimuli to the skin. Activity of muscles beneath the site of skin stimulation was facilitated, and that of other muscles was generally inhibited.[59, 72] Early and late responses were identified. Early responses were likely to cause movement that terminated weight bearing of that limb, and to remain constant, regardless of changes in the location of the stimulus. Late responses were modifiable, and after several trials were adapted to move the limb away from the stimulus[59]; they learned. Skin reflexes of the back and abdomen induced movement away from the stimulus.[72]

Descending Inhibition. The "gate control" theory of pain describes the modulation of sensory nerve impulses by inhibitory mechanisms at and above the spinal level.[84] One of the oldest methods of re-

lieving pain, commonly used in folk-medicine, is "counter-pain" (hyperstimulation analgesia).[86] In a recent controlled study, the application of painfully cold ice massage produced significantly more pain relief than placebo stimulation. Its effectiveness compared well with that of transcutaneous electrical stimulation and acupuncture.[88] The authors concluded that activation of descending analgesia-producing systems would account for the relief of pain.

Trigger Point Inhibition. Application of the vapocoolant spray acts as if the sensory input from the skin turns off the central nervous system feedback mechanism that is sustaining the TP activity. Possible feedback mechanisms are discussed in Chapter 2.

Responses to Stretch and Spray

Ordinarily, a patient is seen for follow-up several days after treatment, or on the next day, if there is unusual urgency.

Good Response. Many patients have been told that their pain is due to a pinched nerve or arthritis, based on radiographic changes in bone. When a good response to myofascial therapy has afforded relief of pain, the operator can say, "I have not changed your bone structure, have I? I eliminated TPs in your muscles. The pain must have been coming from your muscles, not from bones or joints." This encourages patients to pay more attention to their muscles, to avoid reactivating TPs, and to learn how to inactivate them for themselves. As people grow older, on X-ray examination, the majority eventually show the "wear and tear" of osteoarthritis and degenerative disc disease, but many with these changes have no pain. Younger individuals also may have X-ray changes due to degenerative joint disease, without pain.

Poor Response. If, within a few minutes to a few hours following stretch and spray, the patient experiences a severe cramping pain in the general region of treatment, he may have experienced shortening activation of an antagonist muscle.

This reaction of latent TPs in the antagonist to unaccustomed shortening during stretch and spray of the agonist is defined in the Glossary (Chapter 1) under shortening activation, and is described in detail at the end of Section 12 in Chapter 20, and in Section 12 of Chapter 42. It is avoided by systematically treating both the agonist and antagonist groups of muscles, one after the other. The reaction occurs oftener in flexors, like the biceps brachii, finger flexor, and hamstring muscles, than in the extensors. Lengthening treatment of the sternocleidomastoid or quadratus lumborum muscle on one side is likely to activate latent TPs in its contralateral mate. Treatment of the subscapularis may activate TPs in the supraspinatus and infraspinatus muscles. Occasionally, stretch of the abdominal musculature initiates paraspinal cramping.

When the patient returns for the next appointment and complains of "no relief," one must first establish precisely the pattern of the current pain. If the pain for which the patient was treated previously has lessened and this is a new pattern, the pain is usually now coming from less active TPs in other muscles of the myotatic unit. If it is an entirely new pain, it may have originated in a new TP, activated for the first time.

Reasons for Failure

When the patient fails to show lasting improvement after stretch and spray, the following should be considered.

Perpetuating Factors. When active myofascial TPs do not subside after correctly applied stretch and spray, one or more perpetuating factors are usually responsible.

Inadequate Spraying of All Trigger Point Areas. If the spray is applied only to the reference zone where the patient complains of pain, it usually misses the skin overlying the muscle that is causing the pain. When TPs in several widely separated muscles refer pain to the same area, stretching and spraying some, but not all, of these muscles will not secure full relief.

Patient Tense. For effective passive stretch, the patient must voluntarily relax the muscles.

Incorrect Spray Technique. The vapocoolant is less effective if the stream of spray is passed too quickly over the skin, or if the spray bottle is held too close to the skin. The same skin area should not be sprayed so often, or so slowly, that the underlying muscle becomes chilled. The line of spray must be directed over the line of muscle fibers that are under maximum tension so that the skin reflex effects of vapocooling can release them.

Inadequate Stretch Technique. The TPs will persist if insufficient or jerky force is used to passively stretch the muscle. Firm stretch just before spraying can cause painful spasm and seriously impair relaxation.

Incomplete Stretch. Residual tautness remains when the muscle is stretched to less than its **FULL** range of motion. Adjacent muscles often need releasing before this full range can be reached. If stretch is limited by structural impediments, such as an old fracture, osteoarthritis or idiopathic scoliosis,[128] other myofascial therapy will probably be required.

Treatment Afterward. Muscle soreness is greater if the skin is not rewarmed immediately with a hot pack or pad. Recurrence is more likely if the patient then fails to actively move the treated part through its fully shortened and lengthened range of motion to reestablish normal function.

Incomplete Stretch and Spray. Additional cycles of stretch and spray, with rewarming after each, are repeated as long as the range of motion increases significantly with each cycle, or until full range is reached.

Chronicity. Pain recurs when reactivating or perpetuating factors are present, leading to chronicity. However, chronicity *alone* need *not* prevent an immediate response to specific myofascial therapy.

Mennell[89] and Travell[128] also listed reasons for failure.

13. INJECTION AND STRETCH

Comments and Background

Stretch and spray permits one to deal with many more muscles in a shorter period of time than does TP injection. Injection, or a manual pressure technique, must be used when the attachments make it impossible to stretch the muscle, *e.g.* the sternalis. Injection is especially valuable when a few TPs remain that are unresponsive to stretch and spray. Patients with hyperuricemia and gout usually respond better to injection than to stretch and spray.

The following regimen is used for inactivating myofascial TPs by injection:

1. With the patient recumbent, always use a sterile technique to inject the TPs with 0.5% procaine in isotonic saline, until the area becomes non-tender.
2. Immediately after injection, passively stretch the muscle as parallel sweeps of the vapocoolant are directed over it.
3. Apply hot packs for a few minutes to reduce postinjection soreness.
4. Have the patient actively move the muscle through its complete range of motion.
5. If any local TP tenderness or restriction of movement remains, stretch and spray the entire myotatic unit, agonists and antagonists.

Stretch was included in the heading for this section on "Injection and Stretch" to remind the operator that follow-up stretch is important when injecting TPs.[154]

Always have the patient lying down for *any* injection, to avoid psychogenic syncope. When the patient sits in a chair, injections can be hazardous in susceptible individuals.[118, 123]

The presence of epinephrine in the solution significantly increases the hazard of accidental intravenous injection and myotoxicity. Epinephrine should **not** be used when injecting TPs.

Injection is effective using a dry needling technique,[74, 132] isotonic saline,[45] and procaine or other local anesthetic, with or without addition of a steroid.[154] Some commercial isotonic saline contains for bacteriostasis 0.9% benzyl alcohol, which acts as a local anesthetic; it is not classified as a local anesthetic, apparently because of neurotoxicity.[141] Local anesthetics reduce the painfulness of TP injection, as compared with isotonic saline and dry needling.[19] Dentists generally prefer the amide local anesthetics, 2% lidocaine (Xylocaine) or mepivacaine (Carbocaine), in 1.8-ml dental syringes, to 1% or 2% procaine. We recommend 0.5% procaine diluted from 2% with isotonic saline and without epinephrine. If using an amide local anesthetic, lidocaine is much preferred.

Why Procaine?

Procaine, the first of the synthetic local anesthetics, was developed in 1905 by Einhorn to replace cocaine. It has the greatest usage among the short-acting local anesthetics.[53] Longer action may be a disadvantage when injecting TPs; if a nerve is inadvertently injected, the partial sensory block produced by 0.5% procaine wears off in 15–20 minutes, by the time the patient is ready to leave the office. Pain sensation following nerve block reappeared in 19 min after 1% procaine, and in 40 min after 1% lidocaine.[37] Procaine and chloroprocaine have the lowest systemic toxicity of the commonly used local anesthetics.[31]

Procaine has minimal systemic toxicity, absence of local irritation, easy sterilization and reasonable duration of action, at low cost.[140] Procaine is the least myotoxic of the local anesthetics in common use (see the following section). Procaine is the ester of p-aminobenzoic acid and ethanol with a tertiary diethylamino group attached at the other end of the alcohol. It is hydrolyzed rapidly in the blood serum by procaine esterase to p-aminobenzoic acid and diethylaminoethanol.[53] The diethylaminoethanol is an antiarrhythmic agent, but more weakly so than procaine, and is an effective anti-convulsant, although convulsions are one of the toxic effects of the whole procaine molecule.[53] The other product of hydrolysis, p-aminobenzoic acid, is sometimes considered a member of the vitamin B complex because it is needed for the synthesis of folic acid by those bacteria that can produce the vitamin.[53] The potassium salt of p-aminobenzoic acid is sold under the name Potaba as an antifibrotic agent.[104a] It counteracts the effects of sulfonamides on microorganisms[54] and was useful for the treatment of rickettsial disease (Rocky Mountain spotted fever), until more effective antibiotics were discovered.[53] This hydrolysis product of procaine has potent effects of its own and may directly influence myofascial TPs.

Most local anesthetics, including procaine, block nerve conduction by competitively replacing calcium at its membrane binding site.[36] Depolarization of the nerve membrane is essential for the propagation of an action potential and depends on the flow of sodium ions through sodium channels from the inside to the outside of the membrane. Normally, the displacement of calcium from its binding site facilitates the flow of sodium ions across the membrane through the channels. Blockage of this calcium binding site impedes the flow of sodium ions, which prevents depolarization and the propagation of an action potential.[31, 53]

Local anesthetics affect small, usually unmyelinated, fibers before large myelinated nerve fibers and thus block pain perception before voluntary motor control.[53]

Lidocaine, which was synthesized by Löfgren in 1946, is not merely a longer-acting form of procaine. These two agents have different intermediate chains and different aromatic residues.[53] Unlike other amide local anesthetics, lidocaine is an aminoacyl amide. Lidocaine is more effective in a neutral solution; procaine is more potent in an alkaline solution.[36, 111] Procaine was originally recommended for the treatment of malignant hyperthermia[98] before dantrolene sodium (Dantrium) was available[3]; in this condition, lidocaine is contraindicated.[23] Procaine is hydrolyzed in the blood stream; lidocaine is removed from tissues through solubility in fat and is metabolized primarily in the liver.[31] Unlike most local anesthetics, procaine is *not* rapidly absorbed from mucous membranes.[31]

The use of local anesthetics in dentistry and minor surgery generally requires *complete* pain relief for the *full duration* of the painful procedure. Since lidocaine has twice the potency[31] and twice the duration of action of procaine, and is less likely to cause cutaneous allergic reactions,[36] it has largely replaced procaine in minor surgical and dental use. However, for TP injections, only temporary pain relief is required and a strong local vasodilatation effect is desirable.

Both dentists and dermatologists have encountered a relatively high number of syncopal reactions when injecting procaine subcutaneously to obtain skin and mucous membrane anesthesia. Generally, a 27- or 30-gauge needle was used. Even when injecting only intramuscularly for TPs, leakage around the thin needle allowed reflux of anesthetic to the subcutaneous tissues. Some think that episodes of syncope in response to procaine injection can represent an allergic response of the anaphylactic type I. It causes mast cell degranulation, release of histamine and vasomotor syncope secondary to hypotension resulting from capillary dilatation[53] by histamine. We do not see syncope in our myofascial pain patients, who always lie down for injection, nor is it reported in the extensive literature[107a, 112a] that describes the use of procaine for injecting muscles. This suggests that injecting the procaine intramuscularly only, and not subcutaneously, circumvents these allergic syncopal reactions.

Eleven local anesthetics have been approved by the American Dental Association for dental use. Lidocaine, mepivacaine and prilocaine have replaced procaine in dentistry, primarily because of its allergenic properties when injected into mucous membranes or skin. For TP injection, the other eight are either more toxic, or offer no advantage over lidocaine.[91] We recommend 0.5% procaine for the *intramuscular* injection of TPs with a 21- to 23-guage needle, large enough in diameter to minimize reflux to the skin, but do not recommend it for subcutaneous injection.

Dry Needling. In the experience of the senior author, precise dry needling of TPs, without injecting any solution, approaches, but does not quite equal, the therapeutic effectiveness of injecting procaine into TPs. Procaine made one big difference when she tested a series of patients. Without procaine, the treatment was unendurably painful to some patients.[134] In most, the pain lasted for minutes after dry needling, but only seconds after procaine injection. Kraus[71] stated that dry needling is effective, but postinjection pain follows immediately. This difference is more marked with myofascial TPs (in muscles) than with connective tissue TPs in ligaments.

Lewit[74] reported that *accurately localized* dry needling is effective, without quantitatively comparing it to procaine injection. He preferred dry needling to the use of a local anesthetic, because dry needling permitted location of all of the TPs in a region by preserving their telltale pain reaction. The stronger local anesthetics obscure this pain reaction. Dry needling obviously induces no drug reactions. However, dry needling requires the most precise localization of the TPs, and 0.5% procaine, in our experience, does not obscure the local pain reaction of a TP.

Isotonic Saline. Sola and Kuitert[117] treated a series of 100 patients with myofascial TPs by injecting isotonic saline (which also contained a bacteriostatic agent) with multiple needle penetrations in a fanwise pattern. These patients experienced therapeutic results equal to those previously reported with the injection of a local anesthetic. Frost et al.[45] did a controlled, blind comparison between isotonic saline and a long-acting anesthetic, mepivacaine. They injected tender areas of the muscle that showed localized changes in the consistency of the muscle, and from which the patient's pain could be evoked (TPs). Using these TP criteria for the precise localization of the injection, they found that the saline afforded equal, or more pain relief than injection of the same volume of 0.5% mepivacaine.

On the other hand, Hameroff et al.[61] found that injection of the long-acting local anesthetics, bupivacaine and etidocaine, afforded relief for 1-7 days afterward, but that injection of a similar volume of isotonic saline (without bacteriostatic agent), if it had any effect, aggravated the patient's pain. However, although these authors said that they were injecting TPs, they used acupuncture criteria to locate the sites of injection, rather than the TP criteria of this manual. The plain saline solution injected near, but not into, the TPs would, in our experience, be expected to irritate, rather than inactivate them.

Concentration of Procaine Injected. An experiment to test the effectiveness of procaine in concentrations ranging from 0.1% to 2.0% in physiological saline showed no increased anesthesia with concentrations greater than 0.5%.[132] Since the maximum amount of procaine that should be injected at one time is 1 g,[140] this would permit the injection of 200 ml. We find that 40 ml of 0.5% procaine injected intramuscularly during 1/2 hr or longer produces few, if any, central nervous system symptoms. With 0.5% procaine, accidental injection of 2 ml (0.01 gm) into an artery or vein creates no problem, if adequate hemostasis is applied to the vessel. Injection near a nerve with the same strength solution causes only mild sensory loss for a maximum of about 20 min, which is well tolerated if the patient was previously warned that this might happen. These statements are **not** true if the injected solution contains epinephrine, which we do not use and never recommend for the injection of TPs.

Although the 0.5% procaine solution does shorten the duration of pain when the needle contacts a TP, it does not block the referral of pain from the TP at the moment of needle contact. This is important for locating all TPs of a group in one region by probing with a needle. A stronger concentration of procaine or other local anesthetic that obscures this sensitivity of remaining uninjected TPs makes it impossible to insure that all TPs have been inactivated.[125] All of the TPs in a given region should be eliminated before moving on to another area.

Non-analgesic Effects of Procaine. 1. Procaine, like other local anesthetics, causes local arteriolar dilatation.[53] However, thermography showed that subcutaneous injection of procaine solution produced vasodilatation that lasted as long as 24 hr.[47] This indicates a remarkably prolonged action of procaine that would be helpful in reestablishing normal circulation at the site of a TP, if a similar effect occurs in the muscle. Both procaine and lidocaine produce a marked increase in microcirculatory blood flow, but procaine causes greater hypotension,[2] which, if it is due to increased perfusion, may make procaine more effective in relieving any local vasoconstriction at myofascial TPs.

2. Procaine produced a curare-like action on the motor endplate in concentrations of 1:10,000. Harvey[63] injected procaine intraarterially into muscles and produced a partial curarization of the muscle, which could then respond to electrical stimulation with a twitch contraction, but was unable to sustain tetanic contraction. Patients will sometimes say after intramuscular injection with procaine, "Oh, I don't think I can move my arm." When they try, they can move it, but are unable to maintain a strong contraction.

3. Procaine has important effects on the mobility of calcium ions. The intravenous injection of procaine has been recommended for control of the malignant hyperthermia that develops in a few patients who respond abnormally to agents used during anesthesia, usually halothane or succinylcholine.[49, 62, 98] Malignant hyperthermia is thought to be due to an inherited defect of the calcium receptors on certain membranes of the muscle cell, mainly the sarcoplasmic reticulum and the sarco-

lemma. A rapid, uncontrolled release of calcium ions, and/or a failure to recover calcium ions from the myoplasm, causes rigidity due to generalized spontaneous muscular contraction. The resultant uncontrolled metabolism may cause lethal hyperthermia and acidosis.[96]

Procaine effectively blocked halothane initiation of the syndrome in susceptible pigs,[62] and was used successfully to combat a malignant hyperthermia reaction that developed during oral surgery.[98] Meanwhile, dantrolene sodium (Dantrium) has replaced procaine as the drug recommended for treatment of this condition.[23]

In another example of procaine's effect on calcium binding, caffeine has long been known to cause a persistent contracture, or caffeine rigor, of muscle fibers. This rigor is due to enhancement by caffeine of the release of calcium from the sarcoplasmic reticulum and to interference with the rebinding of calcium ions by the sarcoplasmic reticulum.[62, 145] Procaine reverses the effect of caffeine,[62, 146] but lidocaine potentiates it.[120] Since the postulated TP mechanism is similar to this caffeine effect, this action of procaine is another reason for preferring it over lidocaine for injection of TPs.

A third example demonstrates the displacement by procaine of calcium abnormally bound to a cell membrane.[6] The blood of a patient with sickle-cell anemia in remission was "unsickled" by procaine, in vitro. The blood was withdrawn and the erythrocytes exposed to a low concentration of oxygen until they became "irreversibly" sickled. These sickled cells, when placed in a dilute solution of procaine hydrochloride, almost immediately resumed their round shape, which was associated with movement of the calcium from the inside to the outside of the erythrocytes. A similar restoration of shape was produced by the addition of p-aminobenzoic acid to the solution containing the "irreversibly" sickled cells.

4. In dilute solutions that do not totally block nerve conduction, procaine[33] and lidocaine[32] extend the refractory period of peripheral nerve, which markedly reduces its response to high frequency stimulation. This could significantly modify the feedback loop of the postulated TP mechanism.

Myotoxicity of Local Anesthetics. Intra-muscular injection of a 1% or 2% solution of procaine or of lidocaine in rats produced a mild infiltration of neutrophiles, lymphocytes, and macrophages within 24–72 hr.[105] There were no, or at most only occasional, damaged muscle fibers; such fibers were eventually phagocytized. No changes could be detected beyond 7 days, except for a few remaining leucocytes. Perineural injection of the same solutions produced no histological changes within the nerves that had been anesthetized, but a temporary inflammatory reaction developed in 24–72 hr, with nearly complete recovery in 2 weeks. Repeated intramuscular injections of isotonic sodium chloride also caused an inflammatory response.[105] Single intramuscular injections of 2% procaine or isotonic saline caused no muscle necrosis.[25]

The intramuscular injection of longer-acting local anesthetics, like 0.5% dibucaine and 1% tetracaine, produced in the ensuing 24–48 hr moderate infiltration of the muscle with lymphocytes and macrophages as the predominant cells and occasional coagulation (severe) necrosis of the central muscle mass. However, adjacent muscle showed an intensification of eosinophilic infiltration with vacuolization, loss of cross striations, and some phagocytosis of muscle fibers (minimal necrosis). Regeneration of the muscle was complete in about 7 days.

Subcutaneous supramuscular injection (next to, but not into the muscle) of 2% lidocaine, 2% prilocaine or 2% mepivacaine produced moderate inflammation and some muscle damage without nerve damage. Supramuscular injection of 2% procaine produced no histological changes in the adjacent muscle.[115]

Intramuscular injection of 2% lidocaine,[14, 17, 25] cocaine,[17] bupivacaine,[14, 17] and mepivacaine[17] caused muscle necrosis, chiefly of the white muscle fibers.[17] Intramuscular injection of 0.5% bupivacaine destroyed chiefly red muscle fibers.[17]

By 4 days after intramuscular injection of 1.5% and 2% lidocaine in rabbits and mice, any atrophy of the muscle was difficult to measure because of the pronounced inflammatory and degenerative changes in many fibers, with abundant endomysial cellular proliferation. By 16 days after injection, the reaction had subsided leaving centrally located muscle fiber nuclei and small round fibers with significant atrophy, but no fibrosis.[24] Damage to associated tissues and vascular supply was minimal or absent, so that muscle regeneration followed rapidly.[14]

Procaine in 2% solution[17, 24] and 0.5% solutions of lidocaine,[14, 17] cocaine,[17] bupivacaine,[17] mepivacaine,[14, 17] or prilocaine[14] caused *no* such muscle fiber destruction, in contrast to the stronger (2%) concentrations.

Forty-eight hours after intramuscular injection of 3% mepivacaine, the muscle showed extensive necrosis that was specifically related to the increased intracellular concentration of free calcium that it produced. The muscle tissue beneath a subcutaneous injection of the same anesthetic solution exhibited similar, but less extensive damage.[18] Injected supramuscularly, 0.5 ml of 4% prilocaine caused severe muscle necrosis.[15]

The addition of epinephrine increases the destructiveness of the local anesthetic agent to muscle; epinephrine alone also can be destructive. Supramuscular injection of 0.5 ml of epinephrine 1:200,000 in 0.6% saline produced no changes, but more concentrated epinephrine, 1:100,000 in the saline, caused necrosis of surface muscle fibers; and 1:50,000 caused more severe necrosis extending well into the muscle. Addition of epinephrine in strengths of 1:100,000 or greater potentiated the muscle damage caused by local anesthetics.[15] The muscle necrosis caused by supramuscular 2% lidocaine with 1:50,000 epinephrine regenerated completely in 16 days;[15] however, five successive daily injections left evidence of retarded regeneration and microscarring in some areas.[16]

Twenty-four hours after the intramuscular injection of 0.5 ml of 2% lidocaine with 1:100,000 epinephrine into rat gestrocnemius, the muscle was almost totally necrotic. Eighteen hours after the same injection into human sternocleidomastoid muscle, the region of necrosis, which extended along fascial planes, was much more extensive, but the damage was less intense then in the smaller rat muscle. Muscle-enzyme levels in the blood serum increased in both groups and were characteristic of muscle destruction.[153]

Procaine is clearly the least myotoxic of the local anesthetics that are commonly injected intramuscularly. Procainamide, however, after long-term oral administration for cardiac arrhythmias may induce a syndrome that resembles systemic lupus erythematosus with positive antinuclear antibodies.

The muscle necrosis resulting from the injection of a long-acting local anesthetic may be one mechanism for the inactivation of TPs. However, the clinical approach of depending on the extensive muscle necrosis by such a long-acting agent to reduce the precision required in locating a TP is considered undesirable, particularly since it may lead to permanent destruction of muscle fibers and their replacement with fibrous tissue, if the injection is repeated frequently.

Mechanisms of Injection Effect

Several mechanisms may contribute to the inactivation of TPs by injection. (1) The needle may **mechanically disrupt** abnormally functioning contractile elements, or nerve endings which are sensory and motor components of the feedback loop believed responsible for sustaining the TP activity. Cessation of the neuromuscular dysfunction relieves the tautness of the palpable band of muscle fibers and the hyperirritability of the sensory nerves that is responsible for both the referred phenomena and local tenderness. (2) Local **release of the intracellular potassium** due to damage to muscle fibers by the needle also could cause a depolarization block of nerve fibers in areas where extracellular potassium reached sufficient concentration.[132] (3) Fluid that is injected helps to dilute and "**wash out**" any nerve-sensitizing substances. This reduces the irritability of the TP to the extent that it was dependent on such substances. This would tend also to inactivate any neural feedback mechanisms, such as local vasoconstriction, that were maintaining TP activity.[13, 52] (4) Procaine has a **local vasodilatation** effect that would increase circulation at the TP, thereby increasing the local energy supply and the removal of metabolites. (5) A local anesthetic may specifically **interrupt feedback mechanisms** between the TP and the central nervous system. A concentration of procaine and of lidocaine less than that required for total sensory nerve block limits high frequency discharges transmitted by the nerve, which may selectively affect these mechanisms.[32] (6) Depending on which local anesthetic was injected, focal **necrosis** might destroy the TP.[15, 24]

Good[52] proposed in 1950 that injection of procaine interrupted vasoconstriction reflexes and restored local autonomic balance, a mechanism which he thought increased the circulation and eliminated hyperirritability at myalgic spots (TPs).

Adverse Reactions

Adverse reactions to procaine injected intramuscularly may be toxic or allergic. Procaine toxicity is due to an excessively high blood level and must be distinguished from an allergic, or anaphylactic reaction, which is disproportionate to dose. Syncope may be a form of allergic reaction.

Procaine toxicity. This reaction is not likely to appear until a total dose of 1 g is approached, administered within 15 or 20 min. That is 200 ml of a 0.5% solution.[140] Procaine toxicity causes central nervous system excitation, as evidenced by talkativeness, nervousness, and tremulousness, which can progress rapidly to convulsions, unconsciousness and respiratory arrest. Toxicity may present first as drowsiness. The toxicity of procaine is increased by vitamin C deficiency and starvation.[108]

In case of reaction, a tourniquet should be applied to delay absorption if the injection was made into an extremity. Convulsions can be treated with intravenous diazepam or a short-acting barbiturate, such as thiopental; however, the latter is controversial because the barbiturate is also a respiratory depressant.

Respiration is supported using a self-inflating bag with mask or using mouth-to-mouth resuscitation, if necessary. When respiratory distress is present, monitoring the electrocardiogram and keeping a cardiac defibrillator at hand are recommended in case cardiac resuscitation is needed.

One reason that procaine has a lower toxicity than the other local anesthetics may be the anticonvulsant action of the diaminoethanol that is an end product of its hydrolysis by procainesterase.

Allergic Reactions. The symptoms of systemic anaphylaxis may be indistinguishable from those of cardiovascular collapse due to drug toxicity. Anaphylaxis is suspected chiefly by an overwhelming reaction to a minimal dose of procaine. It is treated by epinephrine injection and aggressive support of respiration and circulation. Adrenal corticosteroids can prevent, but do not help to control anaphylactic shock.[36, 53] This allergic reaction may be caused either by the procaine or by a preservative added to its solution.

An allergic response to submucous or subcutaneous procaine apparently occurs oftener than to lidocaine.[40] A systematic study of patients with, and without, a presumptive history of local-anesthetic allergy found positive skin reactions in 42% (25/60) of the patients in the "non-allergic" group. In all cases, the cutaneous reaction followed injection of an ester-type local anesthetic agent, e.g. procaine or chloroprocaine. No allergic skin reactions were observed to amide-type agents, such as lidocaine. Also, 73% of the 11 patients with a history of alleged dental-anesthetic allergy had a positive skin reaction to the ester-type agents, and none to the amide-type agents. None of the subjects showed signs of systemic anaphylaxis after the testing procedure. The cutaneous reactions observed with the ester-type agents were consistent with the frequent observations of dermal reactions described by members of the dental profession when the ester-type agents were the only local-anesthetic drugs available. Since the introduction of the amide-type compounds, such reports have become rare. Patients who are allergic to procaine are likely to be allergic also to the methylparaben preservative commonly used in multiple-dose vials of commercial lidocaine, but not to the lidocaine itself.[40]

These observations may well relate to the higher incidence of syncopal reactions to procaine encountered by dentists and dermatologists when injecting it subcutaneously to anesthetize the skin and the subcutaneous or submucosal tissues. Procaine stimulation of IgE antibody may produce subsequent antigen-induced release of histamine from subcutaneous mast cells, an anaphylactic reaction (type I response).[48] The strong capillary dilatation produced by histamine could account for syncope observed in response to procaine injection, even in the semi-recumbent position.[53] Injection of the procaine intramuscularly apparently circumvents this type of reaction.

Sensitization with antibody of the IgG class, causing a cytotoxic (type II) response,[48] could be responsible for the local inflammatory reaction that creates excessive muscle soreness lasting for a day to a week after injection in some patients. This adverse reaction should be greatly attentuated if a corticosteroid were mixed with the allergenic local anesthetic.

Preinjection Precautions

Recumbent Position. The patient is *always* placed in the recumbent position, not seated or standing, to avoid psychological syncope and the complications of falling, should the patient faint. Recumbency also greatly facilitates locating the TP, since the patient is more comfortable and relaxed. It is then easier to adjust muscle tension so that the bands containing TPs stand out in a background of relaxed muscle fibers.

Syncope is more likely to occur in apprehensive patients; a self-inflating bag with mask to carry out artificial ventilation should be available, in case it is needed. The circulatory arrest observed in one recumbent patient receiving a venipuncture to draw blood was attributed to cardiac arrest by one author,[123] but was interpreted as extreme sinus bradycardia by a cardiologist who reported a similar reaction while an electrocardiographic recording was being made.[118]

Vitamin C and Aspirin. The increased capillary fragility characteristic of a low serum vitamin C level can cause excessive bleeding in muscles injected for TPs. Capillary hemorrhage augments postinjection soreness and leads to unsightly ecchymoses. A frequent source of increased bleeding due to low vitamin C is smoking. Mega-dose vitamin C therapy daily for a week may correct this deficiency. We recommend at least 500 mg of timed-release vitamin C three times daily.

A daily dose of aspirin increases the susceptibility to bleeding.

Solution for Injection. A bacteriostatic agent commonly added to procaine is sodium bisulfite, which is irritating to TPs in muscles and may cause postinjection soreness and pain. Since the 0.5% strength of procaine is not commercially available, it is helpful to buy 2% procaine solution and dilute it with isotonic saline by mixing three parts of saline with one part of procaine. Most bacteriostatic saline for injection contains at least 0.9% benzyl alcohol as the bacteriostatic agent, which is not so irritating to the muscles as sodium bisulfite and has local anesthetic properties of its own.[53, 154]

Selection of Needle. The needle size is important for precise injection of myofascial TPs.

A 22-gauge, 3.8-cm (1½-in) needle is usually used for superficial muscles. In hyperalgesic patients a 25-gauge, 3.8-cm (1½-in) needle may cause less discomfort, but will not provide the clear "feel" of the structures being penetrated by the needle and is marginal as an instrument for mechanically disrupting the TP. When capillary fragility with bleeding is a major concern, or subsequent ecchymosis is especially undesirable, the thinner 25-gauge needle may be preferred. A 27-gauge, 3.8-cm (1½-in) needle is unsatisfactory because it is too flexible; the tip slides around the TP in a taut band, and fewer tactile cues are transmitted by the needle to identify what tissue it is penetrating.

In thick subcutaneous muscles, such as the gluteus maximus or superficial paraspinal muscles, in non-obese persons, a minimum of a 21-gauge, 5-cm (2-in) needle is necessary. When injecting a TP, the needle should be long enough to reach the TP *without indenting the skin with the hub of the needle.* The needle should never be inserted to its full length, because of the embarrassing situation should it break off at the hub and disappear under the skin. A longer needle should be used, or the skin compressed around it, to ensure a stub of needle projecting above the skin surface.

A 21-gauge, 7.6-cm (3-in) needle is generally long enough to reach TPs in the deepest muscles, such as the gluteus minimus and quadratus lumborum, but TPs in these may occasionally require a 8.9-cm (3½-in) needle. This length is available as a 22-gauge disposable spinal needle. The spinal needle is not as effective for TP injection as the hypodermic type because of the spinal needle's flexibility and diamond-shaped tip, which tends to push the

TP aside, rather than to penetrate it. With long slender needles, it is especially important to insert the needle straight and avoid any side pressure that might bend the needle, deflecting the tip an unknown distance to one side.

A needle with a burr at the tip must not be used. When the tip of a disposable needle contacts bone, the impact frequently curls the tip to produce a "fishhook" burr that feels "scratchy" and drags as the needle is drawn through tissues; it causes unnecessary bleeding, and should be replaced immediately. It is especially important to avoid using such a barbed needle when injecting TPs in muscles like the scaleni, which lie near nerve trunks.

Injection Procedure

An aseptic technique is insured by careful cleansing of the skin with a suitable antiseptic, avoiding areas of cutaneous infection, and by use of uncontaminated solutions and of properly sterilized or disposable needles and syringes.

Before injection, the patient is warned that successful needle contact with a TP may produce a flash of distant pain and may cause the muscle to twitch. The patient is asked to note exactly where that pain is felt, permitting an accurate description afterward of the precise pattern of pain referred by that TP. In this way, the operator confirms the referred pain pattern of that TP, and the patient realizes the connection between his or her pain and the TP. This reassures both the operator and the patient as to the importance of inactivating it. Patients learn to welcome this painful harbinger of a successful injection and future relief.

Localizing the TP. Localization of a TP is done mainly by the sense of feel, assisted by patient expressions of pain and by visual observation of LTRs. The TP is identified by palpation as the most tender spot in a palpable band. It is also the most responsive spot for eliciting LTRs. The muscle is placed on sufficient stretch to tauten the muscle fibers containing the TP, but not to cause additional pain. Tautness is necessary to help hold the TP in position so that it does not slide to one side, like a tough vein, as the needle tip encounters it.

When flat palpation is being used, the TP and its taut band can be localized by feeling the band roll back and forth between two fingers (Fig. 3.11A and B). The TP is then fixed for injection by pinning it down between the fingers (Fig. 3.11C). This establishes a plane that passes through the TP midway between the fingers, perpendicular to the skin. The needle can then be inserted precisely in that plane to whatever depth is necessary to impale the TP.

When pincer palpation is used to locate the TP and its band, traction is automatically applied to the muscle fibers as they are rolled between the digits (Fig. 3.6). When located, the TP is held tightly between the thumb and fingertips for injection. This technique is used for muscles like the pectoralis major, latissimus dorsi, long head of the triceps brachii, and sternocleidomastoid. An additional description is found in Section 13 of Chapter 23.

Painless Skin Penetration. Some patients are terribly afraid of the skin pain caused by needle penetration. This fear of the needle is usually acquired in childhood and creates obstacles to a good doctor-patient relationship.[130, 134] Most patients find the skin pain more threatening than the deep, more severe pain of needle contact with the TP. The skin pain is avoidable. A time-honored approach is to substitute a strong, distracting stimulus by stretching, pinching, or slapping the skin just as the needle is inserted; this requires a high degree of coordination and skill to be effective.

In adults, vapocoolant spray provides the simple answer of refrigeration anesthesia,[70, 130, 149] which effectively blocks nerve conduction when the skin temperature falls to 10 C (50 F). After carefully disinfecting the skin with alcohol, one applies the Fluori-Methane spray from a distance of about 45 cm (18 in) for 5 or 6 sec (just short of frosting), and then introduces the needle quickly at the instant when the spray evaporates and leaves the skin dry.[130, 149]

For young children, who dislike the sudden cold impact of the vapocoolant jet stream, a sterile, fluffy, small cotton ball is saturated with vapocoolant until it is dripping wet. *Lightly,* the wetted cotton is held

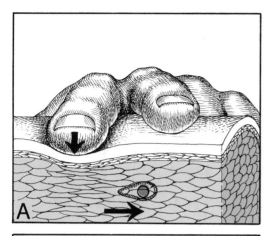

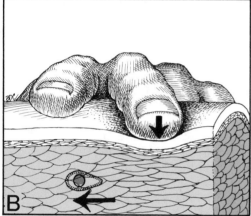

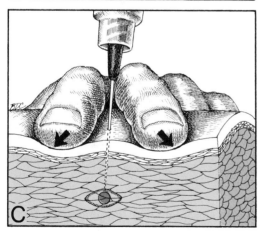

Figure 3.11. Cross-sectional schematic drawing of flat palpation to localize the taut band (*black oval*) and fix the trigger point (*dark red spot*) for injection. *A* and *B*, use of alternating pressure between two fingers to confirm the location of a taut band. *C*, positioning of the band half way between the fingers for injection of the trigger point that lies within the band.

against the skin for about 10 sec, and then removed. *At the instant* that the skin dries, the needle is inserted painlessly.[149]

Three less reliable, but more convenient, techniques that can be combined are: (1) to insert the needle *very quickly* through the skin with a flick of the wrist, (2) to direct it at an acute angle with the skin (not perpendicularly), and (3) to place the skin under marked tension so that the additional tension of the needle penetration is hardly noticeable. The latter may be done by the operator either strongly spreading his or her fingers apart against the skin and inserting a needle between them, or by pinching a fold of the skin between the thumb and fingers and inserting the needle through the tightly folded skin.

The particular technique used is less important than the communication to the patient that the practitioner *cares* and *knows how* to insert the needle painlessly.

Hemostasis. Injecting TPs is a full-time job for both hands. The injecting hand is busy placing the needle and directing the plunger of the syringe for injection. The palpating hand constantly maintains hemostasis and often must fix the TP to help the needle penetrate it. Local bleeding is irritating to the muscle, causes postinjection soreness, may reactivate the TP, and can produce an unsightly ecchymosis. Hemostasis is important.[154] Ecchymosis is usually preventable; when it occurs, only time (assisted by ultrasound) eradicates it.

The fingers of the palpating hand are spread apart, maintaining tension on the skin to reduce the likelihood of subcutaneous bleeding where the needle has penetrated it. Also, during the injection, the fingers exert pressure around the needle tip to provide hemostasis in deeper tissues. When the angle of the needle is changed, the direction of pressure changes. The pressure should be applied *throughout* the injection procedure. As the needle is withdrawn, one finger slides over the track of the needle and instantly applies pressure where it was. If visible bleeding develops, a cold pack is applied and the patient warned of a possible "bruised" spot.

Needling the Trigger Point. Blindly probing an area of diffuse tenderness with no palpable band is generally futile, since the needle then is usually in a pain reference zone, not where the TP is located. Injection in the reference zone is less effective, and any results last for a shorter period, than when the TP is injected.

The precision required to hit the TP with a needle is a difficult skill that requires practice. How good are you at venipuncture? At times the TP in its taut band feels like a tough vein that rolls and slides away from the needle and must be fixed with the palpating fingers. Using flat palpation, as illustrated in Figures 3.11C and 3.12A and B, the needle is inserted between the fingers that have located the TP. The needle penetrates the skin a centimeter or two away from the TP so that the needle can approach it at an acute angle of about 30° to the skin. Adequate tension of the muscle fibers is required to penetrate the TP. The needle should explore both the deep and superficial fibers of the muscle. The syringe is held between fingers of the injecting hand, and thumb pressure is used against the plunger to slowly introduce small amounts of 0.5% procaine solution as the needle advances within the muscle. This assures that the procaine is present to relieve pain at the instant that the needle tip encounters and penetrates the TP.

The palpable band with its TP often feels like hard rubber, which is resistant to penetration and tends to slide to one side.[50] Increased tension of the muscle helps to stabilize the position of the TP to permit precise penetration by the needle, especially for deep TPs which can not be easily fixed in position by palpation.

If an LTR and referred pain were elicited from the TP prior to injection, then both should be observed when the needle penetrates the TP during injection. Otherwise, one has missed the TP; postinjection soreness and incomplete relief result. Following effective needling, most TP characteristics should have disappeared; no LTR, no evoked referred pain, and no spot tenderness should remain.[19, 71] The tense band frequently has relaxed, and is no longer distinguishable by palpation.

When an active TP is contacted by the needle, the patient can usually describe the exact distribution of the referred pain, but only if he or she were alerted beforehand to pay attention to it. Using the needle as a probe, the TP sometimes feels

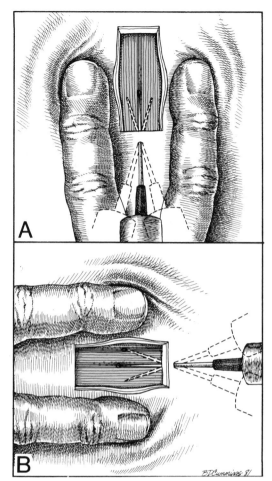

Figure 3.12. Schematic top view of two approaches to the flat injection of a trigger point area (*dark red spot encircled in black*) in a taut band (*closely spaced black lines*). *A*, injection away from fingers, which have pinned down the trigger point so it can not slide away from the needle. *Dotted outline* indicates additional probing to explore for a cluster of trigger points. The fingers are pressing downward and apart to maintain pressure for hemostasis. *B*, injection toward the fingers, with similar finger pressure. Additional trigger points are often found in the immediate vicinity by probing with the needle.

like a dense globule, 2–3 mm in diameter;[50] resistance to penetration helps to identify it,[71] but sometimes no difference in tissue density is detected. Occasionally, TP contact with the needle feels gritty. Whenever a TP is encountered, an additional 0.5–1 ml of procaine solution is injected.

Frequently, multiple TPs are present in one region of muscle. This fact is often recognized when the muscle is palpated for TPs. When one of these TPs has been inactivated, the area is peppered[50] in a fan-like manner,[19] or in a full circle,[71] in an effort to ensure that all remaining TPs in the group are inactivated, as illustrated in Figure 3.12B. After each probing movement, the needle tip must be withdrawn to subcutaneous tissue and redirected before the next movement. When this probing search of the spherical region is completed, the site is palpated for any remaining spots of tenderness. If one is found, it is accurately localized with the fingers and injected. *All* tender spots in that region should be eliminated before leaving it.[148]

To inject TPs in superficial layers of muscle close to the skin, the needle tip can be brought precisely to the TP by first carefully locating the TP with the finger and then, after inserting the needle subcutaneously, pressing it against the finger through the skin to accurately localize it. Finally, the needle tip is directed into the TP by means of this "tactile vision." The same technique is useful when the needle has penetrated a muscle which can be grasped between the fingers (like the pectoralis major, latissimus dorsi, teres major, or triceps brachii) to locate TPs on the side of the muscle opposite the puncture site.

Pneumothorax. The distressing complication of a pneumothorax is avoidable if one NEVER aims the needle at an intercostal space. The patient may sneeze or jump; the operator may startle unexpectedly. As a resident, the senior author found, in her early experience of doing many pleural taps for pleural effusions, that patients consistently reported a salty taste in the mouth whenever the pleura was punctured. The patient might say, "Oh, I can taste the solution." If air is introduced by puncturing the lung, dyspnea, cough, and chest pain characteristic of a pneumothorax follow.

Corticosteroids

We find only two reasons for adding corticosteroid to the procaine solution when injecting TPs. A few patients have symptoms of connective tissue inflammation, as in the "frozen shoulder" (adhesive capsulitis) or bicipital tendonitis, and respond poorly to local treatment, despite correction of all identifiable perpetuating factors. The other patients respond to therapy, but develop excessive postin-jection soreness of the muscles. This may be due partly to an allergic reaction, as discussed above.

We usually give patients belonging to the first group a course of corticosteroid medication by mouth rather than including it in the solution injected to needle TPs. In the past, the senior author has observed that the benefit realized from injected steroid has often appeared in distant muscles as a result of systemic absorption. The response to needling TPs with procaine in this group of patients often improves remarkably during oral steroid therapy. The administration of corticosteroids is discussed below for both groups of patients on page 91.

In *no* case do we recommend long-acting steroids when injecting TPs. Such a preparation of steroid may, by itself, be destructive to muscle fibers,[105] it is generally irritating to nerves, and can produce complications.[55] Use of depot steroids enhances the danger of a systemic cushingoid reaction with repeated injections.

In addition to corticosteroid, one may wish to prescribe 500 mg of sodium p-aminobenzoate (Potaba) daily as an antifibrotic agent for the patients who show evidence of connective tissue inflammation.

Patients have sometimes received steroid injections in joints from other physicians to relieve pain that was referred to the joints from TPs in the muscles. Injecting this reference zone may be helpful, but less so than injecting the guilty TPs.

Postinjection Procedures

Stretch following TP injection is an integral part of that treatment. Zohn and Mennell[154] emphasize that failure to stretch following injection can mean failure of treatment. Kraus[71] devotes the bulk of his therapeutic instructions to stretching and strengthening exercises that are to be done by the patient following injection of myofascial TPs.

As the operator passively stretches the muscle to its full length, it is wise to apply a few sweeps of vapocoolant spray in parallel lines over the muscle and its referred ‚pain pattern, as described above, to relax any remaining tense fibers. This is followed by the application of a hot pack over all TPs that were injected, which markedly reduces postinjection soreness. After a few minutes of this heat application, the patient actively moves the muscle through its full range of motion *several times*, to relieve residual stiffness at full range of motion, to measure the improvement, and to reestablish the patient's awareness of normal function in that muscle.

Lewit[74] noted muscle soreness after dry needling and after a local anesthetic injection, but made no mention of applying heat as part of the treatment. In some patients, postinjection soreness for a few days is merely the unfinished business of a residual tight band of muscle, which may be quickly released by brief passive stretch during a few brushes of vapocoolant spray. The postinjection soreness, *per se*, is not unfavorable if the patient's related pattern of referred pain has been relieved. However, it is wise to let the muscle recover completely from postinjection soreness before injecting its TPs again, which ordinarily requires 3 or 4 days. Soreness is often caused by needling close to, but not into, TPs.

For patients who are troubled by such postinjection soreness, acetaminophen is usually as effective as, and less irritating to the stomach than, aspirin.

If two or three treatments by injection fail to inactivate the TPs in a muscle, repeated injections are rarely the answer. The perpetuating factors that are making the TPs so irritable must be identified and managed.

Reasons for Failure of Injection

1. Injecting a latent TP, not the responsible active TP.
2. Injecting the area of referred pain and referred tenderness, not the TP.[154] This error may provide incomplete, temporary relief, or can aggravate the patient's symptoms.[7]
3. Needling the vicinity of the TP, including needling of the tense band, but missing the TP itself. This tends to irritate, rather than inactivate the TP.[7]
4. Using a needle for injection that was finer than 25 gauge, which allows the tip to slide around the resistant TP.
5. Injecting a solution with an irritating or allergenic bacteriostatic preservative, such as sodium bisulfite; sodium hyposulfite is less irritating.
6. Inadequate hemostasis followed by irritation of the TP due to local bleeding.[154]

7. Overlooking other active TPs in the myotatic unit.
8. Forgetting to have the patient actively move the muscle following injection, so that its full range was not incorporated into daily activities.
9. Omitting regular passive stretch exercises at home, which would have maintained the full length of the muscle.

Ligamentous Sprains

The pain of ankle and wrist sprains can be relieved in most cases by injection with procaine, either with[97] or without epinephrine.[83, 125, 127] Either 0.5%[125] or 1%[83] procaine is effective. Best results are obtained if all of the tender spots in the sprained joint are injected as soon as possible (less than 12 hr) following injury. The joint should be pain free following injection, which should permit normal use of the joint at once, including walking. It should be used in a normal manner to remain free of pain, aided by an elastic support to lighten weight bearing.

13A. ALTERNATIVE TREATMENT TECHNIQUES

This section reviews techniques other than TP injection or stretch and spray that can be used to inactivate myofascial TPs. These other specific myofascial treatments are ischemic compression, massage, stretch without spray, and ultrasound. Moist heat, drug therapy and biofeedback serve as useful adjuncts to more specific treatment. Some physicians report success with transcutaneous electrical stimulation, or galvanic stimulation of the muscle.

Ischemic Compression

The technique that we have described as ischemic compression is essentially what Prudden calls myotherapy.[106] This method, which she developed from the TP concepts of Travell[127] and Kraus,[71] she described in detail for major regions of the body.[106] Ischemic compression applies sustained pressure to the TP with sufficient force and for a long enough time to inactivate it. We termed it ischemic compression because, on release, the skin is at first blanched, and then shows reactive hyperemia. The changes in perfusion of the skin very likely correspond to circulatory changes in the muscle beneath, which was subjected to the same pressure.

Two approaches to ischemic compression are used. As described in the chapters throughout this volume, the first attempts to completely inactivate the TP in one treatment. In the case of recent, moderately active TPs, this is often successful. However, in chronic and very hyperirritable TPs, a second approach, the myotherapy technique,[106] progressively eliminates the TP activity in a succession of small steps that may take days.

To apply ischemic compression, the re-laxed muscle is stretched to the verge of discomfort. Initially, a thumb (or strong finger) is pressed directly on the TP to create tolerably painful, sustained pressure. Treatment is useless if the patient tenses the muscles and so protects the TP from the pressure. As the discomfort tends to abate, pressure is gradually increased by adding a thumb or finger from the other hand, as necessary, for reinforcement (Fig. 3.13). This process is continued up to 1 min with as much as 20 or 30 lb of pressure. If TP tenderness persists, the procedure can be repeated, preferably after a hot pack and active range of motion.

A technique promoted by some chiropractors is similar to myotherapy. It employs pressure for only 7–10 sec, to be repeated as often as several times a day,

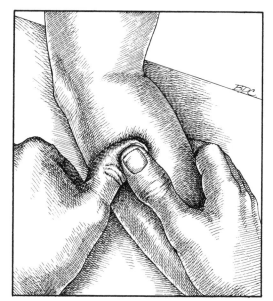

Figure 3.13. Technique for applying ischemic compression to trigger points in the right extensor carpi radialis brevis muscle. Pressure is gradually increased over a period of 30–60 sec until TP tenderness is eliminated.

for as many days as necessary to relieve the spot tenderness in the muscle. Pressure is applied with a finger, thumb, knuckle or elbow, depending on the thickness and depth of the muscle being compressed.

Ischemic compression is especially valuable in muscles that are not suitable for stretch and spray, and in muscles like the infraspinatus and sternalis that are relatively thin and overlie bone.

Digital pressure techniques are useful as self-treatment by the patient. They can be adapted to reach muscles that are otherwise inaccessible in the upper back by substituting a tennis ball for the digits, as described in Section 12 of Chapter 22.

Ischemic compression may fail to afford relief: (1) because the TP is too irritable and requires many applications of pressure; (2) because the operator released pressure, rather than gradually increasing it; (3) when the operator pressed too hard at first, causing excessive pain and autonomic responses with involuntary tensing by the patient; and (4) when the patient has perpetuating factors that continue to make the TPs hyperirritable.

Shiatzu. Shiatzu[65] or acupressure[30] are terms used to describe a pressure version of acupuncture in which the operator applies digital compression in a manner similar to that described above for ischemic compression or myotherapy. The spot for compression, however, is selected not for TP tenderness, but because of its location on an acupuncture chart. The acupressure results are said to be comparable to those obtained by acupuncture at corresponding points. To the extent that the Shiatzu points are located where there is a tender TP, the Shiatzu treatment should yield results comparable to those of ischemic compression. Shiatzu is philosophically quite different from our concept of myofascial TPs, but in practice, the treatments may appear similar.

Massage

If "massage" is employed to relieve TP activity without definition or knowledge of exactly what kind of massage, it is wise to request it only when the TPs are relatively latent and causing minimal referred pain. Vigorous massage of hyperirritable TPs can cause an adverse reaction with marked increase in pain.

Williams and Elkins[150] found massage to

be the single most effective treatment for myalgia (TPs) of the head. Massage was more effective than heat alone, and a firm, heavy, friction type of massage was more effective than the stroking or kneading types. Others considered kneading massage more effective than deep stroking massage in aiding the absorption of substances within the tissues.[11] Williams and Elkins[150] wisely recommended that treatment start with light stroking massage that barely involved the underlying muscular tissue. Then more pressure was added gradually.[150]

The purpose of friction massage is to move the superficial tissues over the underlying structures in order to improve their mobility.[11] This corresponds to the technique of Rolfing (skin rolling) to relieve the subcutaneous tightness of panniculosis (Section 8, above).

Stripping Massage. A successful massage technique in the hands of those therapists who are skilled in its use is a specific stroking massage applied slowly and deeply. The patient must be positioned comfortably so that the muscles to be treated are completely relaxed under moderate stretch. The skin is lubricated, and the thumbs or fingers of both hands are placed at the distal end of the muscle and then slowly slid along the length of the muscle toward the TP, so that the muscle is milked of its fluid content.[103] The digits progress much more slowly, 8 mm/sec (1 in/3 sec), than the usual massage rate of 18 cm/sec (7 in/sec).[11] Pressure is light on the first pass. As the pressure increases on successive passes, a sense of nodular obstruction is encountered at the TP. It feels like a lump, which could be due to damming of blood and other tissue fluids by obstructed blood flow in the region of the TP. The sliding movement continues smoothly over the TP and through the clear area beyond. Repeated strokes with increasing pressure gradually reduce the bumpiness at the TP. By then, the procedure has inactivated the TP, which has become non-tender and no longer refers pain. This technique probably produces ischemia followed by reactive hyperemia behind the massaging fingers.

This technique is specifically *not* the deep friction massage of Cyriax,[38] which he applied *across* the long axis of the muscle fibers.

Another pressure technique is to apply kneading massage in a series of moving circles (epicycles) that overlap the TP, eliminating its spot tenderness with gradually increasing pressure.[150]

Ice Massage. Ice massage is applied by two very different techniques. One is the intermittent use of ice in lieu of the vapocoolant spray as a variation of stretch and spray, described in detail by Zohn and Mennell.[154]

The other technique is a non-specific application of cold stimuli for pain relief. This was tested experimentally in 44 chronic low back pain patients.[88] Gentle ice massage was applied to the back at three sites: in the mid-line of the low back at L_3 and S_1, and at the lateral malleolus of the ankle on the side with the most severe pain. Ice was applied for a maximum of 7 minutes at each site, with a 3-min rest interval between applications, until 30 min had elapsed. Instead of ice, the application of transcutaneous electrical stimulation simultaneously to the same three sites for 30 min was equally effective.

The above non-specific cold application afforded a mean duration of 11 hr of pain relief.[88] As Mennell explained,[90] cold application with stretching of the specific muscle in which the irritable TP is located provides more complete and lasting relief than cold application alone. Mennell warned that excessive use of cold over a muscle decreases its resting length and induces undesirable effects, including shivering and vascular changes that militate against pain relief and healing.[90]

Periosteal Therapy. Periostbehandlung (periosteal therapy) is a rhythmic massage technique applied to bony prominences of the body.[142] Waves of pressure are applied for 2–4 min; each half-wave of increasing or decreasing pressure lasts 4–10 sec. The finger, thumb, or knuckle pressure is applied to the periosteum near painful areas. Pressure is applied in small circles of 5 mm diameter. The pressure massage progresses from the periphery toward the center of periosteal tenderness. The mechanism of pain relief is thought[142] to be distinctly different from that of Druckpunkte (pressure points). Instead, the authors presumed the effects are due to vasomotor reflex changes. The treatment might also affect the activity of TPs in the area, or the induction of a greater pain may help to counter the original pain, as in the hyperstimulation analgesia concept described by Melzack.[86]

Stretch without Spray

Three different stretch techniques can be effective: passive stretch, rhythmic stabilization, and the Lewit technique.

Passive Stretch. It is possible, with a newly activated and only moderately irritable TP, to inactivate it immediately by simply stretching the muscle, without vapocoolant. The muscle must be completely relaxed and then firmly, slowly stretched to the point of moderate pain, gradually restoring its full normal length. Stretching is facilitated by allowing a hot shower to beat on the muscle and on the area of its pain reference zone. Relaxation is improved if the patient sits, rather than stands, under the shower.

Rhythmic Stabilization. The technique for using rhythmic stabilization to increase the stretch range of motion has been described in detail.[26, 68, 112] Alternate contraction of agonist and antagonist muscle groups are resisted by the therapist in a way that keeps the muscles stretched isometrically at the limit of their range. This alternating effort permits gradual lengthening of the affected muscles. This useful technique benefits from reciprocal inhibition, but requires great skill on the part of the therapist.

Nel[99] described a slightly simpler variant of this technique that takes advantage of reciprocal inhibition to help stretch the mandibular elevators. Repeated *active* stretch of the affected muscle against resistance achieves a small gain in range of motion after each effort.

Lewit Technique. Lewit[75] described a technique that combines elements of both passive stretch and rhythmic stabilization. He described it in detail with many illustrations and case reports (in German).[75] The technique is painless and can be remarkably effective. The patient exerts *minimal* voluntary effort to contract the affected muscle that has been stretched to the comfortable limit of its range. The patient holds this contraction for at least 10 sec, while the operator resists the effort isometrically; then the patient relaxes. When *complete* relaxation is realized, the operator passively, *gently* stretches the muscle a little farther, but only if the movement meets no resistance. Specifically those fibers that are short and under tension must be stretched, which requires as much precision as the stretch-and-spray technique. This cycle is repeated until the muscle length no longer increases.

The Lewit technique extends the muscle passively as far as it can lengthen comfortably, then has the patient add a voluntary increment of tension that loads the muscle within the range of comfort and without changing its length. Then, on complete relaxation, the operator takes up the slack induced by the preceding increased tension. We find, for this technique to be effective, that the muscle fibers being stretched by the operator, and the muscle fibers being contracted by the patient must be precisely the same group of muscle fibers that were tensed and shortened by the TP activity. This technique is an effective stretch-without-spray method, but also can be used with vapocooling, if desired.

In effect, the Lewit[75] method substitutes a gentle, voluntary contraction by the patient for the moderately painful, passive stretch by the operator in the stretch-and-spray technique. In many patients, the extra time required by the step-wise Lewit method is unnecessary; stretch and spray allows the muscle to extend to full, normal length more quickly. However, in patients with muscles that are difficult to release, this voluntary contraction step adds two valuable features. First, the patient exerts additional force during the critical phase when a new degree of muscle stretch is being established. This increases the patient's confidence, aids relaxation, and reduces the danger of overstretching the muscle. Second, the patient develops a feel for how to do a self-stretch exercise that is specific to that muscle.

Any of the stretching techniques performed by an operator, passive stretch with or without spray, rhythmic stabilization, and the Lewit technique, require a high degree of manual skill, ample time and close communication between the operator and patient. These treatments can not be done successfully in a hurry.

Ultrasound

Many therapists find the application of ultrasound an effective means of inactivating TPs. One successful technique starts with a setting of 0.5 watt/cm^2, using a slow dwell technique with a circular motion that completes one circle in 1 or 2 sec.[154] The circle is tight enough to provide a small overlap over the TP in the center of the circle. In another technique, the power is first increased to the threshold pain level (to 1.5 watt/cm^2) and then reduced to one-half of that intensity. Over the next 2 to 3 minutes, the intensity is gradually increased with frequent queries as to patient sensations, until the intensity has been increased to, but not beyond the original pain threshold level. Usually, the patient no longer feels pain at this level of stimulation and the TP is less tender and irritable.[100] The Medco-sonlator combines ultrasound with electrical stimulation of sufficient intensity so that the increased current flow through the point of low skin resistance over the TP produces a prickly sensation. This is helpful in locating TPs for those who have not mastered the palpation techniques described in this manual. This electrical stimulation has been reported to be helpful therapeutically, as well as diagnostically.[20, 101]

Heat

Moist hot packs are frequently applied to supine patients for treatment of low back and limb pain of myofascial origin. A moisture-proof electric hot pad with a dampened cloth cover is a convenient source of moist heat. A hot tub bath is another convenient method.[92] Diathermy often intensifies the pain.[92] Moist heat tends to relax the underlying muscles and to diminish the tension on the TPs, thereby reducing referred pain and local tenderness to pressure. The patient's passive or active stretch exercises at home are more effective if performed during or immediately after the application of moist heat.

When a patient experiences reactivation of myofascial TPs that have previously been inactivated, sometimes, but not always, resting the muscle with application of moist heat may allow the muscle to recover within 72 hr without further therapy.

Drug Therapy

In the management of patients with myofascial pain syndromes, one must consider the role of drugs with respect to pain relief, muscular relaxation, sleep, depression, anti-inflammatory action, and adverse side effects.

Pain Relief. Successful management of a myofascial pain syndrome relieves the patient's pain so that strong analgesic medication is no longer needed; this is a major goal of myofascial therapy. At the start of specific treatment, before the patient obtains sustained relief, such medication may be necessary. Relatively small doses of codeine for short periods may suffice.

Aspirin may be helpful.[92] If gastric irritation is a problem, Ecotrin (enteric-coated aspirin), or the 8-hr duration Bayer Timed-release Aspirin, which is available without prescription, may be tolerated. Acetaminophen (Tylenol, and numerous other trade names) causes little gastric irritation and is an effective analgesic in the myofascial syndrome.

If additional relief is required, a wide variety of old and new anti-inflammatory, non-steroidal, analgesic drugs are available, but these have a number of side effects and may not lessen uncomplicated myofascial TP pain before the dystrophic phase.

A combination drug, Esgic, contains butalbital (a barbiturate), caffeine, and acetaminophen. It may enhance the effectiveness of local TP inactivation through reduction of the patient's anxiety and relief of muscle tension pain, especially headache. Since this medication contains caffeine, the patient should limit the intake of other caffeine sources, including coffee, colas, and the many other caffeine-containing analgesic mixtures. A *moderate* amount of caffeine often reduces TP pain, perhaps by vasodilatation in the skeletal muscles, but excess caffeine increases muscle tension and TP irritability.

The placebo effect is one of the potent therapeutic tools available for pain relief. In most controlled studies, between one-quarter and one-third of patients perceive some relief of pain by a placebo; however, this effect is rarely sustained. Any prescribed pill that the patient swallows serves as a symbol of faith in the wisdom and support of the physician, and thus acquires healing potency.[131] Also, some patients clearly show a negative placebo effect; the placebo worsens their symptoms. Placebo effects apply also to therapeutic procedures.

Muscle Relaxants. In our experience, the

muscle relaxants sold for the relief of muscu-loskeletal pain are of limited value to patients suffering from myofascial TPs. In the dosages used to relax muscles, they are prone to release first those muscles that are providing protective splinting. Their relaxation increases the load on, and the TP pain originating in, the primarily affected muscle. Diazepam (Valium) is recommended for relaxation of muscles in reflex spasm following injury and for the management of anxiety disorders. Although it is moderately effective in the myofascial pain syndromes in some patients, its high potential for addiction with long term use has led us to employ other solutions for those with chronic pain problems.

Sleep. Most patients with persistent myofascial TP pain have difficulty sleeping and show abnormal sleep patterns when monitored in a sleep laboratory.[4] In many, it is the referred pain generated by an active TP that disturbs sleep. However, in others the sleep disturbance aggravates the pain.

Moldofsky et al.[94] identify a sleep disorder as a major contributing factor in the musculoskeletal pain that they termed "fibrositis," as defined by Smythe (see Chapter 2). They demonstrated the anomalous presence of alpha-delta sleep in these patients and also in healthy subjects undergoing stage 4 sleep deprivation. In addition, the healthy subjects deprived of stage 4 sleep developed, temporarily, musculoskeletal and mood symptoms comparable to those seen in their chronic pain patients. The authors implicated a lack of brain serotonin as probably responsible for this sleep disorder. Depletion of brain serotonin is associated with the alpha-delta sleep disturbance, and is also associated with increased pain sensitivity in studies on man and animals.[94]

In treating patients with myofascial pain that disrupts sleep, top priority is given to the inactivation of the TPs that are chiefly responsible for insomnia. The patient is shown what sleeping position will minimize myofascial pain and is encouraged to take medication intermittently, as necessary, to obtain restful sleep.

Three antihistamines, which are non-habit-forming, are recommended for better sleep. Dimenhydrinate (Dramamine) and diphenhydramine hydrochloride (Bene-dryl) have a common antihistamine that has a soporific effect on most people. The 50-mg tablet of dimenhydrinate is available without prescription and packs a stronger wallop than a 25-mg capsule of diphenhydramine, which is also available in a 50-mg capsule. The 25-mg dose can usually be repeated during the night, if necessary, without excessive morning hang-over. Generally, sleep medication should be taken $1/2$-hr before retiring.

Promethazine (Phenergan) has a longer duration of action than dimenhydrate, and may be helpful to individuals who fall asleep easily, but have trouble remaining asleep. This antihistamine also has a potent calming effect that is valuable for patients who are anxious. Usually, one 12.5 mg tablet at bedtime suffices.

Anti-inflammatory Agents. Anti-inflammatory agents are recommended in the management of myofascial syndromes in two situations: when the patient experiences excessive muscle soreness after specific myofascial treatment, and when examination indicates connective tissue inflammatory changes and the muscles are refractory to specific myofascial therapy in the absence of any identifiable perpetuating factors.

For the management of TPs refractory to therapy because of connective tissue inflammatory changes, the corticosteroid may be given more effectively by mouth instead of injection. An oral course of short-acting corticosteroid is started with 60 mg daily of prednisone tapered down in a week to 10 mg every other day. This dosage level may be maintained for several weeks as local treatment continues, until all the problem TPs have been inactivated. Improved response to specific myofascial therapy is usually noted within days of starting the oral steroid.

To control excessive post-treatment muscle soreness, 3 cc (12 mg) of dexamethasone, or an equivalent amount of comparable corticosteroid (in a soluble, not delayed release preparation), is mixed with 1 ml of 2% procaine for injection at TP sites, but only after aspirating with the syringe and not drawing blood. Intravenous injection of this solution should be avoided. We include procaine when injecting TPs with coticosteroid to help inactivate and to reduce pain.

Troublemaking Drugs. Small to moderate amounts of caffeine may help to eliminate TPs by increasing vasodilatation in the skeletal musculature. Coffee and/or cola drinks that contain caffeine, when taken in excess of two or three cups, bottles, or cans daily, are likely to aggravate TP activity. A cup of coffee may contain 50–150 mg of caffeine: as a rule, drip coffee contains more than percolated, which contains more than instant. Most of the canned soft drinks contain 30–50 mg of caffeine, except 7up, Sprite, diet 7up, RC-100, *Diet* Sunkist orange, Patio orange, Fanta orange, Fresca, Hires Root Beer and Cragmont cola, which are caffeine free.[34] Many combination analgesic drugs contain caffeine that may add significantly to the total caffeine load without the patient's realizing it, unless the physician analyzes in detail the patient's drug intake.

Regular alcohol consumption may indirectly perpetuate TPs through reduced serum and tissue folate levels. Ingestion of alcohol reduces the absorption of folic acid, while increasing the body's need for it (see Vitamins, in Chapter 4).

The habit of tobacco smoking markedly increases the need for vitamin C, which is poorly stored in the body. The marked capillary fragility associated with low asorbic acid levels greatly increases the tendency for tissue bleeding at injection sites. Injection of TPs in smokers should be postponed until adequate tissue levels of vitamin C are assured (see Vitamins, in Chapter 4).

Biofeedback

Biofeedback alone is not specific myofascial therapy. However, many patients express their anxiety and frustration through general muscular tension, which abuses their muscles. Biofeedback training helps these patients to become aware of unnecessarily sustained contraction of their muscles, and teaches them how to recognize and control the excess tension. Meditation practiced for this same purpose can enhance the patient's ability to reestablish muscular relaxation and emotional tranquility.

Transcutaneous Electrical Stimulation

Transcutaneous electrical stimulation is well established as one means of tempo-rary, sometimes prolonged, pain relief, but it is not a specific myofascial modality, as commonly used. Non-specific relief of pain often helps the patient to regain some muscle function that includes increased mobility and produces a degree of muscle stretching, which otherwise might not occur. One must avoid electrical stimulation of sufficient intensity to cause muscular contractions that tend to aggravate myofascial TP symptoms. Frequently, stimulation is applied to acupuncture points or to reference zones where pain is felt, rather than to TPs where pain originates.

Research is needed to clarify the role of transcutaneous electrical stimulation in the treatment of myofascial pain syndromes.

14. CORRECTIVE ACTIONS

This section reviews what *the patient* must do, or avoid, to achieve lasting recovery; Chapter 4 reviews the perpetuating factors that *the doctor and therapist* must identify and resolve.

Patients must learn respect for their muscles; muscles are designed to contract, relax, and be mobile. They were *not* designed to be held for long periods in sustained contraction or in a fixed position, particularly not in the fully shortened position. Most patients need to apply some myofascial therapy at home, such as moist heat, stretch exercises, and ischemic compression.

Patient Compliance

Patients may fail to perform corrective actions effectively because of over-enthusiasm, misunderstanding or apathy.

Over-enthusiasm: Some patients are hard-driving over-doers who live by the philosophy that if one is good, two must be better, and three much better. They tend to be Spartan and are determined to be a "good sport," performing activities regardless of exhaustion or pain, and refusing to quit. These patients abuse their muscles, rather than respect their normal limitations.

Misunderstanding. People misunderstand instructions, even when written and handed to them (a valuable routine). If something can be misinterpreted, sooner or later it will be. By having the patient *demonstrate* the exercises on return to the office, exactly as performed at home, one learns: (1) what exercise the patient has actually been doing, (2) how the patient has been doing it, and (3) how much improvement in function has occurred, if any. The reason for lack of pain relief may be apparent when one sees how incorrectly the patient had been doing a stretch exercise. This also gives the examiner an opportunity to discuss with the patient the reason for each exercise, specifically what muscle, or muscles are involved, and an opportunity to strongly reinforce skillful, conscientious exercise performance.

When investigating what medications and nutritional supplements patients are taking, drawing a distinction between what they were *told* to take and what they *actually* took is often revealing. Asking "When did you take your folic acid the last time?" or "When do you usually take it?" reveals whether the patient takes it regularly, or whether it is a hit-or-miss operation. Plastic pill boxes with seven separate compartments, each marked for one day of the week, conveniently remind the patient to take the correct medication each day.

Lack of Interest. Frequently, patients have seen many doctors, have been given different diagnoses of their pain and different treatments, none of which afforded significant relief. At first, they have no reason to believe that the new physician will do any better; faith is faltering. These patients need prompt tangible evidence that their pain originates in the muscles, not in the bones and nerves, nor in their head, and that it can respond to myofascial therapy.

Patients with pending disability compensation are likely to be subconsciously ambivalent about losing their pain. Many of these patients are justifiably frustrated with, and distrustful of, the medical profession's ability to identify a cause of their disabling pain that will respond to treatment. Medical pronouncements, based on X-rays, that the patient has "pinched nerves" or "arthritis of the spine," leads to the belief that this is the cause of the pain, a pain without hope of relief except through pain pills, and that disability is permanent.

One approach to this problem of ambiv-alence eliminates these patients by refusing to accept them until the legal reimbursement issue is settled. The other gives the patient an opportunity to reorient life toward function, not disability. One must take the time and effort to establish the myofascial basis of the pain, and then, to educate the patient in its nature and probable response to treatment. Recovery of *function* becomes the primary goal, with *guarded* promises as to pain relief. When successful, as the patient's myofascial TPs are inactivated and pain behavior is replaced by function, the pain complaints also fade.[43] One must treat both the TP sources of pain and chronic pain behavior, which often could have been avoided if the myofascial causes had been recognized initially and treated promptly.

What Activities?

After a treatment session, the patient must understand the kind and dose of activity that is appropriate, and must eliminate or modify habitual movements that are perpetuating their TPs.

Post-treatment Activity. Stretched and injected muscles are likely to be sore for 2 or 3 days following treatment. After that soreness has passed, the patient should experience the full pain relief afforded by the treatment. Strenuous activities should be avoided for at least the period of muscle soreness, and preferably for about a week. That includes playing tennis, gardening, moving furniture and, often, traveling to conventions. On the other hand, the patient is encouraged to use the muscle in a gentle, normal way through its *full* range of motion. The worst activity involves holding the muscle stiffly in a fixed, shortened position.

The patient learns to avoid loading recently injected muscles by substituting less involved muscles, *e.g.* to substitute the uninjected opposite sternocleidomastoid for the one on the treated side, when getting out of bed; or to substitute the brachialis and biceps brachii for the supinator when flexing the elbow.

Perpetuating Movements. When the patient's TPs are extremely hyperirritable, the muscles are *overwhelmed* by the TP activity and are generating pain all of the time, even at rest; almost any activity makes them worse. However, as the muscles improve, when the patient does the wrong thing and pain recurs, an awareness develops as to which activities are now tolerated and which cause pain. This is the *discriminating* phase when the patient can recognize overstress of the muscles and how to avoid it. Any activity that produces pain for more than a few seconds after the effort should be avoided.[92] As all remaining TPs are inactivated, full *recovery* occurs and the patient can do the *normal* things that were done before the pain developed, but not more; he or she never could lift a piano!

In this discriminating stage, the doctor helps the patient decide which aggravating activities are unnecessary and must be eliminated (lifting a paperweight 50 times a day to test whether it still hurts to lift the paperweight), *versus* those which are essential; the latter must be modified so that they are done without damaging stress. The patient learns how to become fully functional within the limits of the state of the muscles.

Patients should learn a few basic rules. NEVER bend over and lift, or pull something, with the back twisted. ALWAYS lift with the knees, holding the back in an erect-forward-facing position. Similarly, NEVER get up from, or sit down in, a chair while leaning forward in the stooped position with the trunk rotated; that is "asking" for low back strain.

To recognize the pain-perpetuating activities, the patient is first alerted as to what kinds of movements are likely to abuse the affected muscles and reactivate their TPs. The patient is asked to report at the next visit any activity that caused referred pain from the stressed muscles, and to note any habitual repetitive movement that would overload those muscles.

When the offending movements are unnecessary, it is a matter of the patient's unlearning a bad habit. When the activity is a necessary one, such as turning the doorknob to open a door, then at least one satisfactory alternate method of performing the activity must be developed; e.g. use the other hand, or rotate the shoulder rather than the forearm, or perhaps lubricate the door latch mechanism.

Some people characteristically make rapid jerky movements. These movements are poorly coordinated and are likely to initiate reflex contraction of muscles and unnecessary stress. Slower, smoother movements must be made habitual.

For patients with acute scalene, serratus anterior or quadratus lumborum TPs (muscles with rib attachments), sneezing or coughing can be exquisitely painful and aggravating to the TPs. The sneeze may be inhibited by promptly biting *high* on the upper lip or by firmly squeezing the upper lip or nostrils to induce distracting pain in the nose area. These painful anti-sneeze stimuli are effective only if started early enough in the sneeze. Otherwise, the patient learns to keep the glottis open during the sneeze to minimize increased intrathoracic pressure and the overload which that imposes on the accessory respiratory muscles.

Students, or other readers, usually place the book on a flat surface or on the lap, bending the head and neck forward to read. This requires that the posterior neck muscles maintain sustained contraction in order to checkrein the heavy weight of the head against gravity. The ensuing neck strain can be avoided by placing the book on a book rack, or by propping it up at eye level. Thus tilted at a convenient angle, it can be read easily when the head is held erect and balanced, without neck strain.

Activity Goals

Not only is WHAT to do important, but also HOW to do it. On performing a task, the patient MUST learn to keep the muscles mobilized, and not held fixed in a contracted position. Muscle fibers need to alternately contract and relax to increase blood flow and replenish their energy supply. Using the motor unit training technique of Basmajian,[9] even a type I motor unit will not sustain a minimal contraction indefinitely, but will drop out and be replaced by another motor unit. When most of the motor units have been recruited and are sustaining moderately high firing rates, even the momentary rest provided by the alternation of motor units becomes inadequate.

Strenuousness of Effort. The patient must avoid using the muscles at maximum effort, when they are most likely to be strained. Lifting, pulling or pushing something should use *less than* maximum strength, always leaving some reserve, especially in the case of muscles susceptible to TPs.

Overload of anterior and lateral neck muscles due to paradoxical breathing must be corrected by learning to synchronize contraction of the diaphragm with contraction of the intercostal muscles (abdominal and chest breathing) (see Section 14 in Chapter 20).

Mobility. Lying still in bed with muscles in a shortened position aggravates their TP activity; being up and doing things helps to mobilize the muscles and reduces TP activity. A mobilizing relaxing activity is rocking in a physiologically well-designed rocking chair, such as the Carolina rocker, with a soft neck pillow.

Muscles need to be stretched to their full range of motion every day. They perform better if activities stretch the muscle when it is *lightly* loaded. The patient should learn to move the part frequently throughout the day in ways that provide gentle stretching, passive or active, of the affected muscles. The forcefulness of stretching should always be within the limits of pain, and should never produce a lasting ache after the stretch.

Travell[133, 134] described the application of these principles to housework.

1. Vary your task each day so as not to overuse any one group of muscles in repetitive work, like ironing for hours at a stretch. Especially, don't combine too many jobs that involve standing and stooping; they place a heavy load on the low back muscles ... To achieve variety of movement, you will have to scramble your housework.

2. Slow your working pace to a speed no faster than your muscles will tolerate. Fatigue of any one of your muscles is a warning signal—learn to pay attention to them ...

3. Cultivate a rhythmn of movement. It discourages the prolonged fixed contraction that tires a muscle, and it encourages pauses during which the working muscles fill up with new blood and fresh fuel. Do your housework as if you were dancing—music helps ...

4. Take short rests frequently. After every hour or less of housework, lie down to rest for a couple of minutes, if only on the floor. The anti-gravity muscles of the neck and back that hold you erect do not relax fully unless your body is supported in a nearly horizontal position ...

5. Don't sit too long in one position. At a movie or the theatre (or watching TV), move around in your seat. At intervals, turn your head from side-to-side and rotate your shoulder blades ... When you drive far, pull off the road every hour and walk around your car two or three times. That doesn't take long. At home, you can sit in a rocker. This constantly changing position prevents resting muscles (electrically silent) from building up the tension (electrical activity) that inevitably occurs when you stay motionless for several minutes or up to one-half an hour, as electromyographic studies have shown.[78]

6. Don't try to lift a heavy piece of furniture by yourself, or to carry large awkward things that extend the leverage length of your arm; the extra leverage multiplies the weight transmitted to your low back muscles. Keep the load close to your body, and just before you lift it, raise your head smartly and look up. That tightens the long spinal muscles and prepares your back for the load.

Relaxation. For relaxation in the sitting position, a well designed chair with adequate lumbar support and the correct height armrests is necessary (see Section 14 in Chapter 42).

When standing or walking, the patient should focus on the floor under the feet, trying to feel the texture and hardness of the rug, linoleum, or concrete with each step. When resting, sensation should be concentrated on the bed that supports the body, on the texture of the sheets, wrinkles, and the shape of the supporting surface. This concentration on the underlying *support* beneath the body directs attention away from the body itself and encourages relaxation. Relaxation is an active process that requires intense concentration.

Training in biofeedback and mind management, like meditation, can help people learn how to relax their muscles.

Between cycles of an exercise, a pause for several deep breaths greatly aids muscular relaxation, permits time for return of circulation, and trains the patient in how to reduce chronic tension of the muscles.

Application of Heat

Allowing the body to become chilled, as by a cold draft across the shoulders, causes muscular contraction and invites activation of TPs. A sweater in the living room by day and an electric blanket at night can make the differences between comfort and pain.

Cold applied to the skin penetrates quickly due to progressive vasoconstriction. Surface heat does not penetrate; the excess heat is quickly carried away by the increased blood flow due to vasodilatation. Prolonged cold over a TP tends to activate it, but prolonged cold applied over the pain reference zone may relieve discomfort by partially anesthetizing sensory nerve function locally.

Whenever the muscles become chilled, especially after exercise, a hot shower or hot bath warms and relaxes them. Professional athletes do not wait after playing competitive sports to run for hot water.

Heat that the patient applies to sore muscles should be moist, not dry. Either a hot wet pack soaked in hot water, or a wet-proof heating pad covered with a damp cloth, serves the purpose. The moist heat is applied over the TP, if its location is known. If a patient with pain asks where to place the moist heat, it is advisable to try several different regions, for approximately 5 min each, to see which location affords the greatest relief. Daily application of moist heat to active TPs can progressively quiet them.

Postural Positioning

Activity Posture. Good posture avoids sustained contraction or prolonged shortening of muscles. Strain of the upper trapezius is lessened by providing armrests that properly support the elbows. These are needed when sitting, reading, telephoning, and driving or riding in a car. Placing the work level low enough so that the shoulders need not be raised to reach it also is important.

Correct Standing and Sitting Posture. The techniques for achieving good posture are presented in detail in Section 14 of Chapter 42.

Reading Position. Tilting the plane of reading glasses, so that the lower rim is against the cheek, allows the patient to read by turning the eyes downward, rather than by bending the neck forward, as is described in Section 7 of Chapter 16 (Fig. 16.4).

When reading, the light should be placed so that the book is well illuminated when it is held straight in front of the reader without the reader having to turn the head. For reading in bed, an overhead light that clips onto the bed, or is mounted on the wall or ceiling, is recommended.

Sleeping Position. Muscles should rest in a neutral or slightly stretched position at night and NEVER be kept in the *fully* shortened position.

The shoulders should not be allowed to creep up toward the ears; correct positioning is helped by tucking the corners of the pillow between the chin and shoulder on each side. When lying on the side, the patient should pull the corner of the pillow around between the lowermost shoulder and chin, to avoid shortening the front-of-the-neck muscles. The patient should use only one comfortable pillow under the head (not under the shoulders) to keep the head and neck in a neutral position, when lying on the back. Tilting the entire bed-frame by elevating the head end of the bed with 3½- to 4-in blocks under its legs creates gentle traction on the neck, especially on the scalene and sternocleidomastoid muscles.

As a rule, lying on the side is most comfortable; lying on the abdomen with the head and neck extended and twisted around sideways is the position most aggravating to neck TPs. Many people with the scalene TP syndrome prefer to lie on the affected side, if the posterior shoulder-girdle muscles will permit weight bearing.

The pillow should be filled with a non-springy material, like feathers or shredded dacron; foam rubber should be discarded. Special pillows designed to maintain the head in a normal alignment with the body, retaining a moderate cervical lordosis, are the Cervipillo designed by Ruth Jackson, MD,[66] and the Wal-Pil-O designed by Lionel Walpin, MD.[144]

The elbows and wrists should not be held sharply flexed at night. A pillow in the axilla, between the arm and chest wall, prevents painful shortening of the muscles in the subscapularis, pectoralis major, latissimus dorsi, triceps brachii, infraspinatus, and teres major and minor TP syndromes. A pillow under the feet lengthens the gastrocnemius/soleus muscles and prevents sustained plantar flexion.

Exercises

An exercise can be designed to produce primarily either stretching, strengthening or conditioning of specific muscles. Exercise to stretch the involved muscles is the key to sustained relief of myofascial pain. Improved conditioning (exercise tolerance or stamina) and increased strength of a group of muscles, achieved through exercise, reduces the likelihood of their developing TPs. However, in most patients with *active* TPs, conditioning and strengthening exercises tend to further activate the TPs, aggravating symptoms. On the other hand, these exercises render latent TPs less prone to reactivation.

The kind of exercise prescribed depends largely on the irritability of the TPs responsible for the pain. When the patient is experiencing **rest pain** for a considerable part of the time, the TPs are very active and rarely respond favorably to anything more than gentle passive stretch and hot packs. At this stage, movement in hot water with rhythmic and gentle, active or passive stretching is relaxing. The object is to unload and stretch the overworked sore muscles; at that stage, active exercise that loads a contracting muscle is not indicated.

Exercise should be regarded as a prescription, much as one prescribes medication. Like a drug, there is a right kind, dose and timing of exercise. The exact exercise to be performed is demonstrated and explained to the patient, who then *does* it to confirm the understanding of the instructions. The rate, number of repetitions, how often in one day and the conditions under which it should be done (not when the muscles are tired or cold) should be spelled out. For any repetitive exercise, whether stretch or strengthening, a pause to relax and breathe should be interposed between each cycle of the exercise. The number of counts during the pause should equal the number required to perform the movement.

As the TPs are inactivated, and rest pain fades, a *carefully graded* exercise program is needed to increase endurance. The program should start with lengthening, not shortening exercises. If an exercise causes pain that lasts after the exercise, it should be postponed. When mild muscular soreness disappears after the first day, the exercise can be repeated on the second day. If soreness lasts into the second day after exercise, the next session should be postponed until the third day and the amount of exercise reduced. If the muscles are still sore on the third day, the exercise should be changed. Also, if the patient on a home program calls to complain of annoying (but not incapacitating) muscle soreness due to an exercise or overenthusiastic activity, he may be told that with rest and moist heat, the postexercise soreness and stiffness should not last longer than 72 hr.

A new exercise should be started on an alternate day schedule, and variety of movement should be emphasized. When TP activity produces only occasional pain in response to movement, the timing of stretch exercises can be raised to a daily schedule, while lengthening exercises for endurance can be replaced by shortening exercises. An exercise that increases referred pain during or after its performance should be stopped.

Patients should avoid activities that produce repetitive muscular loads, such as shovelling snow, raking leaves, vacuum cleaning, painting a wall, or unloading a dishwasher. If such tasks must be performed, then the movements should be varied and sides alternated so that contralateral muscles are used in turn. The number of repetitions of the movement should not exceed 6 or 7 times, with pauses to allow the muscle to rest.

Stretch Exercise. In this manual, stretch exercises are described and illustrated in detail, because they are so important to the recovery from pain due to active TPs and because they are often the only kind of exercise tolerated by hyperirritable TPs. A daily home program of passive stretch exercise that achieves FULL range of motion of the affected muscles helps to insure continued relief. It is important that the patient use an objective measure of the full range of motion, so that any gradual loss is recognized.

Passive stretch is emphasized. Treatment by stretching the muscles to the point of pain flies in the face of intuition, namely, that pain should be avoided. The patient must understand *why* the stretch exercises are necessary and *how* uncomfortable the stretch should be, in order for it to be adequate. Some Spartan individuals assume that "the more pain, the better" and thus aggravate their TPs, rather than inactivate them.

People who are prone to develop TPs do

well to emulate the cat, which rarely tries to walk after sleeping without first stretching its limb muscles. Such active stretching should be accomplished slowly, with a smooth, sustained effort that avoids any jerk at the end.

Active voluntary contraction of the antagonist to assist the stretch may be helpful by inducing reciprocal inhibition of stretch reflexes in the muscle being stretched; however, it will interfere with stretch if it induces cocontraction. More serious, the effort to contract a fully shortened antagonist that harbors latent TPs may activate these and precipitate an acute episode of severe pain. However, if the antagonist has recently been adequately stretched and sprayed, this reaction is unlikely.

A stretch that involves rolling the head around in all directions at full range of motion is hazardous, and is likely to activate TPs when tight shortened muscles are suddenly overloaded at one angle.

Strengthening Exercise. To strengthen a muscle, one needs to hold a *maximal* contraction for only 5 or 10 sec, once a day. Strengthening exercises may be isotonic or isometric. During isotonic exercise, the muscle moves against a relatively constant force. During isometric exercise, the muscle exerts a somewhat variable force in a fixed position. When dealing with muscles that contain myofascial TPs, the movement associated with an isotonic exercise is preferable to the fixed position of the isometric exercise.

A muscle has significantly greater strength and efficiency during a lengthening contraction than during a shortening contraction. A muscle usually shortens as it works; it contracts and becomes shorter. Lengthening contraction occurs when the muscle is overpowered by a greater force than it is producing; its force of contraction resists lengthening. A "sit up" (Fig. 49.11C) requires a shortening contraction; a "sit back" (Fig. 49.11A) produces a lengthening contraction of the same abdominal muscles. A lengthening contraction exerts more force with less energy than does a shortening contraction. It is safer for the patient, initially, to do loading exercises that lengthen, rather than shorten the muscle.

Hill[64] demonstrated the difference in the energy expended by shortening and lengthening contractions in a clear-cut experiment. Two stationary bicycles were directly coupled in opposition so that when subject "X" pedaled one bicycle in the forward direction using shortening contractions, it forced subject "Y" to pedal the other bicycle backward at precisely the same speed, exerting the same force with lengthening contractions. Subject "X" established the speed and subject "Y," the force of resistance. To compensate for individual differences, after suitable rest they reversed directions. At high pedaling speeds, the oxygen consumption of the subject who performed shortening contractions was 6 *times* that of the subject doing lengthening contractions, which agreed with their subjective impressions of the relative effort required.

Strengthening exercises are prescribed with a certain number of repetitions to achieve conditioning. It is important that these exercises be executed smoothly, slowly, rhythmically, and without jerkiness. A *pause* is as important as the movement, and should be equally long; during the pause, deep abdominal breathing helps to reestablish *complete* relaxation.

An example of a lengthening contraction exercise for the biceps brachii and brachialis muscles would be a "chin down," or a "chin up" in reverse. Instead of pulling the body up to bring the chin to the bar, as in a chin up, the patient steps up on a box and lets the arms control the rate at which the body and chin drop away from the bar. A quadriceps lengthening exercise would be a "step down" when going downstairs backwards, as compared to a "step up" when going upstairs forward.

When the patient can do 10 lengthening contractions easily, it is time to replace this exercise with one shortening contraction, which is gradually increased in number on subsequent days. With this approach, the patient is less likely to overload and overstress a weak or tired muscle that harbors TPs. It restores normal muscle function more quickly than a program of limited shortening contractions.

Conditioning Exercise. To condition both the cardiovascular system and a particular set of muscles, the exercise is continued at submaximal strength to the point of fatigue. Swimming, bicycling, tennis, jogging, and jumping rope are examples.

Although not essential for recovery from myofascial TPs, a *regular* conditioning exercise program at least twice a week, or preferably every other day, is strongly recommended for optimal health.

When a warm pool is available, swimming provides excellent exercise for many muscles with minimal hazard of strain. Bicycling is less traumatic than jogging. The least traumatic bicycle exercise is on a machine that the patient pedals from behind, while lying supported in the semi-recumbent position. When riding an upright stationary bicycle, the patient should not hold the handlebars, but should sit up straight and swing the arms from time to time. The trunk-forward, head-up position of bicycling, which is all too common, severely overloads the posterior cervical muscles. Whatever exercise is undertaken, the first efforts should remain *well* within tolerance, by underestimating how much can be done at the start. On the bicycle machine, an increment in either the duration, rate of pedaling or the load (tension) is added *gradually*, one at a time. Overexercise when out of condition is disastrous; when jogging, take a route that allows a shortcut home, if needed.

References

1. Agnew LRC, Aviado DM, Brody JI, et al.: Dorland's Illustrated Medical Dictionary, Ed. 24. W.B. Saunders, Philadelphia, 1965.
2. Altura BM, Altura BT: Effects of local anesthetics, antihistamines, and glucocorticoids on peripheral blood flow and vascular smooth muscle. Anesthesiology 41:197–214, 1974.
3. Austin KL, Denborough MA: Drug treatment of malignant hyperpyrexia. Anesth Intensive Care 5:207–213, 1977.
4. Baker BA: Personal communication, 1981.
5. Baker DM: Changes in the corium and subcutaneous tissues as a cause of rheumatic pain. Ann Rheum Dis 14:385–391, 1955.
6. Baker R, Powars D. Haywood LJ: Restoration of the deformability of "irreversibly" sickled cells by procaine hydrochloride. Biochem Biophys Res Commun 59:548–556, 1974.
7. Bardeen CR: The musculature, Sect. 5. In Morris's Human Anatomy, edited by C.M. Jackson, Ed. 6. Blakiston's Son & Co., Philadelphia, 1921.
8. Bargmann W, Batrawi AM, Beau A, et al.: Nomina Anatomica. Excerpta Medica Foundation, Amsterdam, 1966.
9. Basmajian JV: Muscles Alive, Ed. 4. Williams & Wilkins, Baltimore, 1978 (pp. 103–114, 115–129).
10. Bates T, Grunwaldt E: Myofascial pain in childhood. J Pediatr 53:198–209, 1958.
11. Beard G, Wood EC: Massage: Principles and Techniques. W.B. Saunders, Philadelphia, 1964

(pp. 38–45, 51).
12. Bell WH: Nonsurgical management of the pain-dysfunction syndrome. J Am Dent Assoc 79:161–170, 1969.
13. Bennett BS: Orthopedic problems of aging. J Am Geriatr Soc 9:1086–1091, 1961.
14. Benoit PW: Effects of local anesthetics on skeletal muscle. Anat Rec 169:276–277, 1971.
15. Benoit PW: Reversible skeletal muscle damage after administration of local anesthetics with and without epinephrine. J Oral Surg 36:198–201, 1978.
16. Benoit PW: Microscarring in skeletal muscle after repeated exposures to lidocaine with epinephrine. J Oral Surg 36:530–533, 1978.
17. Benoit PW, Belt WD: Some effects of local anesthetic agents on skeletal muscle. Exp Neurol 34:264–278, 1972.
18. Benoit PW, Yagiela JA, Fort NF: Pharmacologic correlation between local anesthetic-induced myotoxicity and disturbances of intracellular calcium distribution. Toxicol Appl Pharmacol 52:187–198, 1980.
19. Berges PU: Myofascial pain syndromes. Postgrad Med 53:161–168, 1973.
20. Bonica JJ: Management of myofascial pain syndromes in general practice. JAMA 164:732–738, 1957.
21. Boos R: Pannikolose und Pannikulitis. In Fortbildungskurse für Rheumatologie, Der Weichteilrheumatismus, edited by G. Kaganas, W. Müller, and F. Wagenhäuser, Vol. 1. S. Karger, Basel, 1971 (pp. 35–48).
22. Brand PW, Beach RB, Thompson DE: Relative tension and potential excursion of muscles in the forearm and hand. J Hand Surg 6:209–219, 1981.
23. Bronstein SL, Ryan DE, Solomons CC, et al.: Dantrolene sodium in the management of patients at risk from malignant hyperthermia. J Oral Surg 37:719–724, 1979.
24. Brun A: Effect of procaine, carbocaine and xylocaine on cutaneous muscle in rabbits and mice. Acta Anaesthesiol Scand 3:59–73, 1959.
25. Burke GW, Jr., Fedison JR, Jones CR: Muscle degeneration produced by local anesthetics. Va Dent J 49:33–37, 1972.
26. Cailliet, R: Soft Tissue Pain and Disability. F.A. Davis, Philadelphia, 1977 (pp. 160, 161).
27. Ibid. (p. 83).
28. Cardenas DD, Stolov WC, Hardy MS: Muscle fiber number in immobilization atrophy. Arch Phys Med Rehabil 58:423–426, 1977.
29. Cattell McK, Hoagland H: Response of tactile receptors to intermittent stimulation. J Physiol 72:392–404, 1931.
30. Chan P: Finger Acupressure. Ballantine Books, New York, 1975.
31. Chernick WS: Local anesthetics, Chapter 11. In Drill's Pharmacology in Medicine, edited by J.R. DiPalma, Ed. 4, McGraw-Hill, New York, 1971 (pp. 190–193, 196–199).
32. Condouris GA: Local anesthetics as modulators of neural information, In Advances in Pain Research and Therapy, edited by J.J. Bonica, D. Albe-Fessard, Vol. 1. Raven Press, New York, 1976 (pp. 663–667).
33. Condouris GA, Shakalis A: The suppression of

repetitive activity in the axon. *Epilepsia* 10:211–217, 1969.

34. Consumer Reports: Caffeine: how to consume less. *Consumer Reports* 597–599, October, 1981.
35. Copeman WSC, Ackerman WL: "Fibrositis" of the back. *Quarterly J Med* 13:37–51, 1944.
36. Covino BG: Local anesthesia (Part One). *N Engl J Med* 286:975–983, 1972.
37. Covino BG: Local anesthesia (Part Two). *N Engl J Med* 286:1035–1042, 1972.
38. Cyriax JH: Clinical applications of massage, Chapter 7. In *Manipulation, Traction and Massage*, edited by J.B. Rogoff, Ed. 2. Williams & Wilkins, Baltimore, 1980 (pp. 152–155).
39. Dalessio DJ; *Wolff's Headache and Other Head Pain*, Ed. 3. Oxford University Press, New York, 1972 (p. 553).
40. de Jong RH: *Local anesthetics*, Ed. 2. Charles C Thomas, Springfield, Ill. 1977 (p. 273).
41. Dexter JR, Simons DG: Local twitch response in human muscle evoked by palpation and needle penetration of a trigger point. *Arch Phys Med Rehabil* 62:521, 1981.
42. Eisler P: *Die Muskeln des Stammes*. Gustav Fischer, Jena, 1912.
43. Fordyce WE: *Behavioral Methods for Chronic Pain and Illness*. C.V. Mosby, St. Louis, 1976.
44. Friedman M, Dougherty R, Nelson SR, et al.: Acute effects of an aerosol hair spray on tracheal mucociliary transport. *Am Rev Respir Dis* 116:281–286, 1977.
45. Frost FA, Jessen B, Siggaard-Andersen J: A control, double-blind comparison of mepivacaine injection *versus* saline injection for myofascial pain. *Lancet* 1:499–501, 1980.
46. Gardner DA: The use of ethyl chloride spray to relieve somatic pain. *JAOA* 49:525–528, 1950.
47. Gershon-Cohen J: Personal communication, 1965.
48. Gilliland BC: Introduction to clinical immunology, Chapter 61. In *Principles of Internal Medicine*, edited by K.J. Isselbacher, R.D. Adams, E. Braunwald, et al., Ed. 9. McGraw-Hill, New York, 1980.
49. Giosa N: Procaine for malignant hyperthermia *N Engl J Med* 292:869–870, 1975.
50. Gold H, Travell J: Cornell conference on therapy: management of pain due to muscle spasm. *NY State J Med* 45:2085–2097, 1945 (pp. 2095–2096).
51. Good MG: Acroparaesthesia—an idiopathic myalgia of elbow. *Edinburgh Med J* 56:366–368, 1949.
52. Good MG: The role of skeletal muscles in the pathogenesis of diseases. *Acta Med Scand* 138:285–292, 1950.
53. Goodman LS, Gilman A: *The Pharmacological Basis of Therapeutics*, Ed. 4. Macmillan, London, 1970 (pp. 372–376, 382, 1662–1663).
54. Goodman LS, Gilman A: *The Pharmacological Basis of Therepautics*, Ed. 6. Macmillan, New York, 1980 (p. 308).
55. Gottlieb NL, Riskin WG: Complications of local corticosteroid injections. *JAMA* 243:1547–1548, 1980.
56. Gray H: *Anatomy of the Human Body*, edited by C.M. Goss, American Ed. 29. Lea & Febiger, Philadelphia, 1973.
57. Gunn CC: Personal communication, 1982.
58. Gunn CC, Milbrandt WE: Early and subtle signs in low-back sprain. *Spine* 3:267–281, 1978.
59. Hagbarth KE, Finer B: The plasticity of human withdrawal reflexes to noxious skin stimuli in lower limbs. *Prog Brain Res* 1:65–78, 1963.
60. Halkovich LR, Personius WJ, Clamann HP, et al.: Effect of Fluori-Methane spray on passive hip flexion. *Phys Ther* 61:185–189, 1981.
61. Hameroff SR, Crago BR, Blitt CD, et al.: Comparison of bupivacaine, etidocaine, and saline for trigger-point therapy. *Anesth Analg* 60:752–755, 1981.
62. Harrison GG: The effect of procaine and curare on the initiation of anesthetic-induced malignant hyperpyrexia. In *International Symposium on Malignant Hyperthermia*, edited by R.A. Gordon, B.A. Britt, W. Kalow. Charles C Thomas, Springfield, Ill., 1973 (pp. 271–286).
63. Harvey AM; The actions of procaine on neuromuscular transmission. *Bull Johns Hopkins Hosp* 65:223–238, 1939.
64. Hill AV: The mechanics of voluntary muscle. *Lancet* 2:947–951, 1951.
65. Irwin Y, Wagenvoord J: *Shiatzu*. J.B. Lippincott, Philadelphia, 1976.
66. Jackson R: *The Cervical Syndrome*, Ed. 4. Charles C Thomas, Springfield, Ill., 1977 (pp. 310, 311).
67. Kelly M: New light on the painful shoulder. *Med J Aust* 1:488–493, 1942 (Case 2, p. 489).
68. Knott M, Voss DE: *Proprioceptive Neuromuscular Facilitation*, Ed. 2. Harper & Row, New York, 1968 (pp. 97–99).
69. Kraft GH, Johnson EW, LeBan MM: The fibrositis syndrome. *Arch Phys Med* 49:155–162, 1968.
70. Kraus H: The use of surface anesthesia in the treatment of painful motion. *JAMA* 16:2582–2583, 1941.
71. Kraus H: *Clinical Treatment of Back and Neck Pain*. McGraw-Hill, New York, 1970.
72. Kugelberg E, Hagbarth KE: Spinal mechanism of the abdominal and erector spinae skin reflexes. *Brain* 81:290–304, 1958.
73. Laskin DM: Etiology of the pain-dysfunction syndrome. *J Am Dent Assoc* 79:147–153, 1969.
74. Lewit K: The needle effect in the relief of myofascial pain. *Pain* 6:83–90, 1979.
75. Lewit K: Muskelfazilitations- und Inhibitionstechniken in der Manuellen Medizin. Teil II. Postisometrische Muskelrelaxation. *Manuellen Med* 19:12–22, 1981.
76. Liberson WT: Personal communication, 1979.
77. Lloyd DPC: Integrative pattern of excitation and inhibition in two-neuron reflex arcs. *J Neurophysiol* 9:421–438, 1946.
78. Lundervold AJS: Electromyographic investigations during sedentary work, especially typewriting. *Br J Phys Med* 14:32–36, 1951.
79. Macdonald AJR: Abnormally tender muscle regions and associated painful movements. *Pain* 8:197–205, 1980.
80. Maigne R: Low back pain of thoracolumbar origin. *Arch Phys Med Rehabil* 61:389–395, 1980.
81. Margoles MS: Letter to the editor. *Pain* 8:115–117, 1980.
82. McKeag PW: Fibrositis and panniculitis. *Br J Phys Med* 8:107–109, 1933.

83. McLaughlin CW, Jr.: Procaine infiltration in treatment of acute sprains. *Milit Surg* 97:457–460, 1945.

84. Melzack R: *The Puzzle of Pain.* Basic Books, New York, 1973 (pp. 153–190).

85. Melzack R: The McGill pain questionnaire: major properties and scoring methods. *Pain* 1:277–299, 1975.

86. Melzack R: Myofascial trigger points: relation to acupuncture and mechanisms of pain. *Arch Phys Med Rehabil* 62:114–117, 1981.

87. Melzack R, Guite S, Gonshor A: Relief of dental pain by ice massage of the hand. *Can Med Assoc J* 122:189–191, 1980.

88. Melzack R, Jeans ME, Stratford JG, et al.: Ice massage and transcutaneous electrical stimulation: comparison of treatment for low-back pain. *Pain* 9:209–217, 1980.

89. Mennell JM: The therapeutic use of cold. *JAOA* 74:1146–1157, 1975.

90. Mennell J: Spray-stretch for relief of pain from muscle spasm and myofascial trigger points. *J Am Podiatry Assoc* 66:873–876, 1976.

91. Meyers FH, Jawetz E, Goldfien A: *Review of Medical Pharmacology,* Ed. 7. Lange Medical Publications, Los Altos, CA, 1980.

92. Modell W, Travell J, et al.: Treatment of painful disorders of skeletal muscle. *NY State J Med* 48:2050–2059, 1948.

93. Modell W, Travell J, Kraus H, et al.: Relief of pain by ethyl chloride spray. *NY State J Med* 52:1550–1558, 1952.

94. Moldofsky H, Scarisbrick P, England R, et al.: Musculoskeletal symptoms and non-REM sleep disturbance in patients with "fibrositis syndrome" and healthy subjects. *Psychosom Med* 37:341–351, 1975.

95. Morgan GJ Jr.: Panniculitis and erythema nodosum, Chapter 75. In *Textbook of Rheumatology,* edited by W.N. Kelley, E.D. Harris, S. Ruddy, et al., Vol. 2. W.B. Saunders, Philadelphia, 1981 (pp. 1203–1207).

96. Moulds RFW, Denborough MA: Biochemical basis of malignant hyperpyrexia. *Br Med J* 2:241–244, 1974.

97. Nagler JH: Injection treatment of sprains. *Milit Surg* 96:528–529, 1945.

98. Neal HA, Peterson LJ, DeVore M: Survival of an oral surgery patient with malignant hyperthermia. *J Oral Surg* 33:953–960, 1975.

99. Nel H: Myofascial pain-dysfunction syndrome. *J Prosthet Dent* 40:438–441, 1978.

100. Nielsen AJ; Personal communication, 1981.

101. Novich MM: Physical therapy in treatment of athletic injuries. *Tex State J Med* 61:672–674, 1965.

102. Paterson JW, Sudlow MF, Walker SR: Blood-levels of fluorinated hydrocarbons in asthmatic patients after inhalation of pressurised aerosols. *Lancet* 2:565–568, 1971.

103. Patterson WR: Personal communication, 1982.

104. Patton IJ, Williamson JA: Fibrositis as a factor in the differential diagnosis of visceral pain. *Can Med Assoc J* 58:162–166, 1948.

104a. *Physician's Desk Reference.* Medical Economics Company, Oradell, NJ, 1982 (p. 964).

105. Pizzolato P, Mannheimer W: *Histopathologic Effects of Local Anesthetic Drugs and Related Substances.* Charles C Thomas, Springfield, Ill., 1961 (pp. 40, 41, 60, 71).

106. Prudden B: *Pain Erasure: The Bonnie Prudden Way.* M. Evans & Co., New York, 1980 (pp. 18, 19).

107. Rasch PJ, Burke RK: *Kinesiology and Applied Anatomy,* Ed. 6. Lea & Febiger, Philadelphia, 1978 (pp. 46, 47).

107a. Reynolds MD: The development of the concept of fibrositis. *J Hist Med Allied Sci* (In press) 1983.

108. Richards RK: Effects of vitamin C deficiency and starvation upon the toxicity of procaine. *Anesth Analg* 26:22–29, 1947.

109. Rinzler SH, Stein I, Bakst H, et al.: Blocking effect of ethyl chloride on cardiac pain induced by ergonovine. *Proc Soc Exp Biol Med* 85:329–333, 1954.

110. Rinzler SH, Travell J: Therapy directed at the somatic component of cardiac pain. *Am Heart J* 35:248–268, 1948 (p. 250).

111. Ritchie JM, Ritchie BR: Local anesthetics: effect of pH on activity. *Science* 162:1394–1395, 1968.

112. Rubin D: An approach to the management of myofascial trigger point syndromes. *Arch Phys Med Rehabil* 62:107–110, 1981.

112a. Simons DG: Muscle pain syndromes—parts I and II. *Am J Phys Med* 54:289–311, 1975, and 55:15–42, 1976.

113. Simons DG: Electrogenic nature of palpable bands and "Jump Sign" associated with myofascial trigger points. In *Advances in Pain Research and Therapy,* edited by J.J. Bonica, D. Albe-Fessard. Raven Press, New York, 1976 (pp. 913–918).

114. Simons DG, Dexter JR: Unpublished data. [LTR Paper], 1982.

115. Smith ER, Feagans WM, Belt WD, et al.: Tissue reactions to local anesthetic drugs. *Int Assoc Dent Res, Abstract* 684:211, 1969.

116. Sokolov Ye N: *Perception and The Conditioned Reflex.* Macmillan, New York, 1963.

117. Sola AE, Kuitert JH: Myofascial trigger point pain in the neck and shoulder girdle. *Northwest Med* 54:980–984, 1955.

118. Stern S, Keren A: Extreme sinus bradycardia following routine venipuncture. *JAMA* 239:403–404, 1978.

119. Sternbach RA: *Pain Patients.* Academic Press, N.Y., 1974 (pp. 5–11).

120. Strobel GE: Treatment of anaesthetic-induced malignant hyperpyrexia. *Lancet* 1:40, 1971.

121. Taverner D: Alleviation of postherpetic neuralgia. *Lancet* 2:671–673, 1960.

122. Telling WHM: The clinical importance of fibrositis in general practice. *Br Med J* 1:689–692, 1935.

123. Tizes R: Cardiac arrest following routine venipuncture. *JAMA* 236:1846–1847, 1976.

124. Travell J: Rapid relief of acute "stiff neck" by ethyl chloride spray. *J Am Med Wom Assoc* 4:89–95, 1949.

125. Travell J: Basis for the multiple uses of local block of somatic trigger areas (procaine infiltration and ethyl chloride spray). *Miss Valley Med J* 71:13–22, 1949.

126. Travell J: Early relief of chest pain by ethyl chloride spray in acute coronary thrombosis, Case Report. *Circulation* 3:120–124, 1951.

127. Travell J: Pain mechanisms in connective tissue.

In *Connective Tissues, Transactions of the Second Conference, 1951*, edited by C. Ragan. Josiah Macy, Jr. Foundation, New York, 1952 (pp. 90, 92–94, 105, 119, 121).

128. Travell J: Ethyl chloride spray for painful muscle spasm. *Arch Phys Med Rehabil* 33:291–298, 1952.
129. Travell J: Referred pain from skeletal muscle: the pectoralis major syndrome of breast pain and soreness and the sternomastoid syndrome of headache and dizziness. *NY State J Med* 55:331–339, 1955 (pp. 332, 333).
130. Travell J: Factors affecting pain of injection. *JAMA* 158:368–371, 1955.
131. Travell J: Assessment of drugs for therapeutic efficacy. *Am J Phys Med* 34:129–140, 1955.
132. Travell J: Temporomandibular joint pain referred from muscles of the head and neck. *J Prosthet Dent* 10:745–763, 1960.
133. Travell J: Use and abuse of the muscles in housework. *J Am Women's Med Assoc* 18:159–162, 1963.
134. Travell J: *Office Hours: Day and Night*. The World Publishing Company, New York, 1968 (pp. 260, 262, 269, 270, 272, 273, 276, 283).
135. Travell J: Myofascial trigger points: clinical view. *In Advances in Pain Research and Therapy*, edited by J.J. Bonica and D. Albe-Fessard, Vol. 1. Raven Press, New York, 1976 (pp. 919–926).
136. Travell J: Identification of myofascial trigger point syndromes: a case of atypical facial neuralgia. *Arch Phys Med Rehabil* 62:100–106, 1981.
137. Travell J, Bigelow NH: Role of somatic trigger areas in the patterns of hysteria. *Psychosom Med* 9:353–363, 1947.
138. Travell J, Koprowska I, Hirsch BB, *et al.*: Effect of ethyl chloride spray on thermal burns. *J Pharmacol Exp Ther* 101:36, 1951.
139. Travell J, Rinzler SH: Influence of ethyl chloride spray on deep pain and ischemic contraction of muscle. *Fed Proc* 8:339, 1949.
140. Vandam LD: Local anesthetics, I. *N Engl J Med* 263:748–750, 1960.
141. Vandam LD: Local anesthetics, II. *N Engl J Med* 263:963–965, 1960.
142. Vogler P, Kraus H: *Periostbehandlung, Kolonbehandlung: Zwei reflextherapeutische Methoden*. George Thieme, Leipzig, 1975 (pp. 52–69).
143. Voss H: Tabelle der Muskelwichte des Mannes, berechnet und zusammengestellt nach der Untersuchungen von W. Thiele (1884). *Anat Anz* 103:356–360, 1956.
144. Walpin LA: Bedroom posture: the critical role of a unique pillow in relieving upper spine and shoulder girdle pain. *Arch Phys Med Rehabil* 58:507, 1977.
145. Weber A: The mechanism of the action of caffeine on sarcoplasmic reticulum. *J Gen Physiol* 52:760–772, 1969.
146. Weber A, Herz R: The relationship between caffeine contracture of intact muscle and the effect of caffeine on reticulum. *J Gen Physiol* 52:750–759, 1969.
147. Weber EF: Ueber die Längenverhältnisse der Fleischfasern der Muskeln in Allgemeinen. *Berichte über die Verhandlungen der Königlich Sächsischen Gesellschaft der Wissenschaften Zu Leipzig* 3:63–86, 1851.
148. Weeks VD, Travell J: Postural vertigo due to trigger areas in the sternocleidomastoid muscle. *J Pediatr* 47:315–327, 1955.
149. Weeks VD, Travel J: How to give painless injections. In *A.M.A. Scientific Exhibits 1957*. Grune & Stratton, New York, 1957 (pp. 318–322).
150. Williams HL, Elkins EC: Myalgia of the head. *Arch Phys Ther* 23:14–22, 1942.
151. Willis WD, Jr., Grossman RG: *Medical Neurobiology*. C.V. Mosby, Saint Louis, 1973 (p. 103).
152. Wilson TS: Manipulative treatment of subacute and chronic fibrositis. *Br Med J* 1:298–302, 1936.
153. Yagiela JA, Benoit PW, Buoncristiani RD, *et al.*: Comparison of myotoxic effects of lidocaine with epinephrine in rats and humans. *Anesth Analg* 60:471–480, 1981.
154. Zohn DA, Mennell J McM: *Musculoskeletal Pain: Diagnosis and Physical Treatment*. Little, Brown and Company, Boston, 1976 (pp. 126–129, 190–193).

Suppliers

Bayer Timed-release Aspirin, Glenbrook Laboratories, 90 Park Ave., New York, NY 10016

Benadryl, Parke-Davis, 201 Tabor Road, Morris Plains, NJ 07950

Cervipillo, TRU-EZE Mfg. Co., 27635 Diaz, Temecula, CA 92390

Dantrium, Norwich-Eaton Pharmaceuticals, 13–27 Eaton Ave., Norwich, NY 13815

Dramamine, Searle Pharmaceuticals, Inc., Box 5110, Chicago, IL 60680

Ecotrin, Smith Kline & French Laboratories, Menley & James Laboratories, P.O. Box 8082, Philadelphia, PA 19101

Esgic, Gilbert Laboratories, 31 Fairmont Ave., Chester, NJ 07930

Fluori-Methane and ethyl chloride spray, Gebauer Chemical Co., 9410 St. Catherine Ave., Cleveland, OH 44104

Hydrocollator Steam Pack, Chattanooga Corporation, 101 Memorial Drive, Chatanooga, TN 37405

Medco-sonlator, Medco Products Co., Inc., P.O. Box 50070, Tulsa, OK 74150

Phenergan, Wyeth Laboratories, P.O. Box 8299, Philadelphia, PA 19101

Potaba, Glenwood, Inc., 83 N. Summit St. Tenafly, NJ 07670

Rocker, Carolina, P and P Chair Company, Drawer 429, Asheboro, N.C. 27203

Tylenol, McNeil Pharmaceutical, McNeiLab, Spring House, PA 19477

Valium, Roche Laboratories, Nutley, NJ 07110

Wal-Pil-O, RoLoke Co., Box 24DD3, West Los Angeles, CA 90024

CHAPTER 4
Perpetuating Factors

HIGHLIGHTS: **MECHANICAL STRESSES** perpetuate trigger points (TPs) in most patients with persistent myofascial pain syndromes. The most common sources of such physical stress are skeletal asymmetry and disproportion. Asymmetries include a short leg—a 0.5 cm (3/16 in) difference can be critical—and a small hemipelvis. Skeletal disproportions are a long second metatarsal bone (Dudley J. Morton foot) and short upper arms. Other sources of muscular stress, such as misfitting furniture, poor posture, abuse of muscles, constricting pressure on muscles, and prolonged immobility, are frequently significant and nearly always correctable. **NUTRITIONAL INADEQUACIES**, are often crucial perpetuating factors. Low "normal" levels of vitamins B_1, B_6, B_{12} and/or folic acid, are suboptimal, and frequently are responsible when only transitory relief is obtained by specific myofascial treatment of involved muscles. Vitamin C deficiency causes postexercise stiffness and increases bleeding at sites of injection; low levels of this vitamin are the rule in smokers. Vitamin inadequacies are confirmed by measuring blood serum levels; symptoms usually respond to oral supplements. Adequate calcium, potassium, iron, and several trace minerals also are essential for normal muscle function. Borderline anemia is an important factor. **METABOLIC AND ENDOCRINE INADEQUACIES** that commonly perpetuate TPs are hypometabolism due to suboptimal thyroid function, hyperuricemia and hypoglycemia. Apparently, whatever impairs muscle metabolism, including anemia or hypoxia, perpetuates TPs. **PSYCHOLOGICAL FACTORS** that inhibit rapid recovery include depression, tension caused by anxiety, the "good sport" syndrome, secondary gain, and sick behavior. **CHRONIC INFECTION** due to either viral or bacterial disease, and some parasitic infestations, can prevent recovery from myofascial pain syndromes. **OTHER FACTORS**, such as allergy, impaired sleep, radiculopathy and chronic visceral disease, prolong the treatment needed for recovery. The routine **SCREENING LABORATORY TESTS** that are most useful to identify perpetuating factors are serum vitamin levels, a blood chemistry profile, complete blood count with indices, the erythrocyte sedimentation rate, and thyroid hormone levels (T_3 and T_4 by radioimmunoassay).

CLINICAL IMPORTANCE

That it is important to correct perpetuating factors is illustrated by the apocryphal story of the man who stepped in a hole in the sidewalk and broke his leg. He was treated and the bones of his leg healed, but 2 months later he stepped in the same hole and again broke the leg. *No one had patched the hole.* If we treat myofascial pain syndromes without "patching the holes" by not correcting the multiple perpetuating factors, the patient is doomed to endless cycles of treatment and relapse. For patients who have suffered myofascial pain for many months or years, we find it necessary to spend most of our time patching holes. This is *the most important single chapter* in this manual; it concerns the most neglected part of the management of myofascial pain syndromes.

The answer to the question, "How long will the beneficial results of specific myofascial therapy last?," depends largely on what perpetuating factors remain unresolved. In the absence of such factors, the muscle with fully inactivated trigger points (TPs) should be no more susceptible to TP activation than the normal muscle was originally.

One may view perpetuating factors also as predisposing factors, since their presence tends to make the muscles more susceptible to the activation of TPs.

The present chapter concerns the group of mechanical and biochemical factors that perpetuate existing TPs. The previous chapter discussed the common mechanical stresses that initiate TPs by overloading muscles (Section 7), and those that activate latent TPs to cause pain (Section 8). Usually, one stress activates the TP, then other factors perpetuate it. In some patients, these perpetuating factors are so important that their elimination results in *complete* relief of the pain without any local treatment of the muscles.

MECHANICAL STRESS

Three types of mechanical stresses are considered below: structural inadequacies, postural stresses, and constriction of muscle.

Structural Inadequacies

A common structural inadequacy is body asymmetry that creates a difference in the length of the lower limbs. Both a short leg and a small hemipelvis often perpetuate myofascial TPs. Patients with pain aggravated by standing or walking may have a leg-length discrepancy, whereas those with sitting intolerance may have a small hemi-pelvis. Other structural stresses result from the relationship of a long second and a short first metatarsal bone, or from short upper arms in relation to torso height.

Short Leg. A short leg is a frequent and troublesome perpetuator of myofascial TPs, yet one that can be corrected easily. A discrepancy in leg length of 1.3 cm (½ in) may cause no symptoms throughout a lifetime, if myofascial TPs are never activated by some traumatic event. However, a discrepancy of 0.5 cm (³⁄₁₆ in), if uncorrected, can perpetuate myofascial TPs, e.g. in the quadratus lumborum muscle, after TPs have been activated by gross or obscure trauma. Beal[31] noted that the most frequent history of a patient with pain due to a short leg is recurrent backache precipitated by strain.

Leg-length discrepancy occurs frequently. Among 100 asymptomatic soldiers in a study reported by Rush and Steiner,[243] and further analyzed by Beal,[31] 71% had a leg-length difference of at least 0.16 cm (¹⁄₁₆ in); 33% had a difference of more than 0.5 cm (³⁄₁₆ in), and 4% had a difference in leg length of at least 1.1 cm (⁷⁄₁₆ in). In another study,[206] 7% of 72 control (pain-free) patients had a difference of 1.3 cm (½ in) or more. In a group[214] of 1446 schoolchildren between the ages of 5 and 17 years, 80% had a discrepancy of at least 0.16 cm (¹⁄₁₆ in) when measured by an X-ray technique, and 3.4% of them had a difference of 1.3 cm (½ in), or greater. The likelihood of leg-length discrepancy increases with a child's age. In a group of elementary schoolchildren,[157] 75% showed a measurable leg-length difference; this increased to 92% for a group of senior high school students with the same technique of measurement. Compensation generally developed as curvatures of the spine without reduction of the asymmetry.[213] Uncorrected differences tend to grow larger as children become bigger;[157] surprisingly, two studies reported that leg-length differences corrected during childhood often became smaller.[158, 227]

The short leg imposes a strain on the musculature because the muscles attempt to correct the resulting distortions of axial alignment (functional scoliosis) and to maintain the head and shoulders balanced over the feet. A short lower extremity tilts the pelvis down on the same side. *If* there are no other distortions of axial alignment, the lumbar spine is then tilted toward the side of the short leg, and a compensatory scoliosis returns the shoulders toward the midline. In our experience, if the leg-length difference is about 1 cm (⅜ in) or less, the shoulder on the side opposite to the short leg is lower. Judovich and Bates[147] associated this postural relationship with a C-type scoliosis. In this case, raising the left heel elevates the right shoulder.

When the difference in leg length is 1.3 cm (½ in) or more, we find that the shoulder on the same side as the short leg usually sags. The spine then has an S-type scoliosis, and raising the heel on the short side elevates the sagging homolateral shoulder.[147] The muscle that primarily suffers from this axial deviation at the lumbar level is the quadratus lumborum[142, 268, 296] on one or both sides. In our experience, TP involvement of the quadratus lumborum is by far the most commonly overlooked source of low back pain.[296] Furthermore, the tilted shoulder-girdle axis requires constant compensation by neck muscles to maintain the head erect and eyes level.[183] This perpetuates TPs in the scalene, levator scapulae, sternocleidomastoid and upper trapezius muscles, the last two of which often cause headache.[290] The sternocleidomastoid and upper trapezius muscles may induce satellite TPs in the masticatory muscles, which further contribute to headache and facial pain.

Just as a small arc of excursion near the central axis of a seesaw causes a large movement at its ends, a small disparity of 0.6 cm (¼ in) at the hip joints may cause a lowering of the shoulder of about 2.5 cm (1 in) at the full width of the shoulders.[290]

Unfortunately, the linkage between a short leg and the resultant muscular strain is not always simple. Two other conditions may mimic, compensate for, or exaggerate the effects of a short leg. One condition is an abrupt lateral angulation of the lumbar spine, usually between the last lumbar and the first sacral vertebrae, or at the next higher intervertebral joint. In such idiopathic scoliosis, the distortion of vertebral alignment is likely to include a major rotary component.

The other condition is tilting of the sacrum in relation to the pelvis. The sacrum appears to be askew in the pelvis, which can happen when the pelvis is twisted, rotating one iliac bone up and the other down. For whatever reason, as seen on an anteroposterior (AP) radiograph of the pelvis in the standing subject, the base of the sacrum appears tilted at an angle to the horizontal axis of the sacroiliac joints, which passes through the iliac bones. This sacral tilt also causes the lumbar spine to be tipped toward one side when the pelvis appears level.[31, 147, 214]

Thus, the patient may have any combination of three independent deviations: pelvic tilt due to a short leg, angulation of the lumbar spine, or sacral tilt. The relationship between the TP shortening of the quadratus lumborum and each of the last two distortions of axial alignment of the lumbosacral spine have not been critically evaluated. Any or all of these anatomic variations may be strongly influenced by TP shortening of the quadratus lumborum muscle.

A radiographic study of 1446 schoolchildren[214] looked for 14 different combinations of a straight spine, a scoliotic spine, a tilted pelvis due to a short leg, angulation of the lumbar spine, and/or a tilt of the sacrum. By far the most common finding was simply a short leg without lumbar angulation or tilt of the sacrum in the pelvis; it produced a smooth, compensatory, lateral and rotary lumbar scoliosis.

Some authors have described angulation of the lumbar spine as the second-stage compensation, and the sacral tilt as third-stage compensation for the pelvic tilt caused by a short leg.[31] However, the data from the 3-year longitudinal study of more than 1400 schoolchildren mentioned above[214] reported the presence of lumbar angulation and/or sacral tilt in the absence of a short leg, which seriously weakens this progression argument.

Whether or not the short leg should be corrected depends, first, on whether the patient has pain due to myofascial TPs that are being perpetuated by it, and second, on whether the short leg produces a tilt of the pelvis that is not compensated (or is sometimes overcompensated) by a sacral tilt and/or angulation of the lumbar spine. Only if the answer to both questions is yes should the leg-length discrepancy be corrected.

No relation was found[228] in standing subjects, between a short leg and displacement of the center of gravity of the pelvis, nor between a short leg and pelvic rotation.

How Small a Difference in Leg Length Can Be Detected? The answer appears to depend on which method is used for the measurement. Rush and Steiner[243] reported differences in leg length of 0.16 cm (less than ⅟₁₆ in) using a brace to position the subject during radiographic measurement. Pearson, et al.[214] also used a standing radiographic technique, but without fixed positioning, and they reported differences of 0.16 cm (⅟₁₆ in). However, neither presented data on test reproducibility. Klein[157] measured the correction needed beneath one heel to level the posterior superior iliac spines as determined by palpation and concluded that this technique provided a 95% agreement with X-rays when the leg-length difference was 0.6 cm (¼ in) or more.

Ford and Goodman[102] compared dis-

106 Myofascial Pain and Dysfunction: Trigger Point Manual

crepancy in leg length in 443 patients seen for low back pain. They compared an unspecified tape measure technique with a standing anteroposterior X-ray examination, knees extended. All measurements were made to the nearest ¼ in (0.6 cm). The X-ray films were measured at the head of the femur and the top of the ilium. They found that the 7.7% of the patients who had equal leg length by tape measure showed 0.6-cm (¼-in) to 1.9-cm (¾-in) discrepancies by radiography. Conversely, the 2% who showed a *level* pelvis in the standing film, when supine, had as much as a 1.3-cm (½-in) difference by tape measurement from the anterior superior iliac spine to the medial malleolus. Because of these differences in results, the authors recommended that a leg-length discrepancy of less than 0.6 cm (¼ in) be disregarded.

A study[207] of the reproducibility of tape measurements made from the anterior superior iliac spine to the tip of the medial malleolus on the same patients by four observers concluded that a difference of 0.6 cm (¼ in) in leg length is not reliably detectable, but a difference of 1.3 cm (½ in) is meaningful.

Two commonly used techniques for measuring leg-length discrepancy are among the least reliable. One is the tape measure technique just described. The other method measures the longitudinal distance between comparable points on the medial malleoli in the supine patient with the knees straight.[31] This second test is especially vulnerable to error caused by TP shortening of one quadratus lumborum muscle. The patient is non-weight bearing in both tests, and both are subject to distortion introduced by movements at the hip joint, as demonstrated by the leg-lengthening and leg-shortening maneuvers.[46]

Although no test-retest reproducibility measurements were reported except in the tape measure study, radiographic measurement appears to be more accurate than manual methods, if conditions of examination are adequately controlled. The clinical estimation by trial heel lifts of the correction needed to level the hips of the standing patient (described below) appears to be significantly more accurate than supine tape measurement of the discrepancy in leg length.

What Minimum Difference in Leg Length Is Clinically Significant? The answer seems to depend largely on the accuracy with which the discrepancy in leg length was measured.

In the study[243] of 1000 soldiers with backache, whose leg lengths were measured radiographically, using a positioning device and reporting differences as small as 0.1 cm, a discrepancy of 0.5 cm (³⁄₁₆ in) or more was significantly correlated with symptoms and disability. In the study of 443 low-back-pain patients by Ford and Goodman[102] in which they used both a tape measure and a standing radiographic technique, they concluded that a difference of 0.6 cm (¼ in) or more should be corrected by elevating the heel in those patients with low back pain. Using an X-ray technique[147] to determine when the iliac crests were level, the correction of 1 cm (⅜ in) or more alleviated pain along the cervicodorsal and dorsolumbar spine, but not when the pain had a sciatic distribution. The authors[147] warned not to correct a short leg when the lumbar spine tilted away from the short leg.

Stoddard[275] found that 17 of 100 patients with low back pain had 1.3 cm (½ in) or more shortening of one leg, as contrasted with only 8% of symptomless control subjects. Using a tape measure technique, Nichols[206] found that 22% of 180 patients with backache had a leg difference of 1.3 cm (½ in) or more, compared with only 7% of controls, and concluded that such a difference of 1.3 cm (½ in) or more was diagnostically significant.

Hudson, et al.[142] reported an experiment in which one normal subject who had been pain free added a 1.9 cm (¾ in) elevation to the heel of the left shoe. On the third day, the subject experienced aching in the buttocks and after 1 week, tightness and pulling in the dorsolumbar area. After 3 weeks, regular night pain was experienced in these regions. With removal of the elevation, symptoms disappeared in 2 weeks.

Gross[120] queried a group of patients with a short leg, regardless of symptoms, and found that those with a discrepancy of 1.5 cm (⁹⁄₁₆ in) or less did not regard their short leg as a problem, did not wear a lift, and did not feel unbalanced. However, those who had discrepancies of 2.0, 2.5, 3.0, 3.5 cm (¾, 1, 1³⁄₁₆, 1⅜ in) and more responded positively to all of these questions. There was one similarity: the group with a difference of 1.5 cm (⁹⁄₁₆ in) had nearly as much backache as the other groups. The opinions of orthopaedic surgeons queried in this study[120] were rather evenly divided as to whether the minimum discrepancy requiring correction was 1.5, 2.0, 2.5, 3.0, 3.5 or more than 3.5 cm.

In our experience, even in the absence of symptoms, correction of a leg-length disparity of 1.3 cm (½ in) or more is of preventive value; it reduces the likelihood of developing active TPs in the overloaded muscles. When repeated measurements consistently show a discrepancy of 0.5 cm (³⁄₁₆ in) or more in a patient with low back pain, it should be corrected.

Several studies have emphasized the clinical value of correcting the leg-length discrepancy when pain is present. Maigne[186] reported relief of intractable headaches by equalizing leg length with a heel lift. Among 1000 patients routinely screened on admission to an obstetric service,[262] 63 had a clinically evident short leg, confirmed by tape measurement. Of these 63 patients, 53 complained of either low back or flank pain for which no gynecological cause was evident; correction of the disparity in leg length by a compensatory heel lift relieved the pain in 90% of this group. Redler[227] reported that a majority of 42 patients with low back pain were relieved by correcting a 1.3–1.6 cm (½–⅝ in) leg-length discrepancy, which was determined by palpating the iliac crests in the standing patient.

Noteworthy was Redler's observation[227] that 1.3–1.9 cm (½–¾ in) leg-length discrepancies in children between 1½ and 15 years of age were outgrown (disappeared) in 7 of 11 children when leg length was equalized with a heel correction for 3–7 months. This evidence for need of a structural correction in growing children by the temporary addition of a compensatory heel lift was supported in a later 3-year study of elementary, junior and high school boys.[158] Research is needed into the mechanism by which leg-length inequalities in children disappear with correction.

How Does One Detect a Short Leg? When asked, many patients have been told that they had a short leg on a previous examination. Patients may wear a different length of pant-leg, skirt or shoe on one side. These patients often have an uneven gait that cause them to tilt to one side or to sway when walking.[31]

On first observing a patient, body asymmetry may be revealed by a difference in the size of the two halves of the face, by a tilt or lurch to one side when walking,[227] or when the patient assumes a short-leg stance—by standing either with body weight on the short leg and the foot of the long leg forward with the knee slightly flexed[227] or with the long leg placed diagonally at the side.

How Is a Short Leg Measured? When a short leg is suspected in the patient with low back pain, we recommend that the patient first be examined for quadratus lumborum TPs and, if present, that they be inactivated.[263] An attempt to measure leg-length discrepancy in the presence of TP shortening of the quadratus lumborum is likely to produce a misleading result.

The undressed patient stands with the back to the examiner and with both knees straight, preferably facing a full-length mirror. The feet are brought together and an estimate of length difference is made quickly by palpating the iliac crests or posterior superior iliac spines. An approximate correction is placed promptly beneath the short leg, making sure that the patient finds it comfortable. Pages of a pad or small magazine are convenient. The patient is engaged in conversation for a minute or two, and is encouraged to relax and let the weight settle on both feet. As the muscles are relieved of their attempt to compensate for the difference in leg length, they release their protective control and relax. It is then possible to accurately compensate any remaining leg-length inequality by adding correction until the pelvis and shoulders are level and, most importantly, the spine is straight.

To confirm the accuracy of the correction, a millimeter or two of lift may be added to see if the pelvis, and perhaps the shoulders, tip the other way due to overcorrection. Many patients are immediately aware of this unfamiliar strain.

The necessity for the correction is convincingly demonstrated to the patient by removing the correcting heel lift and then calling attention to the body distortion as seen in a full length mirror. When the correction is then briefly transferred to the long leg (doubling the discrepancy) most patients are acutely distressed by the increased crookedness of the body. The correction is quickly returned to the short side to relieve the sense of muscle strain.

Some additional points in the examination are helpful. The arm on the side of the short leg tends to hang away from the body, while the arm on the other side rests against it. Narrowing at the waist and the bulge of the hip appear greater on the side of the long leg. The border of the gluteal fold appears lower on the short side.[147, 262] Skin folds are present or more numerous in the flank of the concave side of the lumbar spine.

The flank skin may be pushed up bilaterally to bring the index fingers of the examiner as close as possible to the uppermost portion of the iliac crests, in order to compare the level on each side.[31, 45, 147, 227, 262] The most prominent bony portion of each ilium posteriorly (posterosuperior iliac spines) may be palpated and accurately located with the thumbs, and then compared visually for levelness.[45, 157, 262] Comparison of the level of the dimples that correspond approximately to the posterosuperior iliac spines is helpful when they are clearly visible. Variation in the levels of these iliac spines is sometimes more clearly revealed by having the patient lean forward 90° at the hips, while sighting across the sacrum to determine any difference in elevation between the two sides.[31, 45]

Similarly, the height of the greater trochanters can be compared.[262] In an obese patient, the trochanter is located by palpating for it while the patient flexes the thigh at the hip.[31]

The patient also may be asked to swing first one foot back and forth, then the other; the foot of the short leg is easily moved with little disturbance in body positioning, whereas swinging the long leg requires upward displacement of the pelvis on that side for the foot to clear the floor.[186]

The lumbar and thoracic spine is examined for scoliosis. If the positions of the spinous processes are difficult to determine, they may be emphasized by asking the patient to lean forward, flexing the spine slightly.

Tilting of the shoulder-girdle axis is often readily apparent in the standing patient. Accurate evaluation of shoulder tilt may be hampered when increased tension of the upper trapezius muscle on one side distorts the silhouette of the shoulders. The position of the scapulae is most accurately determined by palpating the relative levels of their lower poles. A tilt of the shoulder-girdle axis is especially important in patients with head, neck, shoulder-arm, and upper back pain.

When various indicators of disparity in leg length disagree, especially when spinal scoliosis remains after the hips are leveled, the sacrum may be tilted in the pelvis between the ilia, or the lumbar spine may be angulated. Both should be visible on a *standing* anteroposterior X-ray. Twisting of the pelvis due to rotation around its axis through the sacroiliac joints is one possible mechanism for this tilt of the sacrum in the pelvis. Pelvic twist can be detected by palpation[46, 186] and may be corrected by manipulation.[47, 295]

Supine lumbosacral or pelvic radiograms are useless to check leg-length discrepancy. Standing radiograms can significantly improve the accuracy of leg-length determination by direct measurement of the difference at the top of each femoral head, but only if certain critical caveats are observed. A *reliable* horizontal reference marker must be recorded on the film. This can be the edge of the film if it is *always* precisely positioned in a *leveled* cassette. Alternately, a level copper wire or a "U" tube filled with liquid contrast material can be placed in front of the film. The floor where the patient stands must be level and the patient's knees must be *straight*. The bare feet should be placed 8–10 cm (3–4 in) apart to minimize the effects of side sway. Some side sway may be necessary for the patient to relieve the muscle strain without bending a knee. The film should identify whether it was taken with, or without leg-length correction. Films taken without attention to these details of technique can lead to erroneous corrections that aggravate, rather than relieve pain.[31, 209]

Methods of Correcting Leg Length Inequality

The difference in leg length may be corrected temporarily by inserting the same thickness of hard felt (such as orthopaedic felt) with the front edge beveled and cut to fit inside the heel of the shoe. For a permanent correction, a cobbler increases the thickness of the heel on the short side if the heel is low, or cuts down the heel on the long side if the heel is high. With corrections of about 1.3 cm (½ in) or more, the difference should be divided between the two heels. When 1.3 cm (½ in) or more is added to the heel on one side, the sole should also be augmented. The patient with a short foot who does a lot of walking, or who is a compulsive jogger, may require a sole lift of thickness equal to the heel lift.

Discriminating patients are able to feel the reduction in muscle strain when standing, and in heel strike when walking, after the short leg is corrected. Some patients may require several days to adjust to the correction. The patient should never walk in bare feet and should have the bedroom slippers corrected. Walking on slanted surfaces, like a beach, should be avoided, because in one direction the effects of the difference in leg length are increased.

All permanent shoe corrections should be checked for their accuracy.

Small Hemipelvis. Patients with a pelvis that is small in its vertical dimension on one side tend to sit crookedly, leaning toward the small side. They often cross one knee over the other to cantilever up the low side (see Fig. 48.10A). A seesaw effect tilts the pelvis when sitting, if one side of the pelvis is smaller than the other. This tilt is magnified by the normal closeness of the weight-bearing ischial tuberosities. The effects of this tilt on the spine and muscles above the pelvis are comparable to the effects of the pelvic tilt caused by a short leg (see Fig. 48.10B). Since the pelvis is tilted similarly in both standing and sitting positions when the short leg and small hemipelvis are on the same side, the patient suffers the same symptoms whether sitting or standing. The quadratus lumborum is the muscle primarily affected by axial distortions in the lumbar region;[296] the scalene and sternocleidomastoid muscles of the neck are heavily overloaded by tilt of the upper thorax. The small hemipelvis is more neglected than the short leg as a source of spinal distortions that produce chronic muscle strain.

Lowman[184] reported that 20–30% of those examined in an orthopedic practice were found to have a small hemipelvis, which can occur separately or with a short leg, usually on the same side.

For examination, the patient should be seated on a hard, flat surface with the back and buttocks exposed, in a position to be observed from behind. The feet should be supported high enough so that the patient can slip the fingers between the thighs and the front edge of the seat. Examination of the pelvis, back and shoulders is similar to that for a short leg, with specific attention paid to scoliosis, position of the posterior superior iliac spines,[45] the relative heights of the iliac crests, and tilting of the shoulder-girdle axis.

Results of this examination can be confusing if the pelvis is twisted around the horizontal axis through the sacroiliac joints. Such an obliquity is detected by placing the thumbs on the posterior superior iliac spines and resting the hands over the crests of the ilia, pointing each index finger to an anterior superior iliac spine, fingertips at equal distances from the spines bilaterally. The seated patient rocks the pelvis backward, and the relative heights of the anterior and posterior spines are noted on each side of the pelvis. Then the patient rocks the pelvis forward for comparison. When all points on one side are lower than the corresponding points on the other side, regardless of the position of the pelvis, that half of the pelvis is smaller. If, however, one anterior spine dips much lower than the other when the pelvis rocks forward, the pelvis is twisted. This obliquity can, of itself, be a source of pain, and distorts the evaluation of a small hemipelvis; before making a final determination, the obliquity should be corrected as decribed by Bourdillon[47] and by Maigne.[187]

The amount of seated correction for a small hemipelvis is determined by adding increments of lift beneath the ischial tuberosity on the small side until the spine is straightened and the pelvis is leveled with the patient seated on a hard surface. The correction determined on a hard surface must be approximately doubled for a moderately soft chair seat, and tripled for a very soft sofa. Since the torso leans toward the short side, the weight borne on that side is increased, depressing the buttock further into the softer chair seat, as illustrated in Fig. 48.10B and C of Chapter

48. By paying attention to this strain on the muscles, many patients develop a high degree of sensitivity to body balance and learn to avoid this unnecessary seated stress.

For permanent correction, the patient uses a "sit-pad," [184] which we call a "butt lift." This may be a pad of felt of desired thickness sewn into the underwear or placed in a long back pants pocket, or may be a small magazine slipped under the low ischium when sitting. The same effect can be obtained when sitting on either a domed or scooped chair seat by sliding the hips to the side that levels the pelvis. A chair that is used regularly may be fitted with a divided pneumatic seat cushion that permits separate inflation of either half, e.g. the TWIN-REST cushion.*

Soft auto seats are a common source of poor support, which can be remedied by use of a SACRO-EASE† seat insert; usually the wide model BR is used, which provides a stable base on which to sit and firm support for the upper back. The SACRO-EASE may be tilted by placing a book or other material under one side to compensate for pelvic asymmetry. The patient should beware of unwittingly tilting the pelvis by sitting on a wallet in the back pocket,[116] or on a tilted seat in an office chair that lacks coasters under its feet on one side, or on a sideways tilted piano bench; also, the floor or stage may not be level.

Long Second Metatarsal. The patient with a Dudley J. Morton or "classic Greek" foot has a relatively long second and a short first metatarsal bone. This may perpetuate myofascial pain in the low back, thigh, knee, leg, and dorsum of the foot, with or without numbness and tingling.[292] These patients consistently give a history of weak ankles; they say they frequently have turned and sprained these joints, and had difficulty learning to ice-skate.

According to Morton,[197, 198] during normal weight bearing the first metatarsal head should carry half of the body weight; others disagree.[126] When the first metatarsal is relatively short, the second metatar-

sal bears more weight. The foot, balanced on the second metatarsal, rocks as if on a knife edge.[198] To compensate for this, most people modify their gait so that the lateral side of the heel and the medial side of the sole of the shoe show excessive wear. Usually, the foot is slightly externally rotated on heel strike, and during stance phase. The ankle rocks inward (pronates), everting the foot at the ankle, during and after the stance phase. During stance phase, the knee swings in toward the other knee as the thigh internally rotates. The syndrome, as presented by Morton,[197, 198] is well summarized and illustrated by Cailliet.[54]

This gait usually activates myofascial TPs in the posterior gluteus medius muscle, which refer pain to the low back. The rocking foot also strains the peroneus longus muscle, which activates TPs in it that refer pain to the ankle.[294] The taut bands of these TPs may entrap the peroneal nerve against the fibula immediately below its head, producing numbness and tingling across the dorsum of the foot and sometimes motor weakness with foot drop. Extension of TP activity to the posterior gluteus minimus, which externally rotates the thigh at the hip, causes posterior thigh and calf pain. Extension of TPs to the vastus medialis causes medial knee pain[294] and may progress to the buckling knee syndrome.[292] These symptoms mimic radiculopathy, a diagnosis sometimes mistakenly made in these patients.

A study[126] of 3619 Canadian enlisted men who were unselected for symptoms found that 1596 (22%) of their feet had first and second metatarsals of equal length; 2878 (40%) had a first metatarsal shorter than the second by 0.1–1.2 cm; and 2693 (38%) had a first metatarsal longer than the second 0.1–1 cm. The relative length of the metatarsals was measured from the posterior end of the calcaneus to the head of each metatarsal bone.

This syndrome is greatly aggravated by pressure from a shoe that is tight because it is too small or has a tight cap over the toes, and by high heels. Symptoms appear primarily in the shorter leg (which experiences heavier impact) even though both feet have the same disproportion of first and second metatarsal bones.

On physical examination, a relatively long second metatarsal may or may not be

---

* TWIN-REST Cushion, Fashion Able, Rocky Hill, NJ 08553.

† SACRO-EASE, McCarty's Sacro-Ease Division, 3320 Piedmont Ave, Oakland, CA 94611.

identified by a protruding second toe, since the relative lengths of the phalanges of the first and second toes are variable. The most reliable technique is a dorsoplantar radiograph during weight bearing that clearly outlines the bones of the foot. Flexing both the first and second toes at the metatarsophalangeal joints permits visual comparison of the relative positions of each metatarsal head.

Although Morton[197, 198] never specifically claimed that calluses under the second metatarsal head were caused by a long bone, many authors have assumed, because of his detailed description of the weight-bearing changes, that this disproportion was responsible.

In the study of 3619 Canadian enlisted men by Harris and Beath,[126] the authors displayed graphically the concentration of weight borne throughout the plantar surface of the foot and related this to the relative lengths of the first and second metatarsals, as determined by foot X-rays, and to callus formation. Concentration of weight under the central metatarsal heads correlated well with callus formation, but showed no convincing relation to the relative lengths of the first and second metatarsals. Of the 35 feet showing focal concentration of weight bearing under the second to fourth metatarsal heads, 14 (40%) had short first metatarsals and 21 (60%) did not; this was also the percentage of short first metatarsals in the whole study. Apparently, some other factor was chiefly responsible for the formation of callosities under the metatarsal heads of these soldiers.

An American Army study, discussed by Bingham,[126] found that 332 of 10,000 soldiers developed painful feet during 6 months of military training. Thirty-four, or slightly more than 10%, developed symptoms attributed to the long second metatarsal syndrome of Dudley J. Morton. Of this group, 76% were returned to duty by using the shoe insert recommended by Morton.[126]

Morton[197] identified posterior displacement of the sesamoid bone proximal to the head of the first metatarsal as a cause of foot imbalance even when the first metatarsal was not significantly short in relation to the second metatarsal head. The Canadian study,[126] however, was unable to verify a correlation between posterior displacement of the sesamoids and excess weight borne by the heads of the second or the second and third metatarsals.

That the short first metatarsal configuration of the foot introduces a postural distortion that requires extra muscular effort is generally agreed.[126, 197, 198, 292] The physiological mechanisms of compensation are not fully determined. Possibilities include: increased use of the flexor hallucis muscle to increase weight bearing by the first metatarsal head;[126] rocking of the foot toward eversion (pronation with external rotation) of the foot at the ankle, which produces calluses on the medial aspect of the interphalangeal joint of the great toe; inversion (supination with inversion) of the foot, which causes callosities lateral to the head of the fifth metatarsal; and probably others.

Morton[197] recommended correction of the disproportion by inserting into the shoe a leather insole with a leather build-up of 0.3 cm (⅛ in) to 0.5 cm (³⁄₁₆ in) under the head of only the first metatarsal bone. He also added a pad of sponge rubber behind the first to fifth metatarsal heads, which supported the shafts of all five metatarsal bones. We often make the correction more simply by inserting one or two thicknesses of Kiro-Felt* directly under the head of the first metatarsal bone. In addition, often it is necessary to add a felt pad along the medial side of the heel to stabilize the foot in the shoe, since many shoes have a narrow toe and wide heel, compared to the structure of the foot. If the problem is severe enough, and the patient is willing, ankle-high shoes help to support the heel.

We have found that the added support under the short first metatarsal is usually sufficient to relieve the calluses along the sides of the feet, but may not relieve a pressure-callus problem beneath the long metatarsal heads.

Based on the Canadian study,[126] only 2% of that young group had problems with concentrated weight bearing beneath the metatarsal heads (which was highly correlated with callus formation), whereas 40% had short first metatarsal bones. On this basis, one would expect that many

---

* Dr. Scholl's Kiro-Felt, Scholl, Inc., Chicago, IL 60610.

patients with this pressure callus also would have a short first metatarsal bone. Even though the bone disproportion was not primarily responsible for the callus, it would tend to perpetuate it.

To illustrate the usefulness of this Morton correction technique, a 2-year-old child with a Dudley J. Morton type of foot imbalance was toeing-in and frequently falling over his feet. After adding first metatarsal toe pads and medial-side heel fillers, the child at once walked without toeing-in and without tripping.

The Dudley J. Morton foot is unrelated to the metatarsalgia of Morton's neuroma, described by Thomas G. Morton[3] as due to pressure on an interdigital neuroma of the plantar nerve, usually between the third and fourth metatarsal heads.

Surprisingly, TPs in the lower extremity muscles can interact with tense muscles of the head and neck to restrict movement of the latter. Release of tension in the lower extremity muscles, by inactivation of their TPs, such as those perpetuated by a short first, long second, metatarsal relationship, may at once increase a TP-restricted inter-incisal opening of the jaws by 20 or 30%.

Short Upper Arms. Shortness of the upper arms in relation to torso height is a rarely recognized, but not uncommon, source of muscle strain and perpetuation of TPs in the shoulder-girdle musculature. Short upper arms are characteristic of the body structure of the American Indian, but are not limited to this race. If the shoulder-elbow segment of the upper extremity is short in proportion to the rest of the body, when the subject is standing, the elbows do not reach the iliac crests; when the person is sitting, the elbows fail to reach the armrests of the usual chair (Fig. 6.10C). For most adults, the average armrest height from the compressed seat bottom is 22 cm (8½ in), and ranges from 18–25 cm (7–10 in).[83]

This disparity places undue stress on the shoulder-girdle elevators, thus perpetuating TPs in the upper trapezius and the levator scapulae muscles. One must be able to recognize shortness of the upper arms in patients with persistent TPs in these muscles and to make the seating corrections discussed and illustrated in Section 14 of Chapter 6.

Postural Stresses

Here we consider postural stresses due to misfitting furniture, poor posture, abuse of muscles, and immobility.

Misfitting Furniture. Prolonged sitting in a chair not designed for comfort, or in a well-designed chair used for the wrong purpose, quickly tires and strains muscles. Seating should be such that, as the muscles relax and the body tends to sag, correct posture is maintained by the chair and not by sustained effort of the muscles. The chair should do the work.

Travell[291] has listed nine common faults of most household chairs: "No support for your low back; armrests too low or too high; too scooped a backrest in its upper-portion; backrest nearly vertical; backrest short, failing to support your upper back; jackknifing effect at hips and knees; high front edge of the seat, shutting down the circulation in your legs; seat bottom soft in the center, creating a bucket effect which places the load on the outer side of your thighs, rather than on bony points in the buttocks; an excellent chair may be the wrong size for you."[291] Body proportions that are the basis for the design of comfortable chairs have been meticulously detailed.[83] The value of an adequate lumbar support is illustrated in Fig. 42.9E of Chapter 42; auto seats are among the worst offenders in this respect.

Poor Posture. This is another frequent source of chronic muscular strain that perpetuates myofascial TPs. Common examples of poor posture that contribute to continued TP activity are unphysiologic positioning at a desk or work surface (see Fig. 16.4 C and D) and head tilt resulting from poorly adjusted reading glasses (see Fig. 16.4 A and B), as described in Section 14 of Chapter 16.

Reading and copy material should be placed at eye level to avoid sustained forward tilting of the head and to relieve the posterior neck and upper back muscles of prolonged checkreining overload.[286] Correction of a kyphotic, round-shouldered posture when standing (see Fig. 42.9A, B and C, in Chapter 42) and when sitting (see Fig. 42.9 D and E) relieves the upper back and more caudal back muscles, as well as easing chronic shortening of the pectoral

muscles that results from a round-shouldered posture. Standing posture with the
weight on the heels tends to shift the head
forward as a counterweight, resulting in a
loss of the normal cervical and lumbar
lordotic curves.

Disability that continuously influences
posture, such as unilateral deafness or an
old injury that restricts range of motion,
are potent sources of habitual muscle
strain.

Other common sources of postural
strain include malpositioning of the materials with which the subject is working,
such as placing copy flat at one side without a copy stand, writing on the lap, or
using the neck and shoulder muscles to
hold the receiver of the telephone against
the ear.

Abuse of Muscles. People abuse muscles
and thus perpetuate TPs: by poor body
mechanics that render movements need-
lessly stressful, by sustained isometric
contraction or immobility of the muscles,
with too many repetitions of the same
movement, and by excessively quick and
jerky movements.

A common example of *poor body mechanics* is leaning over while twisting
sideways to lift an item from a shelf or the
floor.[286] The same effect is often produced
when a person leans over the sink to brush
the teeth, or stoops forward to get in and
out of a chair (see Fig. 48.12A) instead of
using the sit-to-stand or stand-to-sit technique (see Fig. 48.12B), as discussed in
Section 14 of Chapter 48.

Standing on one leg to put on a skirt or
trousers is likely to strain gluteal and low
back muscles; the person should sit to do
this, or at least lean the weight against a
support. When writing, pressing hard on
the paper with a small-barrelled ball-point
pen held vertically overloads intrinsic
hand muscles; using a felt-tip pen, held
flatter, is less likely to perpetuate TPs.

Troublemaking sources of *sustained
contraction* include reaching up to a typewriter keyboard that is positioned too high,
painting a ceiling, hanging drapes, holding
a chain saw or other power tool in a fixed
position, holding a rope tight on a sailboat,
or merely standing still in one place—
stiffly at military attention, or tensely im-
patient.

A sustained shortened position of the
calf muscles is caused by wearing high
heeled shoes or cowboy boots.

Immobility. Lack of movement, especially when a muscle is in the shortened
position, tends to aggravate and perpetuate
myofascial TPs. This commonly occurs:
when people sleep in a position that places
a muscle in its shortest length; when the
muscle cannot be moved through its full
range of motion due to a fracture, deformity, or articular disease; in individuals who
concentrate on an activity, such as writing
or reading, so intently that they forget to
change position regularly; when patients
have acquired habits of guarding against
movement due to pain; or because they
have been advised to restrict movement of
a part of the body.

A frequent *repetitive movement* can
overload muscles. When patients say, "I
can't do ... without it hurting," they may
be testing to see whether a certain painful
movement can be made without pain. Repeated dozens of times daily, this unconscious testing can serve as the activity
stress that is perpetuating TPs.

Dental malocclusion, bruxism, and emotional tension can interact to overload the
masticatory and neck muscles, perpetuating their TPs and producing much of the
head and face pain of the myofascial pain-
dysfunction syndrome (see Chapter 5).

Some individuals perpetuate myofascial
TPs by **jerkiness of movement.** Rapid
movements that start and stop suddenly
overstress the muscles. Optimal efficiency
is obtained by smoothly coordinated
movements, much as optimal gasoline
mileage is obtained with smooth steady
driving at a moderate pace, without sudden changes in speed. If the same distance
is covered or the same task is performed
at a faster rate, more energy is expended;
the machine is not equally efficient at all
speeds.

Constriction of Muscles

Myofascial TPs are perpetuated by prolonged constricting pressure on a muscle,
e.g. by the pressure from the strap of a
ponderous purse hung over the shoulder,[96]
or by narrow bra straps that support heavy
breasts and groove the upper trapezius.
Constriction by a garter compromises the

gastrocnemius muscle; a bra tight around the chest compresses the latissimus dorsi; a tight shirt collar or necktie, the sternocleidomastoid; and a tight belt around the waist, the paraspinal, abdominal oblique and rectus abdominis muscles. The front edge of a chair seat that is so high the feet do not rest firmly on the floor compresses the hamstring muscles; the hand should slip easily under the thigh, which assures ample clearance between the thigh and the seat.[7]

NUTRITIONAL INADEQUACIES

Nutrients of special concern in patients with myofascial pain syndromes are the water-soluble vitamins B_1, B_6, B_{12}, folic acid, vitamin C; and certain elements, calcium, iron and potassium. These will be considered individually after some general comments.

Extensive material on vitamins is presented here because they are so important to the management of myofascial pain syndromes. Nearly half of the patients whom we see with chronic myofascial pain require resolution of vitamin inadequacies for lasting relief. The complexity of this subject matches its importance. This complexity is increased by the interdependence of certain vitamins on one another, by the individual variations of human enzyme systems, and by the variable responses of individuals to metabolic distress. Although nutritional factors are not mentioned in many chapters of this manual, they **must** be considered in most patients if lasting relief of pain is to be achieved.

A vitamin is a nutrient that plays an essential role in normal body metabolism as a coenzyme to an apoenzyme (that requires the coenzyme to perform its metabolic function), but is not synthesized by the body. A need for better vitamin nutrition appears at *three levels*: vitamin inadequacy, vitamin deficiency, and vitamin dependence.

An apoenzyme that requires a lacking vitamin as a coenzyme will be least affected if the apoenzyme has a high affinity for the vitamin. Enzyme systems in which this affinity is low may be almost completely inactivated by moderate lack of the vitamin. As deficiency progresses, vitamin-dependent enzyme reactions with higher affinities also stop functioning. In

general, the reactions most essential to life tend to be eliminated last.

Vitamin **inadequacy** requires the body to make some degree of metabolic adjustment because the amount of the coenzyme (vitamin) is limited. The patient with a serum vitamin level at the low end of, but within, "normal" limits may show no metabolic evidence of deficiency, yet the level may be inadequate for optimal health. Myofascial pain syndromes are aggravated by inadequate levels of at least four B-complex vitamins, listed above.

Vitamin inadequacy apparently increases the irritability of myofascial TPs by several mechanisms: impairment of the energy metabolism needed for the contraction of muscles and increased irritability of the nervous system. The muscles behave as though neural feedback mechanisms that perpetuate TPs are augmented and as if TP-referred phenomena are intensified.

The vitamin inadequacy becomes a **deficiency** when effects due to impaired function of essential enzymes are grossly apparent, and it has already seriously involved many of the less critical enzyme functions.[23] A vitamin deficiency is established by laboratory evidence of abnormally low serum and tissue values for the vitamin, by excretion of abnormal metabolic products, and by the therapeutic effect of vitamin supplementation.

There is good reason to expect that *normal* serum vitamin levels do not assure *optimal* levels of nutrition. Persons selected as normal controls are seldom screened for the subtle symptoms of vitamin inadequacy, such as chronic pain syndromes, leg cramps, depression or loss of energy. Individuals who typically serve as normal controls were found[17] to have deficient activity of glutamic oxaloacetic transaminase and a deficiency of pyridoxal phosphate in their erythrocytes. In this "normal" group, the tissue stores of this vitamin were depleted to the point of significantly reducing at least one pyridoxal-dependent enzyme function.

This issue of average *versus* optimal vitamin nutrition takes on added significance when the availability of a vitamin coenzyme is related to the production of one of its apoenzymes. A 55–68% increase in the specific activity of erythrocyte glutamic oxaloacetic transaminase after pyridoxine therapy in 10 pyridoxine-deficient patients indicated the biosynthesis of more apoenzyme in response to an adequate supply of coenzyme.[92] Vitamin supplementation may increase the body's production of the enzymes that the vitamin activates.

In a group of 12 elderly subjects who had taken 50–300 mg of pyridoxine daily for at least 1 year,[99] the specific activity of erythrocyte glutamic oxaloacetic transaminase was remarkably constant. However, 5–11 weeks of pyridoxine supplementation were required to reach this same level in pyridoxine-deficient individuals.[99]

The measurement of circulating vitamins per se detects the vitamin inadequacy before biochemical and classical clinical signs appear. For example, the plasma ascorbate level fell to an undetectable level after 41 days of ascorbate depletion, whereas clinical signs of scurvey did not appear for 134 days.[23] Similarly, upon elimination of folate from the diet, it required only 3 weeks for depressed serum folate levels to appear, but 14–18 weeks for a biochemical defect to become apparent, and 20 weeks for the clinical symptoms to develop.[130]

Vitamin **dependence** is observed in only a few individuals who have a congenital deficiency of an enzyme that requires that vitamin as a coenzyme. This defect may require the ingestion of pharmacological, or megadosage, amounts of the vitamin to compensate for the lack of the enzyme that requires that vitamin.[138]

The five *vitamins of special importance* to myofascial pain syndromes are vitamins B_1, B_6, B_{12}, folic acid, and vitamin C. This does not imply that the others are unimportant for optimal health, only that they are less critical for the relief of myofascial TP symptoms; each vitamin fills multiple metabolic roles by serving as an essential coenzyme to several enzyme systems.

Vitamin B_1 (thiamine) is most critical as an energy vitamin and for the synthesis of neurotransmitters; the need for it increases with increased caloric expenditure by the body.

Vitamin B_6 (pyridoxine) is essential to the metabolism of many proteins including several neurotransmitters.

Cobalamins (forms of vitamin B_{12}) are critical for energy and protein metabolism.

Both cobalamins and folates are required for the synthesis of deoxyribonucleic acid (DNA), which is necessary for cell replication. Either a deficiency or an excess of folate increases central nervous system irritability; adequate amounts are essential for normal development of the central nervous system.

From the viewpoint of muscles, vitamin C reduces postexercise stiffness and corrects capillary fragility caused by lack of the vitamin. Adequate tissue levels may be extremely important to the successful management of myofascial pain syndromes in some patients, and are of importance to optimal health in all patients.

Several factors may **cause vitamin insufficiency**: (1) inadequate ingestion of the vitamin, (2) impaired absorption, (3) inadequate utilization, (4) increased metabolic requirement, (5) increased excretion, or (6) increased destruction within the body.[135, 137] Several groups of people are especially vulnerable to vitamin deficiencies: the elderly,[234] pregnant and lactating women,[21] adherents to some cultural dietary customs,[22] substance abusers (most often ethyl alcohol),[135, 314] "crash" dieters and food faddists, the economically disadvantaged, the emotionally depressed,[64] and the seriously ill—a list that adds up to a significant portion of the population. Several of these factors are likely to appear in combination, e.g. among the elderly who are poor, increasing their vulnerability to deficiency.

Vitamin nutrition of the elderly is often caught in a three-way bind: decreased nutritional intake for a number of reasons, decreased absorption that is at least partly due to folate deficiency, and increased need that is caused by the decreasing efficiency of some enzyme systems with age.

The **prevalence of unrecognized hypovitaminosis** is distressingly high. In a randomly selected municipal hospital population,[21] 105 of 120 patients (88%) had abnormally low levels of 1 or more of 11 vitamins; over half the patients were low in 2 or more vitamins. Serum folate was low in 45%; this was the commonest vitamin deficiency. Despite the low blood levels, there was a history of inadequate dietary intake in only 39% of the patients with hypovitaminosis. Moreover, hypovitaminosis was clinically apparent in only 38% of the entire group.[21]

Since the levels necessary for optimal health are unknown and the health cost of vitamin inadequacy (low normal range) is relatively unexplored, the prevalence of such vitamin inadequacy and the toll it exacts appear to be greater than is generally realized.

The *toxicity* of oil-soluble vitamins A, D and E is much greater than that of the water-soluble B-complex group. *Hypervitaminosis A* may cause bone or joint pain and severe throbbing headache, which could be confused with myofascial symptoms related to *hypovitaminosis*.[185]

No toxic effects of thiamine (vitamin B_1) administered by mouth have been reported in man. Rats ingested 100 times their daily requirement for three generations without harmful effects.[204]

Pyridoxine (vitamin B_6) doses of 1 g/kg, more than 10,000 times the daily requirement, were tolerated without ill effects by dogs, rabbits, and rats.[247]

Cyanocobalamin (vitamin B_{12}) in doses 10,000 times the daily requirement was without ill effects,[137] including one patient who had received 1 mg daily by injection for more than 1 year.

Folic acid is the only one of these four B-complex vitamins for which there is evidence of toxicity; if substantiated, this would contraindicate megadosage. Thirteen of 14 normal volunteers on 15 mg daily developed gastrointestinal symptoms or mental changes and sometimes sleep disturbances.[145] However, other investigators reported 15 mg daily as innocuous.[137]

Although megadoses of vitamin C have been identified as theoretically causing cystine and oxalate stones in the urinary tract, it is becoming apparent that patients with normal renal function can tolerate exceptionally high dosage of vitamin C. One patient took 15 g of vitamin C daily for 4 months without ill effects.[306]

When dealing with vitamin requirements, one must recognize the enormous variation in nutritional needs among individuals. For instance, 64 weaning rats of four strains were fed an exclusive diet of white bread. Individual life spans ranged from 6–144 days with weight gains of from 2–212 g. This inborn individuality has a sound biological basis; the evolutionary process could not have taken place without it.[311]

Thiamine (Vitamin B_1)

Discovery. In 1884, Takaki of Japan decreased the disastrous incidence of beriberi in the Japanese navy by adding meat, vegetables and condensed milk to the rice diet of the sailors.[204] By 1912, the therapeutic effectiveness of rice polishings had been demonstrated, and in 1936, Williams and his co-workers announced the chemical structure and synthesis of the active principle, thiamine.[299]

The active form of vitamin B_1 in the body is thiamine pyrophosphate.

Functions. As a critical link in the energy metabolism chain, thiamine is essential for one of the steps required for pyruvate to enter the Krebs citric acid cycle.[175] This step is basic to the oxidative metabolism of glucose. Thiamine also is essential to one step within the Krebs cycle. In anaerobic metabolism, it is a coenzyme for transketolase, which supports glycolytic metabolism and assists in the oxidation of glucose by providing reducing power of plasma in the vicinity of mitochondria.[175]

Thiamine is necessary for the synthesis of two amino acids, isoleucine and valine,[175] that are essential for normal brain function. The brains of animals treated with a thiamine antagonist became deficient in three important amino acid neurotransmitters: γ-aminobutyric acid (GABA), glutamic acid and aspartic acid.[52, 219] The latter two are closely related structurally to isoleucine and valine.

Experimental thiamine deficiency impairs central nervous system function; in rats, it compromised learning[33] and performance of the string test;[29] in kittens and puppies, it impaired the reflex response to impeded breathing during quiet sleep.[226] Thiamine deficiency also impairs the function of both the serotoninergic mossy-fiber afferents to the granule cells of the cerebellar cortex and the serotoninergic terminals in the inferior olive of the medulla, which provides the major source of climbing fiber afferents to the cerebellum. This may account for the ataxia of thiamine deficiency.

Thiamine Inadequacy. We see many patients with thiamine inadequacy as indicated by a low normal, or slightly below normal serum thiamine level. The muscles of these patients have increased susceptibility to myofascial TPs that are resistant to local therapy until the serum thiamine level is raised to the mean normal level, or above. On clinical examination, this insufficiency is most easily detected by using a special Aluminum Alloy Long-period Tuning Fork* that reveals a graded loss of vibratory perception in relation to nerve fiber length, especially in the lower extremity. The threshold for low frequency vibration (128 Hz) is first established at the big toe and ankle, which then is compared sequentially with the threshold at the hand and by air conduction at the ear, without restarting the tuning fork. The threshold for vibratory perception drops progressively at more proximal sites, indicating improved sensation for nerve fibers of shorter length. The greater the discrepancy between the distal and proximal thresholds, the greater the deficiency. Mild elevations of distal thresholds usually return to normal within a few days of intramuscular supplementation with thiamine.

Some thiamine-inadequate and many thiamine-deficient patients have nocturnal calf cramps, mild dependent edema, constipation, fatigue, and decreased vibratory perception in relation to nerve fiber length. When given thiamine parenterally, they promptly lose several pounds by diuresis with resolution of the edema, have softer stools (the body is no longer removing the moisture from the bowel contents to supply the edema), and are relieved of nocturnal calf cramps.

In contrast to the *painful* calf cramps sometimes associated with thiamine deficiency, *painless* contractions of the hand or other muscles may be due to a lack of pantothenic acid, and relieved by its oral supplementation.

Tinnitus may be relieved by a combination of thiamine *and* niacin therapy, but not by one vitamin alone if both are low.

Thiamine Deficiency. The clinical signs and symptoms of thiamine deficiency are distinguished as dry beriberi, wet beriberi, infantile beriberi and deficiencies that result from alcohol abuse.

In a report of three experimental studies of thiamine deficiency,[310] the symptoms

depended on the degree of deficiency and on its duration. In the first study, complete withdrawal of dietary thiamine in 8 subjects for 88–147 days caused a depressed state, paresthesias, giddiness, soreness of the muscles, backache, insomnia, anorexia, nausea and vomiting, and generalized weakness with greatly reduced capacity for muscular work. Blood pressure was lowered and electrocardiographic abnormalities developed. Physical signs of neuropathy did not develop before the study was discontinued because of the severity of symptoms.[310]

A prolonged (6 months) second study reduced thiamine ingestion to 0.22 mg/1000 calories (one-half of the normal requirement). The prolonged thiamine deficit was associated with emotional instability (evidenced by irritability, moodiness, quarrelsomeness, lack of cooperation, agitation, mental depression) and numerous somatic complaints, but again produced no neurological signs, apparently because the deficiency was not severe enough.[310]

The third study[310] imposed severe deficiency on two subjects, allowing periodic partial relief. The subjects received only 0.1 mg of dietary thiamine/1000 calories, augmented by a 1.0-mg test dose of thiamine every 2 weeks of the 17-week study. The previously observed symptoms of dysfunction of the central and peripheral nervous systems preceded by 9 weeks the gross signs of neurologic dysfunction, which appeared in 16 weeks; the latter included disappearance of tendon reflexes and paralysis of the muscles of the thighs and legs.

In one subject who was restricted to one-quarter of the normal requirement of thiamine for 4 months,[95] a temporary fast elevated the blood lactate but not the pyruvate. Both substances were elevated after ingestion of a test meal of glucose.

A patient on a slimming diet abruptly developed alarming motor symptoms and signs after 4 months of severely restricted thiamine intake.[269]

None of these studies demonstrated the classical signs of beriberi, as observed in the Orient. Another study[95] that provided about one-third of the minimum daily requirement of thiamine, with comparable deficits in other B-complex vitamins, caused edema early in the course of the

---

* Aluminum-Magnesium Alloy Tuning Fork, C-128, Cat. No. 251, Arno Barthelmes & Co., Stockacher Str. 116, 7200 Tuttlingen, W. Germany.

deficiency. The edema persisted until thiamine was replaced.

The **dry (neuritic) form of beriberi** is said to develop slowly in patients who eat a marginal diet of approximately 0.2–0.3 mg of thiamine/1000 calories.[246] The limbs of maximum use develop paresthesias, hyperesthesias, patchy anesthesia and weakness. Deep tendon reflexes are at first increased, then decreased, and may become absent. The "heavy feelings" in the legs become stiffness and aching in the muscles. Foot and wrist drop may occur. In the Orient, inability to do the squat test (a deep knee bend) suggests dry beriberi. Decreased attention span and impaired capacity for work are striking.[112, 246, 299]

The **wet (edematous) form** is said to develop when the patient has subsisted on less than 0.2 mg of thiamine/1000 calories.[246] However, other dietary deficiencies also may be contributing to symptoms, despite their prompt reversal with thiamine replacement. Neurologic manifestations of dry beriberi and cardiovascular signs of wet beriberi (dependent edema, cardiac enlargement and an accentuated second pulmonary sound) are observed. Constipation is common, and anorexia may be severe.[246] Unlike congestive heart failure, albumin appears in the urine and the condition fails to respond to digitalis and diuretics.[10] A prompt response to parenteral thiamine, especially if there is a marked diuresis, confirms the diagnosis.

An **infantile** version of beriberi is seen in breast-fed infants of thiamine-deficient mothers, usually between the second and fifth months of life. The mother may be asymptomatic. Weakness may progress until the child, attempting to cry, emits a weak whine or no sound. Death may occur within 24–48 hours unless thiamine treatment is instituted.[10]

The **abuse of alcohol** can lead to signs and symptoms that are a variable composite of three diseases: alcoholism, thiamine deficiency, and liver dysfunction. Not only is the diet of the alcoholic likely to be deficient in thiamine, but the intake of ethyl alcohol seriously reduces thiamine absorption in either the presence[25] or absence[283] of liver disease. The liver disease itself can seriously impair the conversion of ingested thiamine to its active form,

aggravating the thiamine deficiency.[255] The 74% of 43 alcoholic patients who showed enzyme evidence of thiamine deficiency also had gait and oculomotor disturbances; the others did not.[168]

Thiamine Dependence. Maple syrup urine disease is caused by a defect in the branched chain ketoacid decarboxylase complex and results in the excretion of branched-chain ketoacids in the urine. It responds to megadoses of thiamine.[138]

Laboratory Tests. Tests for thiamine include chemical identification, microbiologic assay, erythrocyte transketolase activity, and blood levels of pyruvate and α-ketogluterate.

The photometric thiochrome procedure is the most widely used of the chemical tests for thiamine, but its results are easily distorted by interfering substances.

Lactobacillus viridescens is the most widely employed organism for microbiologic assay, but phytoflagellate *Ochromonas danica* appears to be the most sensitive indicator of thiamine deficiency, especially in the presence of severe liver disease.[23]

Erythrocyte transketolase (ETK) activity decreases in thiamine deficiency and correlates well with clinical symptoms;[38, 182] it should be more than 800 μg hexose/ml/hr.[298] Supplemental information is obtained by the *in vitro* addition of thiamine pyrophosphate to measure its stimulatory effect on transketolase activity. Increased ETK activity with thiamine supplementation indicates either a thiamine deficiency or an increased proportion of young erythrocytes.[285]

The fasting blood pyruvate is elevated above 1.0 mg/dl[298] in patients with thiamine deficiency. Following ingestion of glucose, serum pyruvate peaks in nearly 1 hour due to the disturbed glycogenesis; this is a more specific indicator of thiamine deficiency than increased serum α-keto-glutarate.[50]

Requirement. The need for thiamine is related to caloric intake when this is equal to energy expenditure; the recommended daily allowance (RDA) established for adults by the National Academy of Sciences[202] is 0.5 mg/1000 kcal of energy expended, with a minimum of 1 mg/day for older persons regardless of their activity level. Most adults expend between 1500 and 2500 kcal/day. The RDA is increased for pregnant and lactating women.[202] Normal thiamine reserves usually provide at least 5 weeks protection from severe thiamine deprivation.[314]

Sources. Thiamine is widely distributed in both animal and vegetable foods, but few are rich in it. Lean pork, beans, nuts and certain whole grain cereals are the best sources available; kidney, liver, beef, eggs and fish contain helpful amounts.[112] In cereal grains, the vitamin is present almost exclusively in the germ and hull. Since these are lost in milling and refining, processed grains need to have the thiamine replaced.[10]

Thiamine can be destroyed by heating above 100 C (212 F). It is quickly leached out of foods during washing or boiling.[10] It resists destruction in acid solutions at temperatures up to boiling, but is rapidly degraded in foods fried in a hot pan, foods cooked under pressure (increased temperature), and in an alkaline medium.

The liquid of canned vegetables generally contains only about 30% of the thiamine initially available. Retention in preprocessed meats ranges from 40–85%. Increasing the roasting temperature of beef or pork reduced thiamine content from 62 to 51% of the original. Pasteurization of cow's milk destroys from 3–10% of its thiamine, whereas the additional heat in processing evaporated milk reduces its thiamine by 30%.[10]

Causes of Deficiency. In addition to inadequate ingestion of thiamine, a number of factors can increase the need for the vitamin. Thiamine absorption is impaired by alcohol ingestion,[283] liver injury,[25] magnesium deficiency,[282] tannin in tea,[301] and also antacids. Thus, tea and gastric alkalinizers taken with food, and also alcohol, should be avoided. Vitamin B_1 is destroyed by thiaminase, which is found in a wide variety of fish, and in bracken fern, which grows in upland pastures where it can pose a hazard to foraging animals.[204] Excretion (loss) of thiamine is potentiated by diuretics[112, 302] and probably by regularly drinking large amounts of water, which also causes a diuresis.

Conversion of dietary and synthetic thiamine to thiamine pyrophosphate, the physiologically active form, is seriously compromised in liver disease, which reduces thiamine availability and further aggravates the liver damage.

Overloading the tissues with glucose may precipitate deficiency if the thiamine level is borderline low.[112]

Therapy. Thiamine is available over-the-counter in 10-, 50- and 100-mg tablets. It is also available for injection as Betalin S* in 1-ml ampules, and in 10-ml and 30-ml vials, at a concentration of 100 mg/ml of thiamine. The therapeutic oral dose usually recommended is 10 mg daily for several weeks, or until all evidence of deficiency has disappeared.

When taken in much larger amounts, excess thiamine is excreted in the urine and has no reported human toxicity. Intolerance to oral thiamine is extremely rare; daily doses of 500 mg have been administered for as long as a month without ill effects.[10]

However, in rare instances, intravenous thiamine has produced fatal anaphylactic shock. Most of these reactions occurred in patients who had previously received large doses of thiamine by injection[204]; they apparently developed a hypersensitivity to additives in the injected solution. In animal studies, the toxic intravenous dose varies from 125–350 mg/kg for different species. The toxic oral dose was approximately 40 times higher than the intravenous dose, and was apparently unrelated to its role as a vitamin.[72] If applicable, this would translate to a one-time toxic oral dose of 500,000 mg in man.

In the experience of the authors, the absorption of orally administered thiamine may be inadequate even with a supplement of 100 mg three times daily. Since toxicity is not of concern, there is no known contraindiction to this dosage level. In one study,[283] increasing an oral intake of thiamine above 10 mg increased neither its blood level nor the amounts excreted in the urine, supporting the belief that intestinal absorption of thiamine is likely to be the limiting step.

Injection of thiamine bypasses a mal-

* Betalin S, thiamine hydrochloride injection, Eli Lilly and Company Medical Department, 307 East McCarty St., Indianapolis, IN 46285.

absorption problem, but only a part of each injection is retained. Biweekly intramuscular injections of 100 mg are given for 3 or 4 weeks to bring the serum concentration of this vitamin up to an optimal level; however, smaller doses may be effective.

The intramuscular injection of 1 ml of a 100 mg/ml solution of thiamine hydrochloride is usually intensely painful for about 2 min. Addition of procaine to make a 0.5% solution of the local anesthesic renders the injection less painful; increasing the procaine to a 1 or nearly 2% concentration further reduces the pain, but does not eliminate it completely.[289]

Thiamine seems to potentiate the effectiveness of thyroid hormone. Both are essential to energy metabolism. In our experience, when patients with low thiamine levels and evidence of low thyroid function are given supplemental thiamine, their symptoms of low thyroid function may disappear, and laboratory tests of thyroid function improve without thyroid therapy. Patients already taking a thyroid supplement who receive sufficient thiamine to correct a deficiency of that vitamin may then develop symptoms of excess thyroid hormone, and the dose of thyroid supplement must be reduced.

Conversely, in the presence of thiamine inadequacy, even a small dose of thyroid hormone may precipitate symptoms of acute thiamine deficiency, which, in some respects, mimics thyrotoxicosis and may be misinterpreted as intolerance to the thyroid medication. After the thiamine deficiency has been corrected, the same small dose, and often larger doses, of thyroid hormone are well tolerated.

A thiamine supplement given to thiamine-deficient schoolchildren failed to improve this vitamin deficiency when their diet was also deficient in protein.[22] This may reflect a concurrent deficiency of transport protein for thiamine.

Pyridoxine (Vitamin B₆)

Discovery. In 1934, Szent Györgyi identified a dietary factor that prevents rat acrodynia, a dermatitis on the tail, ears, mouth and paws characterized by edema and scaliness of the skin; later he named this substance vitamin B₆.[216] Pyridoxine occurs as either pyridox*ol*, an alcohol; as pyridox*al*, an aldehyde; or as pyridox-

amine, an amine. These are the dietary precursors of the active coenzyme forms. The precursors are phosphorylated in the body, chiefly in the liver, by pyridoxal kinase to become the active coenzymes, pyridoxal phosphate and pyridoxamine phosphate.[175, 247] The activity of pyridoxal kinase increases as the concentration of pyridoxal phosphate drops, under the control of an unspecified feedback mechanism.[304]

This vitamin proved essential to man when, in the early 1950s, its absence in an infant formula caused an epidemic of convulsions that were curable by pyridoxine injection.[72, 247] In 1968, the National Academy of Sciences recognized its essential nature in human nutrition by assigning it a required daily allowance (RDA).[202]

Functions. Vitamin B₆ is a necessary dietary factor in man, the rat, mouse, pig, dog, chick, turkey and other species, as well as for many microorganisms. After the rumen has developed in cattle, sheep and other ruminants, they no longer require a dietary source of pyridoxine.

Pyridoxal phosphate has been implicated as critical in lipid metabolism because its deficiency causes myelin degeneration in man.[72, 247] Vitamin B₆ deficiency also is characterized by anemia and hormonal imbalance expressed as growth retardation.[87] In pyridoxine deficiency, glutamic oxaloacetic transaminase (GOT) and glutamic pyruvate transaminase (GPT) activity in the blood and its components are reduced.[247]

Deficiency of pyridoxine involves other vitamins. Its deficiency results in reduced absorption and storage of cobalamin, increased excretion of vitamin C, and blocked synthesis of nicotinic acid (niacin). Vitamin B₆ acts synergistically with vitamin E to control the metabolism of unsaturated fats, and with vitamin C in tyrosine metabolism.[87]

More than 60 pyridoxal phosphate-dependent enzymes are known to man. Many of the most important functions of this vitamin concern **amino acid metabolism**. Reactions for which it provides an essential coenzyme include transamination, the reversible transfer of an α-amino group between an amino acid and an α-keto acid; oxidative deamination of an amino acid to an aldehyde; the interconversion of the L and D isomers of an amino acid; decarboxylation; the interconversion of glycine and serine; and the conversion of homocysteine and cystathione to cysteine. Failure of the methionine-to-cysteine pathway leads to homocystinuria. The failure of cystathione conversion leads to cystathioninuria. Pyridoxal phosphate is essential to the cleavage step in the pathway of tryptophan to niacin. Hence, in the absence of an adequate exogenous source of niacin, pyridoxine deficiency enhances the deficiency of niacin.[72]

Although it has no primary effect on metabolism, vitamin B_6 deficiency indirectly influences both anaerobic and aerobic metabolism. Pyridoxal phosphate plays an important conformational or structural role in the enzyme phosphorylase, which is essential to the release of glucose from glycogen for anaerobic metabolism.[87, 175] The product of anaerobic metabolism, pyruvate, is normally the chief substrate for oxidative metabolism in muscle.[175]

The vitamin contributes to aerobic metabolism through the degradation of at least 11 amino acids, making the corresponding α-keto acid analogue of the amino acid available to enter the energy-releasing tricarboxylic acid cycle. Deficiency of pyridoxal phosphate interferes seriously with the disposal of used amino acids, and their reconfiguration for synthesis to new amino acids.[175]

Practically all of the compounds implicated as **neurotransmitters** in the brain are synthesized and/or metabolized with the aid of pyridoxal phosphate. These include dopamine, norepinephrine, serotonin, tyramine, tryptamine, taurine, histamine, γ-aminobutyric acid (GABA), and indirectly acetylcholine.[87] Serotonin is derived, with the help of pyridoxal phosphate, from 5-hydroxytryptophan. Glutamic acid decarboxylase with pyridoxal phosphate catalyzes the formation of GABA, which is a central nervous system inhibitor derived from glutamic acid.[87]

Deterioration of behavior and **mental function** is seen in experimental pyridoxine deficiency. A study[315] showed that pyridoxine-deficient rats were indifferent to food; trembled, were stiff and motionless when handled; startled readily by noises;

and had chattering teeth, as compared with controls. The vitamin B_6-deficient rats required nearly twice the running time and made twice the errors as did control rats on the same diet that, however, included vitamin B_6.

Pyridoxine appears to be necessary for the production of C_1 units from serine, which are required for the biosynthesis of nucleic acids.[16] Deficiency impairs the biosynthesis of ribonucleic acid (RNA), particularly messenger RNA, with subsequent deleterious effects on **cell multiplication**.[260]

Vitamin B_6 is important in the **synthesis** of insulin, growth hormone, follicle-stimulating hormone, luteinizing hormone, aldosterone, glucagon, cortisol, estradiol, testosterone, and epinephrine.[87]

In hemoglobin synthesis, pyridoxal phosphate plays an essential role as a cofactor in the synthesis of porphyrin, which is a part of the hemoglobin molecule.[247] Adults with proven pyridoxine deficiency may show a microcytic hypochromic anemia that fails to respond to iron, but improves dramatically following treatment with small doses of pyridoxine.[72]

Over the past 30 years, animal studies have repeatedly shown that a dietary deficiency of vitamin B_6 results in impairment of both humoral and cell-mediated **immune responses** to particulate antigens and the influenza virus.[16]

In animal studies, vitamin B_6 deficiency suppressed cellular immune competence[233] and increased tolerance to skin grafts from another strain of mouse.[15] The deficiency was demonstrable in vitro. The structure of the thymus was altered, as determined by electron microscopy, and the immunological competence was reduced in the offspring of vitamin B_6-deficient mothers.[233]

An abnormal tryptophan metabolite, xanthurenic acid, is found in the urine of pyridoxine-deficient persons and in the urine of patients with **diabetes**.[72] Rose[236] cited numerous studies that indicate deterioration of glucose tolerance as observed in nearly three-fourths of women taking estrogen-based oral contraceptives; this was reversible by supplementing the diet with vitamin B_6.

Diabetic patients who complained of leg cramps, swelling of the hands, and impaired tactile sensation were relieved of their symptoms while taking 50 mg/day of pyridoxine orally. One patient again experienced the symptoms after 7 weeks without the pyridoxine supplement, but was relieved by resuming vitamin B$_6$ therapy without changing the antidiabetic medication.[93] These data suggest that the vitamin B$_6$ requirement is increased in diabetic patients who excrete xanthurenic acid, and that some of the symptoms ascribed to diabetes, in selected patients may be relieved by supplemental pyridoxine.

During **pregnancy**, the requirement for pyridoxine is markedly increased. Augmenting the basic 2.0 mg RDA of vitamin B$_6$ by 2.5 mg to a total of 4.5 mg daily was not sufficient to raise the blood level of pyridoxal phosphate in pregnant women to that found in nonpregnant women; the metabolic basis for this increased need was not established.[82] Obstetricians have used supplemental pyridoxine to combat the nausea and vomiting of early pregnancy for many years.[93, 247] The senior author has found that one or two intramuscular injections of 100 mg of pyridoxine may promptly terminate these common distressing symptoms of early pregnancy; vitamin B$_6$ therapy also has provided effective prophylaxis against motion sickness in nonpregnant individuals, both adults and children.

Deficiency of vitamin B$_6$ for a year or less had little or no effect on the incidence of **caries** in rhesus monkeys, but more protracted deficiency caused rampant dental caries in the second dentition and had a markedly deleterious effect on the development of the permanent teeth. Long-term studies to assess this effect in man have not been reported.[315]

Which enzymatic functions of vitamin B$_6$ must be lacking to cause increased neuromuscular irritability and perpetuation of TPs has not been established.

Pyridoxine Deficiency. Clear-cut symptoms of pyridoxine deficiency are unusual. Milder, equivocal symptoms appear with inadequate amounts of the vitamin. Three high risk groups that deserve special attention for pyridoxine inadequacy or deficiency are babies born to poorly nourished mothers, the elderly,[86] and women taking an oral contraceptive.[236]

In infants, pyridoxine deficiency is char-

acterized by nervous irritability and convulsions with abnormalities of the electroencephalogram. In an experimental deficiency[267] induced in two infants, the babies ceased to gain weight. Listlessness and convulsions occurred in one after 76 days, and a severe hypochromic, microcytic anemia developed in the other after 140 days, but without central nervous system signs. Two individuals responded quite differently to the same acute pyridoxine deficiency.

Initially, patients on poor diets were observed to have ill-defined central nervous system syndromes of weakness, irritability and nervousness, insomnia, difficulty in walking, loss of "sense of responsibility," and abnormal electroencephalograms. These changes did not respond to treatment with other members of the vitamin B-complex, but were relieved within 24 hours by ingesting pyridoxine. For disorders of the central nervous system, it was at one time advocated that the vitamin be injected intraspinally.[276] Pyridoxine also healed the skin changes of fissuring and dry scaling of the vermilion surface of the lips and angles of the mouth, symptoms which had not responded to riboflavin. Subjects placed on a vitamin B$_6$-deficient diet also developed central nervous system irritability, depression, loss of the sense of responsibility, and electroencephalographic changes. They developed the pellagra-like filiform hypertrophy of the lingual papillae, aphthous stomatitis, and also nasolabial seborrhea with an acneiform papular rash of the forehead.[247]

Six patients[99] selected for symptoms and signs of carpal tunnel syndrome with decreased activity of their erythrocyte glutamic oxaloacetic transaminase (EGOT) were clinically identifiable in a double-blind study by the response of their symptoms to placebo or pyridoxine therapy. Cross-over treatment[91] of another such patient by alternating placebo and pyridoxine produced return of symptoms on placebo, regression of the symptoms of carpal tunnel syndrome with a 2-mg supplement daily, and complete relief with a 100-mg supplement. The median nerve latency improved with pyridoxine treatment.[91] These data indicate that, in some cases, pyridoxine insufficiency can increase the vulnerability of peripheral nerves to entrapment enough to cause the symptoms of a carpal tunnel syndrome.

In a group of 154 patients admitted to the psychiatric unit of a general hospital,[64] the pyridoxine-deficient patients showed a disproportionately high incidence of depression when compared to psychiatric patients without such a deficiency.[180] Iatrogenic vitamin B_6 deficiency due to antituberculosis therapy was associated with psychiatric symptoms of euphoria or depression, loss of control, acute psychotic episodes, and loss of reality testing.[180] A degree of depression and pyridoxine inadequacy are common findings in patients with chronic myofascial pain.

Since vitamin B_6 is required for the conversion of tryptophan to niacin, dermatological lesions of pellagra (niacin deficiency) may result secondarily from vitamin B_6 deficiency, producing mixed symptoms of pyridoxine and niacin deficiencies.[72]

Pellagra has been epitomized by 4 Ds: dermatitis, diarrhea, depression and death.[10] Mild niacin deficiency may show only redness of the tongue, and hypertrophy of its papillae, or their atrophy.[113] These findings, with soreness of the oral mucosa, were observed by Prema and Srikantia[223] in 20% of 2657 low-income women in India. Symptoms were relieved by an oral supplement of 5 mg of riboflavin and 10 mg of pyridoxine daily for 10 days; the pyridoxine probably corrected a niacin deficiency. However, the neurological changes of vitamin B_6 deficiency are not attributable to a secondary lack of niacin because such neurologic changes have not been reported in experimental niacin deficiency.[113] This impression is supported by the fact that patients on isoniazid, an inhibitor of pyridoxal, are likely to develop both skin lesions and a peripheral neuropathy; the skin lesions respond to niacin, but the neuropathy requires treatment with pyridoxine.[100]

Impotence in the male has been ascribed to a deficiency in vitamin B_6 and zinc with return of sexual function after 1 or 2 months of an adequate daily supplement of these nutrients.[216]

Pyridoxine Dependence. The need for very large amounts of pyridoxine occurs when one of the specific enzyme systems that require this vitamin is congenitally incomplete. Megadoses (10 times the RDA, or more) of pyridoxine at least partially compensate for the metabolic abnormality. Dependence is established clinically when both the symptoms and the characteristic abnormal metabolic intermediates recur promptly after resumption of an unsupplemented normal diet. One should expect considerable variability among patients in their need for pyridoxine.[311] Patients with chronic myofascial pain are a select group who show a high prevalence of vitamin inadequacies. Many of these patients do well on large vitamin supplements. One likely explanation for this apparent partial dependence on pyridoxine by a number of patients would be the partial expression of one or more of the genetic enzyme deficiencies described here. This condition would be analogous to the incomplete penetrance of full-blown symptoms often seen in families with inherited myopathies and neuropathies.[49]

The first pyridoxine-dependent disorder to be discovered was the appearance of seizures within the first 2 weeks of life. Convulsions of the infant failed to respond to anticonvulsant drugs, but did respond to pharmacological doses (2–100 mg daily) of pyridoxine.[138, 247]

Another recognized form of dependence is a rare microcytic hypochromic, sideroblastic anemia in the newborn; it is responsive to pharmacological doses of vitamin B_6, but unresponsive to medicinal iron. These infants require from 10 mg to several grams of vitamin B_6 daily, and symptoms recur promptly when this megasupplement is discontinued or reduced to approximately the level of the RDA.

Children *deficient* in vitamin B_6 show abnormal xanthurenic acid excretion in response to a tryptophan load, whereas pyridoxine-*dependent* children, when tested, fail to excrete abnormal amounts of this acid.[138]

After the recognition of **homocystinuria** in 1962, the condition was found to be almost as common as phenylketonuria, occurring once in every 20,000–40,000 births. It must be distinguished from the Marfan syndrome, and is characterized by ectopia lentis of the eye, chest deformity, scoliosis, generalized osteoporosis, recurrent thrombosis in arteries and veins, and in 50% of patients by mental retardation.[264] These patients tend to be tall, and the symptoms are well developed by the age of 10 years. It is diagnosed by the presence of homocysteine in the urine, and is controlled by pharmacological doses of pyridoxine.[138] Pyridoxine, in a daily dose of 500 mg, restored hair pigmentation in a young woman with homocystinuria.[257]

Another metabolically related but much rarer pyridoxine-dependent disorder, **cystathioninuria**, presents with a highly variable clinical picture, ranging from normal to severe mental retardation.[138]

A 1975 study[75] indicates that pyridoxine deficiency and/or dependence is a factor in many **asthmatic** children. Symptoms improved in all children treated with vitamin B_6. Normalization of tryptophan metabolism with pyridoxine therapy in five children indicated a degree of vitamin B_6 dependence (lack of the apoenzyme), rather than a simple dietary deficiency of the vitamin.[75]

Laboratory Tests. In experimental, fulminating deficiency, measurement of circulating serum vitamin B_6 permits detection of the deficit before biochemical and clinical signs appear. Decrease in this blood vitamin level is the earliest warning signal of an acute clinical deficiency. In mild-to-moderate chronic deficiency, the symptoms may depend as much on concomitant secondary deficiencies as on the blood level of pyridoxal phosphate.

Valid assay for the presence of vitamin B_6 requires time and/or special care.[129] A yeast, *Saccharomyces carlsbergensis*, is the test organism commonly used because it is responsive to pyridoxal, pyridoxol, and pyridoxamine. Unlike most other test microorganisms, it is unable to use D-alanine to satisfy its vitamin B_6 requirement. *S. carlsbergensis* is, therefore, suitable for tests on human blood. The yeast *Torulopsis thermophilia* also promises to measure the metabolic activity of all vitamin B_6 components that can be utilized by man.[23, 129]

Recently, an enzymatic method using tryptophanase to assay pyridoxal phosphate directly has been developed which

is accurate, but complex. Unfortunately, the much simpler fluorometric methods are largely unsatisfactory, with the exception of a few that include rigorous purification of the sample to remove interfering substances prior to analysis. Specialized chromatographic procedures employing thin layer electrophoresis are time consuming, but accurate.[129]

In the blood, the assayed level of vitamin B_6 decreases in proportion to decreased intake of the vitamin. The activity of SGOT and SGPT both decrease with pyridoxine deficiency; the latter appears to be more sensitive.[23] The principal metabolic product is 4-pyridoxic acid, which is excreted in the urine together with small amounts of pyridoxal and pyridoxamine. The 4-pyridoxic acid in the urine accounts for 20–40% of the vitamin metabolized daily; what happens to the rest is unknown.[72, 247] Urinary excretion of 4-pyridoxic acid diminishes with low vitamin B_6 intake. However, it accounts for less than half of the pyridoxine intake and is, therefore, not reliable as an indicator of the vitamin B_6 nutritional status.[23] Its continued presence in the urine does not rule out vitamin B_6 deficiency.[299]

Urinary excretion of oxalic acid and xanthurenic acid increases in pyridoxine deficiency. This effect is augmented in pyridoxal-deficient persons from a normal of less than 30 mg to more than 50 mg of xanthurenic acid/24 hrs following the oral administration of 10 mg of L-tryptophan. However, the increase in urinary xanthurenic acid is subject to misinterpretation because it also is increased in riboflavin deficiency.[23]

The alanine-loading test is more specific. In that test, the oral administration of alanine produces a marked rise in blood urea nitrogen in pyridoxine-deficient patients.[93, 114]

Requirement. The 1980 National Research Council RDA for vitamin B_6 was 2.0 mg for adult females and 2.2 mg for adult males, with an additional daily supplement of 0.6 mg for pregnant and 0.5 mg for lactating women. This recommendation was recognized by the Council as barely adequate to prevent clinical evidence of deficiency in the average individual *if* that individual eats no more than the

RDA of protein (0.8 g/kg of body weight).[199] The average American diet exceeds that RDA of protein and the vitamin B_6 requirement rises roughly in proportion to the increase in protein intake,[62, 179] and with age.[202]

Sources. Vitamin B_6 is widely distributed in nature, but not in large amounts. The most available sources of this vitamin include liver and kidney; white meat of chicken; halibut and tuna; English walnuts; soybean flour and navy beans; bananas and avocados. Helpful sources are yeast, lean beef, egg yolk, whole wheat, and milk.[72, 247]

Fresh milk contains 0.6 mg of vitamin B_6/liter (0.14 mg/8 oz serving). Very little is destroyed in milk during processing, but much is lost when milk is exposed to sunlight for more than a few minutes.

The usual synthetic form of vitamin B_6 is pyridoxine hydrochloride, which occurs as white platelets that are readily soluble in water. It is stable in acid solution, but rapidly destroyed by sunlight when in neutral or alkaline solution.[247] This synthetic form is heat stable through most food processing. All three natural forms are stable to heat in acid solutions, but only pyridoxamine is stable to heat in neutral or alkaline solutions. Plant sources contain mainly pyridoxol, whereas animal sources contain both pyridoxal and pyridoxamine as well. Thus, animal sources of vitamin B_6 and the pyridoxine form are less susceptible to loss of the vitamin because of cooking or preserving.[72]

Most of the vitamin B_6 taken orally is well absorbed in the upper intestine by passive transport, where the relatively high pH facilitates absorption. Once absorbed, all three forms of vitamin B_6 are converted to pyridoxal phosphate.

Body stores normally contain about 0.60 mg (0.55–0.66 mg) of pyridoxal phosphate/ 0.45 kilo (1 lb) of body weight. For an 82-kilo (180-lb) individual, the total amount would approximate 108 mg of pyridoxine. Most of it is stored in two tissue compartments. The bulk, 90%, resides in a slow turnover compartment with a half-life of nearly 33 days, representing tightly bound tissue stores. The remaining 10% is held in a fast-turnover compartment with a half-life of about 16 hours. During this time, the exogenous vitamin is either excreted or turned over to the slow compartment for storage. The major part is stored in muscle, liver and blood.[252]

There is a serious question as to whether the microbiological species used in the past for the assessment of bioavailability of vitamin B_6 in foods adequately represented the bioavailability of the vitamin to man. The vitamin's bioavailability, based on the earlier microbiological methods, may have been significantly overestimated, possibly by as much as a factor of two.[118]

Causes of Deficiency. In addition to inadequate dietary intake, tropical sprue and alcohol interfere with its absorption. Several things increase the need for vitamin B_6. Two **antitubercular drugs**, isonicotinic acid hydrazide (INH or isoniazid) and cycloserine, are potent pyridoxine antagonists.[271] Symptoms of pyridoxine deficiency due to INH interaction can be prevented by 50 mg/day of oral pyridoxine.[271] More than this is likely to neutralize the effectiveness of the INH. Cycloserine has produced a high incidence of seizures (nearly 10%). Daily supplementation with 50 mg of pyridoxine greatly reduces this toxic neurologic effect of the drug, but is less helpful in relieving its psychiatric side effects.

The majority of **oral contraceptive** users had abnormal tryptophan metabolism characteristic of pyridoxine deficiency; the estrogenic component of the contraceptive pill was responsible.[236]

Rose[236] reviewed a number of studies that clearly demonstrated an increased requirement for vitamin B_6 in women who took oral contraceptives. Of 80 such "pill" users, 15% had reduced activity of the enzyme alanine aminotransferase, an indicator of vitamin B_6 deficiency. Erythrocyte aspartate aminotransferase also showed frankly subnormal activity in 37% of patients on oral contraceptives, *versus* 13% of controls. Twenty percent of 55 "pill"-medicated women had plasma levels of pyridoxal phosphate equal to, or lower than, the lowest values observed in 77 normal nonuser controls. Among the subjects on a pyridoxine-deficient diet, a daily 2-mg supplement of pyridoxine caused rapid recovery of the indices toward normal in the nonuser control group, but a much slower rate of recovery in the group on oral contraceptives.[236]

Oral contraceptive agents tend to impair glucose tolerance. In one study,[236] 78% of the women taking an oral contraceptive showed impaired glucose tolerance as contrasted with their preuser tests; 13% of the tests became frankly **abnormal**, as in diabetes. However, in another study,[270] 12 women whose oral glucose tolerance had deteriorated while taking oral contraceptives showed significant improvement in the test on a daily supplement of 25 mg of pyridoxine for 4 weeks. Similarly, among 46 oral contraceptive users, supplementation by 20 mg of pyridoxine twice daily for 4 weeks improved the glucose tolerance, but only in the 30% who were considered to be deficient in vitamin B_6.[236]

Depression occurs in about 6% of women taking oral contraceptives. One contributary factor is the increased need for vitamin B_6.[236] A review of the literature[172] showed that depression associated with use of an oral contraceptive was most likely in those patients with a history of previous depression. In a double-blind crossover study of 22 depressed users of an oral contraceptive, the 11 with biochemical evidence of vitamin B_6 deficiency responded clinically to 20 mg of pyridoxine twice daily, whereas the other 11 (nondeficient) users did not respond.[2]

A more recent study[155] of 75 women on a variety of oral contraceptives concluded that a daily supplement of 1–5 mg was inadequate compared to a supplement of 25–100 mg, based on measurements of the specific activity of erythrocyte glutamic oxaloacetic transaminase.

There is no known contraindication to **regularly supplementing** the diet of oral contraceptive users with 5–10 mg of vitamin B_6 daily, except minimal cost; to many individuals, there are important advantages.

The chelating agent, **penicillamine**, is widely used in the treatment of Wilson's disease and sometimes for the reduction of stone formation in cystinuria. The seizures observed in Wilson's disease are at least partly, if not completely, due to the pyridoxine deficiency induced by penicillamine, and they respond to dietary supplementation with 50–100 mg of pyridoxine daily. Such vitamin therapy does not

seem to reduce the other toxic effects of penicillamine.[247]

Among epileptic children taking **anticonvulsants**, 30–60% exhibit various biochemical indices of vitamin B_6 depletion. A pyridoxine supplement of 60–120 mg daily, in addition to the anticonvulsant, eliminated the convulsions. A smaller daily supplement of pyridoxine was not tried.[282]

Supplemental **corticosteroids** increase the need for pyridoxine. The abnormal metabolism that results from the induced pyridoxine deficiency may explain, in part, why patients receiving corticosteroids tend to become insulin resistant and glucose intolerant.[282]

The strong association of pyridoxine deficiency with **excessive alcohol consumption** is widely recognized.[72, 247] The incidence of pyridoxine deficiency, measured by the presence of ring sideroblasts in the bone marrow, is 20–30% in alcoholic populations.[256] However, blood plasma levels of pyridoxal indicate that the incidence of pyridoxine deficiency may be as high as 30–50% in alcoholics *without* liver disease, and 80–100% of alcoholics *with* liver disease.[178]

Pyridoxine deficiency is aggravated in alcoholics: (1) by reduced dietary intake of the vitamin through substitution of alcohol for food, (2) by impaired absorption of the natural dietary forms of vitamin B_6, and (3) by interference with the conversion of vitamin B_6 to the active phosphorylated form by both the alcohol and liver disease. Acetaldehyde, an oxidation product of ethanol, interferes with the metabolism of vitamin B_6 by promoting the degradation of pyridoxal phosphate.[256]

The need for pyridoxine increases during **pregnancy** and lactation; precisely how much is not clear. It is at least the RDA increase of 0.6 mg to 2.6 mg, probably twice that increase, or more, for many women.[82]

The need for vitamin B_6 is increased in **hyperthyroid** patients.[114, 247]

Pyridoxine deficiency often occurs in both dialyzed and nondialyzed *uremic patients*. Based on erythrocyte GOT activity, as many as 70% of these patients are deficient in vitamin B_6, apparently due more to inhibition of pyridoxal kinase activity by uremic toxins than to lower dietary intake. Daily supplements of pyridoxine restored the erythrocyte GOT activity in these deficient patients.[189]

Therapy. Pyridoxine is available over-the-counter in 10- and 50-mg tablets, and in larger amounts by prescription. Parenteral pyridoxine hydrochloride is supplied in vials of 10 and 30 ml in a concentration of 100 mg/ml.* A single intramuscular injection of 100 mg of pyridoxine effectively raises the serum level of the vitamin.

An adequate pyridoxine supplement is needed for individuals who eat marginal or poor diets, those who have relatively high protein intake, pregnant and lactating women, and those on an oral contraceptive. Interactions with other drugs also can be important. Pharmacological doses of vitamin B_6, ranging from 10–100 mg or more daily, are indicated for the pyridoxine-dependent conditions described and are nontoxic.

Cobalamin (Vitamin B_{12})

Discovery. In 1926, Minot and Murphy successfully treated pernicious anemia by feeding the patients liver. Previously, the disease had been invariably fatal.[32] In 1948, the responsible agent, a cobalamin, was finally discovered and crystallized.

Hodgkin won the 1964 Nobel Prize in Chemistry for delineating the structure of this complex molecule. Its central cobalt atom is linked to a variable anionic group. This group is —CN in cyanocobalamin, the common synthetic form; —OH in hydroxocobalamin, the major form in plasma; and —CH_3 in methylcobalamin. At least three other forms are known.[137] It has been officially recommended[85] that the term vitamin B_{12} be reserved specifically for the cyanocobalamin form; "cobalamin" may apply to any of its forms. Methylcobalamin and 5'-deoxyadenosinecobalamin are the only two forms of the vitamin known to be physiologically active.[138] Cyanocobalamin is physiologically inactive and must be converted to other forms, first to be absorbed, and then to be metabolically useful.

Functions. Cobalamins serve numerous essential metabolic functions that include:

(1) deoxyribonucleic acid (DNA) synthesis; (2) regeneration of intrinsic folate, which is also critical to the synthesis of DNA; (3) the transport of folate to, and its storage in, cells; (4) fat and carbohydrate metabolism; (5) protein metabolism; and (6) the reduction of sulfhydryl groups. Since cobalamin and folic acid are required for the synthesis of DNA, both are necessary for normal growth.[137]

Folate deficiency impairs the **synthesis of deoxyribonucleic acid**, causing megaloblastosis in all duplicating cells of the body, most commonly observed in bone marrow cells. The impaired hematopoiesis produces a pancytopenia.

One of the cobalamin-dependent enzymes contributes to **protein synthesis**; it removes a methanol group from methylfolate and delivers it to homocystein, converting it to methionine. A storage of methionine may compromise lipid metabolism. This demethylation of methylfolate also permits **regeneration of tetrahydrofolic acid**, which recycles methylfolate to the body's active folate pool. When a patient suffers from cobalamin deficiency, much of the folate is "trapped" in the metabolically inactive form, methylfolate.[250] This widely accepted "folate trap" hypothesis would explain why the hematologic signs of distress seen in cobalamin deficiency are clinically indistinguishable from those of folate deficiency.[137]

Cobalamin is essential for the **transport** of folate into certain leukocytes and for the **storage** of folate as methyltetrahydrofolate in bone marrow cells.[137] Cobalamin also assists the tissues in their uptake of folic acid. The functions of vitamin B_{12} and folic acid are intertwined in several ways.[67]

The cobalamins are involved in both **fat and carbohydrate metabolism**, since the conversion of methylalanate to succinate is cobalamin-dependent. It has been proposed, but not proved, that the neurological deficits characteristic of cobalamin deficiency are due to compromise of the lipid portion of the lipoprotein myelin sheath surrounding the affected nerve fibers. In both the central and peripheral nervous systems, cobalamin deficiency is associated with inadequate myelin synthesis that leads to, first, demyelination, then ax-

---

* Hexa-Betalin, Pyridoxine hydrochloride injection, Eli Lilly and Company, Medical Department, 307 East McCarty St., Indianapolis, IN 46206.

onal degeneration, and finally neuronal death.[18] Comparable neurologic disease is less frequently caused by folate deficiency.[137] Lesions of the myelinated peripheral nerves due to cobalamin deficiency occur more frequently and earlier than the central nervous system lesions of the myelinated posterior and lateral cords of the spinal column. The latter advanced deficiency is known as subacute combined degeneration, combined system disease, posterior lateral sclerosis, or funicular degeneration.[137]

Cobalamin serves as a **reducing agent** for sulfhydryl groups.[137]

Cobalamin Inadequacy. The symptomatology of a **marginal** amount of cobalamin in the body may be highly variable and difficult to interpret. Nonspecific depression, fatiguability and increased susceptibility to myofascial TPs are likely to predominate. An exaggerated startle reaction to unexpected noise or touch is occasionally a helpful guide. Which of the metabolic pathways that depend on cobalamin are responsible for the increased susceptibility of muscles to TPs when the cobalamin level is low has not been established.

Cobalamin Deficiency. Cobalamin deficiency causes **symptoms** of anemia, such as fatigability, and of neurological dysfunction. Central nervous system symptoms may range from mood changes and depression[235] to confusion, agitation,[137] frank psychosis,[32, 128] and occasionally coma.[165] Tobacco amblyopia and optic atrophy are sometimes seen.[235] Loss of proprioception and pyramidal tract dysfunction are associated with degenerative changes in the dorsal and lateral columns of the spinal cord.[32] Symmetrical neurological symptoms of paresthesias, especially numbness and tingling in the hands and feet, sometimes occur.[137]

Cobalamin deficiency is often associated with constipation, whereas folate deficiency is usually accompanied by diarrhea (sprue-like symptoms).[137]

A few investigations have found evidence for impaired immune function due to cobalamin deficiency.[203]

Examination may reveal **signs** of either augmented, or impaired reflexes at different stages of cobalamin deficiency. Ataxia may progress to spastic paraplegia or flaccid paralysis, depending on whether the dysfunction is due to predominantly upper or lower motor neuron demyelinization; these changes eventually become irreversible.[235] Abnormalities of evoked responses—visual, brain stem auditory, and somatosensory—were found in patients who had sensory loss, motor loss, and cortical dysfunction due to cobalamin deficiency.[166]

With only rare exceptions, symptoms due to tissue depletion of cobalamin were accompanied by a severely depressed serum level of the vitamin.[265]

The peripheral blood shows a pancytopenia,[135] with the development of myeloid megaloblastosis of the bone marrow as a result of either cobalamin or folate deficiency. The circulating blood also contains increased numbers of hypersegmented polymorphonuclear leukocytes; according to the Rule of Fives, more than 5% of the cells have nuclei with five lobes or more.[135]

Although cobalamin deficiency is usually characterized as a macrocytic anemia,[135] and an increase in mean corpuscular volume (MCV) of the erythrocytes *may* be an early indication of that deficiency,[123] that is not necessarily the case. An MCV above 93 fl was a poor index of cobalamin deficiency in a study[265] of 772 patients. Only four of the 101 patients with a low serum cobalamin value in that study had a high MCV; conversely, only 5 of the 45 patients with a high MCV had a low serum cobalamin level. Macrocytosis is a relatively late development and iron deficiency can readily mask this effect of cobalamin deficiency on erythrocyte size.[135]

Because sufficient quantities of folic acid ameliorate the hematologic abnormalities caused by cobalamin deficiency, patients on diets ample in folic acid are likely to develop neurological symptoms before hematological signs, whereas those who are deficient in both folic acid and vitamin B_{12} are likely to show hematologic abnormalities first.[135] The treatment of cobalamin deficiency with folic acid, based on the hematologic response alone, may lead to disaster, because the neurologic abnormalities can progress to irreversible damage while the hematologic picture improves.[135] For the same reasons, a response to *intensive* vitamin B_{12} therapy does not unequivocally establish the diagnosis of cobalamin deficiency; this therapy can reduce some symptoms of a pure folic acid deficiency.[317] For a reliable therapeutic trial, 1 mcg of vitamin B_{12}/day should be used prior to any other vitamin B_{12} administration. Only cobalamin deficiency will exhibit a hematologic response to this small dose of the vitamin.[32]

Urinary excretion of methylmalonic acid, proprionic acid, and acetic acid is increased in cobalamin deficiency.[32, 173] Surprisingly, acute starvation imposed on initially adequate cobalamin levels resulted in *markedly* increased serum levels and increased urinary excretion of cobalamin for several months.[21] Presumably, this remarkable finding was due to loss of protein-binding sites for cobalamin in the liver.

Cobalamin Dependence. Methylmalonic aciduria (with or without homocystinuria) can be due to a large variety of genetic anomalies;[9] in this condition, megadoses of vitamin B_{12}[138] have relieved the failure to thrive after birth, which indicates an abnormal functioning of cobalamin-dependent pathways. Serum cobalamin levels were normal in symptomatic patients who were unable to make 5'-deoxy-adenosine cobalamin. Other individuals with only moderate impairment of one of these metabolic pathways have a need for more than the usual amount of cobalamin and, depending on which cobalamin-dependent enzyme is involved, may or may not show low serum levels of the vitamin.[9]

Laboratory Tests. Only minute amounts of cobalamin, which are measured in picograms (pg), equivalent to micromicrograms, are present in the serum. Normal values range between about 200 and 900 pg/ml. Such small quantities can be measured only by microbiologic assay or radioimmunoassay (RIA). Most popular now for the determination of cobalamins is radioimmunoassay, which uses coated charcoal to separate free from bound cobalamins.[137]

The RIA method tends to exaggerate cobalamin values[85] and, therefore, is likely to yield falsely normal values in cases of deficiency.[77, 164] A number of the standard commercial radiodilution kits are ineffective in screening for cobalamin deficiency.[73] In two studies,[88] some 10% of patients proven to have pernicious anemia by megaloblastic bone marrow and by an abnormal Schilling test had serum cobalamin levels reported well within the normal range. Also, liver disease[137] and poor protein nutrition can increase the reported values deceivingly.[21]

When a cobalamin deficiency has been confirmed, the first- and second-stage Schilling tests indicate whether malabsorption is the cause of the deficiency. In the first stage test, a tracer dose of radiolabeled vitamin B_{12} is administered orally, followed by a flushing dose of unlabeled vitamin B_{12} given intramuscularly. Excretion of radiolabeled cobalamin is measured in the urine. Malabsorption causes decreased urinary excretion of the radioisotope. If the first stage Schilling test indicates malabsorption, the second-stage test repeats the first test with the addition of intrinsic factor (usually bovine) to the oral dose of vitamin B_{12}. Improvement in urinary excretion of labeled vitamin B_{12}, as compared with the first test, shows a lack of intrinsic factor. Intestinal malabsorption is the cause of cobalamin deficiency in almost half of the patients with pernicious anemia. If the second-stage Schilling test fails initially to show a rise in excretion, it should be repeated after 2 months of treatment with parenteral vitamin B_{12}, when impaired intestinal function due to mucosal changes caused by the deficiency will have improved, sometimes allowing the test to return to normal.[135]

When shipping blood for analysis, it is important to remember that heat in the presence of large amounts of vitamin C destroys cobalamin unless it is protected, for instance, by cyanide.[137]

The deoxyuridine-suppression test is helpful in distinguishing between an iron-deficiency, folate-deficiency, and vitamin B_{12}-deficiency anemia. Less suppression occurs when either folate or cobalamin are deficient than when iron is deficient. Normalization of deoxyuridine suppression by adding methylfolate to the culture identifies folate deficiency; normalization by adding hydroxocobalamin, identifies a lack of cobalamin. If both are required, a deficiency of both vitamins exists.[135]

Excretion of increased amounts of methylmalonic acid in the urine is not a very sensitive test, but when positive, it is a reliable metabolic indicator of cobalamin deficiency.[122]

Requirement. The recommended dietary allowance of cobalamins for adults is 3.0 mcg. For pregnant and lactating women, it is increased to 4 mcg.[200]

"Normal" stores of cobalamin range between 1 and 10 mg; the liver contains 50–90% of this total.[137] It is probable that loss occurs only by excretion, mainly in the bile.[137] Most of this is recovered, normally, by an enterohepatic circulation in which 0.6–6 mg of the vitamin excreted daily in the bile is reabsorbed in the ileum.[137] Thus, following total gastrectomy, or after abrupt cessation of adequate treatment of pernicious anemia, a year or more may elapse before deficiency symptoms develop.[32]

Sources. Cobalamins are unique among vitamins, because the only primary food source is from bacteria. The cobalamins are synthesized by certain microorganisms that are found in soil, sewage, water, intestines, or rumen; herbivorous animals depend entirely on microbial sources for their cobalamin.[32] The vitamin is not found in plants unless they are contaminated by microorganisms.[137] The richest food sources are liver, kidney, other animal foods derived from viscera, and shell fish, which siphon large numbers of cobalamin-rich microorganisms. Moderate amounts of cobalamin are present in fish, poultry, egg yolk, and fermented cheeses.[137]

Cobalamins are heat resistant, except in an alkaline medium, to temperatures in excess of 100 C (212 F). Generally, less than 10% of the vitamin is lost in food processing. Except in true vegans (absolute vegetarians who avoid all milk and dairy products), cobalamin deficiency is due to malabsorption or abnormal utilization, not to the diet.[105] However, the voracious uptake of cobalamins by fish tapeworm residing in the human intestine can produce a serious deficiency.

The breast-fed infant of a vegan mother progressed to a comatose state by the age of 9 months, due to cobalamin deficiency.[308]

The complicated mechanism for the absorption of cobalamin begins with the freeing of ingested cobalamins from their polypeptide linkages in food by gastric acid and by gastric and intestinal enzymes. The freed cobalamins form complexes with the intrinsic factor that is produced by normal gastric parietal cells. On reaching a protein receptor on the microvillar membrane of the terminal ileum, in the presence of ionic calcium and at a pH about 6, the cobalamin passes through the mucous membrane into the portal venous blood. There it must join the transport protein, transcobalamin II, which carries it to the liver.

Cobalamins are very poorly absorbed in the absence of intrinsic factor, or in the absence of functional ileal binding and transport sites.[137, 235] In the presence of normal intestinal mucosa, approximately only 1% of any quantity of free vitamin B_{12} is apparently absorbed by diffusion along the entire length of the small intestine.[137]

Causes of Deficiency. The elderly are especially vulnerable to cobalamin deficiency and with it, to pernicious anemia; these become increasingly common beyond the age of 50 or 60 years.[48]

Congenital pernicious anemia is of three types: (1) defective or absent production of intrinsic factor, (2) inadequate ileal absorption of cobalamin, and (3) failure of transcobalamin II transport.[235]

Several additional factors can easily cause cobalamin deficiency: (1) failure to release the protein-bound cobalamin from food in the stomach;[154, 155] (2) impaired absorption caused by gastric antibodies associated with rheumatoid arthritis,[78] or by a primary folic acid deficiency;[135] (3) a structural (surgical) or functional gastric defect, including vagotomy;[277] (4) an ileal defect with inadequate absorption; or (5) pancreatic disease, which prevents optimal absorption of the vitamin from the ileum; and (6) both blocking- and binding-type antibodies, as demonstrated against all major cobalamin binders in the serum. Any one of these can cause a failure of cobalamin transport,[188] e.g. transcobalamin II deficiency.[51] Milder degrees of these abnormalities cause cobalamin inadequacy.

Several **drug interactions** may reduce serum cobalamin levels. Folate is essential for several cobalamin-dependent metabolic steps. Therefore, in the presence of a folic acid deficiency, large doses of folic acid increase the utilization of cobalamin and, when cobalamin reserves are depleted, can precipitate a serious cobalamin deficiency. Other drugs, including neomycin, colchicine, p-aminosalicylic acid, slow-release potassium chloride, biguanide therapy (e.g. metformin),[150, 235, 287] and ethanol have been associated with malabsorption of cobalamin. Persons ingesting large doses of vitamin C for long periods may risk cobalamin deficiency.[135] The reduction in serum cobalamin levels associated with chronic intake of oral contraceptives[305] was not attributable to impaired absorption of cobalamin.[235]

Therapy. If the Schilling test shows abnormal absorption, the cause should be explored. Pernicious anemia may have an autoimmune component that can show two different types of antibody to intrinsic factor.[135] It also may be due to gastric achlorhydria or gastric carcinoma.

Preparations of cyanocobalamin injection USP are ordinarily marketed in solutions containing either 100 or 1000 mcg/ml. Hydroxocobalamin* is retained in the body in greater amounts and for longer periods than cyanocobalamin,[48] and is used widely in Europe.[135] However, hydroxocobalamin is more expensive, and may induce antibodies to plasma cobalamin-binding protein in some patients.[133] We have seen a number of patients whose myofascial syndromes, blood elements and serum cobalamin levels have failed to respond to parenteral cyanocobalamin, but have responded to hydroxocobalamin injected intramuscularly.

No oral preparation of hydroxocobalamin is available for supplementation, but the senior author has administered the injectable solution by mouth in a few cases refractory to cyanocobalamin, with beneficial long-term effects.

Acute therapy customarily involves intramuscular injection of either cyanocobalamin or hydroxocobalamin, 1000 mcg twice weekly for 4 or 5 weeks, followed by a similar maintenance dose monthly, indefinitely.[32] Oral preparations of vitamin B_{12} plus intrinsic factor should not be used for long-term therapy because patients with pernicious anemia are likely to become refractory by developing local intestinal antibodies to the exogenous intrinsic factor.[135]

When a cobalamin deficiency is associated with frank anemia, the patient should be rechecked after 1 month of parenteral vitamin B_{12} therapy for possible folic acid and/or iron deficiency, since the one therapy may unmask another deficiency.[135]

Folic Acid (Folates)

Discovery. Understanding of the overlapping contributions of folic acid and vitamin B_{12} to the etiology of macrocytic anemia evolved slowly. Pteroylglutamic (folic) acid was purified in 1943 by Stokstad and was crystallized from liver in the same year by Pfiffner and associates. By 1948, Angier and his co-workers synthesized it and identified its structure. It then became clear that folic acid was the Wills factor, and the vitamin M previously found in dry brewers' yeast, and also the vitamin B_c of yeast identified in chick experiments.[137]

Chemistry. The term folic acid should be limited to pteroylglutamic acid, rather than applied generically to any member of the folate vitamin family, which consists of tetrahydrofolates. The latter, which are metabolically active, should be referred to as folates.[137] Folic acid is metabolically inactive, and is not found naturally in foods or in the human body in significant concentrations. It occurs as yellow crystals and consists of three parts, a pteridine moiety linked by a methylene bridge to p-aminobenzoic acid, which, in turn, is joined to glutamic acid.

To form folates, various single carbon units may be linked at the N-5 and N-10 positions of folic acid, thus conferring on the folates their multiple roles as single carbon carriers. At least five coenzyme forms of folate are known, as clearly described and illustrated by Herbert.[132] All of these participate in the transfer of a 1-carbon unit necessary for the synthesis of various substrates in the body.[138] The methylated form, methyltetrahydrofolate, is the dominant folate in human serum, and in the liver where it is stored as a polyglutamate.[137] The isolation of the stable folic acid form was the result of oxidation and deconjugation of the naturally occurring folates.

The folates in the tissues are not monoglutamates, but polyglutamates that contain up to six glutamic acid residues linked

---

* AlphaRedisol (hydroxocobalamin) 1000 mcg/ml, Merck Sharp & Dohme, Division of Merck & Co., Inc., Westpoint, PA. 19486.

to the parent compound.[137] Folates from natural food sources are also polyglutamates and may incorporate as many as eight glutamate residues. However, monoglutamates are much more readily absorbed by man.[132, 137]

Functions. The **synthesis of deoxyribonucleic acid** (DNA) requires both cobalamin (vitamin B_{12}) and folate. The disruption of DNA synthesis causes megaloblastosis (giant germinal cells) of any rapidly proliferating cells, including blood-forming elements in the bone marrow and cells lining the gut.[137]

Folate is required for the biosynthesis of pyrimidine nucleotide.[137] The folate trap caused by cobalamin deficiency is considered above under vitamin B_{12}.

Folates are responsible for a number of **single-carbon-unit transfers**, one of which is the biosynthesis of purines. These folate-dependent transfers are responsible for several minor reactions and three major amino acid conversions:[132] histidine to glutamic acid, serine to glycine, and homocysteine to methionine; the latter two conversions also require cobalamin.

Folate is important in the development and normal **function of the brain**. Studies in mice[194] confirm clinical data[253] that folate is critical to development of the brain and essential for its normal functioning after birth. The body normally protects brain folate by concentrating folate in the cerebrospinal fluid[132] to about three times the concentration in the serum;[229] in 6 patients with low serum folate, the cerebrospinal fluid contained two to eight times the concentration in the serum.[40] Furthermore, brain folate levels drop only with deprivation severe enough to have depleted liver folate stores. In mice, the relatively long half-life of brain folate, 5.9 weeks, compared with 1.7 weeks for liver folate, helps to maintain brain folate levels.[194]

Folate contributes to **prostaglandin synthesis**; experiments show that folate deficiency leads to prostaglandin deficiency and folate excess to prostaglandin excess. Prostaglandin synthesis is impaired in schizophrenic patients, while increased prostaglandin synthesis is associated with increased seizure activity in patients with seizures.[140]

Folate Deficiency. The symptoms described by patients with myofascial pain who have marginally low serum folate levels are similar in kind to, but less intense than, many of the symptoms reported by patients with obvious neurologic disorders responsive to folic acid therapy.

Increased muscular irritability and susceptibility to myofascial TPs are commonly observed in patients with low normal (lowest quartile) or subnormal serum folic acid levels. They tire easily, sleep poorly, and feel discouraged and depressed. In our experience, these patients also frequently feel cold and have a reduced basal temperature, as do patients with thyroid hypofunction; their symptoms are often relieved by multivitamin therapy including folic acid. A subnormal serum folate level in time causes megaloblastic hematopoiesis[132] and anemia. The differential diagnosis of anemia is well described by Herbert.[135] Nonspecific symptoms of glossitis,[132, 234] diarrhea,[132, 160] weight loss,[132, 234] irritability,[132] sleeplessness,[132] and forgetfulness[132] are not unusual. Occasionally, patients describe restless legs,[39] diffuse muscular pain,[40] abnormal intellectual functioning,[41] or symptoms of peripheral neuropathy.[42] Evidence of peripheral neuropathy was found in 21% of one group of folate-deficient patients.[261] Similar findings in another group responded to folic acid therapy.[43] Folate deficiency alone can cause signs and symptoms of subacute combined degeneration of the cord, as in vitamin B_{12} deficiency.[42, 121, 217, 218]

Acute experimental deprivation of folate for 6 months[130, 131] produced the following effects: in 3 weeks, low serum folate; in 7 weeks, hypersegmentation of polymorphonuclear leukocytes; in 14 weeks, increased urinary excretion of formiminoglutamic acid; in 18 weeks, low erythrocyte folate and macroovalocytosis; and in 19 weeks, megaloblastic bone marrow and anemia. During the fourth month, sleeplessness and forgetfulness appeared and gradually increased through the fifth month. The mental symptoms disappeared within 48 hours after starting oral folic acid therapy.[130, 131]

A disproportionately high percentage of psychiatric patients are folic-acid deficient.[63, 149, 284] Depression is their most probable psychiatric diagnosis.[63] It now appears that cobalamin deficiency has the greatest impact on the cord and peripheral nerves, whereas folate deficiency is more likely to be associated with mental disorders that concern affect and intellect.[230]

Several studies indicate that folate deficiency can, others that it cannot, impair immune function.[203, 316]

Low serum cholesterol levels were correlated with low serum folate values at or below 6.2 ng/ml in 46 patients, r = 0.58. No such correlation was obtained between cobalamin deficiency and the serum cholesterol level.[36] Low thyroid function of thyroid (but not of pituitary) origin is likely to be associated with an increased serum cholesterol.[146]

Using the recently introduced radioimmunoassay for "true" cobalamin, patients with folate deficiency show a decrease in cobalamin, but an increase in cobalamin analogues. Treatment with folate alone may correct both the low cobalamin and high analogue levels.[258] The impaired intestinal absorption of folate and vitamin B_{12} due to folate deficiency are both improved by folate supplementation.

Folate treatment before conception prevented recurrence of neural-tube defects in babies of 44 women, as compared with six recurrences among the 67 women who did not take the folate supplement.[171]

Folate Dependence. The congenital lack of a specific enzyme that is essential to normal functioning of one of the folate metabolic pathways points up the critical role of folate. **Congenital malabsorption** of folate is unusual, but has been clearly documented.[97, 138, 169, 208, 253] In addition, a specific defect of transport of folate into the cerebrospinal fluid with severe neurological deficits has been reported.[97]

Deficient **dihydrofolate reductase** activity blocks the conversion of folic acid and dihydrofolate to the metabolically active tetrahydrofolate form. These patients respond to folacin, but not to folic acid therapy.[97, 138] Neonates from three families developed megaloblastic anemia within 2–6 weeks after birth due to lack of the enzyme dihydrofolate reductase.[208]

Liver enzyme studies in one group of folate-deficient patients showed markedly decreased activity of **5-methyltetrahydrofolate transferase**.[234]

Patients with **methylenetetrahydrofol-** **ate reductase** deficiency exhibit homocystinuria responsive to folate therapy; in contrast, cystathionine synthase deficiency, which also causes homocystinuria, requires, instead, supplemental vitamin B_6.[97, 138, 208, 240]

Deficiency of **glutamic formiminotransferase** is less rare and blocks the formation of glutamate from histidine[97, 138] causing increased excretion of formiminoglutamate (FIGLU) in the urine.[208, 234] At least three other enzyme deficits are folate-responsive.[208]

These congenital abnormalities in folate-dependent pathways are generally seen initially in children with severe and often irreversible mental retardation and/or megaloblastic anemia. Some are greatly improved by megadoses of folic acid or folacin. Incomplete expression of such congenital enzyme deficiencies can significantly increase the dietary folate requirements of an individual.

Laboratory Tests. Normal human serum contains approximately 7–16 ng/ml of folate in the serum. Such small quantities have been measurable only microbiologically using *Lactobacillus casei* and by radioisotopic assay, first described in 1970; both methods measure 5-methyltetrahydrofolate.[137] Serum folate must be protected against oxidative destruction prior to assay, usually by freezing or by adding ascorbate, which, however, may destroy vitamin B_{12} in storage.[137] Some laboratories measure tissue saturation as erythrocyte folate, which should be more than 150 ng/ml.

The serum or urine may be tested for FIGLU, which appears with folate deficiency. The deoxyuridine suppression test can be applied to bone marrow cells or lymphocytes, which are tested for folate or cobalamin deficiency.[11, 135] Because of their long half-life, peripheral-blood lymphocytes may demonstrate cobalamin or folate deficiency with this test as long as 2 months after treatment has started.

Contrary to expectation, among hospitalized patients, a high mean corpuscular volume (MCV) of 95 cu mm or more had only an 0.18 correlation with folate deficiency, and therefore, would not have been useful to screen for it.[119] In some of the patients, other conditions caused the macrocytosis; or blocked macrocytosis despite the folate deficiency; in other patients, the tissue folate had not yet been sufficiently depleted to produce the macrocytosis.

Iron deficiency can suppress the megaloblastic changes of bone marrow cells and the macrocytosis of erythrocytes usually caused by folate deficiency.[11, 137] This double deficiency of iron and folate is likely in women of childbearing age.[136]

The "folate" trap due to cobalamin deficiency blocks transformation of the metabolically inactive methylfolate, which accumulates and is measured in the serum. Therefore, after starting needed vitamin B_{12} therapy, serum folate levels are likely to drop precipitously as the trapped methylfolate is converted to useable tetrahydrofolates.

Requirement. The recommended dietary allowance is 400 mcg/day of total folacin activity for adults and adolescents. This value is measured as the total pteroylglumatic acid equivalents assayed with the bacterium *L. casei* in extracts of diets treated with conjugase. During pregnancy, this allowance is set at 800 mcg/day and during lactation, 500 mcg/day.[200] Studies showed that the average dietary intake of Canadians was below 400 mcg/day; in the United States the average was 689 mcg/day; these are probably overestimates, as indicated below.[200]

Normal total-body folate stores range from 5–10 mg, of which approximately half is in the liver. Most folate is stored as polyglutamates, which have far greater molecular size and charge than monoglutamates, and probably must be hydrolyzed to monoglutamates to be transported across cell walls, an enzyme-dependent process.[137] In alcoholic subjects on a nearly folate-free diet, megaloblastic hemopoiesis appeared in only 5–10 weeks,[90] as compared to 19 weeks in a nonalcoholic control, in Herbert's classic study.[131] Other experimental low-folate diets produced signs of deficiency in 8–16 weeks depending on the level of initial folate stores.[200]

Sources and Fate. This section considers the dietary sources, absorption, transport mechanisms, and excretion of folates.

The **dietary sources** of folate are leafy vegetables, as the name indicates, and also include yeast, liver and other organ meat, fresh or fresh-frozen uncooked fruit or fruit juice, and lightly cooked fresh green vegetables, such as broccoli and asparagus. Although folates are ubiquitous in nature, being present in nearly all natural foods, they are highly susceptible to oxidative destruction; 50–95% of the folate content of foods may be destroyed in processing and preparation. All folate is lost from refined foods, such as hard liquor and hard candies.[135, 137, 234]

Assessment of the methods used to determine folate in food sources reveals that a large number of factors, identified and unidentified, interact in a complex manner to make it extremely difficult to predict the amount of folate that becomes available to the body. Contradictions between estimated availability of dietary folates and observed serum and tissue deficiency in the same population attest to the overestimation of available folate when the estimate is calculated on the basis of dietary intake.[237]

Folates appear in natural foods almost exclusively as polyglutamates. Before they can be **absorbed**, the polyglutamates must be hydrolyzed to monoglutamate by the enzyme conjugase, which is found in the brush border lining of the proximal jejunum.[74, 137, 239] This hydrolysis is suppressed by specific conjugase inhibitors found in some foods, such as beans and peas; hydrolysis is also inhibited by an acid pH, such as that caused by citric acid in orange juice.[74] Either folate or cobalamin deficiency changes the morphology and function of the mucosal cells of the small intestine so as to perpetuate a deficiency state of either or both of these vitamins.[124]

Active mucosal transport of the normally resultant monoglutamate is required for folate absorption; failure of mucosal transport probably accounts for most instances of folate malabsorption.[137] Intestinal absorption is highly sensitive to pH; maximum transport occurs at pH 6.0, decreasing by half at pH 5.0 or pH 7.0.[239] Metabolic conversion of monoglutamic folate to reduced methylfolate appears to occur within the intestinal wall prior to folate release into the portal circulation.

Synthetic folic acid is well absorbed.[238]

Folate is **transported** by plasma in three fractions: free folate, another loosely bound to low-affinity binders, both in relatively large amounts, and a small fraction bound to high-affinity binders, which are glycoproteins.[137] Delivery of serum methylfolate to marrow and transformed lymphocytes depends on cobalamin.[136]

Of 51 patients with rheumatoid arthritis who were taking aspirin, 71% had abnormally low serum folate levels and abnormally rapid plasma clearance of folic acid due to abnormal binding. The low serum values may have reflected a redistribution, rather than a deficiency of folate.[8]

The enterohepatic circulation transports about 0.1 mg of biologically active folate daily, and is important in maintaining serum folate levels.[137] Folates in the liver and in the cerebrospinal fluid are present in higher concentration than in the serum and must be transported against a concentration gradient. The high concentration in cerebrospinal fluid maintains an increased concentration of folate around the brain, even in states of folate deficiency.[136]

Folate is **excreted** into both the bile and the urine. Most of that excreted in the bile is normally reabsorbed from the duodenum.[234]

Causes of Deficiency. Folic acid deficiency is very prevalent. Population studies have shown that at least half of the Canadians eat less than the recommended dietary allowance of folates, while in the United States, individuals from high-income states showed tissue deficiency in 15% of the white population and in over 30% of the black and Spanish-American groups.[237] Fortunately, the recent taboo against including folic acid in multivitamins for fear it might mask the diagnosis of pernicious anemia due to lack of vitamin B_{12}[94] is giving way to the realization that folic acid deficiency is a more common cause of megaloblastic anemia than is pernicious anemia.[237]

If the prevalence of folate deficiency is so high, especially in vulnerable groups as noted below, how many more individuals must be suboptimal in folate nutrition?

The four commonest causes of folate deficiency are advanced age (an increasing segment of our population), pregnancy or lactation, dietary indiscretion, and drug abuse, most commonly of alcohol.

Many studies[26, 74, 193, 242] show an increased incidence of folate deficiency in the **elderly**. Inadequate diet and small

bowel disorders probably account for more than 90% of the deficiencies. In a study of 210 elderly patients,[193] folate deficiency was found in 24% of those from homes for the aged, in only 7.8% of similar patients from their own homes, and in 5% of a younger control group. Physical disability is seriously underestimated as a cause of impaired nutrition. This situation is compounded by the social isolation, confusion, and interacting drug effects to which the elderly are especially prone.[242]

In addition, Baker and co-workers[26] found an impaired ability of the elderly to absorb folate from dietary sources, compared with their absorption of the monoglutamate, folic acid. Folate deficit itself can induce changes in the epithelial structures and enzyme secretion of the small bowel, which in turn exacerbate folate malabsorption.[135]

A **pregnancy** greatly increases the requirement for folate. In a study of 469 low-income black adults in South Africa, red cell folate levels were deficient in 44% of the pregnant women, in 32% of the nonpregnant women, and in 19% of the men and nulliparous women.[74] One-third of all pregnant women in the world develop a folate deficiency so severe that they have megaloblastic anemia.[135] Among 269 pregnant low-income patients in Gainesville, FL, *15% were deficient* in serum folate (< 3 ng/ml), and *48% were low* in serum folate (3–6 ng/ml), on their first maternity visit.[19] In another study of 174 mothers of low to middle income at parturition,[24] 71% of the 41 patients who took no vitamin supplements had low serum folate levels, and 29% of the 113 patients who did take vitamin supplements received insufficient folate to protect them from deficiency (< 4 ng/ml).

Food fortification with folic acid for populations at risk is practical and would cost only a few cents per person per year.[74]

Although the folic acid levels in the umbilical cord blood of neonates is 2 to 5 times greater than that of the mother,[24] 38% of 37 preterm infants having a birth weight of 2.0 kg or less were deficient in folic acid. Thus, folate deficiency is not just a maternal problem and is especially critical during growth of the nervous system.[279] Another study[27] demonstrated significantly lower folate, cobalamin and panthothenate levels in low birth weight neonates than in babies of normal weight.

Folate deficiency due to **inadequate ingestion** is observed in those who eat mostly starchy foods and little meat or leafy vegetables, often because of limited means. In affluent societies, deficiency is usually considered evidence of blood loss or malabsorption, with the exception of high starch eaters and elderly persons who live alone and subsist on starchy snacks. Also at risk are unsupervised youngsters in large families who eat a folate-deficient diet that they select.[76] Well over a half of alcoholics and nearly half of narcotic addicts are folate deficient, partly because of inadequate ingestion.[135]

Marginal folate deficiency may be discernable only during the winter when intake of the vitamin is lowest. In one study[234] of women who previously had taken an oral contraceptive, decreased plasma and erythrocyte folate levels were found in only those first trimesters of pregnancy occurring during the wintertime.

Use of certain drugs is another common source of folate deficiency. Nine major drug groups have been incriminated. Each is listed with an example: (1) cytotoxic, methotrexate; (2) antimalarial, pyrimethamine; (3) anticonvulsant, diphenylhydantoin; (4) diuretic, triamterene; (5) estrogens, as oral contraceptives; (6) antitubercular, cycloserine; (7) antiinflammatory, aspirin; (8) anti-infective, aromatic diamidine; and (9) abused drugs, of which alcohol is the most frequent offender.[234]

Folic acid analogues, aminopterin in early studies and now methotrexate, have been used as antimetabolites in the therapy of neoplastic disease. They function as folate antagonists by inactivating dihydrofolate reductase, which is necessary to form metabolically active tetrahydrofolate from inactive folic acid and dihydrofolate. One of the hazards of methotrexate therapy is that the effects of excessive dosage cannot be reversed by giving folic acid; a metabolically active form, folinic acid, is required.[55]

Pyrimethamine is effective in the treatment of chloroquine-resistant malaria because of its folate-antagonist affect, which is not selective for the parasite and also inhibits folate metabolism in the host.

Triamterene, used as a diuretic, inhibits the dihydrofolate reductase enzyme, producing a deficiency that is correctable with folinic acid, but only partially correctable with folic acid.[234]

Alcohol is considered here because it involves both inadequate ingestion and malabsorption of folate; other drugs will be discussed in terms of the mechanism by which they cause deficiency. Fifty to 90% of alcoholics are folate deficient.[80, 135] In addition to low intake, this deficiency is due to decreased absorption of natural polyglutamates[125] and to impaired release of folate stores from tissue.[167] However, in alcoholism good absorption of the monoglutamate, folic acid, persisted.[25]

An **impaired absorption** of folate can result from deficiency of either folate or vitamin B_{12}, and from ingesting folates with strongly acid foods.[135] Folic acid supplements also should not be ingested with an antacid. Deficiency due to malabsorption occurs postgastrectomy[234] and in tropical sprue.[135] Treatment of ulcer or colitis with sulfasalazine is associated with an impaired absorption of folate that disappears with cessation of sulfasalazine treatment.[280]

Although one study[210] of 526 women reported that there was no difference in the serum folate level between users and nonusers of oral contraceptives, Streiff[278] found that a group of oral contraceptive users had markedly impaired absorption of natural polyglutamic folates, but could absorb folic acid.

In another study,[307] **impaired utilization** contributed to megaloblastic changes in the epithelium of the uterine cervix. These changes were associated with oral contraceptive therapy and were reversed by supplemental folic acid, but could be related neither to the hematologic findings, to serum folate, nor to cobalamin levels.

Cobalamin (vitamin B_{12}) deficiency impairs folate metabolism partly through the methylfolate-trap mechanism, and also through impaired cell uptake of methyltetrahydrofolate.[234]

Several conditions in addition to pregnancy and lactation can **increase requirements**, such as sickle cell disease in some individuals.[234] The folate deficiency caused by anticonvulsants, such as diphenylhydantoin, phenobarbital and primidone,[115, 159] is ascribed partly to an increased demand for folate,[66, 234] and partly to impaired absorption.[108] However, simply treating 31 patients with a folic acid supplement for 3 months, while they continued the anticonvulsant therapy, markedly reduced their previously normal serum cobalamin, in some cases to the deficiency level.[144] We have seen such a drop in the cobalamin level in our folate-depleted patients after a month or two of folic acid therapy without supplemental parenteral vitamin B_{12}.

Hemodialysis[234] causes **increased excretion** of folate, and so does treatment with methotrexate.[234]

Therapy. The blood changes due to deficiency of either cobalamin or folate can be indistinguishable; the two conditions must be identified by laboratory tests specific for each vitamin, or by a discriminating therapeutic trial.[135] Treating vitamin B_{12} deficiency with folic acid reverses the hematologic changes, but can allow the neurologic deficits to progress disastrously.[94]

Initial therapy for severe folate deficiency *per se* is 1 mg/day of folic acid parenterally for 10 days, followed by the same dose orally, which is usually sufficient to maintain body folate stores in the presence of suboptimal absorption.[135] Oral doses of 5–10 mg/day may be given initially.

The hematological response to treatment of folate deficiency with folic acid appears in 4–7 days,[137] but the increased susceptibility of the skeletal muscles to TPs may require 3 or 4 weeks to subside. If clinical improvement falters after a month or two, serum folate levels should be remeasured to insure that the oral dose was adequately absorbed. After several months of folic acid therapy, cobalamin and vitamin B_6 levels also may increase as intestinal absorption improves.

To distinguish between cobalamin and folate deficiency, the patient may be treated with 100 mcg/day of folic acid, orally if the suspected cause is dietary inadequacy, or parenterally if malabsorption may be present. This dosage produces a maximal hematological response in folate deficiency, but no such response in

patients with cobalamin deficiency.[137] However, large doses of folic acid in cobalamin deficiency, or 500 mcg or more of vitamin B_{12} in folate deficiency, may each produce a hematologic response that can lead to an incorrect diagnosis. Minimal effective therapeutic doses are essential for a discriminating therapeutic test.[317]

Poor hematologic response to folic acid therapy alone may be due to a combined iron and folate deficiency, which often responds dramatically to both iron and folate supplements.

Treatment of sprue with oral tetracycline resulted in marked improvement in serum folate levels due to improved absorption.[161]

Ascorbic Acid (Vitamin C)

This vitamin is of clinical importance to the muscles because it can prevent much postexercise muscle soreness or stiffness; it also corrects the increase in capillary fragility associated with ascorbic acid deficiency, which greatly complicates the injection of TPs.

Discovery: In 1928, Albert Szent-Györgyi isolated a chemical that protects some fruits against discoloration and infection when bruised. The chemical is now known as ascorbic acid, or vitamin C.[59] For its discovery, he won the Nobel Prize in 1937.

Some birds[68] and a few mammals are unable to convert D-glycuronic acid to L-ascorbic acid. Man, monkeys, the guinea pig, and the Indian fruit bat are unable to synthesize ascorbic acid, which makes them dependent on exogenous sources.[174] Three exceptional guinea pigs out of several thousand were apparently able to synthesize it,[109] a capability occasionally observed in this species by other investigators;[177] a few people may possess a similar capability.

Through recorded history, scurvy was the scourge of armies, explorers, and sailors on extended trips without fresh food, until they learned to include an adequate source of vitamin C, such as lime juice, in their diet. On one trip, Vasco da Gama lost 100 of 160 sailors from scurvy.[139]

Functions. Ascorbic acid is involved in a remarkable number of essential body functions, including collagen synthesis, degradation of amino acids, and the synthesis of two neurotransmitters. Also, it is one of the most active reducing agents known to occur naturally in living tissue;[249] it provides a ready source of hydrogen atoms, since it is easily oxidized.[300]

The most abundant protein in mammals is **collagen**. It constitutes nearly one-quarter of the protein in body tissues.[249] The strong reducing action of ascorbic acid is needed for the hydroxylation of the amino acids lysine and proline to form the protocollagen molecule. This function may be assisted by ascorbic acid inhibition of hyaluronidase.[57] At least two other important body components have an amino acid sequence similar to collagen; the Clq subcomponent of complement and the basement membrane of cells.[71, 143]

As an example of its structural importance, the rate of healing of pressure sores was nearly doubled by increasing serum ascorbic levels *within the normal range*, from low normal to high normal levels.[281] The low normal values were clearly suboptimal. Collagen (and therefore vitamin C) is essential for the deposition of calcium phosphate crystals to form bone.[249] In the authors' clinical experience, vitamin C can be important in the treatment of low back pain, presumably because it improves the quality of the connective tissue.

Without vitamin C to provide the collagen needed for a firm vessel wall, the patient experiences marked capillary fragility and easy bruising, with diffuse tissue bleeding following only minor trauma.[249] Scorbutic patients are especially liable to develop postinjection hematomas and ecchymoses, a complication of TP injections that should be avoided.

A 70-kg person on an average diet metabolizes about 400 g of protein/day, of which 100 g of **amino acids** undergo oxidative degradation in a complicated manner that provides the many building blocks for regeneration of protein structures. With no protein ingestion, some 30 g of indigenous protein continues to be oxidatively degraded. Ascorbic acid is essential to the oxidative degradation of two amino acids, phenylalanine and tyrosine.[71, 139, 174] Tyrosinemia of the newborn is correctable by oral ascorbic acid.[139]

This vitamin is required for the synthesis of the essential **neurotransmitters** norepinephrine and serotonin.[71, 139]

Ascorbic acid is **readily oxidized** to dehydroascorbic acid, which retains 80% of its effectiveness, but further oxidation renders it inactive.[249] The vitamin protects the tissue thiol (—SH) group, is needed to convert plasma transferrin to liver ferritin,[71] enhances the absorption of iron in the gastrointestinal tract,[249] and contributes to fatty acid metabolism through the synthesis of carnitine.[205]

In addition, the vitamin contributes to the **stress responses** of the body. Tissue levels in the adrenal gland parallel those of the corticosteroids; both decrease markedly in response to stress.[162] Since ascorbic acid participates in the synthesis of corticosterone and 17-hydroxycorticosterone, adrenal stores of ascorbic acid may be depleted by its release to the circulation, by its utilization for the replacement of corticosteroids, or both.[143, 249]

Ascorbic acid is important to enzymes that protect animals from some toxic substances. It has protected experimental animals against the formation of bladder tumors by 3-hydroxyanthranilic acid and against the hepatotoxic combination of sodium nitrite and aminopyrene.[143]

Increased susceptibility to infectious diseases has been observed consistently among people with scurvy.[139] The claim by Linus Pauling[212] that megadoses of vitamin C protect from the common cold generated much controversy. The immune systems of female children and young female adults are apparently more responsive to ascorbic acid than are those of males.[249] The vitamin does influence the immune system, but its role is not clear.[297] In the authors' clinical experience, ascorbic acid helps to terminate bouts of diarrhea due to food allergy, and to decrease toxicity and trigger-point irritability caused by chronic infection.

In the patient suffering from a cold, after ingestion of 2 g ascorbic acid with 600 mg of aspirin, significant amounts of ascorbic acid entered the leukocytes. Twenty-four days after the respiratory symptoms had disappeared, the leukocytes no longer picked up ascorbic acid in the presence of aspirin.[313] Taken early when the first cold symptoms appear, this combination may help to abort the development of the upper respiratory infection.

There is evidence of decreasing tissue

levels of ascorbic acid with increased age. Damage to membranous cell structures by lipid peroxidation appears to contribute to the deterioration of cells in the absence of ascorbic acid's reductive protection of the tissue thiol groups.[143, 211] Deficiency in guinea pigs caused dystrophic disorganization of muscle structures, including fragmentation of myofilaments, swelling of mitochondria and excessive glycogen.[153] Vitamin C also reverses some of the electrocardiographic changes associated with increasing age.[69] Claims of protection from some cancers by megadoses of vitamin C will probably be substantiated.[58, 59, 61]

The stiffness experienced the day after unusually strenuous exercise is, in our experience, prevented or markedly reduced by 1 g or more of ascorbic acid taken shortly before, or at the time of, the exercise.

Ascorbic Acid Deficiency. In the United States, scurvy, due to inadequate dietary intake of ascorbic acid, is most likely to occur in smokers, alcoholics, older people, infants fed primarily on cow's milk (usually between the ages of 6 and 12 months), food faddists, and psychiatric patients. A series of 35 patients with alcohol-related illness had a 91% prevalence of ascorbic acid deficiency.[20] Antacids oxidize ascorbic acid and should be taken separately so they are not mixed in the stomach.

Scurvy develops after 4–7 months of an insufficient diet.[249] Elderly patients in a chronic disease hospital, on an institutional diet with little fresh fruit, had an average whole blood vitamin C level of only 0.35 mg/dl. Eight ounces of orange juice daily raised the level to 1.52 mg/dl.[65]

Decreased absorption of ascorbic acid is seen in diarrheal diseases, and increased utilization occurs in thyrotoxicosis.

A frequent cause of vitamin C deficiency is cigarette smoking.[37, 56, 143, 205] Either the smoker utilizes more ascorbic acid, or less of the vitamin is available from the same dietary intake.[215]

The symptoms of frank scurvy are easily diagnosed; borderline or subclinical cases are difficult to recognize.[249] Initially, scorbutic patients present with nonspecific symptoms of weakness, lassitude, irritability, and vague aching pains in the joints and muscles. They may complain of weight loss. As the disease progresses, they are aware of easy bruising and even hematomas in the skin and muscles. The gums become swollen, red, and bleed easily. The teeth become loose and may fall out. Gum symptoms develop only in response to contact with irritants (plaque) on the teeth, and are absent in edentulous patients.[249]

Experimentally, the first sign of scurvy was perifollicular hyperkeratotic papules on the buttocks, thighs and legs, later on the arms and back. As the hairs became buried in the papules, petechiae appeared around the lesions.[249]

In advanced scurvy, splinter hemorrhages appear in the distal nail beds. In chronic cases, "woody" edema of the legs develops with pain, hemorrhage and brownish pigmentation, which may advance to a sclerodema-like stage.[249]

In infantile scurvy, bone, joint and muscle involvement dominates the clinical picture.[249]

Laboratory Tests. Determination of plasma L-ascorbic acid, based on its reducing properties, is available through medical laboratories.[139] A simple, lingual screening test for ascorbic acid deficiency has been developed[70, 181, 312] and marketed.*

Requirement. The body pool of ascorbic acid averages about 1500 mg, and the daily rate of metabolism approximates 3% of the existing body pool. At this rate, it would require 45 mg/day to replenish the pool. Without any replacement, a filled body pool is depleted to the scorbutic level in about 2 months.[139]

In the United States, the basic recommended daily allowance is 60 mg, 80 mg for pregnant women and 100 mg for lactating mothers.[200] Some countries recommend a somewhat higher basic daily intake (75 mg in West Germany).[139]

Ordinary farm animals, like horses and pigs, that synthesize ascorbic acid show average plasma concentrations of 0.33–0.40 mg/dl. By comparison, in man the value is stated as[139]:

Well nourished	>1.0 mg/dl,
Adequately nourished	0.6–1.0 mg/dl,
Poorly nourished	0.3–0.6 mg/dl,
Deficient	<0.3 mg/dl.

---

* Lingual Ascorbic Acid Test, Mineralab, Inc. Available through Medical Diagnostic Services, P.O. Box 1441, Brandon FL 33511.

Sources. Ascorbic acid is rapidly oxidized in water to dehydroascorbic acid, which is only 80% as active as ascorbic acid biologically. Further oxidation renders it inactive. Oxidation in solution is accelerated by heat, light, alkalinity, and a metallic iron or copper vessel. This vitamin is highly soluble in water and is often discarded in the pot liquor of cooked foods. Canned tomatoes retain a high percentage of their ascorbic acid content (20 mg/100 g) because of the acid environment.[71]

Excellent potential sources of ascorbic acid that contain more than 100 mg/100 g of *raw* food are broccoli, Brussels sprouts, collards, kale, turnip greens, guava and sweet peppers. Less rich, but valuable, sources of ascorbic acid are cabbage and potatoes, because large amounts of these vegetables commonly are eaten.[139] Citrus fruits are well known to supply vitamin C. The *fresh* juice of a large orange contains about 50 mg of the vitamin; thus 10 oranges would supply 500 mg. However, loss of the vitamin in processing or storage may be large.

Vitamin C is readily absorbed from the upper small intestine; excess is quickly excreted by the kidney, very little *via* other portals. There is no extensive storage. The *maximum* body pool ranges between 1.5 and 5 g,[111] but may be as low as 1 g.[1] The half-life in man ranges from 13–30 days; the larger the intake, the shorter the half-life. Following ingestion, the major portion of the vitamin is excreted through the urine, and also *through the expired air;*[1] the latter pathway is often overlooked. The adrenal cortex is one tissue that is normally richly supplied with ascorbic acid.[139] The human digestive tract absorbs ascorbic acid efficiently at low levels of intake, but becomes less efficient at higher dose levels; approximately 70% of 180 mg, 50% of 1.5 g, and 16% of 12 g is absorbed, respectively. Unabsorbed vitamin C may cause diarrhea due to an osmotic effect.[139]

The concentration of isotope-labeled ascorbic acid in the adrenal gland, liver and kidney closely paralleled the decreasing concentration in the serum during the 24 hr after intravenous injection in rats.[190] Values in the brain and in one muscle continuously increased throughout this period, suggesting that an active transport system was functioning. Another muscle maintained a constant value, indicating that no active transport system was operating in it at that time.[190]

Causes of Deficiency. That cigarette smoking is a major cause of ascorbic acid deficiency was demonstrated in guinea pigs placed on a cigarette smoker for 10 min twice daily.[98] After 28 days, both the smoking and control nonsmoking groups had equal concentrations of ascorbic acid in the liver and testes, but its concentration in the adrenal glands of the "smokers" was 29% less than for the controls and the body weight of the smokers was 30% less.[98]

A study of 17 human volunteers who smoked more than 20 cigarettes/day showed that they required 140 mg of vitamin C daily to maintain a steady state plasma ascorbic acid level compared to a daily intake of only 100 mg of ascorbic acid in nonsmoking controls.[148]

Treatment. Prescription of ascorbic acid can be based on the recommended dietary allowance of 60 mg/day, which will **prevent scurvy,**[200] or on a physiological dose of as much as 500 mg daily, which ensures a **normal metabolic pool** of ascorbic acid to meet emergency demands,[110] or a megadose of 2–8 g/day, which may have additional *nonscorbutic* effects, such as protection from colds and cancer.[58, 61, 139]

The daily dose needed to ensure steady-state saturation levels in the tissues is probably about 450 mg daily, best taken in divided doses.[110] Oral intake beyond tissue saturation should be unnecessary, but the optimal intake required depends on highly variable stress factors. In sickness there is greater tolerance for vitamin C, than in good health; this suggests that megadoses are unnecessary when one is well, yet may be therapeutic when in poor health.[152]

Megadoses are sometimes given in the form of sodium ascorbate powder, which is undesirable because it is so high in sodium; crystalline ascorbic acid and calcium ascorbate contain no sodium. One level teaspoon of the latter powder equals 4 g of ascorbic acid. It can be sprinkled on food or dissolved in juice. Pharmacologic doses are less likely to produce gastric irritation if given in the sustained-release form.

Ascorbic acid exhibits a number of interactions with other vitamins. It apparently is important in the absorption of folic acid and in its conversion to coenzyme form, so that ascorbic acid deficiency in infants between 6 months and 1 year of age may present with the hematologic signs of folic acid deficiency.[212] Scorbutic anemia may be microcytic, due to an associated iron deficiency caused by blood loss, or macrocytic due to associated folic acid deficiency.[249]

The absorption of folic acid is increased by oral supplements of ascorbic acid in the presence of liver disease[35]; however, ingestion of more than 500 mg ascorbic acid/day has been associated with lower serum vitamin B_{12} levels.[249] The increased absorption of some metallic ions produced by supplemental vitamin C is desirable, as in the case of iron, but undesirable in the case of mercury. Ascorbic acid supplementation increases the amount of warfarin required to maintain the same therapeutic effect on blood clotting.[249] Supplemental vitamin C lowers the prothrombin time in patients on warfarin.[84] A daily megadose can cause watery diarrhea[84] that has been misdiagnosed as spastic colon, and a nonspecific urethritis that has unnecessarily led to extensive studies for venereal infection.[101]

The vitamin C requirement in women taking estrogen, or an oral contraceptive agent, may increase 3- to 10-fold, requiring daily amounts of the vitamin up to 500 mg.[249] Increased urinary excretion of vitamin C in man due to high plasma levels produces a mild uricosuric effect, probably because of competition with uric acid for renal tubular reabsorptive transport.[35]

As to side effects of ascorbic acid, no urinary crystallization of oxalic acid or calcium is likely to occur if ingestion of the vitamin is limited to 3–6 g/day. Nausea, abdominal cramps and diarrhea may occasionally be due to an allergic reaction, but are more probably the result of hyperacidity; as stated above, this can often be relieved by prescribing a slow release preparation of ascorbic acid, or by taking the supplement at meals.

Scorbutic symptoms may develop in persons suddenly withdrawn from megadose therapy, just as these symptoms may appear postpartum in babies born to megadose-treated mothers.[306]

For many reasons, patients should be encouraged to stop smoking; the depression of their vitamin C level is only one. Smokers who have stopped smoking should be encouraged to keep their hands

busy. Helpful activities include needlepoint, knitting, or embroidery. Others may prefer to carry a string of beads to run through the fingers when the urge becomes great to smoke. Chewing gum has helped some to quit smoking. Any of these activities carried to excess can abuse the muscles and activate TPs.

Dietary Minerals and Trace Elements

Several minerals, especially calcium, potassium, iron, and magnesium, are needed for normal muscle function. Deficiency of the first three tends to increase the irritability of myofascial TPs. Calcium is essential to muscle for the excitation-contraction mechanism of the actin and myosin filaments. Potassium is needed for rapid repolarization of the nerve and muscle cell membranes following an action potential. Iron is an essential part of the hemoglobin and myoglobin molecules, which transport oxygen to and within the muscle fibers. Magnesium is essential to the contractile mechanism of the myofilaments.

Calcium. Although a recommended daily allowance of 800 mg/day is established for adults,[201] 1000 mg or more of calcium may be needed to maintain mineral and skeletal homeostasis in middle-aged and elderly individuals.[14] A minimum of 1200 mg/day is recommended during gestation and breast feeding.[201] Calcium intakes up to 2500 mg/day do not result in hypercalcemia in normal persons.[14]

A normal value of total serum calcium does not assure adequate calcium nutrition. The physiologic effects of calcium depend on the free ionic calcium; the total calcium, much of which is bound to protein, has no direct correlation with the concentration of serum ionized calcium.[14]

A simple way to meet dietary calcium needs is to eat at least 2 servings daily from the milk group. For those who cannot drink milk because of allergy or lactose intolerance, 30 g (1½ oz) of brick cheese, a carton of yogurt, or 2 cups of cottage cheese suffice. For the many people who are lactose intolerant, calcium may be obtained from milk that is predigested by the enzyme lactase, sold as Lactase*; this hydrolyzes some of the lactose that, undigested, tends to cause diarrhea. Nonfat

---

* Lactase, 25 mg tablets, Rugby Laboratories, Inc., Rockville Centre, NY 11570.

dried milk can be added inconspicuously and acceptably as a dry ingredient in the preparation of foods. A few other foods, such as green leafy vegetables, legumes, canned salmon, clams, oysters, dried fruits and soybean curd (tofu), also supply calcium in the diet.[89] If the patient cannot tolerate dietary sources, a supplement such as calcium phosphate or calcium carbonate should be prescribed, such as Os-Cal† from ground oyster shell, which has vitamin D added. Three 250-mg tablets daily provide 750 mg of elemental calcium and 375 units of vitamin D_2; however, the large 500-mg tablets contain no vitamin D. Adequate absorption of calcium clearly requires sufficient vitamin D, with evidence that fluoride, phosphate, magnesium, and sometimes estrogen are also important for its absorption and utilization.

The importance of calcium to normal membrane function is now unfolding. It plays a critical role in malignant hyperthermia,[127] in the sickling of erythrocytes in sickle cell anemia,[28] and in hypertension.[191, 192] Calcium has long been known to be essential to the transmission of an action potential across the myoneural junction and to normal excitation-contraction of the myofilaments in muscle.[6]

Essential to life, but not as critical for muscle contraction and TP responsiveness, are other elements: zinc, iodine, copper, manganese, chromium, selenium, and molybdenum. In some patients, a close relationship exists between hypomagnesemia, hypocalcemia and hypokalemia. Hypocalcemia that develops as the result of magnesium deficiency improves only with the administration of magnesium as well as calcium.[259] Low serum calcium from this cause will usually return to normal levels within a week after initiating magnesium repletion by oral supplements of antacid or laxative preparations containing magnesium.[259]

Magnesium. The plasma level of magnesium normally varies between 1.5 and 2.1 mEq/liter by the atomic absorption method and is maintained within quite narrow limits.[259] Magnesium plays a key role as a prosthetic group in many essential enzymatic reactions.[259] The recommended daily allowances for magnesium is 350 mg/day for adult men and 300 mg/day for adult women, which is increased to 450 mg/day during pregnancy and lactation.[201] Magnesium toxicity may occur in elderly people who constantly take antacids or laxatives containing magnesium.

In testing the serum of many patients with myofascial pain syndromes for magnesium, the senior author rarely, if ever, found an abnormally low value. A patient with an elevated serum magnesium, however, was likely to have low thyroid function.

Potassium. The normal concentration of serum potassium ranges from 3.5–5.0 mEq/liter. Total body potassium is low in hypothyroidism and high in hyperthyroidism. In addition to aggravating myofascial TPs, potassium deficiency disturbs function of smooth muscle and of cardiac muscle, as shown by an abnormal electrocardiogram.[224]

A diet high in fat, refined sugar and oversalted food is high in sodium, low in potassium, and can lead to potassium deficiency.[216] Diarrhea, laxatives and certain diuretics increase potassium loss. The recommended daily allowance for potassium is at least about 2 g (50 mEq), but more is needed if there are unusual losses.[201] A healthful diet for normal persons is high in potassium and low in sodium. This is not true of those with adrenal insufficiency. Foods particularly rich in potassium are fruits (especially bananas and citrus fruits), potatoes, green leafy vegetables, wheat germ, beans, lentils, nuts, dates, and prunes. The pot liquor of cooked vegetables should be saved and reused to conserve its potassium.

Iron. Patients low in iron are anemic with limited oxygen transport, which impairs energy metabolism of the muscles. The most common cause of iron deficiency is excessive loss of blood with inadequate dietary replacement. Blood loss is likely to be caused by gastric irritation (often due to aspirin), by hemorrhoids, metrorrhagia, or excessive blood donations. The recommended daily allowance is 1.8 mg of *absorbable* iron, rather than total iron. This takes into consideration the nearly 10-fold variability of iron absorption depending on its source and on the composition of the diet.[201]

---

† Os-Cal 250 tablet with vitamin D, Marion Laboratories, Inc., 10236 Bunker Ridge Rd., Kansas City, MO 64137.

The interactions among iron, cobalamins and folates that must be considered when assessing anemia have been summarized under vitamin B$_{12}$ in this chapter, and were extensively reviewed by Herbert.[135] Lean meats, liver and other organ meats, deep-green leafy vegetables, peas and beans, whole-grain cereals or breads, egg yolk, dried fruits, and shell fish are rich in iron.[216] White and colorless foods are low in iron.

Therapeutic Approach to Nutritional Deficiencies

Patients with chronic myofascial pain are a select group which, in our experience, has a remarkably high prevalence of vitamin inadequacies and deficiencies.

When the patient fails to respond to specific myofascial therapy or obtains only temporary relief, vitamin deficiencies must be ruled out as a major contributing cause and, if present, corrected.

Treatment for either folate deficiency or cobalamin (vitamin B$_{12}$) deficiency should not be pursued without establishing the level of, or supplementing, the other vitamins; their symptoms overlap so widely and they interact so strongly that treatment of one may mask or precipitate a deficiency of the other.[135]

A full evaluation of the total vitamin status of the patient is prohibitively difficult because of the many overlapping and nonspecific signs and symptoms of vitamin deficiency, multiple inadequacies, marked individual variations in the daily requirement, multiple causes of inadequacy, and the expense of these laboratory tests. Some laboratories helpfully provide vitamin panels. However, high standards of performance are required at every step to insure meaningful results that reliably tell the state of the patient's vitamin nutrition.

When a full battery of vitamin tests is not available, we find that a complete balanced supplement is a safe and usually effective alternative. Williams[311] recommends ingesting several times the recommended daily allowance of the water-soluble vitamins, but well below any possible toxic levels. One must be careful not to overload the body with the fat-soluble vitamins, particularly vitamin A. The supplement should include close to a recommended daily allowance of the essential minerals. The cost is nominal. This amount is harmless if it is the only supplemental source, and it insures a margin of safety against inadequate levels of essential nutrients.

When the clinical picture indicates a vitamin deficiency or inadequacy, and after blood has been drawn for vitamin assays, if the most rapid relief possible is indicated, intramuscular injections may be given in addition to oral supplements. A mixed injection of 100 mg each of vitamin B$_1$ and B$_6$, 5 mg of folic acid, 1 mg of vitamin B$_{12}$, and 2 mg of procaine is given intramuscularly. Folic acid is sometimes deleted since it is usually well absorbed by mouth in mild to moderate deficiencies. Four or five injections may be required to quickly bring a severely depleted reservoir of these vitamins to a functionally adequate level.

Balanced mixtures of B-complex vitamins are preferred to supplementation with only one or two vitamins; multiple B-complex deficiencies are very common. In addition, the reciprocal interaction among several B vitamins due to the intertwining of their metabolic functions may precipitate deficiency of an unsupplemented vitamin.[135] For this reason, a mixed B complex such as Plebex* may be added to the regimen for intramuscular injection.

An adequate blood level of vitamin C is important to optimal health. It is poorly stored, and its dietary intake is commonly inadequate. We consider it wise to supplement the diet routinely with 500 or 1000 mg of a timed release preparation daily. Ascorbic acid crystals are convenient for patients who need larger amounts because they smoke or have increased capillary fragility. Several grams per day can be sprinkled on the food or dissolved in fruit juice.

METABOLIC, AND ENDOCRINE INADEQUACIES

Clinically, any compromise of the energy metabolism of muscle appears to aggravate and perpetuate myofascial TPs. Anemia has been reviewed under vitamin B$_{12}$ in this chapter. Hypometabolism is covered in depth here because, when pres-

---

* Plebex Injection, Wyeth Laboratories, P. O. Box 8299, Philadelphia, PA 19101.

ent, the results of specific therapy for myofascial pain syndromes can be utterly frustrating until the hypometabolism is corrected; this perpetuating factor is not uncommon. Hypoglycemia is another perpetuating factor related to impaired energy metabolism. The last of this group, gouty diathesis, is a metabolic disturbance not directly related to energy.

Hypometabolism

Hypometabolism, or thyroid inadequacy, describes the condition of someone whose serum levels of thyroid hormones are in the low euthyroid, or just below the "normal" two standard deviation limit. The level of thyroid-stimulating hormone (TSH) may or may not be increased. Clearly hypothyroid patients have thyroid hormone levels below normal and an elevated TSH.[146] Patients referred to us with myofascial pain syndromes often arrive untreated for their slightly low thyroid function because they have only mild symptoms of hypothyroidism and borderline low, or low normal, thyroid tests. Experience has shown that these patients are more susceptible to myofascial TPs;[293] they experience only temporary pain relief with specific myofascial therapy. This increased irritability of their muscles and their poor response to therapy are greatly improved by supplemental thyroid, if they have no other major perpetuating factor.[293] In hyperthyroidism, active TPs are rare; the senior author cannot remember seeing a *hyper*thyroid patient with muscles unresponsive to specific myofascial therapy.

An association was noted[81] between patients diagnosed as hypothyroid and the development of musculoskeletal symptoms of early morning stiffness with pain and weakness of the shoulder girdle. A prospective study of 16 patients[81] with recent onset of rheumatoid arthritis that included a retrospective study of 26 patients diagnosed as having both diseases concluded that subnormal thyroid function may precipitate or exacerbate musculoskeletal symptoms. Reynolds[231] also found that patients with rheumatoid arthritis had significantly more tender points (indicative of myofascial TPs) than a comparable nonarthritic control group, but he did not examine the relation to metabolism.

Another study[309] identified eight patients with symptoms of fibrositis, defined in a way that included disturbed sleep and was compatible with the diagnosis of myofascial TPs. All eight also showed chemical evidence of hypothyroidism, a low T_4 and/or elevated TSH, but with few clinical indications of hypothyroidism. Six of the eight were relieved of their musculoskeletal symptoms by low-dose thyroid administration, and most of them no longer had difficulty sleeping[309]

Our observations and these reports suggest that, at least in some patients, the irritability of myofascial TPs is a sensitive indicator of inadequate thyroid function. It also may reflect a specific vulnerability of the muscles to impaired action of thyroid hormones at the cellular level, a condition that apparently occurs even though the levels of circulating hormone are clearly within normal limits.

This section on hypometabolism considers, in turn, the production of thyroid hormones, their metabolic effects, their concentration in the blood, the measurement of their function, symptoms of thyroid inadequacy, findings on physical examination, laboratory tests, and finally treatment.

Production of Thyroid Hormones. The thyroid hormones are two iodothyronines: tetraiodothyronine (thyroxine; T_4) and triiodothyronine (T_3). The form responsible for most metabolic effects is T_3.[248] The normal thyroid gland produces more T_4 than T_3, in a ratio of 10:1 to 15:1. When thyroid production is forced, as in hyperthyroidism, the gland can increase the relative amount of T_3 to a ratio of 5:1. As much as 98% of the circulating thyroid hormone normally is likely to be T_4 and only 2%, T_3. This occurs because the T_4 is more tightly bound to carrier protein than is the T_3. The carrier is mainly thyroxine-binding globulin (TBG).[146]

The T_4 is converted peripherally to T_3, largely in the liver, kidneys,[273] and skeletal muscles.[248]

Homeostatic levels of the serum iodothyronines are maintained by their release from the thyroid gland in response to TSH from the anterior pituitary gland. The amount of controlling TSH released from the pituitary gland depends on negative feedback control exerted by the serum level of thyroid hormones. The TSH stimulates hormone production by the thyroid gland. The secretion of TSH is stimulated by thyrotropin-releasing hormone (TRH) that is produced in the hypothalamus; TRH also increases the secretion of prolactin.[146, 232]

Thyroid hormone production is likely to be low following exposure of the gland to radiation,[170] as a late sequel of viral or subacute thyroiditis,[146] and after thyroidectomy. Not only is thyroid production likely to wane with advancing age, but the utilization of thyroid hormones at the cellular level may become impaired.

Effects of Thyroid Hormones. The thyroid hormones influence growth, energy production, and energy consumption. Thyroxine (T_4) affects growth by increasing the rate of microsomal protein synthesis through a direct effect on translation that does not require synthesis of RNA. On the other hand, T_3 increases both ribosomal RNA and protein synthesis through an increase in RNA polymerase activity. Thyroxine selectively increases the activity of some enzymes 5–10 times.[232] This helps to explain why adequate thyroid hormone is critical for the replication of many kinds of cells.

The chief product of oxidative phosphorylation is adenosine triphosphate (ATP), the primary source of energy for muscular contraction.[34] The production of ATP by mitochondria is significantly increased when the concentration of T_3 increases. The hormone acts at the inner membrane of the mitochondrion, which is the site of oxidative phosphorylation.[272]

A major mechanism by which T_3 causes increased energy expenditure is the increase of adenosine triphosphatase (ATPase) activity in cell membrane. ATP drives the sodium-potassium pump that maintains gradients of these ions across a cell membrane.[232] These gradients are essential to the excitability of muscle and nerve fibers and apparently have a "vent" system so that, although overactivity of the pump expends additional energy, it does not produce serious hyperpolarization of the membrane.

The increase of pump activity by thyroid hormones provides a potent mechanism for thermogenesis without shivering. It also increases the concentration of intracellular potassium, which agrees with the observation that an initial effect of hyperthyroidism is the accumulation of intracellular potassium.[251] Thyroid influence on this sodium-potassium pump activity is highest in kidney and liver and lowest in spleen and brain. Additional mechanisms of thermogenesis responsive to the thyroid hormones have been reported.[107, 141]

The decoupling of oxidative phosphorylation from ATP synthesis, which at one time was thought to be a major cause of nonshivering thermogenesis by thyroid hormone, appears not to occur at normal levels of thyroid function, but explains some effects of severe hyperthyroidism.[232]

Measurement of Hormone Concentration. The following tests are considered because of their value in helping to identify low thyroid function. Radioimmunoassay (RIA) provides accurate, direct measurement of hormone concentration in the serum: thyroxine (T_4) normally ranges between 4–11 mcg/dl, and triiodothyronine (T_3) ranges about 80–160 mcg/dl. The resin T_3 uptake ($RT_3 U$) normally ranges between 25–35% and corresponds to the percentage of binding sites on thyronine-binding globulin that are occupied, chiefly by T_4. The product of the serum T_4 concentration and the $RT_3 U$ is called the free T_4 index (T_4I) and varies directly with changes in the concentration of free T_4 hormone. The free T_4 theoretically is not affected by changes in the concentration of thyroxine-binding globulin.[146]

Measurement of Hormone Function. The basal metabolic rate (BMR) measures energy expenditure as the rate of oxygen consumption in the basal state. The normal range is approximately −15 to +5%, but this test is of limited diagnostic value because a variety of nonthyroidal factors seriously affect the BMR and make it prohibitively difficult to perform accurately.

Another indicator of energy expenditure in the basal state is basal temperature. This may be measured as either sublingual or axillary temperature on awakening in the morning, while still resting quietly and before stirring or getting out of bed. Normal values for axillary temperature taken for 10 min *by the clock* are given as 36.7 C (98 F) for men and the same for postmenopausal women. For women of childbearing years, it averages 36.4 C (97.5 F) immediately preceding ovulation, which is the value measured for basal temperature, with a peak temperature near 36.9 C (98.5 F) following ovulation.[30] We find that susceptibility of the muscles to TPs is consistently increased when the mean basal temperature is as low as 36.1 C (97.0 F), or lower. It is not clear whether thyroid inadequacy lowers the set point for thermal regulation, or if the mechanisms normally regulating body temperature[44, 53] have decompensated due to the impaired energy production and utilization.

Additional findings that may be warnings of inadequate thyroid function are prolongation of the relaxation phase of the Achilles tendon reflex and an increase in the serum chclesterol.[146]

Symptoms of Inadequate Thyroid Function. Patients with inadequate thyroid function generally present incomplete and moderate to mild symptoms of hypothyroidism. These are easily disregarded if the examiner is not concerned about their importance.

Hypometabolism patients nearly always experience **cold intolerance;** occasionally they are intolerant of both heat and cold. They tend to wear additional clothing (a sweater, jacket, or pullover) when others do not, rarely sweat, and frequently complain of cold hands and, especially, of cold feet.

Characteristically, the **muscular complaints** of the patient with hypometabolism are muscular aches and pains[225] or stiffness of muscles,[146] and those muscles are prone to develop persistent TPs. Chronic fatigue, which may approach lethargy,[146] is noticeable on arising in the morning and is usually worst at midafternoon. These patients are "weather conscious;" muscular pain increases with the onset of cold rainy weather. Inadequate folic acid also depresses the basal temperature, but in this case the muscles are not as weather conscious.

Inadequate metabolism may cause **additional symptoms** that are suggestive of myxedema or, in some patients, just the opposite. The latter are thin, nervous, and hyperactive, as if to keep warm. Constipation is much more likely than diarrhea. Disturbed menses may be evidenced by menorrhagia,[146] amenorrhea, or irregular menses. When due to hypometabolism,

these irregularities are correctable with supplemental thyroid. Hypometabolic patients are likely to suffer from dry, rough skin, which they often mask with an emollient skin cream. Some individuals of this group have difficulty losing weight, which, according to rat experiments,[12] would be aggravated by a thiamine deficiency.

Findings on Physical Examination. Hypometabolic patients are identified by a depressed basal temperature of 36.1 C (97 F) or less. Skin over regions of trauma at the elbows, knees, and behind the heels most clearly show a characteristic dry, scaly roughness. Muscular relaxation after a response of the Achilles tendon is often slow.[146] This is easily tested by having the patient kneel on the seat facing the back of a chair. Hypometabolic patients are subject to myoedema, which is elicited as a local mounding of a muscle in response to a sharp blow, as with a reflex hammer.[245] These phenomena appear to be based on delayed reaccumulation of calcium ions in the endoplasmic reticulum and, therefore, delayed disengagement of the actin and myosin filaments. Clinical electromyography does not reflect these abnormalities.[4]

Laboratory Tests. Serum hormone studies in hypometabolic patients show marginally low T_3 and T_4 levels, usually within the euthyroid range. Thyroid stimulating hormone (TSH) is rarely elevated. The cholesterol value is very likely to be elevated,[36, 156] if this increase is not counteracted by depression of the cholesterol level due to folate deficiency.[146] Vitamin B_{12} deficiency is not reported to affect serum cholesterol.[36] The muscle enzymes, creatine phosphokinase (CPK), serum glutamic-oxaloacetic transaminase (SGOT), lactic dehydrogenase (LDH), and aldolase, are elevated in hypothyroidism,[146] indicating that destruction of muscle structure may occur due to a lack of thyroid hormone. The blood may show increased lymphocytes and monocytes (about 45–50%) and a correspondingly decreased number of polymorphonuclear leukocytes.

Treatment. Before starting treatment with thyroid hormone it is important that the patient have an adequate vitamin B_1 level. Since thyroid increases metabolism, and thiamine requirements are metabolism-dependent, thyroid therapy can convert a vitamin B_1 inadequacy to a severe vitamin B_1 deficiency. If there is doubt, the patient can first be given a sufficient supplement of vitamin B_1 to establish a safe level (25–100 mg, three times daily, for at least 2 weeks before starting thyroid medication). Thiamine in a reduced dosage should be continued during thyroid therapy.

If promptness of relief is critical, initial thyroid therapy with triiodothyronine (T_3; Cytomel*), 12.5–50 mcg daily, provides a response within a few days. A 25-mcg dose corresponds roughly to 65 mg (1 grain) of dessicated thyroid extract.

"Intolerance" to low-dose thyroid therapy repeatedly has been due to aggravated symptoms of vitamin B_1 deficiency. After supplementation with thiamine, administration of the same or larger dose of thyroid medication is well tolerated. Treatment with 100 mcg (0.1 mg) daily of Synthroid† (L-thyroxine; T_4) is equivalent to administering approximately 1 grain of whole thyroid extract, and requires approximately 4–6 weeks to reach its full effect. After a month or more, the clinical situation is reassessed and, if evidence of thyroid inadequacy persists, a small increment (50 mcg daily) is added. Sometimes, the total daily dose must be increased in 50 mcg steps to as much as 300 mcg.

One should be aware that about 200 mcg daily of T_4 supplementation may suppress secretion of thyronine-stimulating hormone (TSH), and thereby much of the body's thyroid hormone production. Sudden withdrawal of the thyroid supplement at a later date can then cause severe exacerbation of the symptoms of low thyroid function. If too much thyroid is administered, the patient develops symptoms of hyperthyroidism. The amount of thyroid to prescribe is the smallest amount that restores normal metabolic function and returns the basal temperature to a normal level.

Hypoglycemia

Myofascial TP activity is aggravated and the response to specific myofascial therapy is reduced or shortened by hypoglycemia. Recurrent hypoglycemic attacks perpetuate myofascial TPs.

The prevalence of hypoglycemia is controversial, largely because the symptoms of hypoglycemia are caused chiefly by increased circulating epinephrine; other conditions, such as anxiety, also increase epinephrine levels, but without hypoglycemia. Clinically, the responses are often indistinguishable.

Two kinds of hypoglycemia are generally recognized, fasting and postprandial; they occur for different reasons, but present the same symptoms.

Symptoms. The initial symptoms of hypoglycemia or of increased epinephrine are usually sweating, trembling and shakiness, a fast heart rate, and a feeling of anxiety. Activation of sternocleidomastoid TPs may cause headache and dizziness. With progressively severe hypoglycemia, due to unusual circumstances, symptoms similar to those of hypoxia develop and are caused by inadequate energy to sustain brain function: visual disturbances, restlessness, impaired speech and thinking, and sometimes syncope.[104]

Fasting Hypoglycemia. Fasting does not cause hypoglycemia in a normal person because the liver releases glucose as the blood glucose starts to fall. Fasting hypoglycemia may result from failure of the liver to release the glucose, failure of the adrenal medulla to produce epinephrine that stimulates the liver to release the glucose, or failure of the anterior pituitary to stimulate the adrenal gland. Liver disease can impair this function of the liver. Alcohol ingestion when glycogen stores in the liver are depleted can precipitate severe hypoglycemia. Rarely, fasting hypoglycemia may be due to the deficiency of an enzyme, such as glucagon.[104]

Postprandial (Reactive) Hypoglycemia. Symptoms of postprandial hypoglycemia typically occur 2 or 3 hours after ingestion of a meal rich in carbohydrates, overstimulating the release of insulin. The insulin triggers a compensatory epinephrine response. The hypoglycemia caused by the insulinemia appears transiently for 15–30 min until it is terminated by the liver's response to an increased epinephrine level. Generally, the epinephrine causes most of the symptoms usually attributed to hypo-

---

* Cytomel, liothyronine sodium (sodium salt of L-triiodothyronine), Smith Kline & French Laboratories, Division of SmithKline Corp., 1500 Spring Garden Street, P. O. Box 7929, Philadelphia, PA 19101.
† Synthroid, levothyroxine sodium, Flint Laboratories, Division of Travenol Laboratories, Deerfield, IL 60015.

glycemia. This form of hypoglycemia is associated with high anxiety levels and is most likely to occur during periods of emotional stress.

An individual who has had part of the stomach removed or other gastric surgery may empty the stomach too rapidly. This, too, causes an abrupt rise in blood glucose level, initiating the same sequence of events and causing the same symptoms. The cause of the patient's symptoms is seen more clearly if the symptoms during a glucose tolerance test are correlated with periodic measurement of both blood glucose and serum insulin levels. In the senior author's experience, when a glucose tolerance test is done to detect fasting hypoglycemia, a positive result (very low glucose value) is more likely to be obtained if the patient exercises, rather than rests, in the intervals between blood samples.

Fasting hypoglycemia appears many hours after eating and tends to persist; postprandial hypoglycemia is self-limited. A reactive hypoglycemia secondary to mild diabetes is most likely to occur between the third and fifth hours of a glucose tolerance test.[104]

An identifiable organic disease process is usually responsible for fasting hypoglycemia, but not for postprandial hypoglycemia. Diagnosis of postprandial or fasting hypoglycemia requires demonstration of the hypoglycemia while the symptoms are present.

Treatment. In either fasting or postprandial hypoglycemia, the fundamental cause should be identified, if possible. For both, symptoms are relieved by eating smaller meals more frequently and by selecting a diet that is low in carbohydrates (75–100 g), high in protein, and includes sufficient fat to maintain caloric requirements. Exercise tends to aggravate hypoglycemia. However, exercise may help to reduce anxiety and, therefore, symptoms that depend on adrenaline release due to anxiety. In addition, patients must remember that coffee, tea, and colas that contain caffeine or theophylline should not be used because they stimulate the release of adrenaline. Alcoholic beverages should be avoided, particularly on an empty stomach. The nicotine in tobacco stimulates the release of adrenaline, so smoking and exposure to cigarette smoke should be eliminated.

Gouty Diathesis

Myofascial TPs and "muscular rheumatism"[117] are aggravated in patients who have hyperuricemia or gout. These patients are susceptible to TPs and when hyperuricemic respond poorly to myofascial therapy, particularly stretch and spray. Gout is a disorder of purine metabolism; the first indication usually is an elevated serum uric acid (>7.0 mg/dl in men, >6.0 mg/dl in women).[151]

Diagnosis. About 5% of asymptomatic hyperuricemic people (by the above criteria) develop acute gouty arthritis, with deposits of crystals of monosodium urate monohydrate in and around the joints, and sometimes in other tissues.[151]

The saturation value of monosodium urate at the pH of serum is about 7.0 mg/dl;[151] it is less soluble in the more acid medium of injured tissue. A more advanced stage of gout with tophi is now rarely seen since the advent of effective drugs for control of hyperuricemia.[151] Symptoms are more likely to occur in patients on a diet with meats high in purines.

A definite diagnosis of gout is made by identifying uric acid crystals in fluid aspirated from inflamed tissue. The crystals also may be obtained from asymptomatic metatarsophalangeal joints in patients who have had symptoms of gouty arthritis with hyperuricemia.[5]

The deposition of calcium pyrophosphate crystals produces symptoms similar to gout, but no metabolite is known to be present in excess in calcium pyrophosphate disease.

Treatment. If hyperuricemia is a probable factor in perpetuating the patient's myofascial TPs, it should be managed according to well-established principles.[151] Many diuretics increase serum uric acid levels. Vitamin C in relatively large amounts (several grams per day) is an effective uricosuric agent.[151]

The TPs of patients with a gouty diathesis respond better to treatment when the hyperuricemia is under control, and better to injection than to stretch and spray.

PSYCHOLOGICAL STRESS

A number of psychological factors can contribute to perpetuation of myofascial

TPs. Most important, the physician must be careful *not to assume* that psychological factors are primary. It is all too easy for the physician to blame the patient's psyche for the inability of the physician to recognize all of the medical and neurophysiological factors that are contributing to the patient's myofascial pain. This wrong assumption can be—and often is—frightfully devastating to the patient. We have so much to learn about pain, especially referred pain!

Patients who misunderstand the nature of their condition may be depressed, may exhibit anxiety tension, or may be victims of the "good sport" syndrome; some may be exhibiting secondary gain and/or sick behavior; a few will evidence conversion hysteria. Each must be diagnosed on its own merits.

Hopelessness

Patients who have been erroneously convinced that their pain is due to untreatable physical factors, such as degenerative joint disease, a "pinched nerve" that is inoperable, or "rheumatism" that they must learn to live with, often live in dread of aggravating their condition by any movement or activity that elicits the pain. The result is that they avoid all painful movements, including those that would stretch the muscles and help them recover function. When their pain is primarily due to myofascial TPs, this excessive restriction of movement and activity aggravates and perpetuates their TPs.

An essential first step with these patients is to convince them that their pain is of *muscular origin* and *treatable*, and that they must understand and respect their muscles. Acceptance of this revises the patients' concept of the prognosis. As they learn what activities to avoid, as well as what they themselves can do to inactivate the TPs, they realize they are gaining control of the sources of their pain. This new confidence in the future of their neuromuscular capability lifts a great load from their shoulders.

Depression

Depression and chronic pain are closely associated,[274] especially when patients have no satisfactory explanation for the cause of their pain, fear how much worse it may become, are convinced that nothing can be done to correct the source of pain, and believe they must accept it on these terms. The depression is partly a product of chronic pain and dysfunction, so that the longer the duration and the greater the intensity of the pain, the greater the depression is likely to be.[103] *Vice versa*, depressed patients are more aware of pain,[254, 274] which contributes to their dysfunction.

The recovery of many patients with myofascial TPs who are also depressed is expedited by combining antidepressant medication with specific myofascial therapy. Tricyclic drugs are most commonly used, but must be prescribed in sufficient dosage to be effective. Relief of depression permits the patient to take more responsibility for the care of their muscles and to engage in the exercises and activities that will help them to recover. These activities, especially under the direction of a therapist, are an effective antidepressant themselves.

Anxiety and Tension

In some individuals, high levels of anxiety are expressed in the form of muscle tension. Many muscles are held in sustained contraction that overloads them and perpetuates myofascial TPs. These patients are easily identified as they sit up stiff and straight, leaning away from the backrest of a chair, maintaining their shoulders in an elevated position, and displaying a tense facial expression. Generally, they are unaware of these expressions of tension. Biofeedback and relaxation therapy can help many of them to discriminate between unnecessarily tense muscles and relaxed ones. They then need to learn conscious techniques of relaxation and how to turn excess tension off. Identifying the major sources of anxiety and emotional tension and adopting the changes in life-style necessary to abate them, may be required to reduce this perpetuating factor enough for lasting relief.

"Good Sport" Syndrome

The "good sport" syndrome is the opposite of hypochondriasis. The "good sport" has a stoical attitude and is determined to ignore pain. He or she charges forth engaging in activities with total disregard of, if not outright defiance of the pain, thereby overloading the muscles and aggravating the TPs.

Good sports often believe that their pain is a sign of "weakness" and that they must push on to demonstrate their mastery of it. They must learn how this abuse of their muscles contributes to their pain, and how new ways of doing things can enable them to safely perform the activities important to them.

Psychological and Behavioral Aspects

A psychologically healthy person finds the functional restrictions imposed by a myofascial pain syndrome frustrating and unrewarding. However, among some persons secondary gain can perpetuate pain behavior. Determining whether the loss of function and the pain behavior is primarily psychological or chiefly neurophysiological can be very difficult and may be necessary only when the patient fails to respond to myofascial therapy. Three questions are helpful.

How effective were the patient's skills in coping with the problems of life prior to the onset of pain? Ineffective coping skills foster disability and respond best to counselling that is function oriented.

Does the patient concentrate on finding ways to do things that circumvent the pain, or focus on reasons why not? The latter suggests that the patient may have a psychological need of the disability.

Is function something the patient tries to do, or only talks about? The latter can represent an emotional need of dysfunction, but not necessarily.

In psychological terms, **primary gain** occurs when neurotic patients *unconsciously* develop psychosomatic symptoms (physically expressed) that tend to relieve their high level of anxiety and tension.[60] In the process secondary gains accrue when *some* patients discover that the privileges of a sick person offer exemption from the normal responsibilities of work and/or mature social interactions; they learn to like the rewards of having pain. These patients also simultaneously realize gratification of other unconscious needs, such as a dependency relationship upon a parent-figure, who may be the physician, a spouse, or other caregiver. Psychiatrists see **secondary gains** as resulting primarily

from psychogenic dysfunction.[60] It is not always that complicated.

Some patients who experience long-standing disabling myofascial pain, not promptly diagnosed and treated, discover advantages that fit this same pattern of secondary gain. The prospect of the beneficial settlement of a law suit or disability claim may loom as a very important secondary benefit to some, but not all, patients. In the presence of neurological or other damage that precludes complete recovery, the financial need is very real. When this issue is discussed openly and the patient's perception of the situation is clearly understood, it usually becomes clear whether the patient considers it in his or her best interest to be as disabled as possible, or to be as functional as possible between now and when the suit is settled.

Sick behavior is behavior that is appropriate to one who is suffering from pain: verbalizations, posturing, taking of medication, restriction of activity, increased rest, etc. In time, these reactions to illness can become a self-perpetuating way of life because of the emotional rewards.[103] Elimination of a TP source of pain can help greatly, but does not automatically reverse this process. The patient, and those with whom he or she lives and interacts closely (including the physician), must replace the reinforcements of the sick behavior with inducements that reinforce normal productive function. The principles of operant conditioning offer a method of treatment in these instances.[103]

Identifying sick behavior that is out of proportion to the pain and suffering experienced by the patient is difficult and hazardous. Only the patient can feel the pain. It is all too easy for the health care professional who is treating the patient to blame treatment failure on psychogenic factors, especially if the only criterion being used is the patient's statement of pain. The objective and semiobjective characteristics of myofascial TPs are most helpful. The answers to two questions also are useful.

What was the level of the patient's function before the event that initiated the pain? A higher level of function is not a realistic goal.

As TPs are inactivated, is the patient resuming activities and responsibilities that he or she had been accustomed to, or looking for reasons why it is not possible to take a step forward in function? The latter response is ominous.

Myofascial pain patients with pending law suits or disability claims are faced with the serious dilemma that any relief of their pain and disability would reduce their chances of receiving remuneration. Since one group of patients intuitively senses that the symptoms are critical to the success of the suits, their minds unconsciously concentrate on an awareness of symptoms rather than on function, whether they intend it or not. How much the patient expects the settlement to mean financially is very important. If it appears to the patient as a major sum, he or she literally can not *afford* to get better. In the management of these patients, it is essential that they understand the nature of their dilemma. They are strongly encouraged to resolve the dilemma before proceeding with therapy.

CHRONIC INFECTION AND INFESTATIONS

Several persistent disease conditions are likely to aggravate myofascial TPs: viral disease, especially herpes simplex; any chronic focus of bacterial infection; and infestations by certain parasites. The mechanism by which these diseases perpetuate myofascial TPs is not clear, but the importance of controlling them to obtain lasting relief from myofascial pain has been demonstrated.[303]

Viral Disease

The activity of myofascial TPs tends to increase during any systemic viral illness; the increased muscle soreness and stiffness may last for several weeks following an acute viral infection, such as the "flu." A common source of increased susceptibility and perpetuation of myofascial TPs is an outbreak of herpes simplex virus type 1. Neither genital herpes (herpes simplex virus type 2) nor herpes zoster seem to aggravate TPs as much as herpes simplex virus type 1.

Diagnosis. Because of its recurrent nature, it is important to identify and control outbreaks of the type 1 herpes virus, which causes the common cold sore, canker sores, and often aphthous mouth ulcers; it also may appear on the skin of the body

or extremities as crops of isolated vesicles filled with clear fluid. The small vesicles develop a reddened areola and form an eczematous patch on the skin,[176] which may remain for several weeks, if untreated. After the small blisters that are filled with watery fluid (never with pus) break, they become crusted red spots.

Lesions have been reported in the esophagus, and symptoms of vomiting and diarrhea strongly implicate gastrointestinal involvement comparable to that of the mouth.

Treatment. No drug is known to cure herpes simplex. However, by using a multipronged attack, one can greatly reduce the frequency and severity of recurrences of herpes simplex virus type 1. This includes medicinal application to the lesions, oral ingestion of niacinamide and Lactinex* and, if necessary, intramuscular injections of human immune serum globulin. Because of the increased irritability of the muscles during an outbreak of herpes simplex virus type 1, it is unwise to inject the muscles for TPs until a few weeks after the herpes attack has subsided. Treated sooner, the muscles respond poorly to local therapy and are prone to excessive post-treatment soreness.

For local treatment of the herpetic dermal and mouth lesions, idoxuridine (Stoxil†) is rubbed into the lesion several times a day. Experience to date suggests, but does not prove, that adenine arabinoside (ara-A, Vira-A§) is useful in cutaneous herpes simplex virus type 1.[176] It is sold as a 3% ophthalmic ointment, which also is rubbed into the lesion two or three times a day. It appears to us that ara-A is as effective as idoxuridine. The package insert notes that ingesting as much as a tube of Vira-A should produce no adverse effects. The newly released Zovirax¶ (acyclo-

* Lactinex Tablets and Granules, Hynson, Westcott & Dunning, Division of Becton Dickinson & Co., Charles & Chase Sts, Baltimore, MD 21201.

† Stoxil, ophthalmic ointment, 0.5%, and ophthalmic solution 0.1%, Smith Kline & French Laboratories, Division of SmithKline Corporation, 1500 Spring Garden St., P. O. Box 7929, Philadelphia, PA 19101.

§ Vira-A, ophthalmic ointment, Parke–Davis Division of Warner–Lambert Company, 201 Tabor Road, Morris Planes, NJ 07950.

¶ Zovirax Ointment 5%, Burroughs Wellcome Co., 3030 Cornwallis Road, Research Triangle Park, NC 27709.

vir), 5% ointment, is promoted for treatment of initial attacks of herpes simplex virus type 2; it also may prove to be effective for type 1 herpes simplex.

In the past, cryotherapy[106] was used for local treatment of the herpetic lesions on lips or skin, and freezing the lesions was accomplished by application of liquid ether or a vapocoolant spray.[244] In recent years, the above antiviral agents have proved effective, and may be conveniently used by the patient as soon as a blister appears.

Administration of niacinamide, 300–500 mg/day, helps the mucous membrane combat the gingivostomatitis of oral herpes simplex (type 1). At the same time, it is important to correct any folic acid deficiency.

Empirically, the symptoms due to extension of herpetic lesions into the small intestine are relieved by taking 1 packet of granules or 3 tablets of Lactinex* 2 or 3 times daily for at least a month, with subsequent reduction in dosage, unless the oral lesions reappear. A course of Lactinex may be needed after antibiotic therapy that might suppress normal intestinal bacteria. Lactinex is a preparation of living *Lactobacilus acidophilus* and *Lactobacillus bulgaricus*. The intestinal component of herpes is an unseen and generally unappreciated site of infection. Lactinex therapy is an important part of the total treatment plan.

The patients who have recurrent episodes of diarrhea associated with outbreaks of oral herpes, also tend not to drink milk. When asked, they are not sure why; they "just don't like it." In fact, they may have a lactose intolerance, and as a result, milk causes diarrhea. It is, therefore, important in these cases to measure their serum *ionized* calcium, which is often low even though the serum *total* calcium is normal. An adequate calcium intake must be provided.

When the patient has a series of herpetic recurrences, or a crop of herpes reactivates TPs, human immune serum globulin can be injected intramuscularly, 0.04 cc/kg (0.02 cc/lb). This usually amounts to a total dose of 2–3 ml/injection. The effectiveness of the viral antibodies from the pooled serum is temporary.

Bacterial Infection

Absorption of bacterial (and viral) toxic products favors the development of active TPs when minor mechanical stress is added.[288] Common locations of chronic bacterial infection are an abscessed tooth, a blocked sinus, and the urinary tract. Such a chronic infection may increase the erythrocyte sedimentation rate, which is a useful screening test. Specific myofascial therapy is unlikely to produce lasting benefits while a focus of chronic infection persists.

Abscessed or Impacted Tooth. The chronic infection of a tooth is suspected from a careful dental history and confirmed by a dental evaluation with an X-ray examination. Impaction of a wisdom tooth can perpetuate TPs in the masticatory muscles, even when local infection is not present.

Sinusitis. Sinusitis is characterized by a sense of fullness in the sinus area, postnasal discharge that may be purulent, and failure of the occluded sinus to transilluminate clearly. If there is an allergic component, the patient is likely to have an eosinophilia. Control of inhalant allergies is generally a prerequisite to a lasting resolution of sinusitis. If there is additional mechanical blockage to sinus drainage as by a deviated nasal septum, this also may require correction in order to cure the sinus infection.

Chronic Urinary Tract Infection. The symptoms of nocturia, dysuria and urgency should arouse the suspicion of a urinary tract infection, especially in female patients. The infection is confirmed by urinalysis and urine culture; it is best managed by the urologist. This specialist can determine the extent of the infection and whether there is incomplete emptying of the bladder, or another cause of the infection.

Infestations

Three infestations are likely to perpetuate myofascial pain symptoms. The fish tapeworm is the worst offender; next is giardiasis. Occasionally amebiasis perpetuates myofascial TPs. The first two tend to impair absorption of nutrients or consume vitamin B_{12}; the third may produce myotoxins that are absorbed.

Fish Tapeworm. The adult worm of *Diphyllobothrium latum* resides in the intestinal lumen; the infestation develops after ingestion of raw infected fish. Infestation is relatively common in a number of foreign countries in temperate climates where it is common practice to eat raw fish, also in Florida, in the northern central United States, and in south-central Canada.

A worm located high in the jejunum may consume 80–100% of ingested labeled vitamin B_{12}, and thus deprive its host of that vitamin.[134] Since the eggs are discharged in large numbers into the stool, they are easily diagnosed by stool examination for ova and parasites.[222]

Giardiasis. The single-celled protozoan, *Giardia lamblia*, is a significant cause of traveler's diarrhea, particularly in the Caribbean countries, Latin America, India, Russia, and the Far East.[221] It is a pear-shaped, flagellated parasite that lives in the human duodenum and jejunum, where it multiplies. It was isolated in 3.8% of stools examined in the United States.

The infestation is often asymptomatic, but may cause nausea, flatulence, epigastric pain, and watery diarrhea with bulky malodorous stools. The acute symptoms are usually limited to a few weeks, but chronic giardiasis can cause malabsorption of carbohydrate, fat and vitamin B_{12}. The lack of vitamin B_{12} perpetuates myofascial TPs.

The diagnosis is made by identifying the cysts in formed feces, or by finding the trophozoites in diarrheal stools, in duodenal secretions, or in jejunal biopsies. In chronic cases, excretion of the organism is often intermittent, and stool specimens must be collected at weekly intervals for 4–5 weeks to exclude this diagnosis.[221]

Amebiasis. Only *Entamoeba histolytica* is pathological among the amebas that parasitize the human intestinal tract. The mature *E. histolytica* lives in the lumen of the large intestine, feeding on bacteria and debris; occasionally it invades the mucosa, causing ulcerations.[220]

Stool surveys reveal the prevalance of this parasite in the United States to be between 1 and 5%, but rates are much higher in tropical areas where the levels of sanitation are low and among groups who spread it by direct fecal-oral contact between sexual partners.[220]

The diagnosis depends on the identification of the organism in the stool or tissue from the large intestine. The laboratory demonstration of this infestation may be difficult and should be performed prior to other diagnostic procedures on the colon. Serological tests using purified antigens are positive in most patients with acute amebic dysentery, but are generally negative in asymptomatic passers of cysts.

These tests should be useful in myofascial pain patients because aggravation of myofascial TPs by *E. histolytica* probably requires tissue invasion. Antibody titers may be elevated for months to years after complete cure.[220] Treatment is difficult and a cure generally requires a combination of drugs.[220]

OTHER FACTORS

Three additional factors, allergic rhinitis, impaired sleep, and nerve impingement, should be considered in the management of myofascial pain syndromes.

Allergic Rhinitis

Many patients with active myofascial TPs, who also have active symptoms of allergic rhinitis, respond only temporarily to specific myofascial therapy. When the allergic symptoms are controlled, the muscle response to local TP therapy usually improves significantly. Hypersensitivity to allergens, with histamine release, seems to act as a perpetuating factor for myofascial TPs.

Koenig, et al.[163] examined 20 "fibrositis" patients with histories that were compatible with a diagnosis of myofascial TPs and tender areas that responded to palpation with a "jump sign." Of the 20 patients, 9 (45%) had convincing histories of either prior or current allergic rhinitis, and 11 of the 20 had positive family histories of allergy. However, none of the 20 patients showed elevated immunoglobulin E levels or an increased total eosinophile count. From this, the authors concluded that it was unlikely that type 1 hypersensitivity played a role in the pathogenesis of fibrositis. We agree that the myofascial pain syndromes are not likely to be activated by an allergy. However, we do find that among a certain number of patients with an active allergic state, the allergy significantly perpetuates the activity of their myofascial TPs. Unfortunately, this study[163] did not address the question, "Does the presence of allergy impede the response to treatment?"

Diagnosis. Allergic rhinitis is characterized by episodic sneezing, rhinorrhea, obstruction of the nasal passages, conjunctival and pharyngeal itching, and lacrimation. Allergic rhinitis predisposes to upper respiratory infection.[13]

The initial diagnosis depends largely on the correlation between exposure to the allergen and appearance of symptoms, both as related to time and place. The peripheral blood and nasal secretions of patients with active allergic rhinitis are rich in eosinophiles. Total serum immunoglobin E is frequently elevated, and the demonstration of antibodies to a specific antigen is critical to an etiologic diagnosis. A number of radioimmune tests are now used.[13]

Skin testing is useful for detecting sensitivity to inhalant allergens, but questionable for food allergens. Food allergies are common and potent,[79] and should be considered as a possible cause of myofascial reactions. Some patients exhibit an idiosyncratic muscle reaction to alcoholic beverages, experiencing an attack of myofascial pain soon after or the day following indulgence.

In most patients, the upper respiratory tract and eyes, the bronchi, the skin, or the joints are the shock organs for allergic reactions. However, in other patients, the skeletal muscles appear to serve as the shock organ for allergies.

Treatment. Most important is avoidance of exposure to the allergen. For inhalant allergies, a room model electrostatic air cleaner is effective, if the air in that room is independent of the air circulating throughout the house. Some portable room models are suitable for use on trips.

Antihistamines effectively control one mediator of allergy, the mast cell-derived reaction, and can be valuable for controlling symptoms of allergic rhinitis. Either Dramamine, 50 mg, or Phenergan, 12.5 or 50 mg, taken shortly before bedtime help to induce sleep. Dramamine is relatively short acting and can be repeated during the night, if needed. These antihistamines are discussed under Drugs on pages 90–92 in Chapter 3.

If antihistaminics provide inadequate control, treatment by hyposensitization can be helpful.[13]

Impaired Sleep

Impaired or interrupted sleep, in our experience, occurs with greater frequency in patients with more severe myofascial pain syndromes. Smythe,[266] in defining "fibrositis," considered disturbed sleep so important that he made it one of four essential diagnostic criteria. Sleep studies[196] in 10 patients with "fibrositis" revealed a decrease in the amount of slow wave activity and intrusion of a rapid alpha rhythm during stages 3 and 4 of sleep. All patients showed an overnight increase in the tenderness of the tender points in their muscles.

In many patients with myofascial TPs, the sleep disturbance can be specifically related to referred pain caused by lying on a TP, or sleeping with an involved muscle in the fully shortened position. Inactivation of the TP permits return to a clinically normal sleep pattern. Other patients are disturbed by noise, which can be corrected with cotton in the ears or suitable ear plugs; or by depression, which should be managed by antidepressent medication as indicated.

However, Moldofsky and Scarisbrick[195] found muscle tenderness and a sense of physical tiredness in the morning in healthy university students when the slow wave non-REM (rapid eye movement) sleep had been disrupted throughout the night. This finding demonstrates the completion of a vicious cycle. The painful muscles interrupt sleep, and disrupted sleep can make the muscles more painful.

History. A careful inquiry as to the precise nature of the sleep disturbance helps to determine what is causing it. Is the difficulty primarily falling asleep, or staying asleep? Anxious and tense patients have trouble falling asleep, depressed patients are likely to awaken during the night. When, during the night, does the patient awaken? This information helps to identify the cause. Was the patient chilly, or in pain? What was the sleeping position? The position helps to identify what TPs may be responsible for pain. Some patients with a severe myofascial pain syndrome can sleep in the sitting position only. How does the patient get back to sleep again? Is the lack of sleep at night compensated by sleep during the day?

Treatment. Inactivation of the TPs that are disrupting sleep holds top priority. If going to sleep is a problem, a warm bath and/or a glass of milk before retiring may help induce sleep (provided the patient likes and digests milk).

An electric blanket is most helpful to prevent chilling of the body and eliminate compensatory muscular contractions to generate heat. The thermostat should be adjusted to slightly above room temperature before retiring by turning the blanket on and the temperature control up, just beyond the "on" click.

Pillow positioning can be the key to restful sleep. When neck and shoulder muscles are involved, the corners of the pillow can be tucked between the ear or chin and the shoulder to prevent tilting of the head and neck to keep the shoulder from riding up against the neck. Excessive neck flexion should be avoided; the pillow should be flat enough to maintain the normal lordotic curve of the cervical spine. An additional small pillow can be positioned to prevent shortening of involved shoulder-girdle and arm muscles during the night. Specific details are described in the individual muscle chapters.

The use of drugs has been mentioned in the previous section, and is discussed on pages 90–92 in Chapter 3.

Nerve Impingement

Both myofascial TP syndromes and radiculopathies are very common. However, one cannot assume that the presence of radiculopathy activated the TPs just because they occurred together in the same individual. The distinction is further clouded by the fact that TPs activated as satellites of the original pain of radiculopathy may refer pain in patterns that mimic the radicular pain.

The two conditions may therefore appear as one in the postdisc syndrome but in reality are separate entities. These patients continue to experience pain following a well performed and truly needed laminectomy. They suffer from continuing activity of myofascial TPs in muscles that refer pain in much the same distribution as that of the previous radicular pain. The postlumbar-laminectomy pain syndrome described by Rubin[241] demonstrates the postdisc syndrome of the lumbar spine.

Recognition and inactivation of the myofascial TPs that remained following a successful laminectomy for nerve root compression has provided complete and lasting relief in many patients.

SCREENING LABORATORY TESTS

The following tests are valuable in the detection of perpetuating factors in patients with chronic myofascial pain, or in any patient with myofascial TPs who responds poorly to specific myofascial therapy. The hematologic profile, blood chemistry profile, and vitamin tests are done routinely. Thyroid tests are done when indicated by history and physical findings.

Hematologic Profile

A normal erythrocyte sedimentation rate helps to eliminate the possibility of a chronic bacterial infection. When elevated, it is nonspecific and may indicate other conditions, such as polymyositis, polymyalgia rheumatica, rheumatoid arthritis, or cancer.

A decreased erythrocyte count and/or low hemoglobin indicates anemia, which tends to make the muscles hypoxic and to increase TP irritability. Anemia can be caused by a folate and/or cobalamin deficiency, each of which additionally increases TP irritability. An increased mean corpuscular volume of >92 fl is suspicious. As it rises from 95 to 100 fl, the likelihood of a folate or a cobalamin deficiency increases.

Eosinophilia may be due to an active allergy, or to infestation with an intestinal parasite, such as *E. histolytica* or a tapeworm.

An increased proportion of mononuclear cells (>50%) may occur because of low thyroid function, or due to active infectious mononucleosis or an acute viral infection.

Blood Chemistry Profile

An automated blood chemistry profile is a useful screening test. Increased serum cholesterol can result from decreased thyroid function, whereas a low serum cholesterol may reflect folate deficiency. Elevated levels of uric acid identify hyperuricemia, which occasionally results in gout. A low serum total calcium suggests a calcium deficiency, but for determination of the adequacy of available calcium, a serum *ionized* calcium measurement is needed.

Low serum potassium can cause muscle cramps and is likely to perpetuate myofascial TPs.

An elevated fasting blood sugar deserves further investigation to rule out diabetes with a 2-hr postprandial blood glucose or a glucose tolerance test. Measurement of nerve conduction velocities can rule out diabetic neuropathy.

Vitamin Determination

Serum levels of vitamins B_1, B_6, B_{12}, folic acid, and vitamin C can be enormously valuable in the rational management of patients with myofascial pain syndromes. Abnormally low levels of any of these vitamins perpetuate TPs. Values in the lower quartile of normal are less than optimal and are highly suspect as perpetuators of myofascial TPs.

Thyroid Tests

The radioimmunoassays for T_3 and T_4 measure the adequacy of hormone production by the thyroid gland. However, basal body temperature provides additional information concerning the adequacy with which the circulating thyroid hormones stimulate metabolism at the cellular level.

References

1. Abt AF, von Schuching S, Enns T: Vitamin C requirements of man re-examined. *Am J Clin Nutr* 12:21–29, 1963.
2. Adams PW, Rose DP, Folkard J, et al.: Effect of pyridoxine hydrochloride (vitamin B₆) upon depression associated with oral contraception. *Lancet* 1:897–904, 1973 (p. 33).
3. Adams RD, Asbury AK: Diseases of the peripheral nervous system, Chapter 377. In *Harrison's Principles of Internal Medicine*, edited by K.J. Isselbacher, R.D. Adams, E. Braunwald, et al., Ed. 9. McGraw–Hill, New York, 1980 (p. 2039).
4. Adams RD, Bradley WG: Other major muscle syndromes, Chapter 383. In *Principles of Internal Medicine*, edited by K.J. Isselbacher, R.D. Adams, E. Braunwald, et al., Ed. 9. McGraw-Hill, New York, 1980 (p. 2071).
5. Agudelo CA, Weinberger A, Schumacher HR, et al.: Definitive diagnosis of gout by identification of urate crystals in asymptomatic metatarsophalangeal joints. *Arthritis Rheum* 22:559–560, 1979.
6. Aidley DJ: *The Physiology of Excitable Cells.* Cambridge University Press, Cambridge, 1971 (pp. 115, 228).
7. Akerblom B: *Standing and Sitting Posture.* A.B. Nordiska Bokhandein, Stockholm, 1948.
8. Alter HJ: Interrelationships of rheumatoid arthritis, folic acid, and aspirin. *Blood* 38:405–416, 1971.
9. Ampola MG, Mahoney MJ, Nakamura E, et al.: Prenatal therapy of a patient with vitamin B₁₂ responsive methylmalonic acidemia. *N Engl J Med* 293:314–317, 1975.
10. Anderson CE: Vitamins, Chapter 3. In *Nutritional Support of Medical Practice*, edited by H.A. Schneider, C.E. Anderson, D.B. Coursin. Harper & Row, Hagerstown, Md. 1977 (pp. 25–27).
11. Anonymous: The deoxyuridine suppression test for the diagnosis of masked or previous folate deficiency. *Nutr Rev* 37:77–80, 1979.
12. Appledorf H, Newberne PM, Tannenbaum SR: Influence of altered thyroid status on the food intake and growth of rats fed a thiamine-deficient diet. *J Nutr* 97:271–278, 1969.
13. Austen KF: Diseases of immediate type hypersensitivity. In *Principles of Internal Medicine*, edited by K.J. Isselbacher, R.D. Adams, E. Braunwald, et al., Ed. 9. McGraw-Hill, New York, 1980 (pp. 345–347).
14. Avioli LV: Calcium and phosphorus, Chapter 7A. In *Modern Nutrition in Health and Disease*, edited by R.S. Goodhart, M.E. Shils, Ed. 6. Lea & Febiger, Philadelphia, 1980 (pp. 298, 305).
15. Axelrod AE: Nutrition in relation to immunity, Chapter 18. In *Modern Nutrition in Health and Diseases*, edited by R.S. Goodhart, M.E. Shils, Ed. 6. Lea & Febiger, Philadelphia, 1980 (p. 585).
16. Axelrod AE: Role of the B vitamins in the immune response. *Adv Exp Med Biol* 135:93–106, 1981.
17. Azuma J, Kishi T, Williams RH, et al.: Apparent deficiency of vitamin B₆ in typical individuals who commonly serve as normal controls. *Res Commun Chem Pathol Pharmacol* 14:343–348, 1976.
18. Babior BM, Bunn HF: Megaloblastic anemias, Chapter 311. In *Harrison's Principles of Internal Medicine*, edited by K.J. Isselbacher, R.D. Adams, E. Braunwald, et al., Ed. 9. McGraw–Hill, New York, 1980 (pp. 1518–1524).
19. Bailey LB, Mahan CS, Dimperio D: Folacin and iron status in low-income pregnant adolescents and mature women. *Am J Clin Nutr* 33:1997–2001, 1980.
20. Baines M: Detection and incidence of B and C vitamin deficiency in alcohol-related illness. *Ann Clin Biochem* 15:307–312, 1978.
21. Baker H, Frank O: Vitamin status in metabolic upsets. *World Rev Nutr Diet* 9:124–160, 1968.

22. Baker H, Frank O, Feingold S, et al.: Vitamins, total cholesterol, and triglycerides in 642 NY City school children. Am J Clin Nutr 20:850–857, 1967.

23. Baker H, Frank O, Hutner SH: Vitamin analyses in medicine, Chapter 20. In Modern Nutrition in Health and Disease, edited by R.S. Goodhart, M.E. Shils, Ed. 6. Lea & Febiger, Philadelphia, 1980 (pp. 612, 621–624).

24. Baker H, Frank O, Thomson AD, et al.: Vitamin profile of 174 mothers and newborns at parturition. Am J Clin Nutr 28:59–65, 1975.

25. Baker H, Frank O, Zetterman RK, et al.: Inability of chronic alcoholics with liver disease to use food as a source of folates, thiamin, and vitamin B6. Am J Clin Nutr 28:1377–1380, 1975.

26. Baker H, Jaslow SP, Frank O: Severe impairment of dietary folate utilization in elderly. J Am Geriatr Soc 26:218–221, 1978.

27. Baker H, Thind IS, Frank O, et al.: Vitamin levels in low-birth-weight newborn infants and their mothers. Am J Obstet Gynecol 129:521–524, 1977.

28. Baker R, Powars D, Haywood LJ: Restoration of the deformability of "irreversibly" sickled cells by procaine hydrochloride. Biochem Biophys Res Commun 59:548–586, 1974.

29. Barclay LL, Gibson GE, Blass JP: The string test: an early behavioral change in thiamine deficiency. Pharmacol Biochem Behav 14:153–157, 1981.

30. Barnes B: Basal temperature versus basal metabolism. JAMA 119:1072–1074, 1942.

31. Beal MC: A review of the short-leg problem. JAOA 50:109–121, 1950.

32. Beck WS, Goulian M: Drugs effective in pernicious anemia and other megaloblastic anemias. Chapter 51. In Drill's Pharmacology in Medicine, edited by J.R. DiPalma, Ed. 4. McGraw–Hill, New York- 1971 (pp. 1062–1074).

33. Bell JM, Stewart CN: Effects of fetal and early postnatal thiamin deficiency on avoidance learning in rats. J Nutr 109:1577–1583, 1979.

34. Bendall JR: Muscles, Molecules and Movement. American Elsevier Publishing Company, New York, 1969. (p. 162).

35. Berger L, Gerson CD, Yü T: The effect of ascorbic acid on uric acid excretion with a commentary of the renal handling of ascorbic acid. Am J Med 62:71–76, 1977.

36. Bezzano G: Effects of folic acid metabolism on serum cholesterol levels. Arch Int Med 124:710–713, 1969.

37. Blum A: Do cigarette smokers need vitamin C supplementation? JAMA 244:193, 1980.

38. Boni L, Kieckens L, Hendrikx A: An evaluation of a modified erythrocyte transketolase assay for assessing thiamine nutritional adequacy. J Nutr Sci Vitaminol 26:507–514, 1980.

39. Botez MI: Folate deficiency and neurological disorders in adults. Med Hypotheses 2:135–140, 1976.

40. Botez MI, Cadotte M, Beaulieu R, et al.: Neurologic disorders responsive to folic acid therapy. Can Med Assoc J 115:217–222, 1976.

41. Botez MI, Fontaine F, Botez T, et al.: Folate-responsive neurological and mental disorders: report of 16 cases. Eur Neurol 16:230–246, 1977.

42. Botez MI, Peyronnard J-M, Bachevalier J, et al.: Polyneuropathy and folate deficiency. Arch Neurol 35:581–585, 1978.

43. Botez MI, Peyronnard J-M, Charron L: Polyneuropathies responsive to folic acid therapy, Chapter 36. In Folic Acid in Neurology, Psychiatry, and Internal Medicine, edited by M.I. Botez, E.H. Reynolds. Raven Press, New York, 1979 (p. 411).

44. Boulant JA: Hypothalamic mechanisms in thermoregulation. Fed Proc 40:2843–2850, 1981.

45. Bourdillon JF: Spinal Manipulation, Ed. 2. Appleton–Century–Crofts, New York, 1973 (pp. 39–43, Figs. 5–10).

46. Ibid. (pp. 42–44, 81).

47. Ibid. (pp. 82–86).

48. Briggs H: Geriatric patients, vitamin B12 and pernicious anemia, and reply. Med J Aust 21:192–193, 1981.

49. Brooke MH: A Clinicians View of Neuromuscular Disease. Williams & Wilkins, Baltimore, 1977.

50. Bueding E, Stein MH, Wortis H: Blood pyruvate curves following glucose ingestion in normal and thiamine-deficient subjects. J Biol Chem 140:697–703, 1941.

51. Burman JF, Mollin DL, Sourial NA, et al.: Inherited lack of transcobalamin II in serum and megablastic anemia: a further patient. Br J Haematol 43:27–38, 1979.

52. Butterworth RF, Hamel E, Landreville F, et al.: Amino acid changes in thiamine-deficient encephalopathy: some implications for the pathogenesis of Friedreich's ataxia. Can J Neurol Sci 6:217–222, 1979.

53. Cabanac M: Temperature regulation. Annu Rev Physiol 37:415–439, 1975.

54. Cailliet R: Foot and Ankle Pain. F.A. Davis Company, Philadelphia, 1968 (p. 94).

55. Calabresi P, Parks RE, Jr.: Alkylating agents, antimetabolites, hormones, and other antiproliferative agents, Chapter 62. In The Pharmacological Basis of Therapeutics, edited by L.S. Goodman, A. Gilman, Ed. 4. Macmillan, New York, 1970 (p. 1361).

56. Calder JH, Curtis RC, Fore H: Comparison of vitamin C in plasma and leucocytes of smokers and non-smokers. Lancet 1:556, 1963.

57. Cameron E: Biological function of ascorbic acid and the pathogenesis of scurvy. Med Hypotheses 2:154–163, 1976.

58. Cameron E, Campbell A, Jack T: The orthomolecular treatment of cancer; III. Reticulum cell sarcoma: double complete regression induced by high-dose ascorbic acid therapy. Chem Biol Interact 11:387–393, 1975.

59. Cameron E, Pauling L: Cancer and vitamin C. Linus Pauling Institute of Science and Medicine, Menlo Park, Calif. 1979.

60. Cameron N: Personality Development and Psychopathology: A Dynamic Approach. Houghton Mifflin, Boston, 1963.

61. Cameron P, Pauling L: The orthomolecular treatment of cancer; I. The role of ascorbic acid in host resistance. Chem Biol Interact 9:273–283, 1974.

62. Canham JE, Baker EM, Harding RS, et al.: Dietary Protein—its relationship to vitamin B6 requirements and function. In Vitamin B6 in Metabolism of the Nervous System. Ann NY Acad

Sci 166:16–29, 1969 (pp. 16–29).

63. Carney MWP: Psychiatric aspects of folate deficiency, Chapter 42. In *Folic Acid in Neurology, Psychiatry, and Internal Medicine*, edited by M.I. Botez, E.H. Reynolds. Raven Press, New York, 1979 (pp. 480–482).

64. Carney MWP, Williams DG, Sheffield BF: Thiamine and pyridoxine lack in newly-admitted psychiatric patients. *Br J Psychiatry 135*:249–254, 1979.

65. Cass LJ, Frederik WS, Cohen JD: Chronic disease and vitamin C. *Geriatrics 9*:375–380, 1954.

66. Chanarin I: Effects of anticonvulsant drugs, Chapter 10. In *Folic Acid in Neurology, Psychiatry, and Internal Medicine*, edited by M.I. Botez, E.H. Reynolds. Raven Press, New York, 1979 (pp. 75, 79).

67. Chanarin I, Deacon R, Perry J, et al.: How vitamin B_{12} acts. *Br J Haematol 47*:487–491, 1981.

68. Chaudhuri CR, Chatterjee IB: L-Ascorbic acid synthesis in birds: phylogenetic trend. *Science 164*:435–436, 1969.

69. Cheraskin E, Ringsdorf WM, Jr.: A relationship between vitamin C intake and electrocardiography. *J Electrocardiol 12*:441, 1979.

70. Cheraskin E, Ringsdorf WM, Jr., El-Ashiry G: A lingual vitamin C test. *Int Z Vitamin Ernahrungsforsch 34*:31–38, 1964.

71. Ciaccio EI: The vitamins, Chapter 62. In *Drill's Pharmacology in Medicine*, edited by J.R. DiPalma, Ed. 4. New York, McGraw–Hill, 1971 (pp. 1293–1294).

72. *Ibid.* (pp. 1282–1284, 1287–1290).

73. Cohen KL, Donaldson RM: Unreliability of radiodilution assays as screening tests for cobalamin (vitamin B_{12}) deficiency. *JAMA 244*:1942–1945, 1980.

74. Coleman N, Herbert V: Dietary assessments with special emphasis on prevention of folate deficiency, Chapter 5. In *Folic Acid in Neurology, Psychiatry, and Internal Medicine*, edited by M.I. Botez, E.H. Reynolds. Raven Press, New York, 1979 (pp. 23–33).

75. Collipp PJ, Goldzier S III, Weiss N, et al.: Pyridoxine treatment of childhood bronchial asthma. *Ann Allergy 35*:93–97, 1975.

76. Conrad ME: Dietary folic acid and iron deficiency among the affluent. *JAMA 214*:1708, 1970.

77. Cooper BA, Whitehead VM: Evidence that some patients with pernicious anemia are not recognized by radiodilution assay for cobalamin in serum. *N Engl J Med 299*:816–818, 1978.

78. Couchman KG, Bieder L, Wigley RD, et al.: Vitamin B_{12} absorption and gastric antibodies in rheumatoid arthritis. *NZ Med J 68*:153–156, 1968.

79. Crook WG: Can what a child eats make him dull, stupid, or hyperactive? *J Learn Disabil 13*:281–286, 1980.

80. Davis RE, Smith BK: Pyridoxal and folate deficiency in alcoholics. *Med J Aust 2*:357–360, 1974.

81. Delamere JP, Scott DL, Felix–Davies DD: Thyroid dysfunction and rheumatic diseases. *J R Soc Med 75*:102–106, 1982.

82. Dempsey WB: Vitamin B_6 and pregnancy, Chapter 12. In *Human Vitamin B_6 Requirements*. National Academy of Sciences, Washington, 1978 (pp. 202, 203).

83. Diffrient N, Tilley AR, Bardagjy JC: *Humanscale*

1/2/3. Massachusetts Institute of Technology Press, Cambridge, 1974 (pp. 19–22).

84. Dipalma JR: Vitamin toxicity. *Am Fam Physician 18*:106–109, 1978.

85. Donaldson RM, Jr.: Serum B_{12} and the diagnosis of cobalamin deficiency. *N Engl J Med 299*:827–828, 1978.

86. Driskell JA: Vitamin B_6 status of the elderly, Chapter 16. In *Human Vitamin B_6 Requirements*. National Academy of Sciences, Washington, 1978 (pp. 252–255).

87. Ebadi M: Vitamin B_6 and biogenic amines in brain metabolism, Chapter 8. In *Human Vitamin B_6 Requirements*, National Academy of Sciences, Washington, 1978 (pp. 129–150).

88. Editorial: Pitfalls in the diagnosis of vitamin B_{12} deficiency by radiodilution assay. *Nutr Rev 37*:313–316, 1979.

89. Editorial Board: Calcium requirements in pregnancy. *Nutrition and the M. D. 8*:4–5, 1981.

90. Eichner ER, Pierce HI, Hillman RS: Folate balance in dietary-induced megaloblastic anemia. *N Engl J Med 284*:933–938, 1971.

91. Ellis J, Folkers K, Watanabe T, et al.: Clinical results of a crossover treatment with pyridoxine and placebo of the carpal tunnel syndrome. *Am J Clin Nutr 32*:2040–2046, 1979.

92. Ellis JM, Kishi T, Azuma J, et al.: Vitamin B_6 deficiency in patients with a clinical syndrome including the carpal tunnel effect. Biochemical and clinical response to therapy with pyridoxine. *Res Commun Chem Pathol Pharmacol 3*:743–757, 1976.

93. Ellis JM, Presley J: *Vitamin B_6: The Doctor's Report*. Harper & Row, New York, 1973 (pp. 74–78).

94. Ellison ABC: Pernicious anemia masked by multivitamins containing folic acid. *JAMA 173*: 86–89, 1960.

95. Elsom KO, Lukens FDW, Montgomery EH, et al.: Metabolic disturbances in experimental human vitamin B deficiency. *J Clin Invest 19*:153–161, 1940.

96. Engle WK: Ponderous-purse disease. *N Engl J Med 299*:557, 1978.

97. Erbe RW: Inborn errors of folate metabolism. *N Engl J Med 293*:753–758, 807–811, 1975.

98. Evans JR, Hughes RE, Jones PR: Some effects of cigarette smoke on guinea-pigs. *Proc Nutr Soc 26*:36, 1967.

99. Folkers K, Watanabe T, Ellis JM: Studies on the basal specific activity of the glutamic oxaloacetic transaminase of erythrocytes in relation to a deficiency of vitamin B_6. *Res Commun Chem Pathol Pharmacol 17*:187–189, 1977.

100. Follis RH, Jr., Van Itallie TB: Pellagra, Chapter 77. In *Harrison's Principles of Internal Medicine*, edited by M.M. Wintrobe, G.W. Thorn, R.D. Adams, et al., Ed. 7. McGraw–Hill, New York, 1974 (p. 429).

101. Fong T: problems associated with megadose vitamin C therapy. *West J Med 134*:264, 1981.

102. Ford LT, Goodman FG: X-ray studies of the lumbosacral spine. *South Med J 59*:1123–1128, 1966.

103. Fordyce WE: *Behavioral Methods for Chronic Pain and Illness*, C.V. Mosby, Saint Louis, 1976 (pp. 72–73).

104. Foster DW, Rubenstein AH: Hypoglycemia, insulinoma, and other hormone-secreting tumors of the pancreas, Chapter 340. In *Principles of Internal Medicine*, edited by K.J. Isselbacher, R.D. Adams, E. Braunwald, *et al.*, Ed. 9. McGraw-Hill, New York, 1980 (pp. 1758–1762).

105. Frader J, Reisman B, Turkewitz D: Vitamin B$_{12}$ deficiency in strict vegetarians. *JAMA* 299: 1319–1320, 1978.

106. Fulhorst HW, Richards AB, Bowbyes J, *et al.*: Cryotherapy of epithelial herpes simplex keratitis. *Am J Ophthalmol* 73:46–51, 1972.

107. Gale CC: Neuroendocrine aspects of thermoregulation. *Annu Rev Physiol* 35:319–430, 1973.

108. Gerson CD, Hepner GW, Brown N, *et al.*: Inhibition by diphenylhydantoin of folic acid absorption in man. *Gastroenterology* 63:246–251, 1972.

109. Ginter E. Ascorbic acid synthesis in certain guinea pigs. *Int J Vitamin Res* 46:173–179, 1976.

110. Ginter E: Chronic marginal vitamin C deficiency: biochemistry and pathophysiology. *World Rev Nutr Diet* 33:104–141, 1979.

111. Ginter E: What is truly the maximum body pool size of ascorbic acid in man? *Am J Clin Nutr* 33:538, 1980.

112. Goldsmith GA: Curative nutrition: vitamins, Chapter 7. In *Nutritional Support of Medical Practice*, edited by H.A. Schneider, C.E. Anderson, D.B. Coursin. Harper & Row, Hagerstown, Md., 1977 (pp. 103–106).

113. *Ibid.* (pp. 108, 109).

114. *Ibid.* (pp. 113–114).

115. Gordon N: Folic acid deficiency from anticonvulsant therapy. *Dev Med Child Neurol* 10: 497–504, 1968.

116. Gould N: Back-pocket sciatica. *N Engl J Med* 290:633, 1974.

117. Gowers WR: Lumbago: its lessons and analogues. *Br Med J* 1:117–121, 1904.

118. Gregory JF, Kirk JR: Vitamin B$_6$ in Foods: assessment of stability and bioavailability, Chapter 5. In *Human Vitamin B$_6$ Requirements*. National Academy of Sciences, Washington, 1978 (pp. 75, 76).

119. Griner PF, Oranburg PR: Predictive values of erythrocyte indices for tests of iron, folic acid, and vitamin B$_{12}$ deficiency. *Am J Clin Pathol* 70:748–752, 1978.

120. Gross RH: Leg length discrepancy: how much is too much? *Orthopedics* 1:307–310, 1978.

121. Guard O, Dumas R, Audry D, Tommasi M, Knopf JF: [Clinical and pathological study of a case of subacute combined degeneration of the cord with folic acid deficiency (author's translation)]. *Rev Neurol (Paris)* 137:435–446, 1981.

122. Hall CA: Pathophysiology of vitamin B$_{12}$. *Pathobiol Annu* 9:257–275, 1979.

123. Hall CA: Vitamin B$_{12}$, deficiency and early rise in mean corpuscular volume. *JAMA* 245: 1144–1146, 1981.

124. Halsted CH: Folate deficiency and the small intestine, Chapter 14. In *Folic Acid in Neurology, Psychiatry, and Internal Medicine*, edited by M.I. Botez, E.H. Reynolds. Raven Press, New York, 1979 (p. 120).

125. Halsted CH, Robles EA, Mezey E: Decreased jejunal uptake of labeled folic acid (^{3}H-PGA) in

alcoholic patients: roles of alcohol and nutrition. *N Engl J Med* 285:701–706, 1971.

126. Harris RI, Beath T: The short first metatarsal, its incidence and clinical significance. *J Bone Joint Surg* 31-A:553–565, 1949.

127. Harrison GG: The effect of procaine and curare on the initiation of anaesthetic-induced malignant hyperpyrexia, Chapter 23. In *International Symposium on Malignant Hyperthermia*, edited by R.E. Gordon, B.A. Britt, W. Kalow. Charles C Thomas, Springfield, Ill., 1973 (pp. 276, 277).

128. Hart RJ, Jr., McCurdy PR: Psychosis in vitamin B$_{12}$ deficiency. *Arch Int Med* 128:596–597, 1971.

129. Haskell BE: Analysis of vitamin B$_6$, Chapter 4. In *Human Vitamin B$_6$ Requirements*. National Academy of Sciences, Washington, 1978 (pp. 61, 67).

130. Herbert V: Experimental nutritional folate deficiency in man. *Trans Assoc Am Phys* 75:307–320, 1962.

131. Herbert V: Biochemical and hematologic lesions in folic acid deficiency. *Am J Clin Nutr* 20:562–569, 1967.

132. Herbert V: Drugs effective in megaloblastic anemias; vitamin B$_{12}$ and folic acid, Chapter 64. In *The Pharmacological Basis of Therapeutics*, edited by L.S. Goodman, A. Gilman, Ed. 4. Macmillan, New York, 1970 (pp. 1431–1441).

133. *Ibid.* (pp. 1414–1431).

134. Herbert V: Malnutrition and the immune response. *Infect Dis* 7: 4–10, 1977.

135. Herbert V: The nutritional anemias. *Hosp Pract* 15:65–89, 1980.

136. Herbert V, Colman N: Hematological aspects of folate deficiency, Chapter 9. In *Folic Acid in Neurology, Psychiatry, and Internal Medicine*, edited by M.I. Botez, E.H. Reynolds. Raven Press, New York, 1979 (pp. 67–72).

137. Herbert V, Colman N, Jacob E: Folic acid and Vitamin B$_{12}$, Chapter 6J. In *Modern Nutrition in Health and Disease*, edited by R.S. Goodhart and M.E. Shils, Ed. 6. Lea & Febiger, Philadelphia, 1980 (pp. 229–255).

138. Hillman RE: Megavitamin responsive aminoacidopathies. *Pediatr Clin North Am* 23:557–567, 1976.

139. Hodges RE: Ascorbic acid, Chapter 6K. In *Modern Nutrition in Health and Disease*, edited by R.S. Goodhart, M.E. Shils, Ed. 6. Philadelphia, Lea & Febiger, Philadelphia 1980 (pp. 259–273).

140. Horrobin DF: Interrelationships between folic acid and prostaglandins in epilepsy, schizophrenia, and peripheral neuropathies, Chapter 44. In *Folic Acid in Neurology, Psychiatry, and Internal Medicine*, edited by M.I. Botez, E.H. Reynolds. Raven Press, New York, 1979 (pp. 489–491).

141. Horwitz BA: Metabolic aspects of thermogenesis: neuronal and hormonal control. *Fed. Proc* 38:2147–2149, 1979.

142. Hudson OC, Hettesheimer CA, Robin PA: Causalgic backache. *Am J Surg* 52:297–303, 1941.

143. Hughes RE: Nonscorbutic effects of Vitamin C: biochemical aspects. *Proc R Soc Med* 70:86–89, 1977.

144. Hunter R, Barnes J, Matthews DM: Effect of folic-acid supplement on serum-vitamin-B$_{12}$ levels in patients on anticonvulsants. *Lancet*

2:666–667, 1969.

145. Hunter R, Barnes J, Oakeley HF, et al.: Toxicity of folic acid given in pharmacological doses to healthy volunteers. *Lancet* 1:61–63, 1970.

146. Ingbar SH, Woeber KA: Diseases of the thyroid, Chapter 335. In *Principles of Internal Medicine*, edited by K.J. Isselbacher, R.D. Adams, E. Braunwald, et al., Ed. 9. McGraw–Hill Book Company, New York, 1980 (pp. 1696, 1698–1699, 1701–1703, 1711).

147. Judovich B, Bates W: *Pain Syndromes*, Ed. 3. F.A. Davis, Philadelphia, 1949 (pp. 46–51, Figs. 31–35).

148. Kallner AB, Hartman D, Hornig DH: On the requirements of ascorbic acid in man: steady-state turnover and body pool in smokers. *Am J Clin Nutr* 34:1347–1355, 1981.

149. Kariks J, Perry SW: Folic-acid deficiency in psychiatric patients. *Med J Aust* 1:1192–1195, 1970.

150. Keiser G, Berchtold P, Bolli P, et al.: Störung der Vitamin-B$_{12}$-Absorption infolge Biguanidtherapie. *Schweiz Med Wochenschr* 100:351–353, 1970.

151. Kelley WN: Gout and other disorders of purine metabolism. Chapter 92. In *Harrison's Principles of Internal Medicine*, edited by K.J. Isselbacher, R.D. Adams, E. Braunwald, et al., Ed. 9. McGraw–Hill, New York, 1980 (pp. 479–486).

152. Kent S: Vitamin C therapy: colds, cancer and cardiovascular disease. *Geriatrics* 33:91–105, 1978.

153. Kim JCS: Ultrastructural studies of vascular and muscular changes in ascorbic acid deficient guinea-pigs. *Lab Anim* 11:113–117, 1977.

154. King CE, Leibach J, Toskes PP: Clinically significant vitamin B$_{12}$ deficiency secondary to malabsorption of protein-bound vitamin B$_{12}$. *Dig Dis Sci* 24:397–402, 1979.

155. Kishi H, Kishi T, Williams RH, et al.: Deficiency of vitamin B$_6$ in women taking contraceptive formulations. *Res Commun Chem Pathol Pharmacol* 17:283–293, 1977.

156. Klein I, Mantell P, Parker M, et al.: Resolution of abnormal muscle enzyme studies in hypothyroidism. *Am J Med Sci* 279:159–162, 1980.

157. Klein KK: A study of the progression of lateral pelvic asymmetry in 585 elementary, junior and senior high school boys. *Am Correct Ther J* 23:171–173, 1969.

158. Klein KK, Redler I, Lowman CL: Asymmetries of growth in the pelvis and legs of children: a clinical and statistical study 1964–1967. *JAOA* 68:153–156, 1968.

159. Klipstein FA: Subnormal serum folate and macrocytosis associated with anticonvulsant drug therapy. *Blood* 23:68–86, 1964.

160. Klipstein FA: Tropical sprue—an iceberg disease? *Ann Int Med* 66:622–623, 1967.

161. Klipstein FA, Schenk EA, Samloff IM: Folate repletion associated with oral tetracycline therapy in tropical sprue. *Gastroenterology* 51:317–332, 1966.

162. Knigge KM, Penrod CH, Schindler WJ: In vitro and in vivo adrenal corticosteroid secretion following stress. *Am J Phys* 196:579–582, 1959.

163. Koenig WC, Jr., Powers JJ, Johnson EW: Does allergy play a role in fibrositis? *Arch Phys Med Rehabil* 58:80–83, 1977.

164. Kolhouse JF, Kondo H, Allen NC, et al.: Cobalamin analogues are present in human plasma and can mask cobalamin deficiency because current radioisotope dilution assays are not specific for true cobalamin. *N Engl J Med* 299:785–792, 1978.

165. Kosik KS, Mullins TF, Bradley WG, et al.: Coma and axonal degeneration in vitamin B$_{12}$ deficiency. *Arch Neurol* 37:590–592, 1980.

166. Krumholz A, Weiss HD, Goldstein PJ, et al.: Evoked responses in vitamin B$_{12}$ deficiency. *Ann Neurol* 9:407–409, 1981.

167. Lane F, Goff P, McGuffin R, et al.: Folic acid metabolism in normal, folate deficient and alcoholic man. *Br J Haematol* 34:489–500, 1976.

168. Langohr HD, Petruch F, Schroth G: Vitamin B$_1$, B$_2$ and B$_6$ deficiency in neurological disorders. *J Neurol* 225:95–108, 1981.

169. Lanzkowsky P: Congenital malabsorption of folate. *Am J Med* 48:580–583, 1970.

170. Larsen PR, Conard RA, Knudsen KD, et al.: Thyroid hypofunction after exposure to fallout from a hydrogen bomb explosion. *JAMA* 247:1571–1575, 1982.

171. Laurence KM, James N, Miller MH, et al.: Double-blind randomised controlled trial of folate treatment before conception to prevent recurrence of neural-tube defects. *Br Med J* 282:1509–1511, 1981.

172. Leeton J: Depression induced by oral contraception and role of vitamin B$_6$ in its management. *Aust NZ J Psychiatry* 8:85–88, 1974.

173. Lehninger AL: *Biochemistry*. Worth, New York, 1970 (p. 430).

174. *Ibid* (p. 204).

175. *Ibid.* (pp. 383, 550).

176. Lerner AM: Infections with herpes simplex virus, Chapter 193. In *Principles of Internal Medicine*, edited by K.J. Isselbacher, R.D. Adams, E. Braunwald, et al., Ed. 9. McGraw–Hill, New York, 1980 (pp. 847–851).

177. Lewis A, Wilson CWM: The effect of vitamin C deficiency and supplementation on the weight pattern and skin potential of the guinea-pig (proceedings). *Br J Pharmacol* 67:457P–458P, 1979.

178. Li T-K: Factors influencing vitamin B$_6$ requirement in alcoholism, Chapter 13. In *Human Vitamin B$_6$ Requirements*. National Academy of Sciences, Washington, 1978 (p. 210).

179. Linkswiler HM: Vitamin B$_6$ requirements of men, Chapter 19. In *Human Vitamin B$_6$ Requirements*. National Academy of Sciences, Washington, 1978 (pp. 282–288).

180. Lipton MA, Kane FJ, Jr.: Psychiatry, Chapter 30. In *Nutritional Support of Medical Practice*, edited by H.A. Schneider, C.E. Anderson, D.B. Coursin, Harper & Row, Hagerstown, Md., 1977 (pp. 468–469).

181. Loh HS: Screening for vitamin C status. *Lancet* 1:944–945, 1973.

182. Lonsdale D, Shamberger RJ: Red cell transketolase as an indicator of nutritional deficiency. *Am J Clin Nutr* 33:205–211, 1980.

183. Lowman CL: The effect of faulty skeletal alignment upon the eyes. *Am J Orthoped Surg* 16:459–492, 1918.

184. Lowman CL: The sitting position in relation to pelvic stress. *Physiother Rev* 21:30–33, 1941.

185. Lui NST, Roels OA: Vitamin A and carotene, Chapter 6A. In *Modern Nutrition in Health and Disease*, edited by R.S. Goodhart, M.E. Shils, Ed. 6. Lea & Febiger, Philadelphia, 1980 (p. 154).

186. Maigne R: *Orthopedic Medicine, A New Approach to Vertebral Manipulation*, translated by W.T. Liberson. Charles C Thomas, Springfield, Ill., 1972 (pp. 192, 292, 390).

187. *Ibid.* (pp. 392–394).

188. Marcoullis G, Parmentier Y, Nicolas J-P: Blocking and binding type antibodies against all major vitamin B_{12}-binders in a pernicious anaemia serum. *Br J Haematol* 43:15–26, 1979.

189. Mark RM, Oyama JH: Nutrition, hypertension and kidney disease, Chapter 33. In *Modern Nutrition in Health and Disease*, edited by R.S. Goodhart, M.E. Shils, Ed. 6. Lea & Febiger, Philadelphia, 1980 (p. 1031).

190. Martin GR: Studies on the tissue distribution of ascorbic acid. *Ann NY Acad Sci* 92:141–7, 1961.

191. McCarron DA: Low serum concentrations of ionized calcium in patients with hypertension. *N Engl J Med* 207:226–228, 1982.

192. McCarron DA, Morris C, Cole C: Dietary calcium and human hypertension. *Science* 217:267–269, 1982.

193. Meindok H, Dvorsky R: Serum folate and vitamin-B_{12} levels in the elderly. *J Am Geriatr Soc* 18:317–326, 1970.

194. Middaugh LD, Grover TA, Zemp JW: Effects of dietary folic acid reduction on tissue folate concentrations and on neurochemical and behavioral aspects of brain function in adult and developing mice, Chapter 24. In *Folic Acid in Neurology, Psychiatry, and Internal Medicine*, edited by M.I. Botez, E.H. Reynolds. Raven Press, New York, 1979 (p. 226, 227).

195. Moldofsky H, Scarisbrick P: Induction of neurasthenic musculoskeletal pain syndrome by selective sleep stage deprivation. *Psychosom Med* 38:35–44, 1976.

196. Moldofsky H, Scarisbrick P, England R, Smythe H: Musculoskeletal symptoms and non-REM sleep disturbance in patients with "fibrositis syndrome" and healthy subjects. *Psychosom Med* 37:341–351, 1975.

197. Morton DJ: *The Human Foot.* Columbia University Press, New York, 1935 (pp. 156–157, Figs. 76, 77).

198. Morton DJ: Foot disorders in women. *J Am Med Wom Assoc* 10:41–46, 1955.

199. National Research Council, Committee on Dietary Allowances: *Recommended Dietary Allowances.* Ed. 9. National Academy of Sciences, Washington, 1980 (p. 46).

200. *Ibid.* (pp. 75–77, 108–110, 117, 118).

201. *Ibid.* (pp. 125–164).

202. *Ibid.* (pp. 84, 85, 99–102).

203. Nauss KM, Newberne PM: Effects of dietary folate, vitamin B_{12} and methionine/choline deficiency on immune function. *Adv Exp Med Biol* 135:63–91, 1981.

204. Neal RA, Sauberlich HE: Thiamin, Chapter 6E. In *Modern Nutrition in Health and Disease*, edited by R.S. Goodhart, M.E. Shils, Ed. 6. Lea & Febiger, Philadelphia, 1980 (pp. 191, 193–196).

205. Nelson PJ, Pruitt RE, Henderson LL, et al.: Effect of ascorbic acid deficiency on the *in vivo* synthesis of carnitine. *Biochim Biophys Acta* 672:123–127, 1981.

206. Nichols PJR: Short-leg syndrome. *Br Med J* 1:1863–1865, 1960.

207. Nichols PJR, Bailey NTJ: The accuracy of measuring leg-length differences. *Br Med J* 2:1247–1248, 1955.

208. Niederwieser A: Inborn errors of pterin metabolism, Chapter 33. In *Folic Acid in Neurology, Psychiatry, and Internal Medicine*, edited by M.I. Botez, E.H. Reynolds. Raven Press, New York, 1979 (pp. 351, 354, 364, 365).

209. Northrup GW: Osteopathic lesions. *JAOA* 71:854–865, 1972.

210. Paine CJ, Grafton WD, Dickson VL, et al.: Oral contraceptives, serum folate, and hematologic status. *JAMA* 231:731–733, 1975.

211. Passeri M: [Preventive role of vitamins in some old age diseases (author's translation)]. *Acta Vitaminol Enzymol* 2:147–62, 1980.

212. Pauling L: *Vitamin C and the Common Cold.* W.H. Freeman, San Francisco, 1970.

213. Pearson WM: Early and high incidence of mechanical faults. *J Osteopathy* 61:18–23, 1954.

214. Pearson WM, Rea FW, Casner VH, et al.: A progressive structural study of school children. *JAOA* 51:155–167, 1951.

215. Pelletier O: Vitamin C status of cigarette smokers and nonsmokers. *Am J Clin Nutr* 23:520–524, 1970.

216. Pfeiffer CC: *Mental and Elemental Nutrients*, Keats Publishing, New Canaan, Conn., 1975 (pp. 146, 251, 280, 281, 469).

217. Pincus JH: Folic acid deficiency: a cause of subacute combined system degeneration, Chapter 39. In *Folic Acid in Neurology, Psychiatry, and Internal Medicine*, edited by M.I. Botez, E.H. Reynolds. Raven Press, New York, 1979 (p. 432).

218. Pincus JH, Reynolds EH, Glaser GH: Subacute combined system degeneration with folate deficiency. *JAMA* 221:496–497, 1972.

219. Plaitakis A, Nicklas WJ, Berl S: Alterations in uptake and metabolism of asparate and glutamate in brain of thiamin deficient animals. *Brain Res* 171:489–502, 1979.

220. Plorde JJ: Amebiasis, Chapter 199. In *Principles of Internal Medicine*, edited by K.J. Isselbacher, R.D. Adams, E. Braunwald, et al., Ed. 9. McGraw-Hill, New York, 1980 (pp. 863–864).

221. Plorde JJ: Minor protozoan diseases, Chapter 205. In *Principles of Internal Medicine*, edited by K.J. Isselbacher, R.D. Adams, E. Braunwald, et al., Ed 9. McGraw-Hill, New York, 1980 (pp. 887–888).

222. Plorde JJ: Cestode (tapeworm) infections, Chapter 213. In *Principles of Internal Medicine*, edited by K.J. Isselbacher, R.D. Adams, E. Braunwald, et al., Ed. 9. McGraw-Hill, New York, 1980 (pp. 916–917).

223. Prema K, Srikantia SG: Clinical grading of lingual lesions in vitamin B-complex deficiency. *Indian J Med Res* 72:537–545, 1980.

224. Randall HT: Water, electrolytes and acid-base balance, Chapter 8. In *Modern Nutrition in Health and Disease*, edited by R.S. Goodhart, M.E. Shils, Ed. 6. Lea & Febiger, Philadelphia, 1980 (pp. 368, 378).

225. Ray, T: What to look for in diagnosing hypothy-

roidism. *Geriatrics* 32:55–59, 1977.
226. Read DJC, Grant SGN, Bishop RO, *et al.*: Defective reflex responses to impeded breathing during quiet sleep or anesthesia in thiamine-deficient kittens and puppies. *Sleep* 3:383–392, 1980.
227. Redler I: Clinical significance of minor inequalities in leg length. *New Orleans Med Surg J* 104:308–312, 1952.
228. Reynolds E, Hooton EA: Relation of pelvis to erect posture; an exploratory study. *Am J Phys Anthropol* 21:253–278, 1936.
229. Reynolds EH: Cerebrospinal fluid folate: clinical studies, Chapter 22. In *Folic Acid in Neurology, Psychiatry, and Internal Medicine*, edited by M.I. Botez, E.H. Reynolds. Raven Press, New York, 1979 (p. 195).
230. Reynolds EH: Interrelationships between the neurology of folate and vitamin B_{12} deficiency, Chapter 46. In *Folic Acid in Neurology, Psychiatry, and Internal Medicine*, edited by M.I. Botez, E.H. Reynolds, Raven Press, New York, 1979 (pp. 504–514).
231. Reynolds MD: Myofascial trigger point syndromes in the practice of rheumatology. *Arch Phys Med Rehabil* 62:111–114, 1981.
232. Robbins J, Rall JE, Gorden P: The thyroid and iodine metabolism, Chapter 19. In *Metabolic Control and Disease*, edited by P.K. Bondy, L.E. Rosenberg, Ed. 8. Saunders, Philadelphia, 1980 (pp. 1333, 1343–1345).
233. Robson LC, Schwarz MR, Perkins WD: Vitamin B_6 and immunity, Chapter 9. In *Human Vitamin B_6 Requirements*. National Academy of Sciences, Washington, 1978 (p. 162).
234. Roe DA: *Drug-induced Nutritional Deficiencies*. AVI Publishing, Westport, Conn., 1976 (pp. 7–17, 72, 73, 79–81, 85, 96–99, 150, 151, 160–167, 215–216, 223–227).
235. *Ibid.* (pp. 72, 83, 120, 217).
236. Rose DP: Oral contraceptives and vitamin B_6, Chapter 11. In *Human Vitamin B_6 Requirements*. National Academy of Sciences, Washington, 1978 (pp. 193–201).
237. Rosenberg IH, Dyer J: The prevalence and causes of folic acid deficiency in the United States, Chapter 4. In *Folic Acid in Neurology, Psychiatry, and Internal Medicine*, edited by M.I. Botez, E.H. Reynolds. Raven Press, New York, 1979 (pp. 19–22).
238. Rosenberg IH, Godwin HA: The digestion and absorption of dietary folate. *Gastroenterology* 60:445–463, 1971.
239. Rosenberg IH, Selhub J, Dhar GJ: Absorption and malabsorption of folates, Chapter 13. In *Folic Acid in Neurology, Psychiatry, and Internal Medicine*, edited by M.I. Botez, E.H. Reynolds. Raven Press, New York, 1979 (pp. 97–99).
240. Rosenblatt DS, Cooper BA: Methylenetetrahydrofolate reductase deficiency: clinical and biochemical correlations, Chapter 34. In *Folic Acid in Neurology, Psychiatry, and Internal Medicine*, edited by M.I. Botez, E.H. Reynolds. Raven Press, New York, 1979 (p. 389).
241. Rubin D: Myofascial trigger point syndromes: an approach to management. *Arch Phys Med Rehabil* 62:107–110, 1981.
242. Runcie J: Folate deficiency in the elderly, Chapter 45. In *Folic Acid in Neurology, Psychiatry,*
and Internal Medicine, edited by M.I. Botez, E.H. Reynolds. Raven Press, New York, 1979 (pp. 493–499).
243. Rush WA, Steiner HA: A study of lower extremity length inequality. *Am J Roentgen Rad Ther* 56:616–623, 1946.
244. Sabin AB: Is topical ether therapy effective for herpes simplex? *JAMA* 238:63, 1977.
245. Salam-Adams M, Bradley GW: Acute and subacute myopathic paralysis, Chapter 379. In *Principles of Internal Medicine*, edited by K.J. Isselbacher, R.D. Adams, E. Braunwald, *et al.*, Ed. 9. McGraw–Hill Book Company, New York, 1980 (p. 2057).
246. Sandstead HH: Clinical manifestations of certain classical deficiency diseases, Chapter 23. In *Modern Nutrition in Health and Disease*, edited by R.S. Goodhart, M.E. Shils, Ed. 6. Lea & Febiger, Philadelphia, 1980 (pp. 686–688).
247. Sauberlich HE, Canham JE: Vitamin B_6, Chapter 6I. In *Modern Nutrition in Health and Disease*, edited by R.S. Goodhart, M.E. Shils, Ed. 6. Lea & Febiger, Philadelphia, 1980 (pp. 219–225).
248. Schimmel M, Utiger RD: Thyroidal and peripheral production of thyroid hormones. *Ann Intern Med* 87:760–768, 1977.
249. Schneider HA, Anderson CE, Coursin DB: *Nutritional support of medical practice*. Harper & Row, Hagerstown, Md., 1977 (pp. 37, 38, 111, 115–118, 131, 436, 450, 480–482).
250. Scott JH, Weir DG: The methyl folate trap. *Lancet* 2:337–340, 1981.
251. Shahawy ME, Tucker R, Wahner H, *et al.*: Hyperthyroidism and Potassium. *JAMA* 217:269, 1971.
252. Shane B: Vitamin B_6 and blood, Chapter 7. In *Human Vitamin B_6 Requirements*. National Academy of Sciences, Washington, 1978 (pp. 115, 122–124).
253. Shapira Y, Zvi AB, Statter M: Folic acid deficiency: a reversible cause of infantile hypotonia. *J Pediatr* 93:984–986, 1978.
254. Sharav Y, Tzukert A, Refaeli B: Muscle pain index in relation to pain, dysfunction, and dizziness associated with the myofascial pain-dysfunction syndrome. *Oral Surg* 46:742–747, 1978.
255. Shaw S, Lieber CS: Nutrition and alcoholism, Chapter 40. In *Modern Nutrition in Health and Disease*, edited by R.S. Goodhart, M.E. Shils. Ed. 6, Lea & Febiger, Philadelphia, 1980 (pp. 1225, 1226).
256. *Ibid.* (p. 1235).
257. Shelley WB, Rawnsley HM, Morrow G III: Pyridoxine-dependent hair pigmentation in association with homocystinuria. *Arch Dermatol* 106:228–230, 1972.
258. Sheppard K, Ryrie D: Changes in serum levels of cobalamin and cobalamin analogues in folate deficiency. *Scand J Haematol* 25:401–406, 1980.
259. Shils ME: Magnesium, Chapter 7B. In *Modern Nutrition in Health and Disease*, edited by R.S. Goodhart, M.E. Shils, Ed. 6. Lea & Febiger, Philadelphia, 1980 (pp. 315, 317).
260. Shils ME: Nutrition and neoplasia, Chapter 38. In *Modern Nutrition in Health and Disease*, edited by R.S. Goodhart, M.E. Shils. Lea & Febiger, Philadelphia, 1980 (pp. 1179, 1180).
261. Shorvon SD, Reynolds EH: Folate deficiency

and peripheral neuropathy, Chapter 37. In *Folic Acid in Neurology, Psychiatry, and Internal Medicine*, edited by M.I. Botez, E.H. Reynolds. Raven Press, New York, 1979 (p. 420).

262. Sicuranza BJ, Richards J, Tisdall LH: The short leg syndrome in obstetrics and gynecology. *Am J Obstet Gynecol* 107:217–219, 1970.

263. Simons DG, Travell J: Common myofascial origins of low back pain. *Postgrad Med* 73:66–108, 1983.

264. Smith LH Jr: Genetic disorders of amino acid metabolism, Chapter 96. In *Harrison's Principles of Internal Medicine*, edited by M.M. Wintrobe, G.W. Thorn, R.D. Adams, *et al.*, Ed. 7. McGraw-Hill, New York, 1974 (p. 595).

265. Smith TJS, Malon RG: Vitamin B$_{12}$ deficiency and early rise in mean corpuscular volume; reply by C.A. Hall. *JAMA* 247:1126, 1982.

266. Smythe HA: Fibrositis and other diffuse musculoskeletal syndromes. In *Textbook of Rheumatology*, edited by W.N. Kelley, E.D. Harris, Jr., S. Ruddy, *et al.*, Vol. 1. W.B. Saunders, Philadelphia, 1981 (p. 489).

267. Snyderman SE, Holt EH, Jr., Carretero R, *et al.*: Pyridoxine deficiency in the human infant. *Am J Clin Nutr* 1:200–207, 1953.

268. Sola AE, Williams RL: Myofascial pain syndromes. *Neurol* 6:91–95, 1956.

269. Sotaniemi KA, Kaarela K: Dry beriberi in a slimmer. *Br Med J* 2:23–31, 1977.

270. Spellacy WN, Buhi WC, Birk SA: The effects of vitamin B$_6$ on carbohydrate metabolism on women taking steroid contraceptives: preliminary report. *Contraception* 6:265–275, 1972.

271. Stead WW: Tuberculosis, Chapter 156. In *Harrison's Principles of Internal Medicine*, edited by M.M. Wintrobe, G.W. Thorn, R.D. Adams, *et al.*, Ed. 7. McGraw-Hill, New York, 1974 (p. 867).

272. Sterling K: Thyroid hormone action at the cell level. *N Engl J Med* 300:117–123, 173–177, 1979.

273. Sterling K, Brenner MA, Saldanha VF: Conversion of thyroxine to triiodothyronine by cultured human cells. *Science* 179:1000–1001, 1973.

274. Sternbach RA: *Pain Patients, Traits and Treatment*, Academic Press, New York, 1974 (pp. 40–51).

275. Stoddard A: *Proceedings of the International Congress of Physical Medicine*. Headley, London, 1955 (p. 260).

276. Stone S: Pyridoxine and thiamine in disorders of the nervous system. *Dis Nerv Syst* 6:1–8, 1950.

277. Streeter AM: Malabsorption of vitamin B$_{12}$ after vagotomy. *Am J Surg* 128:340–343, 1974.

278. Streiff RR: Folate deficiency and oral contraceptives. *JAMA* 214:105–108, 1970.

279. Strelling MK, Blackledge DG, Goodall HB: Diagnosis and management of folate deficiency in low birthweight infants. *Arch Dis Childhood* 54:271–277, 1979.

280. Swinson CM, Perry J, Lumb M, *et al.*: Role of sulphasalazine in the aetiology of folate deficiency in ulcerative colitis. *Gut* 22:456–461, 1981.

281. Taylor TV, Rimmer S, Day B, *et al.*: Ascorbic acid supplementation in the treatment of pressure-sores. *Lancet* 2:544–546, 1974.

282. Theuer RC, Vitale JJ: Drug and nutrient interactions, Chapter 18. In *Nutritional Support of Medical Practice*, edited by H.A. Schneider, C.E.

Anderson, D.B. Coursin. Harper & Row, 1977 (pp. 299, 300, 302).

283. Thomson AD, Baker H, Leevy CM: Patterns of ^{35}S-thiamine hydrochloride absorption in the malnourished alcoholic patient. *J Lab Clin Med* 76:34–45, 1970.

284. Thornton WE, Thornton BP: Folic acid, mental function, and dietary habits. *J Clin Psychiatry* 39:315–319, 322, 1978.

285. Thurnham DI: Red cell enzyme tests of vitamin status: do marginal deficiencies have physiological significance? *Proc Nutr Soc* 40:155–163, 1981.

286. Tichauer ER: Industrial engineering in the rehabilitation of the handicapped. *J Industr Eng* 19:96–104, 1968.

287. Tomkin GH, Hadden DR, Weaver JA, *et al.*: Vitamin B$_{12}$ status of patients on long-term metformin therapy. *Br Med J* 2:685–687, 1971.

288. Travell J: Referred pain from skeletal muscle: the pectoralis major syndrome of breast pain and soreness and the sternomastoid syndrome of headache and dizziness. *NY State J Med* 55:331–339, 1955.

289. Travell J: Factors affecting pain of injection. *JAMA* 158:368–371, 1955.

290. Travell J: Mechanical headache. *Headache* 7:23–29 1965.

291. Travell J: *Office Hours: Day and Night*. The World Publishing Company, New York, 1968 (pp. 270, 284, 285, 301, 302).

292. Travell J: Low back pain and the Dudley J. Morton foot (long second toe). *Arch Phys Med Rehabil* 56:566, 1975.

293. Travell J: Identification of myofascial trigger point syndromes: a case of atypical facial neuralgia. *Arch Phys Med Rehabil* 62:100–106, 1981.

294. Travell J, Rinzler SH: The myofascial genesis of pain. *Postgrad Med* 11:425–434, 1952.

295. Travell J, Travell W: Therapy of low back pain by manipulation and of referred pain in the lower extremity by procaine infiltration. *Arch Phys Med* 27:537–547, 1946.

296. Travell JG: The quadratus lumborum muscle: an overlooked cause of low back pain. *Arch Phys Med Rehabil* 57:566, 1976.

297. Vallance S: Relationships between ascorbic acid and serum proteins of the immune system. *Br Med J* 2:437–438, 1977.

298. Van Itallie TB: Assessment of nutritional status, Chapter 75. In *Harrison's Principles of Internal Medicine*, edited by M.M. Wintrobe, G.W. Thorne, R.D. Adams, *et al.*, Ed. 7. McGraw-Hill, New York, 1974 (p. 419).

299. Van Itallie TB, Follis RH, Jr.: Thiamine deficiency, ariboflavinosis, and vitamin B$_6$ deficiency, Chapter 78. In *Harrison's Principles of Internal Medicine*, edited by M.M. Wintrobe, G.W. Thorn, R.D. Adams, *et al.*, Ed. 7. McGraw-Hill, New York, 1974 (pp. 430–432).

300. Vilter RW: Nutritional aspects of ascorbic acid: uses and abuses. *West J Med* 133:485–492, 1980.

301. Vimokesant SL, Nakornchai S, Dhanamitta S, *et al.*: Effect of tea consumption on thiamin status of man. *Nutr Rep Int* 9:371–376, 1974.

302. Wakabayashi A, Yui Y, Kawai C: A clinical study on thiamine deficiency. *Jpn Circ J* 43:995–999, 1979.

303. Weeks VD, Travell J: Postural vertigo due to

trigger areas in the sternocleidomastoid muscle. *J Pediatr* 47:315–327, 1955.

304. Weiner WJ: Vitamin B₆ in the pathogenesis and treatment of diseases or the central nervous system, Chapter 5. In *Clinical Neuropharmacology*, edited by H.L. Klawans, Vol. 1. Raven Press, New York, 1976 (pp. 107–136).

305. Wertalik LF, Metz EN, LoBuglio AF, *et al.*: Decreased serum B₁₂ levels with oral contraceptive use. *JAMA* 221:1371–1374, 1972.

306. White JD: No ill effects from high-dose vitamin C. *N Engl J Med* 304:1491, 1981.

307. Whitehead N, Reyner F, Lindenbaum J: Megaloblastic changes in the cervical epithelium. *JAMA* 226:1421–1424, 1973.

308. Wighton MC, Mason JI, Speed I, *et al.*: Brain damage in infancy and dietary vitamin B₁₂ deficiency. *Med J Aust* 2:1–3, 1979.

309. Wilke WS, Sheeler LR, Makarowski WS: Hypothyroidism with presenting symptoms of fibrositis. *J Rheumatol* 8:626–631, 1981.

310. Williams RD, Mason HL, Power MH, *et al.*: Induced thiamine (vitamin B₁) deficiency in man. *Arch Intern Med* 71:38–53, 1943.

311. Williams RJ: *Physicians Handbook of Nutritional Science*. Charles C Thomas, Springfield Ill., 1975 (pp. 48, 70–82).

312. Wilson CMW, Kevany JP: Screening for vitamin C status. *Br J Prev Soc Med* 26:53–54, 1972.

313. Wilson CWM, Green M: The relationship of aspirin to ascorbic acid metabolism during common cold. *J Clin Pharmacol* 18:21–28, 1978.

314. Wood B, Breen KJ: Clinical thiamine deficiency in Australia: the size of the problem and approaches to prevention. *Med J Aust* 1:461–462, 464, 1980.

315. Yeh SD, Chow BF: Goodhart RS: Marginal deficiencies of vitamins: 1. in animals, 2. observations in man. *J New Drugs* 1:10–21, 1961.

316. Youinou P, Garre M, Morin JF, *et al.*: Effect of folic acid deficiency on nonspecific immunity (phagocytic activity and nitroblue-tetrazolium reduction). *Pathol Biol* 29:175–178, 1981.

317. Zalusky R, Herbert V, Castle W: Cyanocobalamin therapy effect in folic acid deficiency. *Arch Int Med* 109:545–554, 1962.

PART 1

CHAPTER 5
Head and Neck
Pain-and-Muscle Guide
Introduction to
Masticatory Muscles

HIGHLIGHTS: This chapter is divided into two sections. Section A is a **PAIN GUIDE to INVOLVED MUSCLES** to help the reader determine which muscles to examine, based on the location of the patient's pain. Section B reviews the dental literature, which is replete with references to the **MYOFASCIAL PAIN-DYSFUNCTION SYNDROME.** Then **RECENT ADVANCES** in our understanding of the stomatognathic system are summarized, and the impact of this new information is considered in **RELATION to MYOFASCIAL TRIGGER POINTS.** The **DIFFERENTIAL DIAGNOSIS OF CRANIOMANDIBULAR PAIN** is summarized with emphasis on muscular sources of pain.

Part 1 of this manual is concerned with the muscles of the head and neck that refer pain to these uppermost parts of the body. This first of four parts comprises all of the head muscles and most of the muscles of the neck, including the sternocleidomastoid, trapezius, digastric, suboccipital, and cervical paraspinal muscles. It excludes the scalene and levator scapulae muscles of the neck; they refer pain downward.

Section A

PAIN GUIDE TO INVOLVED MUSCLES

This guide lists the muscles that may refer pain to specific areas of the head and neck, as identified in Figure 5.1. This figure is used by locating the region where the patient has pain. Under that regional heading in the pain guide, the muscles are listed that may refer pain to that anatomic area. The number in parenthesis following each muscle is the chapter number for that muscle; TP stands for trigger point.

The muscles listed in boldface type are likely to refer an essential pain pattern to that area. Regular type identifies the muscles that may refer a spillover pattern to the region.

The muscles are listed so that, in our experience, the higher the muscle stands in the list, the more frequently it is a cause of pain in that area. However, the nature of the examiner's practice influences the selection of patients and, thus, which muscles are involved most often.

PAIN GUIDE

VERTEX PAIN

Sternocleidomastoid (sternal) (7)
Splenius capitis (15)

BACK-OF-HEAD PAIN

Trapezius (TP$_1$) (6)
Sternocleidomastoid (sternal) (7)
Sternocleidomastoid (clavicular) (7)
Semispinalis capitis (16)
Semispinalis cervicis (16)
Splenius cervicis (15)
Suboccipital group (17)
Occipitalis (14)
Digastric (12)
Temporalis (TP$_4$) (9)

TEMPORAL HEADACHE

Trapezius (TP$_1$) (6)
Sternocleidomastoid (sternal) (7)
Temporalis (TPs$_{1,2,3}$) (9)
Splenius cervicis (15)
Suboccipital group (17)
Semispinalis capitis (16)

FRONTAL HEADACHE

Sternocleidomastoid (clavicular) (7)
Sternocleidomastoid (sternal) (7)

Semispinalis capitis (16)
Frontalis (14)
Zygomaticus major (13)

EAR AND TEMPOROMANDIBULAR JOINT PAIN

Lateral pterygoid (11)
Masseter (deep) (8)
Sternocleidomastoid (clavicular) (7)
Medial pterygoid (10)

EYE AND EYEBROW PAIN

Sternocleidomastoid (sternal) (7)
Temporalis (TP$_1$) (9)
Splenius cervicis (15)
Masseter (superficial) (8)
Suboccipital group (17)
Occipitalis (14)
Orbicularis oculi (13)
Trapezius (TP$_1$) (6)

CHEEK AND JAW PAIN

Sternocleidomastoid (sternal) (7)
Masseter (superficial) (8)
Lateral pterygoid (11)
Trapezius (TP$_1$) (6)
Masseter (deep) (8)
Digastric (12)
Medial pterygoid (10)
Platysma (13)
Orbicularis oculi (13)
Zygomaticus major (13)

TOOTHACHE

Temporalis (TPs$_{1,2,3}$) (9)
Masseter (superficial) (8)
Digastric (anterior) (12)

BACK-OF-NECK PAIN

Trapezius (TP$_1$) (6)
Trapezius (TP$_2$) (6)
Trapezius (TP$_3$) (6)
Multifidi (16)
Levator scapulae (19)
Splenius cervicis (15)
Infraspinatus (22)

THROAT AND FRONT-OF-NECK PAIN

Sternocleidomastoid (sternal) (7)
Digastric (12)
Medial pterygoid (10)

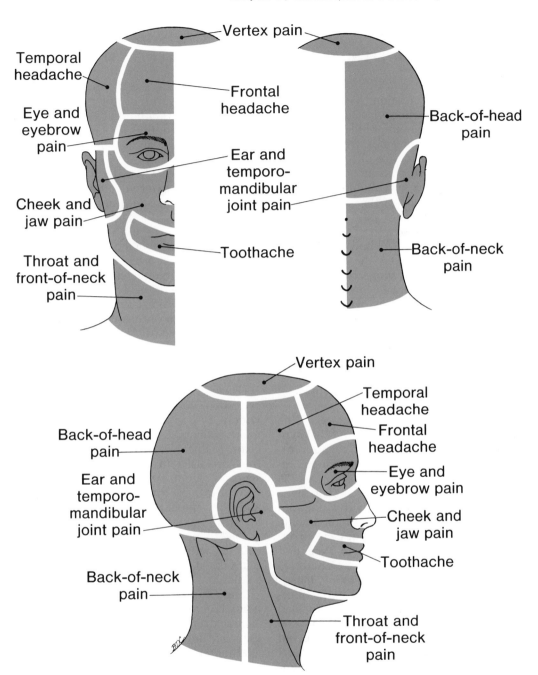

Figure 5.1.   Designated areas in the head and neck region to which pain may be referred by myofascial trigger points. See listing of muscles that refer pain to each of these areas.

Section B

MYOFASCIAL PAIN-DYSFUNCTION SYNDROME

The dental profession has pioneered recognition of the muscular component of the common craniomandibular pain syndromes. These syndromes are frequently associated with evidence of temporomandibular joint (TMJ) dysfunction. As a result, there is now a voluminous dental literature on the role of the skeletal muscles in the myofascial pain-dysfunction (MPD) syndrome and in the TMJ pain-dysfunction syndrome.[77] Mikhail and Rosen[55] have recently reviewed the former. Patients with these syndromes frequently require the management of interacting dental and medical problems, which are best handled if the two professions work together as a team, each fully aware of the expertise provided by the other. This section is intended to inform the non-dentist, health care professional of the expertise among dentists in managing myofascial craniomandibular pain.

The estimate that 20% or more of the population is afflicted with the MPD syndrome is frequently quoted.[60, 79] Supporting this large percentage, a meticulous recent study[87] found that at least 70% of 739 university students were at risk (had signs or symptoms of mandibular dysfunction) and that 5% were in need of immediate treatment. These numbers appear to increase significantly with age. In a group of shipyard workers in Sweden, 30% had *two* or more of the symptoms: clicking, masticatory muscle tenderness, and TMJ tenderness.[35] Among 30 young adults autopsied between the ages of 17 and 38,[36] 10 of 30 temporomandibular joints (33%) showed deviation in form in *all three* anatomical components of the joint. The MPD syndrome is a common, important cause of pain and dysfunction.

In 1969, Laskin[45] proposed the now classical definition of the MPD syndrome. He required the presence of only *one* of the following for its diagnosis: (1) A unilateral pain, ususally in the ear or preauricular area. The pain might radiate to other areas, often increased during the day, and was exacerbated at meal time. (2) Masticatory muscle tenderness. (3) Clicking and popping noises in the TMJ. Joint sounds had to be accompanied by pain or tenderness. (4) Limited opening of the jaws, or deviation of the mandible on opening, but rarely both at the same time. Laskin[45] also required the absence of clinical or radiological evidence of organic changes in the TMJ. There should be no TMJ tenderness when the joint was palpated *via* the external auditory meatus. However, clicking and popping noises in the TMJ are now thought to indicate dysfunction of the disc in the TMJ.[50] *Clearly, patients with any facial pain that extended to the ear or preauricular area, without a demonstrable organic basis, were included in Laskin's definition.* This invited the use of this classification as a catch-all diagnostic category for any patient with facial pain of unknown origin. Many of the characteristics listed above strongly implicate the masticatory musculature as a major source of the pain and dysfunction.

Usage of the terms, TMJ dysfunction syndrome and MPD syndrome, overlaps widely.[55] Clinically, it is often difficult to make a sharp distinction, so we make no effort to differentiate the two terms when they are used in this review. When the scope of symptoms is expanded to include pain anywhere throughout the head, neck and jaws, the expression, *craniomandibular* syndrome, is more appropriate.[26]

To the non-dentist reader, a first encounter with the extensive literature on this subject can be confusing, at times contradictory.[55] As noted by Greene[33] in 1980, "Rarely in the history of dentistry have so many labored for so long, only to end with such extreme disagreement. After more than half a century, the myofascial pain-dysfunction syndrome continues to be one of the most controversial areas in dentistry." We agree with Farrar:[20] this disagreement is more a difference in point of view and emphasis, than a difference in substance.

Periodontists, prosthodontists and oral surgeons each view craniomandibular pain from different perspectives. Periodontists often emphasize the contribution of the muscles and psychophysiological factors. Prosthodontists are likely to emphasize the therapeutic value of prosthetic devices, whereas oral surgeons are prone to view the symptoms in terms of the structural and functional changes associated with the TMJ itself. These lines are seldom clearly drawn in the literature; most authors recognize multiple contributory factors, as is reflected in the 1980 position paper on TMJ disorders of the American Academy of Craniomandibular Disorders.[52] Solberg[86] epitomizes an approach that emphasizes sequence in the appearance of signs and symptoms, while relating the neuromuscular dysfunction to specific morphological and functional disturbances. He reviews spontaneous dislocation and internal derangement of the TMJ, arthralgia, osteoarthrosis, chronic hypomobility, and inflammatory joint disease.

For the benefit of readers who are not already well acquainted with the dental literature, three major points of view are summarized below. Then, newly reported findings are introduced, and the whole picture is related to myofascial trigger-point concepts. The three viewpoints are that: (1) the MPD syndrome is largely of muscular origin; (2) it is a complex psychophysiological phenomenon; and (3) it is due primarily to disturbed occlusal mechanics.

Largely of Muscular Origin

Few authors totally neglect a muscular component when discussing this syndrome; many emphasize muscular symptoms and dysfunction as its primary feature. A number of authors have indicated, as we also believe, that much of the pain associated with the MPD syndrome is myogenic.[7-9, 26, 38, 79, 80] This group emphasizes treatment directed at relieving muscular dysfunction.

Two years after Travell and Rinzler[91] published specific pain patterns for TPs in the masseter and temporalis muscles, Schwartz and Tausig[78] reported a series of patients in whom TMJ pain was relieved by injecting tender masticatory muscles with procaine. A few years later, based on extensive experience in the Columbia University TMJ Clinic, Schwartz[76] attributed the syndrome primarily to the stress of increased muscle tension.

Later, Travell[89] explicitly identified muscles that refer pain and tenderness to the TMJ area and to other parts of the head and face, and muscles that produce symptoms of tinnitus and "stuffiness" of the adjacent ear.

Other authors have stated that initially the muscles responsible for the pain of the MPD syndrome induce masticatory dysfunction.[26] The pain and dysfunction result from myofascial trigger mechanisms[27] in shortened muscles.[37] The stress of increased muscle tension also can cause degenerative joint disease.[76] We agree that these concepts apply to many patients with the MPD syndrome.

The symptoms of the MPD syndrome are sometimes attributed chiefly to muscle *spasm*.[38, 43, 66, 80] Continuous electromyographic (EMG) monitoring of MPD patients confirms increased masseteric EMG activity.[69a] This use of "spasm" appears to us often to be inaccurate and misleading, which contributes to the difficulty in reaching agreement on the MPD syndrome. We regard spasm in a skeletal muscle as involuntary (reflex) motor unit activity of the muscle at rest. The TPs cause increased tension and shortening of local muscle fibers, but in the *absence of motor unit activity*. The use of spasm or myospasm to describe the MPD syndrome derives from the valid observation that the tender muscles are indeed tense and shortened, and sometimes show a modest amount of resting EMG activity. A pain-spasm-pain theory was proposed by Travell and co-workers in 1942 and later embellished by Bayer:[6] painfulness of the skeletal muscle presumably caused that muscle to spasm, which in turn caused more pain, establishing a self-perpetuating cycle. However, when muscles elsewhere in the body are tested, rarely do the muscle fibers in the immediate vicinity of a TP show spontaneous motor unit activity if the muscle is at a comfortable resting length.[41, 84] Experimentally, pain induced by masseter fatigue showed no EMG evidence of associated spasm.[11]

Spontaneous motor unit activity (spasm) does appear in a muscle containing TPs when that muscle is stretched to the point of distressing pain. This response limits the length to which the muscle can be stretched and tends to return it to a shorter, less stressful length. Also, a low level of resting motor unit activity (very mild spasm) can be referred to the pain area from a distant TP in another muscle.[90] Parallel muscles may develop reflex spasm to protect an adjacent, affected muscle from load and stretch. These distinctions are important if one is to understand the nature of the problem in a particular patient. Not all shortened, tender muscles are in spasm; no two patients are exactly alike.

Greene[33] summarized relevant EMG studies. Patients with the MPD syndrome generally have hyperactive muscles of mastication, which respond excessively to stressful stimuli. Abnormal physiological tests, like the disturbed jaw-jerk reflex[34] and abnormal voltage/tension curves,[40] tend to return to normal when pain has been relieved and normal function restored.[33] Experimentally, muscular hyperactivity produced pain similar in location and character to that of the MPD syndrome when normal subjects ground their teeth for 30 min.[43] Masseteric EMG activity was fully monitored in eight patients with MPD syndrome and in five normal controls. Four of these patients showed significantly more EMG activity during the day, and three showed more at night, than did control subjects.[23a] This substantiates the clinical impression of increased muscular activity. The excessive muscular activity and fatigue may have activated latent TPs to cause referred pain. Also, ischemia, which eventually becomes painful, develops when a muscle exerts sustained contraction of approximately 50% of its maximum force. Thus, muscular fatigue alone, when sufficiently severe, becomes painful.

The abnormal habitual movements of bruxism and clenching the teeth are a common component of TMJ dysfunction.[16] The regular, repetitive side-to-side tooth contacts of bruxism differ from the haphazard pattern observed during mastication. It occurs in all stages of sleep, but predominantly in Stage 2. Bruxism at night is often totally beyond the patient's awareness.[28] Clenching and grinding of the teeth also may occur during the daytime. Bruxism and clenching abuse the masticatory muscles, and such overuse is a potent activator and perpetuator of TPs in muscles.

Studies vary as to which masticatory muscles are most likely to be tender. Many, but not all, studies of the MPD syndrome show a greater percentage of tenderness in the medial or lateral pterygoid muscles than in the other muscles of mastication, in both dentulous[29, 57, 81] and edentulous[54] patients. The high prevalence of tenderness reported in the lateral (36%) and in the medial (17%) pterygoid muscles in control subjects, contrasted with only a 0–3% prevalence found in their masseter and temporalis muscles,[81] raises questions as to whether the examining technique for the former muscles is inherently more painful, or whether the pterygoid muscles more commonly harbor latent TPs in people who have not yet developed a clinical pain complaint. More specific evidence of TPs in the muscles, such as evoked referred pain patterns and local twitch responses, should help to answer this question.

Moran and co-workers at Emory University[57] analyzed the records of 236 patients treated for head and neck pain in their MPD Syndrome Clinic. They cited eight other authors who also had found evidence that the lateral pterygoid muscle was specifically responsible for the symptoms of the MPD syndrome: Alderman, Ash, Dawson, Mahan, Ramfjord, Schwartz, Thompson, and Zarb. Dawson[15] explained that occlusal interferences overworked the lateral pterygoid muscle (inferior division) in its effort to center the teeth against the forceful occlusion produced by the mandibular elevator muscles.

Numerous authors accept the muscular origin of the pain associated with the MPD syndrome because of the high percentage of good responses obtained when treatment is focused on the muscles. Several found that injection of the tender muscles with a local anesthetic produced lasting reflief.[18, 37, 78, 89] Biofeedback provided a 62.5% success rate compared with 37.5% for control subjects, who received sham "electrical current" treatments with equal preparation and duration.[17] Treatment directed at relaxing the musculature by teaching awareness of muscles, relaxation exercises, and muscle-relaxing drugs, relieved 77% of 105 patients with the MPD syndrome.[14] Transcutaneous electrical stimulation relieved 95% of patients immediately, and in 86% the relief lasted at least 1 year following treatment.[96]

A Complex Psychological Phenomenon

A psychophysiologic explanation of the MPD syndrome was introduced by Laskin in 1969.[45] He looked beyond the muscular dysfunction and emphasized patient behavior that initiated and perpetuated it. From this point of view, the MPD syndrome depended on interaction of multiple factors much more complicated than a simple cause and effect paradigm.[32] Masticatory muscle involvement has been attributed to one or more of the following causes, the frequency of which was reported by Nel[62] in 127 patients: occlusal disharmony 35%, bruxism 24%, faulty dentures 20%, emotional tension 15%, and dental procedures or miscellaneous causes 6%.

Laskin[45] proposed that the usual mechanism for this syndrome was muscular fatigue induced by habitual clenching or grinding of the teeth, a tension-relieving behavior induced by psychological stress and usually triggered by premature occlusal contacts. Ingle[38] showed that clenching, grinding, or gnashing of teeth in response to stressful life situations caused anxiety or frustration that was more marked in patients with MPD syndrome than in control subjects. Nocturnal monitoring of masseteric EMG activity in bruxers showed marked increases of EMG activity (bruxism) during periods of life situational stress.[75] This disorder, which is initially functional in these cases, ultimately may cause organic changes in the dentition, muscles, and TMJ.[43]

To support a major psychological component of the MPD syndrome, Greene[33] cited studies that showed many personality traits of MPD syndrome patients to be typical of psychophysiological disorders. However, these studies do not resolve whether, initially, the pain distorted the patient's psychological responses, or the psychological distortion heightened the patient's awareness of pain.[23] Shore[83] warned that the symptoms may be primarily *somatopsychic*, rather than psychosomatic: the pain is driving the patient "crazy." We find that the two factors augment each other in many of our patients with myofascial pain, and both need attention.

Patients with the MPD syndrome responded to experimentally induced stress with increased EMG activity in the masseter and frontalis muscles, rather than with increased gastrocnemius EMG activity, skin conductance, or heart rate.[53] They also were reported as being strong placebo reactors; 44% of one group obtained relief from a placebo drug dispensed with positive verbal cues, and 40% were relieved by a sham palatal appliance (false night guard).[53] In another study,[30] 64% responded positively to mock equilibration.

Olson[64] analyzed the psychological factors in patients with MPD syndrome and identified hypernormal, anxious, dependent, hypochondriacal, depressed, neurotic, and psychotic mental states. Depressed patients who remained untreated, or were treated ineffectually for depression, frequently also failed to respond to any treatment of their MPD syndrome.[32] We find this also is true of depressed patients with myofascial TPs in other muscles throughout the body. However, treatment of the depression alone may alleviate, but rarely completely solves, the patient's myofascial pain problem.

Abnormal Occlusal Mechanics

One group of authors focuses on premature occlusal contacts as the major cause of the MPD syndrome. Since the symptoms of this syndrome are often relieved, at least temporarily, by an acrylic resin prosthesis, the approach is then to provide permanent relief by revising the occlusion. Some of these authors are concerned with occlusal disharmony as the primary cause of the muscular dysfunction that produces pain, while others emphasize the signs of disturbed TMJ mechanics.

The *starting point* to be used when determining which tooth contacts are premature as the jaws close is a complicated matter. The obvious answer would seem to be the mandibular rest position, when it is defined as the position of the mandible with the condyles in an unstrained position in a comfortably resting upright patient.[2] This has been attempted clinically by having the patient vocalize a specific letter or word and swallow or, investigationally, by locating the EMG null position of minimum EMG activity. An early EMG study obtained an average resting range of 11.1 mm between the onset of digastric and temporal muscle activity.[24] With modern instrumentation, comparison of clinical and EMG rest positions in 10 subjects resulted in mandibular positions that differed by a mean distance of 7 mm.[74] The mandibular position obtained by either technique may not be a functional position[15] and it is influenced too strongly by common disturbing factors (head position,[73] age, tension and stress) to provide a satisfactory reproducible reference point.[66, 92]

One location of rest position, called myocentric occlusion, was based on the measurement of jaw movement with minimum EMG activity,[39] but it was sensitive to posture and required sophisticated equipment. An EMG "null" technique for medio-lateral positioning of the mandible[70] can be used to identify the musculoskeletal midline location of the mandible. Any EMG method for determining mandibular position is vulnerable to serious error due to the change in jaw position caused by tense TP bands that are free of EMG activity.

Most dentists use centric relation as a starting point, but the definition of this reference position has several variations and for good reason; it is discussed in Section 7 of Chapter 8. Gelb[25] emphasized that centric relation is dynamic and variable, strongly influenced by many factors including dysfunction of the masticatory muscles.

Weinberg[95] distinguished between functional and dysfunctional centric relation, based on the symmetry of placement of the condyles in the middle of each fossa, and on whether any "hit and slide" to centric occlusion can be correlated with displacement of the condyle. He also described several of the commonly used acrylic resin protheses: the maxillary occlusal splint, the Hawley type prothesis, the mandibular anterior repositioning prothesis, and the anterior bite plate.[94] There is also the Tanner appliance.[88]

Schwartz[76] urged that the teeth of patients with the MPD syndrome not be ground until their muscles were no longer shortened and tense. He also found, among more than 1000 patients, that onset of the MPD syndrome often followed grinding of the patient's teeth by a dentist, or the introduction of a restoration.[76]

In his study of 127 patients, Nel[62] observed occlusal disharmony (35%) and faulty dental construction (24%) to be the most common causes of the MPD syndrome. Often a Hawley biteplate produced remarkable relief of pain in 2 or 3 days.[62] Pertes[66] strongly recommended that malocclusion of various types, including excessive freeway space between the teeth, should be corrected orthodontically in youth to prevent subsequent TMJ dysfunction.

Shore[83] presented the TMJ dysfunction syndrome as primarily due to interfering occlusal contacts caused by a tightness of the lateral pterygoid and associated muscles and by disturbed proprioceptive function, (which can be caused also by myofascial TPs; see Section 8 of Chapter 3). Biteplanes, biteplates and splints are used to free the mandible from pathologic occlusion, but may cause iatrogenic dental disease in the process. This is a problem that Shore claimed was greatly reduced by using his Shore Mandibular Autorepositioning Appliance, which was designed to reestablish normal neuromuscular function by approaching the physiological rest position in step-approximations.[83] He emphasized the critical importance of relieving masticatory muscle "spasms" and "negative" proprioception by means of this device before attempting occlusal registration and restorative treatment.

Occlusal disharmony can seriously disturb muscular function. Among 85 patients with masticatory dysfunction, the nocturnal EMG activity of the masseter was significantly correlated with the severity of signs and symptoms of jaw dysfunction, including tooth wear.[12] Relief of such EMG activity by wearing a splint is more variable. In an EMG study of 25 patients with the MPD syndrome, nocturnal masseteric activity was monitored before and during the use of a full arch, maxillary stabilization splint. In half of these patients, EMG activity was significantly reduced by the splint while it was worn, but returned when it was not worn at night. Frequently, pain did not recur coincidental with the EMG activity.[13] This again indicated that the relation between resting EMG activity (spasm) and pain is not direct. The masseter muscles of the other half of the subjects either showed no decrease in activity at night, or showed an increase. The reason for these different responses was not apparent.[13]

Edmiston and Laskin[19] found that the consistency of the sound patterns caused by repeated occlusal contacts were correlated closely with improvement in the symptoms of patients with the MPD syndrome. Another 50 patients with this syndrome were remarkably able to reduce their increased masseteric EMG activity to normal values, at least temporarily, by 3 min of biofeedback. This clearly indicates that most of these patients do not have uncontrollable reflex muscle spasm.[69a] Goharian and Neff[29] reported that the lateral and medial pterygoid muscles were affected on the side of premature occlusal contact, and the masseter and temporalis muscles, on the opposite side. An EMG study of 26 denture wearers, who received examinations before extraction and for 1 year after insertion of dentures, showed marked changes in masticatory muscle activity without development of the MPD syndrome.[88] Together, these studies indicate that the pain of this syndrome may be influenced by the periodontal afferent input originating from premature occusal contacts and that, in some individuals, the neuromuscular control system can adapt itself to major mechanical changes without pain.

Therapeutic results were again used to substantiate a point of view. Surprisingly often, an occlusal prosthesis (splint), which provided a smooth contact surface to replace a premature contact, alleviated the pain of the MPD syndrome, but did not always relieve abnormal muscular activity at night.[13] Of 17 patients with the TMJ syndrome, 84% responded favorably to the occlusal splint.[29] Of 154 patients with the MPD syndrome treated by occlusal adjustment, 64% had total relief of symptoms; an additional 34% had partial relief.[57] Dental surgeons have generally recommended conservative treatment of the MPD syndrome, reserving TMJ surgery for arthritis of the joint.[47, 59]

The reason why an occlusal interference sometimes does, and in other cases does not, cause MPD symptoms is not fully established. A well monitored study of nocturnal masseteric EMG activity in 5 asymptomatic subjects showed that individuals differ widely in their immediate response to an *induced* occlusal interference. Compared to 1 week of baseline values of EMG activity, 10–15 days of induced occlusal disharmony caused a drop in EMG activity in two subjects, no change in two, and an increase in one subject, who had begun to develop muscular discomfort.[4] This suggests that, just as a short leg often perpetuates but rarely activates quadratus lumborum TPs, occlusal disharmony may sustain TP activity rather than initiate it.

RECENT ADVANCES

Temporomandibular Joint Anatomy

New concepts of the mechanics of this joint provide insight into its dysfunctions[85] and how the dysfunctions relate to the masticatory muscles. An articular disc, which is composed chiefly of collagen fibers, is interposed between the head of the condyle and the temporal bone (Fig. 5.2). The surface of the temporal bone that articulates with the condyle is *not* the roof of the articular fossa, but the posterior incline, the crest, and in many persons, also the anterior incline of the articular tubercle or eminence (Fig. 5.3).[48, 66] The bony pressure-bearing surfaces of both the eminencia and the condyle are covered chiefly by collagen fibers, not articular cartilage as in most joints of the body. This makes the interface unusually pliable as the condyle translates from a concave fossa to a convex eminence.[47] The disc divides the TMJ into normally separate superior and inferior cavities. Synovial tissue is confined to the periphery of the two cavities and does not extend over the articular surfaces. The disc is *securely attached to the condyle* at its medial and lateral poles. The condyle carries the disc with it when it translates as the jaws open or close.[46] Hence, marked reconfiguration occurs in both TMJ cavities with translatory movement;[10, 97] this revises the earlier concept that the upper cavity accommodates most of the translatory movement and that the lower cavity functions chiefly as a hinge joint.[66]

The normal attachments of the disc are illustrated in Figure 5.2 and by Perry and

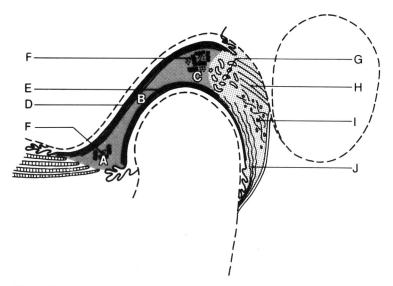

Figure 5.2. Anatomy of the temporomandibular joint in sagittal section. *A*, foot (pes) of the articular disc. *B*, thin, avascular, weight-bearing portion of disc. *C*, thickened posterior portion of disc. *D*, sheet of parallel collagen fibers on the superior surface of the disc that helps to line the superior cavity of the joint. *E*, sheet of parallel collagen fibers on the inferior surface of the disc that partly lines the inferior cavity of the joint. *F*, zones of collagen fibers oriented in three perpendicular directions. *G*, vascular knee region of the disc. *H*, superior (elastin) stratum of the bilaminar zone. *I*, loose areolar connective tissue, vessels and nerves. *J*, inferior (collagen) stratum of the bilaminar zone. (After Parker E. Mahan, reproduced with permission, from W.K. Solberg and G.T. Clark: *Temporomandibular Joint Problems: Biologic Diagnosis and Treatment*, Quintessence Publishing, Chicago, 1980, p. 35.[47])

Marsh.[65] The posterior attachment of the disc, the bilaminar zone, contains a superior stratum of elastin (Fig. 5.2*H*), and an inferior stratum of collagen fibers (Fig. 5.2*J*). Between and in front of these strata is highly vascular areolar tissue (Fig. 5.2*G* and *I*). The upper, elastic stratum attaches posteriorly to the tympanic plate, and is stretched when the condyle and disc translate forward.[68] The lower, collagen stratum attaches posteriorly and inferiorly to the condyle, moving with it and the disc into a position that limits further forward displacement of the disc on the condyle. The disc is thinnest in the region of articulation (Fig. 5.2*B*). Anteriorly, the foot of the disc becomes enlarged, is vascular, and serves, with the upper rim of the pterygoid fovea,[49] as the posterior attachment of the superior division of the lateral pterygoid muscle (Fig. 5.2*A*).[47]

Recent two-cavity arthrographic studies that were pioneered by Wilkes[97] demonstrate the normal functional relationships of the disc to the condyle and to the articular eminence (Fig. 5.3).[10] Initial jaw opening produces chiefly rotary and some translatory motion that involves primarily the inferior joint space.[71] As the jaws open farther, changes in the shape of the contrast medium in the anterior and posterior recesses of the superior and inferior joint spaces identify continuing movement of the disc as the condyle translates.[10, 97]

Muscular Functions

There is reasonable agreement on the main functions of the masticatory muscles, except for the superior division of the lateral pterygoid.

Depression of the mandible activates the digastric,[56, 61, 93] mylohyoid,[56, 93] geniohyoid,[93] and, when translation occurs, the inferior division of the lateral pterygoid muscle.[56, 61]

Elevation of the mandible activates the masseter, medial pterygoid, and tempor-

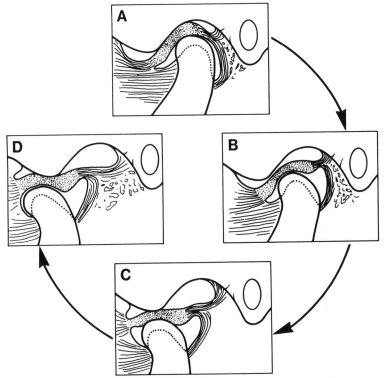

Figure 5.3. Normal temporomandibular joint function during opening movement, as seen by arthrography. The disc is the stippled structure between the condyle below, and the temporal bone above. *A*, mandible in the closed position. *B–D*, progressive stages of opening. The disc slides forward with the condyle as it translates to, and sometimes over, the articular eminence. The superior stratum of the bilaminar zone becomes stretched, the inferior stratum does not. (After D.D. Blaschke, reproduced with permission, from W.K. Solberg and G.T. Clark: *Temporomandibular Joint Problems: Biologic Diagnosis and Treatment*, Quintessence Publishing, Chicago, 1980, p. 73[10])

alis muscles,[56, 61, 93] and the superior division of the lateral pterygoid.[44]

Lateral deviation activates chiefly the posterior portion of the ipsilateral temporalis, the contralateral medial pterygoid,[61, 93] and the inferior division of the contralateral lateral pterygoid muscle.[61] Apparently, either the contralateral[93] or ipsilateral[61] masseter may assist.

Protraction of the mandible activates the medial pterygoid, masseter and suprahyoid muscles,[93] the inferior division of the lateral pterygoid, and sometimes the anterior temporalis muscle.[61]

Mandibular retraction activates the posterior and middle fibers of the temporalis muscle bilaterally,[61, 93] both bellies of the digastric,[61] and sometimes the deep fibers of the masseter.[5]

Until recently, any difference in the functions of the two divisions of the *lateral pterygoid muscle* had been overlooked. Without meticulous dissection from above, the two divisions appear to have nearly the same posterior attachment, and so were assumed to have similar functions. Since the inferior division is more readily accessible to palpation and to intra-oral EMG study, the superior division was neglected. Recent discriminating EMG studies have shown that in the Rhesus monkey,[31, 51] and in man,[44] the two divisions act reciprocally.

The upper division is unusual in three important ways:

1. It attaches to the disc, the movement of which is essential for normal TMJ function. Posteriorly, this division attaches to

the medial anterior margin of the disc and continues posteriorly to attach also to the superior margin of the pterygoid fovea.[42, 47, 49, 67] Thus, we must revise our thinking and apply what we have previously learned about the lateral pterygoid muscle to the inferior division only. The superior division has a newly recognized set of unique functions that are related specifically to disc position.

2. The force exerted by most other muscles in the body is antagonized either by gravity or by another muscle. The force exerted by this masticatory muscle is antagonized by the elastin in the superior stratum of the bilaminar zone located behind the disc in the mandibular fossa (Fig. 5.2). The central nervous system has no control of the counterforce exerted on the upper division of this muscle, and cannot turn it off as it can the muscular antagonists of other muscles. Essentially, the superior division of the lateral pterygoid works against a spring.

3. Recent EMG studies designed to distinguish between the two divisions showed that in the Rhesus monkey,[51] and in man,[44] the two heads act reciprocally. The superior division was found to be active when the mandible closed, but not while it opened.[44, 91] We ordinarily think of muscles as prime movers that contract to shorten the muscle against a load (shortening contraction). Instead, this muscle contracts to retard its extension (lengthening contraction), controlling the backward return of the disc to its rest position as the condyle also glides backward to the posterior slope of the articular eminence. This is a checkrein function similar to that of the paraspinal back muscles when one leans forward at the waist.

The two divisions of this important muscle were formerly assumed to act together.[69] In the older dental literature, the inferior division is the one meant when the lateral pterygoid muscle is referred to without specifying which division. The posterior portion of the inferior division alone attaches to the neck of the mandible, so that during mandibular opening, only this division helps to translate the condyle forward over the eminence. It also contributes significantly to lateral deviation of the mandible.

Condylar Displacement

Posterior superior displacement of the condyle in the fossa of the TMJ is being recognized as one of the abnormalities that may be associated with the MPD syndrome.[50] However, by relating radiographic findings to joint structure, Scheman[82] showed that it was hazardous to draw this conclusion from *conventional* TMJ radiographs; tomograms are more reliable. It is the eminence-condyle relationship, not the fossa-condyle relationship, that constitutes the functional TMJ, as described above.

Conventional radiographs are useful to identify arthritic changes.[47, 82] Special techniques that provide a better indication of displacement of the condyle posteriorly behind the articular disc[58, 63] are recommended when the initial diagnosis is in doubt, or when treatment results are unexpectedly poor.[58, 63] The transcranial lateral oblique view (modified Updegrave technique) and four functional views of the condyle at positions of jaws closed and in 3° of opening should reveal if the condyle is posteriorly displaced.[71]

Disc Displacement

The signs of clicking and locking of the TMJ have been attributed to disc displacement by many authors over the past 7 decades.[22] Not until the recent reports of arthrography did objective evidence substantiate the frequency and importance of disc dysfunction.[10, 97] Farrar and McCarty[22] estimated that 70% of patients with TMJ symptoms have some degree of disc displacement.

A number of authors have demonstrated a strong correlation between clicking and locking of the TMJ with characteristic changes in TMJ arthrograms.[10, 21, 50, 97] Essentially, they agree that clicking occurs when there is partial anterior displacement of the disc, which the condyle must override to reach its normal position for full mouth opening (Fig. 5.4). Blocking of mandibular opening is caused by displacement of the disc so far anteriorly that the condyle is unable to override the normally thick posterior portion of the disc (Fig. 5.2C); the condyle is locked behind the anteriorly dislocated disc (Fig. 5.5).

PART 1

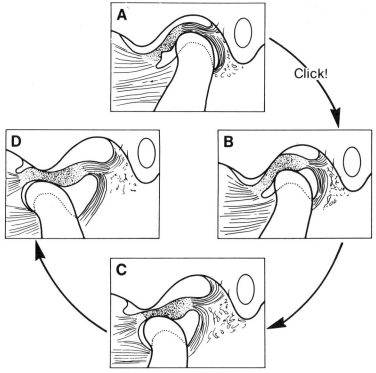

Click!

Figure 5.4. Mechanism of early *click* due to slight anterior displacement of the articular disc. *A*, rest position. *B*, as the condyle begins to translate forward, it must override a thickness of posterior disc material, causing a click. This seats the condyle in the central, thin part of the disc. *C* and *D*, after the click, mandibular opening and translation of the condyle proceed with apparently normal disc mechanics. (After D.D. Blaschke, reproduced with permission, from W.K. Solberg and G.T. Clark: *Temporomandibular Joint Problems: Biologic Diagnosis and Treatment*, Quintessence Publishing, Chicago, 1980, p. 75.[10])

RELATION TO MYOFASCIAL TRIGGER POINTS

The differences of opinion concerning TMJ dysfunction appear to us to result chiefly from differing points of view and overemphasis on only part of the total picture without full consideration of recent advances. Although the signs of TMJ dysfunction and the location of the pain both point to the TMJ as the source of trouble, in fact, such pain is very often referred to the joint from myofascial TPs, chiefly in the lateral pterygoid, sometimes in the medial pterygoid or masseter muscles. Inactivation of TPs in these muscles relieves the pain.

Recognition and treatment of the muscles that have developed TPs can give immediate, but temporary pain relief. Critical perpetuating factors requiring resolution may be single or multiple; they may be mechanical (e.g. malocclusion, a short leg), systemic medical (Chapter 4), or functional (psychological and behavioral). Any of these that are present, plus the myofascial TPs, must be dealt with for complete, lasting relief.

Frequently one stressful activity or event has activated the TPs, but some other factors are perpetuating and reactivating them. Since the initiating event, such as prolonged mouth opening during a dental procedure, is past, it is the major perpetuating factors that must be corrected to maintain improvement.

Clicking and popping of the TMJ during movement of the mandible is generally ascribed either to a displaced disc, or to distortion of the joint surfaces. Shortening of the superior division of the lateral pterygoid muscle due to TP activity would

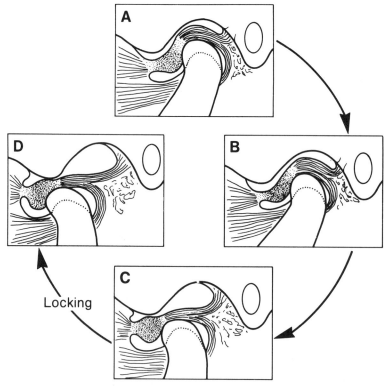

Figure 5.5.   Mechanism of blocking mandibular depression at one point due to marked anterior displacement of the articular disc. *A*, rest position. *B*, as the condyle translates forward, it impinges on the disc, but is unable to ride over it. *C* and *D*, this blocks full forward translation, and thereby, full jaw opening. (After D.D. Blaschke, reproduced with permission, from W.K. Solberg and G.T. Clark: *Temporomandibular Joint Problems: Biologic Diagnosis and Treatment*, Quintessence Publishing, Chicago, 1980, p. 77.[10])

displace the disc anteriorly, which is the displacement reported as responsible for clicking.[10, 50, 97] Distortion of the articular surfaces of the TMJ may be congenital, traumatic or arthritic.

The linkage between these signs of TMJ dysfunction and myofascial TP activity in the superior division of the lateral pterygoid muscle is not firmly established experimentally, but much evidence points to a close relationship. Both divisions of the lateral pterygoid muscle refer pain to the TMJ region. When the superior division develops TPs and shortens, it pulls the disc forward against the unremitting "spring" tension of the elastin. Relief of this referred myofascial pain then requires reduction of muscle tension by inactivating the upper division TPs, through elimination of perpetuating factors and by local treatment directed at that muscle.

Why is the inferior division of the lateral pterygoid muscle so frequently involved? Dawson[15] proposed that it is overworked in the presence of occlusal disharmony by the recurrent necessity to center the teeth against the forceful elevator muscles to correct the displaced bite. In addition, the two divisions of the lateral pterygoid muscle function as an alternating pair; the forcefulness of contraction by the inferior division may be modulated to help maintain the condylar contact in the thinnest part of the disc. In this case, anterior displacement of the disc by tension due to TPs in the superior division of the lateral pterygoid muscle also would tend to overload the inferior division.

A prosthesis that relieves the sensation of a premature contact without disturbing normal craniomandibular mechanics apparently relieves TP activity in both divisions of the lateral pterygoid muscle. This would explain why an occlusal prosthesis eases the pain of the MPD syndrome, but does not relieve the increased EMG activity of the masseter muscle.[39] The splint could reduce TP activity in either the upper or lower division of the lateral pterygoid, thus relieving the pain, while the EMG activity of the masseter could depend primarily on other TPs in the neck muscles.

It should be remembered that the deep layer of the masseter, the medial pterygoid, and the clavicular division of the sternocleidomastoid can *refer* pain to the TMJ region.

DIFFERENTIAL DIAGNOSIS OF CRANIOMANDIBULAR PAIN

The diagnoses to be considered in masticatory pain and dysfunction were recently reviewed clearly and concisely by Solberg.[86] The conditions to be distinguished from myofascial TP syndromes are discussed under Differential Diagnosis in Chapter 2. Muscular sources of craniomandibular pain are covered briefly here.

Muscular Pain and Tenderness

Bell[9] described three myogenous types of craniomandibular pain: local muscle soreness, muscle-splinting pain, and the myofascial pain syndrome. In addition, Solberg describes a form of myositis in one group of patients.[86] Diseases that cause muscle pain are considered in Chapter 2.

The transient, local muscle soreness of the arm, leg and back muscles that is observed the day after unusual exercise is well known and doubtless contributes, at times, to soreness found in the masticatory muscles. Some of the muscle tenderness associated with nocturnal bruxism and daytime clenching may be of this postexercise type. This muscular tenderness subsides spontaneously in a few days, unless reactivated by vigorous exercise.

Muscle-splinting pain is usually part of a complex process. Hemiplegic and brain-injured patients do identify pain that depends on muscle spasm. In these patients, examination shows that the muscle at rest is *strongly* and *persistently* contracted due to neurogenic motor unit activity. The in-creased muscle tension caused by the taut bands associated with myofascial TPs may feel like spasm, but generally, when the subject is relaxed, the resting muscle that harbors TPs shows no motor unit activity. A masticatory muscle, such as the masseter, may be hard and shortened because of tense myofascial TP bands. Its tenderness to palpation may arise from the sensitivity of its own TPs, and/or from tenderness referred by sternocleidomastoid or trapezius TPs. It may also exhibit a modest amount of motor unit activity referred from these distant TPs. A degree of protective masseteric spasm may develop to relieve strain on TPs in its parallel muscle, the temporalis. Recent EMG studies show a dissociation between the electrical activity in masticatory muscles and orofacial pain.[72] Occlusal adjustment relieved pain, but had no consistent effect on EMG activity of the masseter muscles.[3, 13] Seldom is sustained involuntary motor unit activity (spasm) alone responsible for craniomandibular pain, although it may contribute.

Myofascial TPs exhibit distinctive features of marked focal tenderness, palpable bands, characteristic referred pain patterns, other referred phenomena, and local twitch responses—features not found in other conditions, including muscle spasm *per se.*

Dental authorities[86] sometimes diagnose myositis when injection of a local anesthetic into a muscle with myofascial TPs augments, rather than relieves, pain and tenderness. In our experience, most of these patients have one or several perpetuating factors (Chapter 4) that are contributing to the muscular hyperirritability. In a few patients, no such cause can be found, yet they do respond to steroid that is given systemically by mouth, or that is injected with a local anesthetic; this response suggests the presence of an inflammatory component.

Medically, "myositis" denotes an inflammatory reaction of muscle. Adams[1] recognizes two general classes of myositis. In one, no specific causative agent can be found, but the lesion shows histopathologic changes characteristic of inflammation. In the other, a causative agent is identified. The first group includes polymyositis and dermatomyositis, and the second is characterized by infections and infestations. The muscles of the myofascial-pain patients who require anti-inflammatory therapy may have entered the dystrophic phase of the illness, as described in Chapter 2. Myositis should be the term used only if there is histologic evidence of inflammatory changes, not merely muscular hyperirritability; this conforms to the usage of Bell.[9]

References

1. Adams RD: *Diseases of Muscle: A Study in Pathology.* Ed. 3. Harper & Row, Hagerstown, Md. 1975 (pp. 316, 317).
2. Adisman IK, et al.: Glossary of prosthodontic terms. *J Prosthet Dent* 38:70–109, 1977 (p. 99).
3. Bailey JR, Rugh JD: Effect of occlusal adjustment on bruxism as monitored by nocturnal EMG recordings. *J Dent Res* 59, Special Issue A:317, 1980.
4. Barghi N, Rugh JD, Drago CJ: Experimentally induced occlusal disharmonies, nocturnal bruxism and MPD. *J Dent Res* 58, Special Issue A:317, 1979.
5. Basmajian JV: *Muscles Alive,* Ed. 4. Williams & Wilkins, Baltimore, 1978 (p. 385).
6. Bayer H: Die rheumatische Muskelhärte—ein Eigenreflextetanus. *Klin Wochenschr* 27:122–126, 1949.
7. Bell WE: Recent concepts in the management of temporomandibular joint dysfunctions. *J Oral Surg* 28:596–599, 1970.
8. Bell WE: Management of masticatory pain, Chapter 12. In *Facial Pain,* edited by C.C. Alling III and P.E. Mahan, Ed. 2. Lea & Febiger, Philadelphia, 1977 (p. 185).
9. Bell WE: *Orofacial Pains,* Ed. 2. Yearbook Medical Publishers, Chicago, 1979 (pp. 61–66, 100–105, 136, 137, 149–151, 180, 186–209, 260–269, 301–311).
10. Blaschke DD: Arthrography of the temporomandibular joint, Chapter 4. In *Temporomandibular Joint Problems: Biologic Diagnosis and Treatment,* edited by W.K. Solberg and G.T. Clark. Quintessence Publishing, 1980 (pp. 69–91).
11. Christensen LV: Some electromyographic parameters of experimental tooth clenching in adult human subjects. *J Oral Rehabil* 7:139–146, 1980.
12. Clark GT, Beemsterboer PL, Rugh JD: Nocturnal masseter muscle activity and the symptoms of masticatory dysfunction. *J Oral Rehabil* 8:279–286, 1981.
13. Clark GT, Beemsterboer PL, Solberg WK, et al.: Nocturnal electromyographic evaluation of myofascial pain dysfunction in patients undergoing occlusal splint therapy. *J Am Dent Assoc* 99:607–611, 1979.
14. Cohen SR: Follow-up evaluation of 105 patients with myofascial pain-dysfunction syndrome. *J Am Dent Assoc* 97:825–828, 1978.
15. Dawson PE: *Evaluation, Diagnosis, and Treatment of Occlusal Problems.* C.V. Mosby, Saint Louis, 1974 (pp. 18, 48–107).
16. DeSteno CV: The pathophysiology of TMJ Dysfunction and related pain, Chapter 1. In *Clinical Management of Head, Neck and TMJ Pain and Dysfunction,* edited by H. Gelb. W.B. Saunders, Philadelphia, 1977 (p. 15).
17. Dohrmann RJ, Laskin DM: An evaluation of electromyographic biofeedback in the treatment of myofascial pain-dysfunction syndrome. *J Am Dent Assoc* 96:656–662, 1978.
18. Domnitz JM, Swintak EF, Schriver WR, et al.: Myofascial pain syndrome masquerading as temporomandibular joint pain. *Oral Surg* 43:11–17, 1977.
19. Edmiston GF, Laskin DM: Changes in consistency of occlusal contact in myofascial pain-dysfunction (MPD) syndrome. *J Dent Res* 57:27–30, 1978.
20. Farrar WB: To the editor. *J Prosthet Dent* 43:473, 1980.
21. Farrar WB, McCarty WL, Jr.: Inferior joint space arthrography and characteristics of condylar paths in internal derangements of the TMJ. *J Prosthet Dent* 41:548–555, 1979.
22. Farrar WB, McCarty WL, Jr.: The TMJ Dilemma. *J Alabama Dent Assoc* 63:19–26, 1979.
23. Fine EW: Psychological factors associated with non-organic temporomandibular joint pain dysfunction syndrome. *Br Dent J* 131:402–404, 1971.
23a. Finlayson RS, Rugh JD, Dowlick MF: Electromyography of myofascial pain patients and controls in the natural environment. *J Dent Res* 61:277, 1982.
24. Garnick J, Ramfjord SP: Rest position: an electromyographic and clinical investigation. *J Prosthet Dent* 12:895–911, 1962.
25. Gelb H: Evaluation of static centric relation in temporomandibular joint dysfunction syndrome. *Dent Clin North Am* 19:519–530, 1975.
26. Gelb H: Patient evaluation, Chap. 3. In *Clinical Management of Head, Neck and TMJ Pain and Dysfunction,* edited by H. Gelb. W.B. Saunders, Philadelphia, 1977 (p. 75).
27. Gelb H, Tarte J: A two-year clinical dental evaluation of 200 cases of chronic headache: the craniocervical-mandibular syndrome. *J Am Dent Assoc* 91:1230–1236, 1975.
28. Glaros AG, Rae SM: Bruxism: A critical review. *Psychol Bull* 84:767–781, 1977.
29. Goharian RK, Neff PA: Effect of occlusal retainers on temporomandibular joint and facial pain. *J Prosthet Dent* 44:206–208, 1980.
30. Goodman P, Greene CS, Laskin DM: Response of patients with myofascial pain-dysfunction syndrome to mock equilibration. *J Am Dent Assoc* 92:755–758, 1976.
31. Grant PG: Lateral pterygoid: two muscles? *Am J Anat* 138:1–9, 1973.
32. Greene CS: Myofascial pain-dysfunction syndrome: nonsurgical treatment. In *The Temporomandibular Joint,* edited by B.G. Sarnat and D.M. Laskin. Charles C Thomas, Springfield, Ill. 1980.
33. Greene CS: Myofascial pain-dysfunction syndrome: the evolution of concepts, Chapter 13. In *The Temporomandibular Joint.* edited by B.G. Sarnat, and D.M. Laskin. Charles C Thomas, Springfield, Ill. 1980.
34. Griffin CJ, Munro KK: Electromyography of the masseter and anterior temporalis muscles in patients with temporomandibular dysfunction. *Arch Oral Biol* 16:929–949, 1971.

PART 1

35. Hansson T, Nilner M: A study of the occurrence of symptoms of diseases of the temporomandibular joint, masticatory musculature and related structures. *J Oral Rehabil* 2:313–324, 1975.

36. Hansson T, Solberg WK, Penn MK, *et al.*: Anatomic study of the TMJs of young adults. *J Prosthet Dent* 41:556–560, 1979.

37. Ingle JI: The great imposter. *JAMA* 236:1846, 1976.

38. Ingle JI, Beveridge EE: *Endodontics*, Ed. 2. Lea & Febiger, Philadelphia, 1976 (pp. 514–531).

39. Jankelson B: Neuromuscular aspects of occlusion. *Dent Clin North Am* 23:157–168, 1979.

40. Kotani H, Kawazoe Y, Hamada T, *et al.*: Quantitative electromyographic diagnosis of myofascial pain-dysfunction syndrome. *J Prosthet Dent* 43:450–456, 1980.

41. Kraft GH, Johnson EW, LeBan MM: The fibrositis syndrome. *Arch Phys Med Rehabil* 49:155–162, 1968.

42. Krough-Poulsen W: The significance of occlusion in temporomandibular function and dysfunction, Chapter 5. In *Temporomandibular Joint Problems: Biologic Diagnosis and Treatment*, edited by W.K. Solberg and G.T. Clark. Quintessence Publishing, Chicago, 1980 (pp. 98–103).

43. Laskin DM: Myofascial pain-dysfunction syndrome: etiology, Chapter 14. In *The Temporomandibular Joint*, edited by B.G. Sarnat and D.M. Laskin. Charles C Thomas, Springfield, 1980.

44. Lipke DP, Gay T, Gross RD, *et al.*: An electromyographic study of the human lateral pterygoid muscle, Abstract 713. *J Dent Res* 56, *Special Issue B*:B230, 1977.

45. Laskin DM: Etiology of the pain-dysfunction syndrome. *J Am Dent Assoc* 79:147–153, 1969.

46. Mahan PE: Anatomy of the stomatognathic system related to crown and fixed partial prosthodontic therapy, Chapter 15. In *Tylman's Theory and Practice of Fixed Prosthodontics*, edited by SD Tylman and W.F.P. Malone, Ed. 7. C.V. Mosby, Saint Louis, 1978 (pp. 382–390).

47. Mahan PE: The temporomandibular joint in function and pathofunction, Chapter 2. In *Temporomandibular Joint Problems: Biologic Diagnosis and Treatment*, edited by W.K. Solberg and G.T. Clark. Quintessence Publishing, Chicago, 1980 (pp. 33–47).

48. Mahan PE: The stomatognathic system, Chapter 32. In *Clinical Dentistry*, edited by J.W. Clark. Harper & Row, Hagerstown, Md., revised 1980.

49. Mahan PE: Personal communication, 1982.

50. McCarty W: Diagnosis and treatment of internal derangement of the articular disc and mandibular condyle, Chapter 8. In *Temporomandibular Joint Problems*, edited by W.K. Solberg, G.T. Clark. Quintessence Publishing, Chicago, 1980 (pp. 145–168).

51. McNamara JA, Jr.: The independent functions of the two heads of the lateral pterygoid muscle. *Am J Anat* 138:197–206, 1973.

52. McNeill C, Danzig WM, Farrar WB, *et al.*: Craniomandibular (TMJ) disorders—the state of the art. *J Prosthet Dent* 44:434–437, 1980.

53. Mercuri LG, Olson RE, Laskin DM: The specificity of response to experimental stress in patients with myofascial pain dysfunction syndrome. *J Dent Res* 58:1866–1871, 1979.

54. Meyerowitz WJ: Myo-fascial pain in the edentulous patient. *J Dent Assoc South Afr* 30:75–77, 1975.

55. Mikhail M, Rosen H: History and etiology of myofascial pain-dysfunction syndrome. *J Prosthet Dent* 44:438–444, 1980.

56. Møller E: The chewing apparatus: an electromyographic study of the action of the muscles of mastication and its correlation to facial morphology. *Acta Physiol Scand 69 (Suppl 280)*:1–229, 1966.

57. Moran JH, Kaye LB, Fritz ME: Statistical analysis of an urban population of 236 patients with head and neck pain: part III, treatment modalities. *J Periodontol* 50:66–74, 1979.

58. Morgan DH: Mandibular joint pathology: importance of radiographs. *Dent Radiogr Photogr* 43:3–11, 1970.

59. Morgan DH: Dysfunction, pain, tinnitus, vertigo corrected by mandibular joint surgery. *South Calif Dent Assoc J* 39:505–534, 1971.

60. Morgan DH: The great imposter: diseases of the mandibular joint. *JAMA* 235:2395, 1976.

61. Munro RR: Electromyography of muscles of mastication. In *The Temporomandibular Joint Syndrome*, edited by C.J. Griffin and R. Harris. S. Karger, Basel, 1975 (pp. 87–116).

62. Nel H: Myofascial pain-dysfunction syndrome. *J Prosthet Dent* 40:438–441, 1978.

63. Oberg T: Radiology of the temporomandibular joint, Chapter 3. In *Temporomandibular Joint Problems*, edited by W.K. Solberg and G.T. Clark. Quintessence Publishing, Chicago, 1980 (pp. 49–68).

64. Olson RE: Myofascial pain-dysfunction syndrome: psychological aspects, Chapter 15. In *The Temporomandibular Joint*, edited by B.G. Sarnat and D.M. Laskin. Charles C Thomas, Springfield, Ill., 1980.

65. Perry HT, Marsh EW: Functional considerations in early limited orthodontic procedures, Chapter 10. In *Clinical Management of Head, Neck and TMJ Pain and Dysfunction*, edited by H. Gelb. W.B. Saunders, Philadelphia, 1977 (pp. 264–265).

66. Pertes RA: The use of functional appliances in the prevention of the TMJ dysfunction syndrome. *Basal Facts* 3:165–183, 1979.

67. Porter MR: The attachment of the lateral pterygoid muscle to the meniscus. *J Prosthet Dent* 24:555–562, 1970.

68. Rees LA: The structure and function of the mandibular joint. *Br Dent J* 96:125–133, 1954.

69. Reuben B, Laskin DM: Electromyographic analysis of masticatory muscle activity in myofascial pain-dysfunction syndrome. *J Dent Res* 56B:232, 1977.

69a. Riggs RR, Rugh JD, Barghi N: Muscle activity of MPD and TMJ patients and non-patients. *J Dent Res* 61:277, 1982.

70. Robbins JW, Rugh JD: Medio-lateral positioning of the mandible: an electromyographic analysis. *J Dent Res* 60, *Special Issue A*:346, 1981.

71. Rosen LM, Morgan DH: Radiographic procedures, Chapter 7. In *Diseases of the Temporomandibular Apparatus: a Multidisciplinary Approach*, edited by D.H. Morgan, W.P. Hall and S.J. Vamvas. C.V. Mosby, Saint Louis, 1977 (pp. 105, 106).

72. Rugh JD: Psychological stress in orofacial neuro-muscular problems. *Int Dent J* 31:202–205, 1981.
73. Rugh JD, Johnson RW: The effects of head inclination on the relaxed mandibular vertical posture. *J Dent Res* 61:277, 1982.
74. Rugh JD, Drago CJ, Barghi N: Comparison of electromyographic and phonetic measurements of vertical rest position. *J Dent Res 58, Special Issue A*:316, 1979.
75. Rugh JD, Solberg WK: Electromyographic studies of bruxist behavior before and during treatment. *Calf Dent Assoc J* 3:56–59, 1975.
76. Schwartz L: Conclusions of the Temporomandibular Joint Clinic at Columbia. *J Periodontol* 29:210–212, 1958.
77. Schwartz LL: *Disorders of the Temporomandibular Joint.* W.B. Saunders, Philadelphia, 1959.
78. Schwartz LL, Tausig DP: Temporomandibular joint pain—treatment with intramuscular infiltration of tetracaine hydrochloride: a preliminary report. *NY State Dent J* 20:219–223, 1954.
79. Seltzer S: Oral conditions that cause head and neck pain, Chapter 8. In *Pain Control in Dentistry*, J.B. Lippincott, Philadelphia, 1978 (pp. 137–147).
80. Shaber EP: Considerations in the treatment of muscle spasm, Chapter 17. In *Diseases of the Temporomandibular Apparatus*, edited by D.H. Morgan, W.P. Hall, and S.J. Vamvas. C.V. Mosby, Saint Louis, 1977 (p. 235).
81. Sharav Y, Tzukert A, Refaeli B: Muscle pain index in relation to pain, dysfunction, and dizziness associated with the myofascial pain-dysfunction syndrome. *Oral Surg* 46:742–747, 1978.
82. Scheman P: Radiology and radiography of the temporomandibular articulation: Part I. In *Clinical Management of Head, Neck and TMJ Pain and Dysfunction*, edited by H. Gelb. W.B. Saunders, Philadelphia, 1977 (pp. 206–229).
83. Shore NA: *Temporomandibular Joint Dysfunction and Occlusal Equilibration.* Ed. 2, J.B. Lippincott, Philadelphia, 1976 (pp. 193–205, 237–249).
84. Simons DG: Unpublished data.
85. Solberg WK: The troubled temporomandibular joint: new opportunities and challenges in research and clinical management. *Oro Biol* 2:9–12, 1981.
86. Solberg WK: Neuromuscular problems in the orofacial region: diagnosis—classification, signs and symptoms. *Int Dent J* 31:206–215, 1981.
87. Solberg WK, Woo MW, Houston JB: Prevalence of mandibular dysfunction in young adults *J Am Dent Assoc* 98:25–34, 1979.
88. Tallgren A, Holden S, Lang BR, et al.: Jaw muscle activity in complete denture wearers—a longitudinal electromyographic study. *J Prosthet Dent* 44:123–132, 1980.
88a. Tanner HM: The Tanner mandibular appliance. In *Continuum '80 Journal of the L. D. Pankey Institute.* Science and Medicine Publishing Co., New York, 1979 (pp. 23–34).
89. Travell J: Temporomandibular joint pain referred from muscles of the head and neck. *J Prosthet Dent* 10:745–763, 1960.
90. Travell J, Berry C, Bigelow N: Effects of referred somatic pain on structures in the reference zone. *Fed Proc* 3:49, 1944.
91. Travell J, Rinzler SH: The myofascial genesis of pain. *Postgrad Med* 11:425–434, 1952.
92. Troendle R, Troendle K, Rugh JD: Electromyographic and phonetic rest position changes with head posture. *J Dent Res 59, Special Issue A*:494, 1980.
93. Vitti M, Basmajian JV: Integrated actions of masticatory muscles: simultaneous EMG from eight intramuscular electrodes. *Anat Rec* 187:173–189, 1977.
94. Weinberg LA: Treatment prostheses in TMJ dysfunction-pain syndrome. *J Prosthet Dent* 39:654–669, 1978.
95. Weinberg LA: The etiology, diagnosis, and treatment of TMJ dysfunction-pain syndrome. Part II: differential diagnosis. *J Prosthet Dent* 43:58–70, 1980.
96. Wessberg GA, Carroll WL, Dinham R, et al.: Transcutaneous electrical stimulation as an adjunct in the management of myofascial pain-dysfunction syndrome. *J Prosthet Dent* 45:307–314, 1981.
97. Wilkes CH: Arthrography of the temporomandibular joint. *Minn Med* 61:645–651, 1978.

CHAPTER 6
Trapezius Muscle
"The Coat Hanger"

HIGHLIGHTS: The trapezius is tripartite. The upper, middle and lower trapezius fibers can, and often do function independently. Therefore, in several sections of this chapter they are considered separately. **REFERRED PAIN** arises as often from trigger points (TPs) in the upper trapezius as in any muscle of the body. The TPs in the upper trapezius fibers characteristically refer pain along the posterolateral aspect of the neck, behind the ear and to the temple. The TPs in the lower trapezius refer pain mainly to the neck, suprascapular, and interscapular regions. The less common middle trapezius TPs project pain toward the vertebrae and to the interscapular region. **ANATOMICAL ATTACHMENTS** of the paired trapezii form a diamond shape that extends in the midline from the occiput to T_{12} and reaches laterally to the clavicle in front, to the acromion, and to the spine of the scapula behind. **INNERVATION** is provided by the spinal accessory, cranial nerve XI, which supplies mainly motor fibers, and by the second to fourth cervical spinal nerves, which supply mainly sensory fibers to the muscle. **ACTIONS** of the upper trapezius are chiefly elevation of the shoulders and rotation of the glenoid fossa so that the socket of the shoulder joint faces upward. The lower trapezius assists this rotation. The middle trapezius strongly retracts (adducts) the scapula. **SYMPTOMS** are primarily pain referred in characteristic patterns, with little weakness or limitation of motion. **ACTIVATION OF TRIGGER POINTS** in the upper trapezius depends in part on such skeletal variations as a short leg, a small hemipelvis, or short upper arms. Activation also results from the stress of sustained elevation of the shoulders, as when holding a telephone receiver without elbow support, or sitting in a chair with inadequate armrests. Acute trauma, as in a "whiplash" from the side, and chronic trauma, as in compression of the muscle by tight bra straps or a misfitting heavy coat, activate trapezius TPs. **PATIENT EXAMINATION** reveals that active rotation of the head and neck toward the opposite side is painful at nearly full range, and side bending is moderately restricted. **ASSOCIATED TRIGGER POINTS** are often found in the underlying supraspinatus and in the contralateral trapezius muscles. **STRETCH AND SPRAY** are done with the patient seated as the part of the muscle being sprayed is placed on passive stretch. The sweeps of spray are generally applied upward (cephalad) over the involved portion of the muscle, and are continued over the referred pain pattern. **INJECTION AND STRETCH** of the TPs so frequently seen in the upper trapezius are done from the front with the patient supine, whereas the other trapezius TPs are best approached from behind with the patient lying on the opposite side. Trapezius TPs usually respond well to local injection. **CORRECTIVE ACTIONS** for body asymmetry and short upper arms include compensating lifts or pads. Misfitting furniture should be modified or replaced. The muscle should be unloaded of unnecessary stress, and a passive-stretch exercise program instituted to reduce the activity of trapezius TPs.

1. REFERRED PAIN
(Figs. 6.1–6.4)

The authors have found that the trapezius is probably the muscle most often beset by myofascial trigger points (TPs), as have other clinicians.[17, 22, 35, 48, 65] It is a frequently overlooked source of temporal headache.[43] Six TPs with distinctive pain patterns are found in the upper, middle, and lower portions of the trapezius; two TPs are located in each portion. A seventh TP refers a non-painful autonomic response. The TPs are numbered in their approximate order of prevalence.

Trapezius TP_1 is observed the most often of all myofascial TPs in the body. It was clearly the most common in a survey of 200 healthy asymptomatic young adults.[48] This TP_1 area makes a significant contribution to the facial pain of the myofascial pain-dysfunction syndrome, which is widely recognized by the dental profession.[3, 11, 44, 64]

Upper Trapezius Fibers

TP_1 (Fig. 6.1). In our experience, TPs in this area consistently refer pain unilaterally upward along the posterolateral aspect of the neck to the mastoid process, and are a major source of "tension neckache" (Fig. 6.1).[28, 66] The referred pain, when intense, extends to the side of the head, centering in the temple and back of the orbit,[25, 67] and also may include the angle of the jaw.[32, 56, 57, 59, 61, 69] Occasionally, pain extends to the occiput, and

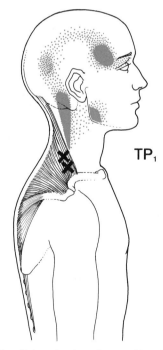

Figure 6.1. Referred pain pattern and location (✕s) of trigger point 1 in the upper trapezius muscle. Solid red shows the essential referred pain zone; stippling maps the spillover zone.

rarely, mild pain is referred to the lower molar teeth. Pain referred from TP_1 may appear in the pinna, but not deep inside the ear. Stimulation of this TP by needling and injection has initiated referred vasomotor effects in the homolateral and opposite ear.[56–58, 60]

Other authors describe a similar post-auricular pain pattern,[12, 23, 39] including one in children.[2] A shoulder component of the pain[13, 24] is to be expected when the underlying supraspinatus muscle also harbors active TPs.[26] Occasional reports[12, 18] associate TP activity of the upper trapezius fibers with symptoms of dizziness or "vertigo," and with dizziness experienced momentarily when the TP is penetrated by a needle during injection. This postural dizziness may be referred directly from the trapezius or, we think more likely, it may result from reflex stimulation of active TPs in the clavicular division of the synergistically related sternocleidomastoid muscle. A comparable secondary extension of referred pain is sometimes seen between related muscle groups in other parts of the body.

When patients had both neck and shoulder pain, Sola and Kuitert[47] found that levator scapulae and infraspinatus TPs were more frequently the cause than were trapezius TPs.

Experimental injection of the upper trapezius with hypertonic saline in 14 normal subjects induced pain at the base of the neck in all but one subject, projected pain to the same side of the face or head in 12 subjects, and decreased the skin temperature that overlapped the area of referred pain in 6 subjects.[50]

TP_2 (Fig. 6.2). The referred pain pattern of this TP lies slightly posterior to the essential cervical reference zone of TP_1, blending with its distribution behind the ear (Fig. 6.2). The location of TP_2 is caudal and posterior to the free border of the upper trapezius.

Lower Trapezius Fibers

TP_3 (Fig. 6.2). This lower trapezius TP refers pain severely to the high cervical region of the paraspinal muscles, to the adjacent mastoid area and to the acromion (Fig. 6.2).[57] It also refers an annoying deep ache and diffuse tenderness over the su-

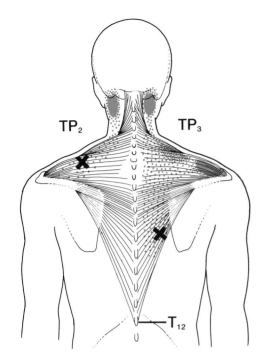

Figure 6.2. Referred pain patterns and locations (×s) of trigger point 2 in the left upper trapezius, and of trigger point 3 in the right lower trapezius. (Conventions are as in Figure 6.1).

prascapular region.[67] This tenderness is described by the patient as a "soreness," and the patient tends to rub the tender region. Such referred diffuse tenderness should not be mistaken for the focal tenderness of a TP. However, TP_1 and TP_2 do often develop as satellites within this zone of pain and tenderness referred from TP_3. These secondary TPs can be distinguished from simple referred tenderness by their palpable bands, local twitch responses, sharply localized spot tenderness, induction of referred pain, and by some restriction of neck rotation to the opposite side.

TP_4 (Fig. 6.3). This TP produces a steady burning pain referred downward along, and medial to, the vertebral border of the scapula.

Middle Trapezius Fibers

TP_5 (Fig. 6.3). From this TP, superficial burning pain is referred medially, between the TP and the spinous processes of the C_7 and T_1 vertebrae.

TP_6 (Fig. 6.4). A trapezius TP that is found near the acromion refers aching

pain to the top of the shoulder, or acromial process.

TP_7 (Fig. 6.4). A superficial TP located within the encircled area in Figure 6.4 can produce a disagreeable "shivery" sensation with pilomotor erection (gooseflesh) on the lateral aspect of the homolateral arm and sometimes also of the thigh, as a referred autonomic phenomenon. The referred activity may be induced merely by stroking the skin over the TP.

2. ANATOMICAL ATTACHMENTS
(Figs. 6.5 and 6.6)

When the right and left trapezius muscles are viewed together from the rear, they form a large diamond shape. Together, the fibers of both upper trapezii are shaped like a coat hanger.

Upper Fibers
(Figs. 6.5 and 6.6)

The upper fibers attach **above** to the medial third of the superior nuchal line. In the midline, they attach to the ligamentum nuchae and to the spinous processes of the

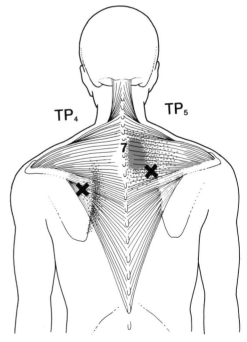

Figure 6.3. Referred pain patterns and locations (×s) of trigger point 4 in the left lower trapezius, and of trigger point 5 in the right middle trapezius. (Conventions are as in Figure 6.1).

PART 1

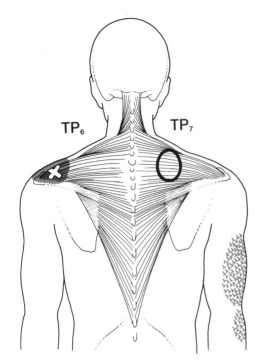

TP₆   TP₇

Figure 6.4. Referred pain pattern and location of trigger point 6 (×) in the left middle trapezius. (Conventions are as in Figure 6.1). Trigger point 7 on the right lies within the *encircled area* of the middle trapezius. The zone to which it refers pilomotor activity, or "gooseflesh," is identified on the right upper extremity by " > " symbols.

C_1 through C_5 vertebrae (Fig. 6.5). *Below* the fibers converge laterally and forward; they attach to the outer third of the clavicle (Fig. 6.6).

Middle Fibers
(Fig. 6.5)

These fibers attach *medially* to the spinous processes and interspinous ligaments of the C_6 through T_3 vertebrae, and *laterally* to the acromion and superior lip of the spine of the scapula (Fig. 6.5).

Lower Fibers
(Fig. 6.5)

These fibers attach *medially* to the spinous processes and interspinous ligaments of the T_4 through T_{12} vertebrae. *Laterally* they ascend and converge onto the tubercle at the medial end of the spine of the scapula just lateral to the lower attachment of the levator scapulae muscle (Fig. 6.5).

Supplemental References

Additional illustrations of this muscle show the back view,[8, 14, 16, 33, 41, 45, 49, 51] the side view,[15, 34, 46, 52] and the anomalous subtrapezius muscle.[8]

3. INNERVATION

Motor innervation of the trapezius is supplied by the spinal portion of the spinal accessory nerve (cranial nerve XI). The trapezius portion of the motor nerve arises within the spinal canal from ventral roots, usually of the first five cervical segments; it ascends through the foramen magnum and exits the skull *via* the jugular foramen to supply, and sometimes to penetrate, the sternocleidomastoid muscle. The nerve then joins a plexus beneath the trapezius.

The plexus is joined by primarily sensory fibers from spinal nerves C_2, C_3 and C_4; it supplies both the motor and sensory innervation to the trapezius muscle.[16, 27]

4. ACTIONS

Summarizing trapezius effects on scapular motions: elevation of the scapula activates the upper and middle trapezius fibers; retraction (adduction) activates all of its fibers; depression employs the lower fibers;[68] and rotation involves chiefly the upper and lower fibers.[42]

Entire Muscle

Acting unilaterally, the trapezius rotates the scapula to direct the glenoid fossa upward,[42] elevates and retracts the scapula, and extends the head and neck while rotating the chin to the opposite side.[7]

Acting bilaterally, the entire muscle assists extension of the cervical and thoracic spine.

Upper Trapezius

Acting unilaterally, this portion of the muscle elevates the shoulder, bends the neck and head laterally toward the same side, and aids in extreme rotation of the head to the opposite side.[1, 7] It usually helps (but can be trained not) to carry the weight of the upper extremity during standing, or to support a weight in the hand with the arm hanging.[1] In conjunction with the levator scapulae and upper

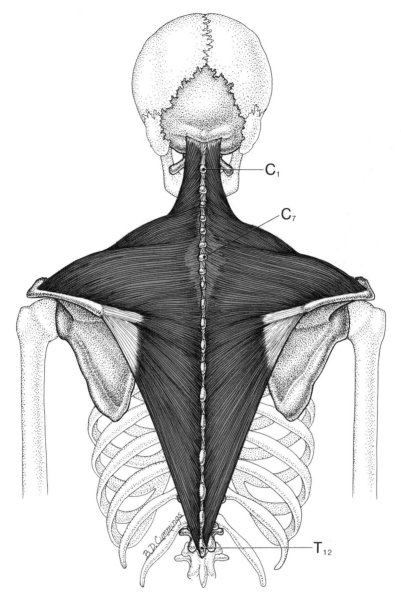

Figure 6.5. Attachments of the right and left trapezius muscles, rear view.

digitations of the serratus anterior, the upper trapezius provides the upper component of the force couple necessary to rotate the scapula, glenoid fossa upward.[1, 20, 42]

Acting bilaterally, the upper fibers may extend the head and neck, but only against resistance.[42, 68] An accessory respiratory function[7] is seriously questioned.[1, 27]

Middle Trapezius

The middle fibers adduct and therefore retract the scapula (i.e., move it toward the midline).[7, 42] They also assist flexion and abduction of the arm at the shoulder, especially near its full range,[42] by helping to rotate the scapula so as to tilt the glenoid fossa upward.[7]

Lower Trapezius

The lower fibers retract the scapula and rotate the glenoid fossa upward by depressing the vertebral border of the scapula; these fibers also assist flexion and abduction of the arm.[1, 42]

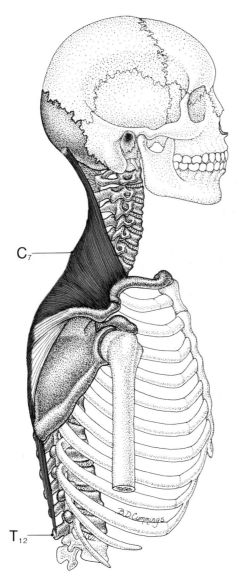

C_7

T_{12}

B.D.Cummings

Figure 6.6. Attachments of the right trapezius muscle, side view.

Typewriting. Lundervold[29-31] studied conditions that increased the electromyographic activity (and therefore the likelihood of activating TPs) in the upper trapezius muscle which he monitored with surface electrodes while his subjects were typewriting. Muscular activity increased markedly when the subject sat in a tense upright posture instead of a relaxed, well-balanced position;[30, 31] sat without a firm back support;[31] typed with the keyboard elevated;[29, 30] was tired;[29] or was untrained.[31] An increased rate of striking one

key increased sharply the amplitude and duration of the bursts of trapezius activity and decreased the silent period between bursts.[31]

Sports. Electromyographic monitoring of the upper, middle, and lower trapezius fibers with surface electrodes was performed during 13 sports activities, including right-handed overhand throws, underhand throws, tennis, golf, and 1-foot jumps in basketball. All records showed the motor unit activity on the left side to be equal to, or greater than, that on the right side, predominantly in the middle and lower trapezius fibers.[4] The recording of the basketball throw showed this effect most strongly. The timing of the response suggested that this strong burst of left-sided activity of the middle trapezius helped to extend rapidly the left upper extremity to balance rotational movement around the long axis of the body, as the right upper extremity approached the end of its forward power stroke.[4]

Driving. While driving an automobile simulator, the upper trapezius contracted only weakly, but more actively than the middle and lower portions of the muscle.[21]

5. MYOTATIC UNIT

The paired trapezius muscles are synergistic for extension of the head, neck, or thoracic spine, and during symmetrical upper extremity activities.

Upper Trapezius

This part of the muscle acts synergistically with the sternocleidomastoid for some head and neck motions. It is an antagonist to the levator scapulae and to the upper digitations of the serratus anterior during scapular rotation. During abduction of the arm, the rotation of the scapula by the trapezius is synergistic with the glenohumeral movement by the supraspinatus and deltoid muscles to produce the "scapulohumeral rhythm."[1, 5]

Middle Trapezius

These nearly horizontal fibers act synergistically with the rhomboid muscles to retract the scapula. By fixing the scapula, they also assist the deltoid, supraspinatus and long head of the biceps brachii in flexion of the arm at the shoulder. These trapezius fibers are antagonists to all but the most caudally directed fibers of the pectoralis major muscle.

Lower Trapezius

These more vertically directed fibers act with the lower part of the serratus anterior to rotate the glenoid fossa of the scapula upward. This function is synergistic with the abductors of the arm, the supraspinatus and deltoid muscles.

6. SYMPTOMS

Upper Trapezius

TP_1. When TP_1 is active, the patient usually has severe posterolateral neck pain, often constant and usually associated with temporal headache on the same side (Fig. 6.1). Occasionally, pain is projected to the angle of the jaw. The patient is likely to be misdiagnosed as having cervical radiculopathy, or atypical facial neuralgia.

TP_2. TP_2 causes similar neck pain, but without headache.

Pain on motion, due to the upper trapezius TPs alone, occurs only when the head and neck are almost fully rotated actively to the opposite side,[56] which contracts the muscle in the fully shortened position. With very active upper trapezius TPs, and with *additional* involvement of the levator scapulae or splenius cervicis muscles, the patient may develop an acute "stiff neck".[37, 53, 55] This also limits rotation of the head toward the same side, which stretches the upper trapezius.

Activity of TP_1 and TP_2 may cause intolerance to the weight of heavy clothing, such as a misfitting heavy overcoat which presses on the trapezius at the angle and back of the neck (coat-hanger muscle), instead of on the acromial processes.

Middle Trapezius

TP_5. TP_5 causes the patient to complain of burning interscapular pain (Fig. 6.3).

TP_6. TP_6 projects referred pain and tenderness over the acromion (Fig. 6.4), making the shoulder intolerant of pressure from a well fitted heavy coat, or from a ponderous purse[9] carried on a shoulder strap.

TP_7. TP_7 may be associated with spontaneous episodes of a "queer shivery feeling" with pilomotor erection (gooseflesh) on the anterolateral surfaces of the homolateral arm, and sometimes of the thigh (Fig. 6.4). The feeling produced by this referred autonomic response is described as "like shivers running up and down the spine" when chalk or a fingernail scrapes a blackboard.

Lower Trapezius

TP_3 and TP_4. TP_3 and TP_4 cause suprascapular, interscapular, acromial, and/or neck pain with little, if any, restriction of neck motion (Figs. 6.2 and 6.3). TP_3 is often the "joker" responsible for persistent upper back and neck pain after the active TPs in the upper trapezius and other shoulder and neck muscles have been eliminated.

7. ACTIVATION OF TRIGGER POINTS

In any part of the trapezius, TPs may be activated by sudden trauma, such as falling off a horse, falling down steps, or suffering a "whiplash" in an auto accident.[28]

Upper Trapezius

Its function of neck stabilization is commonly overloaded by tilting of the shoulder-girdle axis due to a short leg or small hemipelvis (body asymmetry). The short leg tilts the pelvis laterally, which bows the spine into a functional scoliotic curve and, in turn, tilts the shoulders, causing one to sag. The upper trapezius must work constantly to keep the head and neck vertical and the eyes level. A cane 12–15 cm (5 or 6 in) too long tilts the axis of the shoulder girdle and causes a similar trapezius problem by forcing the shoulder up on the side of the cane. A cane is properly fitted if, with the shoulders level, the elbow bends 30–40° with the cane held beside the foot.[19]

The normally minimal antigravity function of the upper trapezius is overstressed by any position or activity in which the trapezius helps to carry the weight of the arm for a prolonged period: telephoning or sitting without armrest support, particularly when the upper arms are congenitally short; holding the forearms up to reach a high typewriter keyboard or drawing board[30]; or sewing on the lap with the elbows unsupported.

The muscle may be strained by obvious acute gross trauma but, more often, it is strained by chronic injury due to overload that is obscure. Such microtrauma can be caused by clothing and accessories, as by pressure from tight narrow bra straps supporting large breasts, by the shoulder strap of a ponderous purse[9] or backpack, or by a heavy coat. It also may be caused by a sustained load in habitual elevation of the shoulders, as an expression of anxiety or other emotional distress, during long telephone calls, playing the violin, or by rotation of the head *far* to one side in a fixed position (holding the head turned to converse with a person seated at the side, or sleeping prone with the head fully rotated).

Other factors may activate upper trapezius TPs. Armrests that are too *high* push the scapulae up and shorten the upper trapezius for long periods. The muscle's accessory function of head rotation can be overstressed by the quick repetitive movement of flicking long hair out of the eyes.

Upper trapezius TPs may be activated by, and remain as sequelae to, cervical radiculopathy.[28]

Middle Trapezius

This part of the muscle also becomes overloaded when the arm is held up and forward for a long time. Sustaining this position also overloads the pectoralis major fibers, many of which develop latent (painless) TP activity that increases their tension, pulling the scapula forward. Then, the antagonistic middle trapezius fibers are overloaded in attempting to counteract this unrelenting protraction of the scapulae ("round-shouldered"). The middle trapezius fibers then develop active TPs that cause pain.

These middle trapezius fibers are subject to strain when the driver of a car holds the hands on top of the steering wheel, again, in a round-shouldered position.

Lower Trapezius

The lower fibers are strained by prolonged bending and reaching forward while sitting (to reach the desk when the knees lack space under its surface) and by supporting the chin on the hand, while resting the elbow on the front of the chest because armrests are missing.[54]

8. PATIENT EXAMINATION

The TPs in the upper and lower fibers of the trapezius can restrict arm abduction at its full range by limiting rotation of the scapula.

Upper Fibers

The patient with an active TP_1 or TP_2 in the upper trapezius, especially the person who has short upper arms or who sits without an armrest, tends to fold the arms across the chest and to cradle the chin in one hand. This patient may be seen to rub the trapezius muscle and to keep moving the head as if trying to stretch the muscle. He or she is likely to assume a habitual posture of bilateral shoulder elevation with a slight tilt of the neck toward the more affected side.

When the trapezius alone is involved, there is minimal limitation of head and neck rotation. The most restricted movement is lateral flexion of the head and neck (side bending) away from the involved upper trapezius. Side bending may be reduced to 45°, or less. Neck flexion is only slightly restricted, as is arm abduction due to the restricted upward rotation of the scapula. Active rotation of the head to the *opposite* side is usually painful at the extreme range of motion, since the muscle contracts strongly in this shortened position. Active rotation to the *same* side is usually pain free, unless either the levator scapulae on the same side, or the opposite upper trapezius, also harbor TPs.

If active TPs also are present in the levator scapulae muscle, head and neck rotation to the painful side is markedly restricted, so that the patient tends to hold the neck stiff and turns the body.

Middle Fibers

The patient tends to become round-shouldered when TPs have developed in the middle trapezius, often secondary to shortening of the antagonistic pectoral muscles caused by their active or latent TPs. The pectoral muscles exhaust the weaker middle trapezius fibers in their futile effort to retract the scapulae to a normal posture.

When the skin overlying an active TP_7 (Fig. 6.4) is lightly stroked, a visible wave of pilomotor activity (gooseflesh), which is an autonomic response, may be seen to spread homolaterally, down the arm and sometimes over the outer aspect of the thigh. The patient is aware of a queer, creeping sensation in the skin.

Lower Fibers

Active TPs in these lower fibers may restrict the last 5 or 10° of cervical and thoracic flexion, and of arm abduction.

9. TRIGGER POINT EXAMINATION
(Fig. 6.7)

Upper Fibers

TP_1. With the patient supine, or possibly seated, the muscle is placed on moderate slack by bringing the ear slightly toward the shoulder on the same side (Fig. 6.7A).

In a pincer grasp, the entire mass of the free margin of the upper trapezius is lifted off the underlying supraspinatus muscle and apex of the lung. Then the muscle is firmly rolled between the fingers and thumb to palpate firm bands and elicit local twitch responses of the bands and to locate the spot tenderness of TP_1. This manual technique has been illustrated previously.[36, 56, 57] Sustained compression of the TP often evokes pain referred to the neck, occiput, and temple, as also observed by Patton and Williamson.[40]

On the other hand, the pain caused by loading the muscle (abducting the arm above 90°) is prevented by firm pressure on the muscle with the palm of the hand during abduction.[24] Some of this pain also may be due to TPs in the underlying supraspinatus muscle, which more directly contributes the power to abduct the arm.

TP_2. This TP may be identified by a similar pincer technique in deeper fibers posterior to TP_1, if the patient has mobile connective tissue. Patients with firmer tissue require flat palpation. TP_2 is located

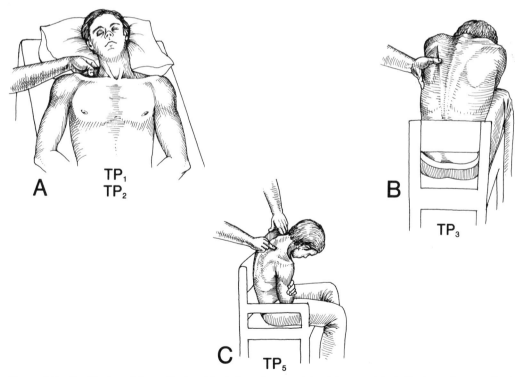

Figure 6.7.   Positioning of the patient and technique for examining trigger points in the trapezius muscle: *A*, trigger point 1 and trigger point 2 in the right upper trapezius, patient supine. *B*, trigger point 3 in the left lower trapezius, patient seated. *C*, trigger point 5 in the right middle trapezius, patient seated.

just superior to the scapula, at about its midline.[28] Webber[63] illustrated the location of TP₂ by "X-2" in Figure 28 of his paper.

Middle and Lower Fibers

To examine the remaining trapezius TPs, the patient sits with the arms folded across the front of the body to protract the scapulae, as in Figure 6.7B and C, and "humps the back" to flex the dorsal spine. Cross-fiber palpation identifies taut bands in the muscle by rolling them against the underlying ribs. The firm bands usually exhibit visible local twitch responses to snapping palpation.

TP₃. This TP lies in the lateral margin (lowest fibers) of the lower trapezius close to where the fibers cross the medial border of the scapula, or sometimes at or below the level of the inferior angle of the scapula (Fig. 6.7B). TP₃ feels like a button or nodule, and is easily missed if the fibers are not placed on a stretch by rotating the scapula upward and forward, as shown.

TP₄. TP₄ is found high in the lower trapezius, over the medial end of the infraspinatus muscle (Fig. 6.3), and is palpated just below the spine of the scapula with the patient positioned as in Figure 6.7C.

TP₅. This TP is located by flat palpation in the superficial, horizontal fibers of the middle trapezius, about 1 cm (1/2 in) medial to the scapular attachment of the levator scapulae (Figs. 6.3 and 6.7C).

TP₆. Finding this less common TP requires flat palpation of the lateral fibers of the middle trapezius over the lateral end of the supraspinatus muscle near the acromion (Fig. 6.4).

TP₇. This infrequent TP lies in the most superficial fibers of the middle trapezius where the fibers cross the levator scapulae muscle (Fig. 6.4). This TP may be stimulated by pinching it through the skin, or it may be stimulated directly by penetrating it with a needle.

Other Trigger Points

When patients have pain and deep tenderness referred to the suprascapular region, but do not have active trapezius TPs, the responsible TPs are likely to be found in the levator scapulae or scalene muscles.

10. ENTRAPMENTS

The greater occipital nerve emerges just below the occiput through the trapezius and underlying semispinalis capitis muscle. The nerve can be entrapped as it emerges through the semispinalis capitis when that muscle becomes taut due to more caudal TPs at the mid-cervical level (see Section 10 of Chapter 16). The trapezius itself has not been found to entrap the nerve, but may contribute a shearing stress.

When the spinal accessory nerve emerges through the sternocleidomastoid muscle, the trapezius muscle may be weakened by entrapment of its motor nerve between taut bands of sternocleidomastoid fibers.[38]

11. ASSOCIATED TRIGGER POINTS

Associated TPs for the upper trapezius are likely to develop in the myotatically related levator scapulae and contralateral trapezius muscles, and also in the homolateral supraspinatus and rhomboid muscles. When the middle trapezius is involved, the pectoral muscles and the paraspinal group in the region of the T₁–T₆ vertebrae commonly contain secondary TPs.

Satellite TPs may appear in the temporalis and occipitalis muscles, which lie within the zones of pain referred from TPs in the upper trapezius. Similarly, satellite TPs often arise in the upper trapezius secondary to TPs in the lower trapezius muscle.

12. STRETCH AND SPRAY
(Fig. 6.8)

Upper Fibers
(Fig. 6.8, TP₁ and TP₂)

TP₁. The patient sits in an armchair and leans back comfortably, with the fingers hooked under the chair seat on each side. This lengthens the trapezius and stabilizes the shoulders. To stretch the fibers containing TP₁, the operator side bends the patient's head toward the opposite side (ear-to-shoulder). For maximum stretch

PART 1

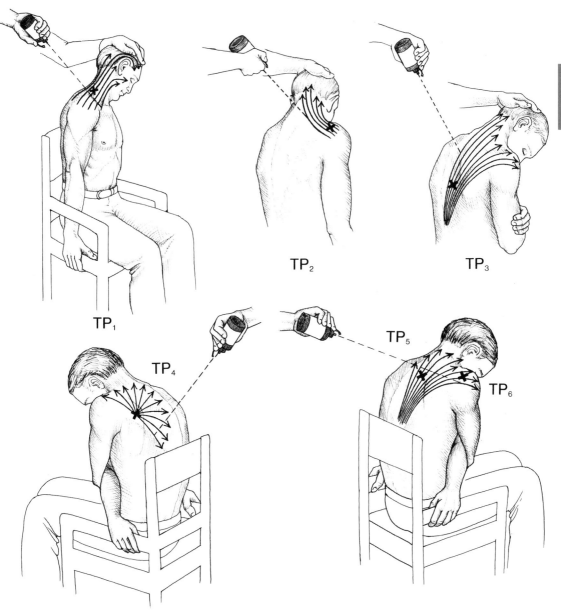

Figure 6.8.   Trapezius stretch positions and spray patterns: for trigger point 1 in the right upper trapezius; for trigger point 2 also in the right upper fibers; for trigger point 3 in the right, and trigger point 4 in the left lower fibers; for trigger point 5 and trigger point 6 in the right middle fibers. If trigger point 7 is active, proceed as for trigger point 6, but extend the spray pattern down the arm to the elbow to cover the zone of "gooseflesh" (referred autonomic effect). Location of trigger points is shown by ×s.

the head is pressed forward to raise the occiput (Fig. 6.8). At the same time, the operator applies the vapocoolant spray in parallel sweeps from the acromion to the mastoid area, behind the ear, around to the temple, and sometimes to the jaw—if that area is included in the patient's pattern of referred pain. Others also have found stretch and spray effective for this muscle.[10, 63, 69]

TP_2. The spray pattern for TP_2 (Fig. 6.8) likewise starts over the TP and extends up the neck over the referred pain pattern. The muscle is stretched by exerting pressure against the head in a slightly more forward direction than for TP_1.

Stretch and spray should always be applied to the contralateral trapezius to prevent activation of any TPs in it due to unaccustomed shortening when the opposite muscle is stretched to its maximum normal length.

The patient should have good elbow support during the rest periods between vapocooling and during hot pack applications; the armrests of the chair should carry the weight of the patient's arm (see Figure 6.10A and D).

Middle Fibers
(Fig. 6.8, TP_5 and TP_6)

To stretch the fibers afflicted with TP_5 or TP_6 (Fig. 6.8), the patient sits with arms folded in front of the body or, for greater stretch, crossed to reach the opposite armrest of the chair. The patient "humps" the back, while taking and holding a deep breath. The operator pushes the shoulder forward to forcefully protract the scapula. Some patients relax better if, instead of crossing their arms, they lean forward and let them drop between the knees. As the spray is applied, the patient is reminded to be "limp" and to "let the head and shoulders hang loosely," to insure complete voluntary relaxation.

The spray is applied over the muscle fibers in an upward direction for TP_5 (Fig. 6.8). For TP_6, the spray follows the direction of the fibers laterally, covering the acromion. Sweeps of the spray should include the referred pain patterns of both TP_5 and TP_6.

For TP_7, the spray is applied as for TP_6, continuing the sweeps down over the lateral aspect of the arm to cover the major "gooseflesh" reference zone.

Lower Fibers
(Fig. 6.8, TP_3 and TP_4)

The patient sits in the armchair, leaning forward with the arms drawn across the body to the opposite arm or armrest in order to separate and protract the scapulae. As the patient "humps" the back (flexes the thoracic spine) and takes a deep breath, the operator presses against the head and, also, against the shoulder, to assist vertebral flexion and scapular protraction within the tolerated limits of pain.

Just before and during this stretch for TP_3 (Fig. 6.8), the spray is applied upward from the T_{12} vertebral attachment of the trapezius, following its fiber direction and fanning out and upward to cover its pain reference zone from the acromion to the occiput.

For TP_4 (Fig. 6.8), the spray is swept fanwise from the vertebral border of the scapula over the infraspinatus region to the acromion, including all of the pain reference zone.

Stretch and spray are applied to the opposite trapezius, which must adjust to the full stretch of its mate, and then also to the antagonist pectoral muscles, which are often involved.

Each stretch and spray is followed promptly by a hot pack to the treated region.

TPs in the lower trapezius fibers respond well to vigorous deep massage and to ischemic compression, which the patient may apply by lying on a tennis ball that is positioned to press on the tender spots.

13. INJECTION AND STRETCH
(Fig. 6.9)

The fibers of the upper trapezius are injected for TPs only if characteristic bands can be palpated and if TP spot tenderness with local twitch responses of the bands can be elicited. Reproduction of the patient's pain by digital compression of the TP accurately localizes at least one source of the symptoms.

Injection is always followed at once by passive stretching, usually during application of vapocoolant, followed by a hot pack.

TP_1, and sometimes TP_2, of the upper trapezius are injected with 0.5% procaine solution from an anterior approach with the patient supine.[57, 59] All other trapezius TPs are injected with the patient lying on the opposite side, with the back toward the operator. Good[13] also found procaine injections in this muscle effective.

To relieve neck and back pain, Trommer and Gellman[62] infiltrated with procaine what they construed to be 15 intracutaneous TPs overlying the upper trapezius. Occasionally, one sees cutaneous TPs that

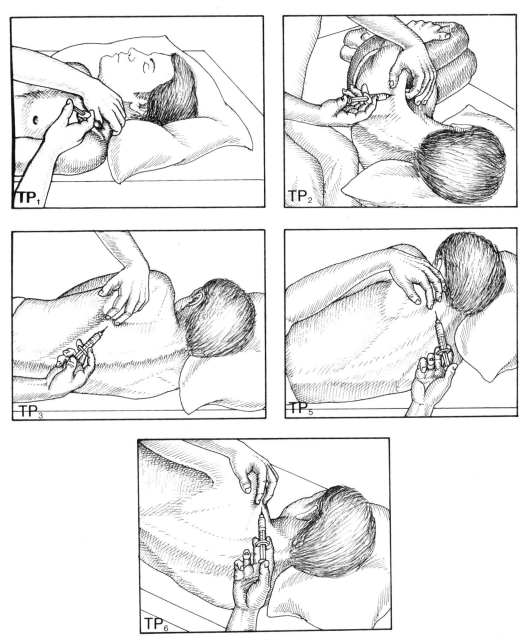

Figure 6.9. Patient position and injection technique for trigger points in the left trapezius muscle. *Trigger point 1*, the patient lies supine for the anterior approach to the upper trapezius, to avoid penetrating the apex of the lung. *Trigger point 2*, the patient lies on the right side for the posterior approach to the left upper trapezius, with the muscle lifted off the apex of the lung. *Trigger point 3*, in the lateral border of the lower trapezius, with the patient lying on the opposite side. The needle is aimed at a rib, to avoid penetrating an intercostal space. *Trigger point 5*, in the middle trapezius close to the medial end of the muscle fibers, with the patient lying on the opposite side. *Trigger point 6*, in the middle trapezius close to the lateral end of its muscle fibers, with the patient lying on the other side.

refer pain like muscular TPs. It also is possible that they relieved the pain by infiltrating the area of referred pain and referred tenderness as described by Weiss and Davis, and by Theobald (References 90 and 82, respectively, under **Somatovisceral Effects**, in Section 6 of Chapter 49). As noted above, pain and tenderness are often referred to this area from TPs in the lower trapezius. In this case, the patient is more likely to experience lasting relief if the active TPs in the lower trapezius that are causing the referred pain are injected, rather than the skin over the upper trapezius where the pain is felt.

Upper Trapezius
(Fig. 6.9, TP_1 and TP_2)

For injection of TP_1, the patient lies supine with the shoulder on the pillow to slacken that part of the muscle (Fig. 6.9). The muscle is held firmly in a pincer grasp to precisely locate the TPs for injection and to lift the muscle off underlying structures. The needle tip is directed upward and remains within the muscle mass that is held between the digits to avoid any possibility of penetrating the apex of the lung.

Except in thin patients, TP_2 is best approached by positioning the patient on the opposite side (Fig. 6.9); the needle is again directed upward away from the lung. To avoid penetrating too deeply when injecting TP_2 in patients with loose skin, the operator's finger can be inserted under the front margin beneath the muscle, between the TP and the chest.

A supraspinatus TP often lies underneath the upper trapezius TP_2, and if it also is penetrated by the needle, the patient may report referred pain felt in the mid-deltoid region.

Middle Trapezius
(Fig. 6.9, TP_5 and TP_6)

The patient lies on the opposite side with the hand placed on the thigh, or between the knees, to stabilize the scapula. TP_5 and TP_6 are quite superficial, so the needle is angled nearly tangent to the skin (Fig. 6.9). Otherwise, these TPs may be missed and underlying structures, even the lung, may be penetrated. Injection of the superficial TP_7 may set off waves of "gooseflesh."

Lower Trapezius
(Fig. 6.9, TP_3)

The patient lies on the opposite side. To locate and inject TP_3, the arm and scapula are swung forward and upward to place the lower trapezius on a moderate stretch

(Fig. 6.9). Care is taken to aim the needle toward an underlying rib, avoiding the intercostal space.

TP_4 overlies the scapula. The scapula is elevated and abducted to stretch the muscle for localization of the TP. To inject this TP, the needle is aligned with the lateral fibers of the muscle and directed toward the shoulder.

14. CORRECTIVE ACTIONS
(Figs. 6.10 and 6.11)

Upper Trapezius

Body Structure. A short leg or small hemipelvis, as described in Section 7 above, must be corrected (see Fig. 48.8C and Fig. 48.9C and D in Chapter 48).

When the patient's upper arms are short in relation to torso height, they do not reach the armrests of most chairs (Fig. 6.10C); this imposes sustained gravity stress on the trapezius muscles. The Boston rocker has high armrests designed for nursing mothers, and is well suited to persons with short upper arms. Fig. 6.10D illustrates another solution. An average armrest height of 21.6 cm (8½ in), measured from the compressed seat, satisfies most people.[6] Pads made from cellulose kitchen sponges or plastic foam may be covered and attached to the armrests, or may be mounted underneath a writing board, which rests on the armrests and raises the board to the desired height for elbow support.

Postural and Activity Stress. No patient with TPs in the upper trapezius should sleep on a foam rubber pillow; its springiness causes vibration that aggravates TP symptoms. When traveling, the patient may take along the nonfoam comfortable pillow from home to avoid this hazard.

Antigravity stress on the upper trapezius in normally proportioned individuals is corrected by selecting chairs with armrests of the correct height to provide elbow support (Fig. 6.10A), or by building up the height of the armrests, if they were designed too low (Fig. 6.10D).[54] Dentists, secretaries, draftsmen, writers and seamstresses, for instance, should arrange their seating to provide suitable elbow support. Every seated person benefits by learning

PART 1

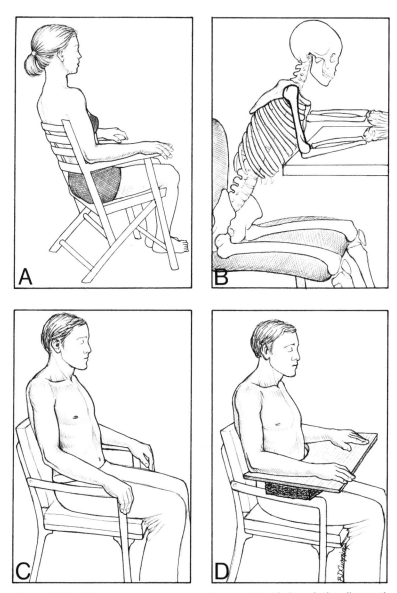

Figure 6.10.   Short upper arms: the problem and its solution. *A*, the elbows of a person with average length of the upper arms are well supported in a properly designed chair; the armrest surface is about 23 cm (9 inches) above the seat bottom. The backrest overlaps the scapulae by several centimeters (an inch or two). *B*, skeleton with short upper arms demonstrates the strained posture that results from that structural inadequacy. *C*, the elbows of the patient with short upper arms are unsupported in another chair similar to that in A. The dangling elbows overload the upper trapezius muscles. *D*, the needed elbow support is obtained by raising the armrest height with cellulose sponges, or plastic foam pads, glued beneath a writing board.

to distinguish between chairs that fit and chairs that enforce poor posture and that abuse the muscles.[54]

Patients who are preoccupied with what they are doing and lose track of time tend to maintain an undesirable posture, such as leaning forward over a desk for a prolonged period while writing. They can relieve muscle tension every 20 or 30 min, without interrupting the train of thought, by setting an interval-timer for that length of time and placing it across the room. Then they must get up, stretch and walk to turn off the buzzer and reset the timer.

For secretaries, a common source of gravity stress is a typewriter keyboard set so high that they hold the shoulders in an elevated position for the fingers to reach the keyboard conveniently. Excessive sustained electromyographic activity of the upper trapezius is eliminated by lowering the typewriter.[29] If the typing table cannot be lowered sufficiently, the height of the seat should be raised until the forearms are horizontal and the trapezius muscles relaxed. Several centimeters (an inch or more) of folded newspapers or a magazine may be placed on the rear two-thirds of the seat bottom; the front third of the seat is not raised, thus avoiding under-thigh compression. This slopes the seat forward and has the advantage of opening the angle at the hips and knees. If this raises the seat so much that the feet no longer rest flat on the floor, a small footrest is required. Typewriter copy should be placed behind the typewriter on a stand sold for this purpose, or on a music stand, directly in front of the typist and behind the typewriter, not at the side. With video terminals, the copy should be placed either above, beneath, or close beside the screen.

For patients who have long conversations on the telephone, an executive (speaker) phone relieves the neck and arm muscles of the strain of holding a handset.

The rotational stress of flicking long hair out of the eyes is readily solved by bobby pins or a haircut.

When conversing, the patient should turn his or her chair to face the visitor, or move the visitor's chair in front of the desk.

When sleeping prone with the head turned to one side, the patient should place a small pillow under the side of the head posteriorly to reduce head and neck rotation. Another pillow placed under the shoulder and chest on the same side as the face further reduces rotation of the neck. A semiprone position, achieved by flexing the knee and hip of the side toward which the face is turned, also helps by partly rotating the torso.

A cane, when positioned beside the leg, should be long enough so that the elbow is bent 30–40°,[19] and does not require fixed elevation of the shoulder and scapula when used.

Constriction. Objectionable pressure on the trapezius by a thin, tight bra strap should be relieved by wearing a wider, nonelastic bra strap, by slipping a plastic shield under the strap to distribute the pressure, or by sliding the strap laterally to rest on the acromion, off the muscle. A strapless bra that constricts too tightly around the ribs may cause comparable pressure activation of TPs in the latissimus dorsi, serratus anterior, or serratus posterior inferior muscles.

A shoulder-strap purse should be slung over the opposite acromion (not resting on the trapezius muscle). The shoulder-strap should be wide and its length adjusted to let the purse fit into the hollow of the waist. This lets the weight of the purse rest partly on the iliac crest when the purse is pressed against the side by the elbow. Occasionally, it is better to hang the purse from a belt.

A heavy coat that rests on the upper trapezius, rather than on the acromial process at the side, should be avoided; shoulder pads inserted in the coat can properly redistribute its weight.

Stretch Exercise. Also helpful to maintain full length of the upper trapezius is the scalenus posterior version of the passive Side-bending Neck Exercise, as illustrated in Figure 20.12B, in Chapter 20.

Active Exercise. Two of the safest general conditioning exercises that help the shoulder muscles, including the trapezius, are swimming and jumping rope while progressing forward. Jogging tends to aggrevate trapezius TPs.

Middle Trapezius

When the arm must be held out in front of the body for a long time, an elbow rest should be devised.

The stretch exercise specifically for this muscle, the Middle-trapezius Exercise, is illustrated in Figure 6.11. The patient is instructed as follows: Lie supine on the floor. Place the elbows, forearms and palms of the hands together in front of the abdomen (Fig. 6.11A). Keep the elbows tightly together as long as possible while raising the forearms over the face (Fig. 6.11B). Then, drop the forearms past the

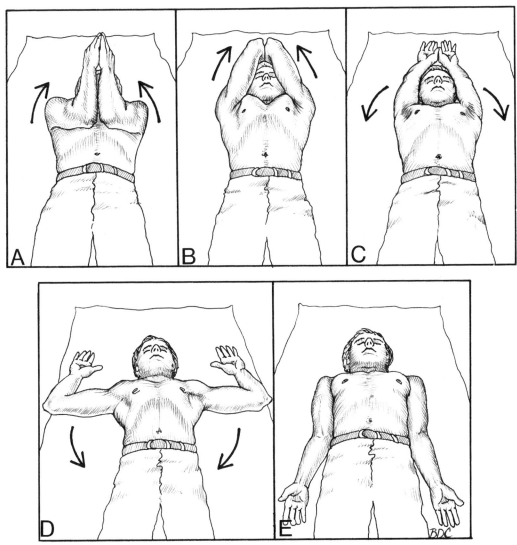

Figure 6.11. Middle-trapezius, Stretch Exercise, designed to stretch the middle and lower parts of the trapezius muscle by fully abducting and rotating the scapulae. Movements progress from *A* through *E*. When completed, the patient pauses, breathes deeply to relax, and repeats the sequence. (See Section 14 for the full description.)

ears to the floor (Fig. 6.11C). Keeping the back of the elbows and wrists in contact with the floor, swing the arms down against the sides of the body (Fig. 6.11D and E). Pause and relax, while taking several slow deep breaths. Repeat the cycle.

The antagonistic pectoralis major fibers usually are in need of stretching when the middle trapezius harbors active TPs. These pectoral fibers are passively stretched by doing the In-doorway Stretch Exercise, (see Fig. 42.10, in Chapter 42). The middle hand position of this exercise specifically stretches the sternal division of the pectoralis major.

Lower Trapezius

Every patient should arrange seated workspace that provides adequate room for the knees underneath the desk or table. The chair should be pulled close enough to the workspace so that the patient can lean back firmly against the backrest; both elbows should rest on the work surface or on short armrests of about the same height as the desk surface.

The exercise for the middle trapezius (Fig. 6.11) also is helpful for at-home stretching of the lower trapezius fibers.

When using a moist heating pad or hot pack for relief of pain referred from TPs in the lower fibers of the trapezius, the patient should apply the heat to the mid-back area where the TPs are located, rather than solely to the suprascapular region and neck where pain is felt.

Supplemental Case Reports

The management of three cases with trapezius TPs is reviewed by the senior author.[53, 58]

References

1. Basmajian JV: *Muscles Alive*, Ed. 4. Williams & Wilkins, Baltimore, 1978 (pp. 186, 189, 191, 193, 356).
2. Bates T: Myofascial pain, Chapter 14. In *Ambulatory Pediatrics II: Personal Health Care of Children in the Office*, edited by M. Green and R.J. Haggerty. W.B. Saunders, Philadelphia, 1977 (pp. 147–148).
3. Bell WE: *Orofacial Pains—Differential Diagnosis*. Denedco of Dallas, Dallas, 1973 (p. 97).
4. Broer MR, Houtz SJ: *Patterns of Muscular Activity in Selected Sport Skills, An Electromyographic Study*. Charles C Thomas, Springfield, Ill., 1967.
5. Cailliet R: *Shoulder Pain*. F.A. Davis, Philadelphia, 1966 (p. 22, Fig. 19).
6. Diffrient N, Tilley AR, Bardagjy JC: *Humanscale 1/2/3*. MIT Press, Cambridge, 1974.
7. Duchenne GB: *Physiology of Motion*, translated by E.B. Kaplan. J.B. Lippincott, Philadelphia, 1949 (pp. 3–5).
8. Eisler P: *Die Muskeln des Stammes*. Gustav Fischer, Jena, 1912 (pp. 344–352, Figs. 43 and 47).
9. Engle WK: Ponderous-purse disease. *N Engl J Med* 299:557, 1978.
10. Gardner DA: The use of ethyl chloride spray to relieve somatic pain. *J Am Osteopath Assoc* 49:525–528, 1950 (Case 4).
11. Gelb H: Patient evaluation, Chapter 3. In *Clinical Management of Head, Neck and TMJ Pain and Dysfunction*, edited by H. Gelb. W.B. Saunders, Philadelphia, 1977 (p. 73).
12. Good MG: What is "fibrositis"? *Rheumatism* 5:117–123, 1949 (pp. 119–121, Fig. 2).
13. Good MG: The role of skeletal muscles in the pathogenesis of diseases. *Acta Med Scand* 138:285–292, 1950 (Fig. 3, Case 2).
14. Grant JCB: *An Atlas of Human Anatomy*, Ed. 7. Williams & Wilkins, Baltimore, 1978 (Fig. 6–30).
15. *Ibid.* (Fig. 9–4).
16. Gray H: *Anatomy of the Human Body*, edited by C.M. Goss, American Ed. 29. Lea & Febiger, Philadelphia, 1973 (p. 446, Fig. 6–33; pp. 447, 448, 876, 944, 945).
17. Gustein M: Diagnosis and treatment of muscular rheumatism. *Br J Phys Med* 1:302–321, 1938 (pp. 310, 311).
18. Gutstein-Good M: Idiopathic myalgia simulating visceral and other diseases. *Lancet* 2:326–328, 1940.
19. Hoberman M: Crutch and cane exercises and use, Chapter 10. In *Therapeutic Exercise*, edited by J.V. Basmajian, Ed. 3. Williams & Wilkins, 1978 (p. 239).
20. Inman VT, Saunders JB, Abbott LC: Observations on the function of the shoulder joint. *J Bone Joint Surg* 26:1–30, 1944 (p. 25, Fig. 31; pp. 26, 27).
21. Jonsson S, Jonsson B: Function of the muscles of the upper limb in car driving, I–III *Ergonomics* 18:375–388, 1975 (p. 381).
22. Kelly M: Some rules for the employment of local analgesic in the treatment of somatic pain. *Med J Aust* 1:235–239, 1947.
23. Kelly M: The relief of facial pain by procaine (novocaine) injections. *J Am Geriatr Soc* 11:586–596, 1963 (Table 1, Fig. 4, Case 3).
24. Kelly M: New light on the painful shoulder. *Med J Aust* 1:488–493, 1942 (Cases 1 and 2).
25. Kraus H: *Clinical Treatment of Back and Neck Pain*. McGraw-Hill, New York, 1970 (p. 98).
26. Lange M: *Die Muskelhärten (Myogelosen)*. J.F. Lehmanns, München, 1931 (p. 129, Fig. 40b; p. 93, Case 3; p. 118, Case 15; p. 130, Case 21).
27. Lockhart RD, Hamilton GF, Fyfe FW: *Anatomy of the Human Body*, Ed. 2. J.B. Lippincott, Philadelphia, 1969 (pp. 318, 321).
28. Long C, II: Myofascial pain syndromes: Part II—Syndromes of the head, neck and shoulder girdle. *Henry Ford Hosp Med Bull* 4:22–28, 1956.
29. Lundervold A: Occupation myalgia. Electromyographic investigations. *Acta Psychiatr Neurol* 26:360–369, 1951.
30. Lundervold A: Electromyographic investigations during sedentary work, especially typewriting. *Br J Phys Med* 14:32–36, 1951.
31. Lundervold AJS: Electromyographic investigations of position and manner of working in typewriting. *Acta Physiol Scand* 24:Supplementum 84, 1951 (pp. 26, 27, 94, 95, 97, 126, 129).
32. Marbach JJ: Arthritis of the temporomandibular joints. *Am Fam Phys* 19:131–139, 1979 (p. 136).
33. McMinn RMH, Hutchings RT: *Color Atlas of Human Anatomy*. Year Book Medical Publishers, Chicago, 1977 (Fig. 111).
34. *Ibid.* (Fig. 35).
35. Melnick J: Trigger areas and refractory pain in duodenal ulcer. *NY State J Med* 57:1073–1076, 1957.
36. Michele AA, Davies JJ, Krueger FJ, Lichtor JM: Scapulocostal syndrome (fatigue-postural paradox). *NY State J Med* 50:1353–1356, 1950 (p. 1355, Fig. 4).
37. Modell W, Travell JT, Kraus H, Hardy JD: Contributions to *Cornell Conferences on Therapy*. Relief of pain by ethyl chloride spray. *NY State J Med* 52:1550–1558, 1952.
38. Motta A, Tainiti G: Paralysis of the trapezius associated with myogenic torticollis. *Ital J Orthop Traumatol* 3:207–213, 1977.
39. Pace JB: Commonly overlooked pain syndromes responsive to simple therapy. *Postgrad Med* 58:107–113, 1975 (Fig. 4).
40. Patton IJ, Williamson JA: Fibrositis as a factor in the differential diagnosis of visceral pain. *Can Med Assoc J* 58:162–166, 1948 (Case 1).

PART 1

41. Pernkopf E: *Atlas of Topographical and Applied Human Anatomy*, Vol 2. W.B. Saunders, Philadelphia, 1964 (p. 33, Fig. 27).
42. Rasch PJ, Burke RK: *Kinesiology and Applied Anatomy*, Ed. 6. Lea & Febiger, Philadelphia, 1978 (pp. 146–150).
43. Rubin D: An approach to the management of myofascial trigger point syndromes. *Arch Phys Med Rehabil* 62:107–110, 1981.
44. Sharav Y, Tzukert A, Refaeli B: Muscle pain index in relation to pain, dysfunction, and dizziness associated with the myofascial pain-dysfunction syndrome. *Oral Surg* 46:742–747, 1978.
45. Sobotta J, Figge FHJ: *Atlas of Human Anatomy*, Ed. 9, Vol. 1. Hafner, New York, 1974 (p. 142).
46. *Ibid.* (pp. 141, 169, 192).
47. Sola AE, Kuitert JH: Myofascial trigger point pain in the neck and shoulder girdle. *Northwest Med* 54:980–984, 1955.
48. Sola AE, Rodenberger ML, Gettys BB: Incidence of hypersensitive areas in posterior shoulder muscles. *Am J Phys Med* 34:585–590, 1955.
49. Spalteholz W: *Handatlas der Anatomie des Menschen*, Ed. 11, Vol. 2., S. Hirzel, Leipzig, 1922 (pp. 302, 303, Fig. 380).
50. Steinbrocker O, Isenberg SA, Silver M, *et al.*: Observations on pain produced by injection of hypertonic saline into muscles and other supportive tissues. *J Clin Invest* 32:1045–1051, 1953 (Fig. 2).
51. Toldt C: *An Atlas of Human Anatomy*, translated by M.E. Paul, Ed. 2, Vol. 1. Macmillan, New York, 1919 (Fig. 507).
52. *Ibid.* (Fig 534).
53. Travell J: Rapid relief of acute "stiff neck" by ethyl chloride spray. *J Am Med Wom Assoc* 4:89–95, 1949 (Cases 2 and 4).
54. Travell J: Chairs are a personal thing. *House Beautiful*, pp. 190–193, (Oct.) 1955.
55. Travell J: Temporomandibular joint pain referrd from muscles of the head and neck. *J Prosthet Dent* 10:745–763, 1960 (Figs. 1 and 2).
56. Travell J: Mechanical headache. *Headache* 7:23–29, 1967 (Fig. 1).
57. Travell J: Symposium on mechanism and management of pain syndromes. *Proc Rudolf Virchow Med Soc* 16:128–136, 1957 (Figs. 1 and 2).
58. Travell J: Basis for the multiple uses of local block of somatic trigger areas (procaine infiltration and ethyl chloride spray). *Miss Valley Med J* 71:13–22, 1949 (Case 3).
59. Travell J: Pain mechanisms in connective tissues. In *Connective Tissues, Transactions of the Second Conference, 1951*, edited by C. Ragan. Josiah Macy, Jr. Foundation, New York, 1952 (pp. 94–96, Figs. 28 and 29).
60. Travell J, Bigelow NH: Role of somatic trigger areas in the patterns of hysteria. *Psychosom Med* 9:353–363, 1947.
61. Travell J, Rinzler SH: The myofascial genesis of pain. *Postgrad Med* 11:425–434, 1952.
62. Trommer PR, Gellman MB: Trigger point syndrome. *Rheumatism* 8:67–72, 1952 (Case 7).
63. Webber TD: Diagnosis and modification of headache and shoulder-arm-hand syndrome. *JAOA* 72:697–710, 1973 (Fig. 28, No. 2).
64. Wetzler G: Physical therapy, chap. 24. In *Diseases of the Temporomandibular Apparatus*, edited by D.H. Morgan, W.P. Hall and S.J. Vamvas. C.V. Mosby, St. Louis, 1977 (p. 355).
65. Williams HL, Elkins EC: Myalgia of the head. *Arch Phys Ther* 23:14–22, 1942 (p. 19).
66. Winter Z: Referred pain in fibrositis. *Med Rec* 157:34–37, 1944.
67. Wyant GM: Chronic pain syndromes and their treatment. II. Trigger points. *Can Anaesth Soc J* 26:216–219, 1979 (Case 1, Fig. 1).
68. Yamshon LJ, Bierman W: Kinesiologic electromyography: II. The trapezius. *Arch Phys Med Rehabil* 29:647–651, 1948.
69. Zohn DA, Mennell J McM: *Musculoskeletal Pain*. Little, Brown & Company, Boston, 1976 (Figs. 7-4B and 9-12).

CHAPTER 7
Sternocleidomastoid Muscle
"Amazingly Complex"

HIGHLIGHTS: The sternocleidomastoid muscle frequently contains multiple trigger points (TPs) in either its sternal or clavicular division, or both. **REFERRED PAIN** from the two divisions presents quite different patterns. In each division, TPs also evoke different autonomic phenomena or proprioceptive disturbances. The sternal division may refer pain to the vertex, to the occiput, across the cheek, over the eye, to the throat, and the sternum. With clavicular division TPs, patients commonly experience frontal headache and earache, whereas sternal division TPs give rise to eye and face pain likely to be diagnosed as "atypical facial neuralgia." Referred autonomic phenomena from the sternal division involve the eye and sinuses, while from the clavicular division they are more likely to concern the forehead and ear, including proprioceptive dizziness related to posture and disturbed equilibrium. **ACTIONS** of one muscle alone include rotating the face to the opposite side and lifting it toward the ceiling. Together, the paired sternocleidomastoid muscles flex the head and neck and act as auxiliary muscles of inspiration. **SYMPTOMS** of postural dizziness and imbalance may prove even more incapacitating than the head pain referred from TPs in this muscle. **ACTIVATION OF TRIGGER POINTS** is usually due to mechanical overload, often caused by structural inadequacies of the body, or by paradoxical breathing. **TRIGGER POINT EXAMINATION** is simplified by the ease with which the fingers can encircle both divisions in order to minutely examine the muscle for palpable bands, tender TPs and local twitch responses. **STRETCH AND SPRAY** are effective when the precise technique has been mastered. **INJECTION AND STRETCH** are relatively simple and safe when properly done, but sometimes produce afterpain and distressing referred autonomic and proprioceptive phenomena. **CORRECTIVE ACTIONS** to secure lasting relief usually require identification of, and structural compensation for, congenital body inadequacies, such as, a short leg, a small hemipelvis, or short upper arms. Lasting relief also may require the modification of daily activities, for example, telephoning.

1. REFERRED PAIN (AND CONCOMITANTS)
(Fig. 7.1)

The sternal and clavicular divisions have their own characteristic referred pain patterns and concomitants.[49, 50, 53] As a rule, neither division refers pain to the neck; both refer pain to the face and cranium. The face pain referred from trigger points (TPs) in this muscle is frequently the basis for the diagnoses of "atypical facial neuralgia,"[53] tension headache,[18, 25] and cervicocephalalgia.[27] The pain and the autonomic or proprioceptive components referred from TPs in this muscle are widely recognized by the dental profession as a significant component of the common complaint, myofascial pain-dysfunction syndrome.[32, 37]

The pain pattern referred from the sternocleidomastoid muscle in children is similar to that in adults.[3]

Williams and Elkins[60] remarked that myalgia of the head is accompanied by circumscribed tender regions in the neck muscles at their attachments to the cranium. We occasionally find TPs at the mas-

PART 1

toid attachment of the sternocleidomastoid. They reported inducing referred head pain by applying digital pressure to these tender muscles and by injecting hypertonic salt solution into them, location unspecified.

Sternal Division
(Fig. 7.1A)

An active TP in the *lower end* of the sternal division refers pain downward over the upper portion of the sternum (Fig. 7.1A). This is the only downward reference of pain from this muscle.[49, 53] True trigeminal facial neuralgia is not accompanied by sternal pain, which, when also present, suggests the sternocleidomastoid myofascial syndrome.

When an unusual TP is activated in the lowest part of the sternal division, where that division may merge with a slip of the inconstant sternalis muscle, the TP is associated with a paroxysmal dry cough that can be precipitated by mechanical stimulation of the TP.

At the *mid-level* of the sternal division, TPs refer pain homolaterally, arching across the cheek (often in finger-like projections) and into the maxilla, over the supraorbital ridge and deep within the orbit.[61] Pain may be referred on the same side to the external auditory canal.[56, 62] The quality of the pain is described by patients to be aching as in the deep pain defined by Kellgren.[23] The TPs along the inner margin at the mid-level of this division refer pain to the pharynx and to the back of the tongue during swallowing,[5] which causes "sore throat," and to a small round area at the tip of the chin.[53] Marbach[28] shows a similar pattern that includes the cheek, temporomandibular joint and mastoid areas.

In the *upper end* of the sternal division, TPs refer pain to the occipital ridge behind, but not close to the ear, and to the vertex of the head like a skull cap, with scalp tenderness in the pain reference zone.

Autonomic concomitants of TPs in the sternal division relate to the homolateral eye and nose.[49, 53] Eye symptoms include excessive lacrimation, reddening (vascular engorgement) of the conjunctiva, apparent "ptosis" (narrowing of the palpebral fissure) with normal pupillary size and reactions, and visual disturbances. The "ptosis" is due to spasm of the orbicularis oculi muscle, rather than to weakness of the levator palpebrae muscle. The spasm is caused by increased excitability of motor units within the reference zone of sternal division TPs. The patient may have to tilt the head backward to look up, because of inability to raise the upper eyelid. Visual disturbances include not only blurring of vision,[47, 49] but also dimming of perceived

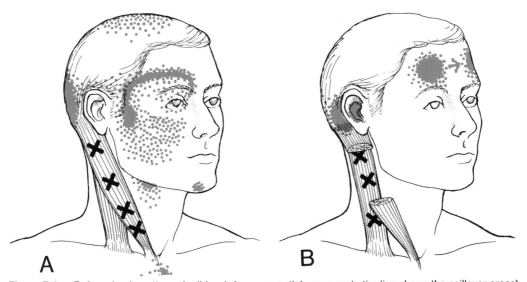

Figure 7.1.   Referred pain patterns (*solid red* shows essential zones and *stippling* shows the spillover areas) with location of corresponding trigger points (**X**s) in the right sternocleidomastoid muscle. *A*, the sternal (superficial) division. *B*, the clavicular (deep) division.

light intensity.[54] Sometimes coryza and maxillary sinus congestion develop on the affected side.

One reliable patient reported a crackling sound in the homolateral ear, which was reproduced by pinching the superficial fibers of the sternal division at its mid-level.

In our experience, unilateral deafness in a few patients with no complaint of tinnitus, has been traced to TPs in the sternocleidomastoid muscle. Wyant[61] attributed tinnitus in one patient to TPs in either the sternocleidomastoid, upper trapezius or cervical paraspinal muscles. Travell[49] has noted the association of unilateral tinnitis with a TP in the deep division of the masseter muscle.

Clavicular Division
(Fig. 7.1B)

At the *mid-level* of this division, TPs refer pain to the frontal area; when severe, the pain extends across the forehead to the other side (crossed reference).[48, 49] The *upper part* of this division is likely to refer pain homolaterally deep into the ear and to the posterior auricular region, and sometimes refers poorly localized pain to the cheek and molar teeth on the same side (Fig. 7.1B).[53]

Proprioceptive concomitants of TPs in the clavicular division[47, 58] relate chiefly to spatial disorientation. Patients complain of postural dizziness (in the form of a disagreeable movement or sensation within the head),[24] and less often of vertigo (the sensation of objects spinning around the patient, or *vice versa*).[47, 58] During severe attacks,[58] syncope following sudden turning of the head may be due to stretch-stimulation of active TPs in the clavicular division. Episodes of dizziness lasting from seconds to hours are induced by a change of position which requires contraction of the sternocleidomastoid muscle, or which places it on a sudden stretch. Disequilibrium may occur separately from, or be associated with postural dizziness; it may cause sudden falls when bending or stooping, or ataxia (unintentional veering to one side when walking with the eyes open).[46] The patient is unable to relate the vertigo or dizziness to a particular side of the head, even though it can be shown to depend on trigger mechanisms in only one sternocleidomastoid muscle. Postural re-

sponses are exaggerated in some patients; when looking up, they feel as if they will "pitch over backwards," and when glancing down, they tend to fall forward. The illusion of a tilted bed is not rare. Nausea is common, but vomiting is infrequent. Dimenhydrinate (Dramamine) may relieve the nausea, but not the dizziness.

Good[16] attributed symptoms of dizziness to TPs in either the sternocleidomastoid or the upper trapezius muscles. We have observed this symptom only from the former, although both muscles are commonly involved together.

These symptoms apparently derive from a disturbance of the proprioceptive contribution of this neck muscle to body orientation in space.[11] In man, it is probably the chief muscular source of proprioceptive orientation of the head.[48] Experiments in monkeys[9, 10] established that the proprioceptive function of the labyrinths is confined to orienting the head in space, while the neck proprioceptive mechanisms are concerned with orienting the head in relation to the body. Abolition of either of these systems produces spatial disorientation that is similar in form and magnitude.[10]

When objects of equal weight are held in the hands, the patient with unilateral TP involvement of the clavicular division may show dysmetria by underestimating the weight of the object held in the hand on the same side as the affected sternocleidomastoid muscle. Inactivation of the responsible TPs promptly restores weight appreciation by this test. Apparently, the afferent discharges from these TPs disturb central processing of proprioceptive information from both the upper limb and the neck muscles.

Active TPs in the clavicular division also can refer the autonomic phenomena of localized sweating and vasoconstriction (blanching) to the frontal area of referred pain.

2. ANATOMICAL ATTACHMENTS
(Fig. 7.2)

Caudally the sternocleidomastoid muscle consists of two divisions: the sternal (medial and more superficial) and the clavicular (lateral and deeper). *Cephalad* the two divisons blend to form a common attachment (Fig. 7.2). The relative size of the

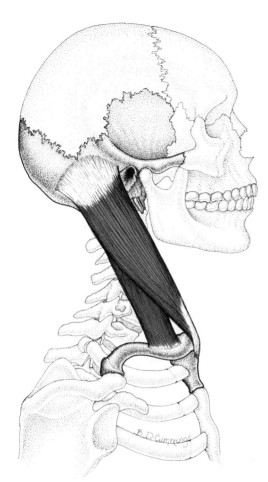

Figure 7.2. Attachments of the sternocleidomastoid muscle.

two divisions and the space between them at the clavicle are variable.

Sternal Division

These fibers attach **below** to the anterior surface of the manubrium sterni. They attach **above** to the lateral surface of the mastoid process and to the lateral half of the superior nuchal line of the occipital bone (Fig. 7.2).

The variable sternalis muscle may extend downward over the anterior chest, appearing like a continuation of the sternal division of the sternocleidomastoid (see Chapter 44).

Clavicular Division

This section attaches **below** to the superior border of the anterior surface of the clavicle along its medial third. It attaches

above to the same bony structures as does the sternal division (Fig. 7.2).

Supplemental References

The authors illustrate this muscle well in the front view,[30, 40, 43] in the side view,[14, 17, 29, 39, 42, 44] and from the rear.[41] The sternocleidomastoid is presented in cross section in Figure 7.6C, of this chapter, in Figure 16.9 of Chapter 16, and by others.[9]

3. INNERVATION

The spinal portion of cranial nerve XI (spinal accessory), which supplies the sternocleidomastoid muscle, arises within the spinal column from the ventral roots (motor fibers) of the upper five cervical segments. Probably only the higher cervical segments innervate the sternocleidomastoid. The motor nerve fibers ascend through the foramen magnum and then descend through the jugular foramen where they form a plexus with fibers from the anterior primary divisions of the second, and sometimes of the third, cervical nerve.[14] These latter cervical nerve fibers to the muscle are primarily sensory.

Central connections of the spinal nerve fibers include the pyramidal tract and the medial longitudinal fasciculus, for the coordination of head and eye movement.[17]

4. ACTIONS

Both Muscles Together

1. Acting bilaterally, the sternocleidomastoid muscles flex the neck and pull the head forward, bringing the chin onto the chest,[2, 21, 35] unless the head is strongly extended initially.[13]

2. On upward gaze, they checkrein hyperextension of the neck. They also resist forceful backward movement of the head, which can occur when an unprotected passenger is riding in an auto that is struck from the rear (whiplash).

3. Together with the trapezius, the two muscles help to stabilize and fix the position of the head in space when the mandible moves during talking and chewing.

4. By strongly lifting the upper anterior rib cage, they act as important auxiliary muscles of inspiration,[2, 8, 13, 21, 35] but only when the head and neck are in the erect or hyperextended position, and not when the neck is flexed.

PART 1

5. Clinically, they participate in the act of swallowing[5] (see Sternocleidomastoid Compression Test in Section 8 of this chapter) although this was not confirmed electromyographically.[2]

6. They contribute to spatial orientation, weight perception, and motor coordination. Experimental loss of sensory input at C_1, C_2, and C_3 results in spatial disorientation, imbalance and motor incoordination in monkeys and baboons.[9, 11]

One Muscle

1. Acting unilaterally, the sternocleidomastoid muscle rotates the face toward the opposite side and tilts it upward.[2, 21, ,35]

2. Acting with the upper trapezius, it side-bends the cervical column, drawing the ear down to the shoulder on the same side.[2, 21, 35]

3. Acting with the scalene and trapezius muscles of the same side, it helps to compensate for the head tilt that is due to tilting of the shoulder-girdle axis, which, in turn, is often caused by the functional scoliosis associated with a short leg or small hemipelvis.

Sports

During *right*-handed sport activities, the greatest electromyographic activation of the sternocleidomastoid was seen in the *left* muscle during the tennis serve, a golf swing, and during a jump on one foot in volleyball.[6]

5. MYOTATIC UNIT

One sternocleidomastoid muscle is synergistic with its homolateral upper trapezius during active lateral bending of the head and neck toward the same side, and also when they checkrein lateral bending toward the opposite site.

Together, both sternocleidomastoid muscles in their entirety are synergistic in checkreining hyperextension of the head and neck. Likewise, they are synergistic with the scalene muscles bilaterally during vigorous chest breathing (inspiration).

The sternal division on each side acts as an antagonist to the opposite muscle for head rotation.

The platysma, a skin muscle that over-

lies the sternocleidomastoid, does not appear to be functionally related to it.

6. SYMPTOMS

Contrary to expectation,[25] neck pain and stiffness are not features of sternocleidomastoid TPs.[7, 45] The patient may complain of "soreness" in the neck on rubbing these muscles, but the symptom is often disregarded, sometimes because the TP tenderness is mistakenly attributed to lymphadenopathy ("glands"). Surprisingly, this patient prefers to lie on the side of the sore muscle if a pillow is adjusted to support the head so that the area of referred tenderness in the face does not bear weight. This muscle may add an additional component to the "stiff neck" syndrome,[45] which is primarily due to TP activity in the levator scapulae, posterior cervical and trapezius muscles. "Tension headache" is the diagnosis often given to the patient with the myofascial pain syndrome of the sternocleidomastoid.[11, 25] The patient may be aware of ipsilateral sweating of the forehead, reddening of the conjunctiva and tearing of the eye, rhinitis, and "ptosis." Blurred, or possibly double vision, are sometimes reported; the pupils react normally. For the referred pain distribution and concomitants of sternocleidomastoid TPs, see Section 1.

Rarely do sternocleidomastoid TPs cause a complaint of restricted neck movement, although some limitation at the extremes of neck rotation, flexion and extension may be noted on careful examination.

Sternal Division

Pain referred from the sternal division may occur independently of pain referred from the clavicular division.[53] Sternal division pain involves chiefly the cheek, temple and orbit, as described in Section 1.

Autonomic phenomena referred from TPs in this division, such as profuse tearing of the eye, is more distressing to some patients than the pain. Rather than blurring and dimming of vision, the patient may be most aware of a visual disturbance when viewing strongly contrasting parallel lines, such as a venetian blind. Narrowing of the palpebral fissure is usually a prominent feature on the side of the active TPs in the sternal division.

Clavicular Division

Any one of the three major symptoms produced by TPs in the clavicular division, namely, frontal headache, postural dizziness or imbalance, and dysmetria (disturbed weight perception)[19] may dominate the clinical picture. The dizziness is postural and occurs with changing loads on the muscle. Hyperextension of the neck and overstretching of the muscle, caused by lying without a pillow on a hard X-ray or examining table, may precipitate an attack of dizziness. Active TPs in the clavicular division may contribute to seasickness or car sickness. Patients may complain of a "sick stomach" with nausea and anorexia that leads to a poor diet. The patient is likely to experience dizziness when turning over in bed at night, and should learn to roll the head on the pillow without lifting the head. During the day, transient loss of equilibrium is likely to follow vigorous quick rotation of the head and neck. During an acute attack of this postural dizziness, a person suddenly cannot drive his car. It veers, too. This may be a significant undocumented factor in traffic accidents.[52] Loss of equilibrium also may follow sustained tilting of the head to one side, as when holding a telephone receiver to the ear, or bird-watching with binoculars. The disturbed proprioception causing postural dizziness may be more disabling than the head pain referred from this muscle.

Symptoms may appear in any combination, or all appear together.

In a few patients, hearing was impaired unilaterally due to active TPs in the clavicular division on the same side. Tinnitus has not been found to originate from TPs in the sternocleidomastoid, but is likely to originate in TPs high in the deep division of the masseter muscle.

7. ACTIVATION OF TRIGGER POINTS
(Fig. 7.3)

Sleeping on two pillows (for example, to improve "sinus drainage") flexes the neck and shortens the sternocleidomastoid muscles, which tends to activate their TPs. If the head must be elevated, it is advisable to place blocks under the legs at the head of the bed to tilt the bed frame, rather than to use extra pillows (see Chapter 20).

Mechanical Stress

Sternocleidomastoid TPs are usually activated during an acute episode of mechanical overload, for instance, by protracted neck extension in overhead work (painting a ceiling, writing on a blackboard, hanging curtains, sitting in a front-row seat in a theater with a high stage); by overuse in sports (wrestling); or by accidental injury (a fall on the head, "whiplash" in an automobile crash).

One common source of chronic postural stress on the sternocleidomastoid muscles is severe deformity or injury that restricts upper extremity movement and requires awkward compensatory neck positioning. The other is a structural inadequacy, such as a short leg or small hemipelvis, both of which produce a functional scoliosis and shoulder-girdle tilting (see Fig. 48.8 in Chapter 48). The sternocleidomastoid muscles, in conjunction with the scalene muscles, are overloaded by the necessity for compensation of the resultant tilt of the shoulder-girdle axis, in order to maintain normal head position and to level the eyes.

Reading in bed with a light placed at one side (Fig. 7.3B) chronically strains the sternocleidomastoid because the muscle on one side must carry most of the weight of the rotated head. Cocking the head to avoid the reflection of overhead lights from contact lenses or eyeglasses,[51] or to improve hearing in one-ear deafness, has been a critical stress factor in some patients.

Paradoxical breathing, or a chronic cough (of emphysema or asthma) overloads this accessory muscle of respiration.

Patients may overstress the sternocleidomastoid by the hauling and pulling associated with horseback riding and the handling of horses.

Compression of the muscle by a tight shirt collar or necktie activates its TPs.

Hangover Headache

The "morning-after" hangover headache from alcoholic overindulgence may represent referred pain from active sternoclei-

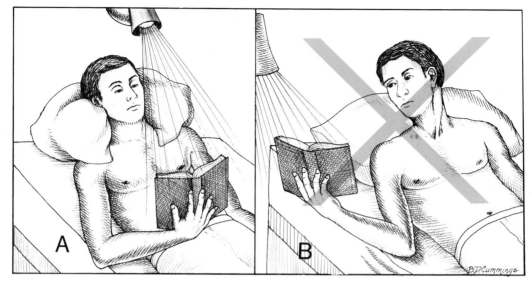

Figure 7.3.   Strain of the left sternocleidomastoid muscle by head positioning. *A*, correct lighting and head support when reading in bed. *B*, incorrect positioning which places sustained stress on the left sternocleidomastoid muscle.

domastoid TPs.[45] This hangover pain may be quickly relieved by stretch and spray of the affected muscles.

Spinal Tap Headache

The leakage of cerebrospinal fluid, which occasionally follows a spinal tap or myelogram, may cause irritation of brain stem structures that activates sternocleidomastoid TPs. These TPs may then cause chronic headache for weeks, months or years, which, regardless of duration, can be relieved by inactivating the responsible myofascial TPs.

Chronic Infection

Any focus of chronic infection, such as sinusitis or a dental abscess, should be eliminated. Herpes simplex (oral) recurrent infection may be a stubborn perpetuator of TPs in the neck and masticatory muscles.

8. PATIENT EXAMINATION

The patient with headache due to active sternocleidomastoid TPs has minimal restriction of the active range of head and neck motion. Flexion may be slightly restricted (lacking about one fingerbreadth between the chin and the sternum). With sufficiently active TPs, rotation is limited by about 10° to the opposite side, without

pain. The contracting muscle is inhibited reflexly by the stretched sternocleidomastoid on the opposite side.

When examining the standing patient with active sternocleidomastoid TPs, and the discrepancy in the length of the lower extremities is less than 6 mm (¼ in), the shoulder opposite to the short leg usually sags, whereas in patients with 1.2 cm (½ in) or more of leg-length disparity, the shoulder usually droops on the same side as the short leg.

Signs of autonomic concomitants may be evident in the pain reference zones, as noted in Section 1. The patient with dizziness and disequilibrium due to TPs in the clavicular division has neither a Romberg's sign nor nystagmus. With this type of myofascial disequilibrium, the patient cannot walk in a straight line toward a point across the room where he fixes his gaze. He veers to one side, usually to the side of the active TPs in the clavicular division.

One man, wearing a stereophonic headset, was aware of markedly decreased hearing in the right ear, on the same side as the active sternocleidomastoid TPs. He found that turning the face fully to the right, and then dipping the chin to the shoulder (raising the mastoid process), restored his hearing to normal, as he passively stretched the tensed sternocleidomastoid muscle on the side of his impaired hearing. This hearing loss apparently was due to TP-induced reflex disturbance of function of the tensor tympani muscle on the same side.

When objects of equal weight are placed in the hands of a patient with unilateral clavicular division TPs that are sufficiently active, the object hefted on the affected side is perceived as lighter.[19] A difference in weight perception may not be apparent when TP involvement of the sternocleidomastoid muscles is bilateral, as is often the case.

At midlevel of the sternal division, the TPs responsible for "sore throat" (referred pharyngeal pain during swallowing) shows a positive Sternocleidomastoid Compression Test. To perform this test, the sternocleidomastoid muscle is held firmly in a pincer grasp, as for examination, and the tender region immobilized by steadily compressing the belly of the muscle while the patient swallows.[5] Pressure also may be effectively applied over the muscle by picking up the largest fold of skin possible overlying and parallel to the muscle, and squeezing the skin very firmly while the patient swallows. If TPs are responsible for the throat pain, and if the muscle or skin are held tightly enough, swallowing becomes pain free.

The patient may cough in response to palpation of a TP near the sternal attachment of the muscle. The complaint of a persistent dry, tickling cough should alert one to examine the patient at and below both sternal attachments for this "cough" TP.

Differential Diagnosis

The head pain referred from sternocleidomastoid TPs is readily mistaken for vascular headache or atypical facial neuralgia.[53] The pain from sternocleidomastoid TPs can mimic true trigeminal neuralgia in distribution, and the arthritic pain of the sternoclavicular joint.[36]

Unlike Ménière's disease, symptoms and signs arising from myofascial TPs in the clavicular division are rarely associated with unilateral deafness, but not with tinnitus. The patient shows a normal calorimetric test and a negative Romberg's sign. Pupils are normal. There is no nystagmus, and no neurological deficit. Nystagmus

and a positive Romberg's sign should alert one to a possible neurological lesion. Consciousness is unimpaired. These features distinguish the myofascial syndromes from more serious conditions like tic douloureux, Ménière's disease, cerebellopontine tumors, intracranial vascular lesions, inflammation of the labryrinth, hemorrhage into the pons, and petit mal epilepsy. The symptom of vertigo usually implies neurological disease and causes the sensation of the patient's spinning, or of the environment revolving around the patient.[12] It should be distinguished from postural dizziness; the latter is a nonspecific feeling of disorientation, as some patients say, a "swimmin' in the head." The patient's imbalance due to myofascial TPs may mimic ataxia.

Dizziness due to vestibular disease is identified by nystagmus and other tests of vestibular function. The non-vestibular sources of dizziness include: ear wax that touches the tympanic membrane; stenosis of the internal carotid artery, which may be detected by listening for a bruit over the bifurcation of the carotid artery, or higher in the neck; hypertension; intracranial aneurysm or tumor; or a subclavian steal syndrome with reverse vertebral artery flow. Dizziness has been reported as an early sign of multiple sclerosis in children;[27] as a side effect of quinine,[57] and from drugs other than quinine; as the result of postural hypotension due to excessive dosage of antihypertensive medication,[59] or due to adrenocortical insufficiency with failure of the orthostatic reflex response. The patient's blood pressure should be taken supine, sitting and standing.

The facial grimace of *tic* douloureux clearly distinguishes this neurological disease from atypical facial neuralgia and from pain due to TPs in the sternal divsion of the sternocleidomastoid.[53]

When autonomic symptoms are due to myofascial TPs in the sternal division, the absence of miosis and enophthalmus, and the presence of a ciliospinal reflex rule out a Horner's syndrome. The eye symptoms must be distinguished also from paralysis of the extraocular muscles and from conversion hysteria.

The symptoms of "stiff neck"[26, 45, 51] due to myofascial TPs, which develop in otherwise normal muscles during or after childhood, are easily distinguished from congenital torticollis, which is characterized by fibrosis and structural shortening of one sternocleidomastoid muscle from infancy.[22, 31] Spasmodic or paroxysmal torticollis (wry neck) is a clonic or tonic contraction of cervical muscles due to organic disease of the central nervous system, or possibly to conversion hysteria. Symptomatically, this condition merges into torsion dystonia of the neck, and the muscles involved become hypertrophied. Spasmodic torticollis may be inhibited by exerting slight pressure against the jaw on the side to which the head is rotated. Dystonic movement ceases during sleep. Clonic jerks are particularly common in hysterical patients.[4] Spasmodic torticollis in infancy[38] and spasmus nutans[20] are described as self-limited conditions of infancy or childhood, characterized by a head tilt that is strongly suggestive of sternocleidomastoid TP dysfunction and may include a significant myofascial component.

9. TRIGGER POINT EXAMINATION
(Fig. 7.4)

For examination of the sternocleidomastoid muscle, the patient may be seated (Fig. 7.4A), or supine (Fig. 7.4B). The muscle is slackened somewhat by tilting the patient's head so as to bring the ear toward the shoulder on the symptomatic side (Fig. 7.4B) and, if necessary, by turning the face slightly away from the muscle to be examined. The muscle is grasped firmly between the thumb and fingers, separating it from the underlying structures in the neck (as in Fig. 7.6C). The digits first encircle the entire muscle near its mid-belly and then examine separately the deep and superficial divisions for palpable bands,[25] deep tenderness, and local twitch responses. Snapping a band between the fingers at the TP regularly produces a visible twitch response, which is seen as a slight jerk of the head, if it is free to move. The TPs may lie close to the upper or lower attachments, at the mid-level of either division, or at all levels of the muscle. Both divisions must be examined thoroughly.

A prickling sensation in the face, over the mandible, which is the characteristic referred response of TPs in the overlying platysma muscle, may inadvertently be triggered while palpating the sternocleidomastoid muscle. This may startle and concern the patient, especially if this unexpected sensation is not explained (see Fig. 13.1 in Chapter 13).

10. ENTRAPMENTS

When the spinal accessory nerve (cranial nerve XI) penetrates the sternocleidomastoid muscle en route to the trapezius muscle, myogenic torticollis due to contracture of the sternocleidomastoid muscle can cause paresis of the trapezius muscle on the same side.[33]

11. ASSOCIATED TRIGGER POINTS

When TPs are present in one sternocleidomastoid muscle, they usually are found in the opposite muscle. The scalene muscles also tend to develop TPs, especially if the sternocleidomastoid has been affected for a considerable period of time, usually several weeks. If the neck motion (rotation) is "stiff," TPs may be present in the levator scapulae, trapezius, splenius cervicis, and other posterior neck muscles.[45]

An anomalous sternalis muscle may develop satellite TPs as a result of primary TPs in the lower end of the sternal division. Such satellite TPs in the sternalis refer pain deep under the sternum and across the upper pectoral region to the arm on the same side. The pectoral muscles, in turn, may develop another set of satellite TPs. The masseter, temporalis, orbicularis oculi and frontalis muscles tend to develop satellite TPs, since they also lie within pain reference zones of the sternocleidomastoid muscle TPs.

12. STRETCH AND SPRAY
(Fig. 7.5)

The patient sits comfortably and relaxed in a low-backed firm-seated armchair with the fingers of each hand hooked under the chair seat. A small hemipelvis, if present, should be corrected by leveling the patient's pelvis with a butt lift before starting treatment (see Fig. 48.9D in Chapter 48). When multiple neck muscles harbor TPs, stretch and spray are applied first to the

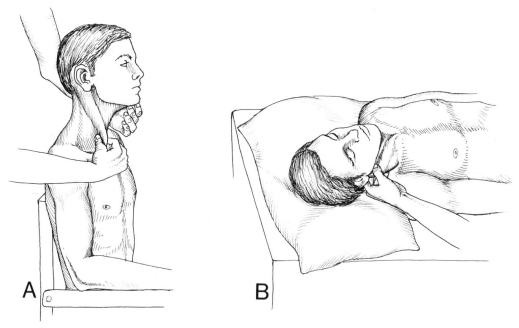

Figure 7.4. Examination of the sternocleidomastoid muscle may be done with the patient seated or supine. *A*, examination of the lower end of the sternal division, with the patient seated. *B*, examination of the deeper clavicular division, with the patient supine and the head tilted toward the same side, to slacken the muscle and permit the examiner to lift it off the underlying structures.

trapezius and levator scapulae muscles, so as to insure sufficient range of head and neck rotation to permit a full passive stretch of the sternal division of the sternocleidomastoid. It may be necessary to alternate treatment between the clavicular division of the sternocleidomastoid and the scalene muscles in order to obtain the full range of motion and maximal length of the muscle. To help the patient relax the neck muscles, the patient's head may be cradled in the operator's hand, with the head resting against the operator's arm or chest. The patient is encouraged to rest the weight of the head on the operator and to use abdominal breathing, which also assists relaxation.

The clavicular division of the muscle is gradually stretched by bending the head and neck backward and rotating it so that the face turns toward the opposite side (Fig. 7.5*A*), as also illustrated by Zohn and Mennell.[62] Pressure to increase the stretch is applied within the patient's ability to remain relaxed. Immediately preceding and during this passive stretching, the vapocoolant spray is applied in slow parallel sweeps from the muscle's lower at-

tachment on the clavicle, upward to its upper attachment on the mastoid process and occiput. The sweeps are continued behind the ear and across the forehead to cover the pain reference zones.[52]

The sternal division of the muscle is passively stretched by first turning the head toward the same side (Fig. 7.5*B*). Then, at full rotation, the chin is tipped downward to the shoulder. This movement elevates the occiput and mastoid process to secure maximal stretch on the muscle (Fig. 7.5*C*). While thus stretching the sternal division, sweeps of the spray are applied upward from the sternal attachment around the neck, covering the muscle to the mastoid region and occiput (Fig. 7.5*C*). Each rotation is carefully coordinated with a sweep of the spray to stay ahead of the loss of access to the skin over the muscle due to closure of neck space as the head rotates (Fig. 7.5*C*). The sweeps are extended to cover all sternocleidomastoid pain reference zones (Fig. 7.5*D*).

Holding the head rotated in the fully stretched position should be limited to only a few seconds. This position may

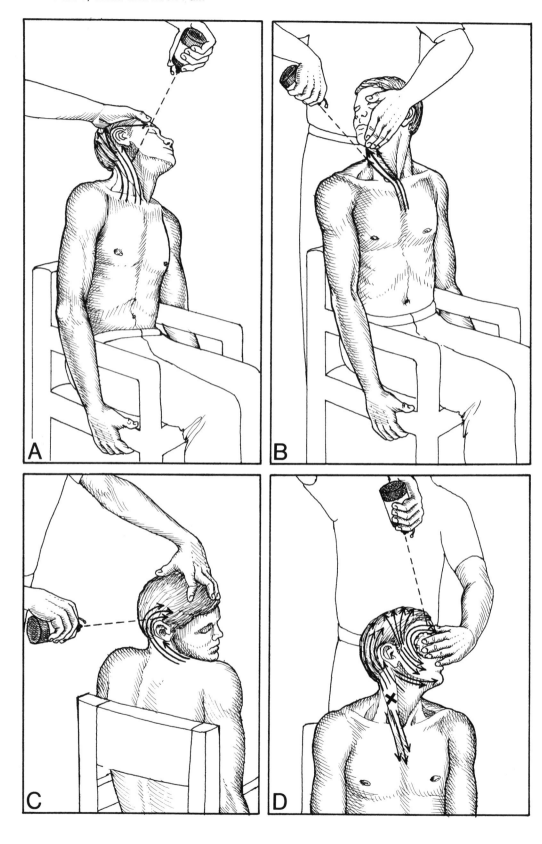

occlude an atherosclerotic vertebral artery at the base of the skull and, if held too long, can cause dimming of vision and dizziness.

For the deep-ear pain reference, one sweep should cross and enter the auditory canal, after warning the patient first. In 1902, Politzer[34] recommended brief spraying of the tympanic membrane with ethyl chloride for relief of pain due to acute otitis media.

Stretch and spray are always applied to both the right and left sternocleidomastoid muscles. The increased range of head rotation achieved by releasing the sternocleidomastoid on one side is likely to induce reactive cramping of the suddenly shortened contralateral muscle. This can cause afterpain and dizziness, due to activation of latent contralateral TPs by this unaccustomed shortening. Also, a few sweeps of the spray are applied downward over the sternal and pectoral areas while the patient inhales deeply. If this is not done, palpation or treatment of very irritable TPs in the sternocleidomastoid muscles may activate pre-existing latent TPs in the sternalis and pectoralis muscles and, within minutes or hours, produce an attack of chest pain.

After stretch and spray, hot packs are applied at once over treated muscles. When sternocleidomastoid TPs are hyperirritable in the acute post-traumatic stage, the muscles should be relieved of load by support without immobilization; a Thomas plastic collar may be worn upside down for a chin rest, or a soft collar may be worn loosely. There should be room for head rotation, with space at the side for the chin when looking around.

13. INJECTION AND STRETCH
(Fig. 7.6)

The sternocleidomastoid TPs often react to injection therapy with head pain and more local soreness than do other muscles, perhaps because of the multiplicity of TPs,

some of which remain active in spite of treatment, or because of the strong autonomic influence of its TPs. Injection of TPs should be undertaken only after maximum benefit has been obtained for that patient by stretch and spray of the muscle. After injection, the patient should plan to rest in bed and apply moist hot packs at home. If the patient must take a trip, or is committed to activity immediately afterward, then it is wise to stretch and spray the muscle and to defer its injection. The muscle on ONE SIDE only is injected during a visit. On the second side, TPs should be injected only after any reaction to the previous injection has subsided, and if a good result was obtained.

For injection, the patient lies supine (Fig. 7.6). The muscle is slackened by tilting the ear toward the shoulder on the affected side with the face turned slightly upward and to the opposite side; the pillow is placed under the shoulder of the same side to lift the chest and further slacken the muscle. The entire muscle should be encompassed by the examiner's thumb and fingers and lifted off the underlying blood vessels, nerves and scalene muscles (Fig. 7.6C).

The course of the external jugular vein is outlined by blocking the vein with a finger just above the clavicle. If the midlevel of the muscle is being injected, the vein can be shifted either laterally or medially by the finger to avoid penetrating it. The vein is illustrated in Figure 12.5A in Chapter 12, and in Figure 20.8A in Chapter 20.

A 22- to 25-gauge needle, preferably 24 gauge, that is 3.8 cm (1½ in) long, is selected. Penetration of the needle into the TP at the precise point of maximal tenderness is confirmed by a local twitch response and by projection of the predicted pattern of referred pain.

Through a single skin puncture, multiple needlings with continuous injection of 1 or 2 ml of 0.5% procaine solution can be car-

---

Figure 7.5.   Stretch positions and spray patterns for the right sternocleidomastoid muscle. The direction of the sweeps is shown by the arrows. *A,* clavicular division. *B,* sternal division, initial stretch position. *C,* sternal division, concluding stretch by tilting the face downward. *D,* completing coverage of distant pain reference zones with the vapocoolant spray to include the forehead bilaterally and the homolateral cheek, occiput, ear, submandibular region and sternum, and also the top of the head, if this region is part of the patient's pattern of pain.

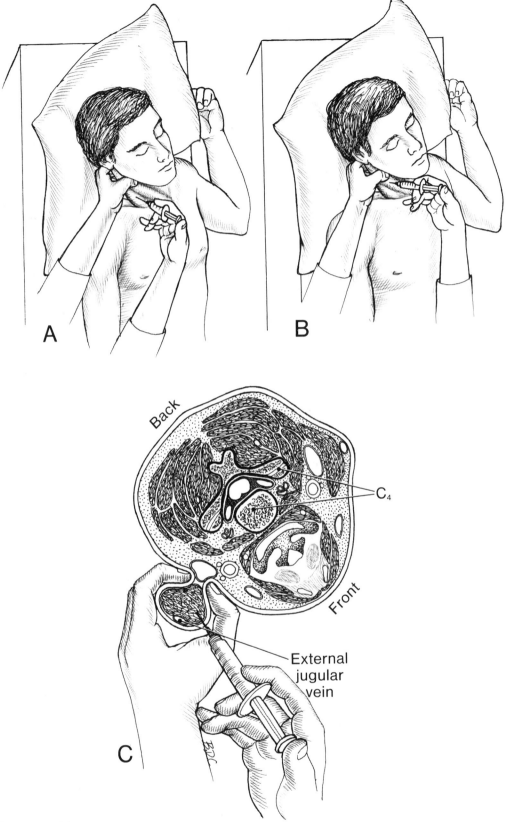

Figure 7.6. Injection of the right sternocleidomastoid muscle, with the patient supine, head tilted toward the same side and the face turned away. *A*, mid-portion of the clavicular (deep) division. *B*, mid-portion of the sternal (superficial) division. *C*, injection seen in anatomical cross section, at the level of the 4th cervical vertebra.

ried out until pain and twitch responses are no longer elicited by the probing needle.[24, 48] Then, with the needle held just under the skin, the muscle can be palpated for any residual firm bands that still harbor TPs, which are still tender and capable of local twitch responses. If such TPs are present, further probing with the needle should inactivate them. Usually, TPs in the superficial, more medial sternal division are inactivated first (Fig. 7.6B), then the TPs in the deeper and more posterior clavicular division (Fig. 7.6A).

Hemostasis at the injection site is applied by compressing the injected muscle between the fingers *during* and *after* the injection to avoid bleeding. Ecchymosis is unsightly and increases postinjection soreness. If the patient smokes, or is exposed to smoke, the diet should be supplemented with ascorbic acid, four daily doses of 500 mg each, for a few days before injection.

After injection, a hot pack is applied over the muscle at once, while the patient lies on the treated side with a pillow between the head and shoulder to lift the chin and place the sternocleidomastoid muscle in a neutral position (see Fig. 7.7C). After a few minutes of moist heat, the muscle is checked again for tenderness and local twitch responses.

The muscle is then stretched and sprayed essentially as in Fig. 7.5. If spot tenderness in the muscle has not been eliminated, ischemic compression with the muscle on a partial stretch is employed to inactivate residual TPs while some local procaine effect remains.

The patient is taught how to load the uninjected opposite sternocleidomastoid muscle when lifting the head to rise from the supine position. Turning the face to the same side relieves the recently injected muscle of possible strain until the local tissue soreness from needling has disappeared, which may require several days.

After the treatment, a soft cervical collar, worn loosely, may be helpful to support the head and inhibit sudden rotary and side motions while riding in a car as a passenger. Otherwise, a pillow may be placed between the patient's head and the car window to support the head from the side and to rest the sternocleidomastoid muscle.

At home after the treatment, the patient should relax in bed and, using a hot moist pack (or a wetproof heating pad with a dampened cover), lie in the most comfortable position. The patient should apply the hot pack on retiring at night. A mild analgesic, such as acetaminophen, two tablets (0.325 g each) two or three times daily, may reduce postinjection discomfort. Strenuous activity should be avoided for a few days.

Subsequently, with similar precautions, TPs in the contralateral sternocleidomastoid muscle may be injected, if indicated.

Occasionally, during the injection of TPs at or above the mid-level of the sternocleidomastoid muscle, the patient may describe a numbness in the face, which involves tissue deeper than the skin. The patient can still feel light touch, heat and cold, and also may feel a prickling pain in the angle of the jaw, cheek and pinna of the ear. These symptoms may be due to procaine infiltration of the posterior branch of the greater auricular nerve, which loops around and traverses the face of the sternocleidomastoid muscle.[1] If this nerve is blocked by 0.5 procaine solution, the sensation of numbness disappears in 15 or 20 min, as the local anesthetic effect dissipates.

It is rarely necessary to infiltrate the inferior end of the clavicular division of the muscle. If so, it must be kept in mind that this location overlies the apex of the lung and, therefore, must be injected with care to avoid penetrating the lung and causing a pneumothorax.

14. CORRECTIVE ACTIONS
(Fig. 7.7)

Posture and Activity Stress

When a person sits up from the supine position facing forward, the sternocleidomastoid muscles flex the neck and lift the head, which heavily loads them. The patient should be taught, when lifting the head, to turn it and unload the affected muscle by using the opposite, less involved sternocleidomastoid. Similarly, the patient may wish to rotate the head slightly when doing a Sit-back or Sit-up Exercise. When turning over in bed at night, the patient should roll the head on the pillow, **not** lift the head. With bilateral involvement, the patient may need to get out of bed by backing up from the prone position, thus avoiding overload of these anterior muscles on either side.

A small pillow behind the neck produces moderate (normal) cervical lordosis, and a side pillow limits head rotation at night. The patient should tuck the corner of the pillow between the shoulder and chin (Fig. 7.7, *A* and *C*), NOT under the shoulder (Fig. 7.7 *B* and *D*). The latter arrangement causes prolonged shortening of the anterior neck muscles on one side during sleep.

Postural strain is avoided by training patients to straighten their posture and to hold the head erect, not projected forward, when sitting and standing (see Fig. 42.9 in Chapter 42). When standing, the patient transfers the body weight from the heels toward the balls of the feet and leans forward from the ankles; the head then acts as a counterweight and the body automatically assumes a more erect position. The shoulders should hang loosely.

Revision of the patient's chair may be required to eliminate a headrest that pushes the occiput forward. A lumbar pillow is often essential to restore both the normal lumbar and cervical curves.

Nearsightedness should be corrected, since it favors a head-forward posture, which shortens the sternocleidomastoid muscles.

The muscles supporting the head are abused when the bed lamp is placed at one side of the bed (Fig. 7.3*B*). The light should be located directly overhead, either on the headboard (Fig. 7.3*A*), or suspended from the ceiling.

The patient should hold the telephone receiver in one hand, not between the head and shoulder, and at intervals, use the opposite hand to hold the receiver (not changing ears); this varies the tilt of the head. If a patient does much telephoning, an executive (speaker) telephone is recommended, instead of a handset.

Swimming the crawl stroke is hazardous, especially if breathing is done by turning the head to the opposite side from that of the affected sternocleidomastoid muscle, which contracts it strongly in the shortened position.

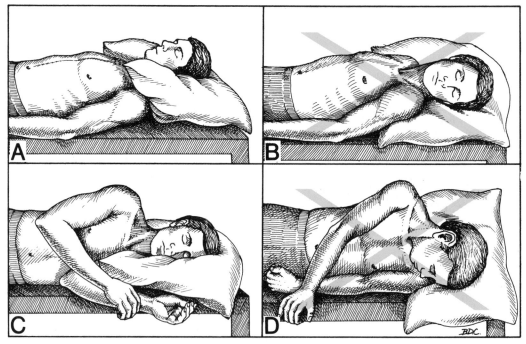

Figure 7.7. Positioning of the pillow for relief of the sternocleidomastoid myofascial syndrome. *A, correct* position, patient supine with the corners of the pillow tucked between the chin and shoulders. *B, wrong* position, patient supine, with the pillow *under* the shoulders. *C, correct* position, patient side-lying, with the pillow between the head and shoulder. *D, wrong* position, patient side-lying, with the chin in the hollow of the shoulder and the pillow under the shoulder, placing the sternocleidomastoid and scalene muscles in a shortened position.

The patient should **not** do head-rolling exercises; they readily over-stretch affected muscles, catching them off guard.

Activities that require prolonged neck extension in overhead work overload the checkrein function of the sternocleidomastoid muscles.

Body Asymmetry

The head stabilization function of these muscles is abused by the seesaw tilting of the shoulder-girdle axis when a short leg and/or small hemipelvis is not corrected by suitable lifts (see Figs. 48.8 and 48.9 in Chapter 48).

Pillow

At night, this muscle is especially vulnerable to the jiggling, vibratory movements caused by a foam rubber pillow, often prescribed to eliminate feather allergens. Symptoms may recur within a day or two with reactivation of sternocleidomastoid TPs, if the patient again sleeps on a bouncy foam pillow. The comfortable home pillow should go along on trips, whenever possible.

Constriction

Pressure on the sternocleidomastoid muscles and activation of TPs may be caused by tightness of the shirt collar. The examiner's finger should fit comfortably inside the collar, not only when the patient is looking straight ahead, but also when the head is turned, which increases the diameter of the neck inside the collar. Constriction also can be caused by cinching the necktie too tightly.

Chronic Infection

Sources of chronic infection, as listed in Chapter 4, must be eliminated.

Exercise

For a home stretch-exercise, the patient does the Side-bending Neck Exercise, by bringing the ear to the shoulder first on one side, then on the other, while lying supine (see Fig. 20.12 in Chapter 20). When performing the In-doorway Stretch Exercise for pectoralis TPs, the patient who also has sternocleidomastoid TPs, must not project the head forward, but should keep it erect by looking up slightly. Look-ing down shortens the sternocleidomastoid muscles, aggravating their TP activity.

The patient should breathe with the chest and diaphragm correctly coordinated, not in a paradoxical manner (see Fig. 20.13 in Chapter 20). The habit of correct abdominal breathing should be established by an exercise program, if the patient has this problem.

Supplemental References, Case Reports

The total management of patients with sternocleidomastoid TPs is detailed in case reports by the senior author.[47, 53, 55, 58]

References

1. Alberti PWRM: The greater auricular nerve. *Arch Otolaryngol* 76:422–424, 1962.
2. Basmajian JV: *Muscles Alive*, Ed. 4. Williams & Wilkins, Baltimore, 1978 (pp. 356, 398).
3. Bates T: Myofascial pain, Chapter 14. In *Ambulatory Pediatrics II. Personal Health Care of Children in the Office*, edited by M. Green and R.J. Haggerty. W.B. Saunders, Philadelphia, 1977 (pp. 147–148).
4. Brain WR, Walton JN: *Brain's Diseases of the Nervous System*, Ed. 7. Oxford University Press, New York, 1969 (pp. 517, 541–543).
5. Brody SI: Sore throat of myofascial origin. *Milit Med* 129:9–19, 1964.
6. Broer MR, Houtz SJ: *Patterns of Muscular Activity in Selected Sports Skill*. Charles C Thomas, Springfield, Ill., 1967.
7. Brudny J, Grynbaum BB, Korein J: Spasmodic torticollis: treatment of feedback display of the EMG. *Arch Phys Med Rehabil* 55:403–408, 1974.
8. Campbell EMJ: Accessory muscles, Chapter 9. In *The Respiratory Muscles, Mechanics and Neutral Control*, edited by E.M.J. Campbell, E. Agostoni, J.N. Davis, Ed. 2. W.B. Saunders, 1970 (pp. 183–186).
9. Carter BL, Morehead J, Wolpert SM, *et al.*: *Cross-Sectional Anatomy*. Appleton-Century-Crofts, New York, 1977 (Sects. 9–21).
10. Cohen LA: Body orientation and motor coordination in animals with impaired neck sensation. *Fed Proc* 18:28, 1959.
11. Cohen, LA: Role of eye and neck proprioceptive mechanisms in body orientation and motor coordination. *J Neurophysiol* 24:1–11, 1961.
12. Denny-Brown DE: Neurologic aspects of vertigo. *N Engl J Med* 241:144, 1949.
13. Duchenne GB: *Physiology of Motion*, translated by E.B. Kaplan. J.B. Lippincott, Philadelphia, 1949 (p. 479).
14. Eisler P: *Die Muskeln des Stammes*. Gustav Fischer, Jena, 1912 (pp. 235, 239).
15. Gilbert GJ: The medical treatment of spasmodic torticollis. *Arch Neurol* 27:503–506, 1972.
16. Good MG: Senile vertigo caused by curable cervical myopathy. *J Am Geriatr Soc* 5:662–667, 1957.
17. Gray H: *Anatomy of the Human Body*, edited by C.M. Goss, American Ed. 29. Lea & Febiger, Philadelphia, 1973 (pp. 395, 396, 946, 960).

18. Gutstein M: Diagnosis and treatment of muscular rheumatism. *Br J Phys Med* 1:302–321, 1938 (p. 311).

19. Halpern L: Biological significance of head posture in unilateral disequilibrium. *Arch Neurol Psychiatr* 72:160–180, 1954 (Case 3).

20. Hoefnagel D, Biery B: Spasmus nutans. *Dev Med Child Neurol* 10:32–35, 1968.

21. Hollinshead WH: *Functional Anatomy of the Limbs and Back*, Ed. 4. W.B. Saunders, Philadelphia, 1976 (pp. 101, 377).

22. Horton CE, Crawford HH, Adamson JE, et al.: Torticollis. *South Med J* 60:953–958, 1967.

23. Kellgren JH: Deep pain sensibility. *Lancet* 1:943–949, 1949.

24. Kraus H: *Clinical Treatment of Back and Neck Pain*. McGraw-Hill, New York, 1970 (pp. 97, 104, 105).

25. Lange M: *Die Muskelhärten (Myogelosen)*. J.F. Lehmanns, München, 1931 (pp. 88, 89, Fig. 30).

26. Llewellyn LJ, Jones AB: *Fibrositis*. Rebman, New York, 1915 (pp. 201, 203).

27. Long C, II: Myofascial Pain Syndromes: Part II—Syndromes of the head, neck and shoulder girdle. *Henry Ford Hosp Med Bull* 4:22–28, 1956 (p. 23).

28. Marbach JJ: Arthritis of the temporomandibular joints. *Am Fam Physician* 19:131–139, 1979 (Fig. 9D).

29. McMinn RMH, Hutchings RT: *Color Atlas of Human Anatomy*. Year Book Medical Publishers, 1977 (p. 35).

30. *Ibid.* (pp. 37, 108).

31. Middleton DS: The pathology of congenital torticollis. *Br J Surg* 18:188–204, 1930.

32. Mikhail M, Rosen H: History and etiology of myofascial pain-dysfunction syndrome. *J Prosthet Dent* 44:438–444, 1980.

33. Motta A, Trainiti G: Paralysis of the trapezius associated with myogenic torticollis. *Ital J Orthop Traumatol* 3:207–213, 1977.

34. Politzer A: *A textbook of Diseases of the Ear*, Ed. 4. Lea Bros & Co., Philadelphia, 1902 (p. 642).

35. Rasch PJ, Burke RK: *Kinesiology and Applied Anatomy*. Lea & Febiger, Philadelphia, 1967 (pp. 231, 233, 258).

36. Reynolds MD: Myofascial trigger point syndromes in the practice of rheumatology. *Arch Phys Med Rehabil* 62:111–114, 1981 (Tables 1 and 2).

37. Sharav Y, Tzukert A, Refaeli B: Muscle pain index in relation to pain, dysfunction, and dizziness associated with the myofascial pain-dysfunction syndrome. *Oral Surg* 46:742–747, 1978.

38. Snyder CH: Paroxysmal torticollis in infancy. *Am J Dis Child* 117:458–460, 1969.

39. Sobotta J, Figge FHJ: *Atlas of Human Anatomy*, Ed. 9, Vol. 1. Hafner Division, Macmillan, New York, 1974 (p. 174).

40. *Ibid.* (pp. 242, 246).

41. *Ibid.* (p. 169).

42. Sobotta J, Figge FHJ: *Atlas of Human Anatomy*, Ed. 9, Vol. 3. Hafner Division of Macmillan, New York, 1974 (p. 242).

43. Spalteholz W: *Handatlas der Anatomie des Menschen*, Ed. 11, Vol. 2. S. Hirzel, Leipzig, 1922 (p. 270).

44. Toldt C: *An Atlas of Human Anatomy*, translated by M.E. Paul, Ed. 2, Vol. 1. Macmillan, New York, 1919 (p. 292).

45. Travell J: Rapid relief of acute "stiff neck" by ethyl chloride spray. *J Am Med Wom Assoc* 4:89–95, 1949.

46. Travell J: Pain mechanisms in connective tissue. In *Connective Tissues, Transactions of the Second Conference, 1951*. Josiah Macy, Jr. Foundation, New York, 1952 (pp. 86–125).

47. Travell J: Referred pain from skeletal muscle: pectoralis major syndrome of breast pain and soreness and sternomastoid syndrome of headache and dizziness. *NY State J Med* 55:331–339, 1955.

48. Travell J: Symposium on mechanism and management of pain syndromes. *Proc Rudolf Virchow Med Soc* 16:128–136, 1957 (pp. 4, 5, Figs. 2, 3).

49. Travell J: Temporomandibular joint pain referred from muscles of the head and neck. *J Prosthet Dent* 10:745–763, 1960.

50. Travell J: Mechanical headache. *Headache* 7:23–29, 1967.

51. Travell J: *Office Hours: Day and Night*. The World Publishing Company, New York, 1968 (p. 271).

52. *Ibid.* (pp. 293–294).

53. Travell J: Identification of myofascial trigger point syndromes: a case of atypical facial neuralgia. *Arch Phys Med Rehabil* 62:100–106, 1981.

54. Travell J, Bigelow NH: Role of somatic trigger areas in the patterns of hysteria. *Psychosom Med* 9:353–363, 1947.

55. Travell J, Rinzler SH: Pain syndromes of the chest muscles: Resemblance to effort angina and myocardial infarction, and relief by local block. *Can Med Assoc J* 59:333–338, 1948 (pp. 334, 335, Case 2).

56. Travell J, Rinzler SH: The myofascial genesis of pain. *Postgrad Med* 11:425–434, 1952.

57. Webber TD: Diagnosis and modification of headache and shoulder-arm-hand syndrome. *JAOA* 72:61–74, 1973 (p. 8, Figs. 20–23).

58. Weeks, VD, Travell J: Postural vertigo due to trigger areas in the sternocleidomastoid muscle. *J Pediatr* 47:315–327, 1955.

59. Williams HL: The syndrome of physical or intrinsic allergy of the head: myalgia of the head (sinus headache). *Proc Staff Meet Mayo Clinic*, 20:177–183, 1945.

60. Williams HL, Elkins, EC: Myalgia of the head. *Arch Phys Ther* 23:14–22, 1942.

61. Wyant GM: Chronic pain syndromes and their treatment. II. Trigger points. *Can Anaesth Soc J* 26:216–219, 1979 (Patient 1, and Fig. 1a).

62. Zohn DA, Mennell J McM: *Musculoskeletal Pain: Diagnosis and Physical Treatment*. Little, Brown & Company, Boston, 1976 (Figs. 9–12, 7-4C).

CHAPTER 8
Masseter Muscle
"The Trismus Muscle"

HIGHLIGHTS: **REFERRED PAIN** from trigger points (TPs) in the superficial layer of the masseter muscle may be projected to the eyebrow, maxilla, mandible anteriorly, and to the upper or lower molar teeth, which become hypersensitive to pressure and temperature change. In the deep layer of the muscle, TPs refer pain deep in the ear and to the region of the temporomandibular joint (TMJ). **ANATOMICAL ATTACHMENTS** of the masseter are located, above, on the zygomatic arch and maxilla and, below, on the outer surface of the ramus and angle of the mandible. **ACTIONS** of the masseter (superficial fibers) are primarily to elevate the mandible, and for the deep fibers to retrude it. **SYMPTOMS** of active TPs in this muscle are chiefly pain and trismus (marked restriction of opening of the jaws). *Unilateral tinnitus* may be a symptom of TPs high in the *deep* portion of the muscle. **ACTIVATION OF TRIGGER POINTS** results from gross trauma, the microtrauma of bruxism or chronic overwork, acute overload, occlusal imbalance, and holding the mandible in other than a rest position for prolonged periods. **PATIENT EXAMINATION** reveals restriction of the mandibular opening to two-thirds, or less, of the normal aperture (at least 45 mm for women and 50 mm for men). The jaws admit a tier of no more than two knuckles between the incisor teeth, instead of the normal three knuckles. **TRIGGER POINT EXAMINATION** requires that the jaws be propped open slightly. This places the masseter fibers on sufficient stretch to make the taut bands and TP spot tenderness palpable. **ASSOCIATED TRIGGER POINTS** are likely to develop in the ipsilateral temporalis and medial pterygoid muscles, and in the contralateral masseter muscle. Masseter TP activity is often a satellite manifestation of sternocleidomastoid TPs, and may be secondary to TMJ arthropathy. **STRETCH AND SPRAY** are done best by having the patient pull forward and then down on the mandible, or by propping the jaws open as wide as possible, as with the cardboard cylinder of the spray bottle. Meanwhile, sweeps of spray are directed upward over the muscle and its referred pain pattern. The seated, or supine patient can assist by pulling forward and then down on the mandible, stretching the masseter while the operator applies the spray. **INJECTION AND STRETCH** at the mid-level of the muscle employ a pincer grasp, with one digit localizing a TP in the superficial portion from inside the mouth and another digit pressing from the outside. Other masseter TPs are palpated and injected against underlying bone. **CORRECTIVE ACTIONS** include the avoidance of mouth breathing and exhaustive chewing; avoidance of clenching and grinding of teeth; the regular use of passive self-stretch exercises that sometimes incorporate reciprocal muscle inhibition; the elimination of premature tooth contacts; and the inactivation of related TPs in muscles of the neck or other distant parts of the body.

---

1. REFERRED PAIN
(Fig. 8.1)

Superficial Layer

Myofascial trigger points (TPs) in the superficial layer of the masseter muscle refer pain mainly to the lower jaw, molar teeth and related gums, and to the maxilla.[34, 80–82] When located in the anterior border and *upper* part of this layer, TPs refer pain to the upper molar teeth, adjacent gums, and maxilla.[34, 80] The maxillary pain is often described by the patient as "sinusitis" (Fig. 8.1*A*). When the TPs are

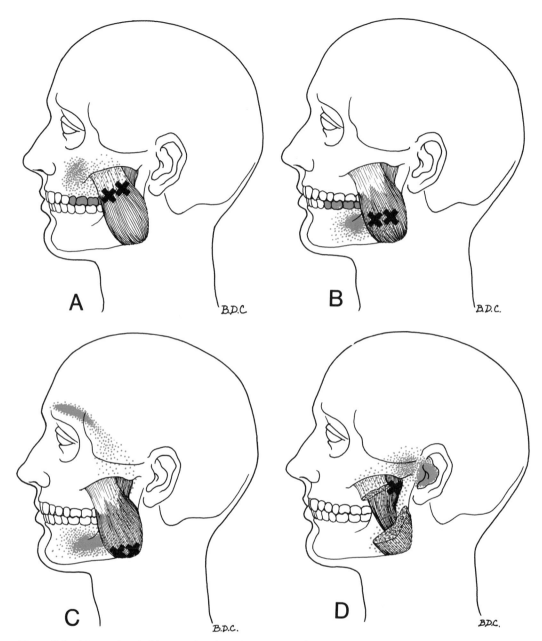

Figure 8.1.   The ×s locate trigger points in various parts of the masseter muscle. *Solid red* shows essential referred pain zones, and the *stippled areas* are spillover pain zones. *A,* superficial layer, upper portion. *B,* superficial layer, mid-belly. *C,* superficial layer, lower portion. *D,* deep layer, upper part—just below the temporomandibular joint.

located just *below* the mid-belly of the muscle, they refer pain to the lower molar teeth and mandible (Fig. 8.1*B*).[80, 86] From TPs along the lower edge of the mandible close to its angle, pain is projected in an arc that extends across the temple and over the eyebrow; it also is referred to the lower jaw (Fig. 8.1*C*).[31, 80–82] A masseter TP at the gonial angle may refer pain preauricularly in the region of the TMJ.[69] Prolonged pain responses to a thermal stimulus to a tooth may indicate a pulpitis, whereas sensitivity to percussion and pressure can result from inflammation of

PART 1

the periodontal ligament.[58] Referred pain and tenderness from TPs in the masseter (or temporalis) muscle may cause tooth hypersensitivity to any or all stimuli: occlusal pressure, percussion, heat, and cold.

Deep Layer

The TPs in the underlying deep layer of the masseter muscle which lie over the ramus of the mandible are likely to refer pain diffusely to the mid-cheek area in the region of the lateral pterygoid muscle and sometimes of the TMJ. When a TP is found at a very precise point close to the posterior zygomatic attachment of the deep portion of the masseter, it is likely to refer pain deep into the ear, as in Fig. 8.1D.[7, 20, 50, 55, 80, 81] The latter TP also may cause tinnitus in the adjacent ear.[80] The tinnitus may be set off by pressure on the TP, or may be constant, but the patient may be unaware of its presence until it is stopped by inactivation of the TP. Stretching the jaws wide open may also either activate, or interrupt the tinnitus. The tinnitus is usually described as a "low roaring" and is not associated with the deafness and vertigo of a central neurological lesion.

Prevalence

Among the masticatory muscles, the masseter very frequently harbors TPs. In one study of 56 patients with the myofascial pain-dysfunction syndrome, the superficial portion of the masseter was the most commonly involved muscle, and the deep masseter was the fifth.[10] In another study of 277 patients with TMJ pain-dysfunction, 81% complained of pain. Of these patients with pain, the masseter was the second most commonly involved muscle (70% of that group); the lateral pterygoid was tender in 84% of the pain group.[26] Sharav and associates[60] observed that the masseter had the second highest prevalence of active TPs, namely, 69% of 42 patients with the myofascial pain-dysfunction syndrome, following lateral pterygoid TPs which were found in 83% of the patients. However, in another study, the masseter was the least commonly involved.[27] Solberg and coauthors[71] observed tenderness in the superficial masseter with limited mouth opening four times as often in subjects who reported awareness of bruxism as in those who did not.

Experimental Studies

Kellgren[31] experimentally induced referred pain from the masseter muscle in a normal subject by injecting 0.1 ml or 6% saline solution into its fibers just above the angle of the mandible. This procedure caused "toothache" of the upper jaw, pain in the region of the TMJ, and pain in the external auditory meatus.[31]

During maximum voluntary tooth clenching, electromyographic changes in the masseter correlated well with the onset of fatigue and the moment of muscle exhaustion, but did not relate to the onset of muscle pain.[12] This supports our understanding that the pain of which patients complain is more likely to be referred from TPs than due to spasm with excessive motor unit activity.

2. ANATOMICAL ATTACHMENTS
(Fig. 8.2)

Both superficial and deep layers of the masseter attach *above* to the zygomatic process of the maxilla and to the zygomatic arch (Fig. 8.2). *Below* the superficial layer attaches to the external surface of the mandible at its angle and to the inferior half of its ramus; the deep layer attaches to the superior half of the ramus,[24, 61] and may extend to the angle of the mandible.[17]

Supplemental References

The masseter muscle has been clearly illustrated in cross section,[21, 66] from the front,[64] from the side,[16, 22, 65, 72, 77] from below,[67, 76] and from behind.[73] The superficial portion has been shown with overlying structures (nerves and parotid gland).[23, 37] The fibers of the deep portion have been illustrated separately.[17, 66, 78]

3. INNERVATION

The masseter muscle is innervated by the masseteric nerve that arises from the anterior branch of the mandibular division of the trigeminal nerve (cranial nerve V).[25]

4. ACTIONS

The chief action of the muscle is to elevate the mandible and close the jaws, as during clenching into centric occlusion.[6, 24, 46, 85] The deep fibers also retrude the mandible.[6]

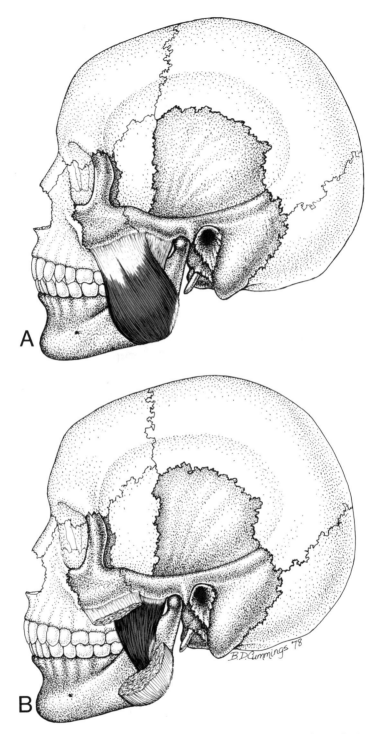

Figure 8.2.   Attachments of the masseter muscle. *A,* superficial layer. *B,* deep layer, with the superficial layer removed.

Electromyographically, the superficial portion of the masseter participated during simple protrusion in approximately one-third of 536 tests, but not during retrusion and depression.[17]

Normally, activity of the masseter is not required to maintain the mandibular rest position.[6] Generally, the masseter and temporalis muscles function closely together, with only minor differences in motor unit activity. The temporalis is more likely to respond for mandibular balance and posture control; the masseter is used for greater closing force.[74] During chewing of hard or soft foods, the masseter always responded before the temporalis.[6] In the mandibular rest position, the masseter showed little difference in electrical activity between the sitting and supine postures, but the temporalis activity was markedly affected by this change of position.[41]

One objective test demonstrated the modulation of reflex activity by active TPs in the masticatory muscles. A silent period of about 24 msec interrupts masseteric motor unit activity during jaw clench when a jaw-jerk response is produced by a tap on the chin,[5, 9] or by a tap on a tooth.[6] The silent period results primarily from stimulation of the receptors in the periodontal ligament, which surrounds the teeth.[9] The duration of the silent period was clearly increased among patients with severe symptoms of the myofascial pain-dysfunction syndrome,[35, 63] and was decreased following successful treatment.[60]

5. MYOTATIC UNIT

Synergists of the superficial layer of the masseter for mandibular elevation are the contralateral masseter and, bilaterally, the temporalis, medial pterygoid[6] and superior division of the lateral pterygoid muscles. Antagonists include the geniohyoid, omohyoid, and hypoglossus muscles, the anterior belly of the digastric, and the inferior division of the lateral pterygoid.

Synergistic with the deep layer of the masseter for retrusion of the mandible is the posterior portion of the temporalis. It is antagonized chiefly by the lower division of the lateral pterygoid muscle.

6. SYMPTOMS

Pain, as described in Section 1, is the major complaint. In many instances, "temporomandibular joint" symptoms are related to incoordination and increased "spasm" (tension) of the masticatory muscles, rather than to derangement of the joint itself.[26] Active TPs in the deep portion of the masseter can mimic the TMJ pain of rheumatic disease;[50] then, the masseter and lateral pterygoid are the muscles most likely to be involved.[10, 26, 60] Restriction of

jaw opening (trismus) is greater when the TPs are located in the superficial layer of the masseter than when they occur in the deep layer of the muscle. Surprisingly, the patient is often unaware of restriction, if the jaws open wide enough to bite a sandwich.[79]

Unilateral tinnitus may be associated with TPs in the upper posterior portion of the deep layer of the muscle. This symptom may be due to referred motor unit activity of the stapedius muscle of the tympanic membrane, which lies within the pain reference zone of these TPs. Spasm of the stapedius muscle could cause an oscillation of the middle ear ossicles. Unilateral tinnitus also may arise from TMJ intracapsular disease[59] and could be explained by the fascial connection between the TMJ and the middle ear.[48] If the tinnitus is bilateral, one should suspect a systemic, rather than a myofascial cause. However, the deep layer of the masseter can become involved bilaterally, giving rise to bilateral tinnitus. In this case, unilateral fluctuation in its intensity is likely to occur. Tinnitus may be due to a high serum salicylate level; drug-induced tinnitus is usually bilateral and dose-dependent,[42] not predominantly unilateral, as is typical of deep masseter TPs. Impairment of hearing is not a feature of masseteric TP activity.

Complex symptoms and overlapping patterns of facial pain may be referred from multiple TPs in the head and neck muscles, and can be more easily traced to the individual muscles producing each part of the total pattern, if the distribution of pain is sketched on a body form for each patient, as described by Bell[8] and as recommended by Melzack.[38]

7. ACTIVATION OF TRIGGER POINTS

Activity Stress

Masseteric TPs may be activated to cause pain and trismus by sustained or repetitive overwork, e.g., bruxism, the microtrauma of thumb sucking late in childhood, chewing gum incessantly, prolonged clamping of the jaws on the mouthpiece of a pipe or cigarette holder,[36] or biting off thread by a seamstress; by sudden forcible contraction of the masseter muscle, as in cracking nuts or ice between the teeth; by occlusal disharmony, especially with decreased vertical dimension due to worn natural teeth, loss of posterior teeth, worn denture teeth, or resorption of alveolar bone; and by mouth breathing (through a surgical mask, or due to nasal airway obstruction), which requires contraction of the masticatory muscles to hold the jaws open slightly, often with mandibular retrusion.

The masseter muscles are among the first to contract in persons who are in a state of extreme emotional tension, intense determination or desperation,[86] and they often remain contracted for abnormally long periods in patients who develop the temporomandibular pain-dysfunction syndrome.[87] The significant contribution of emotional stress and tension bruxism to TP pain has been well demonstrated in specific cases.[8] Unfortunately, the emotional component of pain is sometimes overemphasized, to the neglect of the myofascial TP contribution to internal derangements of the TMJ.[39]

Occlusal Disharmony

Sustained electrical activity (spasm) of a muscle under what would normally be rest conditions is likely to activate TPs in it. On this basis, the increase in the resting contractile activity of the masticatory muscles due to abnormal positioning of the mandible reinforces the clinical observation that occlusal disharmony can be a major factor in the activation of myofascial TPs in the masseter and temporalis muscles.[19]

In order to establish which teeth are making the premature contacts that constitute occlusal disharmony, a starting position must be established from which the jaws are closed in centric occlusion. Starting positions commonly considered are rest positions and centric relation.

Rest position. This may be determined clinically or electromyographically. As noted under Abnormal Occlusal Mechanics in Section B of Chapter 5, the clinical rest position of the mandible, as determined clinically by first having the patient vocalize and swallow,[62] is not easily reproduced; it is influenced by head position, age, tension and stress.[47]

The numerous reports of minimum or zero motor unit activity of the masseter and temporalis muscles in the mandibular rest position[29, 49, 62, 75] do not resolve: (1) how much misinformation may be introduced by inadequate amplification and a high noise level of the amplifiers used;[49] (2) the difference between the clinically obtained position and the EMG null position;[52, 53] (3) the ambiguity of what muscles contribute EMG activity to the surface pickup electrodes, and of what contribution the unmonitored medial pterygoid muscle is making; and (4) what contribution the tension of taut bands caused by myofascial TPs is making to mandibular position without contributing to the EMG recording. Using low-noise, high-gain amplifiers, Rugh and Drago[52] observed that the mean vertical dimension (mouth opening) for 10 normal subjects at electromyographic (EMG) null was at least three times larger than at the clinical rest position. Neither technique has gained widespread acceptance, and most dentists employ centric relation as the starting position.

Centric relation. This position is officially defined in three forms.[1] One definition is the most retruded position of the mandible from which it can make unstrained lateral excursions.[1] Another is the terminal hinge position (hinge axis) of the mandible.[57] That the mandible rotates without any translation in this position has been questioned.[30] The appropriateness of using centric relation, when determined in either of these ways to locate abnormal occlusal contacts, has been seriously challenged; centric relation was never encountered during chewing and swallowing in a study of 400 subjects.[29] There are also variations in the descriptions of how to position the jaws in centric relation.[13, 32, 45, 83] Also, condylar placement at rest and abnormal muscular activity may be additional critical factors in the interpretation of centric relations.[83]

The decision as to which definition of centric relation to use can be critical when it is the reference position from which faulty occlusal positions and abnormal occlusal contacts are determined as the mandible moves into centric occlusion. It is *not* described as simply the most retruded position of the mandible, but close to it. In practice, it is a position obtained through manipulation of the mandible of a *relaxed* patient. Thus, it is an operational maneuver that is not easily reduced to a few words. Detailed instructions by Dawson[13] describe a backward motion of the mandible with an upward rotary thrust that should, in patients with normal TMJ structure, seat the condyle superiorly in the thin portion of the intra-articular disc along the posterior slope of the articular eminence. This is the anatomical and functional position for predominantly hinge-axis rotation of the mandible. From this position, the patient then closes the jaws to centric occlusion. Locating a "normal" position of centric relation requires the development of considerable manipulative skill and may be impossible in many patients with active TPs in the masticatory muscles. Recognizing this, the multiplicity of definitions and techniques is understandable.

Centric occlusion. This is the position of jaw closure with full tooth contact and is defined as "the centered contact position of the occlusal surfaces of the mandibular teeth against the occlusal surfaces of the maxillary teeth",[1] or the customary position of the mandible when the teeth are in maximum intercuspation.[57] As the mandible shifts from the rest position to centric occlusion, the level of electrical activity of the masseter consistently increases.[49, 62]

Other Factors

Other factors that may activate latent TPs in the masseter muscle include prolonged over-stretching during a dental procedure; immobilization of the mandible in the closed position (by the head halter during continuous neck traction, or by wiring the jaws shut); the direct trauma of an accident; chronic pulpal or periodontal inflammation;[58] TMJ arthropathy; activation of satellite TPs by primary TPs in the sternocleidomastoid that refer pain to the masseteric region; and emotional distress.[56]

8. PATIENT EXAMINATION
(Fig. 8.3)

Marked restriction of mandibular vertical opening is evident on examination, although the patient may not be aware of it. Unilateral masseter TPs tend to deviate the mandible toward the affected side.

Knowledge of the normal maximal interincisal distance (measured as clearance between the incisor teeth) is needed to determine restriction of opening. Table 8.1 shows a larger average maximal opening in men than in women, and in three groups screened to eliminate those with masticatory dysfunction,[2, 3, 80] than in two unscreened groups of nonpatients.[4, 71] From her data, Travell[80] selected a 50-mm interincisal opening for men, and a 45-mm opening for women as the lower limit of normal for individuals of average height. Travell's[80] mean values were 4.3 mm larger than Agerberg's[3] for 16-year-old boys and the same as Agerberg's[3] for the 16-year-old girls, and were 3.5 mm larger than Agerberg's[2] male, and 2.0 mm larger than his female students. The screened students were medical students and student nurses,[80] naval cadets, dental and dental assistant students.[2] The two unscreened non-patient groups were students being enrolled in the student health service of the University of California at Los Angeles[71] and a randomly sampled one-third of the 3500 70-year-old inhabitants of Gothenburg, Sweden.[4]

The difference in mean values between the two screened groups may have been due largely to the rigor with which subjects who had latent TPs were eliminated from the two groups. Travell screened out all subjects who had *ever* experienced *any* headache, facial, or neck pain, who had any history of head or neck trauma, and who had *any* tenderness of the masticatory muscles on careful palpation.[80] Agerberg[2] screened 16-year-olds and students who had no known head trauma, TMJ luxation, or pain in or around the TMJ. The students were unaware of any present or past functional disorders of the masticatory system.[2] Palpation of the masticatory musculature and TMJs of the 16-year-olds produced no pain.[3] Among the students, palpation of the masticatory muscles and the TMJ joints produced no *severe* pain. Active maximal movements of the mandible produced no pain and showed no *great* deviations or irregularities.[2]

This effect of latent TPs was demonstrated by selecting a group of individuals who were unable to pass the Three-knuckle Test and who had no pain or known TMJ dysfunction at that time. After briefly stretching and spraying their masseter, medial pterygoid, and temporalis muscles, each subject could pass the test.

Table 8.1
Maximum interincisal opening and its lower limit of normal among men and women free of masticatory system signs and symptoms, and among unselected subjects some of whom had masticatory signs and symptoms.

	Men				Women				Source
	No.	Mean	Low Range	Mean −2 S.D.[a]	No.	Mean	Low Range	Mean −2 S.D.[a]	
		mm	mm	mm		mm	mm	mm	
Sign and Symptom-free									
16-year-olds	42	54.7	38	37.1	40	52.8	44	41.8	Agerberg[3]
Students	69	59	50		81	53	45		Travell[80]
Students	102	55.5	42	41.3	103	51.0	39	39.6	Agerberg[2]
Unselected									
70-year-olds	77	49.1		35.9	90	47.4		34.6	Agerberg and Österberg[4]
Students	369	54.4		40.1	370	50.9		37.5	Solberg et al.[71]

[a] Mean minus two standard deviations.

On further questioning, most of this group had a history of headaches or head and neck trauma. The rapidity with which the ruler measurement of interincisal opening was taken could easily have made a difference of a few millimeters; the digastric muscle tired quickly when holding maximal opening against the overwhelmingly more powerful elevators. Travell took the measurement quickly to catch the initial maximum aperture.

The unscreened mean and minimum values were smaller than the screened values, as would be expected. Agerberg[2] reported a significant correlation ($r = 0.35$, $p < 0.05$) between the maximal mouth opening and body height in men, but not in women. None of these opening measurements included vertical overbite.

Establishing the *truly unrestricted* (optimum health and function) interincisal opening is essential if one is to know when some restriction of mouth opening exists. Either active *or latent* TPs in the extremity and trunk muscles significantly restrict full lengthening of these muscles. We find the same to be true of the masticatory muscles.

A simple and convenient test is based on the observation that a tier of the first three knuckles (second, third and fourth digits) of the nondominant hand normally fits between the upper and lower incisor teeth (Fig. 8.3), if the masticatory muscles are free of TPs. This Three-knuckle Test was first reported by Dorrance[15] in 1929. However, in a population unscreened for subjects with masticatory symptoms and tender masticatory muscles, only a tier of the distal three finger *phalanges* (not knuckles) fitted between the incisor teeth of many subjects.[4] Many of those with latent TPs in the mandibular elevator muscles were unable to pass the more rigorous Three-knuckle Test; with very few exceptions, those free of TPs can pass it.

When active or latent TPs are present in the masseter muscles, the opening usually admits a tier of only two knuckles. Severe restriction by masseter TPs may limit the opening to one and one-half knuckles.

Measurement of the interincisal opening by forcing three knuckles between the teeth, or pushing the cardboard wedge between the teeth forces the mouth open slightly and results in a measurement sev-

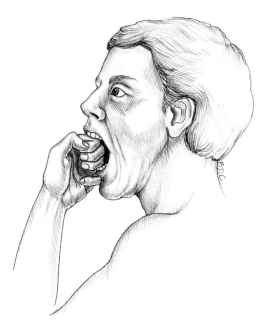

Figure 8.3. Three-knuckle Test. The fully opened jaws should admit the first three knuckles (non-dominant hand) in a tier between the incisor teeth of individuals with normal joint and bone structures and without demonstrable myofascial trigger points.

eral millimeters larger than that obtained with the usual Boley gauge or a millimeter rule used without exerting pressure.

It is a remarkable fact that TP activity in leg muscles due to a Dudley J. Morton foot,[43, 44] or TP activity in certain neck or shoulder-girdle muscles (sternocleidomastoid, trapezius, scalene, and pectoral) restricts mouth opening. Inactivation of TPs in these non-masticatory muscles can markedly increase the maximal interincisal opening, at once.

Anterior displacement of the articular disc and postoperative trismus due to activation of TPs in the medial pterygoid muscle also may restrict jaw opening severely, but temporalis or lateral pterygoid TPs usually limit it only minimally.

9. TRIGGER POINT EXAMINATION
(Fig. 8.4)

To examine the masseter for TPs, the jaws are propped open far enough to tauten the muscle just within the limit of pain. Palpation of TPs is done either by pressing the muscle against the mandible or, for the anterior portion of the superficial layer, by squeezing the muscle in a pincer grip with one digit placed inside and another outside the cheek (Fig. 8.4).[28] Tenderness of the masseter muscle at the gonial angle is disclosed by flat palpation and is significantly associated with bruxism.[71]

TPs in the deep layer of the masseter are located by palpation against the posterior portion of the ramus and along the base of the zygomatic buttress. Pressure on a TP in the upper posterior portion of the deep layer may activate unilateral tinnitus.

10. ENTRAPMENTS

The pterygoid venous plexus, which lies between the temporalis and the lateral pterygoid muscles and between the two pterygoid muscles, drains the temporalis muscle *via* the deep temporal vein and drains the infraorbital region *via* the orbital vein.[25] The plexus empties primarily into the maxillary vein. Entrapment of the maxillary vein may occur due to masseter TPs where it emerges between the masseter and the mandible.[68]

Engorgement of the deep temporal vein and pterygoid plexus favors bleeding and ecchymosis after injection of TPs in the temporalis muscle.

The increased firmness of taut bands

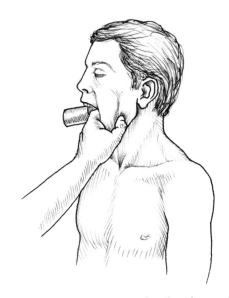

Figure 8.4. Pincer method for locating trigger points in the superficial portion of the masseter muscle. The muscle is stretched to its maximum non-painful length by a prop between the upper and lower teeth.

due to TPs in the masseter muscle may restrict venous flow from the infraorbital subcutaneous tissues. This engorgement of the orbital vein produces puffiness ("bags") beneath the eye on the affected side, and thus narrows the palpebral fissure. Narrowing of the fissure also may be caused by spasm due to activation of satellite TPs in the orbicularis oculi muscle, which lies in the pain reference zone of TPs in the sternal division of the sternocleidomastoid muscle.

11. ASSOCIATED TRIGGER POINTS

The main synergists of the masseter, *i.e.*, the temporalis and medial pterygoid muscles, tend to develop secondary TPs, as does the contralateral masseter.

Masseter TPs also may originate as satellites due to increased motor unit activity secondary to TPs in the sternal division of the sternocleidomastoid muscle.

In time, the digastric and the inferior division of the lateral pterygoid tend to develop active TPs, because of the increased demands placed on them as antagonists to the taut masseter fibers.

12. STRETCH AND SPRAY
(Figs. 8.5 and 8.6)

To inactivate TPs in the masseter muscle, the jaws are propped open with the muscles on a tolerable stretch. For this purpose, the cardboard cylinder from the nozzle of the vapocoolant spray bottle can act as a prop, or a small dental bite block may be placed horizontally between the incisor teeth (Fig. 8.5*A*). A wider opening is obtained by moving the prop back between the premolar, or molar teeth, closer to the TMJ. For a still larger opening, the prop may be cut down on a slant (Fig. 8.6) and inserted vertically between the incisor teeth (see Fig. 9.4, in Chapter 9). The tooth mark at maximal opening may be used as the patient's guide to the progress made during treatment.

Parallel sweeps of vapocoolant are directed upward over the muscle, from the mandible over the cheek, and over the pain reference zones in the temple and forehead (Fig. 8.5*A* and *B*), as also described by Bell.[8] The seated patient's head is tilted backward against the operator to reduce postural reflex tension in the masticatory muscles[40] and to prevent the vapocoolant

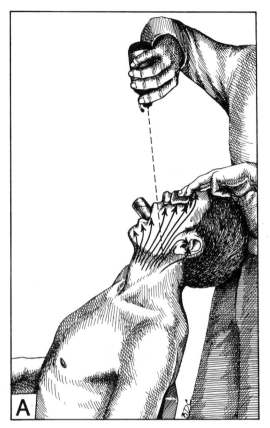

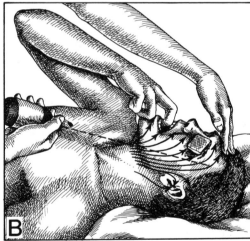

Figure 8.5. Stretch position and spray pattern (*arrows*) for trigger points in the masseter muscle. *A,* patient seated. For smaller or larger jaw openings, a cardboard prop may be cut on a slant, as in Fig. 8.6, and inserted as shown in Fig. 9.4, Chapter 9. *B,* supine patient applying self-stretch during vapocooling by the operator.

liquid from trickling into the eye; it is wise to cover the eye with an absorbent pad. The masseter muscles on *both* sides of the

PART 1

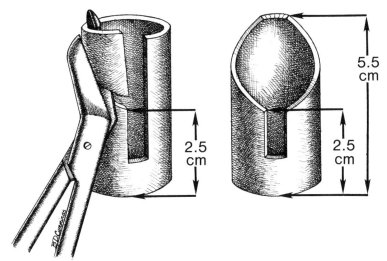

5.5 cm

2.5 cm

2.5 cm

Figure 8.6. Method of making a prop by cutting the cardboard cylinder that slips over the nozzle of each vapocoolant-spray bottle. The variable-height prop is used to adjust the degree of jaw opening, and to record the maximum opening between the incisor teeth (see Fig. 8.10).

face should be sprayed, since both are stretched and there is almost always some degree of bilateral TP involvement.

After removal of the prop, an increase in the mandibular range of active motion is measured by a change in the tooth mark (see Fig. 8.10), and the masseter is again palpated for residual TP tenderness. After rewarming the skin with a hot pack, stretch and spray may be repeated if restriction of opening or spot tenderness remains. The patient should yawn to open the jaws as wide as possible.

The effectiveness of stretch and spray is often improved by letting the patient do the passive stretching. Instead of having the jaws propped open, the patient inserts two fingers of one hand behind the lower incisor teeth and, with the thumb hooked behind the mandible under the chin, pulls the mandible forward and downward to *fully* open the jaws, while the operator applies the spray (Fig. 8.5B). This passive self-stretch may be effective when static stretch by the prop fails. The self-stretch is best done with the patient supine, to eliminate postural reflexes. Rat experiments support the clinical observation that head position and tonic neck reflexes strongly influence the masticatory muscles, including the masseter.[18] Additional release of muscle tension may be achieved by having the patient actively try to open the mouth while passively self-stretching

as above, thereby reciprocally inhibiting the stretched elevator muscles.

The patient must maintain the new range of motion by active and passive stretch exercises daily at home.

13. INJECTION AND STRETCH
(Fig. 8.7)

If the immediate response to stretch and spray is not satisfactory, injection of the masseter TPs usually inactivates them.[8] The mid-belly TPs are most effectively localized by pincer palpation just below the inferior border of the zygoma with the jaws propped open (Fig. 8.4) so that they can be fixed between the digits (Fig. 8.7A) for injection, either intraorally or extraorally. The TPs near the ends of the superficial layer are localized by flat palpation with the jaws propped open. For injection, the caudal group of TPs is fixed against the underlying mandible, and the upper group, against the base of the zygomatic buttress (Fig. 8.7B). A 2.5-cm (1-in), 23-gauge or 24-gauge needle is convenient. A 27-gauge needle is so fine that it slides around the TP without hitting it, just as it would around a tough vein.

To localize the TPs in the deep portion of the masseter for injection, the jaws are propped wide open, and the depression just below the knob-like head of the mandible is palpated in front of the external

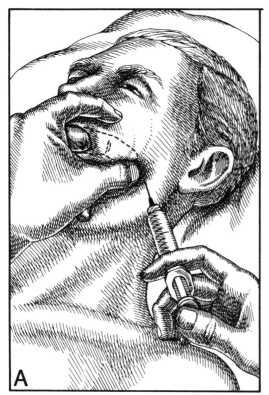
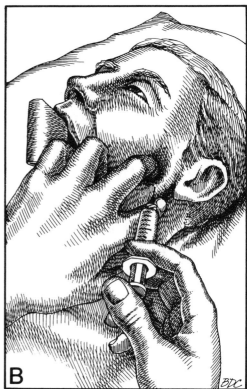

Figure 8.7. Injection of trigger points in the masseter muscle. *A*, mid-belly of the superficial portion, using pincer palpation to localize the trigger points for injection. *B*, deep portion of the muscle, using flat fixation of the trigger point.

auditory meatus. The deep masseter overlies the posterior portion of the ramus of the mandible.

The injection is followed with bilateral stretch and spray to inactivate any residual TPs, and then a hot pack is applied over the masseter on each side of the face.

14. CORRECTIVE ACTIONS
(Figs. 8.8–8.10)

Activity Stress

The patient should develop awareness of mandibular posture, avoid exhaustive chewing, and make the changes necessary to insure nose, rather than mouth, breathing. Habits of "clenching" the teeth should be revised by the pipe smoker and those who abuse their mandibular elevators, as in cracking hard candy or nuts with the teeth, and by constantly chewing gum. Bruxist behavior should be identified and treated.[53] These sources of excessive loading can also injure the TMJ itself.[70]

Occlusal Disharmony

As explained in Section 7, repetitive premature occlusal contacts and interferences may be the result of, or the cause of, myofascial TP activity in the masseter and other masticatory muscles. An occlusal splint or orthopaedic appliance that eliminates the stimulus of occlusal interference and provides needed occlusal stability may be invaluable for temporarily relieving pain referred from masticatory muscles. Using this pain-free time to inactivate the masticatory TPs helps to restore normal muscle balance and to return the articular discs to their normal position, *before* making a permanent occlusal correction. Improperly fitted occlusal splints may, in time, cause adverse tooth movement; placement of the condyles in an abnormally retruded position separates the molar teeth and allows them to supererupt and may be associated with the onset of the pain-dysfunction syndrome.[54]

For effective treatment of patients with the resultant myofascial pain-dysfunction syndrome, an understanding of myofascial TPs, TMJ function, and occlusal equilibration is essential. This may require closely coordinated dental and medical management,[14] since the lasting inactivation of myofascial TPs in the masticatory muscles often requires both dental procedures and medical expertise to eliminate perpetuating factors of systemic and mechanical origin, including the neck region and, sometimes, the lower extremities. Often overlooked causes are low thyroid function, anemia, vitamin deficiencies, electrolyte disorders, depression, a short leg, or painful feet due to the unstable Dudley J. Morton foot structure.[44] One vitamin-deficiency cause of tinnitus may be relieved by supplements of both niacinamide and thiamine.

Other Perpetuating Factors

During prolonged neck traction, the patient should wear a dental splint that eliminates premature contacts, provides mandibular stability, and reduces mandibular elevator shortening.

During a long dental procedure that requires wide opening of the mouth, periodic relief for the stretched muscles and sedation of the patient help to prevent subsequent TP trismus. Preliminary examination for latent TPs and treatment with stretch and spray prior to the procedure provide additional insurance against acute trismus.

Organic intracapsular TMJ diseases that, themselves, cause pain or distort normal joint mechanics, can perpetuate masseter TPs.

A chronic focus of infection may be a contributory factor, especially if the erythrocyte sedimentation rate and white blood cell count are elevated on repeated testing.

Life stress and tension anxiety that lead to jaw clenching and bruxism should be managed by reducing emotional strain and improving the patient's coping behavior. Wearing a nocturnal occlusal splint reduces bruxism associated with high-stress life situations.[53]

Contributory TPs in the sternocleidomastoid, trapezius, and other distant muscles, including those in the lower extremities, should be inactivated. Muscles that refer pain to the region of the masseter are likely to activate satellite TPs in that muscle; the primary TPs must be eliminated for sustained relief.

Exercises

Passive and active self-stretch exercises after hot packs to the face are useful. Application of vapocoolant by self-spray during self-stretch is more effective for those patients who can learn the technique, and who can relax well. A family member may be taught to apply the Fluori-Methane* spray.

The passive Mandibular Self-stretch Exercise for the masseter (Fig. 8.8) starts with the patient seated at a sink. The patient: (1) warms the face with hot wet towels or hydrocollator packs (Fig. 8.8A); (2) supports the forehead with one hand at the sink while gradually, firmly pulling the mandible forward with the other, being careful not to jerk it suddenly (Fig. 8.8B); (3) pulls the lower jaw down, as well as forward (Fig. 8.8C); (4) holds the jaw in this stretch position, perhaps to a count of five; and (5) completes the cycle by gradually releasing the pull, closing the lower jaw, and relaxing. The cycle is repeated five or six times per exercise session, which should be performed daily until complete relief is obtained, or on alternate days if poststretch stiffness or soreness is a problem.

To do self-stretch and self-spray (Fig. 8.9), the supine patient performs the passive self-stretch with one hand, while applying sweeps of the vapocoolant spray with the other hand in the pattern shown, avoiding the eye, which should have a protective cover.

An active-assisted exercise, which is a form of rhythmic stabilization,[11, 51] applied to the mandibular elevator muscles helps to overcome restriction of opening. Myofascial TPs limit jaw aperture primarily by shortening of the mandibular elevator muscles due to taut muscular bands associated with the TPs. Direct attempts to stretch the muscles by simply forcing the mouth open produces severe pain and

---

* Gebauer Chemical Company, Cleveland, Ohio 44104.

PART 1

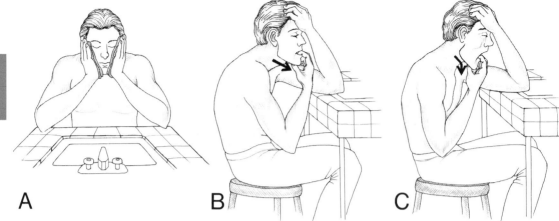

A   B   C

Figure 8.8.   The seated passive Mandibular Self-stretch Exercise for the masseter is performed at a sink in three steps. *A,* hot packs are applied to the face. *B,* two fingers are inserted behind the lower incisor teeth, while the thumb grasps the chin to pull the lower jaw forward. *C,* full stretch is achieved by pulling the jaw downward while continuing to pull it forward.

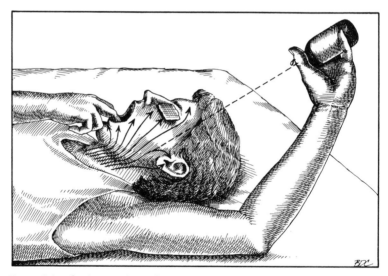

Figure 8.9.   Supine passive self-stretch and self-spray for trigger points in the masseter muscle.

reflex spasm that further aggravates the muscle tension; this must be avoided. Instead, the patient is taught a three-step resistive exercise that alternates between opening and closing efforts with the mouth open wide. It starts with the application of gentle resistance held for 10 sec as the patient actively, gently tries to close the mouth while it is held wide open by the hand of the operator or of the patient. Next, the patient relaxes as hand pressure is released. Then, the patient tries to open the mouth as wide as possible with gentle assistance from the hand, slightly increas-

ing the range of motion. Finally, an active opening effort of the patient is resisted by the hand.[33] This last step, which has been recommended as a separate exercise, invokes reciprocal inhibition.[84] The three steps are repeated at least three times, or until no further gain in range of motion is realized. The patient then opens and closes the mouth through the maximal active range of motion several times without resistance.

Yawning is strongly recommended as a home exercise. It is an active stretching movement that is accompanied by strong

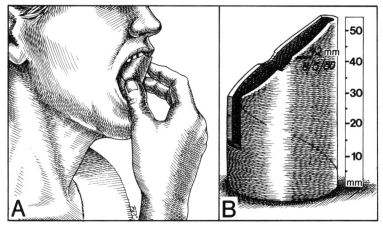

Figure 8.10.   Use of the cardboard prop as a measure. *A*, the patient places the prop between the incisor teeth of the fully opened jaws and bites down so as to indent the prop. *B*, the dent made by the upper tooth is marked so that the patient can measure the mouth opening and compare it for future progress in the home stretch-program.

reflex inhibition of the mandibular elevators.

These stretch procedures must be applied cautiously in the presence of radiographic evidence of TMJ arthropathy.

Conclusion

Since patients are unable to judge accurately their maximum jaw opening within the functional range, an objective measure of progress is important if the patient is to reach *full* range of motion on a home exercise program. Achieving full range and maximum stretch of the muscles greatly reduces the likelihood of recurrence of the TP pain and tension. To measure the jaw aperture, the patient opens the mouth as wide as possible, places the slanted prop (Fig. 8.6) between the upper and lower incisor teeth, and bites down on it (Fig. 8.10A). The level of the tooth indentation is marked (Fig. 8.10B) and dated. The patient repeats this procedure every day or two, so that progress can be judged by the successive marks on the prop. The minimum goal is an aperture that admits a tier of the first three knuckles of the non-dominant hand, as in Fig. 8.3.

Bell[8] details the importance of dealing with multiple contributory factors. He recommends reduction of life situational stress and development of a positive mental attitude; an occlusal splint temporarily relieves occlusal disharmony until the muscles are free of TP tension, when re-sidual malocclusion should be corrected. In addition, correction of nutritional deficiencies and use of stretch exercises help to insure continued normal functioning of the muscles treated for TPs.

Supplemental References, Case Reports. A detailed case report of acute trismus following a dental procedure described prompt pain relief and gradual increase of jaw opening from 15 mm to 51 mm by repeated injections of 0.5% procaine solution into TPs in the masseter and lateral pterygoid muscles.[79, 80]

Another patient experienced tinnitus and "stuffiness" of the ear due to TPs in the deep division of the masseter muscle. Procaine injection of the responsible TPs permanently eliminated those symptoms.[80]

References

1. Adisman IK, *et al.*: Glossary of Prosthodontic terms. *J Prosthet Dent* 38:70–109, 1977 (p. 75).
2. Agerberg G: Maximal mandibular movements in young men and women. *Swed Dent J* 67:81–100, 1974.
3. Agerberg G: Maximum mandibular movements in teen-agers. *Acta Morphol Neerl Scand* 12:79–102, 1974.
4. Agerberg G, Österberg T: Maximal mandibular movements and symptoms of mandibular dysfunction in 70-year-old men and women. *Swed Dent J* 67:147–164, 1974.
5. Bailey JO, Jr., McCall WD, Jr., Ash MM, Jr.: Electromyographic silent periods and jaw motion parameters: quantitative measures of temporomandibular joint dysfunction. *J Dent Res* 56:249–253, 1977.

6. Basmajian JV: *Muscles Alive*, Ed. 4. Williams & Wilkins, Baltimore, 1978 (pp. 101, 385, 388).
7. Bell WE: *Orofacial Pains—Differential Diagnosis*. Denedco of Dallas, Dallas, Texas, 1973 (p. 94, Fig. 10-1, Case 5).
8. Bell WH: Nonsurgical management of the pain-dysfunction syndrome. *J Am Dent Assoc* 79:161–170, 1969 (Cases 3 and 5).
9. Bessette RW, Mohl ND, Bishop B: Contribution of periodontal receptors to the masseteric silent period. *J Dent Res* 53:1196–1203, 1974.
10. Butler JH, Folke IEA, Bandt CL: A descriptive survey of signs and symptoms associated with the myofascial pain-dysfunction syndrome. *J Am Dent Assoc* 90:635–639, 1975.
11. Cailliet R: *Soft Tissue Pain and Disability*. F.A. Davis, Philadelphia, 1977 (p. 160).
12. Christensen LV: Some electromyographic parameters of experimental tooth clenching in adult human subjects. *J Oral Rehabil* 7:139–146, 1980.
13. Dawson PE: *Evaluation, Diagnosis, and Treatment of Occlusal Problems*. C.V. Mosby, Saint Louis, 1974 (pp. 48–107).
14. Domnitz JM, Swintak EF, Schriver WR, et al.: Myofascial pain syndrome masquerading as temporomandibular joint pain. *Oral Surg* 43:11–17, 1977.
15. Dorrance GM: New and useful surgical procedures; the mechanical treatment of trismus. *Pa Med J* 32:545–546, 1929.
16. Eisler P: *Die Muskeln des Stammes*. Gustav Fischer, Jena, 1912 (p. 198).
17. *Ibid.* (p. 204).
18. Funakoshi M, Amano N: Effects of the tonic neck reflex on the jaw muscles of the rat. *J Dent Res* 52:668–673, 1973.
19. Gelb H: Evaluation of static centric relation in the temporomandibular joint dysfunction syndrome. *Dent Clin North Am* 19:519–530, 1975.
20. Gelb H: Patient evaluation, Chapter 3. In *Clinical Management of Head, Neck and TMJ Pain and Dysfunction*, edited by H. Gelb. W.B. Saunders, Philadelphia, 1977 (p. 82, Fig. 3–4).
21. Grant JCB: *An Atlas of Human Anatomy*, Ed. 7. Williams & Wilkins, Baltimore, 1978 (Figs. 7-2, 7-105).
22. *Ibid.* (Fig. 7-68).
23. *Ibid.* (Fig. 7-16).
24. Gray H: *Anatomy of the Human Body*, edited by C.M. Goss, American Ed. 29. Lea & Febiger, Philadelphia, 1973 (p. 389).
25. *Ibid.* (p. 686).
26. Greene CS, Lerman MD, Sutcher HD, Laskin DM: The TMJ pain-dysfunction syndrome: heterogeneity of the patient population. *J Am Dent Assoc* 79:1168–1172, 1969.
27. Hansson T, Nilner M: A study of the occurrence of symptoms of diseases of the temporomandibular joint, masticatory musculature and related structures. *J Oral Rehabil* 2:313–324, 1975.
28. Ingle JI, Beveridge EE: *Endodontics*, Ed. 2. Lea & Febiger, Philadelphia, 1976 (p. 520).
29. Jankelson B: Neuromuscular aspects of occlusion. *Dent Clin North Am* 23:157–168, 1979.
30. Jankelson B: Personal communication, 1982.
31. Kellgren JH: Observations on referred pain arising from muscle. *Clin Sci* 3:175–190, 1938 (p. 180).
32. Levy PH: Clinical implications of mandibular re-

positioning and the concept of an alterable centric relation. *Dent Clin North Am* 19:543–570, 1975.
33. Lewit K: Muskelfazilitations- und Inhibitionstechniken in der Manuellen Medizin, Teil II and Teil III. *Manuelle Medizin* 19:12–22, 40–43, 1981.
34. Marbach JJ: Arthritis of the temporomandibular joints. *Am Fam Physician* 19:131–139, 1979 (Fig. 9F).
35. McCall WD, Jr., Goldberg SB, Uthman AA, Mohl ND: Symptom severity and silent periods: preliminary results in TMJ dysfunction patients. *NY State Dent J* 44:58–60, 1978.
36. McInnes B: Jaw pain from cigarette holder. *N Engl J Med* 298:1263, 1978.
37. McMinn RMH, Hutchings RT: *Color Atlas of Human Anatomy*. Year Book Medical Publishers, Chicago, 1977 (p. 35).
38. Melzack R: The McGill pain questionnaire: major properties and scoring methods. *Pain* 1:277–299, 1975.
39. Millstein-Prentky S, Olson RE: Predictability of treatment outcome in patients with myofascial pain-dysfunction (MPD) syndrome. *J Dent Res* 58:1341–1346, 1979.
40. Mohl ND: Head posture and its role in occlusion. *NY State Dent J* 42:17–23, 1976.
41. Møller E, Sheik-Ol-Eslam A, Lous I: Deliberate relaxation of the temporal and masseter muscles in subjects with functional disorders of the chewing apparatus. *Scand J Dent Res* 79:478–482, 1971.
42. Mongan E, Kelly P, Nies K, et al.: Tinnitus as an indication of therapeutic serum salicylate levels. *JAMA* 226:142–145, 1973.
43. Morton DJ: *The Human Foot*. Columbia University Press, New York, 1935.
44. Morton DJ: Foot Disorders in Women. *J Am Med Wom Assoc* 10:41–46, 1955.
45. Moss ML: A functional cranial analysis of centric relation. *Dent Clin North Am* 19:431–442, 1975.
46. Moyers RE: An electromyographic analysis of certain muscles involved in temporomandibular movement. *Am J Orthod* 36:481–515, 1950.
47. Pertes RA: The use of functional appliances in the prevention of the TMJ dysfunction syndrome. *Basal Facts* 3:165–183, 1979.
48. Pinto O: A new structure related to the temporomandibular joint and the middle ear. *J Prosthet Dent* 12:95, 1962.
49. Ramfjord SP: Temporomandibular joint dysfunction; dysfunctional temporomandibular joint and muscle pain. *J Prosthet Dent* 11:353–374, 1961.
50. Reynolds MD: Myofascial trigger point syndromes in the practice of rheumatology. *Arch Phys Med Rehabil* 62:111–114, 1981.
51. Rubin D: An approach to the management of myofascial trigger point syndromes. *Arch Phys Med Rehabil* 62:107–110, 1981.
52. Rugh JD, Drago CJ: Vertical dimension: a study of clinical rest position and jaw muscle activity. *J Prosthet Dent* 45:670–675, 1981.
53. Rugh JD, Solberg WK: Electromyographic studies of bruxist behavior before and during treatment. *Calif Dent Assoc J* 3:56–59, 1975.
54. Schwartz L: Conclusions of the temporomandibular joint clinic at Columbia. *J Periodontol* 29:210–212, 1958.
55. Schwartz LL: Ethyl chloride treatment of limited, painful mandibular movement. *J Am Dent Assoc*

48:497–507, 1954 (Case 4).

56. Schwartz RA, Greene CS, Laskin DM: Personality characteristics of patients with myofascial pain-dysfunction (MPD) syndrome unresponsive to conventional therapy. *J Dent Res* 58:1435–1439, 1979.

57. Seibly WS, James RA: Gnathology treatment, Chapter 15. In *Diseases of the Temporomandibular Apparatus*, edited by D.H. Morgan, W.P. Hall, and S.J. Vamvas. C.V. Mosby, St. Louis, 1977 (pp. 215, 216).

58. Seltzer S: Dental conditions that cause head and neck pain, Chapter 7. In *Pain Control In Dentistry: Diagnosis and Management*. J.B. Lippincott, Philadelphia, 1978 (pp. 105–136).

59. Shaber EP: Personal communication, 1981.

60. Sharav Y, Tzukert A, Refaeli B: Muscle pain index in relation to pain, dysfunction, and dizziness associated with the myofascial pain-dysfunction syndrome. *Oral Surg* 46:742–747, 1978 (p. 744).

61. Shore NA: *Temporomandibular Joint Dysfunction and Occlusal Equilibration*. J.B. Lippincott, Philadelphia, 1976 (pp. 61, 62).

62. Shpuntoff H, Shpuntoff W: A study of physiologic rest position and centric position by electromyography. *J Prosthet Dent* 6:621–628, 1956.

63. Skiba TJ, Laskin DM: Masticatory muscle silent periods in patients with MPD syndrome. *J Dent Res* 55:B249 (Abst 748), 1976.

64. Sobotta J, Figge FHJ: *Atlas of Human Anatomy*, Ed. 9, Vol. 1. Hafner Division of Macmillan, New York, 1974 (p. 178).

65. *Ibid*. (p. 183).

66. *Ibid*. (p. 185).

67. *Ibid*. (p. 188).

68. Sobotta J, Figge FHJ: *Atlas of Human Anatomy*, Ed. 9, Vol. 3. Hafner Division of Macmillan, New York, 1974 (p. 211).

69. Solberg WK: Personal communication, 1981.

70. Solberg WK: The troubled temporomandibular joint: new opportunities and challenges in research and clinical management. *ORO-BIO* 2:9–12, 1981.

71. Solberg WK, Woo MW, Houston JB: Prevalence of mandibular dysfunction in young adults. *J Am Dent Assoc* 98:25–34, 1979.

72. Spalteholz W: *Handatlas der Anatomie des Menschen*, Ed. 11, Vol. 2. S. Hirzel, Leipzig, 1922 (p. 264).

73. *Ibid*. (p. 267).

74. Staling LM, Fetchero P, Vorro J: Premature occlusal contact influence on mandibular kinesiology. In: *Biomechanics V-A*, edited by P.V. Komi. University Park Press, Baltimore, 1976 (pp. 280–288).

75. Staling LM, Gigliotti R: Application of neuromuscular function to determine occlusion and rest by visualizing masticatory muscle potentials. *J Balto Coll Dent Surg* 27:58–64, 1972.

76. Toldt C: *An Atlas of Human Anatomy*, translated by M.E. Paul, Ed. 2, Vol. 1. Macmillan, New York, 1919 (p. 293).

77. *Ibid*. (p. 302).

78. *Ibid*. (p. 303).

79. Travell J: Pain mechanisms in connective tissue. In *Connective Tissues, Transactions of the Second Conference, 1951*, edited by C. Ragan. Josiah Macy, Jr. Foundation, New York, 1952 (pp. 114, 115).

80. Travell J: Temporomandibular joint pain referred from muscles of the head and neck. *J Prosthet Dent* 10:745–763, 1960 (pp. 748, 750, 752–756).

81. Travell J: Mechanical headache. *Headache* 7:23–29, 1967 (p. 27, Fig. 7).

82. Travell J, Rinzler SH: The myofascial genesis of pain. *Postgrad Med* 11:425–434, 1952 (p. 427).

83. Weinberg LA: The etiology, diagnosis, and treatment of TMJ dysfunction-pain syndrome. Part II: differential diagnosis. *J Prosthet Dent* 43:58–70, 1980.

84. Wetzler G: Physical therapy, Chapter 24. In *Diseases of the Temporomandibular Apparatus*, edited by D.H. Morgan, W.P. Hall, and S.J. Vamvas. C.V. Mosby, St. Louis, 1977 (pp. 349–353, Fig. 24-2C).

85. Woelfel JB, Hickey JC, Stacey RW, *et al.*: Electromyographic analysis of jaw movements. *J Prosthet Dent* 10:688–697, 1960.

86. Wolff HG: *Wolff's Headache and Other Head Pain*, revised by D.J. Dalessio, Ed. 3. Oxford University Press, 1972 (p. 550).

87. Yemm K: Temporomandibular dysfunction and masseter muscle response to experimental stress. *Br Dent J* 127:508–510, 1969.

CHAPTER 9
Temporalis Muscle
"Temporal Headache and Maxillary Toothache"

HIGHLIGHTS: **REFERRED PAIN** from trigger points (TPs) in the temporalis muscle extends mainly over the temporal region, to the eyebrow, the upper teeth, and occasionally to the maxilla and the temporomandibular joint (TMJ); TPs also refer tenderness and hypersensitivity of the upper teeth to heat and cold. **ANATOMICAL ATTACHMENTS** are chiefly, above, to the temporal bone and to fascia in the temporal fossa and, below, to the coronoid process of the mandible. **ACTIONS** of this muscle are primarily to close the jaws. The posterior and middle fibers bilaterally retrude the mandible; acting unilaterally, they deviate the mandible to the same side. **SYMPTOMS** are pain over the temporal area, often hypersensitivity and aching of the upper teeth, and sometimes patients are aware of premature tooth contact. **ACTIVATION OF TRIGGER POINTS** may be due to long periods of jaw immobilization (open or closed), bruxism, clenching of teeth, occlusal disharmony, exposure to a cold draft over the fatigued muscle, and direct trauma to the muscle. Temporalis TPs also may develop secondarily as satellites of primary sternocleidomastoid or upper trapezius TPs. **PATIENT EXAMINATION** reveals an abnormal Three-knuckle Test (usually admitting only 2½ knuckles) and sometimes malocclusion of the teeth. **TRIGGER POINT EXAMINATION** of this muscle first requires that the mandible be propped open 2–3 cm (about 1 in), near the mid-position of its range. The TPs are usually found in a horizontal line about one fingerbreadth above the zygomatic arch. **STRETCH AND SPRAY** are accomplished with the patient's head oriented horizontally (looking up) and with the patient applying passive self-stretch to open the jaws as wide as possible, while the operator directs the vapocoolant spray over the muscle and its pain reference zones. **INJECTION AND STRETCH** are effective, but injection should avoid the temporal artery. **CORRECTIVE ACTIONS** call for the elimination of systemic perpetuating factors, and for a home program, which includes the Mandibular Self-stretch Exercise, an active-resistive exercise of the mandibular elevators, exaggerated yawning and supine self-stretch with self-spray. Malocclusion that remains after occlusal splint therapy and inactivation of TPs should be corrected.

1. REFERRED PAIN
(Fig. 9.1)

Headache due to active trigger points (TPs) in the temporalis muscle is common,[50] and is described as pain felt widely throughout the temple, along the eyebrow, behind the eye, and in any or all of the upper teeth.[34, 44, 45, 47] Temporalis TPs also may refer hypersensitivity to percussion and to moderate temperature changes into any or all of the upper teeth on the same side, depending on the TP location.[44, 45] Myofascial TPs in the temporalis TP$_1$ region lie in the anterior portion of the muscle (Fig. 9.1A) and refer pain forward along the supraorbital ridge[51] and downward to the upper incisor teeth.[25, 36, 44, 49] The TP$_2$ and TP$_3$ regions lie in the intermediate portions of the muscle (Figs. 9.1B and C) and refer pain upward in finger-like projections to the mid-temple area and downward to the intermediate maxillary teeth on the same side.[4, 6, 25, 36, 44, 49, 55] In the pos-

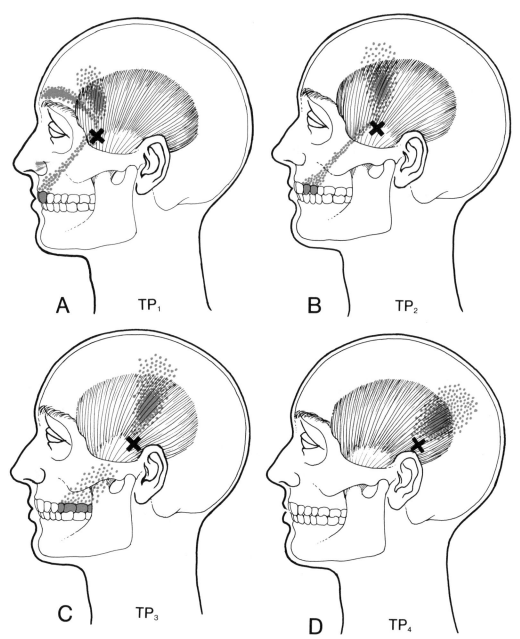

Figure 9.1   Referred pain patterns from trigger points (✕s) in the left temporalis muscle (essential zone *solid red*, spillover zone *stippled*). *A*, anterior "spokes" of pain arising from the anterior fibers (trigger point one region). *B* and *C*, middle "spokes" (trigger point two and trigger point three regions). *D*, posterior supra-auricular "spoke" (trigger point four region).

terior section, active TPs in the TP_4 region refer pain backward and upward (Fig. 9.1D).[44] Fibers of the temporalis deep in the TP_3 region, like the deepest masseter fibers, may refer pain to the maxilla and the TMJ.[6, 44]

Deep tenderness may be found in each of these pain reference zones even when the corresponding TPs are latent (clinically silent with respect to pain). Sometimes toothache with hypersensitivity of the upper teeth to ordinary stimuli (biting, heat, cold) is the chief complaint, rather than headache.[44]

Wolff[53] studied the vascular response and neuromuscular changes in 10 non-headache subjects, 10 headache subjects when headache-free, and 10 headache subjects during right temporal "muscle contraction" headache. An autonomic component was clearly demonstrated by the differences in the measured amplitude of the temporal artery pulse wave. In the non-headache group, its amplitude averaged 12 mm; in the headache group without headache, 8.3 mm; and during temporal headache, only 4.6 mm. Motor unit activity in the temporalis muscle during temporal headache was increased in frequency and was 10 times the amplitude of the activity in the same muscle in headache-prone subjects when having a headache, than when free of headache. Wolff[53]

surmised that muscular contraction caused the pain by means of ischemia, whereas we think of this motor unit activity and pain in the temporalis muscle as referred phenomena, probably from TPs in the sternocleidomastoid or trapezius muscles.

2. ANATOMICAL ATTACHMENTS (Fig. 9.2)

The temporalis muscle attaches **above** to the bone and fascia in the temporal fossa, superior to the zygomatic arch (Fig. 9.2).

Below it attaches to the coronoid process of the mandible and along the anterior

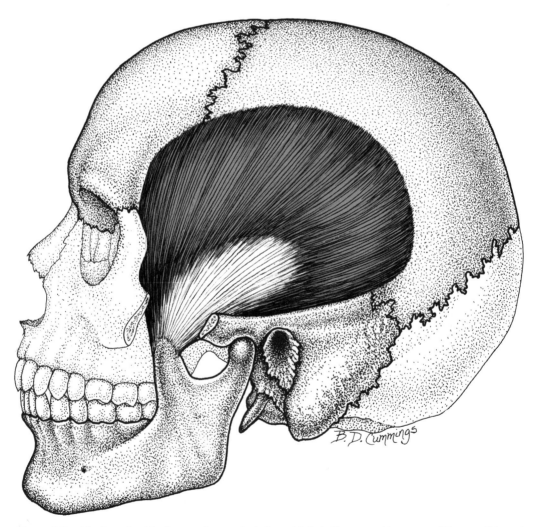

Figure 9.2   Attachments of the temporalis muscle, below, chiefly to the coronoid process of the mandible and, above, to the temporal bone. The anterior fibers (trigger point one region) are nearly vertical and posterior fibers (trigger point four region), nearly horizontal. The zygomatic arch has been removed.

edge of the mandibular ramus, extending almost to the last molar tooth.[18] Temporalis fibers also may attach to the medial surface of the coronoid process.[22] The temporalis fibers fan out anteroposteriorly from the coronoid process to form three functionally distinct groups. The anterior fibers are nearly vertical, the middle fibers oblique, and the posterior fibers nearly horizontal.[29]

Supplemental References

Anatomy textbooks illustrate this muscle from the lateral view.[11, 17, 18, 40, 41, 43]

3. INNERVATION

The temporalis muscle is supplied by the anterior and posterior deep temporal nerves, which branch from the anterior division of the mandibular portion of the trigeminal nerve (cranial nerve V).

4. ACTIONS

All fibers of the temporalis muscle contribute to its primary function of elevation (closure) of the mandible. The posterior fibers, in addition, are important for retrusion and lateral deviation of the mandible to the same side.

When the mandible is closed and the jaws are clenched tightly in centric occlusion, the temporalis is activated before the masseter,[31, 32, 52] and all parts of the muscle are involved.[29] Closure to incisor bite (anterior occlusion) involves mainly the anterior temporal fibers.[31] With normal dentition, gentle closure activates mainly the anterior fibers,[31] or the anterior and middle fibers.[3] If the subject is edentulous and wearing dentures, all three parts of the temporalis contract equally.[3]

The posterior, much more than the middle or anterior, fibers are consistently activated during retraction (retrusion) of the mandible.[3, 29, 31, 52] Bruxism with a posterior thrust of the mandible strongly involves these posterior fibers.[1]

Lateral movements to the same side regularly activate the temporalis,[3] particularly its middle and posterior, more than its anterior fibers;[52] these lateral movements always involve the posterior fibers if the lower jaw is not protruded at the same time. Protrusion conflicts with the retraction function of, and therefore inhibits activity of, the posterior temporalis fibers.[29]

The temporalis muscle was generally inactive during protraction (protrusion),[3, 52] but was active in 5% of efforts,[29] probably to counteract the depressor effect of the primary protruder, the inferior division of the lateral pterygoid muscle.

The important question of whether temporalis motor units normally show activity at rest is clearly resolved only in the supine position, when no activity is observed.[24] The presence of resting motor unit activity in the erect subject is controversial;[3, 48] activity is reported as greater in the posterior than in the anterior fibers.[3, 31] Basmajian[3] states that the temporalis alone is the muscle responsible for keeping the mandible in the rest position during upright posture. Yemm[54] found no activity in repeated recordings of three temporalis muscles in seated subjects at rest with head and trunk erect. These differing conclusions could result from the variation in the rest position, differences in the degree of anxiety-induced muscle tension, variations in electrode technique, head position, the presence or absence of occlusal disharmony and of latent TPs in the masticatory musculature.

Unlike most deep tendon reflex responses, which are simple biphasic potentials, the jaw jerk of the masseter and temporalis muscles has a three-component response. The first component is the usual monosynaptic reflex with a latency of approximately 7.5 msec and a duration of 10 msec. The second component is a silent period of approximately 10 msec, followed by a polysynaptic reflex with a latency of approximately 27 msec. This tripartite response resembles the blink reflex in form, but not in its neural pathways.[31]

5. MYOTATIC UNIT

Synergists of the temporalis for mandibular elevation include, ipsilaterally: the masseter, the superior division of the lateral pterygoid, and the medial pterygoid muscles. Contralaterally, the synergists are the same muscles plus the temporalis.

Antagonists are the inferior division of the lateral pterygoid, anterior digastric, omohyoid and mylohyoid muscles.

6. SYMPTOMS

Patients complain of head pain, as described in Section 1, but are rarely aware of any restriction of jaw opening, which is usually reduced only by 5–10 mm (about ⅜ in). Thus, ordinary mandibular movement does not cause pain. The patients may say, "My teeth don't meet right." They usually have intermittent toothache, with or without hyperalgesia of one or more upper teeth.[44] These referred phenomena can explain the fruitless extraction of a painful and hypersensitive, but healthy, tooth.[45]

7. ACTIVATION OF TRIGGER POINTS

Occlusal Imbalance

A premature occlusal contact is likely to activate, or perpetuate temporalis TPs. As discussed more fully under the corresponding heading in Chapter 8, an interfering occlusal contact may increase the electrical activity of the masticatory muscles.[33] In one study, premature cuspid contact on the left side increased motor unit activity more for the temporalis than for the masseter, and more on the left than on the right side.[13]

Vertical Dimension

When the space between the teeth is abnormally large or small in the upright position with the muscles at rest, the masticatory muscles must compensate. Too large a vertical dimension overloads the masseter, temporalis and medial pterygoid muscles. This can activate and perpetuate TPs in them.[27, 37]

Trauma and Immobilization

Temporalis TPs may be activated: by bruxism and clenching the teeth; by direct trauma to the muscle, as from a fall on the head, impact from a golfball or baseball, or by an auto accident, if the head is thrown against the side of the car; by a long period of jaw immobilization in a dental chair for an extensive dental procedure; or by continuous cervical traction for neck pain without an occlusal splint, a situation which usually immobilizes the closed mandible. In the latter case, the iatrogenic temporalis TPs may then add the symptoms of facial pain, toothache and secondary malocclusion to the original complaint of neck pain or headache. Sometimes, the neck traction was ordered

for neck pain and headache that were caused by primary TPs in the upper trapezius, a situation in which traction provides no relief.

Activity Stress

Bruxism may cause, or result from, temporalis TPs. In either case, the overuse of the muscle aggravates these TPs. Restlessness of the masticatory muscles can depend on increased neuromuscular irritability due to folic acid deficiency. This restlessness may be expressed as bruxism and is similar to that induced by folate deficiency in the biceps femoris and calf muscles, known as "restless legs."[8]

Excessive gum chewing or jaw clenching may activate, and is likely to perpetuate, masticatory muscle TPs.

The wearing of a surgical face mask or a court reporter's dictating mask favors mouth breathing and retraction of the mandible, resulting in the development of TPs in the temporalis and other masticatory muscles.

Other Factors

Especially when the patient is tired, temporalis TPs may be activated by a cold draft over the muscle, e.g. a stream of cold air from a ventilator or airconditioner, or wind through an open car window.[44] Persons with low-normal serum levels of thyroid hormones (T_3 and T_4 by radioimmunoassay (RIA)), as well as those clearly hypothyroid, are particularly vulnerable to such muscle cooling.

The temporalis muscle TPs may be activated as satellites when they lie within the pain reference zone of active TPs in the upper trapezius and sternocleidomastoid muscles. Active TPs in lower extremity muscles also may cause a significant reduction of maximal interincisal opening, and thus may influence masticatory muscle function.

8. PATIENT EXAMINATION

Among patients with either a myofascial pain-dysfunction or a TMJ pain-dysfunction syndrome, the temporalis muscle was the second,[10, 38] or third,[19, 23] most commonly involved of the masticatory muscles, after the masseter and lateral pterygoid. In these studies, the temporalis was involved in one-third to nearly two-thirds of the patients.

The patient performs the Three-knuckle Test (see Fig. 8.3 in Chapter 8) by attempting to place a tier of the proximal interphalangeal joints of the first three fingers of the non-dominant hand between the upper and lower incisor teeth. Usually, about 2½ knuckles of jaw opening is reached if the temporalis, but not the masseter, muscle is involved. Masseter tension restricts opening more severely. When the posterior fibers of the temporalis harbor active TPs, the mandible may show zigzag deviation during opening and closing of the mouth.

Grating sounds detected by stethoscopic examination over the TMJ during chewing movements, or crepitus felt over the joint, may indicate intracapsular derangement that calls for expert dental and TMJ examination. The patient may have a disc erosion, seating bone on bone, or may have arthritic destruction of joint surfaces.[16]

The presence of TPs in a muscle is not associated with atrophy of that muscle, but in the masticatory muscles appears to produce degenerative, TMJ disease by the strain the TP-tension produces on the joint elements.[14]

Silent Period Changes

The silent period is a normal interruption of electrical activity in the mandibular elevators during moderate jaw-clench. It is the response to initial tooth contact during an open-and-close clenching cycle, or follows the tooth contact that results from a reflex jaw-jerk response.[31, 32]

Several phenomena were abnormal in patients with TMJ pain-dysfunction syndrome: (1) the silent period was usually absent or, when present, prolonged.[30] A prolonged silent period was more likely to appear for the masseter than for the temporalis muscle in one study,[20] but *vice versa* in another.[39]; and (2) of 24 patients with TMJ dysfunction, 23 showed abnormal continuation of the temporalis or masseter motor unit activity during the open phase of the chewing cycle, more frequently in the temporalis than the masseter.[26] The causal relationship of these electrophysiological abnormalities to TMJ dysfunction and to myofascial TPs is not clear; specific data relating these measurements to the TP activity of individual muscles and to other signs of TMJ dysfunction are needed.

Differential Diagnosis

Polymyalgia Rheumatica. The head pain of polymyalgia rheumatica is distinguished from that due to temporalis and trapezius TPs by the more extensive distribution of the *bilateral* polymyalgia pain, which usually includes the shoulders,[7] often the neck, back, upper arms, and thighs;[21] by the increased erythrocyte sedimentation rate, usually of at least 50 mm/hr and even 100 mm/hr, which is evidence of inflammation with increases in fibrinogen and in the α_2-globulin fraction; and by anemia due to blocked utilization of iron.

Polymyalgia rheumatica is rarely seen below the age of 50; it usually occurs in men and women of 60 or more years.[21] Myofascial TP syndromes are seen at any age, especially in the most active, middle years. In polymyalgia rheumatica, the duration of morning stiffness exceeds 1 hr, depression and/or weight loss are often present, the upper arms are tender bilaterally,[7] and the teeth are not painful. In myofascial syndromes, morning stiffness usually lasts less than 1 hr; pain is primarily unilateral or, if bilateral, its distribution is not symmetrical; and depression is due to the life situation caused by the pain.

Polymyositis. This disease is most likely to present as *painless* proximal muscle weakness and to show elevation of serum enzymes including aldolase, creatine kinase, lactate dehydrogenase, aspartate aminotransferase, alanine aminotransferase, the isoenzymes creatine kinase MB, and lactate dehydrogenase isoenzymes 2 and 3.[28]

Giant Cell Arteritis. Nearly 50% of patients with polymyalgia rheumatica have been shown to have associated giant cell arteritis with headache and fever, and the threat of consequent blindness when the cranial arteries are involved.[12] Temporal arteritis is demonstrable by biopsy. However, recognition of giant cell arteritis can be difficult.[42] Both polymyalgia rheumatica and giant cell arteritis are remarkable for their prompt response to oral corticosteroid therapy and for their poor response to other measures.[2, 21] The polymyalgic and myofascial syndromes both cause morning stiffness without muscle atrophy, but only myofascial TPs cause the specific referred pain patterns on compression of tender spots and induce local twitch responses on snapping palpation.

9. TRIGGER POINT EXAMINATION
(Fig. 9.3)

The jaws must be propped *partly* (not fully) open to place the muscle fibers on the degree of stretch required to optimize the palpation of the temporalis TPs. When the jaws are closed and the muscle is fully shortened, its palpable bands are much more difficult to feel; they are less tender, and the local twitch response to snapping palpation may be unobtainable. When the cardboard cylinder that caps each Fluori-Methane* spray nozzle is turned sidewise, it makes a convenient jaw-prop for the examination of this muscle (Fig. 9.3). The anterior and intermediate parts of the muscle are palpated through the skin just above the upper border of the zygomatic arch (Fig. 9.1) for firm bands of temporalis fibers that exhibit deep tenderness (TP_1–TP_3); TPs in the TP_4 region of the posterior fibers are found above the ear, as illustrated in Figs. 9.1 and 9.3, and by Burch.[9] Examination of the temporalis for TPs is not complete until its insertion on the inner surface of the coronoid process has been palpated from within the mouth. The technique is the same as that for examining the inferior division of the lateral pterygoid muscle (see Section 9, Chapter 11) except that pressure is directed outward against the coronoid process, rather than inward toward the pterygoid plate. Across-the-fiber snapping palpation elicits local twitch responses that are *felt* more readily than seen in this muscle.

10. ENTRAPMENTS

The temporalis muscle is not known to cause nerve entrapment.

11. ASSOCIATED TRIGGER POINTS

Temporalis muscle TPs are likely to be associated with TPs in the ipsilateral mas-

---

* Fluori-Methane, distributed by Gebauer Chemical Co., Cleveland, OH 44104.

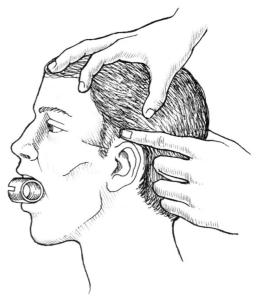

Figure 9.3 Examination of the posterior (trigger point four) portion of the temporalis muscle. For all portions, the jaws should always be propped open several centimeters to place the muscle on moderate stretch. This accentuates the firm bands of muscle fibers, increases the spot tenderness of the trigger points to pressure, and increases the likelihood of the local twitch response of a taut band to snapping palpation.

seter (deep division) and in the contralateral temporalis muscle. Less commonly, either or both the medial and lateral pterygoid muscles may be involved, sometimes bilaterally.

Satellite TPs often develop in the temporalis muscle because it lies within the pain reference zones of the frequent upper trapezius and sternocleidomastoid TPs.

12. STRETCH AND SPRAY
(Figs. 9.4 and 9.5)

To stretch and spray the temporalis muscle, the supine position is preferable. However, the patient may sit in a low-backed armchair (Fig. 9.4), (or dental chair) reclining the head backward against the operator, or headrest, to tilt the face upward and reduce postural reflexes.[15, 24] The patient is encouraged to relax.

The mouth is propped open at the limit of tolerance, using a jaw clamp, or a slanted cardboard cylinder (see Fig. 8.6 in Chapter 8). When the patient bites down on the cylinder, the dent made by the incisor teeth serves as a rough measure of

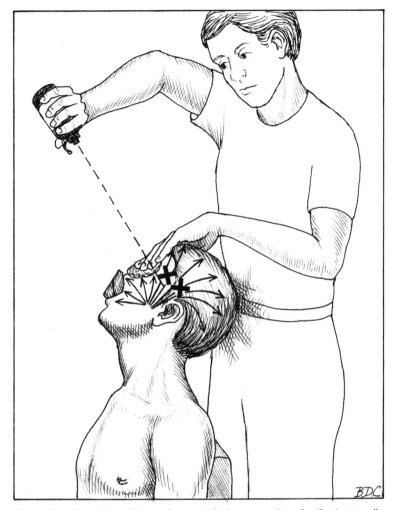

Figure 9.4 Stretch position and vapocoolant spray pattern for the temporalis muscle. Trigger points are indicated by ✕s. The mandible is depressed as far as possible by a slanted cardboard prop. The seated patient leans the head back almost horizontally against the operator to eliminate postural antigravity reflexes.

jaw opening, which the patient can see and use for later comparison.

While the temporalis muscle is thus stretched by the prop, the vapocoolant spray is applied from the attachment of the muscle on the coronoid process upward to cover the muscle fibers and all referred pain areas.[44] The patient's eyes are protected with cotton; the backward tilt of the head prevents the irritating vapocoolant liquid from running into the eyes. Stretch and spray should be applied bilaterally, over *both* temporalis muscles. A resultant increase in the jaw opening may be detected by the Three-knuckle Test, or measured again with the tooth-marked prop.

After a hot pack application to the face, stretch and spray may be repeated. This may be done several times at 5-min intervals (rewarming each time) until the patient's three knuckles fit in a tier between the margins of the incisor teeth. The minimum normal opening for persons of average stature is close to 45 mm in adult women, and 50 mm in adult men.[44]

Stretch and spray also may be applied to the temporalis muscles with the patient providing passive self-stretch in the supine position while the operator applies the spray (Fig. 9.5). Thus, the patient practices the technique of self-stretch to be used at home. To do this, the patient inserts two fingers behind the lower incisor teeth with

PART 1

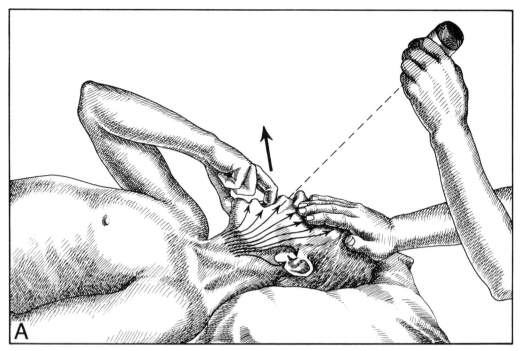

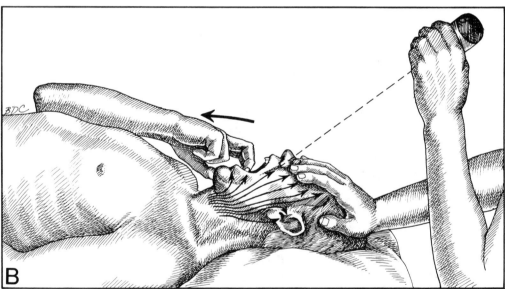

Figure 9.5   Self-stretch, during vapocooling of the temporalis muscle and other elevators of the mandible, with the patient lying supine. *A*, first step, the patient pulls the mandible upward in protrusion. *B*, second step, the patient then pulls the mandible down and also forward, to open the jaws as wide as possible. This two-step procedure can be used as a passive self-stretch exercise at home and should be followed by a hot pack.

the thumb under the chin, and, by pulling the mandible forward and then downward, applies a gradually increasing temporalis passive stretch. The Fluori-Methane* spray is applied by the operator (or

the patient) in upward sweeps in the directions illustrated in Fig. 9.5. This supine technique may be effective when stretch and spray fails in the seated patient, even though the head is tilted backward, almost horizontally.

Therapy of the temporalis muscle for TPs is not complete until all active TPs in

_____

* Fluori-Methane, distributed by Gebauer Chemical Co., Cleveland, OH 44104.

the upper trapezius and sternocleidomastoid muscles also have been inactivated. The TPs in the latter neck muscles can indirectly restrict mandibular opening.

13. INJECTION AND STRETCH
(Fig. 9.6)

Before injecting temporalis TPs, the operator first eliminates any TP tension in the masseter muscle to avoid bleeding in the temporal region. Tautness of masseter fibers can entrap venous drainage from the temporalis muscle (see Section 10, Chapter 8). If the masseter tension is not released, the patient is more likely to develop a large ecchymosis and a "black eye" following the temporalis TP injection; the patient should be warned of this possibility.

The lower jaw may be held open, as for examination (Fig. 9.3). The temporal artery should be identified by its pulsations, and avoided (Fig. 9.6). Using a sterile technique, the needle is directed away from the artery, or angled under it, to avoid puncturing it, as also noted by Bell.[5] After locating the temporalis TPs by palpation, one finger is placed on the artery to continuously monitor its location, while other fingers localize and fix the TP for injection.

A 2.5-cm (1-in), 23- or 24-gauge needle is used to inject the TPs with a local anesthetic in an upward direction between the fingers. A 27-gauge needle is too flimsy. We recommend 0.5% procaine without epinephrine for intramuscular injection. Alternatively, the 2% lidocaine is much preferred to the 3% mepivacaine supplied in the convenient 1.8-ml dental syringes (see Section 13, Chapter 3). Immediately after the injection, maximal passive stretch of the muscle is carried out while applying vapocoolant spray bilaterally. A hot pack follows, then active range of jaw motion. If the range of opening is still restricted, stretch and spray to the temporalis muscles may be repeated bilaterally, after rewarming, to achieve an additional increment of jaw opening.

The upper trapezius and sternocleidomastoid muscles should be checked for

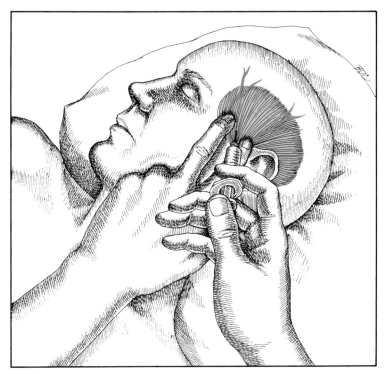

Figure 9.6 Injection of a trigger point in the trigger point one, trigger point two or trigger point three regions (*light red*) of the temporalis muscle. The temporal artery (*red*) is avoided. A finger is placed on the pulsating artery to continuously monitor its location, while other fingers localize the trigger point in a taut band and fix it for injection.

active TPs. These TPs are likely to refer pain to the temple. If present, they should be inactivated.

14. CORRECTIVE ACTIONS

Occlusal Disharmony

Malocclusion due to premature occlusal contact should be alleviated immediately with an occlusal splint. This eliminates a major perpetuator of masticatory muscle TPs. With few exceptions, correction of malocclusion by permanent reconstructive dental procedures should be deferred until the TPs in the temporalis and other masticatory muscles have been inactivated.

Exercise Program

The patient learns how to passively stretch the temporalis in the supine position by doing the Mandibular Self-stretch Exercise daily (see Fig. 8.8 in Chapter 8). Before this exercise is done, the patient applies a hot pack over the temporalis muscle, covering the side of the head and face, for 10–15 min before retiring at night.

When the patient is comfortable with this passive exercise, the next step is an active-resistive exercise of the mandibular elevators, which helps to overcome restricted motion through reciprocal inhibition (see Section 14, Chapter 8). If the posterior fibers of the temporalis muscle are involved, causing the mandible to deviate on opening, the patient must modify this exercise: the patient firmly stretches the jaw muscles during lateral movement by placing one hand against the opposite maxilla and the other hand against the ipsilateral side of the mandible. The lower jaw is pushed away from the side toward which it deviates, while the patient *assists* the motion with the jaw muscles for most effective stretch. The mandible is gently restored to the starting position before pressure is fully released. To use this as a strengthening and reconditioning exercise, the patient *resists* the same motion. When full relief is obtained, the exercises may be reduced to two or three times weekly.

Some patients are able to learn self-stretch and self-spray for the temporalis muscle, done *supine*, similar to the technique described for the masseter (see Fig. 8.9 in Chapter 8).

The patient is encouraged to induce a wide-open yawn as a regular exercise; the reflex inhibition helps to obtain greater stretch of the temporalis muscle.

Postural Stress

The activation of TPs during a prolonged dental procedure may be prevented by taking breaks for active movement, or occasional application of vapocoolant spray over the muscle while it is passively stretched by propping the mouth open.

Prolonged maximal shortening of the muscle during sleep may be prevented by a "night guard" or occlusal splint with a flat occlusal plane, which keeps the upper and lower teeth a few millimeters apart and can relieve bruxism. This is especially helpful during periods of high stress.[35] A dental splint also should be used during prolonged cervical traction, especially in the patient who has a history of headache.

Body asymmetry and the resultant functional scoliosis should be corrected by appropriate lifts, since this postural stress may activate TPs in the neck muscles that cause satellite TPs in the masticatory muscles.

The habit of mouth breathing should be corrected by eliminating contributory factors, such as nasal obstruction.

Activity Stress

Prolonged restriction of opening by a face mask should be relieved by occasional removal of the mask and stretching of the jaw muscles.

The patient should avoid cold drafts that blow directly on the temple by wearing a night cap, protective hood, or scarf.

The patient should be persuaded to stop chewing gum, eating caramels, biting a pen or pencil, chewing tough meat, and cracking nuts or ice with the teeth.

Other Actions

The patient should be checked for evidence of reduced thyroid function, other metabolic disorders, and nutritional deficiencies, any of which may increase neuromuscular irritability, as described in Chapter 4. Elimination of TP activity in the muscles of the neck, and even of the lower extremities, may be critical for *complete* lasting relief of myofascial pain and dysfunction of the masticatory muscles.

PART 1

Supplemental Reference, Case Report

The diagnosis and management of a patient with temporalis involvement is given in a case report by Travell.[46]

References

1. Adams SH, II: Personal communication, 1981.
2. Atkins SD: Giant cell arteritis—a systemic spectrum including temporal arteritis and polymyalgia rheumatica. *J. Fam Pract* 7:1109–1116, 1978.
3. Basmajian JV: *Muscles Alive*, Ed. 4. Williams & Wilkins, Baltimore, 1978 (pp. 101, 185–186, 380–384).
4. Bell WE: *Orofacial Pains—Differential Diagnosis*. Denedco of Dallas, 1973 (p. 94, Fig. 10-1).
5. Bell WE: Management of masticatory pain. Chapter 12. In *Facial Pain*, edited by C.C. Alling III and P.E. Mahan, Ed. 2. Lea & Febiger, Philadelphia, 1977 (pp. 185, 188).
6. Bell WH: Nonsurgical management of the pain-dysfunction syndrome. *J Am Dent Assoc* 79:161–170, 1969 (pp. 165, 169, Case 5).
7. Bird HA, Esselinckx W, Dixon ASTJ, et al.: An evaluation of criteria for polymyalgia rheumatica. *Ann Rheum Dis* 38:434–439, 1979.
8. Botez MI, Fontaine F, Botez T, et al.: Folate-responsive neurological and mental disorders: report of 16 cases. *Eur Neurol* 16:230–246, 1977.
9. Burch JG: Occlusion related to craniofacial pain. Chapter 11. In *Facial Pain*, edited by C.C. Alling III, P.E. Mahan, Ed. 2. Lea & Febiger, Philadelphia, 1977 (pp. 169, 170).
10. Butler JH, Folke LEA, Bandt CL: A descriptive survey of signs and symptoms associated with the myofascial pain-dysfunction syndrome. *J Am Dent Assoc* 90:635–639, 1975.
11. Eisler P: *Die Muskeln des Stammes*. Gustav Fischer, Jena, 1912 (p. 204).
12. Ettlinger RE, Hunder GG, Ward LE: Polymyalgia rheumatica and giant cell arteritis. *Annu Rev Med* 29:15–22, 1978.
13. Franks AST: Masticatory muscle hyperactivity and temporomandibular joint dysfunction. *J Prosthet Dent* 15:1122–1131, 1965 (p. 1126).
14. Freese AS: Myofascial trigger mechanisms and temporomandibular joint disturbances in head and neck pain. *NY State J Med* 59:2554–2558, 1959 (Fig. 1).
15. Funakoshi M, Amano N: Effects of the tonic neck reflex on the jaw muscles of the rat. *J Dent Res* 52:668–673, 1973.
16. Gelb H: Patient evaluation, Chapter 3. In *Clinical Management of Head, Neck and TMJ Pain and Dysfunction*, edited by H. Gelb. W.B. Saunders, Philadelphia, 1977 (pp. 73–116).
17. Grant JCB: *An Atlas of Human Anatomy*, Ed. 7. Williams & Wilkins, Baltimore, 1978 (Fig. 7-70).
18. Gray H: *Anatomy of the Human Body*, edited by C.M. Goss, American Ed. 29. Lea & Febiger, Philadelphia, 1973 (p. 387, Fig. 6-5).
19. Greene CS, Lerman MD, Sutcher HD, et al.: The TMJ pain-dysfunction syndrome: heterogeneity of the patient population. *J. Am Dent Assoc* 79:1168–1172, 1969.
20. Griffin CJ, Munro RR: Electromyography of the masseter and anterior temporalis muscles in patients with temporomandibular dysfunction. *Arch Oral Biol* 16:929–949, 1971.
21. Healey LA: Polymyalgia rheumatica, Chapter 50. In *Arthritis and Allied Conditions*, edited by J.L. Hollander and D.J. McCarty, Jr., Ed. 8. Lea & Febiger, Philadelphia, 1972 (pp. 885–889).
22. Johnstone DR, Templeton McC: The feasibility of palpating the lateral pterygoid muscle. *J Prosthet Dent* 44:318–323, 1980.
23. Kaye LB, Moran JH, Fritz ME: Statistical analysis of an urban population of 236 patients with head and neck pain. Part II. Patient symptomatology. *J Periodontol* 50:59–65, 1979 (p. 61).
24. Møller E, Sheik-Ol-Eslam A, Lous I: Deliberate relaxation of the temporal and masseter muscles in subjects with functional disorders of the chewing apparatus. *Scand J Dent Res* 79:478–482, 1971 (p. 481).
25. Marbach JJ: Arthritis of the temporomandibular joints. *Am Fam Physician* 19:131–139, 1979 (p. 137, Fig. 9E).
26. McCall WD Jr, Goldberg SB, Uthman AA, Mohl ND: Symptom severity and silent periods: Preliminary results in TMJ dysfunction patients. *NY State Dent J* 44:58–60, 1978.
27. Morgan DH: Personal communication, 1981.
28. Morton BD, Statland BE: Serum enzyme alterations in polymyositis. *Am Soc Clin Pathol* 73:556–557, 1980.
29. Moyers RE: An electromyographic analysis of certain muscles involved in temporomandibular movement. *Am J Orthod* 36:481–515, 1950.
30. Munro RR: Electromyography of the masseter and anterior temporalis muscles in the open-close-clench cycle in temporomandibular joint dysfunction. In *The Temporomandibular Joint Syndrome*, edited by C.J. Griffin and R. Harris, Vol. 4 of *Monographs in Oral Science*. S. Karker, Basel, 1975 (pp. 117–125).
31. Munro RR: Electromyography of the muscles of mastication. In *The Temporomandibular Joint Syndrome*, edited by C.J. Griffin and R. Harris, Vol. 4. of *Monographs in Oral Science*. S. Karger, Basel, 1975 (pp. 87–116).
32. Munro RR, Basmajian JV: The jaw opening reflex in man. *Electromyography* 11:191–206, 1971.
33. Ramfjord SP: Dysfunctional temporomandibular joint and muscle pain. *J Prosthet Dent* 11:353–374, 1961.
34. Rubin D: An approach to the management of myofascial trigger point syndromes. *Arch Phys Med Rehabil* 62:107–110, 1981.
35. Rugh JD, Solberg WK: Electromyographic studies of bruxist behavior before and during treatment. *Calif Dent Assoc J* 3:56–57, 1975.
36. Shaber EP: Considerations in the treatment of muscle spasm, Chapter 16. In *Diseases of the Temporomandibular Apparatus*, edited by D.H. Morgan, L. R. House, W.P. Hall, and S.J. Vamvas, Ed. 2. C.V. Mosby, St. Louis, 1982 (p. 281, Fig. 16-2B).
37. Shaber EP: Personal communication, 1981.
38. Sharav Y, Tzukert A, Refaeli B: Muscle pain index in relation to pain, dysfunction, and dizziness associated with the myofascial pain-dysfunction syndrome. *Oral Surg* 46:742–747, 1978 (Table 1).
39. Skiba TJ, Laskin DM: Masticatory muscle silent

periods in patients with MPD syndrome. *J Dent Res* 55:B249 (Abst 748), 1976.

40. Sobotta J, Figge FHJ: *Atlas of Human Anatomy*, Ed. 9, Vol. 1. Hafner Division of Macmillan, New York, 1974 (p. 185).

41. Spalteholz W: *Handatlas der Anatomie des Menschen*, Ed. 11, Vol. 2. S. Hirzel, Leipzig, 1922 (p. 265).

42. Strachan RW, How J, Bewsher PD: Masked giant-cell arteritis. *Lancet* 1:194–196, 1980.

43. Toldt C: *An Atlas of Human Anatomy*, translated by M.E. Paul, Ed. 2, Vol. 1. Macmillan, New York, 1919 (p. 306).

44. Travell J: Temporomandibular joint pain referred from muscles of the head and neck. *J Prosthet Dent* 10:745–763, 1960 (pp. 748–749, Figs. 3, 13).

45. Travell J: Mechanical headache. *Headache* 7:23–29, 1967 (p. 26).

46. Travell J: Identification of myofascial trigger point syndromes: a case of atypical facial neuralgia. *Arch Phys Med Rehabil* 62:100–106, 1981.

47. Travell J, Rinzler SH: The myofascial genesis of pain. *Postgrad Med* 11:425–434, 1952 (p. 427).

48. Vitti M, Basmajian JV: Muscles of mastication in small children: an electromyographic analysis. *Am J Orthod* 68:412–419, 1975.

49. Wetzler G: Physical therapy, Chapter 24. In *Diseases of the Temporomandibular Apparatus*, edited by D.H. Morgan, W.P. Hall, and S.J. Vamvas. C.V. Mosby, St. Louis, 1977 (pp. 356, Fig. 24-4).

50. Williams HL: The syndrome of physical or intrinsic allergy of the head: myalgia of the head (sinus headache). *Proc Staff Meet Mayo Clin* 20:177–183, 1945 (p. 181).

51. Williams HL, Elkins EC: Myalgia of the head. *Arch Phys Ther* 23:14–22, 1942 (pp. 18, 19).

52. Woelfel JB, Hickey JC, Stacey RW, *et al.*: Electromyographic analysis of jaw movements. *J Prosthet Dent* 10:688–697, 1960.

53. Wolff HG: *Wolff's Headache and Other Head Pain*, revised by D.J. Dalessio, Ed. 3. Oxford University Press, 1972 (pp. 538, 539).

54. Yemm R: The question of "resting" tonic activity of motor units in the masseter and temporal muscles in man. *Arch Oral Biol* 22:349, 1977.

55. Zohn DA, Mennell J McM: *Musculoskeletal Pain: Diagnosis and Physical Treatment*. Little Brown & Company, Boston, 1976 (Fig. 9–12).

CHAPTER 10
Medial (Internal) Pterygoid Muscle
"Ache inside the Mouth"

HIGHLIGHTS: **REFERRED PAIN** from this muscle projects vaguely to the back of the mouth and pharynx, below and behind the temporomandibular joint (TMJ), and deep in the ear. **ANATOMICAL ATTACHMENTS** of the medial pterygoid to the angle of the mandible and to the lateral pterygoid plate form a sling with the masseter muscle to suspend the mandible. **ACTIONS** are primarily to elevate the mandible and to laterally deviate it to the opposite side; it also can assist protrusion of the mandible. **SYMPTOMS** caused by active trigger points (TPs) in this muscle are difficulty in swallowing and painful, moderately restricted, jaw opening. **ACTIVATION OF TRIGGER POINTS** is often secondary to lateral pterygoid involvement and to occlusal imbalance. The muscle is rarely involved alone. **PATIENT EXAMINATION** usually reveals contralateral deviation of the incisal path as the jaws are opened and closed, with restriction of opening. **TRIGGER POINT EXAMINATION** should include palpation from inside and outside the mouth. **STRETCH AND SPRAY** are usually successful if active TPs in other masticatory muscles and in the neck muscles have been inactivated first. **INJECTION AND STRETCH** may be approached from inside or outside the mouth, but may not be necessary after stretch-and-spray treatment. **CORRECTIVE ACTIONS** include use of an occlusal splint, inactivation of masticatory TPs, equilibration of the dentition if occlusal disharmony persists, and self-stretch exercises.

1. REFERRED PAIN
(Fig. 10.1)

The medial pterygoid muscle refers pain in poorly circumscribed regions related to the mouth (tongue, pharynx, and hard palate), below and behind the TMJ, including deep in the ear, but not to the teeth (Fig. 10.1).[5, 39, 40] Other authors have reported pain referred to the retromandibular and infra-auricular area,[4, 7, 13] including the region of the lateral pterygoid muscle, the floor of the nose, and the throat.[30] Patients describe pain from the medial pterygoid as being more diffuse than the pain referred from trigger points (TPs) in the lateral pterygoid muscle.

Stuffiness of the ear may be a symptom of medial pterygoid TPs. In order for the tensor veli palatini muscle to dilate the Eustachian tube, it must push the adjacent medial pterygoid muscle and interposed fascia aside; in the resting state, the presence of the medial pterygoid helps to keep the Eustachian tube closed. Tense myofascial TP bands in the medial pterygoid muscle may block the opening action of the tensor veli palatini on the Eustachian tube producing barohypoacusis (ear stuffiness). Medial pterygoid tenderness was confirmed in all 31 patients who were examined and who had this symptom.[1]

2. ANATOMICAL ATTACHMENTS
(Fig. 10.2)

The medial pterygoid and the masseter muscles together suspend the angle of the

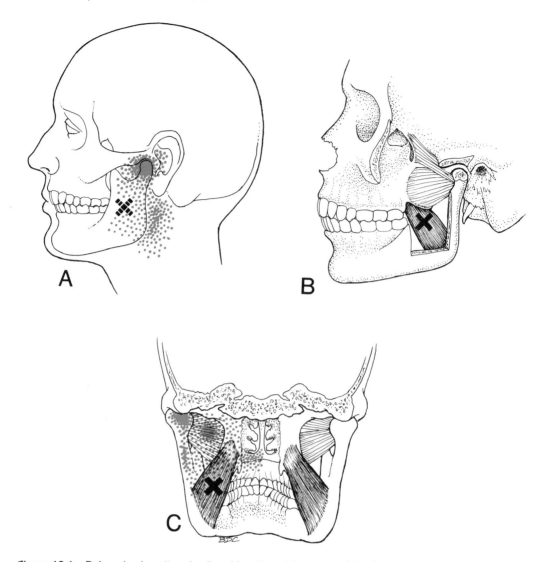

Figure 10.1   Referred pain pattern (*red*) and location of the responsible trigger point (✕) in the left medial pterygoid muscle. *A*, external areas of pain to which the patient can point. *B*, anatomical cut-away to show the location of the trigger point area in the muscle, which lies on the inner side of the mandible. *C*, coronal section of the head through the temporomandibular joint, looking forward, showing internal areas of pain.

mandible, like a sling. The bulk of the medial pterygoid attaches **above** to the medial (inner) surface of the lateral pterygoid plate, and lies partly under the inferior division of the lateral pterygoid muscle (Fig. 10.2A).

A slip of the medial pterygoid often attaches to the lateral surface of the palatine bone, passing over the lateral surface of the lateral pterygoid plate, and thus covers the lower end of the inferior division of the lateral pterygoid muscle. From the side view, this gives the erroneous impression

that the entire medial pterygoid attaches to the lateral (outer) surface of the lateral pterygoid plate.[21]

The medial pterygoid muscle attaches **below** by a short aponeurosis to the lower border of the ramus to the mandible, close to the angle of the mandible (Fig. 10.2B).

Supplemental References

Other authors illustrate this muscle in the lateral (side view),[17, 21, 33, 35, 38] in medial view (from inside the mouth),[16, 22, 34] in rear view (from inside the mouth),[11, 23, 36, 37] and

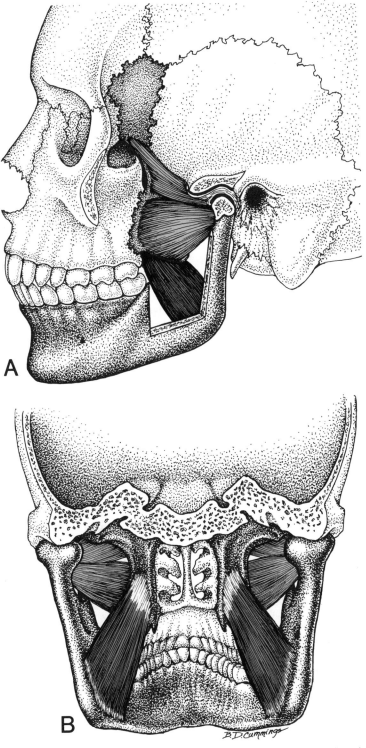

Figure 10.2 Attachments of the medial pterygoid muscle (*dark red*) and its relation to the lateral pterygoid muscle (*light red*). *A*, lateral view showing the medial pterygoid muscle beneath the mandible. Part of the mandible and the zygomatic arch have been removed. *B*, coronal section of the skull just behind the temporomandibular joint, looking forward inside the mouth. The medial pterygoid muscle attaches, above, to the medial (inner) surface of the lateral pterygoid plate of the sphenoid bone and, below, to the medial surface of the mandible, above its angle.

in cross section.[10, 15] One lateral view also shows the overlying pterygoid venus plexus.[35]

3. INNERVATION

The muscle is supplied by the medial pterygoid nerve which arises from the common, fused portion of the mandibular division of the trigeminal nerve (cranial nerve V).

4. ACTIONS

Bilaterally, the medial pterygoid muscles help to elevate the mandible (close the jaws) in concert with the masseter and temporalis muscles.[2, 3, 17, 19, 43] The medial pterygoid activity is increased if the mandible also is protruded while it is being elevated.[24] Acting unilaterally, the medial pterygoid muscle deviates the mandible toward the opposite side.[2, 3, 19, 43]

The medial pterygoid becomes electromyographically active during simple protrusion of the mandible, especially if the jaws are only slightly apart,[3] but of less intensity if the mandible is voluntarily depressed.[24] Protrusion by the medial pterygoid would be inhibited during mandibular depression since this muscle is a major antagonist to the opening motion and only an assistant to the lateral pterygoid for protrusion of the mandible.

5. MYOTATIC UNIT

Acting bilaterally, the medial pterygoid muscles function synergistically with the masseter and temporalis muscles to close the jaws; and they act as antagonists to the inferior division of the lateral pterygoid and the digastric muscles, which open the jaws. Bilaterally, the medial pterygoid muscles are synergistic with the lateral pterygoid muscles for protrusion of the mandible.

Each medial pterygoid is synergistic with its neighboring lateral pterygoid muscle when deviating the mandible toward the opposite side. As a result, both pterygoid muscles on one side act as antagonists to their counterparts on the other side for lateral deviation of the mandible.

6. SYMPTOMS

Patients describe pain referred from TPs in this muscle as shown in Fig. 10.1 and as described in Section 1. This pain is increased by attempts to open the mouth wide, by chewing food, or by clenching the teeth. Patients also may complain of soreness inside the throat and of painful swallowing. When attempting to swallow, they extend the neck and push the tongue forward, apparently trying to overcome a restriction in the forward movement of the mandible.

7. ACTIVATION OF TRIGGER POINTS

Occlusal Imbalance

Involvement of the medial pterygoid muscle can be secondary to the muscular dysfunction that results from TPs in the lateral pterygoid muscle; TPs in both these muscles are activated by occlusal disharmony, which is discussed in more detail in Section 7 of Chapter 8. The importance of an interfering occlusal contact is demonstrated by the return of more normal muscle function and by pain relief in response to occlusal splint therapy.[27] This is achieved by an occlusal appliance, such as, the Hawley biteplate,[25] the Shore mandibular autorepositioning appliance,[32] the Gelb mandibular orthopaedic repositioning appliance,[14] or the Tanner appliance, to mention several. Each has its protagonists.

The medial pterygoid muscle on one side may develop active TPs because of the increased stress imposed on it by TP activity in, and distorted function of, the corresponding muscle on the opposite side.

Activity Stress

Sucking of the thumb after infancy or excessive gum chewing may activate TPs in this muscle. Occlusal interference, bruxism (lateral grinding of the teeth), clenching of teeth, anxiety and emotional tension are common activating factors.

A less common cause is trismus due to medial pterygoid spasm, activated reflexly by cellulitis in the pterygomandibular space.[7]

8. PATIENT EXAMINATION

The mandibular opening is usually obviously restricted,[5] so that the jaw aperture barely admits two knuckles (see Three-knuckle Test, Chapter 8).

PART 1

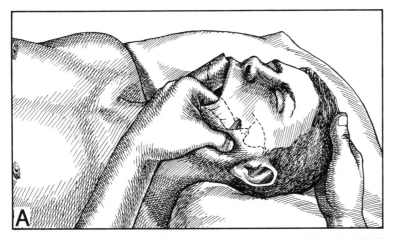

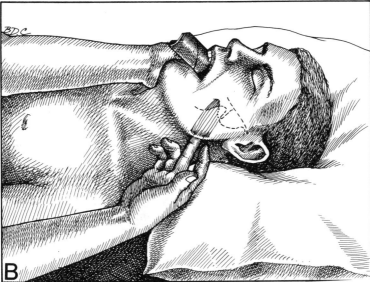

Figure 10.3   Examination of the medial pterygoid muscle. *A*, intra-oral palpation behind the last molar tooth, with the muscle and the ramus of the mandible between the palpating digits. The mouth is securely propped open, since the index finger is in a vulnerable position between the molar teeth. *B*, extra-oral palpation of the muscle along the inner surface of the mandible, at its angle.

During opening of the jaws, unilateral involvement of the medial pterygoid muscle is variously reported as deviating the mandible toward the opposite side,[5] to the same side, or not at all.[28] We find that deviation due mainly to shortening of this muscle is most marked to the contralateral side as the mandible approaches the maximum mouth opening. The side to which the mandible deviates depends greatly on how severely other protruding, retruding, and lateral-deviating muscles are involved; one medial pterygoid muscle rarely develops TPs alone.

9. TRIGGER POINT EXAMINATION
(Fig. 10.3)

A prop is inserted between the incisor teeth to open the jaws as wide as is comfortable in order to place the medial pterygoid fibers on moderate tension. To palpate the medial pterygoid from outside the mouth, the head is tilted slightly to improve access to the muscle. One finger examines the inner (medial) surface of the mandible by pressing upward at its angle (Fig. 10.3B).[8,45] The firm mass, approximately 1 cm (⅜ in) above the angle of the mandible, just within reach of the finger, is the mandibular end of the muscle.

Palpation of the mid-belly of the muscle is performed intra-orally with the mouth propped open (Fig. 10.3A). The pad of the palpating index finger faces outward and slides over the molar teeth until it encounters the bony edge of the ramus of the mandible, which lies behind and lateral to the position of the last molar tooth, as also illustrated by others.[13, 20, 29]

Palpating the muscle against the mandible through the pharyngeal mucosa is likely to make the patient gag. The gag reflex is greatly reduced if, during examination, the patient either exhales fully or takes a deep breath,[1] and holds it during examination. Rolling the tip of the tongue as far as possible down the throat behind the molar teeth on the opposite side further inhibits the gag reflex. The harder the patient forces the tongue backward and down the throat, the less sensitive the reflex becomes.

Just posterior to the bony edge of the ramus, the finger encounters a vertical muscular mass, the medial pterygoid muscle. It is clearly identified by having the patient alternately clench and relax against a block placed between the teeth while the operator indents the mass with the finger. When the medial pterygoid harbors active TPs, pressure on it elicits exquisite tenderness, revealing the precise location of a TP.

If there is concern for the safety of the examining finger, a finger of the examiner's other hand can push from the outside to pouch some of the patient's opposite cheek between the back teeth. The patient will now bite his own cheek before biting the finger.

Studies have repeatedly shown that in patients with the myofascial pain-dysfunction syndrome this muscle, which is seldom involved alone, is less likely to be tender than are most of the other masticatory muscles.[9, 12, 18, 31]

10. ENTRAPMENTS

No neurovascular entrapments due to TPs in this muscle have been identified.

11. ASSOCIATED TRIGGER POINTS

The medial pterygoid usually develops TPs in association with myotatically re-

lated muscles, especially the lateral pterygoid and masseter, as noted in Section 5.

12. STRETCH AND SPRAY
(Fig. 10.4)

In our experience, the medial pterygoid usually responds well to stretch and spray; it rarely requires injection, unless the patient has chronically "frozen" or dystrophic jaw musculature. Passive stretch may be applied while the patient is seated comfortably, and has the jaws propped open at a tolerable stretch (Fig. 10.4A), as described in Chapter 8. Sweeps of vapocoolant spray are applied from the neck below and behind the mandible, upward over the cheek, beneath the ear, and over the temporomandibular joint.

Additional relaxation and a greater degree of stretch may be obtained when the patient lies supine and applies self-stretch, by placing two fingers behind the lower incisor teeth and the thumb under the chin, then by pulling the mandible forward and down to open the jaws fully (Fig. 10.4B). Self-stretch helps apprehensive patients to accept this treatment. Meanwhile, the operator applies the spray to the same skin areas, as above. It is wise to apply spray to the opposite medial pterygoid that also is being stretched. It is not necessary to spray the mucous membrane inside the mouth. A hot pack is applied promptly over the cooled skin.

Schwartz and Tausig[28] present illustrative case reports of stretch-and-spray therapy.

An effort is made to avoid unnecessary inhalation of the spray vapor by the supine patient. Inhalation should be avoided, even though Fluori-Methane spray is applied. If ethyl chloride spray is being used (which is not recommended) and the patient is supine, it is absolutely essential that the heavy vapor does not pool around the patient's face. Ethyl chloride is a rapidly acting, potentially lethal, general anesthetic; Fluori-Methane is not a general anesthetic.

Ultrasound is more effective, if directed at the TPs, rather than at the pain reference zones. For this muscle, it may be applied behind the gonial angle of the mandible because of its depth of penetration,[25] or intra-orally.

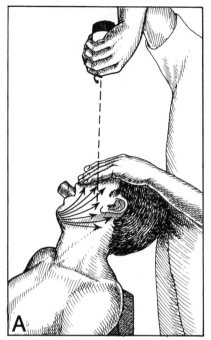

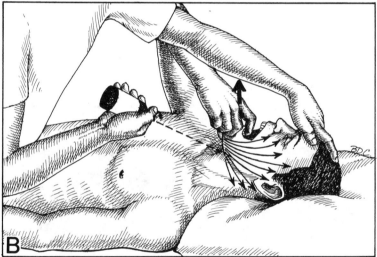

Figure 10.4 Stretch positions and spray pattern (*arrows*) for the left medial pterygoid muscle. *A*, seated, with the head tilted back against the operator and the patient's jaws propped open. *B*, self-stretch while supine, for better relaxation; the patient pulls the mandible forward and down to fully depress the mandible during application of the vapocoolant spray, with bracing of the patient's forehead by the operator. A pad should protect the eye.

13. INJECTION AND STRETCH
(Fig. 10.5)

The medial pterygoid rarely requires injection of its TPs, since they respond well to stretch and spray, provided that active TPs in other masticatory muscles have been inactivated first. On the other hand,

Gelb[14] reports that intra-oral injection of active TPs in the medial pterygoid relieves pain arising from TPs in other muscles on that side of the face. Masticatory muscles tend to breed secondary and satellite TPs among themselves.

The muscle may be approached for injection from either inside, or outside the

PART 1

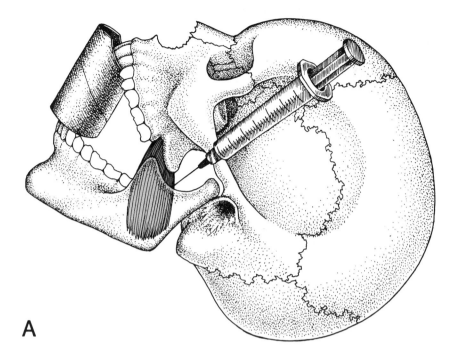

A

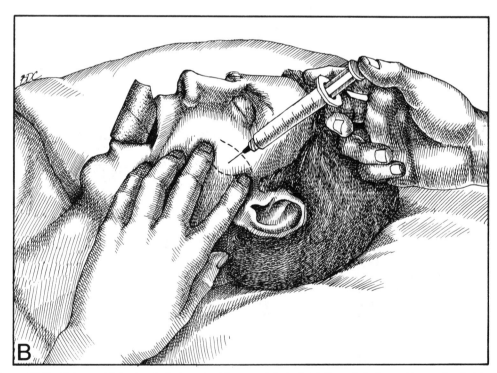

B

Figure 10.5   Extra-oral injection technique for trigger points in the left medial pterygoid muscle. *A*, lateral view showing access to the muscle through the space above the mandibular notch between the coronoid process and the condyle of the mandible. The jaws must be propped wide open. *B*, injection through the opening above the mandibular notch. *C*, lateral view of the injection technique to show the level of the section in Part *D*. To reach the medial pterygoid muscle using this approach, the needle must penetrate to a depth greater than that of the pterygoid plate. *D*, coronal section of the head, located just behind the needle insertion, looking forward. Note that the medial pterygoid attaches to the underside of the pterygoid plate, and the lateral pterygoid muscle attaches to the outer surface of the plate.

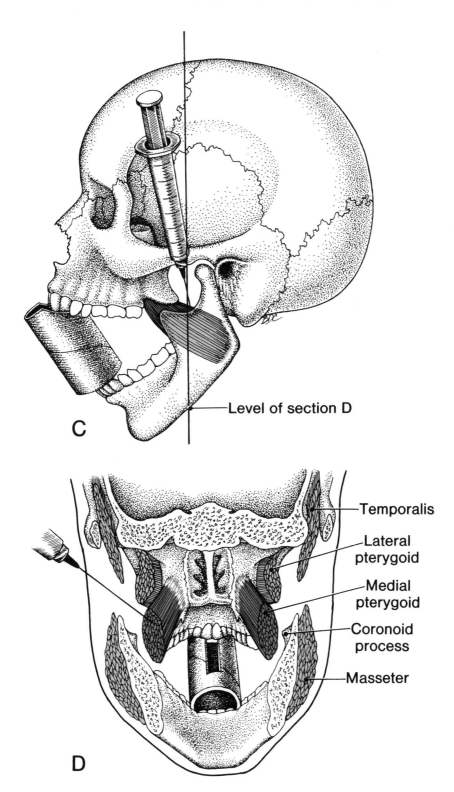

Level of section D

C

Temporalis

Lateral
pterygoid

Medial
pterygoid

Coronoid
process

Masseter

D

Figures 10.5 *C* and *D*.

mouth. To inject the muscle through the skin of the supine patient[6, 39] the mouth is propped open as wide as can be tolerated in order to lower the mandibular notch. After disinfection of the skin, the vapocoolant, Fluori-Methane spray, is applied for cutaneous local anesthesia to eliminate the pain of the needleprick,[41] as described in Section 13, Chapter 3. The needle is inserted between the condyle and the coronoid process, and is directed caudally along the vertical axis of the ramus of the mandible, as in Fig. 10.5. Examination of a skull is helpful to visualize clearly the path of the needle and the depth of penetration required to enter the belly of the muscle deep to the level of, and posterior to, the lateral pterygoid plate.

No major arteries or nerves lie in this path of the needle in the immediate vicinity of the medial pterygoid muscle. The needle, however, must traverse the extensive network of the pterygoid venous plexus, which lies superficial to the lateral pterygoid muscle[35] and is a potential source of bleeding. This injection should be avoided in patients who have an abnormal bleeding tendency, as occurs with low levels of ascorbic acid, or with anticoagulant medication.

To inject the muscle from inside the mouth, the TP is located by palpation and injected directly through the pharyngeal wall, as illustrated by Gelb.[14] A hyperactive gag reflex makes it difficult to use the intra-oral route.

14. CORRECTIVE ACTIONS

Premature Tooth Contacts

A first approach to premature tooth contacts and/or bruxism is a trial with an occlusal splint and inactivation of TPs in the masticatory muscles. If occlusal disharmonies persist, occlusal equilibration may be required for prolonged relief.[14, 32] However, irreversible tooth reconfiguration should wait until TPs in the masticatory muscles have been eliminated.[7, 32]

Exercise Therapy

The patient should first be instructed in a self-stretch, passive, jaw-opening exercise performed while supine, like the movement used for the self-stretch and operator-spray technique shown in Fig.

10.4B. As the muscle lengthens and becomes less painful, the patient can progress to active, resistive, and facilitatory exercises for jaw opening and for lateral deviation, as described and illustrated by Wetzler.[44] The lateral deviation exercise for the lateral pterygoid is equally applicable to the medial pterygoid muscle.

Other Measures

Mechanical and reflex perpetuating factors, such as, active TPs in the neck, shoulder-girdle, and sometimes even in the lower-extremity muscles, should be eliminated. Common nutritional perpetuating factors are critically important, as discussed in Chapter 4.

Factors that increase anxiety and emotional tension, including depression, should be identified and alleviated, if possible.

Any chronic infection, especially in the head and neck region, should be treated; recurrent oral herpes simplex infection should be controlled.

If the patient continues to have difficulty in swallowing, after inactivation of medial pterygoid TPs, the sternocleidomastoid (Chapter 7), the digastric (Chapter 12), and possibly the longus capitis and longus colli muscles, should be examined for TPs. The latter can be palpated behind the posterior pharyngeal wall through the open mouth and may be inactivated by stretch and spray (see Fig. 7.5 in Chapter 7, and Fig. 16.7 in Chapter 16), or by the application of 1.0 watt/cm^2 of ultrasound to the muscles.[26]

Until the dysphagia is relieved, swallowing a tablet or capsule is facilitated by placing the medication *underneath* the tip of the tongue, behind the lower front teeth; from there, when the head is erect, the medication follows the bolus of liquid being swallowed.[42] When the tablet is placed on *top* of the tongue, as is customary, the tongue presses it against the roof of the mouth where it may stick during swallowing.

References

1. Adams SH II: Personal communication, 1981.
2. Bardeen, CR: The musculature, Sect. 5. In *Morris's Human Anatomy*, edited by C.M. Jackson, Ed. 6. Blakiston's Son & Co., Philadelphia, 1921 (p. 377).

3. Basmajian, JV: *Muscles Alive*, Ed. 4. Williams & Wilkins, Baltimore, 1978 (pp. 386–390).
4. Bell WE: Clinical diagnosis of the pain-dysfunction syndrome. *J Am Dent Assoc* 79:154–160, 1969 (p. 158).
5. Bell WE: Nonsurgical management of the pain-dysfunction syndrome. *J Am Dent Assoc* 79:161–170, 1969 (p. 165).
6. Bell WE: Management of masticatory pain, Chapter 12. In *Facial Pain*, edited by C.C. Alling, III, P.E. Mahan, Ed. 2. Lea & Febiger, Philadelphia 1977 (p. 189, Fig. 12-5).
7. Bell WE: *Orofacial Pains—Differential Diagnosis*, Ed. 2. Yearbook Medical Publishers, Chicago, 1979 (pp. 193, 242, 252).
8. Burch JG: Occlusion related to craniofacial pain, Chapter 11. In *Facial Pain*, edited by C.C. Alling, III, P.E. Mahan, Ed. 2. Lea & Febiger, Philadelphia, 1977 (p. 171, Fig. 11-10).
9. Butler JH, Folke LEA, Bandt CL: A descriptive survey of signs and symptoms associated with the myofascial pain-dysfunction syndrome. *J Am Dent Assoc* 90:635–639, 1975.
10. Eisler P: *Die Muskeln des Stammes*. Gustav Fischer, Jena, 1912 (Fig. 25).
11. *Ibid.* (Fig. 26).
12. Franks AST: Masticatory muscle hyperactivity and temporomandibular joint dysfunction. *J Prosthet Dent* 15:1122–1131, 1965 (p. 1126).
13. Gelb H: Patient evaluation, Chapter 3. In *Clinical Management of Head, Neck, and TMJ Pain and Dysfunction*, edited by H. Gelb. W.B. Saunders, Philadelphia, 1977 (pp. 85, 96, Fig. 3-14).
14. Gelb H: Effective management and treatment of the craniomandibular syndrome, Chapter 11. In *Clinical Management of Head, Neck and TMJ Pain and Dysfunction*, edited by H. Gelb. W.B. Saunders, Philadelphia, 1977 (pp. 299, 301, 302, 309, 314, Fig. 11-6I).
15. Grant JCB: *An Atlas of Human Anatomy*, Ed. 7. Williams & Wilkins, Baltimore, 1978 (Fig. 7-82).
16. *Ibid.* (Fig. 7-89).
17. Gray H: *Anatomy of the Human Body*, edited by C. M. Goss, American Ed. 29. Lea & Febiger, Philadelphia, 1973 (p. 389, Fig. 6-6).
18. Greene CS, Lerman MD, Sutcher HD, *et al.*: The TMJ pain-dysfunction syndrome: heterogeneity of the patient population. *J Am Dent Assoc* 79:1168–1172, 1969.
19. Hollinshead WH: *Functional Anatomy of the Limbs and Back*, Ed 4. W.B. Saunders, Philadelphia, 1976 (p. 376).
20. Ingle JI, Beveridge EE: *Endodontics*, Ed. 2. Lea & Febiger, Philadelphia, 1976 (Fig. 11-12B).
21. McMinn RMH, Hutchings RT: *Color Atlas of Human Anatomy*. Year Book Medical Publishers, Chicago, 1977 (p. 38).
22. *Ibid.* (p. 45).
23. *Ibid.* (p. 50).
24. Moyers RE: An electromyographic analysis of certain muscles involved in temporomandibular movement. *Am J Orthod* 36:481–515, 1950 (pp. 484, 490, 502).
25. Nel H: Myofascial pain-dysfunction syndrome. *J Prosthet Dent* 40:438–441, 1978 (pp. 440, 441).
26. Palchick Y: Personal communication, 1981.
27. Perry HT Jr.: Muscular changes associated with temporomandibular joint dysfunction. *J Am Dent Assoc* 54:644–653, 1957.
28. Schwartz LL, Tausig DP: Temporomandibular joint pain—treatment with intramuscular infiltration of tetracaine hydrochloride: a preliminary report. *NY State Dent J* 20:219–223, 1954 (Cases 3, 4 and 5).
29. Seltzer S: Oral conditions that cause head and neck pain, Chapter 8. In *Pain Control in Dentistry*, J.B. Lippincott, Philadelphia, 1978 (Fig. 8-12).
30. Shaber EP: Considerations in the treatment of muscle spasm, Chapter 17. In *Diseases of the Temporomandibular Apparatus*, edited by D.H. Morgan, W.P. Hall, S.J. Vamvas. C.V. Mosby, St. Louis, 1977 (p. 250).
31. Sharav Y, Tzukert A, Refaeli B: Muscle pain index in relation to pain, dysfunction, and dizziness associated with the myofascial pain-dysfunction syndrome. *Oral Surg* 46:742–747, 1978.
32. Shore NA: *Temporomandibular Joint Dysfunction and Occlusal Equilibration*, Ed. 2. J.B. Lippincott, Philadelphia, 1976 (pp. 237, 238).
33. Sobotta J, Figge FHJ: *Atlas of Human Anatomy*, Ed. 9, Vol. 1. Hafner Division of Macmillan, New York, 1974 (pp. 184, 186).
34. *Ibid.* (p. 187).
35. Sobotta J, Figge FHJ: *Atlas of Human Anatomy*, Ed. 9, Vol. 3. Hafner Division of Macmillan, New York, 1974 (p. 211).
36. Spalteholz W: *Handatlas der Anatomie des Menschen*, Ed. 11, Vol. 2. S. Hirzel, Leipzig, 1922 (p. 267).
37. Toldt C: *An Atlas of Human Anatomy*, translated by M.E. Paul, Ed. 2, Vol. 1. Macmillan, New York, 1919 (p. 295).
38. *Ibid.* (p. 307).
39. Travell J: Temporomandibular joint pain referred from muscles of the head and neck. *J Prosthet Dent* 10:745–763, 1960 (pp. 749, 750, Fig. 5).
40. Travell J: Mechanical headache. *Headache* 7:23–29, 1967 (pp. 26, 27).
41. Travell J: *Office Hours: Day and Night*. World Publishing Company, New York, 1968 (pp. 296–297).
42. Travell JG: Nonstick trick for pill swallowing. *Patient Care* 9:17, 1975.
43. Vamvas SJ: Differential diagnosis of TMJ disease, Chapter 13. In *Diseases of the Temporomandibular Apparatus*, edited by D.H. Morgan, W.P. Hall, S.J. Vamvas. C.V. Mosby, St. Louis, 1977 (p. 190).
44. Wetzler G: Physical therapy, Chapter 24. In *Diseases of the Temporomandibular Apparatus*, edited by D.H. Morgan, W.P. Hall, S.J. Vamvas, C.V. Mosby, St. Louis, 1977 (pp. 348–353, Fig. 24-2B).
45. Whinery JG: Examination of patients with facial pain, Chapter 10. In *Facial Pain*, edited by C. C. Alling III, P.E. Mahan, Ed. 2. Lea & Febiger, Philadelphia, 1977 (p. 159).

CHAPTER 11
Lateral (External) Pterygoid Muscle
"TMJ-dysfunction"

HIGHLIGHTS: The lateral (external) pterygoid muscle is frequently the key to understanding and managing the temporomandibular joint (TMJ) dysfunction syndrome and related craniomandibular disorders. Active trigger points (TPs) in this muscle disturb the position of the mandible and its incisal path during opening and closing of the jaws. REFERRED PAIN from TPs in this muscle is felt strongly in the TMJ and in the maxilla. ANATOMICAL ATTACHMENTS and functions of the two divisions of the lateral pterygoid muscle are distinctly different. The superior division attaches, in front, to the sphenoid bone and, behind, to the articular disc and capsule of the TMJ. The inferior division attaches, in front, to the lateral pterygoid plate and, behind, to the neck of the mandible. The ACTION of the superior division pulls the articular disc forward and checkreins its backward movement, thus assisting mandibular elevation; that of the inferior division protrudes and depresses the mandible with lateral deviation to the opposite side. SYMPTOMS include pain in the region of the TMJ and maxilla, and neuromusculoskeletal dysfunction of the chewing apparatus. ACTIVATION OF TRIGGER POINTS may result from decreased vertical dimension and from occlusal disharmony that, in turn, can be aggravated by TP activity in this muscle. PATIENT EXAMINATION shows slight restriction of jaw opening, a distorted incisal path, and often occlusal abnormality. TRIGGER POINT EXAMINATION differs for the anterior and posterior parts of both the superior and inferior divisions of this muscle, is difficult, and requires knowledge of the regional anatomy. STRETCH AND SPRAY of this muscle are severely limited by the bone structure. INJECTION AND STRETCH, therefore, are frequently needed. Injection of TPs in this muscle is difficult because of their protected position behind the zygomatic arch and coronoid process of the mandible. CORRECTIVE ACTIONS may initially depend on an occlusal splint and, then, if needed after TP inactivation, restoration of a normal occlusal pattern and condyle-disc relationship. A home exercise program for improving masticatory muscle function, and the elimination of stress factors insure continued relief.

1. REFERRED PAIN
(Fig. 11.1)

The lateral (external) pterygoid muscle refers pain deep into the TMJ[3, 5, 15, 52, 65, 66] and to the region of the maxillary sinus (Fig. 11.1).[52, 65, 66] The pain is strongly associated with functional disorders of that joint.[14, 52] In our experience, TPs in this muscle are the chief myofascial source of referred pain felt in the TMJ area. The syndrome is easily mistaken for the pain of TMJ arthritis.[49]

No distinction has been drawn as to the patterns of pain referred from the two divisions of this muscle; it is sometimes difficult to be sure which division the needle has penetrated.

Pain referred to the teeth has not been

260

PART 1

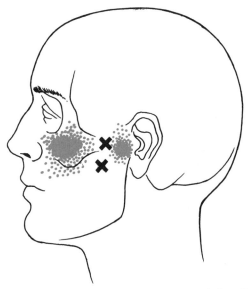

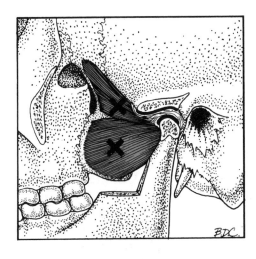

Figure 11.1. The referred pain pattern (dark *red*) of trigger points (×s) in the left lateral pterygoid muscle (lighter red). See caption of Figure 11.2 for anatomical notes.

traced to TPs in the lateral pterygoid muscle.

2. ANATOMICAL ATTACHMENTS
(Fig. 11.2)

The two divisions of the lateral pterygoid muscle lie deep to, and largely behind, the zygomatic arch and the coronoid process of the mandible. There is full agreement that **anteriorly** the *superior* division attaches to the infratemporal crest and to the inferior lateral surface of the great wing of the sphenoid bone, while the *inferior* division attaches to the lateral surface of the lateral pterygoid plate (Fig. 11.2).[1, 12, 20, 59-61]

The precise attachments **posteriorly** at the mandibular end are not so well known. Several anatomists make no distinction between the posterior attachments of the two divisions.[20, 31, 59] The fibers of the *inferior* division slant diagonally upward and are generally said to attach to the condylar neck and ramus of the mandible just below the joint.[1, 12, 24, 45, 61] Examining 42 joints by the superior approach, Porter[48] found that some fibers of the inferior division also attach to the medial portion of the condyle.

The fibers of the *superior* division slant diagonally downward and backward toward the TMJ. Although variable, the **an-**terior attachment is more likely to be lower, as in Figure 11.2, than as in Figure 11.1, producing a more horizontal force vector on the disc.[34] Their **posterior** attachment is generally misunderstood. According to several anatomists, the posterior attachments of this division include not only the ligament of the joint capsule and articular disc, but also the upper one-third of the front of the neck of the condyle.[1, 12, 61] One author[24] specifically dissected 10 muscles in five human cadavers to determine precisely where the fibers of the two divisions attach to the mandible; another[48] dissected 42 cadavers. In all these dissections, the *superior* division attached posteriorly only to the capsular ligament and articular disc, and *not* to the neck of the condyle. Perry and Marsh[45] illustrated each muscular attachment at the joint in vertical section and made this same distinction. Apparently, when a few fibers of the superior division occasionally attach below the capsular ligament, they are exceptional and of negligible functional importance.

Rarely, the lateral pterygoid may fuse with the temporalis muscle, but fibers of the two divisions of the lateral pterygoid do not fuse with each other.[1]

It is helpful to remember that the anterior attachments of the *medial* pterygoid

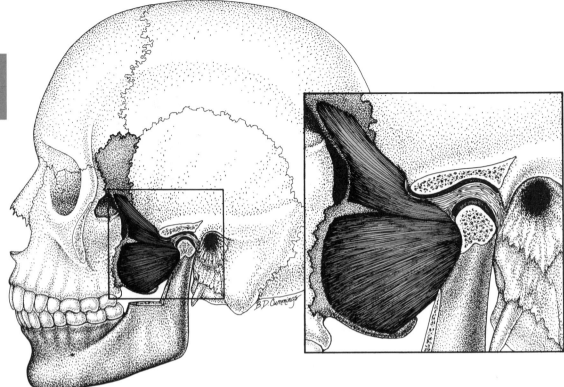

Figure 11.2   Attachments of the lateral pterygoid muscle. The zygomatic arch and superficial portion of the temporomandibular joint have been removed to show the attachments of the superior division to the articular disc and joint capsule. The inferior division attaches to the neck of the condyle, on the mandible. The condyle normally articulates with the posterior surface of the articular tubercle, or eminentia.

muscle and the inferior division of the *lateral* pterygoid muscle are separated by the pterygoid plate (see Fig. 11.5*C* and *D*); the medial pterygoid fibers attach to the medial surface of the plate, and the inferior division of the lateral pterygoid, to the lateral surface of the plate.[31]

The condyle of the mandible must glide forward over the posterior surface of the articular tubercle (eminence) to open the jaws fully, which explains the double-cavity structure of the TMJ with an intermediate articular disc (Fig. 11.2).[20] This articular disc consists of collagen fibers, not cartilage.[35] (See Chapter 5, Fig. 5.2, for structural details of the TMJ.)

Supplemental References

The lateral pterygoid muscle is clearly illustrated from the side,[1, 12, 18, 20, 31, 39, 58–60, 62, 64] from the rear,[61, 63] in cross section,[10, 13, 17] and in sectional side view.[45]

3. INNERVATION

Both divisions are innervated by the lateral pterygoid nerve from the anterior division of the mandibular branch of the trigeminal nerve (cranial nerve V).[20] The buccal and lingual nerves also may contribute filaments to this muscle.[1]

4. ACTIONS

Although authors in the past have referred to the actions of *the* lateral pterygoid muscle, one must now think of its two divisions as, functionally and anatomically, two separate reciprocating muscles. The functions ascribed to the "lateral pterygoid" muscle in the past are those of the *inferior division* which might be called more appropriately, the *inferior lateral pterygoid muscle.* Its functions include: opening the jaws, protrusion of the mandible by the muscles on both sides acting together, and lateral deviation of the mandible to the opposite side by one muscle acting unilaterally.[1, 2, 20, 23, 60, 67] Confirming the first three functions electromyographically by placing a needle in the inferior division *via* the oral route, Moyers[44] observed earlier onset of, and more vigorous motor unit activity in, the inferior division than in the digastric muscle during mandibular opening. The inferior division became active during closure only if the movement was combined with protrusion. Activation of this division by lateral movement of the mandible to the opposite side increased if the mandible was simultaneously depressed.

In the past, failure to make a functional distinction between the two divisions of the lateral pterygoid muscle has led to inconsistent and contradictory statements as to whether this muscle opens or closes the jaws.[40] Electromyographically, the two divisions are antagonists in Rhesus monkeys[40] and in man.[19, 30] Additional studies in man with fine wire electrodes indicate that the two heads function reciprocally during both vertical and horizontal mandibular movements.[34] Anatomically,[11] biomechanically,[19] and electromyographically,[30, 40] the *superior division* exerts forward traction on the articular disc at the level of the condylar head during closure of the jaws. Overactivity or TP shortening of the superior division fibers, therefore, displaces the articular disc forward and impedes its return to its normal position on closure of the jaws (Figs. 5.2–5.5 in Chapter 5). On the other hand, the *inferior division* pulls the condylar head forward and down so that the condyle can translate over the posterior surface of the eminence, a movement essential for full opening.

Myofascial TPs in either division of the lateral pterygoid muscle can be the cause, or the result, of premature contacts.[67] Needle-electrode study of the inferior division shows this muscle to be the most active in positioning the mandible during ipsilateral clench as the teeth are forced together by other muscles.[69] The medial pterygoid and both divisions of the lateral pterygoid participate in the lateral and closing movements when grinding food between the molar teeth.[1, 67]

A few muscle spindles are reported in the lateral pterygoid (division not specified), but in a much lower concentration per gram of muscle than in the other primary muscles of mastication.[29, 37] This masticatory muscle, therefore, may have less active stretch reflexes than the others.

5. MYOTATIC UNIT

The two divisions of the lateral pterygoid act alternately when the jaws are opened and closed. To depress the mandible, the lower division acts synergistically with the digastric and other suprahyoid muscles.[1, 30, 40, 67] During elevation of the mandible, the superior division of the lateral pterygoid becomes active with the masseter and temporalis muscles.[30, 40] Mandibular protrusion is assisted slightly by the superficial layer of the masseter and by the medial pterygoid,[67] and by the anterior fibers of the temporalis muscle.[1] Mandibular movements to the opposite side are assisted by the ipsilateral medial pterygoid, contralateral masseter, and anterior fibers of the contralateral temporalis muscle.[57, 67]

The inferior divisions of the paired lateral pterygoid muscles act synergistically for protrusion, but electromyographically are antagonistic to each other for lateral movements of the mandible.[22, 44, 69]

6. SYMPTOMS

Most patients with the myofascial pain-dysfunction (MPD) syndrome suffer primarily from a muscular disorder, such as that caused by active TPs in the lateral pterygoid muscle.[25] Severe pain in the TMJ region is commonly referred from TPs in the lateral pterygoid, the medial pterygoid, or the deep layer of the masseter. The pain projected to and felt in the TMJ,[49] as well as malocclusion due to TP tension with shortening of the muscles, often have caused treatment to be misdirected to the joint and teeth, with frustrating results. This happens when the critical role played by TPs in the lateral pterygoid and other masticatory muscles has been ignored.

Severe pain referred to the maxilla, with the autonomic concomitant of excessive secretion from the maxillary sinus, may likewise be misdiagnosed as sinusitis, so that the patient describes the pain as a "sinus attack."

Myofascial pain on chewing tends to be proportional to the vigor of movement.[5] Clicking sounds in the TMJ area, which are now attributed to an anteriorly displaced articular disc,[7, 38] may result from dysfunction of the lateral pterygoid muscles.[36] Although the opening between the jaws is reduced when only the lateral pterygoid muscle harbors active TPs, the decrease in range may not be sufficient for the patient to be aware of it.

The *pain* associated with malocclusion, or occlusal disharmony, is often due to involvement of the masticatory muscles, especially the lateral pterygoid,[6, 46, 50–52] but the *malocclusion* itself also may be due to internal TMJ derangement or advanced arthritis of this joint.

It is not clear whether degenerative arthritic changes in the TMJ with their grinding, clicking sounds and crepitus are a result of, or one of the causes of TP activation in the lateral pterygoid muscle. They seem to intensify each other. The presence of structural changes in the joint may be demonstrated by tomograms, computerized tomography, arthrograms, and modified Updegrave transcranial lateral oblique radiograms.

7. ACTIVATION OF TRIGGER POINTS

Lateral pterygoid TPs may develop as satellites in response to TP activity of the neck muscles, especially the sternocleidomastoid, which, in turn, may be activated by the mechanical stress caused by a short leg or a small hemipelvis.

Occlusal Activation

Malocclusion with premature occlusal contact can be a major etiologic factor in the activation of lateral pterygoid TPs. As discussed more fully in Chapter 8, Section 7, an interfering occlusal tooth contact increases contractile activity of the lateral pterygoid, and should be investigated as an initiating and perpetuating cause of these masticatory TPs.

Activity Stress

Bruxism may be either the cause, or the result of lateral pterygoid TPs, and contributes strongly to the overuse of this muscle.

It can be seriously overloaded by excessive gum chewing, by playing a wind instrument with the mandible fixed in protrusion, and by maintaining mandibular side pressure to hold a violin in playing position.

8. PATIENT EXAMINATION

When only the **inferior division** of the lateral pterygoid muscle is affected, there is a slight decrease in jaw aperture that prevents the entry of a tier of three knuckles between the incisor teeth (see Fig. 8.3, the Three-knuckle Test, in Chapter 8), and lateral excursion of the mandible is reduced toward the opposite side, away from the involved muscle. When the patient slowly opens and closes the jaws, the midline incisal path of the mandible deviates; it wobbles back and forth. The most marked deviation from the mid-line during movement is usually away from the side of the more affected lateral pterygoid muscle. Involvement of other masticatory muscles, especially the medial pterygoid, also can contribute to this finding. Lateral pterygoid function is practically eliminated by having the patient slide the tip of the tongue backward along the roof of the mouth to the posterior border of the hard palate, which stops translation of the condyles across the eminentia. If the incisal path straightens out when the mouth is opened in this way, it is chiefly lateral pterygoid dysfunction that is causing the muscular imbalance; if the incisal path still zigzags, other muscles and/or a TMJ derangement are responsible, and the abnormality may or may not also involve the lateral pterygoid.

In our experience and that of many other authors, the lateral pterygoid muscle (inferior division) is strongly implicated in the myofascial or TMJ pain-dysfunction syndromes. The muscle was also tender to palpation more frequently (75–100% of these patients) than any other masticatory muscle in studies of nearly 300 patients.[14, 21, 28, 41] Some authors found that other muscles were tender more frequently than the lateral pterygoid, but it was still tender in 31% of 56 patients,[9] and in 20% of 42 patients.[53] These lower values may reflect the difficulty in palpating this muscle, or differences in the patient populations.

Shortening of the inferior division of one lateral pterygoid muscle displaces anteriorly the mandibular condyle to which it attaches, causing premature contact of the anterior teeth on the opposite side and malocclusion of the posterior teeth on the same side. Little pain is experienced in this displaced resting position, but closing the teeth fully usually induces pain referred to the TMJ on the same side as the involved lateral pterygoid muscle. Vigorous closure increases the pain. Insertion of a tongue blade between the molar teeth on the painful side often eliminates the pain on vigorous clenching. This result strongly implicates the inferior division of the lateral pterygoid muscle on the painful side.[5]

Auditory symptoms associated with dysfunction of the intra-articular disc in the TMJ may be explained by the tiny ligament that connects the malleus ossicle of the middle ear to the medio-postero-superior part of the capsule, the interarticular disc, and the sphenomandibular ligament.[47]

The degree to which TPs in the **upper division** of the lateral pterygoid are responsible for the forward displacement of the intra-articular disc that is associated with clicking, and for posterior superior displacement of the condyle, is not yet firmly established, but deserves investigation. Drawing a clear distinction between the effects of TPs in the upper and lower divisions is critical to a full understanding of these relationships.

9. TRIGGER POINT EXAMINATION
(Fig. 11.3)

To examine *intraorally* for TP tenderness at the anterior attachment of the inferior division of the lateral pterygoid muscle, the finger presses backward as far as possible along the vestibule that forms the roof of the cheek pouch. The mouth is opened about 2 cm (¾ in) and the mandible deviated laterally to the side being examined to improve the clearance, as the finger is squeezed between the maxilla and the coronoid process, along the roots of the upper molar teeth. Several authors have described and illustrated this technique.[8, 26, 41, 54] The handle end of a dental mirror or other blunt instrument is said to substitute for the finger if the space is too tight,[27, 32] but may produce a stronger stimulus. After sliding the finger along the outer side of the cul-de-sac to reach as high as possible along the inner surface of the coronoid process, the examiner presses inward toward the lateral pterygoid plate (see Figs. 11.2 and 11.3B). This pressure reveals *exquisite* tenderness if active TPs are present in this part of the lateral pterygoid muscle.[15] TP tenderness of temporalis muscle fibers attaching to the medial aspect of the coronoid process (lateral to the finger or probe) are distinguished from tenderness of lateral pterygoid fibers (medial to the finger or probe) by the patient's response to the direction of pressure.[27]

With the jaws closed, the lateral pterygoid muscle is inaccessible to *external* palpation; then the superior division lies beneath the zygomatic arch, and the inferior division, beneath the ramus of the mandible. With the jaws separated about 3 cm (1⅛ in) a more posterior portion of the inferior division and also of the superior division may be approached externally through masseter fibers and through the opening between the mandibular notch and the zygomatic arch (Fig. 11.3). One must first identify and inactivate any TP tenderness in the masseter fibers in the area to be examined. With the mouth propped open, in thin persons with suitable bony structure, tenderness elicited by pressure directed upward and slightly forward may indicate active TPs in the mid-portion of the superior division. Tenderness to pressure directed downward and forward toward the mouth may indicate TPs in the mid-portion of the inferior division. When TP tenderness is present in the masseter, its tense bands are readily palpable, but TP bands in the underlying lateral pterygoid muscle are too deep to be distinguished by more than their local tenderness and possibly their referred pain response to pressure.

10. ENTRAPMENTS

The buccal nerve, which arises from the anterior division of the mandibular branch of the trigeminal nerve (cranial nerve V), usually passes between the two divisions of the lateral pterygoid muscle,[20, 63] but sometimes through the superior division.[18] It innervates the buccinator muscle, the

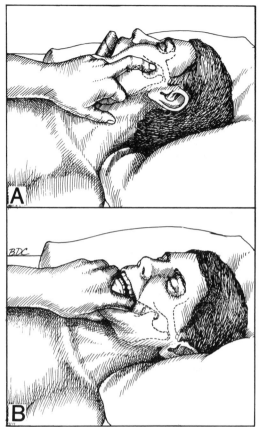

Figure 11.3 Examination of the left lateral pterygoid muscle. *A*, the mandible is propped open widely to palpate the posterior end of each division of the muscle, which lies under the masseter muscle. Palpation is through the aperture between the mandibular notch and the zygomatic process (*dotted lines*). *B*, intra-oral palpation to press on the lower end of the inferior division by slipping a finger into the uppermost rear corner of the cheek pouch and pressing inward. The jaws should be open about 5–8 mm (about ¼ in) to let the fingertip squeeze beneath the coronoid process.

skin of the cheek overlying it, the adjacent mucous membrane of the mouth, and part of the gum. Tautness of the lateral pterygoid muscle fibers due to active TPs, theoretically, could entrap this nerve to cause buccinator weakness with numbness and paresthesias in the distribution of the nerve. Mahan,[33] in discussing this, describes such a weird tingling of the cheek area in a number of patients.

11. ASSOCIATED TRIGGER POINTS

When the inferior division of the lateral pterygoid muscle harbors active TPs, its antagonists are likely to develop associated TPs. Most vulnerable is its chief antagonist for lateral motion of the mandible, the medial pterygoid muscle on the opposite side. Next are its antagonists for protrusion, the deep masseter and posterior temporalis fibers on the same side.

12. STRETCH AND SPRAY
(Fig. 11.4)

It may be possible to stretch both divisions of the lateral pterygoid muscle a few millimeters by forcibly retruding the mandible as far as possible against the restraining ligaments, without opening the mouth appreciably. This maneuver will stretch the upper division only to the extent that the disc is retruded with the mandible. We find only occasional benefit from this maneuver.

To stretch and spray this muscle, the patient lies supine, which inhibits antigravity reflexes and encourages full relaxation of the masticatory muscles. The operator, or the patient, gently but firmly passively retrudes the mandible while rocking it from side to side and holding the jaws open only a few millimeters (Fig. 11.4). At the same time, the vapocoolant spray is applied over the length of the muscle toward its pain reference zone, forward and/or backward depending on the location of the pain. Stretch and spray are followed promptly by hot packs and active range of motion. Better results may be obtained by TP injection.

13. INJECTION AND STRETCH
(Fig. 11.5)

Since stretch of the lateral pterygoid muscle is limited by restraining ligaments and bone, and since the muscle is not accessible for ischemic compression, it is frequently necessary to inject its TPs. The anterior portion of the inferior division is relatively easily reached *via* the intraoral approach, as described and illustrated by Gelb.[16] The superior division is not accessible from inside the mouth. In our hands, this approach to the inferior division is rarely necessary, but may be simpler and more direct if one is accustomed to injecting within the mouth. Extraoral injection of either division requires knowledge of the anatomy, because of the difficulty in palpating the muscle; there are numerous

PART 1

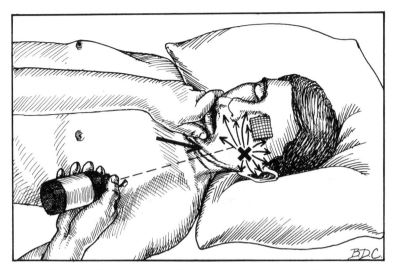

Figure 11.4   Stretch and spray technique for the lateral pterygoid muscle. Only a few millimeters of stretch are obtainable beyond the rest position of the mandible. The mandible is fully retruded passively as vapocoolant is applied from the trigger point, covering the muscle and pain patterns. The gauze protects the eye from misdirected vapocoolant.

neighboring nerves and vessels. The technique is well illustrated by Bell.[5] The critical importance of this muscle as a major source of TMJ pain makes it worthwhile to develop the skill necessary to inject it.

In the absence of a history of allergic reactions to procaine, the use of 0.5% procaine in isotonic saline, rather than a long-acting local anesthetic, reduces the likelihood of adverse reactions. Even if a nerve or blood vessel is penetrated, the dilute procaine is rapidly degraded by procainesterase as the drug enters the blood stream. Lidocaine (Xylocaine) 2%, or mepivacaine (Carbocaine) 3%, have been used successfully, but require care to avoid intravascular injection (see Section 13 in Chapter 3). Epinephrine-containing solutions are NOT used.

All portions can be injected extraorally through the sigmoid notch. Since the entire muscle cannot be palpated directly, the needle must be oriented by visualizing the relation of the muscle and it TPs to adjacent structures. Examination of a skull, in conjunction with the drawings of Figures 11.2 and 11.5, helps to establish a clear three-dimensional image of the lateral pterygoid muscle and its landmarks.

Externally, it must be injected through the masseter and deep to the ramus of the mandible. The volume of the space occupied by the lateral pterygoid muscle is limited by bony structures on all sides, which places a premium on locating the TPs as precisely as possible so as to inject a minimum volume. To avoid traversing this region with a dull needle, one disposable needle is used to penetrate the rubber stoppers of the vials, and a fresh needle for injection. The needle should be replaced immediately if it contacts bone solidly, and whenever it feels as if the tip had a burr which "catches" or "scratches," instead of gliding smoothly through the tissue. A 3.8-cm (1½-in) 22- to 24-gauge needle is adequate. A thinner needle is more likely to miss blood vessels, but is much harder to position accurately and slides right past the TPs.

When injecting this muscle with a local anesthetic other than 0.5% procaine, it is critically important not to inject while passing to or from the muscle while the needle is traversing the pterygoid plexus and to aspirate for evidence of blood in the syringe before injecting.

To inject the *posterior* portion of *either division* of the muscle, the jaws are propped open 22 to 30 mm (about 1 in), with the patient supine. The open space of the mandibular notch is bounded by the zygomatic arch above, the coronoid process in front and the mandibular condyle behind. The needle is inserted through the notch, directed nearly perpen-

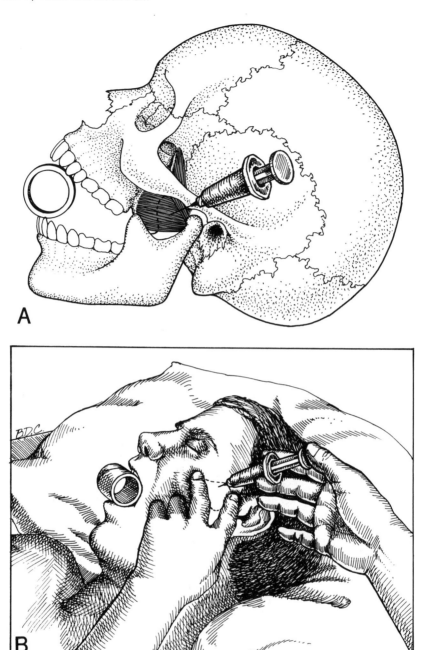

Figure 11.5 Injection technique for the inferior division of the left lateral pterygoid muscle (*dark red*). *A*, lateral view of its anatomical relationships when the jaw is propped open. The needle reaches the inferior division through the bony aperture above the mandibular notch, between the coronoid process, in front, and the condyle of the mandible, behind. *B*, surface markings, same injection as in *Part A. Dotted lines* outline the palpable bony margins of the aperture. *C*, frontal section of the head at the level of needle penetration (level of cross section shown in *Part D*). This view looks forward through the open mouth. The condylar neck of the mandible obscures part of the needle which penetrates the inferior division of the muscle. The medial pterygoid muscle (*light red*) lies in the foreground and attaches to the inner surface of the pterygoid plate. *D*, cross section showing needle penetration through the masseter and temporalis muscles (*light red*) in front of the condylar neck of the mandible above the mandibular notch (level of cross section shown in *Part C*). The needles reach the anterior and posterior portions of the inferior division of the lateral pterygoid muscle (*dark red*).

PART 1

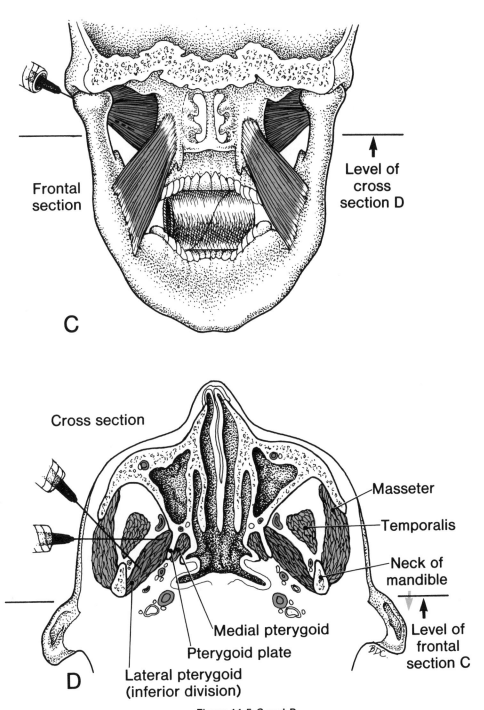

Frontal
section

Level of
cross
section D

C

Cross section

Masseter

Temporalis

Neck of
mandible

Level of
frontal
section C

Medial pterygoid

Pterygoid plate

D   Lateral pterygoid
(inferior division)

Figure 11.5 *C* and *D*.

dicular to the surface, and slightly posteriorly. When directed upward beneath the zygomatic arch, the needle reaches the superior division. When directed down-

ward toward the angle of the mandible, it reaches the inferior division.

To inject the *anterior* portion of the *superior* division, the jaws are propped wide open, and the needle is inserted just anterior to the TMJ, below the zygomatic arch (Fig. 11.5A); then it is directed anteriorly and upward toward, but short of, the orbit, and parallel to the fiber direction of the superior division, as illustrated by Bell.[4] These lateral pterygoid fibers can be reached only after the full depth of the masseter muscle has been penetrated. The depth to the sphenoid bone is established by contacting it gently with the needle tip; the sphenoid bone forms the floor of the space within which the muscle lies.

To inject the *anterior* portion of the *inferior* division, the needle is inserted just below the condyle at the level of the neck of the mandible and is directed toward the roots of the upper molar teeth (Fig. 11.5A and B). The full depth of the anterior portion of the muscle can be established by contacting the pterygoid plate, which is *outlined* in Fig. 11.5A.

Important signs of effective treatment are the return of the normal range of jaw opening, linearity of the incisal path during opening and closing, non-tenderness of the lateral pterygoid muscle to palpation, and cessation of the patient's referred pain.

14. CORRECTIVE ACTIONS

Occlusal Disharmony

First, the lateral pterygoid and other masticatory muscles are rendered nontender and their normal range of motion restored by inactivating their TPs and by the application of an occlusal splint, such as the Shore mandibular autorepositioning appliance.[55] By eliminating the increased muscle tension that distorts mandibular positioning, it then becomes possible to check for occlusal disharmonies that would contribute significantly to stress overload of these muscles, especially those contacts that restrict forward gliding of the mandibular teeth.

In assessing occlusal disharmony, head and body posture greatly influence tooth contact patterns.[42] Electromyographic feedback can be a useful adjunct.[56]

It also is important to check for TPs in the sternocleidomastoid muscle of the neck that refer pain to the region of the lateral pterygoid muscle and, thereby, can induce satellite TPs in it.

Activity Stress

Bruxism is increased by premature occlusal contact and by increased emotional tension and anxiety. Both should be treated.

Regular chewing of gum should be discontinued.

Body Asymmetry

Tilting of the pelvis caused by disparity in leg length or by a small hemipelvis, as described in Section 14, Chapter 48, should be corrected.[43]

Central Nervous System Hyperirritability

Suboptimal levels of vitamins B_1, B_6, B_{12}, or folic acid are likely to act as perpetuating factors (see Chapter 4) in the MPD syndromes. Inadequate levels of one or more of these vitamins can aggravate bruxism through increased central nervous system and neuromuscular irritability, as can emotional stress also.

Exercise

Both divisions of the lateral pterygoid muscle are passively stretched by maximal retrusion of the mandible, which is the specific stretch for the inferior division. The supine patient rests the head against a firm support, relaxes the jaw muscles (preferably after several minutes of application of a hot pack), and grasps the point of the chin with one hand, while gently, but firmly, pushing the mandible backward and upward with the teeth separated by only a few millimeters. A gentle sideways rocking motion is added to this push to insure maximum retrusion. Then, the patient should practice full active range of motion by maximally protruding and retruding the mandible, without manual assistance.

Rhythmic stabilization self-stretch is performed by the patient's grasping the mandible by the fingers and thumb, inside and outside the mouth, then slowly and smoothly, but firmly, pulling it forward until the muscles feel tight. Alternate, gentle, rhythmic protrusive and retrusive efforts are resisted by the hand. This contraction of the antagonists of the lateral pterygoid helps to reciprocally inhibit reflex spasm of the muscle in response to stretch.

Strengthening   and   conditioning   the

muscle requires active resistive exercises. The patient is taught to protrude the mandible against resistance, and then to move the mandible to each side also against resistance, but especially to the side away from the involved muscle. These exercises are illustrated by Wetzler.[68]

Opening the jaws as far as possible without translation and in maximum voluntary retrusion should stretch the upper division of the lateral pterygoid muscle slightly. This is performed by opening the mouth while retruding the mandible and preventing condylar translation by placing the tip of the tongue against the roof of the mouth, as far back as possible. While holding the tongue in place, the mouth is then alternately opened and closed about 20 or 25 mm (nearly 1 in), as described by Marbach.[36]

Since the elevator muscles of mastication usually become secondarily involved together with the lateral pterygoid, maximal-opening exercises aid in restoring normal function of the entire temporomandibular apparatus (see Section 14, Chapter 9).

References

1. Bardeen CR: The musculature, Sect. 5. In *Morris' Human Anatomy*, edited by C.M. Jackson, Ed. 6. Blakiston's Son & Co., Philadelphia, 1921 (p. 377, Fig. 377).
2. Basmajian JV: *Muscles Alive*, Ed. 4. Williams & Wilkins, Baltimore, 1978 (pp. 386, 387).
3. Bell WE: Clinical diagnosis of the pain-dysfunction syndromes. *J Am Dent Assoc* 79:154–160, 1969 (p. 158).
4. Bell WE: Management of masticatory pain, Chapter 12. In *Facial Pain*, edited by C.C. Alling III, P.E. Mahan, Ed. 2. Lea & Febiger, Philadelphia, 1977 (p. 189, Fig. 12-4).
5. Bell WE: *Orofacial Pains—Differential Diagnosis*, Ed. 2. Year Book Medical Publishers, Chicago, 1979 (pp. 85, 200–203, Figs. 7-8, 7-9).
6. Bell WH: Nonsurgical management of the pain-dysfunction syndrome. *J Am Dent Assoc* 79:161–170, 1969.
7. Blaschke DD: Arthrography of the temporomandibular joint, Chapter 4. In *Temporomandibular Joint Problems*, edited by W.K. Solberg, G.T. Clark. Quintessence Publishing, Chicago, 1980 (pp. 69–91).
8. Burch JG: Occlusion related to craniofacial pain, Chapter 11. In *Facial Pain*, edited by C.C. Alling III, P.E. Mahan, Ed. 2. Lea & Febiger, Philadelphia, 1977 (pp. 170, 174, Fig. 11-5).
9. Butler JH, Folke LEA, Bandt CL: A descriptive survey of signs and symptoms associated with the myofascial pain-dysfunction syndrome. *J Am Dent Assoc* 90:635–639, 1975.
10. Carter BL, Morehead J, Wolpert SM, *et al*: *Cross-Sectional Anatomy*. Appleton-Century-Crofts, New York, 1977 (Sects. 9–11).
11. Christensen FG: Some anatomical concepts associated with the temporomandibular joint. *Ann Aust Coll Dent Surg* 2:39–60, 1969.
12. Eisler P: *Die Muskeln des Stammes*. Gustav Fischer, Jena, 1912 (p. 212, Fig. 24).
13. *Ibid*. (Fig. 25).
14. Franks AST: Masticatory muscle hyperactivity and temporomandibular joint dysfunction. *J Prosthet Dent* 15:1122–1131, 1965 (p. 1126).
15. Gelb H: Patient evaluation, Chapter 3. In *Clinical Management of Head, Neck and TMJ Pain and Dysfunction*, edited by H. Gelb. W.B. Saunders, Philadelphia, 1977 (pp. 83, 85, 96, Fig. 3–15).
16. Gelb H: Effective management and treatment of the craniomandibular syndrome, Chapter 11. In *Clinical Management of Head, Neck and TMJ Pain and Dysfunction*, edited by H. Gelb. W.B. Saunders, Philadelphia, 1977 (p. 301, Fig. 11-6G and H).
17. Grant JCB: *An Atlas of Human Anatomy*, Ed. 7. Williams & Wilkins, Baltimore, 1978 (Fig. 7-105).
18. *Ibid*. (Fig. 7-80).
19. Grant PG: Lateral pterygoid: two muscles? *Am J Anat* 138:1–10, 1973.
20. Gray H: *Anatomy of the Human Body*, edited by C.M. Goss, American Ed. 29. Lea & Febiger, Philadelphia, 1973 (pp. 389, 920, Fig. 6-6).
21. Greene CS, Lerman MD, Sutcher HD, *et al*.: The TMJ pain-dysfunction syndrome: heterogeneity of the patient population. *J Am Dent Assoc* 79:1168–1172, 1969.
22. Hickey JC, Stacy RW, Rinear LL: Electromyographic studies of mandibular muscles in basic jaw movements. *J Prosthet Dent* 7:565–570, 1975.
23. Hollinshead WH: *Functional Anatomy of the Limbs and Back*, Ed. 4. W.B. Saunders, Philadelphia, 1976 (p. 376).
24. Honee GLJM: The anatomy of the lateral pterygoid muscle. *Acta Morphol Neerl Scand* 10:331–340, 1972.
25. Ingle JI: "The great imposter". *JAMA* 236:1846, 1976.
26. Ingle JI, Beveridge EE: *Endodontics*, Ed. 2. Lea & Febiger, Philadelphia, 1976 (p. 520, Fig. 11-12).
27. Johnstone DR, Templeton McC: The feasibility of palpating the lateral pterygoid muscle. *J Prosthet Dent* 44:318–323, 1980.
28. Kaye LB, Moran JH, Fritz ME: Statistical analysis of an urban population of 236 patients with head and neck pain. Part II. Patient symptomatology. *J Periodont* 50:59–65, 1979.
29. Kubota K, Masegi T: Muscle spindle supply to the human jaw muscle. *J Dent Res* 56:901–909, 1977.
30. Lipke DP, Gay T, Gross RD, Yaeger JA: An electromyographic study of the human lateral pterygoid muscle (Abstract 713). *J Dent Res Special Issue B* 56:B230, 1977.
31. Lockhart RD, Hamilton GF, Fyfe FW: *Anatomy of the Human Body*, Ed. 2. J.B. Lippincott, Philadelphia, 1969 (p. 157, Fig. 266).
32. Mahan PE: Differential diagnosis of craniofacial pain and dysfunction. *Alpha Omegan* 69:42–49, 1976.
33. Mahan PE: The temporomandibular joint in function and pathofunction, Chapter 2. In *Temporomandibular Joint Problems*, edited by W.K. Solbert and G.T. Clark, Quintessence Publishing,

Chicago, 1980 (pp. 33–47).

34. Mahan PE: Personal communication, 1981.

35. Mahan PE, Kreutziger KL: Diagnosis and management of temporomandibular joint pain, Chapter 13. In *Facial Pain*, edited by C.C. Alling III, P.E. Mahan, Ed. 2. Lea & Febiger, Philadelphia, 1977 (pp. 201–204).

36. Marbach JJ: Therapy for mandibular dysfunction in adolescents and adults. *Am J Orthod* 62:601–605, 1972.

37. Matthews B: Mastication, Chapter 10. In *Applied Physiology of the Mouth*, edited by C.L.B. Lavelle. John Wright and Sons, Bristol, 1975 (p. 207).

38. McCarty W: Diagnosis and treatment of internal derangements of the articular disc and mandibular condyle, Chapter 8. In *Temporomandibular Joint Problems*, edited by W.K. Solberg, G.T. Clark, Quintessence Publishing, Chicago, 1980 (pp. 145–168).

39. McMinn RMH, Hutchings RT: *Color Atlas of Human Anatomy*. Year Book Medical Publishers, Chicago, 1977 (p. 38).

40. McNamara, JA, Jr.: The independent functions of the two heads of the lateral pterygoid muscle. *Am J Anat* 138:197–206, 1973.

41. Meyerowitz WJ; Myofascial pain in the edentulous patient. *J Dent Assoc S Afr* 30:75–77, 1975.

42. Mohl N: Head inposture and its role in occlusion. *Int J Orthod* 15:6–14, 1977.

43. Morton DJ: Foot disorders in women, *J Am Med Wom Assoc*, 10:41–46, 1955.

44. Moyers RE: An electromyographic analysis of certain muscles involved in temporomandibular movement. *Am J Orthod* 36:481–515, 1950.

45. Perry HT, Marsh EW: Function considerations in early limited orthodontic procedures, Chapter 10. In *Clinical Management of Head, Neck and TMJ Pain and Dysfunction*, edited by H. Gelb. W.B. Saunders, Philadelphia, 1977 (p. 264).

46. Perry HT Jr.: Muscular changes associated with temporomandibular joint dysfunction. *J Am Dent Assoc* 54:644–653, 1957.

47. Pinto OF: A new structure related to the temporomandibular joint and middle ear. *J Prosthet Dent* 12:95–103, 1962.

48. Porter MR: The attachment of the lateral pterygoid muscle to the meniscus. *J Prothet Dent* 24:555–562, 1970.

49. Reynolds MD: Myofascial trigger point syndromes in the practice of rheumatology. *Arch Phys Med Rehabil* 62:111–114, 1981.

50. Schwartz LL, Tausig DP: Temporomandibular joint pain—treatment with intramuscular infiltration of tetracaine hydrochloride; a preliminary report. *NY State Dent J* 20:219–223, 1954.

51. Schwartz LL: Ethyl chloride treatment of limited, painful mandibular movement. *J Am Dent Assoc* 48:497–507, 1954.

52. Shaber EP: Considerations in the treatment of muscle spasm. In *Diseases of the Temporomandibular Apparatus*, edited by D.H. Morgan, W.P. Hall, S.J. Vamvas, C.V. Mosby, St. Louis, 1977 (pp. 237, 249, 250).

53. Sharav Y, Tzukert A, Refaeli B: Muscle pain index in relation to pain, dysfunction, and dizziness associated with the myofascial pain-dysfunction syndrome. *Oral Surg* 46:742–747, 1978.

54. Shore NA: Temporomandibular joint dysfunction: medical-dental cooperation. *Int Coll Dent Sci Ed J* 7:15–16, 1974.

55. Shore NA: *Temporomandibular Joint Dysfunction and Occlusal Equilibration*, Ed. 2. J.B. Lippincott, Philadelphia, 1976 (pp. 238–249).

56. Shpuntoff H: Biofeedback electromyography and inhibition release in myofascial pain dysfunction cases. *NY J Dent* 47:304–309, 1977.

57. Silverman SI: Kinesiology of the temporomandibular joint. *Arch Phys Med Rehabil* 41:191–194, 1960.

58. Sobotta J, Figge FHJ: *Atlas of Human Anatomy*, Ed. 9, Vol. 3. Hafner Division of Macmillan, New York, 1974 (pp. 212, 213).

59. Sobotta J, Figge FHJ: *Atlas of Human Anatomy*, Ed. 9, Vol. 1. Hafner Division of Macmillan, New York, 1974 (pp. 184, 186).

60. Spalteholz W: *Handatlas der Anatomie des Menschen*, Ed. 11, Vol. 2. S. Hirzel, Leipzig, 1922 (p. 266).

61. *Ibid.* (p. 267).

62. Toldt C: *An Atlas of Human Anatomy*, translated by M.E. Paul, Ed. 2, Vol. 1. Macmillan, New York, 1919 (p. 307).

63. *Ibid.* (p. 295).

64. Toldt C: *An Atlas of Human Anatomy*, translated by M.E. Paul, Ed. 2, Vol. 2. Macmillan, New York, 1919 (p. 865).

65. Travell J: Mechanical headache. *Headache* 7:23–29, 1967 (pp. 26–27).

66. Travell JG: Temporomandibular joint pain referred from muscles of the head and neck. *J Prosthet Dent*, 10:745–763, 1960 (pp. 746, 749, 753).

67. Vamvas SJ: Differential diagnosis of TMJ disease, Chapter 13. In *Diseases of the Temporomandibular Apparatus*, edited by D.H. Morgan, W.P. Hall, S.J. Vamvas. C.V. Mosby, St. Louis, 1977 (p. 190).

68. Wetzler G: Physical therapy, Chapter 24. In *Diseases of the Temporomandibular Apparatus*, edited by D.H. Morgan, W.P. Hall, S.J. Vamvas, C.V. Mosby, St. Louis, 1977 (pp. 350, 351, Fig. 24-2).

69. Woelfel JB, Hickey JC, Stacey RW, *et al*: Electromyographic analysis of jaw movements. *J Prosthet Dent* 10:688–697, 1960.

CHAPTER 12
Digastric Muscle
"Pseudo-sternocleidomastoid Pain"

HIGHLIGHTS: **REFERRED PAIN** and tenderness from trigger points (TPs) in the posterior belly of the digastric muscle are projected to the upper part of the sternocleidomastoid muscle. When this referred pain persists after inactivation of sternocleidomastoid TPs, it is commonly, and mistakenly, attributed to the latter muscle, so that the pain referred from TPs in the posterior belly deserves to be called "pseudo-sternocleidomastoid" pain. The anterior belly of the digastric projects pain to the four lower incisor teeth. **ANATOMICAL ATTACHMENTS** of the digastric are, above, close to the symphysis of the mandible for its anterior belly, and to the mastoid notch for its posterior belly. Below, the bellies join end-to-end in a common tendon at the hyoid bone. **ACTIONS** of both bellies of this muscle are to assist depression and retrusion of the mandible. The **MYOTATIC UNIT** includes the inferior division of the lateral pterygoid as its synergist for opening the jaws. The powerful elevators of the mandible are its antagonists for closing the jaws. **ACTIVATION OF TRIGGER POINTS** in the digastric commonly occurs as a result of TPs in the antagonistic masseter muscle, and is often due to the added stress of habitual mouth-breathing. **STRETCH AND SPRAY** of the posterior belly require that the hyoid bone be laterally deviated to the opposite side and stabilized, while the head is rotated to move the mastoid process away from the hyoid bone, thus lengthening the posterior belly; the spray is applied from front to back. The anterior belly is stretched by extending the neck and head with the jaw protruded and nearly closed, while the spray is swept upward. **INJECTION AND STRETCH** are performed under direct tactile control of the palpating fingers. **CORRECTIVE ACTIONS** include ischemic compression self-applied directly to the TPs, and passive stretch exercises. Measures should be taken to stop the habit of mouth-breathing, to stop retrusive bruxing, and to correct persistent malocclusion.

1. REFERRED PAIN
(Fig. 12.1)

Each belly of the digastric muscle has its own referred pain pattern. Pain arising from trigger points (TPs) in the posterior belly (Fig. 12.1A) radiates into the upper part of the sternocleidomastoid muscle,[3] to the throat in front of that muscle under the chin, and sometimes extends onto the occiput. Occipital pain is likely to be associated with referred "soreness" and tenderness, which may activate satellite TPs in the occipital portion of the occipitofrontalis muscle.

Head and neck pain have been attributed to both the stylohyoid muscle and the posterior belly of the digastric.[23] These two muscles lie close together, have similar functions, and are difficult to distinguish by palpation.

Less frequently, the pain is referred from TPs in the anterior belly of the digastric to the four lower incisor teeth and the alveolar ridge below them (Fig. 12.1C). The responsible TP is located just under the tip of the chin in the anterior belly of the digastric muscle on either side (Fig. 12.1B).

2. ANATOMICAL ATTACHMENTS
(Fig. 12.2)

Below the anterior and posterior bellies of the digastric muscle (Fig. 12.2) are

273

PART 1

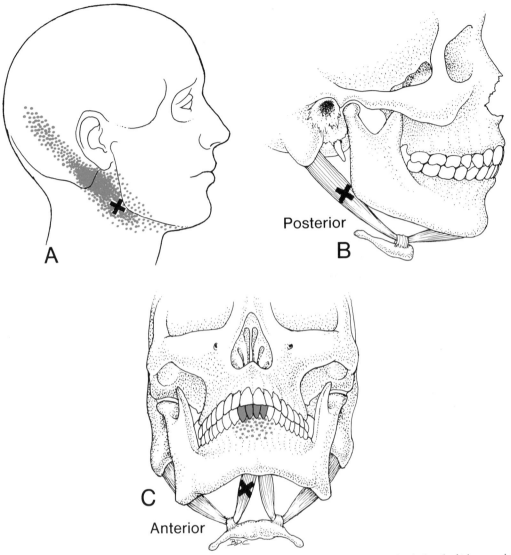

Figure 12.1.   Referred pain patterns (essential portion, *solid red*; spillover portion, *stippled red*) of trigger points (× s) in the right digastric muscle. *A* and *B*, posterior belly, side view. *C*, anterior belly, front view.

united end-to-end by a common tendon that attaches to the hyoid bone through a fibrous loop or sling. ***Behind and above*** the posterior belly attaches to the mastoid notch deep to the attachments of the longissimus capitis, splenius capitis and sternocleidomastoid muscles on the mastoid process. In ***front and above*** the anterior belly attaches to the inferior border of the mandible, close to its symphysis.

The common tendon perforates the stylohyoid muscle, which lies near the front half of the posterior belly of the digastric.

The common tendon of the digastric connects to the hyoid bone either directly by bands, or by sliding through a fibrous loop.[1]

Supplemental References

Anatomy textbooks illustrate both bellies of the digastric muscle in level side view[12, 20, 22] and as seen from below in side view,[1, 5, 10, 16, 21] from inside the mouth,[6] and from the front.[15] The relationship between the muscle and underlying neurovascular structures is clearly illustrated in

PART 1

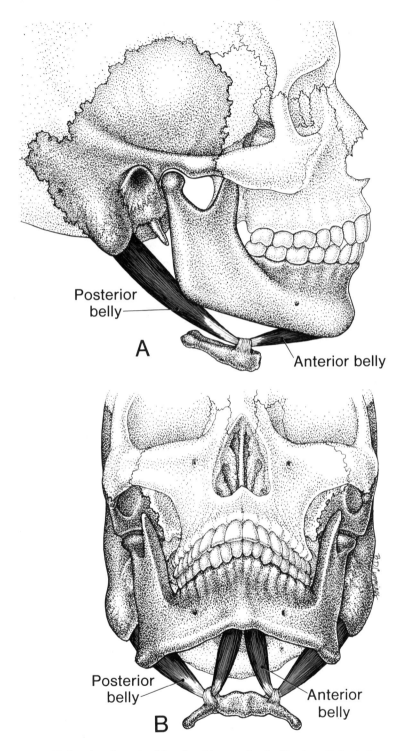

Posterior
belly

A

Anterior belly

Posterior
belly

B

Anterior
belly

Figure 12.2.   Attachments of the digastric muscle. *A*, side view. *B*, front view.
The posterior belly attaches, above, to the mastoid notch and, below, by the
muscle's common tendon to the hyoid bone. The anterior belly attaches, above,
to the mandible at the point of the chin and, below, by the common tendon to the
hyoid bone.

a side view.[9, 17] The anterior belly is seen in detail from the side[18] and from below.[7] The posterior belly is seen in detail from the side[8] and from behind.[19]

3. INNERVATION

The anterior belly of the digastric is supplied by the mylohyoid nerve from the alveolar branch of the posterior division of the mandibular third of the trigeminal nerve (cranial nerve V). The posterior belly is innervated by a branch of the facial nerve (cranial nerve VII).

4. ACTIONS

When the hyoid bone is fixed, the digastric muscle assists in depressing the mandible to open the mouth.[1, 2, 10, 15, 20] With the mandible fixed, the muscle elevates the hyoid bone.[1, 10, 15, 20] Together, the right and left digastric muscles assist in retruding the lower jaw.[1, 2] During mandibular depression, motor unit activity of the anterior belly follows that of the inferior division of the lateral pterygoid. The digastric appears to be less important than the lateral pterygoid for initial opening of the jaws, but is essential for maximum depression, or forced opening.[2] Digastric activity is inhibited during depression of the mandible if the mandible is protruded at the same time, which logically would inhibit the retraction function of the muscle. The digastric is always active during mandibular retrusion.[13] The right and left digastric muscles nearly always contract together, not independently.[2] Coughing, swallowing and retrusion of the mandible strongly recruit the digastric muscles.[2, 24]

The digastric muscle was electromyographically active in 85% of records while the mandibular elevators were reflexly inhibited by tooth contact.[14]

One major difference is reported in the actions of the two bellies of the digastric muscle. The hyoid bone is displaced dorsally by the posterior belly, but cephalad and ventrally by the anterior belly.[1, 10, 20]

The location of their attachments should make the anterior belly better suited for mandibular opening, and the posterior belly better suited for mandibular retrusion. Together, both bellies of one muscle exert a lateral-deviation force,[1] the effect of which is seen clinically, but only occasionally electromyographically.[13]

5. MYOTATIC UNIT

Muscles synergistic with the anterior belly of the digastric for opening the jaws (depressing the mandible) include the inferior division of the lateral pterygoid, and the infrahyoid strap muscles. For retrusion of the mandible, synergists of the entire muscle are the posterior fibers of the temporalis and the deep portion of the masseter.

Antagonists to its jaw-opening action are the mandibular elevators: the masseter, the temporalis, the medial pterygoid and the superior division of the lateral pterygoid.

6. SYMPTOMS

The distribution of pain is described in Section 1. The patient also has difficulty in swallowing. Pain referred from the posterior belly usually becomes apparent after inactivation of TPs in the sternocleidomastoid muscle. Then, pain and soreness persist in the upper part of the sternocleidomastoid muscle, which remains diffusely and moderately tender to palpation, but free of taut bands and local twitch responses. The TPs in the posterior belly of the digastric muscle account for these "pseudo-sternocleidomastoid" findings.

7. ACTIVATION OF TRIGGER POINTS

Activation of TPs in the digastric muscle may be secondary to myofascial dysfunction of muscles in its myotatic unit.

Overload due to bruxing, by retruding the mandible, and due to mouth-breathing (one sign of which is inward, rather than outward, flaring of the nostrils during inspiration) predisposes to activation of TPs in the digastric muscle. Mouth-breathing may result from mechanical blockage (as by nasal polyps), structural distortion (deviated septum) of the nasal passages, sinusitis, or recurrent allergic rhinitis.

A mechanical source of irritation, which may contribute to the activation of TPs in the posterior belly of the digastric and in the medial pterygoid muscle, is an elongated styloid process, the "Eagle syndrome."[11] The patient with this structural problem complains of pain in the angle of the jaw on the side of involvement, and also may have symptoms of dizziness and visual blurring with "decreased" vision on the same side, probably due to sternocleidomastoid TPs. Pressure of the process against the carotid artery during extreme rotation of the head (chin on top of the shoulder) may cause pain and dizziness. The abnormal elongation of the styloid process by calcification of the stylohoid ligament is palpable from inside the mouth.[11] It may be necessary to remove the excess calcium surgically to provide relief.

8. PATIENT EXAMINATION

Involvement of the posterior belly of the digastric muscle tends to pull the mandible toward the same side. This loads, and may help to activate, TPs in the antagonistic fibers of the opposite posterior temporalis and of the opposite masseter's deep division; tautness of these antagonists may nearly balance the mandibular deviation induced by the digastric. If the contralateral muscles are cleared of active TPs, the mandible is then free to deviate to the side of the affected posterior belly of the digastric muscle. If deviation is due solely to posterior digastric TPs, the mandible is pulled over as the jaws start to separate, but with further opening, it returns to the midline.

One test of anterior digastric TP involvement as a source of lower incisor tooth pain is to ask the patient to pull the corners of the mouth down vigorously enough to tense the anterior neck muscles. When positive, this **Anterior Digastric Test** activates the toothache and implicates the anterior belly of at least one digastric muscle.

9. TRIGGER POINT EXAMINATION
(Fig. 12.3)

The posterior belly of the digastric is examined with the patient supine and the head extended, in order to enlarge the space for palpation between the neck and the angle of the mandible. This belly (and the stylohyoid muscle) are palpated (Fig. 12.3A) by rubbing across the direction of the fibers behind the angle of the mandible,[4] and by sliding the finger upward toward the ear lobe along the anterior border of the sternocleidomastoid muscle, while pressing inward against the underlying neck muscles. The initial pressure on active TPs in the posterior belly elicits exquisite local tenderness; sustained pres-

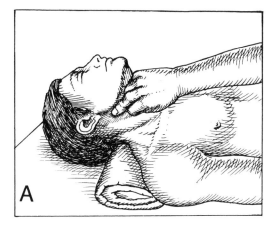
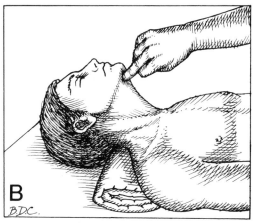

Figure 12.3. Examination of the digastric muscle. *A,* posterior belly: palpated between the angle of the jaw and the mastoid process, against the underlying neck structures. *B,* anterior belly: the head is tilted back and the neck extended, with the jaws closed, to stretch the muscle as it is palpated against the underlying soft tissues.

sure may reproduce the patient's more distant neck and head pain.

The anterior belly of the digastric muscle is examined with the patient supine, the head tilted back and the neck extended (Fig. 12.3B), by palpating the soft tissues just beneath the point of the chin on either side of the midline. A tender button-like thickening of the muscle belly may be felt at the TP.

10. ENTRAPMENTS

No neurovascular entrapments are attributed to TP activity in this muscle.

11. ASSOCIATED TRIGGER POINTS

Active TPs in the posterior belly of the digastric are a common problem when trismus due to masseter tension has been present for a long time. These digastric TPs rarely occur when only the neck muscles and not those of mastication are involved.

With posterior digastric involvement, TPs also may occur in the retrusion synergists: the posterior fibers of the temporalis and the deep fibers of the masseter, often on the opposite side.

With anterior digastric involvement, other TPs are likely to develop in the antagonistic masseter on the same side.

12. STRETCH AND SPRAY
(Fig. 12.4)

To stretch the posterior belly of the digastric muscle, the patient leans the head back against the operator in a relaxed position with the teeth nearly approximated (Fig. 12.4B). For passive stretching of the right posterior digastric, the patient's head is turned toward the right to swing the mastoid process away from the hyoid bone. The head and neck are extended to increase the distance between the chin and the hyoid bone, tensing the anterior belly in case the common tendon is free to slide through a sling at the hyoid bone. The operator further increases tension on the posterior belly by pressing the hyoid bone down and toward the left. Meanwhile, parallel sweeps of vapocoolant spray are applied upward over the length of the muscle and over its referred pain pattern (Fig. 12.4B).

To stretch the anterior belly of the digastric (Fig. 12.4A), the head is tilted backward, with the mandible protruded in a nearly closed position. At the same time, the spray is swept upward over the length of the muscle and beyond, to include the skin covering the painful lower teeth; the patient should hold the breath, or exhale, to avoid inhalation of the spray vapor.

In both bellies of the digastric muscle, TPs are responsive to ischemic compression (see Section 12 of Chapter 3 for the technique).

13. INJECTION AND STRETCH
(Fig. 12.5)

If TP sensitivity persists after stretch and spray, and after ischemic compression, with the patient supine, either the posterior or anterior belly of the muscle

may be fixed between the fingers and its TPs injected (Fig. 12.5B). When injecting the posterior digastric, it is wise not to penetrate the external jugular vein which is readily identified by blocking the vein lower in the neck (Fig. 12.5A). During injection with a 3.8-cm (1½-in) 22-gauge needle, one finger is used to displace the vein, while the taut band containing the tender TPs is localized between two fingers for tactile guidance of the needle. The internal carotid neurovascular bundle lies beneath the muscle. It must be avoided by palpating the size of the muscle to begin with, and then by injecting within the confines of the muscle; the needle is directed posteriorly, as illustrated.[9, 17]

When injecting these TPs, no effort is made to distinguish the posterior belly of the digastric from the stylohyoid muscle.

Needle penetration of the TP in the posterior belly of the digastric may cause a flash of pain over the occipital region, if that spillover pattern is part of the patient's pain complaint.

To inject TPs in the anterior belly, the head and neck of the patient are extended, and the TP spot tenderness in the taut subcutaneous muscle fibers is localized between two fingers of the palpating hand for injection.

After injection, stretch and spray are repeated at once, followed by a hot pack over the muscle.

14. CORRECTIVE ACTIONS

The patient learns to apply ischemic compression, or "pressure massage," on the TPs. The patient must understand the concept of referred pain and learn exactly where to press on the posterior belly of the digastric muscle deep to the angle of the mandible, rather than on the sternocleidomastoid muscle where the "soreness" of the referred tenderness is felt.

The patient should do a self-stretch, jaw-protruding passive exercise, lying supine. If the mandible deviates to one side during active opening and closure, the patient should rhythmically resist deviation, pushing the mandible to the opposite side with the hand while the jaws are less than half open. This rhythmic stabilization exercise helps to stretch the tight posterior belly of the digastric muscle.

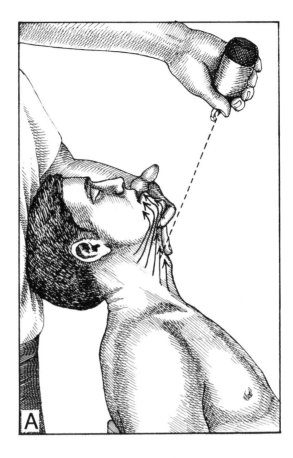

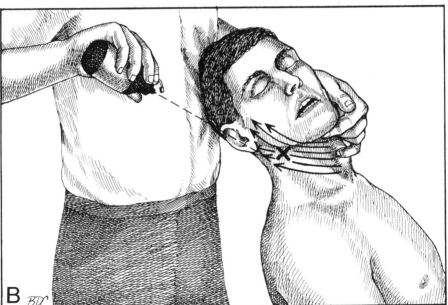

Figure 12.4.   Stretch position and spray patterns (*arrows*) for the diagastric muscle. *A*, anterior belly. *B*, posterior belly (trigger point at ×).

PART 1

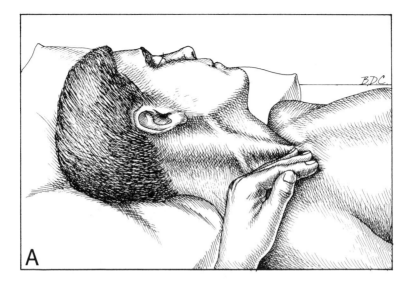

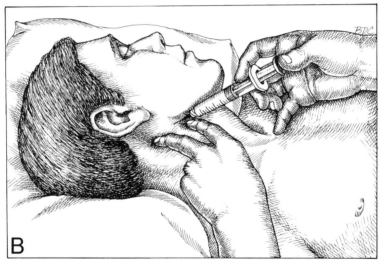

Figure 12.5. Injection of the posterior belly of the digastric muscle. *A*, manual occlusion of the external jugular vein to demonstrate its path near the angle of the jaw. *B*, injection of the muscle belly using the index finger to displace the external jugular vein to one side. The middle finger presses against the sterno-cleidomastoid muscle on the posterior side of the digastric, and the posterior belly is fixed between the two fingers.

Steps should be taken to stop retrusive bruxism and to restore breathing through the nose, rather than through the mouth. The latter favors retrusion of the mandible.

Malocclusion may require permanent correction when symptoms persist after the masticatory TPs have been inactivated.

References

1. Bardeen, CR: The musculature, Sect. 5. In *Morris's Human Anatomy*, edited by C.M. Jackson, Ed. 6. Blakiston's Son & Co., Philadelphia, 1921 (pp. 378, 379).

2. Basmajian JV: *Muscles Alive*, Ed. 4. Williams & Wilkins, Baltimore, 1978 (pp. 101, 361, 386).
3. Bell WH: Nonsurgical management of the pain-dysfunction syndrome. *J Am Dent Assoc* 79:161–170, 1969.
4. Burch JG: *Occlusion related to craniofacial pain*, Chapter 11. In *Facial Pain*, edited by C.C. Alling III and P.E. Mahan, Ed. 2. Lea & Febiger, Philadelphia, 1977 (p. 171, Fig. 11-11).
5. Eisler P: *Die Muskeln des Stammes*. Gustav Fischer, Jena, 1912 (p. 275, Fig. 34).
6. Grant JCB: *An Atlas of Human Anatomy*, Ed. 7. Williams & Wilkins, Baltimore, 1978 (Fig. 7-89).
7. *Ibid.* (Fig. 9-26).
8. *Ibid.* (Fig. 7-70).
9. *Ibid.* (Fig. 9-21).

10. Gray H: *Anatomy of The Human Body*, edited by C.M. Goss, American Ed. 29. Lea & Febiger, Philadelphia, 1973 (p. 396, Fig. 6-10).
11. Kelly RJ, Jackson FE, DeLave DP, *et al.*: The Eagle syndrome: hemicrania secondary to elongated styloid process. *US Navy Med* 65:11–16, 1975.
12. McMinn RMH, Hutchings RT: *Color Atlas of Human Anatomy*. Year Book Medical Publishers, 1977 (p. 40).
13. Moyers RE: An electromyographic analysis of certain muscles involved in temporomandibular movement. *Am J Orthod* 36:481–515, 1950 (pp. 485, 487, 489, 491, 505, 506, 554).
14. Munro RR, Basmajian JV: The jaw opening reflex in man. *Electromyography* 11:191–206, 1971 (p. 205).
15. Sobotta J, Figge FHJ: *Atlas of Human Anatomy*, Ed. 9, Vol. 1. Hafner Division of Macmillan, New York, 1974 (p. 172).
16. *Ibid.* (p. 185).
17. Sobotta J, Figge FHJ: *Atlas of Human Anatomy*, Ed. 9, Vol. 3. Hafner Division of Macmillan, New York, 1974 (pp. 243, 245).
18. *Ibid.* (pp. 210, 213).
19. *Ibid.* (p. 248).
20. Spalteholz W: *Handatlas der Anatomie des Menschen*, Ed. 11, Vol. 2. S. Hirzel, Leipzig, 1922 (p. 271).
21. Toldt C: *An Atlas of Human Anatomy*, translated by M.E. Paul, Ed. 2, Vol. 1. Macmillan, New York, 1919 (p. 292).
22. *Ibid.* (p. 297).
23. Williams HL: The syndrome of physical or intrinsic allergy of the head: myalgia of the head (sinus headache). *Proc Staff Meet Mayo Clin* 20:177–183, 1945 (p. 181).
24. Woelfel JB, Hickey JC, Stacey RW, *et al*: Electromyographic analysis of jaw movements. *J Prosthet Dent* 10:688–697, 1960.

PART 1

CHAPTER 13
Cutaneous—I: Facial Muscles
(Orbicularis Oculi, Zygomaticus Major and Platysma)

"Facial Expression"

HIGHLIGHTS: The orbicularis oculi, zygomaticus major, and platysma muscles serve as examples of trigger point (TP) involvement, which may be found in any of the muscles of facial expression. **REFERRED PAIN** to the nose is rarely caused by TPs in any muscle except the orbicularis oculi. The zygomaticus major refers pain in an arc close to the side of the nose and up to the forehead. The platysma refers a prickling sensation over the lower jaw. **ANATOMICAL ATTACHMENTS** at both ends of these skin muscles are usually to subcutaneous fascia; only rarely do they attach to bony structures. **ACTION** of the orbicularis oculi is to close the eye, of the zygomaticus major to draw the corner of the mouth upward and backward, as in smiling, and of the platysma to tense the skin of the anterior neck and to pull the corner of the mouth downward. **ACTIVATION OF TRIGGER POINTS** in these skin muscles often occurs because the muscles lie in the pain reference zones of TPs in the sternocleidomastoid and masticatory muscles. **TRIGGER POINT EXAMINATION** requires careful exploration of the subcutaneous tissue, using pincer (simultaneous intra- and extra-oral) palpation when possible, and flat palpation when necessary. **STRETCH AND SPRAY** are usually effective for the platysma, but not for the other two muscles. **INJECTION AND STRETCH** require precise injection into the TPs to afford relief for all three muscles. **CORRECTIVE ACTION** for these skin muscles is chiefly the inactivation of the primary TPs in other muscles responsible for these satellite foci of hyperirritability.

1. REFERRED PAIN
(Fig. 13.1)

Orbicularis Oculi
(Fig. 13.1A)

This is one of the few muscles from which trigger points (TPs) refer pain to the nose (Fig. 13.1A); no muscle is known to refer pain to the tip of the nose. Less intense pain may be felt in the cheek close to the nose and over the upper lip, homolaterally.[16]

Zygomaticus Major
(Fig. 13.1B)

The TPs in this muscle refer pain in an arc that extends along the side of the nose and then upward over the bridge of the nose to the mid-forehead (Fig. 13.1B).[16]

Platysma
(Fig. 13.1C)

Active TPs in the platysma usually overlie the sternocleidomastoid muscle, and refer a strange prickling pain to the skin over the lateral surface of, and just

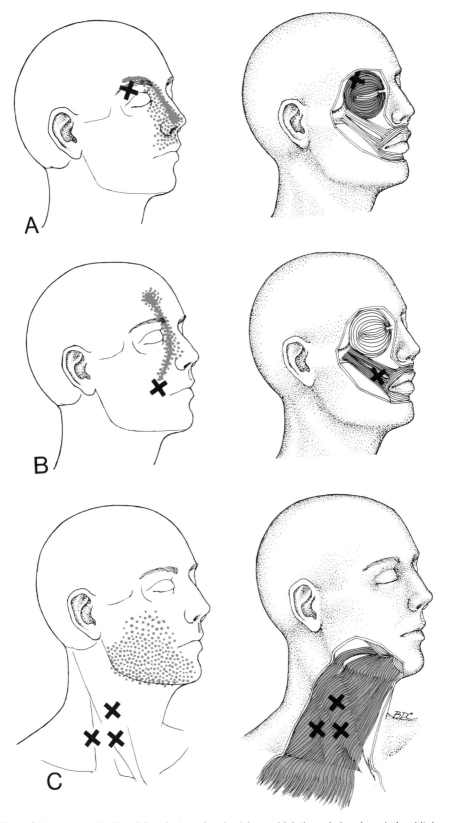

Figure 13.1. Pain patterns (*red*) and the trigger points (×s) from which the pain is referred. *A*, orbital portion of the right orbicularis oculi muscle. *B*, right zygomaticus major muscle. *C*, right platysma muscle.

below, the mandible on the same side (Fig. 13.1C). A platysma TP just above the clavicle may refer hot prickling pain across the front of the chest.

2. ANATOMICAL ATTACHMENTS (Fig. 13.2)

The fibers of these cutaneous muscles lie within the subcutaneous tissues.

Orbicularis Oculi

This muscle has a palpebral portion contained in the eyelids, and an orbital portion surrounding the lids. Fibers of both portions follow a circular path around the palpebral fissure (Fig. 13.2). Fibers of the orbital portion form bony attachments along the superior medial part of the orbit

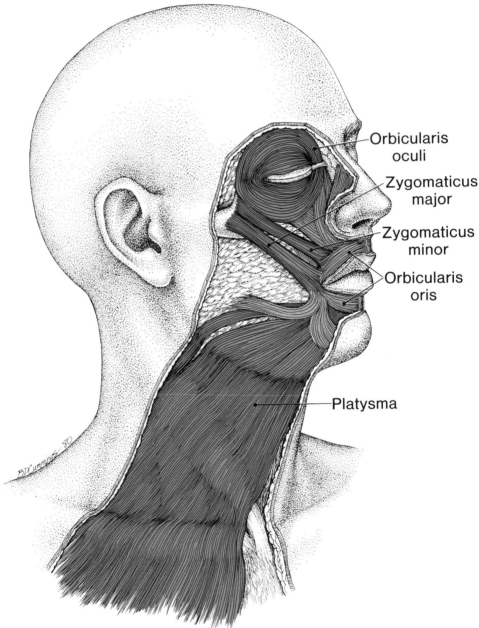

Figure 13.2.   Attachments of selected facial muscles and face-related cutaneous muscles. Three muscles are *dark red*: the orbicularis oculi, the zygomaticus major, and the platysma. The palpebral portion of the orbicularis oculi covers only the eyelids; the remaining fibers are the orbital portion. The zygomaticus major reaches from the zygoma to the corner of the mouth. The platysma connects the skin muscles near the mouth to the subcutaneous fascia of the upper chest. The orbicularis oris is *light red*.

and attach medially to a short fibrous band, the medial palpebral ligament. The fibers circle around the palpebral fissure in concentric curves.[6]

Zygomaticus Major

This muscle of mouth control attaches *above* to the malar surface of the zygomatic bone; and *below* to the angle of the mouth where it blends with fibers of the orbicularis oris (Fig. 13.2).[7]

Platysma

The fibers of the platysma muscle lie in the subcutaneous fascia of the lower face and neck (Fig. 13.2). *Above* many of its fibers interlace with the orbicularis oris while other fibers attach to the corner of the mouth, to other facial muscles, and to the lower margin of the mandible; *below* the fibers attach to the subcutaneous fascia of the upper thorax.[1, 8, 11]

Supplemental References

Other authors have clearly illustrated the orbicularis oculi,[4, 10, 12, 13, 15] the zygomaticus major,[4, 9, 12, 13, 15] and the platysma.[1, 5, 14, 15]

3. INNERVATION

All three muscles are supplied by the facial nerve (cranial nerve VII), which supplies the motor fibers and deep facial sensation.[17]

4. ACTIONS

Orbicularis Oculi

Activation of only the palpebral portion of the orbicularis oculi produces gentle, but rapid closure of the eye, as in blinking; additional activation of the orbital portion produces strong closure of the eye which throws the skin into folds at the lateral angle of the eyelid.[2, 6] Paralysis of the orbicularis oculi abolishes tight closure of the eye, which threatens the cornea with devastating dehydration and may interfere with the drainage of tears, causing them to spill over the lower lid.[9] Electromyographically, the eye normally closes gently by allowing the upper lid to drop passively without muscular contraction.

Zygomaticus Major

This muscle draws the angle of the mouth upward and backward, as in smiling and laughing,[2, 7] or saying, "Whee."

Platysma

Contraction of the platysma muscle pulls the angle of the mouth downward and the thoracic skin upward.[8] Also, as confirmed by electromyography, the muscle becomes active when widening the aperture of the already open jaws, but not during swallowing or during neck movements.[3] It corresponds to the neck muscle that horses use to shake off flies.

5. MYOTATIC UNIT

Closure of the upper lid by the orbicularis oculi is antagonized by the levator palpebrae muscle.

The zygomaticus major muscle is assisted by the parallel zygomaticus minor, which also is known as the zygomatic head of the quadratus labii superioris.

The platysma TPs apparently develop in relation to involvement of the sternocleidomastoid muscle, which it overlies in parallel.

6. SYMPTOMS

Patients report pain as described in Section 1.

Individuals with myofascial dysfunction of the orbicularis oculi muscle may complain of "jumpy print." When reading type with strong black and white contrast, the letters seem to jump, making it difficult to focus on them.

Prickling pain due to platysma TPs feels like multiple pinpricks. The sensation is not like the tingling caused by an electric current, a feature which usually denotes a neurologic origin. Patients who experience this prickling pain in the face in combination with headaches from TPs in the sternocleidomastoid muscle are often greatly concerned and baffled, as are their physicians.

7. ACTIVATION OF TRIGGER POINTS

Habitual frowning, squinting (due to photophobia or astigmatism), or TPs in the sternal division of the sternocleidomastoid muscle, which refer pain to the orbit, may activate TPs in the orbicularis oculi muscle.[16]

Myofascial dysfunction of the masticatory muscles that is severe enough to cause trismus may activate TPs in the zygomaticus major muscle.

Platysma TPs are activated secondarily

by TPs in the sternocleidomastoid-scalene family of muscles.

8. PATIENT EXAMINATION

Activation of TPs in the orbicularis oculi muscle may produce a unilateral narrowing of the palpebral fissure that resembles the ptosis of Horner's syndrome, but without the change in pupillary size. When upward gaze is tested, these patients tilt the head backward, because they can not raise the upper eyelid sufficiently to look up.

The zygomaticus major muscle may restrict the normal 45 to 50 mm jaw opening by 10 or 20 mm; the restriction can be released by inactivating the TPs in this muscle.

9. TRIGGER POINT EXAMINATION

Orbicularis Oculi

The TPs in the upper orbital portion of this muscle are found by flat palpation, by running the tip of the examining finger crosswise over the muscle fibers that lie above the eyelid, just beneath the eyebrow and against the bone of the orbit.

Zygomaticus Major

The patient relaxes, either sitting or supine; the jaws are propped open as wide as is comfortable. Most of the length of the muscle can be palpated for spot tenderness by pincer grasp, placing one digit inside the cheek and one outside (see Fig. 13.4A). The palpable band is appreciated chiefly by the outside finger. See Figure 13.1B for location of the TPs in this muscle.

Platysma
(Fig. 13.3)

Local twitch responses are not observed in the previous two muscles, probably because it is difficult to put them on sufficient stretch. However, the twitch response of the band is likely to be seen and felt during examination of the platysma. The patient tips the head back far enough to tauten the muscle, and then the examiner pinches successive lines of skin across the muscle fibers (Fig. 13.3) approximately 2 cm (1 in) above the clavicle. Rolling the skin and platysma between the digits usually sets off the referred prickling sensation in the face (Fig. 13.1C).

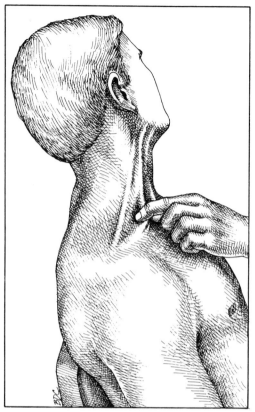

Figure 13.3. Rolling the skin of the neck between the thumb and fingers tests for the presence of active trigger points in the platysma muscle.

10. ENTRAPMENTS

No nerve entrapments have been observed due to active TPs in these muscles.

11. ASSOCIATED TRIGGER POINTS

The sternocleidomastoid, scalene and masticatory muscles on the same side often harbor active TPs, and platysma TPs are rarely, if ever, seen in the absence of such TPs in one of these other muscles.

12. STRETCH AND SPRAY

Orbicularis Oculi

Stretch and spray of this muscle are unsatisfactory because of difficulty in obtaining adequate stretch, and of keeping the liquid out of the eye. Since the muscle is so superficial, repeated cutaneous application of a penetrating local anesthetic, such as Quotane ointment,* over its TPs

---

*Quotane ointment (dimethisoquin) manufactured by Smith, Kline & French, Philadelphia, PA 19101.

PART 1

may inactivate them. This use for relief of myofascial pain is neither approved, nor disapproved, by the United States Food and Drug Administration.

Zygomaticus Major
(Fig. 13.4A)

Either sitting or supine, the patient relaxes, with a prop between the jaws to open them as wide as is comfortable. The fibers of the zygomaticus major muscle are lengthened by pulling the cheek outward with one finger, as shown in Fig. 13.4A. While the operator maintains tension on the muscle fibers, the spray is applied upward over the muscle and then over the distribution of the referred pain. However, it is difficult to obtain an adequate stretch of this long slack muscle, so that stretch and spray may be ineffective.

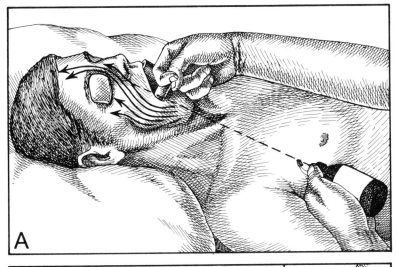

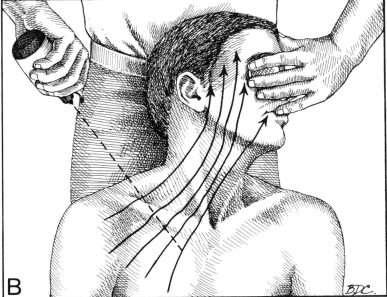

Figure 13.4.   Stretch position and spray patterns (*arrows*) for two skin muscles. *A*, the zygomaticus major. The fingers pull the corner of the mouth down and forward, away from the zygoma. The patient is instructed to hold the breath, or to exhale, as the operator protects the eye and applies vapocoolant to the cheek and nose area as shown. *B*, platysma muscle. The head and neck are extended and the face turned to the opposite side, as the spray is applied upward.

Platysma
(Fig. 13.4*B*)

With the patient seated, and the arm on the same side anchored, the operator presses against the head so as to extend and laterally flex the head and neck. The spray travels upward along the line of the platysma fibers, covering the muscle and its referred pain pattern with parallel sweeps of the vapocoolant. If, on reexamination, the TPs still show signs of activity, a TP is firmly pinched, and the pressure maintained to produce ischemic compression for a minute or two, until the TP often is fully inactivated.

13. INJECTION AND STRETCH

Orbicularis Oculi

Locate the TPs in this muscle by focal tenderness in a taut band palpated in the upper arc of the orbital portion of the muscle (Fig. 13.1*A*). A 16-mm (⅝-in), 25- or 26-gauge needle is used to inject the TPs with 0.5% procaine in isotonic saline. The patient should be warned that ecchymosis may develop in the injected area, causing a "black eye."

Zygomaticus Major
(Fig. 13.5)

Injection of the TPs in this muscle usually is more effective than treatment by stretch and spray. A pincer grasp holds the TP between the digits (as during examination) for injection of the taut band at its most tender point under tactile guidance (Fig. 13.5).

Platysma

Injection is rarely required to clear this muscle of active TPs.

One may accidentally encounter a TP in the platysma and evoke the referred prickle when injecting the underlying sternocleidomastoid muscle. The patient may react with alarm to the unexpected prickling sensation in the face caused by the needle-stimulation of the TP, until its cause is explained.

Injection in each case is followed by passive stretching and a hot pack.

14. CORRECTIVE ACTIONS

Any TPs in muscles that are likely to refer pain to the same side of the face,

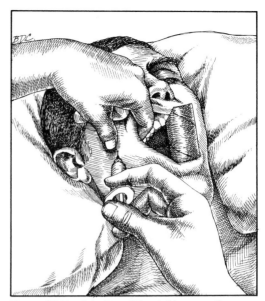

Figure 13.5.   Injection of the right zygomaticus major muscle, using pincer grasp to localize the trigger points between the digits.

such as the masticatory, sternocleidomastoid and upper trapezius muscles, should be inactivated.

The "jumpy print" symptom due to orbicularis oculi TPs has been temporarily alleviated by placing a screen of clear plastic over the print to reduce its contrast, and has been eliminated by injecting the active TPs in the orbicularis oculi.

Following treatment of the platysma muscle, and of associated TPs in muscles of the head and neck, regular passive stretching exercises and resumption of full activity should prevent recurrence of the platysma TPs.

References

1. Bardeen CR: The Musculature, Sect. 5. In *Morris's Human Anatomy*, edited by C.M. Jackson, Ed. 6. Blakiston's Son & Co., Philadelphia, 1921 (pp. 364, 365).
2. Basmajian JV: *Muscles Alive*, Ed. 4. Williams & Wilkins, Baltimore, 1978 (pp. 393, 410).
3. *Ibid.* (p. 397).
4. Grant JCB: *An Atlas of Human Anatomy*, Ed. 7. Williams & Wilkins, Baltimore, 1978 (Fig. 7–15).
5. *Ibid.* (Fig. 9-3).
6. Gray H: *Anatomy of the Human Body*, edited by C.M. Goss, American Ed. 29. Lea & Febiger, Philadelphia, 1973 (p. 381).
7. *Ibid.* (p. 383).
8. *Ibid.* (p. 390).
9. Hollinshead WH: *Anatomy for Surgeons*, Ed. 2, Vol. 1, The Head and Neck. Harper & Row, Hagerstown, 1969 (pp. 334, 335).

10. *Ibid.* (pp. 109, 338).
11. Hollinshead WH: *Functional Anatomy of the Limbs and Back*, Ed. 4. W.B. Saunders, Philadelphia, 1976 (pp. 372–374).
12. McMinn RMH, Hutchings RT: *Color Atlas of Human Anatomy.* Year Book Medical Publishers, Chicago, 1977 (pp. 34–36).
13. Sobotta J, Figge FHJ: *Atlas of Human Anatomy*, Ed. 9, Vol. 1. Hafner Division of Macmillan, New York, 1974 (pp. 169, 178, 181).
14. *Ibid.* (p. 168).
15. Toldt C: *An Atlas of Human Anatomy*, translated by M.E. Paul, Ed. 2, Vol. 1. Macmillan, New York, 1919 (pp. 290, 300, 302).
16. Travell J: Identification of myofascial trigger point syndromes: a case of atypical facial neuralgia. *Arch Phys Med Rehabil* 62:100–106, 1981 (Fig. 5).
17. Willis WD, Grossman RG: *Medical Neurobiology.* C.V. Mosby, Saint Louis, 1973 (p. 366).

PART 1

CHAPTER 14
Cutaneous—II: Occipitofrontalis
"Scalp Tensors"

HIGHLIGHTS: **REFERRED PAIN** from trigger points (TPs) in the frontalis belly of the occipitofrontalis muscle projects locally over the forehead. Pain from TPs in the occipitalis belly is projected to the back of the head and through the cranium to the back of the orbit ("behind the eye"). **ANATOMICAL ATTACHMENTS** of these epicranial muscle bellies are, above, to the galea aponeurotica. Below, the frontalis attaches to the skin of the forehead, and the occipitalis to the occipital bone. **ACTION** of these muscles is to wrinkle the forehead; the occipitalis assists the frontalis. **ACTIVATION OF TRIGGER POINTS** in the frontalis belly may arise from direct trauma, or secondarily as satellites from TPs in the clavicular division of the sternocleidomastoid muscle, or from the over-load stress of habitually wrinkling the forehead. **TRIGGER POINT EXAMINATION** is easily accomplished by flat palpation of the muscle against the underlying skull for taut bands, TP tenderness, and local twitch responses. **ENTRAPMENT** of the supraorbital nerve can be caused by TPs in the frontalis muscle. **STRETCH AND SPRAY** are usually unsatisfactory for these muscles, but ischemic compression is remarkably effective. **INJECTION AND STRETCH** of TPs in these scalp muscles require a finer needle than for most muscles. **CORRECTIVE ACTIONS** include training the patient to avoid prolonged, intense frowning or wrinkling of the forehead and the inactivation of primary TPs in the clavicular division of the sternocleidomastoid muscle.

1. REFERRED PAIN
(Fig. 14.1)

Frontalis
(Fig. 14.1A)

The trigger points (TPs) of the frontalis belly evoke pain that spreads upward and over the forehead on the same side (Fig. 14.1A). The referred pain remains local, in the region of the muscle, like that from TPs in the deltoid muscle.

Occipitalis
(Fig. 14.1B)

"Fibrositic nodules" or "myalgia" (used in the sense of myofascial TPs) of the occipitalis belly are a recognized source of headache.[10, 24] Occipitalis tenderness was found in 42% of 42 patients with ipsilateral face and head pain associated with the myofascial pain-dysfunction syndrome.[14]

Active TPs in the occipitalis belly (Fig. 14.1B) refer pain laterally, diffusely over the back of the head and through the cranium, causing intense pain deep in the orbit. Kellgren[10] reported that the injection of hypertonic saline into normal occipitalis muscle gave rise to "earache." Cyriax[3] similarly injected muscles and fascia of the head and neck to map referred pain patterns. He found that injection into the galea aponeurotica between the frontalis and occipitalis bellies referred pain homolaterally behind the eye, in the eyeball,

PART 1

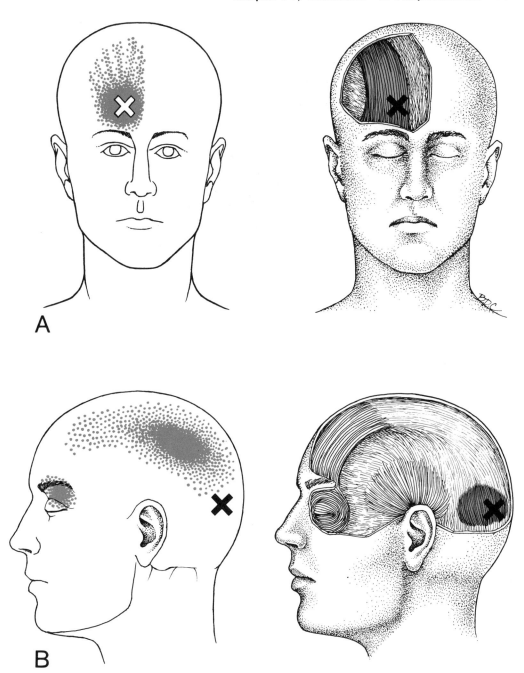

Figure 14.1.   Pain patterns (*red*) referred from trigger points (×s) in the occipitofrontalis muscle. *A,* right frontalis belly. *B,* left occipitalis belly.

and in the eyelids. These referred pain patterns were later confirmed clinically by Williams.[24]

2. ANATOMICAL ATTACHMENTS
(Fig. 14.2)

The major cutaneous muscle of the scalp (the epicranial muscle) is the occipitofron-

talis, which has two bellies, the frontalis anteriorly, and the occipitalis posteriorly. These attach *above* to one large, flat tendinous sheet, the galea aponeurotica, which covers the vertex. The galea is firmly connected to the skin, but slides over the periosteum[19] (Fig. 14.2).

The frontalis belly attaches *below and*

PART 1

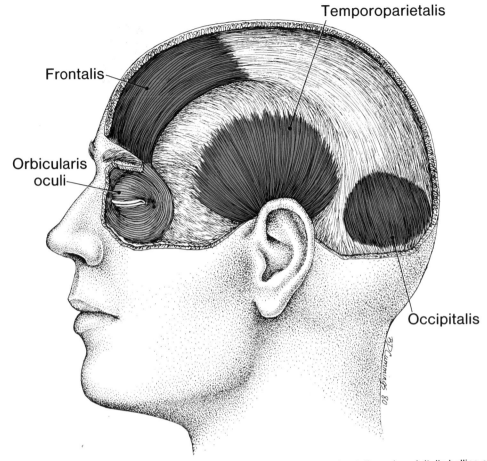

Figure 14.2. Attachments of the left epicranial muscles (*dark red*): the frontalis and occipitalis bellies of the occipitofrontalis muscle, and also the temporoparietalis muscle. Each connects above to the tendinous galea aponeurotica. Below, the frontalis attaches to the skin near the eyebrow; the occipitalis anchors to bone along the superior nuchal line, and the temporoparietalis to the skin above the ear. The cutaneous orbicularis oculi muscle is shown in light red.

in front to the skin over the eyebrow, where it interdigitates with the orbicularis oculi muscle. The occipitalis belly attaches *below and behind* to the superior nuchal line of the occipital bone.[1, 8]

Supplemental References

The frontalis has been illustrated by other authors in side view,[1, 7, 8, 16] from above,[5] from in front,[12, 15, 19, 20] in cross section,[17] and from the side with associated vessels and nerves.[18]

The occipitalis has been illustrated in side view,[1, 4, 8, 13, 16, 22] from behind,[6, 21] and from the side with associated vessels and nerves.[18]

3. INNERVATION

The epicranial muscle is supplied by the facial nerve (cranial nerve VII).

4. ACTIONS

The frontalis belly raises the eyebrow and wrinkles the forehead[9]; acting bilaterally, this produces an expression of surprise or attention.[8] The occipitalis and frontalis, acting together, further retract the skin of the forehead, opening the eyes widely in an expression of horror. This shifts the scalp toward the occiput, which makes the hair stand up, because the hair bulbs in the frontal region slant backward.[1] The occipitalis anchors and retracts the galea posteriorly, so that the frontalis can more effectively pull against it; this action gives rise to the combination name of the occipitofrontalis muscle.

Because the frontalis is associated with the increased muscle tension of anxiety, it is commonly monitored for biofeedback. Contrary to some statements in the literature, all electrical activity in the frontalis ceases at complete rest in normal subjects.[2]

5. MYOTATIC UNIT

The frontalis and occipitalis bellies function as synergists in tandem. The frontalis may contract with, or independently of, the perpendicularly placed corrugator muscle, which shortens the eyebrows in a frown.

The frontalis and procerus, which pulls the medial end of the eyebrow down, are antagonists.[2]

6. SYMPTOMS

The chief symptom is pain, as described in Section 1. The patient with occipitalis TPs cannot bear the weight of the back of the head on the pillow at night because of the pain induced and must lie on the side.

The deep aching occipital pain caused by occipitalis TPs must be distinguished from the more superficial scalp tingling and hot prickling pain due to entrapment of the greater occipital nerve by the posterior cervical muscles. The patient with pain referred from myofascial TPs finds, as a rule, that moist heat provides relief. The patient with head pain due to nerve entrapment cannot tolerate heat, but prefers the cold of an ice pack.

7. ACTIVATION OF TRIGGER POINTS

In the frontalis, TPs are likely to develop as satellites of TPs in the clavicular division of the sternocleidomastoid muscle, which refer head pain to the frontal region. Frontalis TPs also may be activated by work overload, especially in tense people with great mobility of facial expression, people who persistently use the frontalis to maintain a worried, frowning expression, or an expression of attention with raised eyebrows and wrinkled forehead.

Occipitalis TPs are likely to occur in patients with decreased visual acuity and/ or with glaucoma, due to persistent, strong contraction of the forehead and scalp muscles. These TPs may likewise be activated as satellites of posterior cervical TPs, which refer pain and tenderness to the occipital region.

8. PATIENT EXAMINATION

No specific sign of this myofascial syndrome has been noted on examination. The patient tends to frown a lot.

9. TRIGGER POINT EXAMINATION

An active TP in the frontalis belly is identified by flat palpation as spot tenderness above the medial end of the eyebrow (Fig. 14.1A).

An active TP in the occipitalis belly lies in a small hollow just above the superior nuchal line approximately 4 cm (1½ in) lateral to the midline (Fig. 14.1B); spot tenderness is located by flat palpation. This location was published in 1915 as the site of tender "nodules" found in chronic cervical fibrositis.[11]

10. ENTRAPMENTS

Active TPs in the medial half of the frontalis belly apparently can entrap the supraorbital nerve. This entrapment produces a unilateral frontal "headache" with primarily neuritic, rather than myofascial pain characteristics. The symptoms are relieved by inactivating (injecting) the apparently responsible frontalis TPs.

11. ASSOCIATED TRIGGER POINTS

Active TPs in the frontalis belly are often found as satellites in association with longstanding TPs in the clavicular division of the sternocleidomastoid muscle on the same side.

In patients with occipital aching pain, those muscles which refer pain to the occiput, including the posterior digastric, should be checked for TP tenderness and for induction of pain referred to the occiput.

12. STRETCH AND SPRAY

The frontalis responds poorly to stretch and spray, since the muscle is so difficult to stretch. It does respond well to ischemic compression and to the application of a topical local anesthetic, Quotane ointment.* Because Quotane ointment is both fat and water miscible, it penetrates more deeply than do most topical analgesics. Cutaneous application over frontalis TPs

---

* Quotane ointment (dimethisoquin) is manufactured by Smith, Kline & French, Philadelphia, PA 19101.

may eliminate the headache within about 5 min. With repeated applications, the TP activity tends to recur less frequently and with less intensity, so that the frontalis headaches gradually fade away. Patients appreciate this self-control of pain without the use of analgesic pills.[23] This use of Quotane ointment for relief of myofascial pain is neither approved, nor disapproved, by the United States Food and Drug Administration.

For treatment of the occipitalis belly, the same measures may be used. In addition, massage[3, 24] and large doses of niacin[24] have been recommended.

13. INJECTION AND STRETCH

The frontalis muscle fibers are thin and very superficial, which makes its TPs difficult to locate with the needle tip. To inject it, a 2.5-cm (1-in), 24- or 25-gauge needle is directed across the muscle fibers (parallel to the eyebrow), nearly tangent to the skin.

The occipitalis belly is thicker than the frontalis and may require a 2.5-cm (1-in), 22-gauge needle. Injection of these posterior TPs is technically more satisfactory since they lie in a small hollow which holds sufficient muscle mass to receive the needle. However, considerable probing of the area may be necessary to locate them.

14. CORRECTIVE ACTION

For occipitofrontalis involvement, the patient must avoid persistent frowning and vigorous wrinkling of the forehead. In addition, for prevention of recurrences of TP activity, the patient should learn to use ischemic compression of the TPs.

Any related TPs in the clavicular division of the sternocleidomastoid and posterior neck muscles should be inactivated.

References

1. Bardeen CR: The Musculature, Sect. 5. In *Morris's Human Anatomy*, edited by C.M. Jackson, Ed. 6. Blakiston's Son & Co., Philadelphia, 1921 (pp. 364, 371, Fig. 372).
2. Basmajian JV: *Muscles Alive*, Ed. 4. Williams & Wilkins, Baltimore, 1978 (p. 394).
3. Cyriax J: Rheumatic headache. *Br Med J* 2:1367–1368, 1938.
4. Eisler P: *Die Muskeln des Stammes*. Gustav Fischer, Jena, 1912 (p. 170, Fig. 18).
5. *Ibid*. (p. 184, Fig. 20).
6. Grant JCB: *An Atlas of Human Anatomy*, Ed. 7. Williams & Wilkins, Baltimore, 1978 (Fig. 5-33).
7. *Ibid*. (Fig. 7-15).
8. Gray H: *Anatomy of the Human Body*, edited by C.M. Goss, American Ed. 29. Lea & Febiger, Philadelphia, 1973 (pp. 379, 380).
9. Hollinshead WH: *Functional Anatomy of the Limbs and Back*, Ed. 4. W.B. Saunders, Philadelphia, 1976 (p. 374).
10. Kellgren JH: Observations on referred pain arising from muscle. *Clin Sci* 3:175–190, 1938 (p. 181).
11. Llewellyn LJ, Jones AB: *Fibrositis*. Rebman, New York, 1915 (Fig. 32 opposite p. 210).
12. McMinn RMH, Hutchings RT: *Color Atlas of Human Anatomy*. Year Book Medical Publishers, 1977 (p. 34).
13. *Ibid*. (p. 35).
14. Sharav Y, Tzukert A, Refaeli B: Muscle pain index in relation to pain, dysfunction, and dizziness associated with the myofascial pain-dysfunction syndrome. *Oral Surg* 46:742–747, 1978.
15. Sobotta J, Figge FHJ: *Atlas of Human Anatomy*, Ed. 9, Vol. 1. Hafner Division of Macmillan, New York, 1974 (p. 178).
16. *Ibid*. (pp. 181, 185).
17. Sobotta J, Figge FHJ: *Atlas of Human Anatomy*, Ed. 9, Vol. 3. Hafner Division of Macmillan, New York, 1974 (p. 68).
18. *Ibid*. (p. 210).
19. Spalteholz W: *Handatlas der Anatomie des Menschen*, Ed. 11, Vol. 2. S. Hirzel, Leipzig, 1922 (p. 260).
20. Toldt C: *An Atlas of Human Anatomy*, translated by M.E. Paul, Ed. 2, Vol. 1. Macmillan, New York, 1919 (p. 300).
21. *Ibid*. (p. 266).
22. *Ibid*. (p. 302).
23. Travell J: *Office Hours: Day and Night*. The World Publishing Company, New York, 1968 (pp. 296–297).
24. Williams HL: The syndrome of physical or intrinsic allergy of the head: myalgia of the head (sinus headache). *Proc Staff Meet Mayo Clin* 20:177–183, 1945 (p. 181).

CHAPTER 15
Splenius Capitis and Splenius Cervicis Muscles

"Ache Inside the Skull"

HIGHLIGHTS: **REFERRED PAIN** from trigger points (TPs) in the splenius capitis appears in the vertex of the head, and from the splenius cervicis is projected upward to the occiput, diffusely through the cranium, intensely to the back of the orbit, and sometimes downward to the shoulder girdle and to the angle of the neck. **ANATOMICAL ATTACHMENTS** of the splenii are, below, to the spinous processes of the lower cervical and upper thoracic vertebrae. Above, the splenius cervicis attaches to the transverse processes of the upper cervical vertebrae, and the splenius capitis attaches to the mastoid process of the skull. The splenius cervicis and capitis lie superficial to the semispinalis capitis and other paraspinal muscles, deep to the trapezius, and posterior and medial to the levator scapulae. **ACTIONS** of the splenii are to extend the head and neck, and to rotate them, turning the face toward the same side. **SYMPTOMS** of head and neck pain with homolateral blurring of vision can be due to active TPs in the splenius cervicis and splenius capitis muscles. **ACTIVATION OF TRIGGER POINTS** in these muscles is often due to sudden direct trauma, or caused by holding the head and neck in a forward, crooked position for a prolonged period. These neck muscles are especially vulnerable when they are tired and the overlying skin is exposed to a cold draft. **PATIENT EXAMINATION** reveals moderate restriction of head and neck flexion and rotation to the same side. These myofascial symptoms are clearly distinguished from the neurological disease, spasmodic torticollis. **TRIGGER POINT EXAMINATION** requires that the relation of the splenii to adjacent muscles be kept clearly in mind. Most of their course lies between and beneath other muscles. **ASSOCIATED TRIGGER POINTS** are commonly found in the levator scapulae, upper trapezius, and sternocleidomastoid muscles, and in the posterior cervical musculature. **STRETCH AND SPRAY** of the splenius capitis are performed mainly with an up-stroke pattern of the vapocoolant. These TPs also respond to ischemic compression and deep massage. The splenius cervicis is sprayed in both an up-sweep and a down-sweep pattern. **INJECTION AND STRETCH** of the splenius capitis should be avoided because of the underlying, unprotected vertebral artery. The splenius cervicis usually responds well to this therapy. **CORRECTIVE ACTIONS** include the elimination of perpetuating sources of muscle strain, and the performance of daily passive self-stretch of the splenii.

1. REFERRED PAIN
(Fig 15.1)

A trigger point (TP) in the splenius capitis muscle refers pain to the vertex of the head on the same side (Fig. 15.1A).[4, 18, 31–33]

A TP in the upper end of the splenius cervicis (Fig. 15.1B—pattern on the *left* figure) refers a diffuse pain through the inside of the head focussing severely behind the eye on the same side, and sometimes refers pain to the scalp over the occiput.[29] A TP in the lower portion of the splenius cervicis at the angle of the neck (Fig. 15.1B—pattern on the *right* figure) refers pain upward and to the base of the neck,

PART 1

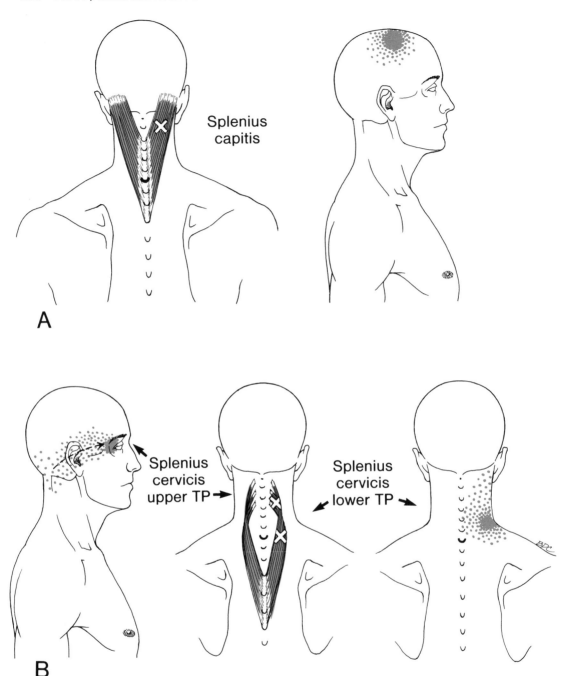

Figure 15.1   Trigger points (×s) and referred pain patterns (*red*) for the right splenius capitis and splenius cervicis muscles. A, the splenius capitis trigger point, which overlies the occipital triangle. B, the upper splenius cervicis trigger point (figure on the *left*) refers pain to the orbit. The black, *dash line* and *arrow* indicate that the pain seems to shoot through the inside of the head to the back of the eye. The lower splenius cervicis trigger point (figure on the *right*) refers pain to the angle of the neck. The *middle* figure shows upper and lower splenius cervicis trigger points.

within the upper part of the pain pattern of the levator scapulae.

In addition to pain, an upper splenius cervicis TP may cause blurring of near vision in the homolateral eye, without dizziness or conjunctivitis. This symptom has resolved immediately and completely with inactivation of the responsible TP.

PART 1

2. ANATOMICAL ATTACHMENTS
(Fig. 15.2)

Splenius Capitis

Below this muscle attaches in the midline to the fascia over the spinous proc- esses of the lower half of the cervical spine and of the first three or four thoracic vertebrae (Fig. 15.2). *Above and laterally* its fibers attach to the mastoid process and to the adjacent occipital bone underneath the attachment of the sternocleidomastoid muscle.[14]

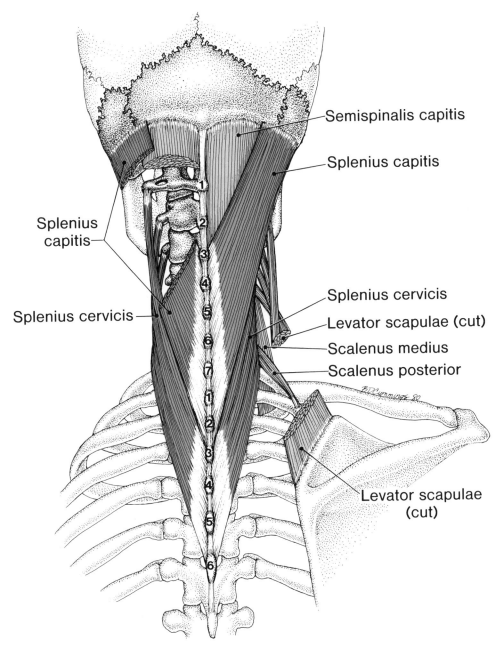

Figure 15.2. Attachments of the right splenius capitis muscle (*upper dark red*), and of the right splenius cervicis muscle (*lower dark red*). Adjacent muscles are shown in *light red*. The levator scapulae (*right side*, cut) crosses over the upper part of the splenius cervicis, with which it has common attachments to the transverse processes of the upper cervical vertebrae. The trapezius muscle (not shown) covers much of both splenii.

Splenius Cervicis

This muscle lies to the lateral side and caudal to the splenius capitis. The splenius cervicis, like the capitis, attaches **below** in the midline to the spinous processes; the cervicis fastens from the T_3 to T_6 vertebrae. The muscle connects **above** to the posterior tubercles on the transverse processes of the upper two or three cervical vertebrae. On these posterior tubercles, the cervicis forms the most posterior of a triple attachment with the levator scapulae in the middle and the scalenus medius in front.

Bilaterally, the paired splenius cervicis and splenius capitis muscles each form a "V" shape.[41]

Supplemental References

The splenius capitis has been illustrated by other authors as seen from behind,[7, 12, 22, 24, 27] from the side,[8, 13, 23, 28] and in cross section.[11]

The splenius cervicis is presented from behind.[12, 22, 24, 27]

3. INNERVATION

Both muscles are innervated by lateral branches of the dorsal primary divisions of spinal nerves C_2–C_4, frequently also C_1, sometimes C_5, and rarely C_6.[9]

4. ACTIONS

Splenius Capitis

A sophisticated study using implanted fine-wire electrodes in 15 subjects determined that the splenius capitis showed strong activity bilaterally during extension of the head and neck, and unilaterally during rotation of the face to the same side.[3] The splenius capitis showed no activity at rest in the upright balanced position, and did *not* become active during lateral flexion of the head and neck.[3, 25]

When the face is rotated to one side with the chin tilted upward, the splenius capitis muscles on *both* sides work vigorously; apparently, the one on the same side rotates the head and neck, while the opposite muscle extends the head and neck.[25]

Early stimulation experiments on an unspecified splenius muscle described lateral inclination and extension with rotation of the head to the stimulated side.[6] Subsequent authors attributed extension and lateral flexion of the head and neck to activity of one splenius capitis muscle,[6, 14, 20] and attributed extension of the head and neck to its bilateral contraction.[14, 15, 20] A significant lateral flexion function is highly questionable.

Splenius Cervicis

No electromyographic data specific to the splenius cervicis muscle were found. Most authors attribute rotation and side-bending of the cervical spine to contraction of one muscle and extension of the neck to the action of both muscles bilaterally.[14, 20] Others identify only rotation and extension.[2, 15]

5. MYOTATIC UNIT

Synergists of the splenii capitis and cervicis for extension of the head and neck are the posterior cervical group as a whole, especially the semispinalis capitis and cervicis muscles acting bilaterally. Antagonists for extension are the anterior cervical and sternocleidomastoid muscles. The synergist for rotation to the same side is the levator scapulae, while on the opposite side the synergists are the upper trapezius, the semispinalis capitis, the deep paraspinal muscles and the sternocleidomastoid. The antagonists to the splenii capitis and cervicis for rotation are the muscles contralateral to the above synergists.

6. SYMPTOMS

Patients with active splenius capitis TPs usually present with a primary complaint of pain referred close to the vertex, as described in Section 1.

Patients with splenius cervicis TPs complain primarily of pain in the neck, cranium and eye; they may complain also of a "stiff neck,"[17, 19, 29] because rotation of the head and neck is limited by pain. However, the patient experiences less restriction of rotation with only splenius cervicis involvement than with only levator scapulae involvement. Simultaneous TP activity in both the levator and splenius muscles may almost completely block head rotation to that side. Involvement of the splenius cervicis may become apparent because of residual pain and stiffness following elimination of TP activity in the levator scapulae.

Pain in the orbit and blurring of vision are disturbing symptoms referred homolaterally to the eye from TPs in the upper part of the splenius cervicis muscle.

7. ACTIVATION OF TRIGGER POINTS
(Fig. 15.3)

Postural Stress

Postural stresses that overload extension or rotation of the head and neck are likely to initiate and perpetuate splenius cervicis TPs. Clinical examples include bird-watching through binoculars, seated in a position that extends the neck to compensate for a strong thoracic kyphosis (Fig. 15.3), assuming a similar head-back posture while playing the accordion, and working at a desk with the head turned to one side and projected forward. In addition, TPs in either, or both, the splenius capitis and splenius cervicis may be activated by falling asleep with the head and neck bent in a crooked position, as with the head on the armrest of a sofa without an adequate pillow. A cold air conditioner or cool draft blowing on the exposed neck, together with muscular fatigue, greatly increase the likelihood of activation of these neck-muscle TPs.

One patient developed a splenius capitis syndrome after acquiring contact lenses[30]. He held his head in a cocked position at his desk to avoid reflections on the glasses from overhead lights. Adjustments in neck posture to see through the middle section of trifocal lenses may have the same result.

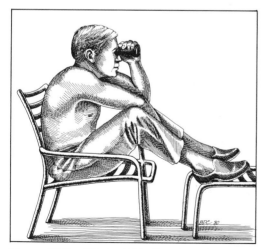

Figure 15.3. "Bird-watching" posture that strains the splenius cervicis muscles.

Activity Stress

Pulling or hauling on a rope while projecting the head forward may activate TPs in the splenii.

Other Factors

The activation of both splenius cervicis and levator scapulae TPs may occur with marked skin cooling, for example, exposure to a breeze when a person relaxes in a wet bathing suit in the shade (even on a warm day) after the fatigue of swimming, without additional stress.

These muscles are susceptible to the trauma of a rear-end collision in an automobile followed by a sudden stop,[21] especially if the head and neck are somewhat rotated at the time of impact.

8. PATIENT EXAMINATION

The patient shows painful restriction of active head rotation to the same side. Flexion of the chin onto the chest may lack one or two finger widths. One is likely to uncover the splenius cervicis TP involvement when the pain and restricted rotation improve, but fail to clear up, after TPs in the levator scapulae muscle have been inactivated.

Myofascial TP involvement of the splenii, levator scapulae, upper trapezius and sternocleidomastoid muscles must be distinguished from spasmodic torticollis (wry neck),[1, 10] which is a neurological condition characterized by paroxysmal or clonic contractions of the involved muscles, especially the sternocleidomastoid. The latter also may exhibit tonic spasm. In spasmodic torticollis, hypertrophy of the muscles develops, associated with fibrotic change and permanent contracture. In contrast, the apparent shortening and tautness of a muscle due to myofascial TPs in that muscle does not cause hypertrophy, and presents a steady resistance to stretch without paroxysmal or clonic contractions. Spasmodic torticollis, like the dystonias, appears to have a central nervous system origin,[10] and the irritable focus in the brain may be treated surgically.[1, 4, 5]

The differential diagnosis of "stiff neck" of myofascial origin[29] is discussed further in Section 8, Chapter 7 and in Section 6, Chapter 19.

9. TRIGGER POINT EXAMINATION

Splenius Capitis

Splenius capitis TPs can be identified by flat palpation, and are usually found where this muscle lies subcutaneously, within the upper portion of the muscular triangle bounded by the trapezius behind, the sternocleidomastoid in front, and the levator scapulae below.[2, 26] Williams[32] located this TP at the insertion of the splenius capitis muscle on the mastoid process and in the portion of the muscle just distal to this attachment.

Splenius Cervicis
(Fig. 15.4)

As viewed from behind, the upper trapezius covers much of the splenius cervicis on its medial side,[22] and the levator scapulae covers much of the muscle when viewed from its lateral side.[23] To palpate

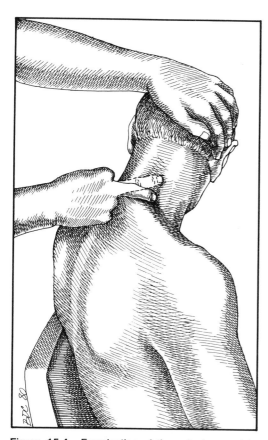

Figure 15.4. Examination of the splenius cervicis muscle. The lower finger (*solid lines*) palpates the lower trigger point. The *dash line* finger (*above*) palpates the upper trigger point.

the cervicis, therefore, the patient's head and neck are flexed toward the side being examined, thus slackening the upper trapezius and levator scapulae. The operator displaces the free border of the upper trapezius medially, and presses the levator scapulae anterolaterally, to permit palpation of the splenius cervicis directly beneath the skin.

The lower TP is palpated just above the angle of the neck (Fig. 15.4).[22] The head and neck are rotated to the opposite side as necessary to stretch the splenii to the desired degree of tautness for palpation of their TPs. The upper TP is located by sliding the finger cephalad along the line of the splenius cervicis fibers between the upper trapezius and levator scapulae muscles (Fig. 15.4). The splenius cervicis lies just posterior to the lower cervical transverse processes, which are clearly palpable in some patients. Kelly[16] described the location of a TP that lies in the angle between the upper ends of the trapezius and sternocleidomastoid muscles, which referred pain in the distribution we recognize as characteristic of the upper end of the splenius cervicis muscle.

10. ENTRAPMENTS

The authors are not aware of any nerve entrapment due to involvement of these muscles.

11. ASSOCIATED TRIGGER POINTS

Active TPs rarely appear in the splenii muscles alone; either or both the levator scapulae and the posterior cervical muscles also are usually involved.

12. STRETCH AND SPRAY
(Fig. 15.5)

These muscles generally are stretched and sprayed sequentially with their synergists as part of one treatment. Tightness of one muscle may prevent full stretch of one or the other of the synergistic parallel units.

The patient is seated and the axis of the shoulder girdle is checked to be sure that it is horizontal. If not, the pelvis is leveled and the spine straightened by adding a butt lift under the ischial tuberosity on the side of the small hemipelvis (see Fig. 48.10, Chapter 48).

PART 1

Splenius Capitis
(Fig. 15.5A)

The patient sits in a comfortable arm-chair with good elbow support, so that he or she can relax the shoulder-girdle muscles while leaning against the chair back. The patient's head is rotated 20° or 30° toward the opposite side while the head is gently pressed forward and sideways to the opposite side, slightly more laterally than forward (Fig. 15.5A), in the same manner as pictured by Zohn and Mennell.[34] At the same time, the vapocoolant spray is swept upward over the muscle and occiput to the vertex.

If well coordinated and relaxed, the patient may obtain more effective stretch by using his own hand to grasp the back of the head, turn the face to the other side, and pull the head down in the direction of the face, while the operator applies the spray. The patient thus learns exactly how to stretch this muscle at home.

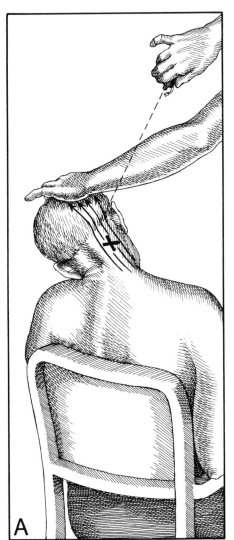
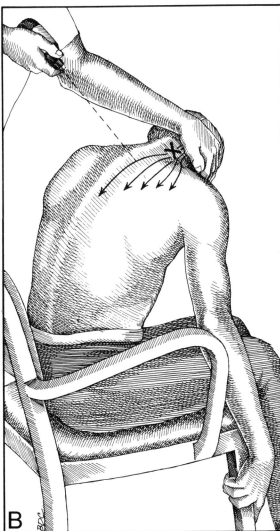

Figure 15.5. Stretch position and spray patterns for trigger points (×s) in the right splenius capitis and splenius cervicis muscles. The head and cervical spine are rotated and pressed toward the opposite side, while both are flexed. *A,* splenius capitis: head movement on top of the neck post brings the ear toward the front of the shoulder, while the spray is applied in an up-sweep pattern to the vertex. *B,* splenius cervicis: pressure is applied to emphasize neck movement, while the spray is applied, first in a down-sweep pattern, then in an up-sweep pattern toward the eye.

Splenius Cervicis
(Fig. 15.5B)

With the patient seated as above, the stretch is started by letting the weight of the head drop forward with the face turned 30° or 40° toward the opposite side. The patient's head is pressed into more forward than lateral flexion, to stretch this rotator and extensor of the neck. To cover the muscle and its pain reference zones (Fig. 15.1B), the spray follows first a down-sweep pattern (Fig. 15.5B), and then sweeps up as far as the eyebrow. The eye should be protected. Then, the patient latches the fingers over the back of the cranium (not shown) and pulls it forward and down with the head turned so as to stretch the splenius cervicis, while the operator applies the spray. This teaches the patient the stretch exercise to be done at home while seated under a hot shower.

A hot pack over the treated muscles promptly follows stretch and spray.

13. INJECTION AND STRETCH
(Fig. 15.6)

Splenius Capitis

Due to the proximity of the underlying loop of the vertebral artery, injection of this TP is to be avoided. This muscle's TPs are inactivated by stretch and spray and by ischemic compression.

Splenius Cervicis

The patient lies on the opposite side, with the head supported on a pillow between the cheek and shoulder, without bending or rotating the head and neck. The TP is located by palpation, as described in Section 9. When injecting the upper TP in the splenius cervicis, the needle is inserted precisely, below and lateral to, the posterior occipital triangle, through which passes the vertebral artery (see Fig. 16.4, Chapter 16). Even outside the triangle, if the needle penetrates too deeply, it may pass between the vertebral transverse processes, which encircle the vertebral artery (see Fig. 16.6, Chapter 16).

The splenius cervicis muscle lies medial and deep to the levator scapulae. Its lower TP is located between the lower end of the splenius capitis and the levator scapulae muscles (Fig. 15.6A), and is best injected with the needle directed from lateral to medial, while the needle point is kept posterior to the plane of the transverse processes (Fig. 15.6B). In this approach, the needle enters the splenius cervicis beneath the anterior border of the upper trapezius muscle.

If the patient is being treated for a "stiff neck," any TPs in the levator scapulae should be injected at the same time as those in the splenius cervicis.

14. CORRECTIVE ACTIONS

Postural Stress

As patients become aware that certain activities, like bird-watching and accordion playing, initiate and perpetuate splenius TPs, they learn to avoid the postural strain by straightening their posture, keeping the head and neck erect and the thoracic spine extended.

Body asymmetry due to a short leg or small hemipelvis should be corrected. A long cane should be avoided. When typing, the patient learns to place copy and reading material on a steno stand or music stand directly in front of the eyes, rather than flat on the desk at one side; this avoids the repetitive muscular strain of turning the head to read. Neck strain is avoided also by not sleeping with the head and neck in a crooked position.

Reflections on eyeglasses and contact lenses can be managed by changing the relative position of the light source or by using tinted lenses. Trifocal eyeglasses should not be worn by patients susceptible to splenius cervicis TPs.

Activity Stress

If hauling on a rope cannot be avoided, the patient should learn to pull it without tensing the neck muscles.

Other Factors

Chilling the skin of the neck, especially when the muscles are fatigued, often activates TPs in posterior neck muscles. The patient learns to keep the neck warm by sleeping in a high-necked sleeping garment, by wearing a turtle-neck sweater or scarf during the waking hours, and by avoiding cold drafts.

Exercise Therapy

The patient places these muscles on a passive stretch, as described in Section 12,

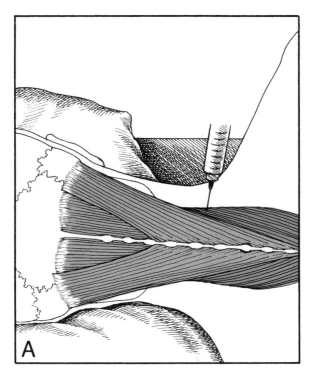

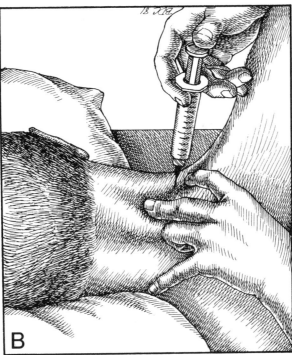

Figure 15.6. Injection of the lower trigger point area in the splenius cervicis muscle (*dark red*). *A*, location where the needle penetrates the muscle. *B*, injection of trigger point as diagrammed in *Part A*. The middle finger presses the splenius capitis (*light red*) to one side; the index finger presses the levator scapulae out of the way to the other side.

by latching the fingers behind the head while seated on a stool under a hot shower. As the splenius tautness releases slightly in response to the sustained pressure, the patient takes up the slack with small increments of increased downward pull on the head. This passive stretch exercise is similar to that illustrated in Figure 16.7 in Chapter 16, but adds some head and neck rotation to the flexion. After release of the stretch, the patient moves the head and neck through a full range of active motion for the specific muscles stretched. If parallel fibers remain sore and taut, the Seated-shower Exercise is repeated, changing the angle of pull to stretch them.

Swinging the head around at the full range of motion ("head rolling") can seriously *overload* adjacent lines of taut muscle fibers, and worsen the condition. Therefore, the patient should stretch the muscles in one direction at a time, release the tension, turn the head slightly, and then pull to stretch in the next direction.

References

1. Adson AW, Young HH, Ghormley RK: Spasmodic torticollis. *J Bone Joint Surg* 28:299–308, 1946.
2. Bardeen CR: The musculature. Sect. 5. In *Morris's Human Anatomy*, edited by C.M. Jackson. Ed. 6. Blakiston's Son & Co., Philadelphia, 1921 (p. 447).
3. Basmajian JV: *Muscles Alive*, Ed. 4. Williams & Wilkins. Baltimore, 1978 (p. 399).
4. Cooper IS: *Parkinsonism. Its Medical and Surgical Therapy.* Charles C Thomas, Springfield, Ill., 1961 (pp. 224–228).
5. Cooper IS: Cryogenic surgery of the basal ganglia. *JAMA* 181:600–604, 1962.
6. Duchenne GB: *Physiology of Motion*, translated by E.B. Kaplan. J.B. Lippincott, Philadelphia, 1949 (p. 513).
7. Eisler P: *Die Muskeln des Stammes.* Gustav Fischer. Jena, 1912 (Figs. 51, 53, 55).
8. *Ibid.* (Fig. 52).
9. *Ibid.* (p. 396).
10. Foltz EL, Knopp LM, Ward AA Jr: Experimental spasmodic torticollis. *J Neurosurg* 16:55–67, 1959.
11. Grant JCB: *An Atlas of Human Anatomy*, Ed. 7. Williams & Wilkins, Baltimore, 1978 (Fig. 5-24).
12. *Ibid.* (5–27).
13. *Ibid.* (9–5).
14. Gray H: *Anatomy of the Human Body*, edited by C.M. Goss. American Ed. 29. Lea & Febiger, Philadelphia, 1973 (p. 403).
15. Hollinshead WH: *Functional Anatomy of the Limbs and Back*, Ed. 4. W.B. Saunders, Philadelphia, 1976 (pp. 225, 226).
16. Kelly M: The relief of facial pain by procaine (novocaine) injections. *J Am Geriatr Soc* 11:586–596, 1963 (Cases 1 and 2).
17. Llewellyn LJ, Jones AB: *Fibrositis.* Rebman, New York, 1915 (p. 209, Fig. 210 opposite p. 210).
18. Marbach JJ: Arthritis of the temporomandibular joints. *Am Fam Physician* 19:131–139, 1979 (Fig. 9C).
19. Modell W, Travell JT, Kraus H, Hardy JD: Contributions to *Cornell Conferences on Therapy.* Relief of pain by ethyl chloride spray. *NY State J Med* 52:1550–1558, 1952 (p. 1551).
20. Rasch PJ, Burke RK: *Kinesiology and Applied Anatomy*, Ed. 6. Lea & Febiger, Philadelphia, 1978 (p. 236).
21. Rubin D: An approach to the management of myofascial trigger point syndromes. *Arch Phys Med Rehabil* 62:107–110, 1981.
22. Sobotta J, Figge FHJ: *Atlas of Human Anatomy*, Ed. 9, Vol. 1. Hafner Division of Macmillan, New York, 1974 (pp. 142, 144).
23. *Ibid.* (pp. 169, 185).
24. Spalteholz W: *Handatlas der Anatomie des Menschen*, Ed. 11. Vol. 2. S. Hirzel, Leipzig, 1922 (pp. 308).
25. Takebe K, Vitti M, Basmajian JV: The functions of semispinalis capitis and splenius capitis muscles: an electromyographic study. *Anat Rec* 179:477–480, 1974.
26. Toldt C: *An Atlas of Human Anatomy*, translated by M.E. Paul, Ed. 2, Vol. 1. Macmillan, New York, 1919 (p. 266).
27. *Ibid.* (p. 268).
28. *Ibid.* (p. 277).
29. Travell J: Rapid relief of acute "stiff neck" by ethyl chloride spray. *J Am Med Wom Assoc* 4:89–95, 1949 (p. 91 Fig. 3. p. 93 Case 3).
30. Travell J: *Office Hours: Day and Night.* The World Publishing Company, New York, 1968 (p. 271).
31. Travell J, Rinzler SH: The myofascial genesis of pain. *Postgrad Med* 11:425–434, 1952 (p. 427).
32. Williams HL: The syndrome of physical or intrinsic allergy of the head: myalgia of the head (sinus headache). *Proc Staff Meet Mayo Clin* 20:177–183, 1945.
33. Wyant GM: Chronic pain syndromes and their treatment. II. Trigger points. *Can Anaesth Soc J* 26:216–219, 1979 (Case 2, Table 1).
34. Zohn DA, Mennell J McM: *Musculoskeletal Pain: Diagnosis and Physical Treatment.* Little, Brown, Boston, 1976 (p. 127, Fig. 7-4A).

CHAPTER 16
Posterior Cervical Muscles

Semispinalis Capitis, Semispinalis Cervicis, and Multifidi

"Pain in the Neck"

HIGHLIGHTS: The muscles of the back of the neck lie in four layers of increasing depth: (1) the trapezius; (2) the splenius capitis and cervicis; (3) the semispinalis capitis, semispinalis cervicis, and longissimus capitis; and (4) the multifidi, rotatores, and small suboccipital muscles which connect the occiput with the first two cervical vertebrae. The first and second layers are presented in Chapters 6 and 15. The posterior cervical muscles, which are covered in this chapter, comprise the third layer and the underlying multifidi and rotatores of the fourth layer. The remainder of the fourth layer, the suboccipital group or the "skull-movers" are presented in Chapter 17. Trigger points (TPs) are found at three levels in the posterior cervical group of muscles. **REFERRED PAIN** from the TP$_1$ area at the C$_4$, C$_5$ level, the commonest location, travels strongly upward to the suboccipital region, and downward over the neck and upper part of the shoulder girdle; the TP$_2$ area, a few centimeters lower, refers pain over the posterior occiput; the TP$_3$ area in the superior portion of these muscles is felt in a band-like pattern projected above the orbit. **ACTIONS** of the posterior cervical muscles are primarily extension and rotation of the head and neck. **SYMPTOMS** due to active TPs in these muscles are pain, marked restriction of head and neck flexion, and less severe restriction of extension and rotation of the head and neck. **ACTIVATION OF TRIGGER POINTS** is usually caused by sustained partial neck flexion when reading, writing, or sewing; by holding a stooped posture; or by gross trauma. **TRIGGER POINT EXAMINATION** reveals tenderness to palpation and frequently also elicits the predictable referred pain pattern. **ENTRAPMENT** of the greater occipital nerve is commonly caused by tension due to TP$_1$ at the level of the C$_4$ or C$_5$ vertebra, several centimeters below where the nerve penetrates the semispinalis capitis muscle. **STRETCH AND SPRAY** require coordination of the direction of passive stretch with the path of the spray so that the vapocoolant covers the groups of fibers under maximum stretch. This therapy for these muscles often gives dramatic improvement in the range of motion, similar to stretch and spray of the hamstring muscles. **INJECTION AND STRETCH** of the posterior cervical muscles may be required for relief, but injection entails hazards and must avoid the vertebral artery. **CORRECTIVE ACTIONS** include improved posture and a passive-assisted, Neck-stretch Exercise while seated under a hot shower.

1. REFERRED PAIN
(Fig. 16.1)

A different referred pain pattern is observed for each of the three trigger point (TP) areas (Fig. 16.1A). The common TP$_1$ location lies above the base of the neck at the C$_4$, C$_5$ level. The TPs in this area refer

pain and tenderness upward to the sub-occipital region and sometimes down the neck to the upper vertebral border of the scapula (Fig. 16.1B) in adults[16, 41, 43] and in children.[3] These TPs may lie as deep as the semispinalis cervicis and multifidus muscles.

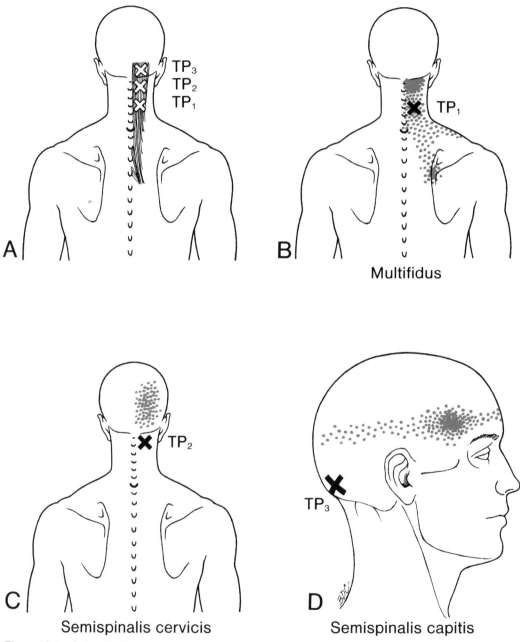

Figure 16.1. Referred pain patterns (*red*) and their trigger points (✕s) in the medial posterior cervical muscles. *A*, three major trigger point locations. *B*, TP$_1$ lies deep at the C$_4$ or C$_5$ level in the multifidi or rotatores; it is the posterior cervical trigger point most commonly found and often leads to entrapment of the greater occipital nerve. *C*, TP$_2$ in the third-layer semispinalis cervicis. *D*, the uppermost TP$_3$ in the semispinalis capitis.

PART 1

Activity of TP$_2$, located 2–4 cm (1–2 in) below the occiput, refers pain over the occiput and toward the vertex (Fig. 16.1C).

TP$_3$ lies just below the occipital ridge at the insertion of the semispinalis capitis. Its referred pain travels forward like a band that half encircles the head and reaches its maximum intensity in the temple and forehead over the eye (Fig. 16.1D). This TP does not refer pain to the neck. Infrequently, TPs in the posterior cervical muscles below the occiput may refer pain to the hands and feet bilaterally, or to the body below the shoulder on the same side.[40]

The referred pain patterns from all three locations were reproduced by the injection of hypertonic salt solution into these posterior cervical muscles.[5, 42]

2. ANATOMICAL ATTACHMENTS
(Figs. 16.2 and 16.3)

The four layers[33] of the posterior cervical muscles alternate direction, suggesting the plies of a tire (Fig. 16.2).

The most superficial, the upper trapezius fibers, converge above, tending to form a "∧", or roof-top shape. The next deeper, the splenius fibers, converge below to form a "∨" shape. The semispinalis capitis fibers of the third layer lie nearly vertical, parallel with the spine. All of the remaining, deepest fibers return to the "∧"

Layer	Muscle	Fiber Direction
1	Trapezius	
2	Splenii	
3	Semispinalis capitis	
	Semispinalis cervicis	
4	Multifidi	
	Rotatores	

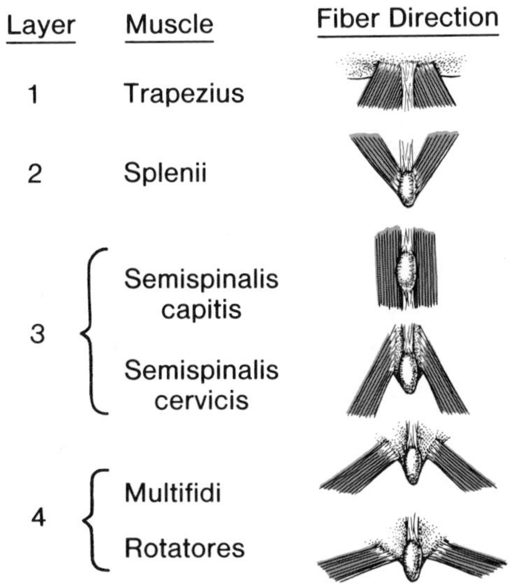

Figure 16.2. The changes in direction of successively deeper fibers in the four layers of the posterior cervical muscles.

shape. These include the more deeply placed semispinalis cervicis of the third layer and the multifidi and rotatores fibers, which constitute the fourth layer. The angle becomes progressively flatter (more obtuse) as successively deeper fibers span fewer segments.

Knowledge of this fiber arrangement is helpful in order to stretch and spray these muscles effectively.

Semispinalis Capitis and Semispinalis Cervicis

The semispinalis capitis muscle overlies the semispinalis cervicis. Both attach **below** to the transverse processes of the thoracic vertebrae, T$_1$ to T$_6$, and sometimes T$_7$ (Fig. 16.3). The semispinalis capitis also attaches below to the transverse processes of cervical vertebrae C$_3$ to C$_6$ and often has a tendinous inscription that runs across the muscle opposite the C$_6$ vertebra, most marked where the fibers come from the thoracic vertebrae. **Above** the semispinalis capitis attaches to the occiput between the superior and inferior nuchal lines, while the cervicis (illustrated in Fig. 48.4, Chapter 48) attaches to spinous processes of the C$_2$ to C$_5$ vertebrae.[13] The fibers of the semispinalis cervicis cross four or five vertebrae.[1] The longissimus capitis has common thoracic attachments below with the semispinalis capitis (T$_1$ to T$_6$), but connects, above, to the skull just lateral to the semispinalis capitis, so that both muscles have similar actions; the longissimus capitis is treated in this manual as part of the semispinalis capitis.

Multifidi and Rotatores

The cervical multifidi attach **above** to the spinous processes of vertebrae C$_2$ to C$_5$. They attach **below** to the articular processes of the last four cervical vertebrae, C$_4$ to C$_7$; its fibers cross two to four vertebrae (Fig. 16.3).

The cervical rotatores have comparable attachments, but are shorter and connect adjacent or alternate vertebrae (Fig. 16.3). Since they lie immediately beneath the multifidi and have essentially the same functions, the rotatores are considered as part of the multifidi in this manual.

Supplemental References

Other authors have illustrated the semispinalis capitis as seen from be-

PART 1

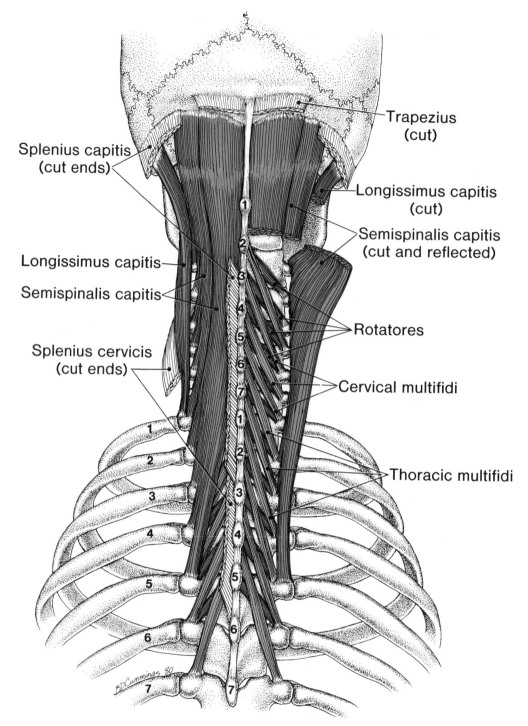

Figure 16.3. Attachments of the posterior cervical muscles. **Left side**, the fibers of the longissimus capitis and semispinalis capitis muscles (*medium red*) lie almost vertically, between the skull and the thoracic vertebrae. The semispinalis cervicis is not shown here (see Fig. 48.4, Chapter 48). It is intermediate between the semispinalis capitis and multifidi in depth, fiber length, and angulation of fibers. **Right side**, the deepest layer, the multifidi (*light red*) and rotatores (*dark red*). They travel diagonally to form, bilaterally, the roof-top "∧" shape.

hind[7, 10, 23, 28, 30, 36] and from the three-quarters rear view.[8] They have portrayed the semispinalis cervicis from behind[7, 24, 29, 36] and from the three-quarters rear view.[35] They have shown the multifidi from behind,[9, 24, 29, 31] from a three-quarters rear view,[35] and from the side.[11] They presented the rotatores as seen from behind,[9, 12, 32] and from the side.[11]

3. INNERVATION

The semispinalis capitis is supplied by branches of the posterior primary divisions of the first four or five cervical nerves. The semispinalis cervicis and the deeper posterior cervical muscles are supplied by branches of the posterior primary divisions of the third to sixth cervical nerves.[35]

4. ACTIONS

Semispinalis Capitis

Electrical stimulation of the semispinalis capitis produced head extension and slight inclination to the same side, but not *neck* extension.[6] Based on other considerations, other authors also identified the extension function.;[1, 13, 22, 25] some identified lateral flexion to the same side[1, 25] and one, head rotation to the opposite side.[13] The last function is questionable.

A sophisticated electromyographic study of strengthening exercises,[22] using fine-wire electrodes in 15 subjects, reported that the semispinalis capitis muscle responded vigorously during extension of the head and neck but, with training, electrical silence could be achieved while the head and neck were held in the erect, balanced position. Electrical activation of these muscles in support of the head appeared only during body activity that disturbed the balance of the head on the body.[22] Also, no electromyographic activity was observed in this muscle during lateral flexion of the head, and during head rotation. The semispinalis cervicis responded similarly, but less reliably.[22]

No study was found which specifically examined the slightly forward, flexed head posture commonly assumed for reading. The exercise data[22] strongly suggest that the semispinalis capitis consistently, and the semispinalis cervicis at times, provide the checkrein function during even slight flexion of the neck, which has been so well demonstrated for the erector spinae muscles at the lumbar level.[2] Abuse of this checkrein activity is a major cause of the frequently observed chronic strain of the posterior cervical muscles.

Semispinalis Cervicis

This muscle is reported to extend the cervical spine,[13, 25] to rotate the spine to the opposite side,[13, 25] and to produce lateral flexion of the spine.[25]

Multifidi and Rotatores

No description of the functions of this group of muscles specifically for the cervical area was found, but they have been identified generally as extensors of the spine, as lateral flexors of the spine to the same side, and as rotators of the spine to the opposite side.[13, 25]

The multifidi were identified as contributing especially to lateral flexion of the spine.[25] These deeper muscles are said to contribute also to positional adjustments between vertebrae, rather than to movements of the spine as a whole.[15]

5. MYOTATIC UNIT

Semispinalis Capitis

For extension of the head, *synergists* of the semispinalis capitis include, bilaterally, the semispinalis cervicis, the deep occipital muscles that lie vertically, the superficial trapezius, splenius capitis, and longissimus capitis. *Antagonists* include the head flexors, especially the sternocleidomastoid muscles acting bilaterally.

Semispinalis Cervicis

For extension of the neck, *synergists* of the semispinalis cervicis are the erector spinae, the splenius cervicis bilaterally, the longissimus cervicis, the semispinalis capitis, and the levator scapulae bilaterally, plus the multifidi acting bilaterally. *Antagonists* are the anterior neck muscles, including the strap muscles and longus colli.

For rotation of the neck, the semispinalis cervicis functions *synergistically* with the opposite splenius cervicis and levator scapulae, and with the homolateral multifidi and rotatores.

Multifidi and Rotatores

The multifidi are primarily synergistic with the semispinalis capitis for extension of the neck, and the deep rotatores are primarily synergistic with the semispinalis cervicis for rotation. Additional synergists and antagonists are the same as those listed above under the semispinalis cervicis.

6. SYMPTOMS

Patients complain of pain, as described in Section 1. They are also likely to complain of tenderness over the back of the head and neck, so that pressure from the weight of the head on a pillow at night quickly becomes intolerable. They usually experience some degree of painfully restricted motion of the neck in all directions, especially head and neck flexion.

With entrapment of the greater occipital nerve, as a sequel to prolonged activation of TP_1 (Fig. 16.1), in addition to pain, patients complain of numbness, tingling and burning pain in the scalp over the homolateral occipital region ("occipital neuralgia"). They may have received anesthetic blocks of the greater occipital nerve, with relief only for the duration of the local anesthetic effect. Prior to the development of the nerve entrapment, these patients prefer local heat for relief of the referred occipital aching pain; as the pain becomes neurogenic, they cannot bear heat, and prefer cold. They look for an ice-bag to relieve the burning occipital pain.

7. ACTIVATION OF TRIGGER POINTS
(Fig. 16.4)

Postural Stress

Reading or working at a desk with the neck in sustained flexion commonly activates posterior cervical TPs. This position may be assumed because: (1) the lenses of the eyeglasses have too short a focal length (Fig. 16.4C); (2) the frames of the eyeglasses are adjusted improperly (Fig. 16.4A); (3) the chair has inadequate or no lumbar support; (4) the location of work equipment, such as a typewriter, is physiologically incorrect[34]; (5) the tension caused by TPs in the pectoralis major muscles[39] increases thoracic kyphosis (see Fig. 42.7, Chapter 42); or (6) the patient is emotionally depressed.[4]

Excessive cervical extension at night tends to activate these TPs by placing the posterior cervical muscles in the shortened position. This posture occurs when lying on the back on too hard a mattress without a pillow, or when a too hard, poorly fitted pillow is placed under the shoulders and neck.

Trauma

The trauma of a fall on the head from a horse, an automobile accident, or diving into the bottom of a swimming pool commonly produces forceful neck flexion and muscle strain without fracture. The strain activates TPs in these muscles.

Other Factors

Too tight a bathing cap or a heavy overcoat with a tight collar may compress the posterior cervical muscles, impair their blood flow and activate their TPs, as is described for the trapezius muscle in Chapter 6.

A patient with a long supple neck is more prone to develop active TPs in the posterior cervical muscles than one with a short stocky neck because of the greater leverage placed on the muscles.

A skin TP was reported that referred pain from 2 cm (¾ in) above the left iliac crest to the area of the spinous process of the C_7 vertebra.[27] It is not known whether cutaneous TPs can induce secondary TPs in the muscles that lie within their pain reference zone, as do myofascial TPs. If so, skin TPs would be another source for activation of posterior cervical TPs.

Increased nerve irritability due to entrapment, as in spinal radiculopathy, can be a significant factor in the activation of these cervical TPs.

8. PATIENT EXAMINATION

The patients with posterior cervical TPs often hold the head and neck upright with the shoulders high[42]; they may hold the head with the face tilted up somewhat[42] and tend to suppress the bobbing and nodding movements of the head that ordinarily accompany talking.

The patient usually shows marked restriction of head and neck flexion, which can be three fingerbreadths (5 cm) short of the chin reaching the sternum. Marked restriction of head and neck rotation and of side bending usually are due to involvement of associated neck muscles. Generally, extension is slightly restricted.

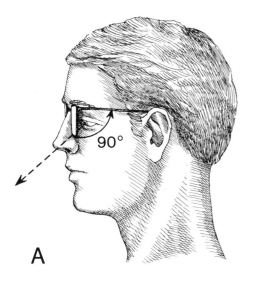

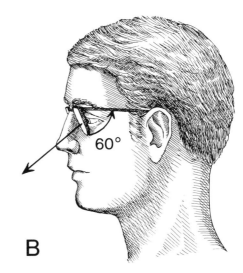

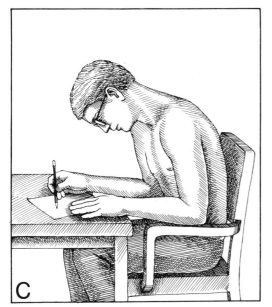

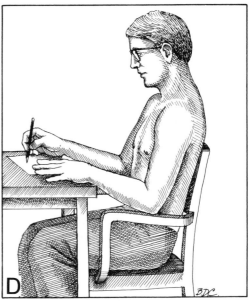

Figure 16.4. Causes and corrections of unnecessary load on the posterior cervical muscles. *A,* view obstructed by the lower rim of the eyeglasses, which must be compensated by a forward tilt of the head in order to read. *B,* unobstructed view for reading with the head in an erect, balanced position, after the axis of the lens has been tilted downward 30° or more, to bring the lower rim against the cheek. *C,* sustained spine flexion while working at a low desk, causing checkrein overload of the posterior cervical muscles. The overload is due partly to short focal-length lenses and rim obstruction to the line of vision. Additionally, too low an armrest for adequate elbow support creates a drag on the upper trapezius muscle; lack of lumbar support in the backrest favors reversal of the normal lordotic curve; and the low table top increases flexion of the spine. *D,* good posture of subject in a chair with adequate elbow support at a higher table that provides knee room. The subject also is making better use of the backrest, but needs additional lumbar support. All of these contribute to a balanced head position.

If involvement of the posterior cervical muscles is mainly one-sided and the head and neck are flexed, these muscles on the painful side may be seen to stand out like a rope from the skull to the level of the shoulder-girdle.

Differential Diagnosis

Cervical radiculopathy can activate TPs in the posterior cervical muscles that become self-perpetuating, a common cause of cervical postlaminectomy pain syndromes.[26] Since both may occur at the same time, each condition must be diagnosed on its own merits. Cervical radiculopathy from C_4–C_8 rarely fails to cause limb signs or symptoms. Posterior cervical TPs do not. Cervical radiculopathy is much more likely to show a positive **Sperling test**, spinal compression applied as downward pressure on the head with the upright cervical spine slightly extended. Positive electrodiagnostic findings are very helpful in identifying cervical radiculopathy.

9. TRIGGER POINT EXAMINATION

In our experience, TP_1 is the most commonly encountered of the posterior cervical TPs, TP_2 is the next most frequent, and TP_3 the least common.

We find that slight flexion of the head and neck enhances band tautness and TP tenderness in posterior neck muscles that are relaxed by providing head support in the seated or the side-lying position. All three posterior cervical TP locations (Fig. 16.1) are best examined by flat palpation. Lange[18] recommended that for examination of the posterior cervical muscles the patient be placed prone on the examining table with a pad, or small pillow, under the forehead to keep the neck straight.

To the examiner, TP_1 feels like a large, deep, lumpy mass of muscle which must be pressed very firmly to elicit referred pain. This TP_1 is usually found a centimeter or two from the midline at the C_4 or C_5 level. Deep tenderness, on examination, is much less intense than would be expected from the severity of the pain referred by this TP. Pressure applied to TP_2 or TP_3 elicits marked local tenderness and frequently induces the referred pain pattern characteristic of that TP,[42] but rarely induces a detectable local twitch response.

10. ENTRAPMENT
(Fig. 16.5)

The greater occipital nerve is the medial branch of the dorsal primary division of the second cervical nerve. This cervical nerve emerges beneath the posterior arch of the atlas above the lamina of the axis (Fig. 16.5). It then curves around the lower border of the obliquus inferior muscle, which it crosses before penetrating the semispinalis capitis and trapezius muscles near their attachments to the occipital bone.[10] From there, the nerve remains subcutaneous.[14, 20] Entrapment symptoms apparently develop when TP activity in the semispinalis capitis produces taut bands of muscle fibers that compress the nerve as it penetrates the muscle.

The symptoms associated with entrapment of the greater occipital nerve are described in Section 6. They are often relieved by inactivation of TP_1, which usually responds well to local procaine injection.

11. ASSOCIATED TRIGGER POINTS

Since the more longitudinal posterior cervical muscles commonly function in bilateral pairs, involvement of one side soon leads to at least some involvement of the contralateral muscles. Both the synergists and antagonists mentioned in Section 5 are likely to develop secondary TPs.

The erector spinae muscles, which extend onto the thorax, are also likely to become involved. The segmental level of TP involvement often can be identified by a flattened spot in the normally smooth curvature of the thoracic spine; when tested by forward flexion, one spinous process does not stand out as it should. This restriction of motion may respond well to stretch and spray of the deep paraspinal muscles at the level of the flattening.

When patients continue to complain of suboccipital pain and soreness, especially near the mastoid process, active TPs should be sought in the posterior belly of the digastric muscle and in the upper medial corner of the infraspinatus muscle on the same side as the pain. These TPs cause little restriction of motion and are easily overlooked.

12. STRETCH AND SPRAY
(Figs. 16.6 and 16.7)

Patients who complain of neck "stiffness" generally have restricted head and neck movements in several directions due to a combination of involved muscles.[37, 38] Range of motion is tested for flexion, extension, rotation, and side bending. As a rule, stretch and spray are applied first to the muscles that are causing the greatest restriction of movement. When

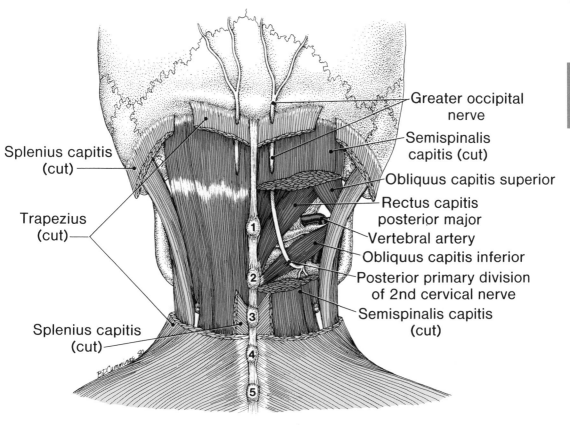

Splenius capitis (cut)

Trapezius (cut)

Splenius capitis (cut)

Greater occipital nerve

Semispinalis capitis (cut)

Obliquus capitis superior

Rectus capitis posterior major

Vertebral artery

Obliquus capitis inferior

Posterior primary division of 2nd cervical nerve

Semispinalis capitis (cut)

Figure 16.5. Course of the second cervical nerve, which becomes the greater occipital nerve and then penetrates the semispinalis capitis (*light medium red*) and trapezius muscles (*light red*) to continue beneath the scalp. Entrapment can occur where the nerve passes through the semispinalis muscle. Note the vertebral artery (*dark red*) in the sub-occipital triangle, which is bounded by the rectus capitis posterior major and the obliqui capitis superior and inferior muscles (*dark medium red*).

movement is severely restricted in all directions, it is usually best to first restore flexion, then side bending, rotation and, finally, extension. The degree of involvement of individual muscle groups must be assessed for each patient and the overlapping functions of these muscles considered.

Because of the multiple contributions of several muscles to movement in one direction, stretch and spray, slowly with unidirectional parallel sweeps,[21] usually releases that movement only partially; the adjacent, nearly parallel, muscle fibers also must be stretched and sprayed. After one round of stretch and spray to release all directions of restricted movement, and rewarming, it is often necessary to apply a second or third round to achieve complete restoration of movement.

When stretching and spraying the neck

muscles to improve flexion, first the sub-occipital (see Fig. 17.4A, Chapter 17) and the high cervical muscles (Fig. 16.6A) are treated, next the long-fibered low cervical and high thoracic muscles (Fig. 16.6B), and then the low thoracic and lumbar muscles (see Fig. 48.5, Chapter 48) are stretched and sprayed.

It helps to visualize clearly the location and direction of the muscle fibers being passively stretched. This procedure stretches primarily the longitudinal paraspinal muscles, which include the rectus capitis posterior minor (see Fig. 17.2, Chapter 17), the semispinalis capitis (Fig. 16.2), and the longissimus capitis, cervicis, and thoracis muscles (see Fig. 48.3, Chapter 48).

To complete the release of head and neck flexion, other neck muscles that combine extension with rotation also must be stretched and sprayed. This requires a

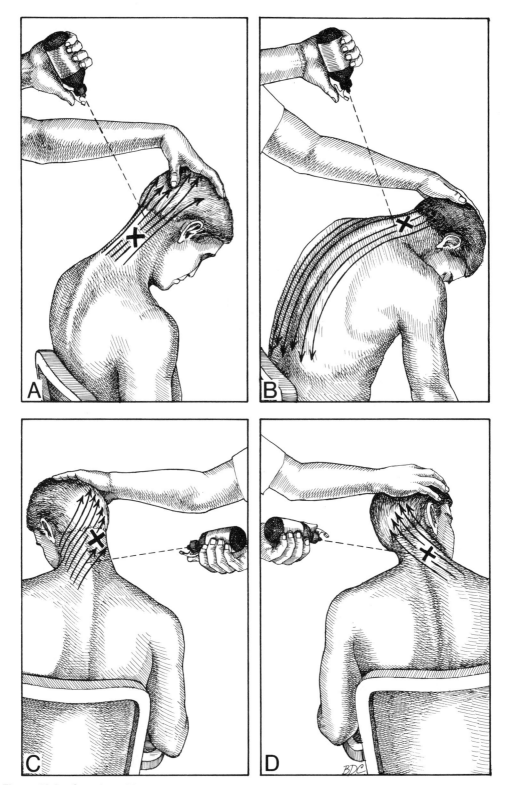

Figure 16.6. Stretch position and spray pattern (*arrows*) for trigger points (×s) in the posterior cervical muscles, primarily on the right side. *A*, upper cervical stretch for the semispinalis capitis muscles bilaterally, using straight flexion with an up-sweep pattern. *B*, lower posterior cervical and upper thoracic longissimus stretch bilaterally, with the down-pattern of spray application. *C*, stretch of the ''v'' diagonal muscles on the right and the ''∧'' diagonal fibers on the left, by firmly flexing the head and neck while applying gentle side pressure and turning the face to the left. The skin over the muscles being stretched is covered with an up-pattern of the vapocoolant. *D*, passive stretch primarily of the right ''∧'' diagonal and left ''v'' diagonal muscles by strongly flexing the head and neck, while turning the face toward the right and pulling the neck post gently to the left.

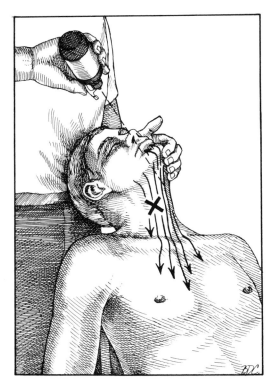

Figure 16.7. Stretch position and spray pattern (*arrows*) for a trigger point (**×**) in the anterior neck muscles. When these muscles are taut and shortened, they overload the antagonistic posterior cervical muscles. This treatment also prevents a shortening reaction of the anterior neck muscles during or following full stretch and lengthening of the posterior group.

flexion and rotation stretch, in one direction for the "v" oriented splenii (Fig. 16.6*C*), in the other direction for the "∧" oriented trapezius, semispinalis cervicis, multifidi, and rotatores muscles (Fig. 16.6*D*)

Posterior Neck Muscles

To stretch and spray the longitudinal posterior cervical muscles, the patient sits in an armchair that supports the elbows, and has a seat low enough to prevent excessive pressure under the thighs. The hips are moved forward slightly to better recline the trunk against the backrest. The patient lets the head and neck hang forward, relaxed. The operator gently presses the head farther forward and downward in midline flexion while the vapocoolant is applied upward over the back of the neck and head (Fig. 16.6*A*). Next the patient is asked to slump forward (Fig. 16.6*B*) as the

operator continues forward pressure on the head and neck and applies a down-spray pattern bilaterally to cover the long paraspinal muscles from the occiput to the lower thorax. The entire spine flexes until the head hangs as close to the knees as possible. This stretch is facilitated if the patient takes a deep breath to "hump the back" (see Fig. 48.5, Chapter 48).

To stretch and spray the right "v" diagonal posterior neck muscles, the head is firmly flexed and rotated with the face to the opposite side so as to stretch the right splenii capitis and cervicis (Fig. 16.6*C*). For the right "∧" diagonal posterior neck muscles, the head is firmly flexed and the face turned to the same side to stretch the right upper trapezius, semispinalis capitis and cervicis, multifidi, and rotatores (Fig. 16.6*D*). During this stretch, vapocoolant is applied bilaterally in a diagonal upsweep pattern that follows the line of the stretched fibers on *both* sides of the neck (Fig. 16.6*C* and *D*), because stretch of "v" diagonal muscles on the right also stretches "∧" diagonal muscles on the left, and *vice versa*.

Anterior Neck Muscles

If, after inactivating the TPs in the posterior cervical muscles by stretch and spray, neck flexion still lacks a full range of motion by one fingerbreadth between the chin and sternum, the trouble may lie in the anterior neck muscles that flex the neck. As the head and neck are extended, the spray is applied bilaterally over the anterior cervical and hyoid-attached muscles in down-sweeps from the chin over the clavicles to the sternum (Fig. 16.7). The patient should then be able to bring the chin firmly against the chest.

This application to the anterior neck is also important to prevent shortening reactions due to activation of TPs in the antagonistic anterior cervical muscles. Anterior stretch and spray should include the clavicular divisions of the sternocleidomastoid muscles, bilaterally.

To relieve patients who speak with a hoarse voice because of active TPs in the laryngeal muscles, the head is tilted back to stretch the anterior neck muscles. While the patient sings and holds a note ("Ahhh—"), the vapocoolant spray is swept upward from the sternum and clavicles covering the laryngeal region, then to the chin and mastoid area bilaterally. Clearing of the tone may occur during the few parallel sweeps of the spray over the skin.

13. INJECTION AND STRETCH
(Figs. 16.8 and 16.9)

If, after stretch and spray, less than the full range of neck flexion has been achieved, if one still finds spot tenderness in the posterior cervical muscles, and if their referred pain patterns persist, TP injection should be considered. Injection of posterior cervical muscles also was described and illustrated by Kraus.[17]

TP_1

When injecting this TP, it feels as though, to reach it, one must penetrate a third layer of muscle, the semispinalis capitis, after first passing through the trapezius and splenius capitis muscles. The TP is usually encountered at least 2 cm (¾ in)

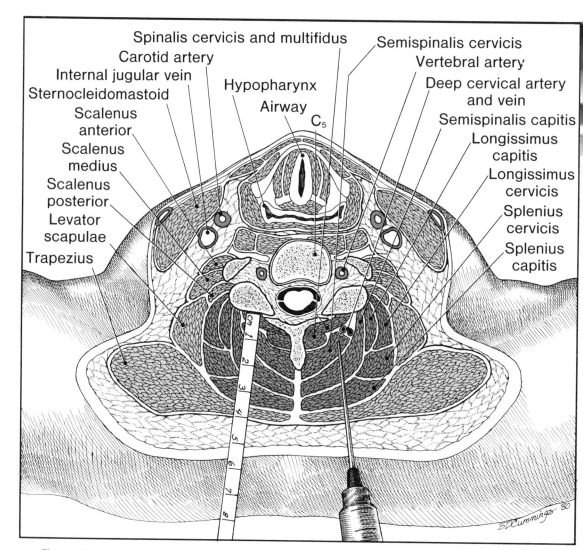

Spinalis cervicis and multifidus
Carotid artery
Internal jugular vein
Sternocleidomastoid
Scalenus anterior
Scalenus medius
Scalenus posterior
Levator scapulae
Trapezius

Hypopharynx
Airway
C_5

Semispinalis cervicis
Vertebral artery
Deep cervical artery and vein
Semispinalis capitis
Longissimus capitis
Longissimus cervicis
Splenius cervicis
Splenius capitis

Figure 16.8. Cross section of the neck through the C_5 vertebra, which corresponds to the level of TP_1. The bony parts of the vertebra are stippled black and are outlined by a *dark line surrounding black stipples.* The ruler shows that the 5-cm (2-in) needle cannot penetrate the full depth of the posterior cervical muscles without compression of the skin. The vertebral artery is surrounded by the vertebral transverse processes. It travels anterior to, and along the lateral border of the posterior cervical muscles. Paraspinal muscles and major blood vessels are *dark red*; other muscles are *light red*.

PART 1

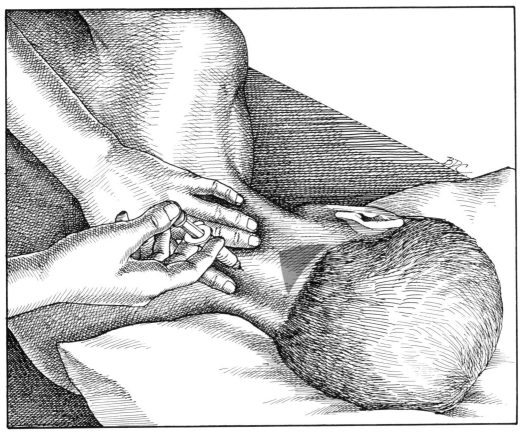

Figure 16.9.   Injection of the TP_1 area in the left posterior cervical muscles at the C_4 or C_5 level. The *red color* locates the suboccipital triangle that is not injected, so as to avoid the unprotected vertebral artery. Figure 16.5 shows the boundries of the triangle.

beneath the skin, and may lie beyond the reach of a 3.8-cm (1½-in) needle. A 5-cm (2-in) needle may be needed (Fig. 16.8). Frequently, the semispinalis cervicis and multifidi underneath the semispinalis capitis also contain TPs that require injection. This means needle penetration to about 5 cm (2 in), nearly halfway through the diameter of the neck (Fig. 16.8), to reach the deepest paraspinal muscles. The TPs in the posterior cervical muscles are usually bilateral, and eventually it may be necessary to inject both sides. A common mistake is failure to inject deeply enough because of the possibility of penetrating the vertebral artery or dura mater of the spinal cord. These are significant concerns, so these deep TPs should not be injected by beginners and never in a hurry.

The vertebral artery lies several centimeters anterior and somewhat lateral to the multifidi (Fig. 16.8). Although much of

it is surrounded by the bony transverse processes of the vertebrae, it is conceivable that one could reach the artery between vertebrae. Therefore, when the depth of the laminae has been established by needle contact at 1 cm lateral to the edge of a spinous process, needle penetration is limited to that depth whenever the needle is inserted 2 cm or more lateral to the spinous process of a vertebra.

In some patients, the cervical spinal cord may not be covered by bone between vertebrae as far as 1 cm lateral to the edge of a cervical spinous processes. Penetration of the dura in this space is avoided by establishing the depth of the laminal at 1 cm lateral to the lateral edge of a cervical spinous process, and not inserting the needle to a greater depth when it is directed medially.

The pain response to injection may seem out of proportion to the tenderness elicited by palpation, because of the depth of the TPs. Following injection, passive stretch during vapocooling and a hot pack are applied. Immediate restoration of full neck flexion often results, but the scalp pain and hyperesthesia of occipital nerve entrapment may last from a few days to several weeks, diminishing gradually.

TP$_2$

This TP is located in the semispinalis cervicis and lies immediately over the vertebral artery. Thus, it should NOT BE INJECTED. Instead, stretch and spray, ischemic compression, and deep massage should be employed.

TP$_3$

After confirming that pain is originating from this TP located in the semispinalis capitis, the tender area may be injected by angling the needle upward, directing it toward the occipital bone, not below the bony margin. This avoids the vertebral artery, which lies just caudal to the skull (Fig. 16.5).

Atlas

Lewit[19] describes the treatment of headache of cervical origin by manipulation of the cervical spine and by dry needling of TPs along the dorsal surface of the posterior arch of the atlas. These may be fascial, rather than myofascial TPs.

Vertebral Artery

Injections of TP$_3$, if properly done, are sufficiently far above, and those of TP$_1$ sufficiently far below, the suboccipital triangle to miss the vertebral artery. The artery is easily encountered with a needle as the vessel emerges from its path through the transverse processes of the vertebrae to enter the cranial vault (Figs. 16.5 and 16.9).

The triangle is bounded by the rectus capitis posterior major and the obliqui capitis inferior and superior (see Fig. 17.5, Chapter 17).

A number of disturbing experiences have occurred when injecting deeply in the region of TP$_2$ over the artery. One report[40] was based on the impression that numbness, tingling, and weakness which developed in the opposite arm during the TP injection may have been due to vertebral artery spasm and spinal cord or brain ischemia. Months later, the patient, apparently malingering, was receiving compensation for the complaints while working full time elsewhere, without evident disability. Apparently, the symptoms had cleared up spontaneously.

A second patient, previously unreported, during posterior cervical TP injection, developed similar contralateral arm symptoms, which suggested cerebral or spinal cord ischemia. The symptoms disappeared spontaneously in 3 days.

A third patient developed similar symptoms of persistent tingling and pain in the contralateral upper extremity during this TP injection, and was reexamined meticulously 3 days following the onset. He was found then to have marked activation of TPs in the scalene muscles on the side of the symptoms. Inactivation of these scalene TPs by procaine injection promptly eliminated the upper extremity pain, without recurrence through several years of follow-up. Latent scalene TPs may have developed as satellites of the posterior cervical muscles on the contralateral side, which were activated during the initial period of contralaterally referred pain.

14. CORRECTIVE ACTIONS
(Fig. 16.10)

Postural Stress

Chronic strain activates posterior cervical TPs as these muscles checkrein the weight of the head when it is held in partial flexion for prolonged periods. Corrections include: (1) A reading stand or adjustable music stand to change the angle of, and to raise, reading or work materials. This permits eye-level contact and avoids sustained flexion of the head and neck. (2) Eyeglasses with adequate focal length so that the patient can see clearly with the head held in a balanced upright position. A new prescription for longer focal length lenses ("card playing glasses") should be obtained. (3) Selection of bifocal insets that are large, fully half the height of the entire lens, for close work, such as, reading or sewing. (4) Adjustment of eyeglass frames so that the lower portion of the rim does not occlude the line of sight on looking down (Fig. 16.4C). (5) Exercising on a standing bicycle by sitting upright with the arms swinging freely or placed on the hips,

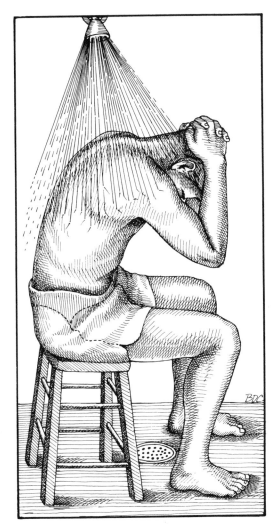

Figure 16.10. Seated Under-shower Stretch Exercise for the posterior cervical muscles. These muscles are stretched by the weight of the head and by the weight of the arms. The fingers are locked behind the occiput, while complete relaxation of the posterior neck muscles is helped by the impact of the hot water. The patient should move the head slowly, exploring flexion, side-bending, and rotation in turn, to locate taut bands that need gentle stretching.

and *not* hunched over holding handlebars that do not steer the machine. (6) Placement of a cloth roll or pillow behind the lumbar spine in a chair, to maintain the normal lumbar lordotic curve and straighten any functional thoracic kyphosis. (7) Inactivation of pectoralis major or minor TPs that induce a similar kyphotic posture. These last two corrections permit the erect head and neck to assume a balanced relaxed position over the tho-

racic spine (see Fig. 42.7, Chapter 42). In summary, the patient must establish a balanced-head posture.[34]

Excessive cervical extension at night is corrected by obtaining a slightly softer (non-sag) mattress, or by using a small soft neck pillow that comfortably supports the normal cervical curve. The round small neck pillow (Cervipillo) designed by Ruth Jackson[16] is well suited to this purpose. A jiggly foam rubber pillow must be discarded and replaced with one filled with a non-springy material, like feathers or shredded dacron.

Other Factors

The neck muscles of patients with posterior cervical TPs may be particularly vulnerable to chilling and should be kept covered at night by a turtle-neck sweater worn in bed, or by a scarf wrapped around the neck. Similarly, the neck must be protected from cold drafts during the day. Long hair offers natural protection against this cold exposure.

To temporarily relieve neck strain after an acute exacerbation when riding in a car or working at a desk, one may prescribe a soft collar to be worn loosely as a *chin rest.* It is NOT tightly adjusted for immobilization of the neck, but applied loosely. For instance, a Thomas plastic collar may be worn upside down and loosely enough to allow space for head rotation and to look down at the sides, yet tight enough to support the chin in the neutral position of the head.

Exercise Therapy

The Under-shower Stretch Exercise, which is performed while seated on a stool under a hot shower (Fig. 16.10), is very effective. The patient latches the fingers over the occiput and lets the weight of the arms pull the head down and forward, passively stretching the posterior cervical muscles. The head is released and turned to a new angle before stretching a different line of muscle fibers.

The patient may place a 2 kg (5 lb) sandbag on the head during periods of the day for posture training.[4]

Head-rolling exercises, or other movements which turn the head while in the fully flexed or extended positions, should be avoided.

PART 1

References

1. Bardeen CR: The musculature, Sect. 5. In *Morris's Human Anatomy*, edited by C.M. Jackson, Ed. 6. Blakiston's Son & Co., Philadelphia, 1921 (p. 452).
2. Basmajian JV: *Muscles Alive*, Ed. 4. Williams & Wilkins, Baltimore, 1978 (pp. 282, 288).
3. Bates T: Myofascial pain, Chapter 14. In *Ambulatory Pediatrics II: Personal Health Care of Children in the Office*, edited by M. Green and R.J. Haggerty, W.B. Saunders, Philadelphia, 1977 (Fig. 14-1, p. 148).
4. Cailliet, R: *Soft Tissue Pain and Disability*, F.A. Davis, Philadelphia, 1977 (pp. 131–133).
5. Cyriax J: Rheumatic headache. *Br Med J* 2:1367–1368, 1938.
6. Duchenne GB: *Physiology of Motion*, translated by E.B. Kaplan. J.B. Lippincott, Philadelphia, 1949 (p. 534).
7. Eisler P: *Die Muskeln des Stammes*. Gustav Fischer, Jena, 1912 (pp. 401, 404, Figs. 56, 57).
8. *Ibid.* (p. 405, Fig. 58).
9. *Ibid.* (p. 426, Figs. 59, 61).
10. Grant JCB: *An Atlas of Human Anatomy*, Ed. 7. Williams & Wilkins, Baltimore, 1978 (Figs. 5-27, 5-33).
11. *Ibid.* (Fig. 5-36).
12. *Ibid.* (Fig. 5-31).
13. Gray H: *Anatomy of the Human Body*, edited by C.M. Goss, American Ed. 29. Lea & Febiger, Philadelphia, 1973 (pp. 406, 407).
14. *Ibid.* (p. 949, Figs. 12-28).
15. Hollinshead WH: *Functional Anatomy of the Limbs and Back*, Ed. 4. W.B. Saunders, Philadelphia, 1976 (p. 230).
16. Jackson R: *The Cervical Syndrome*, Ed. 3. Charles C Thomas, Springfield, Ill., 1977 (pp. 310–314).
17. Kraus H: *Clinical Treatment of Back and Neck Pain*. McGraw-Hill, New York, 1970 (pp. 104, 105).
18. Lange M: *Die Muskelhärten (Myogelosen)*. J.F. Lehmanns, Müchen, 1931 (pp. 48, 49, Fig. 12).
19. Lewit K: Pain arising in the posterior arch of the atlas. *Eur Neurol* 16:263–269, 1977.
20. Lockhart RD, Hamilton GF, Fyfe FW: *Anatomy of the Human Body*, Ed. 2. J.B. Lippincott, Philadelphia, 1969 (pp. 169, 274, Fig. 278).
21. Modell W, Travell JT, Kraus H, Hardy JD: Contributions to Cornell Conferences on Therapy. Relief of pain by ethyl chloride spray. *NY State J Med* 52:1550–1558, 1952.
22. Pauly JE: An electromyographic analysis of certain movements and exercises: 1. Some deep muscles of the back. *Anat Rec* 155:223–234, 1966.
23. Pernkopf E: *Atlas of Topographical and Applied Human Anatomy*, Vol. 2. W.B. Saunders, Philadelphia, 1964 (Fig. 30).
24. *Ibid.* (Fig. 35).
25. Rasch PJ, Burke RK: *Kinesiology and Applied Anatomy*, Ed. 6. Lea & Febiger, Philadelphia, 1978 (pp. 240, 241).
26. Reynolds MD: Myofascial trigger point syndromes in the practice of rheumatology. *Arch Phys Med Rehabil* 62:111–114, 1981.
27. Sinclair DC: The remote reference of pain aroused in the skin. *Brain* 72:364–372, 1949 (p. 372, table).
28. Sobotta J, Figge FHJ: *Atlas of Human Anatomy*, Ed. 9, Vol. 1. Hafner Division of Macmillan, New York, 1974 (pp. 144, 146).
29. *Ibid.* (p. 148).
30. Spalteholz W: *Handatlas der Anatomie des Menschen*, Ed. 11, Vol. 2. S. Hirzel, Leipzig, 1922 (pp. 308, 311).
31. *Ibid.* (p. 312).
32. *Ibid.* (p. 313).
33. Takebe K, Vitti M, Basmajian JV: The functions of semispinalis capitis and splenius capitis muscles: An electromyographic study. *Ant Rec* 179:477–480, 1974.
34. Tichauer ER: Industrial engineering in the rehabilitation of the handicapped. *J Ind Eng* 19:96–104, 1968 (p. 98 Fig. 2, p. 99 Table 2).
35. Toldt C: *An Atlas of Human Anatomy*, translated by M.E. Paul, Ed. 2, Vol. 1. Macmillan, New York, 1919 (p. 272).
36. *Ibid.* (p. 270).
37. Travell J: Rapid relief of acute "stiff neck" by ethyl chloride spray. *J Am Med Wom Assoc* 4:89–95, 1949.
38. Travell J: Pain mechanisms in connective tissue. In *Connective Tissues, Transactions of the Second Conference, 1951*, edited by C. Ragan. Josiah Macy, Jr. Foundation, New York, 1952 (pp. 119, 120).
39. Travell J: Referred pain from skeletal muscle: the pectoralis major syndrome of breast pain and soreness and the sternomastoid syndrome of headache and dizziness. *NY State J Med* 55:331–339, 1955.
40. Travell J, Bigelow NH: Role of somatic trigger areas in the patterns of hysteria. *Psychosom Med* 9:353–363, 1947 (p. 361, Figs. 7, 8).
41. Travell J, Rinzler SH: The myofascial genesis of pain. *Postgrad Med* 11:425–434, 1952.
42. Wolff, HG: *Wolff's Headache and Other Head Pain*, revised by D.J. Dalessio, Ed. 3. Oxford University Press, New York, 1972 (pp. 549, 554).
43. Zohn DA, Mennell J McM: *Musculoskeletal Pain: Diagnosis and Physical Treatment*. Little, Brown & Company, Boston, 1976 (p. 191, Fig. 9-12).

CHAPTER 17
Suboccipital Muscles

Recti Capitis Posteriores Major and Minor, Obliqui Inferior and Superior

"Headache Ghosts"

HIGHLIGHTS: **REFERRED PAIN** from these muscles is "ghostly" in the poor definition of the deep head pain that radiates from the occiput to the orbit and because of the lack of distinction between symptoms produced by the trigger points (TPs) of the suboccipital muscles and those of the overlying posterior neck muscles. **ANATOMICAL ATTACHMENTS** of these four muscles reach the occiput, the posterior arch of the atlas, the spinous process of the axis, and the transverse process of the atlas. Three of these suboccipital muscles frame the posterior occipital triangle, which encloses the exposed transverse loop of the vertebral artery. **ACTIONS** of these four deeply placed, bilateral suboccipital muscles are to extend, rotate and tilt the head to the same side. **ACTIVATION OF TRIGGER POINTS** is caused, in these muscles, by abuse of the checkrein function during sustained head flexion, by abuse of the extension function during sustained upward head tilt, and by abuse of rotation as a result of sustained head rotation and tilt of the skull. The suboccip-

ital muscles are prone to develop active TPs as satellites of TPs in other neck muscles, and from chilling the neck when the muscles are fatigued. **PATIENT EXAMINATION** reveals restriction of head flexion, rotation, and/or side-bending at the *top* of the neck post. **TRIGGER POINT EXAMINATION** reveals only tenderness to pressure on the deep suboccipital muscles through the overlying semispinalis capitis and trapezius. By palpation, it is rarely possible to distinguish TPs in the individual suboccipital muscles. **STRETCH AND SPRAY** are first applied to the other neck muscles that are likely to be responsible for activating secondary TPs in the suboccipital group. Stretch and spray of the suboccipital muscles must consider all actions, using an up-sweep pattern followed by ischemic compression and deep, vigorous massage. **INJECTION AND STRETCH** are not recommended because of the adjacent exposed vertebral artery. **CORRECTIVE ACTIONS** include the elimination of stress factors and a stretch exercise program at home.

---

1. REFERRED PAIN
(Fig. 17.1)

These four paired muscles are the most deeply-placed just below the base of the skull. Their trigger points (TPs) refer head pain that seems to penetrate inside the

skull, but is difficult to localize. Pain referred from these muscles has been called "indurative headaches."[10] Patients are likely to describe it as "all over," but on careful questioning, it extends forward unilaterally to the occiput, to the eye and the forehead, with a ghostly lack of clearly definable limits (Fig. 17.1). The pain does not have the straight-through-the-head quality of pain referred from the splenius cervicis muscle.

Hypertonic saline injected into the suboccipital muscles produced pain felt deeply in the head, and described as "headache."[8]

2. ANATOMICAL ATTACHMENTS
(Fig. 17.2)

Three of these short suboccipital muscles connect the first two cervical vertebrae with the occipital bone,[4, 7] and the fourth, the obliquus capitis inferior, connects the upper two cervical vertebrae with each other (Fig. 17.2).

Rectus Capitis Posterior Minor

This short, nearly vertical muscle converges **below** to attach to the tubercle on the posterior arch of the atlas. It spreads **above** along the medial half of the inferior nuchal line of the occiput just above the foramen magnum.[4]

Rectus Capitis Posterior Major

The fibers of this muscle skip the atlas and attach **below** to the spinous process of the axis. **Above** they fan out, attaching to the rest of the inferior nuchal line of the occiput, lateral to the rectus capitis posterior minor.

Obliquus Capitis Superior

These "oblique" fibers lie almost vertical. They attach **below** to the transverse process of the atlas, and **above** between the superior and inferior nuchal lines of the occiput laterally, beneath the lateral part of the semispinalis capitis muscle.[3, 4]

Obliquus Capitis Inferior

This oblique head rotator is the only suboccipital muscle that does not fasten to the skull, but connects the first two cervical vertebrae (the atlas and axis). **Medially and below** it attaches to the spinous process of the axis. **Laterally and above** it fastens to the transverse process of the atlas.[3, 4]

Suboccipital Triangle

This triangle is bounded by three suboccipital muscles: the two obliques and the rectus capitis posterior major. The triangular space is covered by the semispinalis capitis muscle and is filled largely with fibrofatty tissue. The vertebral artery (Fig. 17.2) traverses this space, and the greater occipital nerve (see Fig. 16.4, Chapter 16) crosses the ceiling of the triangle.

Supplemental References

The suboccipital muscles have been well illustrated in posterior[2, 3, 5, 6, 13, 14, 16] and in side views.[15]

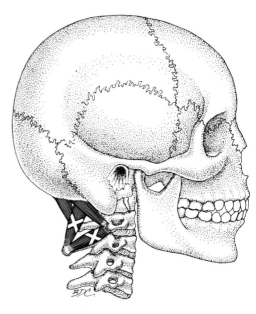

Figure 17.1.   Referred pain pattern (*red*) of trigger points (×s) in the right suboccipital muscles (*medium red*).

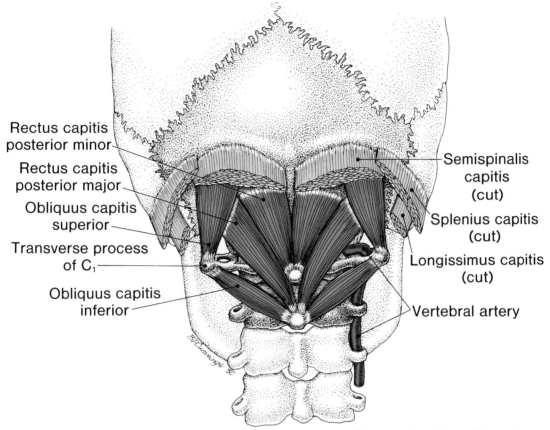

Rectus capitis
posterior minor

Rectus capitis
posterior major

Obliquus capitis
superior

Transverse process
of C₁

Obliquus capitis
inferior

Semispinalis
capitis
(cut)

Splenius capitis
(cut)

Longissimus capitis
(cut)

Vertebral artery

Figure 17.2. Attachments of the suboccipital muscles (medium red). The most lateral three of these four muscles define the suboccipital triangle. This triangle surrounds the transverse portion of the vertebral artery (dark red) and should be avoided when injecting TPs in the posterior neck muscles. The more superficial overlying muscles are *light red*.

3. INNERVATION

The suboccipital muscles are supplied by branches of the dorsal primary division of the suboccipital (first cervical) nerve.

4. ACTIONS
(Fig. 17.3)

The first two joints at the top of the spinal column are highly specialized joints to provide head mobility. The first provides flexion-extension (rocking) and side-bending (tilting) movements, and the second provides head rotation. The suboccipital muscles specifically control movement at these two joints.

The atlantooccipital joint allows about 10° of flexion and 25° of extension.[1] The suboccipital muscles that connect the atlas with the skull across this joint, the rectus capitis posterior minor and the superior oblique, function as extensors of the head.[4]

Figure 17.3 graphically summarizes the actions of these muscles.

The atlantoaxial joint provides 45° of rotation to either side.[1] The two suboccipital rotators, the inferior oblique muscle, which connects the axis to the atlas, and the rectus capitis posterior major, which connects the axis to the skull, rotate the head toward the side of muscular activity. Only the rectus capitis posterior major provides both extension and rotation.[4]

A lateral tilt function is not mentioned for the suboccipital muscles in many texts.[4, 6, 7, 13] However, one would expect, from its anatomical attachments, that the superior oblique should tilt the head to the same side, and clinical observations support this impression.

The muscle drawings of Figure 17.5 (see Section 12) identify *in red* the muscle stretched by each position shown. The drawings also can help to visualize the

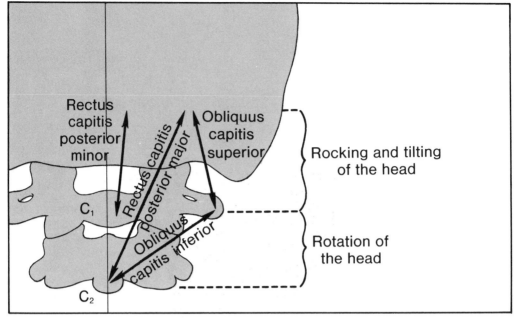

Figure 17.3.   Graphic summary of the actions of the right suboccipital muscles.

opposite movement produced by contraction of each muscle.

5. MYOTATIC UNIT

For extension, the major synergist of the suboccipital muscles is the semispinalis capitis. Antagonists for extension are the longus capitis and rectus capitis anterior.

For rotation, the major synergists are the splenius capitis on the same side and the sternocleidomastoid on the opposite side. The major antagonists for rotation are the contralateral mates to the two synergists.

6. SYMPTOMS

Pain evoked by TPs in the suboccipital muscles blurs indistinguishably with pain referred from the semispinalis. It is rarely, if ever, that the suboccipital muscles develop TPs without associated involvement of other major posterior cervical muscles. Patients complain of distressing headache caused promptly when the weight of the occiput presses against the pillow at night. Pain from the suboccipital muscles tends to be more deeply seated in the upper neck region, and to be located more laterally than that experienced from the posterior cervical muscles. Patients often poke around with their fingers at the base of the skull, locating "a sore spot right there."

7. ACTIVATION OF TRIGGER POINTS

Since these muscles are largely responsible for rocking the skull on top of the neck post, they are likely to develop TPs when checkreining flexion, or when maintaining extension while the subject looks upward.

If upward gaze is maintained by tilting the entire cervical spine, the checkrein function of the sternocleidomastoid muscles is abused. If, instead, a person rocks the head on top of the cervical spine, the suboccipital extensors are strained by prolonged contraction. The checkrein function of the suboccipital extensors is overloaded by sustained forward flexion of the head and neck due often to problems with the visual apparatus: maladjusted eyeglass frames, uncorrected nearsightedness, lenses with too short a focal length, and the use of trifocal lenses which require excessively fine adjustment of head position. People who use inverted eyeglasses to do fine overhead work, with their bifocals above rather than below, are in serious trouble with head-positioning the rest of the time if they do not have a second pair of bifocals arranged in the conventional manner.

The rotation and head-tilt functions may be overused by sustained awkward head positions, as when avoiding the glare from a strong light source that reflects off the inside of the eyeglass lenses, or by prolonged typing while reading copy with the pages placed flat on the desk at one side of the typewriter.

Chilling the back of the neck, while holding tired neck muscles in a fixed position, is a major contributor to the activation of TPs in these muscles.

The suboccipital muscles are a common TP source of post-traumatic headache.[12]

8. PATIENT EXAMINATION
(Fig. 17.4)

Activation of TPs in the suboccipital muscles produces relatively minor restriction of the range of motion of the head and neck. When only the TP residue in the suboccipital muscles remains untreated, flexion (Fig. 17.4B) and side bending (Fig. 17.4C) are restricted by one or two finger-breadths. Flexion-rotation is reduced 10° or 15° (Fig. 17.4D). On examination for head mobility, the examiner feels increased resistance at the top of the neck post sooner than normal, causing early movement of the cervical vertebrae.

9. TRIGGER POINT EXAMINATION

Examination by flat palpation elicits deep tenderness without evidence of palpable bands or local twitch responses. Induction of referred pain by pressure on suboccipital TPs is difficult.

10. ENTRAPMENTS

No nerve entrapment has been observed that was thought to be due to TPs in these muscles.

11. ASSOCIATED TRIGGER POINTS

When the suboccipital muscles harbor TPs, many of the major groups of neck muscles also are involved, including the posterior cervical, trapezius, sternocleidomastoid, and sometimes the splenii. No simple relations of these to the suboccipital muscles have been observed, since these muscles tend to function as complex myotatic units.

12. STRETCH AND SPRAY
(Fig. 17.5)

The head must be tilted on top of the neck post in specific directions to stretch either those muscles that extend the head (Fig. 17.5A), the ones that tilt it to one side (Fig. 17.5B), or those that rotate it (Fig. 17.5C). In each case, the line of spray should extend upward well above the hair line. With thick hair, the effectiveness of the vapocoolant spray may be increased by separating the hairs to make a track through them. A roll of bandage is handy to tie up long hair and lift it off the neck. A wig should be removed.

The stretch-and-spray procedure should be followed by a hot pack which adequately covers the lower occiput, as well as the posterior neck region. This is important, but may be difficult because the patient frequently does not want the hair to get wet, and the pack tends to slide down.

Ischemic compression may be useful to inactivate TPs in the suboccipital muscles close to their attachments on the occiput. Very *deep* message is required to penetrate the overlying trapezius, semispinalis, and splenius capitis muscles.[12] The suboccipital triangle, which the vertebral artery transverses horizontally, should be avoided if massage in that area causes any symptoms suggestive of brain ischemia.

13. INJECTION AND STRETCH

Active TPs in the suboccipital muscles are frequently satellites of other TPs, such as the lowest ones in the semispinalis capitis muscle, which refer pain to the suboccipital area. Repeated applications of stretch and spray with deep massage generally are effective in eliminating suboccipital TP irritability. Daily application of 2 watts/cm^2 of ultrasound with a moving head technique is helpful, but usually requires 2 weeks of treatment to produce results. If these fail, and injection is regarded as necessary, due consideration must be given to the proximity of the vertebral artery and to the untoward results of local injection in this region, as described in Section 13, and as illustrated in Fig. 16.9, Chapter 16. For example, immediately after injection in the upper posterior cervical region, a patient became unresponsive, then developed grand mal seizures, but recovered fully.[11] The age and potential susceptibility of the patient to cerebral ischemia should be weighed seriously in making this decision.

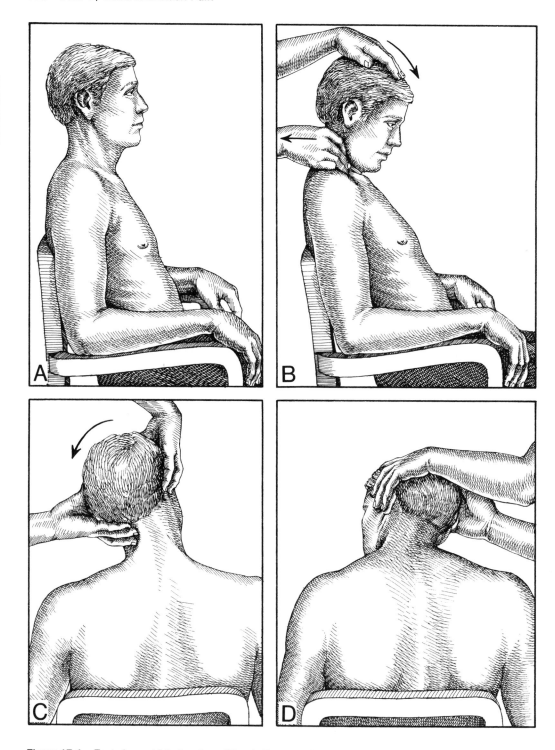

Figure 17.4. Tests for restricted motion of the skull on top of the neck post due to taut suboccipital muscles. Restricted movement of the head on the neck is found by stabilizing the cervical spine and noting early motion between successively lower cervical vertebrae, below the atlantoaxial joint. *A*, resting seated position, *B*, testing flexion requires that one hand stabilize the middle of the neck to determine at what spinal level flexion is taking place. *C*, testing side tilt of the head. *D*, testing diagonal stretch of the right rectus capitus posterior major.

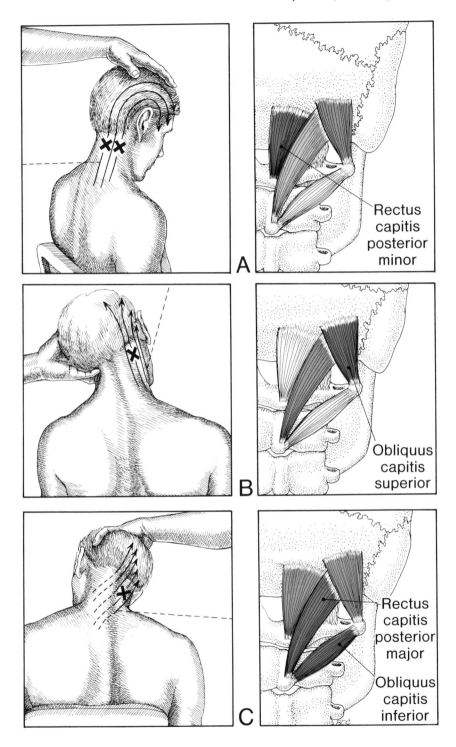

PART 1

Figure 17.5.   Stretch position and up-spray patterns for trigger points in the right suboccipital muscles. The *dark red* indicates which muscles are strongly stretched by each position; *light red*, indicates those muscles only partially stretched. *A*, flexion of the head on top of the neck post stretches the extensor muscles; *B*, side-tilt stretches the muscles contributing to lateral flexion at the top of the neck post. The fingers exert pressure to prevent bending of the neck below the suboccipital region. *C*, rotation with flexion stretches muscles that combine the extension and rotation functions.

It may be necessary to inject above the hairline, after separating the hair and scrubbing and soaking the skin with antiseptic solution. The TP to be injected is identified by the restriction of motion that it causes and by spot tenderness to deep palpation. A clear mental image of its relation to the vertebral artery must be formulated; for injection, the needle is directed away from the artery (Fig. 17.2, and also as seen in Fig. 16.4, Chapter 16).

Dry needling along the posterior arch of the atlas has been recommended, described, and illustrated.[9]

Any TP injection should be followed promptly by passive stretch, usually with vapocooling, and then a hot pack.

14. CORRECTIVE ACTIONS

For patients who develop active TPs in the suboccipital muscles, it is critically important to keep this part of the neck warm by wearing the hair long, or by wearing a turtle-neck sweater indoors and a hood that covers the head and neck outdoors. Nightwear rarely provides a collar high enough to cover the suboccipital area adequately; therefore, the patient should wear something like an old-fashioned nightcap, a soft hooded jacket, or tie a scarf under the chin with the large part of the scarf turned to the rear to protect the suboccipital skin from cooling.

Sustained upward gaze with the head tilted up must be avoided by revising the individual's activity to whatever extent is necessary. For example, a stage director learned to direct from farther back in the theater, and not from the front row where he was below the level of the actors on the stage.

Sustained and strained positions of the head are reduced: (1) by avoiding use of trifocals; (2) by using lenses with adequate focal length (card-playing glasses) to allow the head to rest in a balanced upright position on top of the neck post; (3) by rearranging the location of the patient, or the room lighting, to eliminate glare reflected from the inside of the lenses (alternately, the inside of the lenses may be coated against glare, if repositioning of lights is not practical); and (4) by placing copy material in front of the patient on a vertical stand, not flat at one side.

The patient should learn how to relax the neck muscles, and to do a passive self-stretch exercise while *seated* on a stool or chair under a hot shower. The stretch is assisted by pulling the head down with the hands clasped behind the occiput and by humping the upper back (see Fig. 16.7, Chapter 16). A series of passive stretches should be applied separately in unidirectional movements (no head rolling) with successive degrees of head rotation and tilt to fully stretch *all* of the suboccipital muscles. Passive stretching should be followed by active full range of motion, contracting and stretching muscles in both the agonist and antagonist directions. This cycle of movements is repeated slowly without jerking, several times.

Patients with suboccipital TPs find that a cervical collar is more annoying and irritating than helpful, due to its direct pressure on these muscles. In contrast, patients with sternocleidomastoid TPs find a *loose* collar helpful, even though this muscle is extremely tender.

Supplemental References

Travell[17] reported the management of a patient with an unusual referred pain pattern from suboccipital TPs. The patient also showed evidence of conversion hysteria.

References

1. Cailliet R: *Soft Tissue Pain and Disability*, F.A. Davis, Philadelphia, 1977 (pp. 107–110).
2. Eisler P: *Die Muskeln des Stammes.* Gustav Fischer, Jena, 1912 (Fig. 63, p. 433).
3. Grant JCB: *An Atlas of Human Anatomy*, Ed. 7. Williams & Wilkins, Baltimore, 1978 (Figs. 5-34, 5-35).
4. Gray H: *Anatomy of the Human Body*, edited by C.M. Goss, American Ed. 29. Lea & Febiger, Philadelphia, 1973 (pp. 408, 409).
5. *Ibid.* (Fig. 6-15, p. 408, Fig. 12-28, p. 949).
6. Hollinshead WH: *Anatomy for Surgeons*, Ed. 2, Vol. 1, *The Head and Neck.* Harper & Row, Hagerstown, 1968 (Fig. 1-51, pp. 80, 81).
7. Hollinshead WH: *Functional Anatomy of the Limbs and Back*, Ed. 4. W.B. Saunders, Philadelphia, 1976 (p. 228).
8. Kellgren JH: Observations on referred pain arising from muscle. *Clin Sci* 3:175–190, 1938 (pp. 180, 210, 212).
9. Lewit K: The needle effect in the relief of myofascial pain. *Pain* 6:83–90, 1979.
10. Llewellyn LJ, Jones AB: *Fibrositis.* Rebman, New York, 1915 (Fig. 32 opposite p. 210).
11. Rubin D: Personal communication, 1979.

12. Rubin D: An approach to the management of myofascial trigger point syndromes. *Arch Phys Med Rehabil* 62:107–110, 1981.

13. Sobotta J, Figge FHJ: *Atlas of Human Anatomy,* Ed. 9, Vol. 1. Hafner Division of Macmillan, New York, 1974 (pp. 148, 150).

14. Spalteholz W: *Handatlas der Anatomie des Menschen,* Ed. 11, Vol. 2. S. Hirzel, Leipzig, 1922 (p. 314).

15. Toldt C: *An Atlas of Human Anatomy,* translated by M.E. Paul, Ed. 2, Vol. 1. Macmillan, New York, 1919 (pp. 278, 279).

16. *Ibid.* (pp. 270, 271).

17. Travell J, Bigelow NH: Role of somatic trigger areas in the patterns of hysteria. *Psychosom Med* 9:353–363, 1947 (Case 3, pp. 360, 361).

PART 1

PART 2

CHAPTER 18
Upper Back, Shoulder and Arm Pain-and-Muscle Guide

INTRODUCTION TO PART 2

This second part of THE TRIGGER POINT MANUAL includes the muscles of the upper back, shoulder, and arm that refer pain downward into the torso and upper extremity. It includes: the scalene and levator scapulae neck muscles; all the muscles that attach to the scapula; all the muscles that cross the glenohumeral joint, and the anconeus, which is included as an extension of the triceps brachii muscle.

PAIN GUIDE TO INVOLVED MUSCLES

This guide lists the muscles that may be responsible for pain in the areas shown in Figure 18.1. The muscles most likely to refer pain to each specific area are listed below under the name of that area. One uses this chart by locating the name of the area that hurts and then by looking under that heading for all the muscles that are likely to cause the pain. Then, reference should be made to the individual muscle chapters; the number for each follows in parenthesis.

In a general way, the muscles are listed in the order of the frequency in which they are likely to cause pain in that area. This order is only an approximation; the selection process by which patients reach an examiner greatly influences which of their muscles are most likely to be involved. Boldface type indicates that the muscle refers an essential pain pattern to that pain area. Normal type indicates that the muscle refers a spillover pattern to that pain area. TP stands for trigger point.

PAIN GUIDE

UPPER-THORACIC BACK PAIN

Scaleni (20)
Levator scapulae (24)
Supraspinatus (21)
Trapezius (TPs$_2$ and TP$_3$) (6)
Trapezius (TP$_5$) (6)
Multifidi (48)
Rhomboidei (27)
Splenius cervicis (15)
Triceps brachii (TP$_1$) (32)
Biceps brachii (30)

BACK-OF-SHOULDER PAIN

Deltoid (28)
Levator scapulae (19)
Scaleni (20)
Supraspinatus (21)
Teres major (25)
Teres minor (23)
Subscapularis (26)
Serratus posterior superior (45)
Latissimus dorsi (24)
Triceps brachii (TP$_1$) (32)
Trapezius (TP$_3$ and TP$_6$) (6)
Iliocostalis thoracis (48)

BACK-OF-ARM PAIN

Scaleni (20)
Triceps brachii (TP$_1$ and TP$_3$) (32)
Deltoid (28)
Subscapularis (26)
Supraspinatus (21)
Teres major (25)
Teres minor (23)
Latissimus dorsi (24)
Serratus posterior superior (45)
Coracobrachialis (29)
Scalenus minimus (20)

MID-THORACIC BACK PAIN

Scaleni (20)
Latissimus dorsi (24)
Levator scapulae (19)
Iliocostalis thoracis (48)
Multifidi (48)
Rhomboidei (27)
Serratus posterior superior (45)
Infraspinatus (22)
Trapezius (TP$_4$) (6)
Trapezius (TP$_5$) (6)
Serratus anterior (46)

FRONT-OF-SHOULDER PAIN

Infraspinatus (22)
Deltoid (28)
Scaleni (20)
Supraspinatus (21)
Pectoralis major (42)
Pectoralis minor (43)
Biceps brachii (30)
Coracobrachialis (29)
Sternalis (44)
Subclavius (42)
Latissimus dorsi (24)

FRONT-OF-ARM PAIN

Scaleni (20)
Infraspinatus (22)
Biceps brachii (30)
Brachialis (31)
Triceps brachii (TP$_5$) (32)
Supraspinatus (21)
Deltoid (28)
Sternalis (44)
Scalenus minimus (20)
Subclavius (42)

PART 2

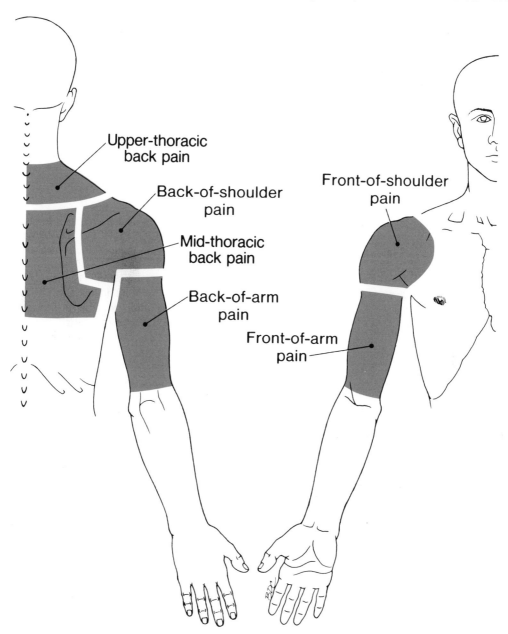

Figure 18.1   The designated areas (*red*) within the upper back, shoulder, and arm that may encompass pain referred there by myofascial trigger points. See text for listing of muscles that may refer pain to each area.

CHAPTER 19
Levator Scapulae Muscle
"Stiff Neck"

PART 2

HIGHLIGHTS: When a patient suffers from a "stiff neck" (markedly limited rotation), trigger points (TPs) in the levator scapulae muscle are usually responsible. **REFERRED PAIN** from the levator scapulae concentrates in the angle of the neck and along the vertebral border of the scapula. It may project to an area posterior to the shoulder joint. **ANATOMICAL ATTACHMENTS** are to the transverse processes of the first four cervical vertebrae above, and to the superior angle of the scapula below. **ACTIONS** at the scapula elevate the scapula and rotate the glenoid fossa downward. Actions at the cervical end of the muscle assist rotation of the front of the neck to the same side and can assist extension of the neck. **ACTIVATION OF TRIGGER POINTS** is most likely to occur because of sustained elevation of the shoulders or due to cramped positioning, particularly when the muscle is fatigued and exposed to cold. **PATIENT**

EXAMINATION reveals primarily restriction of neck rotation. **TRIGGER POINT EXAMINATION** by palpation of the muscle as it emerges from beneath the trapezius at the angle of the neck discloses its most important TP, which may be difficult to locate. Palpation just above the angle of the scapula often locates a second TP. **STRETCH AND SPRAY** require careful coordination of the direction of stretch with sweeps of the spray. The spray application first matches the forward pressure on the head used to stretch the nearly longitudinal fibers, and then is redirected with rotary pressure to stretch the diagonal lateral fibers. **INJECTION AND STRETCH** require careful positioning of the patient and often needling at both TP sites to be successful. **CORRECTIVE ACTIONS** call for relief of muscular strain and for regular passive stretching of the muscle at home, preferably while the patient is seated under a hot shower.

1. REFERRED PAIN
(Fig. 19.1)

The levator scapulae is one of the most commonly involved shoulder-girdle muscles. In a study of these muscles in 200 normal young adults, Sola et al.[22] found latent trigger points (TPs) in more levator scapulae muscles (20% of subjects) than in any other muscle except the upper trapezius. In a clinical study of active TPs,[21] the levator scapulae was the most commonly involved shoulder-girdle muscle.

At both locations shown in Fig. 19.1, TPs project pain to their essential reference zone at the angle of the neck,[23] with a spillover zone along the vertebral border of the scapula,[27] and to the shoulder posteriorly.[10, 26, 28] The lower TP may project pain to the inferior angle of the scapula.

This "stiff neck" muscle, when involved, consistently limits neck rotation due to pain on movement. If the TPs are active enough, they refer severe pain at rest.

2. ANATOMICAL ATTACHMENTS
(Fig. 19.2)

The fibers of the levator scapulae attach **above** to the transverse processes of the first four cervical vertebrae (posterior tubercles of the C_3 and C_4 transverse processes); and **below** to the vertebral border of the scapula between the superior angle and root of its spine (Fig. 19.2).

The twist of the muscle fibers is rarely noted or illustrated.[8, 24] The C_1 digitation is superficial to the others and passes more vertically to the vertebral border of the scapula. The C_4 digitation lies deepest and

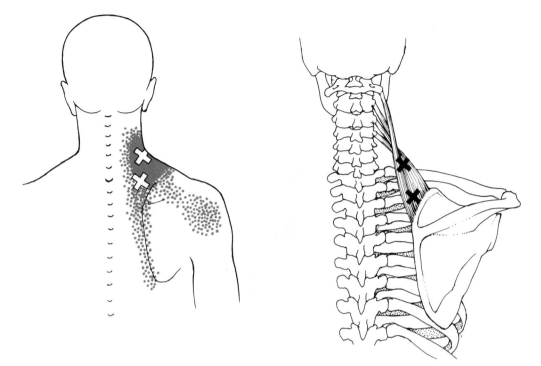

Figure 19.1.   Consolidated referred pain pattern of the two trigger point locations (**✕s**) for the right levator scapulae muscle. The essential pain pattern is *solid red*, and the spillover pattern is *stippled red*.

passes diagonally to a lateral attachment on the superior angle of the scapula.

Supplemental References

Other authors have illustrated the muscle as seen from the front,[3, 20] the side,[4, 19, 25] and from behind.[5, 6, 8, 17, 24]

3. INNERVATION

The levator scapulae is supplied by branches of the third and fourth cervical nerves *via* the cervical plexus and sometimes, in part, by fibers from the dorsal scapular nerve derived from the C_5 root.[7]

4. ACTIONS

One levator scapulae muscle, when anchored at the neck, first helps to rotate the scapula, facing the glenoid fossa downward, and then elevates this bone as a whole.[7, 18] When the scapula is anchored, one muscle helps to complete neck rotation to the same side.[7] Both muscles acting together checkrein neck flexion.

In conjunction with the upper trapezius and uppermost fibers of the serratus anterior, the levator scapulae helps to elevate the scapula, for example, when shrugging the shoulders, when supporting weight directly on the shoulder girdle (hod carrier or postman), and when lifting a weight with the upper extremity.[1, 18] The levator scapulae, rhomboidei major and minor, and the latissimus dorsi together rotate the glenoid fossa of the scapula downward. This pulls the inferior angles of the scapulae together posteriorly.[1, 9]

5. MYOTATIC UNIT

Muscles which are synergistic with the levator scapulae, and which may develop active TPs in association with it, are the splenius cervicis and the scalenus medius. The splenius cervicis is located deep to the levator scapulae and attaches, above, to the posterior tubercles *behind* this muscle. The scalenus medius is attached, above, to the posterior tubercles in *front* of the muscle. These two synergistic muscles attach, below, to the rib cage, rather than to the scapula.

Antagonists to the elevator function of the levator scapulae are the lowest fibers of the serratus anterior and the latissimus dorsi. The latter, however, is a synergist for scapular rotation and attaches to the humerus, rather than to the scapula.

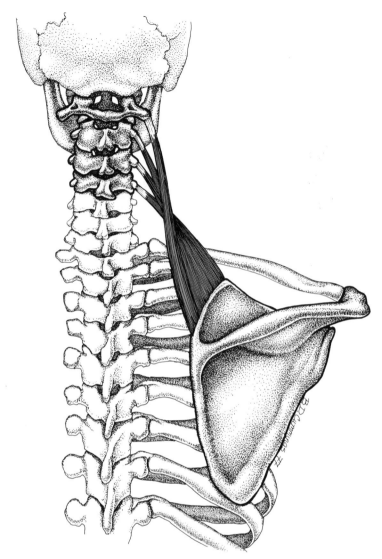

Figure 19.2   Attachments of the levator scapulae muscle.

6. SYMPTOMS

With severe involvement of the levator scapulae alone, patients complain of pain at the angle of the neck and of a painfully "stiff neck." The diagnosis of the scapulocostal syndrome[2, 12, 13] emphasizes the referred pain symptoms arising from the levator scapulae. The diagnosis of the "stiff neck syndrome," or torticollis[23, 26] emphasizes the restriction of range of motion, since tension in the levator scapulae is a common cause of neck stiffness.[23, 26] (see Chapter 7, for the differential diagnosis of torticollis.) Patients with active TPs in the levator scapulae are unable to turn the head to the same side, and must turn the body instead to look behind.

7. ACTIVATION OF TRIGGER POINTS
(Fig. 19.3)

Postural Stress

Patients are likely to develop the levator scapulae type of "stiff neck" because of occupational stresses, such as, typing with the head and neck turned to look toward the side of the typewriter; making long telephone calls; and talking, at length, with the head turned toward someone sitting at one side.[2] Another activating stress is sleeping with the neck in a tilted position that shortens the levator scapulae, as on a sofa with the head on the armrest without adequate pillow support, or in an uncomfortable airplane seat when the muscle is fatigued and exposed to a cold draft. Rec-

shortens the muscle bilaterally, which encourages activation of its latent TPs. Walking with a cane that is too long, so that it forces unnatural elevation of one shoulder, tends to activate TPs in the levator scapula on the same side (Fig. 19.3).

Activity Stress

Overexercise, such as playing vigorous tennis or swimming the crawl stroke when out of condition, or repetitive rotation of the head as in "spectator neck," which is caused by sitting near the net beside a tennis court and turning the head and neck to follow the ball back and forth, can initiate this syndrome.

Infection

During the prodromal stage of an acute upper respiratory infection, the levator scapulae is vulnerable to activation of its TPs by mechanical stresses that are usually well within its tolerance. This susceptibility to ordinary loads may start a day or two before the full blown symptoms of a head cold or sore throat appear, and may last for several weeks thereafter. The stiff neck often begins during an attack of oral herpes simplex.

8. PATIENT EXAMINATION

The patient tends to hold the neck rigid, looking sideways by turning the eyes or body, but NOT the neck. The head may be tilted slightly toward the involved side.[26] With active upper trapezius TPs, the patient moves the neck frequently trying to stretch the trapezius, whereas levator scapulae involvement reduces such neck movement.

Neck rotation is markedly restricted as the face turns toward the side of the pain. The degree of restriction depends upon the severity of involvement. When both sides are involved, as commonly occurs, rotation is restricted in both directions. Neck flexion is blocked only at the end of the movement; extension is unaffected.

There is minimal limitation of shoulder motion; full abduction of the arm is limited by some restriction of scapular rotation. The Hand-to-shoulder-blade Test is normal (see Fig. 22.4). The Mouth Wraparound Test (see Fig. 22.3) is restricted chiefly by the lack of head rotation.

If rotation of the neck is unrestricted, active TPs in the levator scapulae are un-

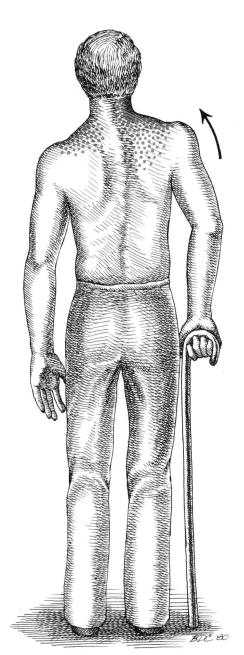

Figure 19.3 Activation primarily of right levator scapulae trigger points, and secondarily of other muscles on the left, by walking with a cane that is too long, held in the right hand. The patient's resultant pain distribution is shown in *red*.

reational stress while gazing fixedly at a stage or movie screen also can precipitate the problem. Psychological stress, which produces a "weight-of-the-world-on-my-shoulders" reaction or a tense, hostile, aggressive posture, also may be contributory.[2] Sitting in a chair with armrests that are too high elevates the scapulae and

PART 2

likely. If the patient's head is strongly tilted to one side (wry neck), sternocleidomastoid TPs are more likely to be responsible than are levator scapulae TPs.

9. TRIGGER POINT EXAMINATION
(Fig. 19.4)

The levator scapulae develops TPs in two locations: a primary TP area at the angle of the neck where the muscle emerges from beneath the anterior border of the upper trapezius;[11, 13, 26] and a secondary TP area just cephalad to the attachment of the muscle to the superior angle of the scapula.[11, 12, 13, 16] For the anatomical relations of this muscle, see Figure 20.7 in Chapter 20. Sola and Williams[23] reported locating the lower TP by electrical stimulation, which produced pain referred to the neck and back of the head. Michele et al.[12] in an initial article, described in great detail how to locate the lower TP, but did not identify the muscle in which it was located. Later, Michele and Eisenberg[13] identified both the upper and lower levator scapulae TPs as such, and illustrated how to palpate the upper TP as the prime source of the scapulocostal syndrome.

The primary TP in the levator scapulae at the angle of the neck is best palpated with the patient comfortably seated and the hips far enough forward on the chair seat to place the weight of the upper torso against the backrest. Both the levator scapulae and upper trapezius muscles are slackened slightly by supporting the elbows on the armrests, using small pillows, if needed. The laxity permits the examiner's fingers to push the upper trapezius backward so as to uncover and straddle the levator scapulae (Fig. 19.4A). The face and neck are gently turned toward the opposite side to tauten and lift the levator scapulae against the palpating fingers. The increased tension may raise the sensitivity of the TP enough so that sustained pressure on it reproduces its referred pain pattern. Successful palpation depends upon slackening the upper trapezius sufficiently to reach the upper TPs within the belly of a tautened levator scapulae muscle.

To locate the lower TP, the patient may be seated, or lying on the opposite side (Fig. 19.4B). Palpation across the fibers of the muscle is applied about 1.3 cm (½ in) above the superior angle of the scapula.

The tense TP bands are exquisitely tender to pressure, but local twitch responses and referred pain are not readily elicited from this lower TP area, which is covered by the trapezius. This TP is located by rocking the fingers back and forth across the muscle so that they straddle it.

10. ENTRAPMENTS

No nerve or vascular entrapments have been recognized as due to TPs in this muscle.

11. ASSOCIATED TRIGGER POINTS

In the "stiff neck" syndrome, the splenius cervicis also is likely to be involved. When TPs in the levator scapulae are very active, it is wise to check also the scalenus posterior and iliocostalis cervicis muscles for TP activity. Contrary to what might be expected, rhomboid TP activity is rarely associated with levator scapulae involvement.

12. STRETCH AND SPRAY
(Figs. 19.5 and 19.6)

Prior to treatment, X-ray films of the cervical spine should be inspected to detect any condition that would preclude vigorous neck flexion and rotation.

The patient sits relaxed in an armchair, with the pelvis level, and with the fingers hooked under the chair seat or a rung to hold down the scapula (Fig. 19.5). Alternatively, an assistant may stabilize the scapula. Pressure from the operator's hand against the head rotates the face about 30° toward the opposite side. The vapocoolant is sprayed downward in parallel sweeps over those fibers as illustrated by the medial spray lines in Figure 19.5A, and as previously described.[14, 26] Next, forward pressure stretches the most vertical fibers of the levator scapulae (Figure 19.5A) as the spray is continued. The force is then redirected to exert nearly lateral pressure in order to stretch the diagonal twisted fibers. The spray traces the lateral lines in Figures 19.5A and B. The entire neck post is pressed and bent laterally, not just the skull on top of it.

An alternate stretch technique, suggested by Nielsen,[15] is useful if an assistant is not available. It provides a strong counter force on the shoulder and scapula,

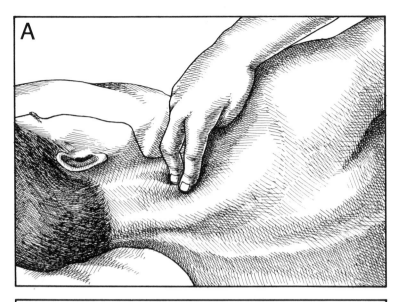

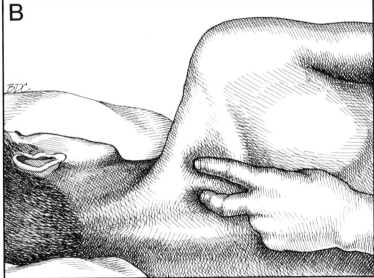

Figure 19.4. Examination of the levator scapulae muscle, patient supine. *A*, pressing the free border of the upper trapezius aside with the index finger to straddle the tense muscle and localize the upper trigger point between the fingers. *B*, straddling the lower trigger point just cephalad to the muscle's attachment to the superior angle of the scapula.

which is usually essential for success. The operator places an elbow in front of the patient's acromion, while pressing the patient's head forward and to the opposite side with the hand of the same arm (Fig. 19.6). Stretch and spray are applied to each set of levator scapulae fibers, as described above. Unless the more horizontal fibers also are stretched and sprayed, the patient is not likely to obtain total relief from the TPs in this muscle.

This is frequently a tight area that is difficult to release by stretch and spray. Parallel myotatic muscles, including the splenius cervicis, scalenus medius, scalenus posterior, and the posterior cervical muscles, must be released to achieve a full stretch on the levator scapulae. If the scalene muscles require stretch and spray, it also is desirable to stretch and spray the upper pectoralis major fibers, since their TPs may cause disagreeable chest pain

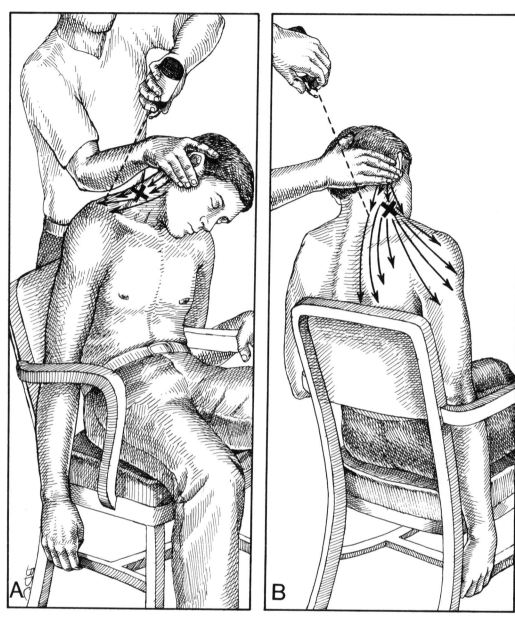

Figure 19.5. Stretch technique and spray pattern (*arrows*) for trigger points in the left levator scapulae muscle, patient seated. *A*, stretch of the diagonal fibers, as seen from in front. *B*, stretch of the most vertical fibers, as seen from behind.

and are often involved as a result of scalene TP activity.

Sometimes the antagonistic neck muscles also must be stretched and sprayed to coax the levator scapulae to lengthen. This stretch of the levator scapulae may allow the serratus anterior muscle on the same side to shorten more than usual, activating its latent TPs and causing a painful reactive cramp with chest pain. This problem is prevented, or readily relieved, by stretching and spraying the serratus anterior muscle (see Chapter 46).

If the pain shifts to the other side of the neck, the procedure has uncovered a lesser, but significant, degree of TP activity

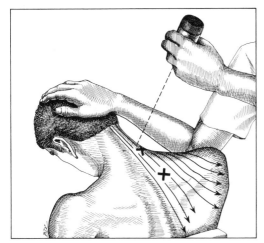

Figure 19.6. Alternate stretch technique for trigger points (×s) in the right levator scapulae muscle. The patient's head is pressed forward and toward the opposite side while the operator's elbow presses the shoulder down and back from the front. The spray pattern (*arrows*) is essentially the same as in Figure 19.5.

in the contralateral levator scapulae, which requires application of the same procedures to that muscle.

13. INJECTION AND STRETCH
(Fig. 19.7)

The lower TP, at the scapular attachment of the levator scapulae, is more readily located, but the upper TP is the critical one and is usually more active and hypersensitive. Injection of the upper TP may eliminate the lower one, but not *vice versa*. Injection of only the lower TP may aggravate the pain referred from the upper TP.

To inject the upper TP, the patient lies on the opposite side, with the back toward the operator and the body angled across the treatment table, placing the shoulder closer than the hips to the near edge of the table. A pillow between the chin and lower shoulder supports the head. The patient rests the top upper extremity on the side,

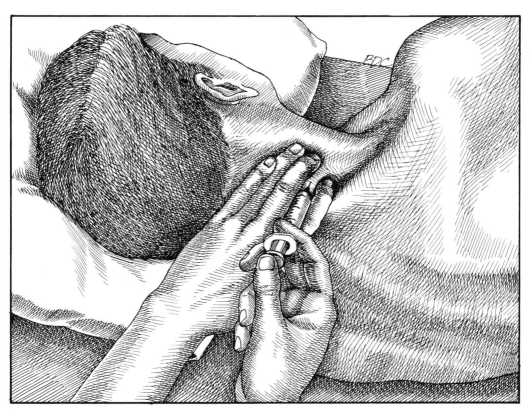

Figure 19.7. Injection of the upper trigger point in the right levator scapulae at the base of the neck where the muscle emerges from beneath the upper trapezius.

with the elbow bent to balance it. The operator presses aside the free upper border of the trapezius muscle and palpates the levator scapulae as it emerges from beneath the trapezius (see Fig. 20.7, Regional Anatomy, Chapter 20 and Fig. 16.8, Cross Section, Chapter 16). The TP (the spot of maximum tenderness in the taut muscle fibers) is fixed against the cervical spine (Fig. 19.7) for injection. The needle is directed upward and medially toward the underlying transverse process of the vertebra. It should be aimed at a sufficiently shallow angle to insure its remaining outside the thoracic cage, as illustrated in Figure 19.7. The injection of this TP also can be made from in front of the patient, as suggested by Figure 19.4A.

If soreness persists in the lower TP, it is injected next, just above the scapular attachment of the levator scapulae. The scapula is protracted by having the patient, who is lying on the opposite side, bend forward in a "round-shouldered" posture to stretch and thin out the overlying trapezius. Palpation of TPs just above the superior angle of the scapula is done by moving the finger transversely across the fibers of the muscle. The fingers of one hand localize the band containing the TPs. For injection, a 3.8-cm (1½-in), 22-gauge needle is directed upward just above the scapular border. Needle insertion at this shallow tangential angle avoids passing it between the ribs where it might cause a pneumothorax.

Injection is followed by stretch and spray, hot packs and, finally, active range of motion.

14. CORRECTIVE ACTIONS

The patient learns to passively stretch the relaxed levator scapulae muscle by using external force, while seated under a hot shower on a chair or stool that has a low backrest. Thus seated, the patient relaxes the neck muscles as much as possible and pulls the head down with the contralateral hand to obtain the stretch effects of Figure 19.5 and 19.6, while the hot water beats on the neck. The scapula must be stabilized by hooking the fingers of the homolateral hand under the stool. A slow steady stretch without jerking is applied in those directions in which the muscle feels tight and restricted. Standing under a hot shower is less effective than sitting, because of postural reflexes that inhibit muscular relaxation. Some patients achieve an effective passive stretch by latching the fingers across the back of the occiput and letting the head hang forward so that it carries the weight of the relaxed arms. This is repeated with varying degrees of head rotation.

If the patient sits at a desk when talking with visitors, he or she should turn the chair (not the head) to face the visitor squarely, or rearrange the furniture so that the visitor's chair is in front of the desk.

To avoid posterior cervical and levator scapulae strain when reading, writing or typing, myopia must be corrected by eyeglasses with a sufficiently long focal length. Material to be read should be in focus when placed upright on a bookholder, steno stand, or music stand. The use of one of these book supports relieves sustained neck flexion. For a card player, one pair of eyeglasses should be adjusted for focus at arms' length, "card-playing glasses."

If the typewriter is too high, but cannot be lowered, and the typist's chair provides inadequate adjustment, 2 or 3 cm (about an inch) or so of folded newspapers, or a magazine, may be placed on the rear two-thirds of the seat bottom. The front one-third of the seat is not raised, to avoid compression of the thighs and to open the angles at the hips and knees. The backrest should provide adequate lumbar support (see Fig. 42.9E, Chapter 49).

The patient should apply a hot pack or a moist heating pad to the TP areas, especially at the end of the work day or on retiring.

When in bed, the patient's pillow should be positioned to avoid shortening and cramping of the muscle (see Fig. 7.7, Chapter 7).

If a cane is used, its length should provide a level shoulder-girdle axis, during walking.

References

1. Basmajian JV: *Muscles Alive*, Ed. 4. Williams & Wilkins. Baltimore, 1978 (pp. 191, 192).
2. Cailliet R: *Neck and Arm Pain*. F.A. Davis, Philadelphia, 1964 (p. 97).
3. Eisler P: *Die Muskeln des Stammes*. Gustav

Fischer, Jena, 1912 (Fig. 49).

4. *Ibid.* (Figs. 50, 52).

5. *Ibid.* (Fig. 51).

6. Grant JCB: *An Atlas of Human Anatomy*, Ed. 7. Williams & Wilkins, Baltimore, 1978 (Figs. 5–26, 6–30).

7. Gray H: *Anatomy of the Human Body*, edited by C.M. Goss, American Ed. 29. Lea & Febiger, Philadelphia, 1973 (p. 449).

8. Hollinshead WH: *Anatomy for Surgeons*, Ed. 2, Vol. 3, *The Back and Limbs*. Harper & Row, New York, 1969 (p. 312, Fig. 4–36).

9. Hollinshead WH: *Functional Anatomy of the Limbs and Back*, Ed. 4. W.B. Saunders, Philadelphia, 1976 (p. 103).

10. Kraus H: *Clinical Treatment of Back and Neck Pain*. McGraw-Hill, New York, 1970 (p. 98).

11. Llewellyn LJ, Jones AB: *Fibrositis*. Rebman, New York, 1915 (p. 210, Fig. 32).

12. Michele AA, Davies JJ, Krueger FJ, Lichtor JM: Scapulocostal syndrome (fatigue-postural paradox). *NY State J Med* 50:1353–1356, 1950 (p. 1355, Fig. 4).

13. Michele AA, Eisenberg J: Scapulocostal syndrome. *Arch Phys Med Rehabil* 49:383–387, 1968 (pp. 385, 386, Fig. 4).

14. Modell W, Travell JT, Kraus H, Hardy JD: Contributions to Cornell Conferences on Therapy. Relief of pain by ethyl chloride spray. *NY State J. Med* 52:1550–1558, 1952 (p. 1551).

15. Nielsen AJ: Personal communications, 1979.

16. Pace JB: Commonly overlooked pain syndromes responsive to simple therapy. *Postgrad Med.* 58:107–113, 1975 (p. 110).

17. Pernkopf E: *Atlas of Topographical and Applied Human Anatomy*, Vol. 2. W.B. Saunders, Philadelphia, 1964 (Fig. 28).

18. Rasch PJ, Burke RK: *Kinesiology and Applied Anatomy*. Lea & Febiger, Philadelphia, 1967 (p. 154–156).

19. Sobotta J, Figge FHJ: *Atlas of Human Anatomy*, Ed. 9, Vol. 1. Hafner Division of Macmillan, New York, 1974 (p. 169).

20. *Ibid.* (p. 176).

21. Sola AE, Kuitert JH: Myofascial trigger point pain in the neck and shoulder girdle. *Northwest Med* 54:980–984, 1955.

22. Sola AE, Rodenberger ML, Gettys BB: Incidence of hypersensitive areas in posterior shoulder muscles. *Am J Phys Med* 34:585–590, 1955.

23. Sola AE, Williams RL: Myofascial pain syndromes. *Neurol* 6:91–95, 1956 (p. 93, Fig. 1).

24. Toldt C: *An Atlas of Human Anatomy*, translated by M.E. Paul, Ed. 2, Vol. 1. Macmillan, New York, 1919 (p. 269).

25. *Ibid.* (pp. 277, 293).

26. Rapid relief of acute "stiff neck" by ethyl chloride spray. *J Am Med Wom Assoc* 4:89–95, 1949 (pp. 91–93, Fig. 3, Case 1).

27. Travell J, Rinzler SH: The myofascial genesis of pain. *Postgrad Med* 11:425–434, 1952.

28. Zohn DA, Mennell J McM: *Musculoskeletal Pain: Diagnosis and Physical Treatment*. Little, Brown & Company, Boston. 1976 (Fig. 9–12).

PART 2

CHAPTER 20
Scalene Muscles
"The Entrappers"

HIGHLIGHTS: Scalene trigger points (TPs) and their associated thoracic outlet entrapment syndrome are often *overlooked* sources of pain in the shoulder-girdle and upper extremity. **REFERRED PAIN** from all three of the major scalene muscles can radiate anteriorly, laterally or posteriorly. Anteriorly, persistent aching pain is referred through the pectoral region; laterally, it is referred down the front and back of the arm, skipping the elbow to the radial forearm, and extending to the thumb and index finger. On the left side, this pain is easily mistaken for angina pectoris during activity or at rest. Posteriorly, pain is referred to the upper vertebral border of the scapula. **ANATOMICAL ATTACHMENTS:** above, all scalene muscles attach to transverse processes of the cervical vertebrae; below the scalenus anterior and scalenus medius attach to the first rib, and the scalenus posterior, to the second rib. **ACTIONS** of the scalene muscles stabilize the cervical spine against lateral movement and elevate the first and second ribs to assist inspiration. **SYMPTOMS** may be primary myofascial pain, or secondary sensory and motor disturbance due to neurovascular entrapment. Pain on the radial side of the hand indicates a referred myofascial source; pain on its ulnar side with puffiness of the hand suggests brachial plexus and subclavian vein entrapment. **ACTIVATION OF TRIGGER POINTS** occurs by pulling, lifting and tugging; by overuse of these accessory inspiratory muscles as in coughing; and by chronic muscle strain due to a tilted shoulder-girdle axis caused by body asymmetry with a short leg or small half-pelvis. **PATIENT EXAMINATION** is assisted, diagnostically, by the Finger-flexion Test, the Scalene Range-of-motion Test and the Scalene-relief Test. **TRIGGER POINT EXAMINATION** by flat palpation readily locates most scalene TPs against the underlying transverse processes of the vertebrae. **ENTRAPMENT** of the lower trunk of the brachial plexus is commonly due to TP tautness of the scalenus anterior and the scalenus medius. This entrapment causes ulnar pain, tingling, numbness, and dysesthesia. TP activity in the scalenus anterior often causes hand edema. **STRETCH AND SPRAY** employ neck side bending with self-stretch of the scalene in the supine position, while the operator applies down sweeps of vapocoolant spray over the muscle and its pain reference zones. **INJECTION AND STRETCH** may be necessary for complete relief, but must be done with full understanding of, and respect for, local anatomy. **CORRECTIVE ACTIONS** are usually essential for continued relief and require daily passive side bending by doing the Neck-stretch Exercise, correction of body asymmetry, relief of respiratory overload, and elevation of the head of the bed to tilt the entire bed frame and create gentle traction on the scalene muscles during sleep.

---

1. REFERRED PAIN
(Fig. 20.1)

Active trigger points (TPs) in any one of the anterior, medial, or posterior scalene muscles may refer pain anteriorly to the chest, laterally to the upper extremity, and posteriorly to the medial scapular border and adjacent interscapular region (Fig. 20.1A).[20, 42, 45]

Anteriorly, persistent aching pain is referred in two fingerlike projections over the pectoral region down to about the nipple level[43]; this pattern commonly originates in the lower part of the scalenus medius or scalenus posterior.

PART 2

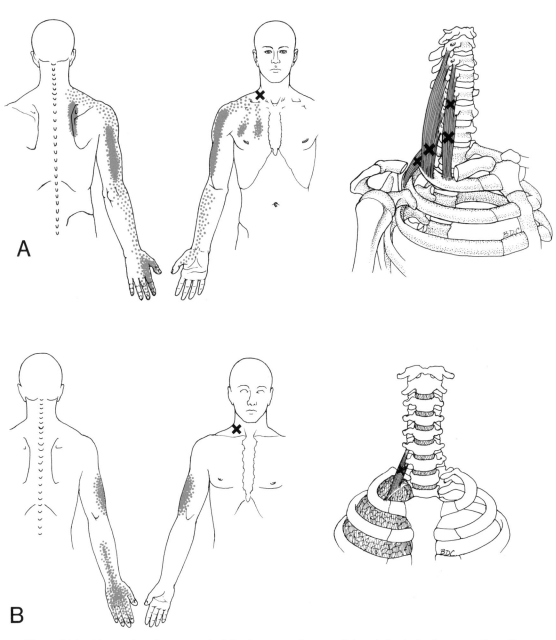

Figure 20.1. Composite pain patterns (*solid red* areas are the essential, and *stippled red* areas are the spillover pain reference zones) with location of trigger points (×s) in the right scalene muscles. *A*, scalenus anterior, medius and posterior. Some trigger points may have only one essential reference zone. *B*, scalenus minimus.

Scalene pain referred to the anterior shoulder region is not described as deep in the joint, as is the pain referred from the infraspinatus muscle. Scalene pain extends down the front and back of the arm (over the biceps and triceps). The referred pain skips the elbow and reappears in the radial side of the forearm, the thumb, and the index finger. This upper extremity pattern arises from TPs in the upper part of the scalenus anterior and from the scalenus medius. On the left side, this referred pain may be mistaken for angina pectoris since TP pain may occur during activity or at rest.

In an upper extremity amputee, this referred pattern of upper extremity pain produced severe phantom limb pain that was relieved by the senior author by inactivation of the scalene TPs. Sherman[28] lists elimination of TPs as one treatment for relief of phantom limb pain.

Posteriorly, pain is commonly referred from TPs in the scalenus anterior to the back, over the upper half of the vertebral border of the scapula and to the adjacent interscapular region.

Experimental injection of 0.2 to 0.5 ml of a 6% solution of sodium chloride into the scalenus anterior in seven subjects evoked referred pain primarily in the shoulder region in all subjects, pain down the arm in one, and a superficial hyperesthesia radiating upward over the neck in two.[35]

The less frequently seen pain referred from TPs in the scalenus minimus projects strongly to the thumb (Fig. 20.1*B*). This pain covers the lateral aspect of the arm from the deltoid insertion to the elbow but skips the elbow to cover the dorsum of the forearm, wrist, hand and all five digits, accenting the thumb. Periods of myofascial pain may be associated with what the patient calls "numbness" of the thumb without demonstrable hypoesthesia to cold or touch.

2. ANATOMICAL ATTACHMENTS
Figs. 20.2 and 20.3)

Scalenus Anterior
(Fig. 20.2)

The anterior scalene muscle attaches *above* to the anterior tubercles on the transverse processes of vertebrae C_3 to C_6; *below* it attaches by a tendon to the scalene tubercle on the inner border of the first rib (Fig. 20.2).[14] Vertebra C_7 is unlikely to have an anterior tubercle unless an anomalous slip of the scalenus anterior or a scalenus minimus muscle requires it.

Scalenus Medius
(Fig. 20.2)

The scalenus medius is the largest of the scalene muscles and attaches *above* to the posterior tubercles on the transverse processes usually of vertebrae C_2 through C_7 (sometimes to the processes of only the 4th and 5th vertebrae).[2] The muscle slants diagonally and attaches *below* to the cranial surface of the first rib, anterior and lateral to the groove for the subclavian artery (Fig.

20.2 and also Fig. 20.9). A slip of the muscle sometimes extends to the second rib.

Scalenus Posterior
(Fig. 20.2)

This muscle attaches *above* to the posterior tubercles on the transverse processes of the lowest two or three cervical vertebrae, and *below* to the lateral surface of the second, and sometimes of the third rib. The scalenus posterior crosses the first rib posterior to the scalenus medius and deep to the levator scapulae muscle (Figs. 20.2 and 20.7).

Scalenus Minimus
(Fig. 20.3)

All the scalene muscles are variable in their attachments and fiber arrangements. The most variable is the scalenus minimus, which occurred on at least one side of the body in one-half to three-quarters of the bodies studied.[3, 9] This muscle usually extends *above* to the anterior tubercle on the transverse process of vertebra C_7, sometimes also of C_6. *Below* it attaches to the pleural dome and beyond to the inner border of the first rib, which lies behind the scalenus anterior and behind the groove for the subclavian artery (Fig. 20.3 and also Fig. 20.9).[14] The pleural dome, or cupola, is strengthened by Sibson's fascia and anchored by this fascia to the anterior tubercle of C_7 and to the inner border of the first rib. The scalenus minimus reinforces this fascia and can be a strong, thick muscle.[9, 15]

The scalenus minimus passes behind and beneath the subclavian artery to attach to the first rib, whereas the anterior scalene muscle passes over and in front of the artery (see Fig. 20.9).[9]

Omohyoid Muscle
(see Fig. 20.7)

The omohyoideus has two bellies connected by a central tendon. The inferior (caudal) belly attaches to the cranial border of the scapula between its superior angle and the coracoid process, close to this process. The belly passes forward and up to the attachment of the central tendon on the clavicle; from there, the superior

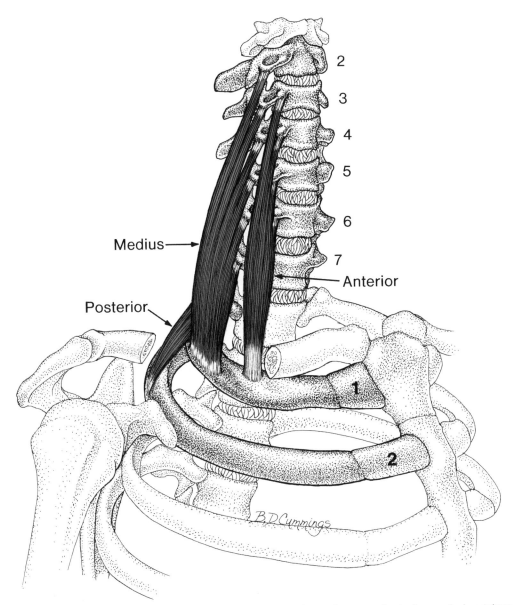

Figure 20.2. Oblique view of the attachments of the three major scalene muscles to the cervical vertebrae and to the first and second ribs. The clavicle has been cut and the section that overlies the scalene muscles removed.

belly travels up and attaches to the hyoid bone (see Fig. 20.7).[17]

Supplemental References

As seen from the front, other authors have illustrated the scalenus anterior,[9, 14, 21, 30, 33, 37] the scalenus medius,[9, 10, 14, 30, 33, 37] the scalenus posterior,[10, 14, 30, 33, 37] and the scalenus minimus muscles.[9, 13] The three major scalene muscles were shown from the side.[32, 36] The posterior view was used

for the scalenus medius[31] and the scalenus posterior.[31, 38]

The three major scalene muscles are seen in cross section at the C_5 level in Figure 16.8.

3. INNERVATION

All the scalene muscles are innervated by motor branches of the anterior primary divisions of spinal nerves C_2 through C_7,

PART 2

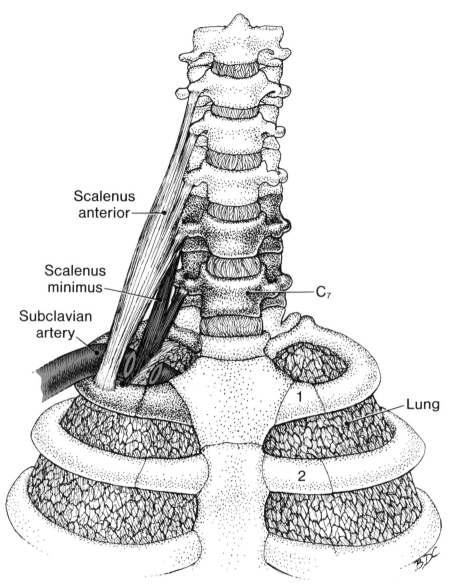

Scalenus
anterior

Scalenus
minimus

Subclavian
artery

C₇

1

Lung

2

Figure 20.3. Anterior view of the attachments of the scalenus minimus muscle, which lies *behind* the subclavian artery (cut), whereas the scalenus anterior lies *in front of* it, more laterally. Note how high into the neck the dome of the pleura extends, where it is vulnerable to needle penetration.

according to the segmental level of muscular attachment.

4. ACTIONS

Fixed From Below

Acting unilaterally, the scalene muscles serve as prime movers for lateral flexion of the cervical spine[25] and, when stimulated, flex the head obliquely forward and sideways.[7] Acting bilaterally, the anterior scalene muscles assist in neck flexion.[14] The much flatter angle of the scalenus posterior makes it especially suited to stabilizing the base of the neck by preventing, or controlling, side sway, in a manner similar to the lowest diagonal fibers of the quadratus lumborum muscle at the base of the lumbar spine.

Fixed From Above

Clearly, the scalene muscles are important auxiliary muscles of inspiration and are more commonly used for respiration than are the sternocleidomastoid muscles;[6, 20] electromyographic evidence supports a primary, not just an accessory inspiratory function.[4, 8] Scalenotomy causes an immediate decrease in the vital capacity, but considerable recovery occurs later.[6] When present, the scalenus minimus, too, should function as an accessory muscle of inspiration, which may explain its hypertrophy in some persons. The scalene muscles help to support and elevate the upper rib cage when one carries, lifts or pulls heavy objects, probably unnecessarily.

5. MYOTATIC UNIT

The scalene muscles on one side are synergistic with each other. The chief anatomical difference between the scalenus anterior and the scalenus medius is the anterior-posterior displacement of their attachments. The fibers of the scalenus posterior and scalenus minimus attach low on the neck post and lie more nearly horizontal than the other two muscles.

Elevation of the chest (vigorous inspiration) also is assisted by both divisions of the sternocleidomastoid muscle.

The upper trapezius,[6] levator scapulae, and omohyoid muscles are synergistic for elevation of the shoulder and help to lift the weight of the shoulder girdle off the chest wall. They assist the scalene muscles by relieving downward pressure on the thorax that would encumber inspiration. The pectoralis minor muscle also has a synergistic myotatic function with the scalene muscles for elevation of the ribs when the scapula is stabilized.[6]

The contralateral scalene muscles are antagonists for stabilization and lateral flexion of the neck.

6. SYMPTOMS

Referred pain from the scalene muscles, especially from the scalenus anterior, is very frequent among the shoulder and upper extremity pain syndromes.[20] Nearly half of several classes of physical therapy students had tender scalene muscles due to latent TPs on at least one side.[23] This is higher than the 11% prevalence reported by Sola et al.[34] in a population of Air Force inductees.

The scalenus anticus (anterior) syndrome was identified in early papers by pain in the anterior or posterior aspect of

the arm and at the upper medial border of the scapula, as well as by the tenderness of the muscle to palpation.[20, 22, 24] Later, Travell et al.[41] reported signs of venous obstruction, vasomotor changes and, if the syndrome was severe, evidence of arterial insufficiency and compression of the motor and sensory nerves of the affected arm. Ochsner et al.[24] attributed the symptoms of the syndrome to contraction and spasm of the muscle, which abnormally elevated the first rib. This was confirmed by the finding, in all operated cases, of an overdeveloped, spastic, and stiffened scalenus anterior muscle with sudden and marked descent of the first rib following surgical division of the muscle. We agree that this explains the neurovascular entrapment in many patients.

Relief of pain by infiltrating the scalene muscles was used by Adson[1] as a diagnostic test to distinguish the scalenus anterior syndrome from structural causes of cephalobrachialgia. After an initial wave of enthusiasm for scalenotomy following Adson's report, interest waned as emphasis shifted to the carpal tunnel syndrome and to radiculopathy from nerve root compression by a protruded cervical disc. As overenthusiasm for these diagnoses fades, the abundant evidence that the scalenus anterior tension causes serious compressive syndromes in many patients is gaining attention. The so-called "reflex" spasm of the scalenus anterior muscle that results from compression of a cervical nerve root may produce neurocirculatory signs that overshadow the typical clinical features of discogenic disease.[18]

On the other hand, entrapment of a muscle's nerve may activate TPs in the muscle. Scalene tautness, due to self-perpetuating myofascial TPs, is likely to persist following cervical disc surgery and also must be eliminated for lasting relief of symptoms.

The back, "shoulder," upper extremity, and chest pain patterns characteristic of scalene TPs are described in Section 1. When the patient complains of pain in the upper back just medial to the superior angle of the scapula, the most likely myofascial source is a scalene TP. Patients speak of their "shoulder" pain while rubbing the upper half of the arm. Sleep is often disturbed by pain; when night pain is severe, the patient is likely to sleep sit-

PART 2

ting up on a sofa, or propped up on pillows, for relief. This helps to prevent the shortening of the scalene muscles that occurs when the patient lies flat and the chest rides up around the neck.

Neurological symptoms of numbness and tingling in the hand (chiefly in the ulnar distribution) and the unexpected dropping of objects from the hand result from entrapment of the lower trunk of the brachial plexus as it leaves the thorax by hooking over the first rib.

Edema of the hand, when present, appears diffusely distal to the wrist, particularly over the bases of the four fingers and dorsum of the hand. Patients are likely to experience puffiness of the dorsum of the hand, stiffness of the fingers, and tightness of rings on fingers, especially in the morning on awakening. This is due to scalene TPs and may be caused by entrapment of the subclavian vein and/or lymph duct as they pass in front of the scalenus anterior. The puffiness disappears later in the day. The associated stiffness of the fingers is not due solely to the edema, but also to myofascial tautness of the finger extensors. A test for this stiffness is illustrated later in Fig. 20.6.

Scalene TP activity alone causes minimum restriction of neck rotation, whereas active TPs in the levator scapulae and splenius cervicis muscles markedly limit cervical rotation.

Differential Diagnosis

When taut and shortened, the anterior and middle scalene muscles are likely to entrap part of the brachial plexus at the thoracic outlet. Pain is then experienced on the *ulnar* side of the hand with dysesthesias and objective sensory impairment. However, pain referred from scalene TPs is experienced on the *radial* side of the forearm and hand, without objective sensory loss. When scalene TPs are very active, both referred and entrapment pain may be present.

The pain in the areas of the glenohumeral joint and the finger joints, pain that is referred from scalene TPs, easily leads to the misdiagnosis of rheumatic disease.[26]

The costoclavicular syndrome[11] is manifested when the patient retracts the shoulders in a military stance (brace) and compresses the neurovascular bundle between the clavicle and the first rib. The scapulocostal syndrome is discussed under Section 6, Chapter 19.

The pectoralis minor syndrome (hyperabduction syndrome) is reviewed in Chapter 43. Its neurovascular entrapment symptoms may be indistinguishable from those of scalene entrapment. The two sites of entrapment may coexist.

Symptoms of neurovascular compression at the thoracic outlet can be aggravated, or caused, by a cervical rib. Cervical ribs have been classified as (1) reaching some distance beyond the transverse process, but not to the first rib; (2) having a free end touching the first rib; (3) an almost complete rib, with a distinct fibrous band that connects the free end of the cervical rib to the cartilage of the first thoracic rib; and (4) a complete rib with a true cartilage that unites with that of the first thoracic rib.[1] Osseous ribs are identified by palpation and X-ray visualization. A cartilaginous cervical rib is suspected radiographically by a long C_7 vertebral transverse process that is at least as broad as the T_1 process.[1] Frequently, patients with cervical ribs are fearful of "pinching something" and, therefore, immobilize themselves; this aggravates their myofascial pain problems. These patients may, or may not, continue to have symptoms due to the cervical rib after myofascial TP activity has been eliminated.

Tension headache has been associated with TPs in the upper portion of the scalenus anterior.[20] In our experience, the pain is referred from secondary TPs in the sternocleidomastoid muscle, TPs which have developed as part of the myotatic unit of the scalene muscles.

The differential diagnosis of the scalenus anterior syndrome also should include the carpal tunnel syndrome, subacromial bursitis, incomplete supraspinatus tendon rupture, rotator cuff tendinitis, cervico-dorsal sympathalgia, Raynaud's disease, brachial neuritis,[24] cervical disc compression of nerve roots, a tumor in the neck, and intrathoracic disease.

7. ACTIVATION OF TRIGGER POINTS

Scalene TPs may be activated by *pulling or lifting*, especially with the hands at waist level, as in swinging a scythe, when hauling ropes in sailing, when handling and riding horses, in a tug-of-war, competitive swimming,[12] or in carrying awkwardly large objects; by overuse of these *accessory respiratory* muscles in paradoxical breathing, hard paroxysms of coughing due to pneumonia, bronchitis, asthma or emphysema, and quadraplegia; by sleeping with the *head and neck low* when the head of the bed is slightly lower or level with the foot of the bed (a thick rug placed only under the foot of the bed); by a *tilted shoulder-girdle axis* due to a short leg when standing, to a small hemipelvis when seated, due to loss of an upper extremity, or due to idiopathic scoliosis; by an awkward *leaning position* assumed when seated in order to compensate for short upper arms that do not reach the armrests of most chairs, or assumed because of an awkward positioning of the head.[40]

Scalene TPs are often activated secondary to TPs in the sternocleidomastoid muscle, with which the scalene muscles form a myotatic unit. The severe "stiff neck" syndrome of the levator scapulae muscle sometimes includes active scalene TPs.[39]

8. PATIENT EXAMINATION
(Figs. 20.4–20.6)

Patients with the scalene myofascial syndrome tend to move the arm and neck restlessly, as if trying to relieve a "sore" muscle. Lateral bending of the neck to the opposite side is usually restricted by at least 30°. Neck rotation is painful only at the extreme range of motion to the same side, especially when the chin is then dipped down toward the shoulder, as described below for the Scalene-cramp Test. Scalene involvement alone causes little or no restriction of motion at the glenohumeral joint, and pain is not significantly increased by tests of shoulder motion. However, abduction at the shoulder may be limited by associated TPs in the pectoral muscles.

Scalene-cramp Test
(Fig. 20.4)

To perform this test, the patient rotates the head fully to the side of the pain and actively pulls the chin down into the hol-

low above the clavicle by flexing the head (Fig. 20.4). This strongly contracts the scalene muscles, activates their TPs, and evokes their pattern of referred pain. If the patient is in severe pain at the time, the test may not be positive because the patient does not perceive the additional pain caused by the test. In this situation, the Scalene-relief Test (below) may be helpful.

Scalene-relief Test
(Fig. 20.5)

Referred pain of the scalenus anterior syndrome is relieved by elevation (flexion) of the arm and clavicle.[24] The Scalene-relief Test makes use of this fact. The patient places the painful forearm across the forehead while raising and pulling the shoulder *forward* to lift the clavicle off the underlying scalene muscles and brachial plexus (Fig. 20.5C). Pain relief, when it occurs, ensues within a few minutes. The two fingers in Fig. 20.5 *A* and *B* demonstrate how the test increases clearance behind the clavicle, relieving pressure on a taut and tender scalene "clothes line." None of the positions in Figure 20.5 should have any marked effect on pain due to cervical radiculopathy.

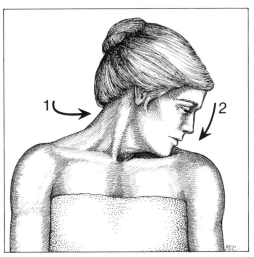

Figure 20.4. The Scalene-cramp Test elicits pain from active trigger points in the left scalene muscles. *1,* the head rotates fully to the left side. *2,* the chin dips into the hollow behind the clavicle. The pain caused by this hard contraction of scalene muscles with active trigger points is referred to a distance, as illustrated in Figure 20.1.

PART 2

Finger-Flexion Test
(Figure. 20.6)

To be valid, this test of finger flexion must be performed with the metacarpophalangeal (MCP) joints actively held straight, in full extension. This position requires forceful contraction of the extensor digitorum muscle, but the tightly closed fist does not. The test is normal when the fingertips can firmly touch the volar pads of the MCP joints (Fig. 20.6A). If one or more sections of the extensor digitorum muscle harbor active TPs, each corresponding finger fails to flex completely. Fig. 20.6B shows a positive test for TPs in the extensor of the index finger. Voluntary hyperextension of the MCP joints strongly loads the finger extensors, increasing the activity of these TPs. This TP activity apparently reflexly limits simultaneous end-finger flexion by reciprocal inhibition of the finger flexors.

The test also is positive when active TPs are present in the scalene muscles. In this case, all four fingertips fail to touch the

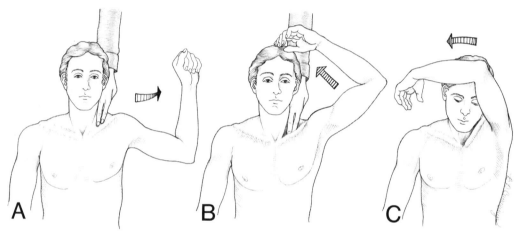

Figure 20.5.   The scalene-relief Test helps to identify the source of referred pain caused by clavicular pressure on active trigger points in the scalene muscles. *A,* fingers demonstrate tightness of the space between the clavicle and scalene muscles. *B,* the fingers demonstrate the increased clearance behind the clavicle provided by raising the shoulder and arm. *C,* clearance beneath the clavicle is maximized by swinging the shoulder forward, which protracts the scapula and pivots the clavicle forward and upward to fully relieve clavicular pressure on thoracic outlet structures. Pain relief by this test should occur within a few minutes.

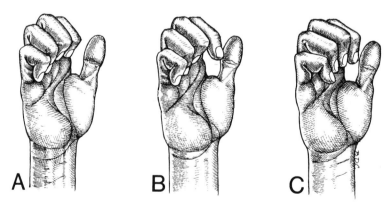

Figure 20.6.   Finger-flexion Test. *A,* normal. With the proximal phalanges extended, *all* fingertips press tightly against the metacarpophalangeal joints. *B,* positive extensor digitorum test. Incomplete index finger flexion indicates a trigger point in that part of the extensor digitorum muscle which attaches to the index finger, or in the extensor indicis. *C,* positive scalene test. Incomplete flexion of all fingers indicates more general involvement of the extensor digitorum muscle, which occurs when scalene trigger points are active on the same side.

palm (Fig. 20.6C). However, there is no difficulty in making a tight fist, when the MCP joints are allowed to flex. Apparently, TPs in the extensor digitorum communis are activated secondarily, as satellite TPs, because they lie within the pain reference zone of primary scalene TPs.

A positive test is not simply due to edema, since this test of the function of the finger muscles is frequently restored to normal immediately after stretch and spray of the involved scalene muscles. Furthermore, edema is more likely to occur only with involvement of the scalenus anterior, whereas TPs in any of the scalene muscles that are actively referring pain and tenderness to the forearm may be responsible for an abnormal Finger-flexion Test.

Other Tests

A positive response to any of the above three tests helps to establish a primary myofascial component of the patient's pain. The Adson manuever[1, 5] helps to identify a neurovascular component of the patient's symptoms. Adson's original description called for the patient to take a long breath, elevate his chin, and turn it to the affected side, while seated upright, arms resting on the knees. This maximally elevated the first rib, compressing the neurovascular bundle against the elevated rib and the taut muscle. A diminution or obliteration of the radial pulse, or a change in blood pressure, established a positive test. Initially called the "Vascular Test," a positive response was considered a strong indication for scalenotomy.[1]

The military stance (or military brace) produces neurovascular effects due to costoclavicular compression, or due to further tension on an already taut, constricting pectoralis minor muscle.

Cervical Rib

A cervical rib is a well known nonmyofascial source of the thoracic outlet compression syndrome. This additional rib is palpated at the level of the clavicle as a bulge where one would expect to find the groove between the anterior and middle scalene muscles, where the rib extends toward them from the transverse process. The rib appears in the triangle between the neck and the clavicle, leaving a narrow gap through which to palpate the first rib. An osseous rib is confirmed by visualization in an X-ray film. The presence of a cartilaginous cervical rib is suggested radiographically by an abnormally wide and long C_7 transverse process (as long or longer than that of T_1).

9. TRIGGER POINT EXAMINATION (Figs. 20.7 and 20.8)

In the authors' experience, the scalene muscles harbor active TPs in the following order of frequency: anterior, middle, posterior, and minimus. The TPs in the scalenus anterior are found by palpating the muscle beneath the posterior border of the clavicular division of the sternocleidomastoid muscle (Fig. 20.7). The posterior sternocleidomastoid border is approximated by locating and occluding the external jugular vein with finger pressure just above the clavicle (Fig. 20.8A). This vein usually crosses the scalenus anterior muscle at about the level of its active TPs. The groove between the anterior and middle scalene muscles is distinguishable at Erb's point, in the space behind the clavicle, where the pulsating subclavian artery passes between these two muscles and crosses over the first rib (Fig. 20.7). The fingers of one hand straddle the scalenus anterior to establish its location, while the other hand palpates and precisely localizes taut bands and TP tenderness and induces referred pain.(Fig. 20.8B).

The scalenus medius lies deep, anterior to the free border of the upper trapezius (Fig. 20.7). It can be palpated against the posterior tubercles of the transverse processes of the vertebrae.

The scalenus posterior is more difficult to reach. It lies more horizontal than, and dorsal to, the scalenus medius. It passes beneath the levator scapulae, which must be pushed aside at the point where the levator scapulae emerges from beneath the anterior free border of the upper trapezius (Fig. 20.7).

Scalenus minimus TP activity is usually discovered only after inactivation of TPs in the other scalene muscles. Involvement of this variable muscle is then recognized by residual tenderness deep to the midportion of the scalenus anterior (see Section 2).

A scalene TP is located by the ropy

PART 2

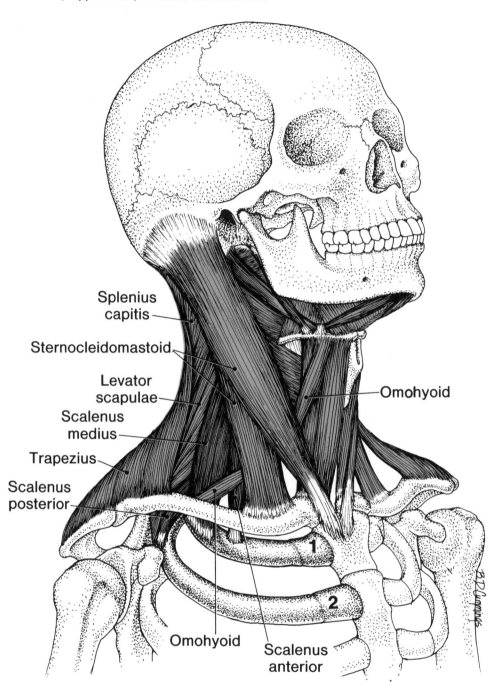

Figure 20.7. Neighboring muscles (*medium red*) that are useful landmarks in locating the scalene muscles (*dark red*).

feeling of the band of muscle in which it lies; by exquisite tenderness, which is greatest at the TP; and by the characteristic referred pain that sustained pressure on the TP usually evokes. Scalene local twitch responses are seldom visible.

Whenever active scalene TPs are present, the area on the chest just below the clavicle in the middle of the infraclavicular fossa is tender to pressure. This **Scalene Test point** overlies, or is slightly medial to, the pectoralis minor muscle. The sensitivity to pressure may be due solely to referred tenderness from the scalene TPs, or it may be related to TPs in the pectoralis musculature. If the pectoral muscles are

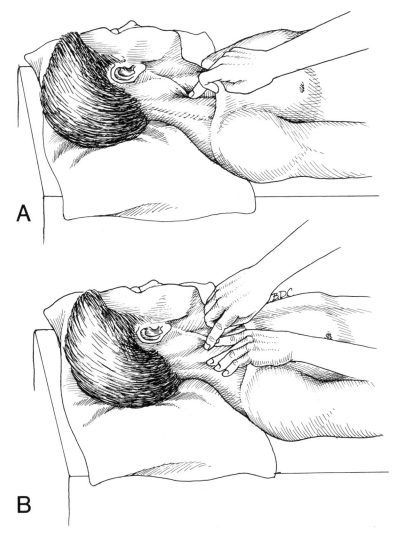

Figure 20.8. Palpation of the anterior and middle scalene muscles. *A*, the posterior border of the clavicular division of the sternocleidomastoid muscle is identified by palpation. The external jugular vein is occluded so that it stands out and can be pressed aside to expose the anterior border of the scalenus anterior at the level of its usual TPs. *B*, fingers of the left hand straddle both the scalenus anterior and scalenus medius muscles. The right index finger approaches the groove between these two muscles at the level of the upper TP in the scalenus medius.

not involved, this spot tenderness promptly disappears following elimination of scalene TP activity.

Omohyoid Muscle

When this muscle develops TPs and becomes tense, it can act as a constricting band across the brachial plexus.[34] Because the tense muscle stands out prominently when the head is tilted to the other side, it is easily mistaken for the upper trapezius or a scalene muscle. When the omohyoid

harbors TPs, it can prevent full stretch of the trapezius and scalene muscles, and therefore also must be released.

10. ENTRAPMENTS
(Fig. 20.9)

Myofascial Thoracic Outlet Compression

The brachial plexus and subclavian artery emerge from the thorax through the thoracic outlet between the scalenus anterior and scalenus medius muscles. The

PART 2

slit-like opening of the outlet is formed at its upper end by the separation of the anterior and posterior tubercles of the transverse processes, since the scalenus anterior fibers attach to the anterior tubercles and the scalenus medius fibers attach to the posterior tubercles. Each cervical root emerges beneath and between the tubercles. At the exit of the thoracic outlet, the subclavian artery and the lower trunk together emerge across the first rib between the attachments of these two sca-

lene muscles onto the first rib (Fig. 20.9), behind and below the clavicle. The subclavian artery may occasionally pass through and divide the scalenus anterior muscle.

Scalene-produced entrapments in the region of the thoracic outlet may involve the nerves, arteries, veins, and lymph ducts. Clinically, one observes that, as the scalenus anterior becomes taut and shortened due to TP activity, the muscle is more likely to entrap the subclavian vein than the subclavian artery, and it is likely

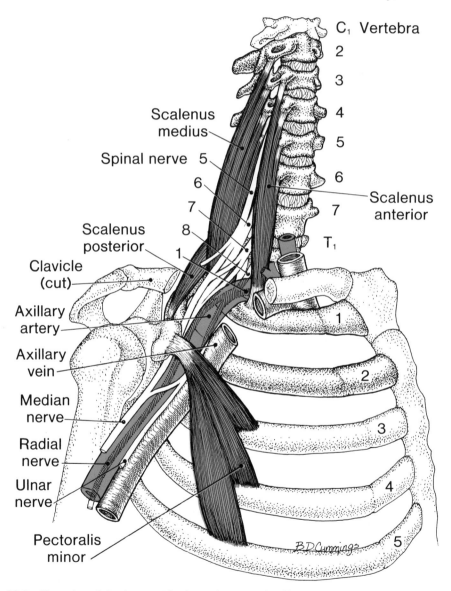

Figure 20.9. Thoracic outlet entrapment by the scalene muscles. The neurovascular bundle is spread out to show the relations of its component parts. A portion of the clavicle has been removed. The brachial plexus and axillary artery emerge above the first rib and behind the clavicle between the scalenus anterior and scalenus medius muscles. The spinal nerves are numbered on the *left*, the vertebrae on the *right*. The T$_1$ nerve lies dorsal to and beneath the subclavian artery.

also to cause pressure on the lower trunk of the brachial plexus. When the scalenus medius develops TPs and becomes taut, it entraps chiefly the lower trunk of the plexus.

Nerve Compression

The brachial plexus emerges between the anterior and middle scalene muscles, then passes downward across the rib attachment of the scalenus medius (Fig. 20.9). The scalene syndrome of brachial plexus compression leads to neuropathy with neurological signs and symptoms chiefly in the ulnar distribution.[19, 27, 41] Entrapment of the lower trunk of the brachial plexus affects nearly all fibers of the ulnar nerve, and some fibers of the median nerve. Patients with this lower trunk compression complain chiefly of numbness, tingling, and dysesthesias in the 4th and 5th digits, ulnar side of the hand, and occasionally of the forearm. Patients show mild hypoesthesia to light touch, pinprick and temperature change in the little finger.

The lower trunk is formed from spinal nerves C_8 and T_1. The T_1 nerve exits the spinal foramen between the first and second thoracic vertebrae, and courses cephalad to hook over the first rib where its fibers and those of the C_8 spinal nerve are wedged between the subclavian artery and the rib attachment of the scalenus medius. When TP activity in the scalenus anterior or medius elevates the first rib, fibers of the lower trunk must angulate more sharply over it. This angulation also wedges the subclavian artery more tightly against the lower trunk.

The Adson manuever (see Section 8) tests the susceptibility of the neurovascular bundle to compression by tensing the anterior scalene most strongly and by elevating the first rib. A variation of the original test, done by rotating the face toward the unaffected side, is more likely to be positive if the scalenus medius or posterior muscle is involved, than if the scalenus anterior is tautened. Identification of which muscles are involved is easily confirmed by palpating each for TPs.

Another type of nerve entrapment produced by the scalenus medius is the pressure exerted by taut TP bands when spinal nerves C_5 and C_6 pierce the scalenus medius instead of passing between it and the scalenus anterior.[13]

Electrodiagnostically, the junior author finds that the compression of the lower trunk caused by scalene TPs slows conduction at the site of entrapment with a variable degree of slowing of the ulnar motor conduction velocity through the Erb's point-to-axilla segment. The distal ulnar sensory latency and ulnar F-wave latency are consistently prolonged. These nerve conduction signs, and the rare finding of spontaneous potentials on needle electromyography of the ulnar-innervated muscles at rest, indicate that this myofascial entrapment usually causes a degree of neuropraxia (loss of conduction only at the site of compression), but rarely axonotmesis (axonal degeneration).

Venous or Lymphatic Obstruction

Edema of the fingers and dorsum of the hand, associated with entrapment of the subclavian vein and/or lymph drainage due to scalene TPs, was noted above in Section 6. Impairment of venous return is due to compression of the subclavian vein by the firm, shortened scalenus anterior muscle behind it, the first rib below it, and the clavicle in front of it. The lymphatics of the upper extremity drain through the subclavian trunk to enter the venous circulation via the thoracic duct at the junction of the internal jugular and subclavian veins,[13] or indirectly into the jugular lymphatic trunk.[16] This lymph channel, the subclavian trunk, is as susceptible as the subclavian vein to compression by a taut scalenus anterior muscle since it, too, must squeeze through the same narrow space in front of the muscle between the first rib and the clavicle. Of the three structures surrounding the space through which the subclavian vein passes, only the scalenus anterior has resilience, which it loses when the muscle develops TPs. Shortening of either the anterior or middle scalene muscles by TP activity tends to lift the first rib against the clavicle, intensifying compression of the vein (Fig. 20.9).

Reflex suppression of peristaltic contractions of the lymph duct due to scalene TP activity may contribute to the edema.

Arterial Compression

Entrapment of the axillary artery is more often due to TP activity and tautness of the pectoralis minor (see Chapter 43) than to TP activity of the scalene muscles.

PART 2

The artery also may be entrapped by cos-toclavicular compression, which is often aggravated by poor posture. Since pectoralis TPs are likely to be associated with scalene TPs, the arterial flow may suffer a double entrapment: where the subclavian artery emerges from the thorax wedged between the first rib and the tendon of the scalenus anterior, and where the axillary artery hooks beneath the pectoralis minor muscle (Fig. 20.9).

Angulation and compression of the neurovascular bundle is greatly aggravated by extension of the bundle over a cervical rib.

11. ASSOCIATED TRIGGER POINTS

The scalenus anterior and medius muscles are often involved together. If the scalenus minimus harbors active TPs, all four scalene muscles usually are affected. The sternocleidomastoid muscle, which is also an important part of the myotatic unit for accessory inspiration, is likely to become involved if the scalene TPs have been active for a considerable period of time.

Active TPs in the scalenus medius have been reported in association with TPs in the upper trapezius, sternocleidomastoid and splenius capitis muscles.[44]

Satellite TPs may develop in several of the areas to which the scalene muscles refer pain. Both the pectoralis major and minor muscles commonly develop TPs in regions that correspond to the scalene pattern of anterior chest pain. Satellite TPs in the long head of the triceps brachii correspond to the scalene pattern of posterior arm pain. Although the dorsal forearm is a less common site of scalene pain, secondary TPs tend to develop in the brachioradialis, extensores carpi radialis and extensor digitorum muscles.

When TPs in the lateral part of the brachialis muscle are induced as satellites of scalene TPs, both the brachialis and scalene muscles refer pain to the thumb, making this digit especially painful.

12. STRETCH AND SPRAY
(Fig. 20.10)

If the patient is treated in the seated position, the operator first makes sure that the pelvic- and shoulder-girdle axes are level. A small hemipelvis is corrected by a butt lift under the small side to straighten the spine and level the patient's shoulders. This is essential for relaxation of overloaded neck muscles. The patient slides the hips forward slightly on the chair seat, leans back comfortably against the backrest, and hooks the fingers under the seat of the chair to anchor the scapula and rib cage on the side to be stretched. The other arm may rest in the lap or on the armrest, hand limp (Fig. 20.10). The patient is encouraged to relax and let the shoulders drop.

In an alternate approach, the patient lies supine with instructions to do passive self-stretch of the scalene muscles as described for the Side-bending Neck Exercise in Section 14 (see Fig. 20.12). At the same time, the spray is applied as described below, over the scalene muscle being stretched and then over the full referred pain pattern. This position makes it more difficult to spray the upper back and scapular pain reference zone, but usually provides more relaxation and effective stretch, and also trains the patient in the self-stretch technique for home use.

Scalenus Anterior

To stretch this muscle after a few initial sweeps of spray, the head and neck of the seated patient is tilted toward the opposite side and the head is pressed in a posterolateral direction. Meanwhile, the vapocoolant is applied along the lines of the scalenus anterior fibers and over the referred pain pattern of the chest (Fig. 20.10A). Then the spray again is swept over the muscle to the front and back of the arm and continued downward to include the thumb and index finger (Fig. 20.10B). Finally, the spray is again directed downward over the muscle and continued over the upper back to cover the referred pain area around the upper and medial borders of the scapula.

Scalenus Medius and Scalenus Posterior

To stretch the scalenus medius, the seated patient's head and neck are turned and tilted as for the scalenus anterior, but the head and neck are now pressed toward the contralateral shoulder (Fig. 20.10B). To stretch the scalenus posterior, the head and neck are not turned, and are pressed in an anterolateral direction along the lines

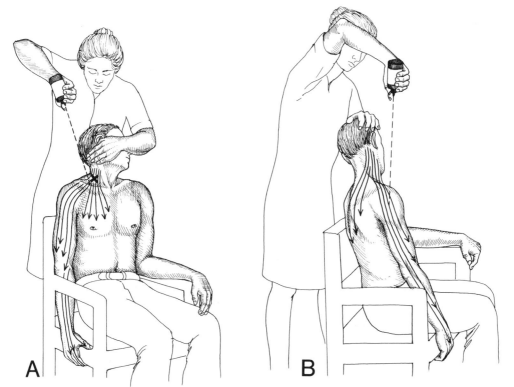

Figure 20.10. Stretch positions and spray pattern for the right scalene muscles. *A*, front view of the stretch position for the scalenus anterior showing the anterior part of the spray pattern. *B*, side view of the stretch position for the scalenus medius with pressure applied toward the opposite shoulder, showing the posterior part of the spray pattern. The total spray pattern should be used for each of these muscles. The patient's stabilizing hand is moved to the front of the seat bottom if this facilitates relaxation.

of the scalenus posterior fibers. If the patient's head is cradled between the operator's hand and body, vertical neck traction can be applied simultaneously. This feeling of support and the release of pressure on cervical structures usually helps the patient to relax the neck muscles.

The spray follows the direction of the muscle fibers being stretched. As a scalene muscle is covered with parallel sweeps of the spray, sweeps are carried over the pain reference zones of each of the three scalene muscles, concentrating especially on those areas where the patient has been experiencing spontaneous pain. However, a greater range of neck motion, and therefore more complete and lasting relief, usually occurs if *all* parts of the composite referred pain pattern (Fig. 20.1) are vapocooled. Stretch and spray are followed at once with hot packs.

Tenderness at the scalene test point below the clavicle, described in Section 9,

should have disappeared with *complete* release of the scalene muscles, if the pectoralis major or minor are not also involved.

To fully lengthen the scalene muscles, it is often necessary, first, to release parallel muscles that are tautened by TPs and which also restrict side bending of the neck. One must consider the upper trapezius and both the clavicular and sternal divisions of the sternocleidomastoid muscle. Less frequently, a tense omohyoid muscle stands out under the skin like a rope as it stretches over other neck structures to attach on the acromion. The omohyoid is stretched by tilting the head to the opposite side and retracting the scapula while applying downsweeps of spray over the muscle. Adson relieved pain and dysesthesia resulting from pressure on the brachial plexus due to this taut band of muscle by surgically sectioning the omohyoid.[1]

Stretch and spray of the scalene muscles should be applied bilaterally to avoid activating latent TPs that might cause reactive cramping on the untreated side. Stretching a muscle on one side of the neck post causes unaccustomed sudden shortening of its partner on the other side. This shortening may activate latent TPs in the partner. If such new and severe contralateral pain ensues, it should be treated by immediate stretch and spray of the reacting shortened muscles.

As a rule, patients sleep most comfortably lying on the side of the involved scalene muscles. If TPs in the posterior scapular musculature, e.g. the infraspinatus, prevent this, these TPs must be inactivated so that the patient can sleep comfortably on the preferred side.

13. INJECTION AND STRETCH
(Fig. 20.11)

Scalenus Anterior and Medius

Long[20] recommended injection with procaine for relief of myofascial pain due to TPs in the scalene muscles. A recent study did not find the pain relief obtained by infiltrating the scalenus anterior with 1.0% lidocaine helpful in predicting the results of scalenotomy[29]. However, the final therapeutic effect of the injection was not studied, and injection was not directed specifically to TPs.

For injection of TPs in the anterior and middle scalene muscles, the patient should lie supine and turn the head slightly away from the side to be injected (Fig. 20.11). Both the head and the shoulder on the side of the TPs are elevated slightly by a pillow to slacken the sternocleidomastoid and trapezius muscles. The most common TP in the scalenus anterior is found either under, or slightly anterior to the external jugular vein (Fig. 20.8). The operator's free hand presses the clavicular division of the sternocleidomastoid muscle and jugular vein aside, and palpates the tense muscular bands for tender points that reproduce the patient's pain complaint. Several individual muscle bands that contain active TPs are usually palpable. A band is pinned down between the index and middle fingers to localize it for injection and to provide hemostasis during and after injection. The needle is inserted well above the apex of the lung, which ordinarily extends about 2.5 cm (1 in) above the clavicle.[13] *All scalene injections are made at least 3.8 cm (1½ in) above the clavicle.* The underlying transverse processes are identified and the needle angled up toward them (Fig. 20.11). Active scalene TPs are found as high as

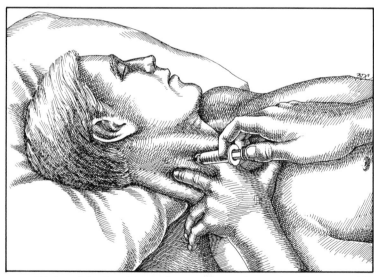

Figure 20.11.   Injection of the scalenus medius, patient supine. Fingers straddle the middle scalene muscle with the index finger in the groove between the scaleni anterior and medius muscles to locate the brachial plexus. The needle is directed toward the dorsal side of a cervical transverse process to avoid the nerve plexus.

PART 2

halfway between the clavicle and the mastoid process.

The vertical groove between the anterior and middle scalene muscles is identified, and the needle kept on either side of it to avoid the brachial plexus. Farther cephalad, at the level where one injects the scalene TPs, the groove is often more difficult to clearly distinguish unless one has followed it up from the first rib. Two fingers straddle the muscle to be injected. The needle is angled in front of (ventral to) the groove to inject the scalenus anterior and behind (dorsal to) it to inject the scalenus medius.

As seen from the operator's side view of the neck, if the needle strays too deep, too caudad, and a little too far in front, the stellate ganglion or sympathetic trunk may be anesthetized, producing a transient Horner's syndrome. The stellate ganglion usually lies ventral to the origin of the first rib at the junction of its head and neck.[15]

The roots of spinal nerves C_4 to C_7 and the lower trunk of the brachial plexus emerge through the slit between the anterior and middle scalene muscles and then cross in front of the lower portion of the scalenus medius (Fig. 20.9). Care and patience are needed to inject the TPs in the multiple thin bands of involved scalenus medius muscle above the level of these nerves. The patient should be warned of possible transient numbness and weakness of the arm due to infiltration of the nerve trunks by the local anesthetic. Scalene TPs often refer sharp intense pain to the arm and hand when penetrated by the needle; this symptom need not be due to needle contact with nerve fibers. A 2.5-cm (1-in), 23- or 24-gauge needle may be used. After injection, pressure is maintained for hemostasis; bleeding within the scalene muscles causes local irritation and marked afterpain.

Scalenus Posterior

To inject the scalenus posterior, the patient lies on the opposite side with the back toward the operator and the face turned slightly to slacken the upper trapezius, which is pushed aside (Fig. 20.7 shows why); the technique is similar to that described by Kraus.[19] The levator scapulae muscle is located as it emerges

from beneath the trapezius at the root of the neck (Fig. 20.7). The scalenus posterior is then found just beneath and anterior to the levator scapulae. The scalenus posterior TPs are approached from behind. Because of its submerged position among other muscles, a 22-gauge, 3.8-cm (1½-in) needle is used. To avoid introducing the needle between the ribs, it is directed tangential to them and medially. The scalenus posterior can be injected readily through the same skin puncture as that used to inject the upper TP of the levator scapulae. When a scalenus posterior TP is encountered, the patient usually reports pain referred to the region of the triceps brachii muscle.

For TPs in any of these scalene muscles, injection is followed by stretch and spray, a hot moist pack, and active side-bending movements to full range on both sides, while the patient is supine.

Scalenus Minimus

The scalenus minimus TPs, as a rule, are not inactivated by stretch and spray. Local injection is indicated if local tenderness and referred pain characteristic of TPs in the scalenus minimus persist and the other scalene muscles are free of TPs. The minimus may be injected through the same skin puncture that is used for the lower TP of the scalenus anterior. The needle is inserted at least 3.5 cm (1½-2 in) above the clavicle, straight in rather than upward, through the scalenus anterior toward a transverse process. The needle passes through the empty space above the subclavian artery before it encounters the scalenus minimus muscle. A 3.8-cm (1½-in), 23-gauge needle is used. Following the injection, stretch and spray, and a hot pack are applied.

14. CORRECTIVE ACTIONS
(Figs. 20.12 and 20.13)

In most patients, multiple factors contribute to the activation and reactivation of scalene TPs. Elimination of one factor may result in some improvement. Identification and correction of all major causal factors, together with local treatment of the affected muscles, in our experience, provides lasting relief.

PART 2

PART 2

Bed Elevation

The head of the patient's bed is raised by placing blocks, 8 or 9 cm (3–3½-in) high, under the legs at the head-end of the bed to tilt the bed frame. Additional correction is required if a rug lies under the foot-end, but not under the head of the bed.

The bed frame tilted with the head up prevents the chest from riding up around the neck at night and creates mild steady traction on the scalene muscles. If the chest rides up, these muscles are placed in a cramped position of sustained shortening, which impedes venous drainage and lymph flow, as evidenced by hand edema in the morning. Usually, scalene TPs can *not be permanently extinguished* without this elevation of the head of the bed.

The patient may sleep on two pillows to try to obtain the same effect, or to improve "sinus drainage." The result is increased pain; two pillows do elevate the patient's head, but also flex the neck, which creates anterior scalene shortening and aggravates scalene TP symptoms.

Pillow

The patient should use only one soft comfortable pillow of the right thickness to keep the head and neck in a neutral position. The corner of the pillow is bunched up between the neck and shoulder when the patient lies on the affected side, to prevent tilting of the head and sustained shortening of the involved scalene muscles.

A foam rubber pillow should be discarded. The jiggle of the head and neck on a springy pillow aggravates scalene TPs. The patient with allergies may select a foam rubber pillow to avoid allergenic fillers, and should be warned against this. Sensitive patients may wish to carry their "safe" home pillow with them on trips.

When lying on the back, the patient should pull the corner of the pillow forward between the shoulder and the cheek on each side. This insures that the shoulder rests on the bed, not on the pillow, and that the cervical spine is in line with the thoracic spine. This pillow position supports the head in the midline, and encourages bilateral scalene relaxation (see Fig. 7.7A).

Body Warmth

Chilling the body, especially when resting, reduces peripheral blood flow and can lead to increased skeletal muscle irritability. In bed, an electric blanket is invaluable. It is helpful in the living room, also, when sitting or lying on a sofa in cold climates, during inclement weather, or when the thermostat is set low.

If the bedroom is drafty, a high-necked sweater or warm scarf should be worn in bed. Such neck protection is often helpful on airplane flights.

The patient should apply a moist heating pad over the scalene TPs on the front of the neck for 10–15 min before going to sleep at night.

Seating and Lighting

The patient should provide and use an appropriate elbow rest, especially on the affected side, when sitting and reading, writing, sewing, driving, riding in a car, or telephoning. The telephone receiver should be held in the hand on the unaffected side, with occasional change of hands (not ears) on long calls. An executive (speaker) phone eliminates the problem of holding the telephone receiver for a long time. Use of the shoulder to hold the handset is not recommended for these patients.

The light should shine directly on reading material from overhead and *not* from the affected side, causing the head to be turned that way. For those who read in bed, a light that clips on the head of the bed or is attached anywhere overhead may be essential to recovery.

Stretch Exercises

Also critical to recovery of many of these scalene patients is daily passive stretching of their scalene muscles at home, by doing the Side-bending Neck Exercise (Fig. 20.12). With the patient lying supine, first the shoulder of the side to be stretched is lowered and anchored by placing the hand under the buttock (Fig. 20.12A). The patient must learn to reach across to the ear with the hand of the opposite side, pulling the head and neck so as to tilt it to the opposite side, while concentrating on relaxation of the neck

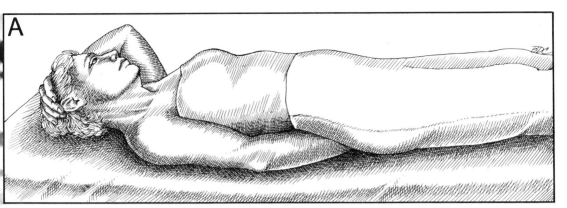

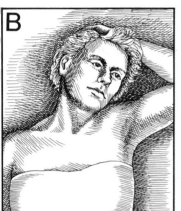
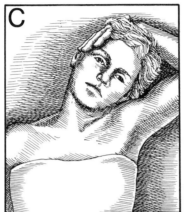
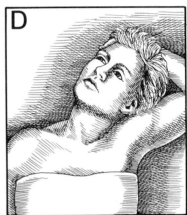

Figure 20.12. The Side-bending Neck Exercise is performed bilaterally, with the patient supine. Each position passively stretches one of the three major scalene muscles. The exercise should always be done bilaterally. *A*, the hand on the side to be stretched is anchored under the buttock. *B*, to stretch the scalenus posterior, the face is turned toward the direction of pull. *C*, the face looks forward to stretch the scalenus medius. *D*, the face is turned away from the direction of pull to stretch the scalenus anterior.

muscles. The ear is pulled smoothly down toward the shoulder, while the degree of head rotation determines which of the three major scalene muscles is placed on stretch.

To stretch the scalenus posterior (Fig. 20.12B), the patient turns the face toward the pulling arm. To stretch the scalenus anterior, the patient turns the face away from the pulling arm. For the scalenus medius, the patient looks straight up at the ceiling, or slightly toward the pulling arm. The patient concentrates the stretch on those directions in which the muscles feel tightest and holds each stretch for a slow count of six to give the stretched muscles time to release, and to take up any slack that develops. The head is returned to the neutral mid-position. A pause, with deep abdominal breathing between each pas-

sive stretch, helps to reestablish complete muscular relaxation. The exercise should always be done bilaterally. It is more effective if performed after a hot pack across the front of the neck has warmed the skin over the scalene muscles for 10–15 min.

An effective active scalene exercise is the Scalene-cramp Test (Fig. 20.4), which provides true rotation without lateral bending or tilting. The head is turned as far as it can rotate to one side and the chin then dipped to the shoulder. The head is returned to neutral, and the patient breathes deeply. The cycle is repeated in the opposite direction. This alternately stretches and actively contracts the scalene muscles. About four cycles are performed daily. This is useful as an active range of motion follow-up to the passive Side-bending Neck Exercise.

Respiration
(Fig. 20.13)

Paradoxical respiration is a common source of abuse and overload of the scalene muscles and is frequently used by patients who avoid abdominal protrusion to improve the appearance of their figure. They often complain that they are "always out of breath," or that they "run out of breath" when talking on the telephone.

Contraction of the diaphragm pushes the abdominal contents down toward the pelvis, causing protrusion of the abdomen and increased lung volume in the lower chest during inhalation. Normal resting inhalation coordinates contraction of the diaphragm with expansion of the *lower* thorax and elevation of the rib cage, all of which increase lung volume. In paradoxical respiration, these chest and abdominal functions oppose each other; the patient exhales with the diaphragm while inhaling with the thoracic muscles, and *vice versa*. Consequently, a normal effort produces inadequate tidal volume, and the accessory respiratory muscles of the *upper* chest, including the scalene muscles, overwork to exchange sufficient air. This muscular overload results from the failure to coordinate the different parts of the respiratory apparatus.

The patient who breathes paradoxically must learn to synchronize abdominal and chest breathing if they are to relieve the scalene overload (Fig. 20.13). To do this, the supine patient breathes through the open mouth, with one hand placed on the abdomen and one on the chest, and identifies the paradoxical pattern while taking a deep breath (Fig. 20.13*A*). This paradoxical pattern moves air between the upper and lower chest, but moves little through the airway. To learn abdominal breathing, the patient exhales fully with one hand on the chest and the other on the abdomen (Fig. 20.13*B*). Abdominal respiration alone is most easily learned if the patient holds the chest fixed in the collapsed, rather than the expanded position (Fig. 20.13*C*), and concentrates on breathing by alternately contracting the diaphragm and abdominal muscles without expanding the upper chest, or elevating the sternum. It may help the patient to think of expanding the "lateral bellows" (the lateral T_{10}, T_{11}, T_{12} rib cage), which expands during full diaphragmatic inspiration. When this is achieved, the patient then learns to coordinate both costal and diaphragmatic respiration during inhalation (Fig. 20.13*D*) and exhalation (Fig. 20.13*B*). The patient should note the closeness of the hands during exhalation and their separation during inhalation; the hands move up and down *together*. Positional feedback from the hands is often needed for a patient to learn this technique.

The patient should practice *coordinated* breathing at intervals throughout the day and on retiring. Taking each breath to the count of 4 "in," and a count of 4 "out," then a pause, "hold-and-relax" for a count of 4 improves pacing and provides rhythm. The patient should become aware of using this coordinated breathing throughout the day.

Two additional training techniques can be useful. To reinforce coordinated chest and abdominal breathing while sitting upright, the patient sits in a chair with a firm flat seat, slowly rolls forward on the seat by tilting the front of the hips down (exaggerating the lumbar lordosis), and draws in a slow deep breath. This separates the anterior chest from the symphysis pubis, making it easy and natural to contract the diaphragm and protrude the abdomen while inspiring. Then, by rocking backward on the hips (abdominal curl movement) during slow exhalation, the lumbosacral spine approaches kyphosis which closes the anterior abdominal opening and automatically forces the abdominal contents inward and up against the diaphragm, assisting diaphragmatic relaxation.

If the patient is unable to grasp the concept of abdominal breathing, strapping a belt tightly around the upper chest while the patient does the exercise illustrated in Fig. 20.13*C*, helps to enforce diaphragmatic respiration only, so that the patient learns to recognize what that movement feels like. More simply, lying prone on a firm surface inhibits chest breathing and assures predominantly abdominal respiration.

Some means must be found to teach synchronized respiration.

Muscle Strain

Body Asymmetry. The tilted shoulder-girdle axis, caused by the functional scoliosis associated with a short leg and/or a

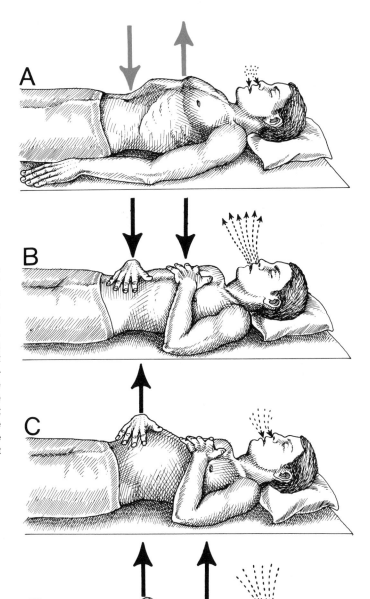

PART 2

Figure 20.13. Learning normal, instead of paradoxical respiration. The patient is trained to become aware of the respiratory mechanism by feeling the position and movement of the hands. *A*, erroneous paradoxical breathing (*red arrows*): abdomen in, chest out. *B*, first step, complete exhalation. *C*, then inhalation, using the diaphragm only by protruding the abdomen and keeping the chest collapsed. *D*, finally, synchronize deep respiration by moving the chest and abdomen in and out together.

small hemipelvis, places chronic strain on the scalene muscles, which must help to straighten the neck tilt in order to level the eyes. An uncorrected leg length or pelvic discrepancy of as little as 1 cm (⅜ in), sometimes less, can perpetuate scalene TPs despite all other efforts in management. For identification and correction of these asymmetries, see Chapter 4 and Section 14 in Chapter 48.

Body Mechanics. The patient must avoid carrying awkward packages that require lifting with the arms extended out in front, or hauling, pulling or tugging strenuously. Whenever undertaking any such vigorous effort, the patient must learn to reduce consciously the neck-muscle tension caused by elevating the shoulders and projecting the head forward. Scalene strain due to increasing intra-abdominal pressure when closing the glottis, as when straining during lifting or defecation, may be reduced by panting through the open mouth and dropping the shoulders, which protects the scalene muscles.

When turning over in bed, the patient should *roll* the head without lifting it off the pillow.

Appropriate medical management should be employed to reduce excessive demands on the auxiliary muscles of respiration caused by coughing and sneezing, e.g. in patients with bronchitis, pneumonia, emphysema, asthma, sinusitis, and allergic rhinitis. Severe attacks of coughing may be controlled with adequate antitussive medication and by teaching the patient to suppress the cough reflex.

The patient with active scalene TPs, who has been instructed to do the In-doorway Stretch Exercise (see Fig. 42.10) because of active TPs in other muscles, should start with the arms-high position and avoid the arms-down position until the scalene muscles are TP and symptom free.

Postural Strain. The lower rims of eyeglasses often occlude the line of vision for writing or reading when the head is held in the balanced erect position. The person then tilts the head forward and down to see clearly over the lower rims, causing persistent shortening of the anterior neck muscles and strain of the posterior neck muscles. The correction for this, by tilting the plane of the eyeglasses, is illustrated in Fig. 16.4.

Patients with active scalene TPs who have a unilateral hearing impairment are often refractory to treatment because they persistently rotate the head and neck to face the "good ear" toward the speaker. The patient should turn the body, not just the head, and should take other measures to improve the hearing (e.g. a hearing aid), if possible.

Cervical Rib

The patient with a cervical rib is especially prone to develop entrapments and pain due to TPs in the scalene muscles. This condition can sometimes be managed conservatively by eliminating the increased scalene tension due to TP activity. Then the patient should be encouraged to engage in normal, but reasonable, physical activities. Many patients suffer needless disability due to constant guarding for fear of neurovascular compression by the extra rib, which sometimes can be relieved by restoring full scalene muscle length.

The patient with a cervical rib should do the In-doorway Stretch Exercise (see Fig. 42.10) only with the hands in the high position, never with the hands in the horizontal or low positions, to avoid momentary compression of the neurovascular bundle across the extra rib.

References

1. Adson AW: Cervical ribs: symptoms, differential diagnosis and indications for section of the insertion of the scalenus anticus muscle. *J Int College Surg* 16:546–559, 1951 (p. 548).
2. Bardeen CR: The Musculature. Sect. 5. In *Morris's Human Anatomy*, edited by C.M. Jackson, Ed. 6. Blakiston's Son & Co., Philadelphia, 1921 (p. 388).
3. *Ibid.* (p. 389).
4. Basmajian JV: *Muscles Alive. Their Functions Revealed by Electromyography*, Ed. 4. Williams & Wilkins, Baltimore, 1978 (p. 340, 356).
5. Cailliet, R: *Soft Tissue Pain and Disability*, F.A. Davis, Philadelphia, 1977 (p. 144).
6. Campbell EJM: Accessory muscles. In *The Respiratory Muscles: Mechanics and Neural Control*, edited by E.J.M. Campbell, E. Agostoni, J.N. Davis, Ed. 2. W.B. Saunders, Philadelphia, 1970 (pp. 181–183, 186).
7. Duchenne GB: *Physiology of Motion*, translated by E.B. Kaplan. J.B. Lippincott, Philadelphia, 1949 (p. 511).
8. *Ibid.* (pp. 479–480).
9. Eisler P: *Die Muskeln des Stammes*. Gustav Fischer, Jena, 1912 (pp. 308–310, Figs. 39, 40).
10. *Ibid.* (Fig. 41).
11. Falconer MA, Weddell G: Costoclavicular compression of the subclavian artery and vein, relation to the scalenus anticus syndrome. *Lancet* 2:539–544, 1943.
12. Frankel SA, Hirata I, Jr.: The scalenus anticus syndrome and competitive swimming. *JAMA* 215:1796–1798, 1971.
13. Grant JCB: *An Atlas of Human Anatomy*, Ed. 7. Williams & Wilkins, Baltimore, 1978 (Figs. 9-46, 9-83).
14. Gray H: *Anatomy of the Human Body*, edited by C.M. Goss, American Ed. 29. Lea & Febiger, Philadelphia, 1973 (Fig. 6-12).
15. *Ibid.* (p. 400–401).
16. *Ibid.* (pp. 1020, 1136).
17. *Ibid.* (pp. 703, 750).
18. Hollinshead WH: *Anatomy for Surgeons*, Ed. 2, Vol. 1, *The Head and Neck*. Harper & Row, Hagerstown, 1969 (pp. 551–554).
19. Kraus H: *Clinical Treatment of Back and Neck Pain*. McGraw-Hill, New York, 1970 (pp. 104, 105).

PART 2

20. Long C: Myofascial pain syndromes: part 2—syndromes of the head, neck and shoulder girdle. *Henry Ford Hosp Med Bull* 4:22–28, 1956.
21. McMinn RMH, Hutchings RT: *Color Atlas of Human Anatomy.* Year Book Medical Publishers, Chicago, 1977 (p. 189).
22. Naffziger HC, Grant WT: Neuritis of the brachial plexus mechanical in origin. The scalenus syndrome. *Surg Gynecol Obstet* 67:722–730, 1938.
23. Nielsen AJ: Personal communication, 1980.
24. Ochsner A, Gage M, DeBakey M: Scalenus anticus (Naffziger) syndrome. *Am J Surg* 28:669–695, 1935.
25. Rasch PJ, Burke RK: *Kinesiology and Applied Anatomy,* Ed. 6. Lea & Febiger, Philadelphia, 1978 (pp. 233, 258).
26. Reynolds MD: Myofascial trigger point syndromes in the practice of rheumatology. *Arch Phys Med Rehabil* 62:111–114, 1981 (Table 1).
27. Rubin D: An approach to the management of myofascial trigger point syndromes. *Arch Phys Med Rehabil* 62:107–110, 1981.
28. Sherman RA: Published treatments of phantom limb pain. *Am J Phys Med* 59:232–244, 1980.
29. Sivertsen B, Christensen JH: Pain relieving effect of scalenotomy. *Acta Orthop Scand* 48:158–160, 1977.
30. Sobotta J, Figge FHJ: *Atlas of Human Anatomy,* Ed. 9, Vol. 1. Hafner Division of Macmillan, New York, 1974 (pp. 169, 176).
31. *Ibid.* (p. 144).
32. *Ibid.* (p. 162).
33. Sobotta J, Figge FHJ: *Atlas of Human Anatomy,* Ed. 9, Vol. 3. Hafner Division of Macmillan, New York, 1974 (p. 83).
34. Sola AE, Rodenberger ML, Gettys BB: Incidence of hypersensitive areas in posterior shoulder muscles. *Am J Phys Med* 34:585–590, 1955.
35. Steinbrocker O, Isenberg SA, Silver M, et al.: Observations on pain produced by injection of hypertonic saline into muscles and other supportive tissues. *J Clin Invest* 32:1045–1051, 1953.
36. Toldt C: *An Atlas of Human Anatomy,* translated by M.E. Paul, Ed. 2, Vol. 1. Macmillan, New York, 1919 (pp. 277, 293).
37. *Ibid.* (p. 298).
38. *Ibid.* (p. 269).
39. Travell J: Rapid relief of acute "stiff neck" by ethyl chloride spray. *J Am Med Wom Assoc* 4:89–95, 1949.
40. Travell J: *Office Hours: Day and Night.* The World Publishing Company, New York, 1968 (pp. 271–272).
41. Travell J, Rinzler S, Herman M: Pain and disability of the shoulder and arm, treatment by intramuscular infiltration with procaine hydrochloride. *JAMA* 120:417–422, 1942.
42. Travell J, Rinzler SH: The myofascial genesis of pain. *Postgrad Med* 11:425–434, 1952 (p. 428).
43. Webber TD: Diagnosis and modification of headache and shoulder-arm-hand syndrome. *JAOA* 72:697–710, 1973 (p. 706, Fig. 30).
44. Wyant GM: Chronic pain syndromes and their treatment. II. Trigger points. *Can Anaesth Soc J* 26:216–219, 1979 (Patients 1 and 2).
45. Zohn DA, Mennell J McM: *Musculoskeletal Pain: Diagnosis and Physical Treatment.* Little, Brown and Company, Boston, 1976 (p. 192, Fig. 9–13).

PART 2

CHAPTER 21

Supraspinatus Muscle

"Subdeltoid Bursitis Mimicker"

HIGHLIGHTS: **REFERRED PAIN** from trigger-points (TPs) in this muscle is felt as a deep ache in the mid-deltoid region of the shoulder and usually extends part way down the arm. The pain also may concentrate at the lateral epicondyle and, rarely, may extend to the wrist. **ANATOMICAL ATTACHMENTS** are to the supraspinatus fossa, medially, and to the greater tubercle of the head of the humerus, laterally. **ACTIONS** of this muscle are to abduct the arm and to pull the head of the humerus inward toward the glenoid fossa. Its **MYOTATIC UNIT** includes the middle deltoid and upper trapezius as synergists for abduction. **SYMPTOMS** are chiefly referred pain which is aggravated by forceful abduction of the arm at the shoulder and by passive stretching when adducting the arm behind the back. Patients report difficulty in reaching up above the shoulder, and may experience pain at night that disturbs sleep. **ACTIVATION OF TRIGGER POINTS** is likely to result when heavy objects are carried with the arm hanging down, or when lifted above shoulder height. **PATIENT EXAMINATION** demonstrates reduced range of motion in the Hand-to-shoulder Blade Test and the Mouth Wraparound Test. **TRIGGER POINT EXAMINATION** of the medial TP area by flat palpation elicits definite tenderness, but the lateral TP area, adjacent to the acromion, is so deeply placed that firm palpation may reveal only minimal tenderness. **ASSOCIATED TRIGGER POINTS** may be found in the infraspinatus and upper trapezius, the anterior and middle deltoid, and in the antagonistic latissimus dorsi. **STRETCH AND SPRAY** begin with the patient seated and the hand placed as high as tolerable behind the back, while a stream of vapocoolant spray is applied from the medial to the lateral direction over the muscle fibers and referred pain pattern. **INJECTION AND STRETCH** are carried out with the patient lying on the opposite side, and the needle directed into one of the three TP areas: the medial, more superficial part of the muscle; the lateral, deeply placed muscular area; or the tendon located laterally beneath the acromion. **CORRECTIVE ACTIONS** include the avoidance of continued overload of the muscle, and the use of a stretch exercise at home while seated under a hot shower.

1. REFERRED PAIN
(Fig. 21.1)

When active trigger points (TPs) are present in the supraspinatus muscle, a deep ache is felt around the shoulder; the pain concentrates in the mid-deltoid region. This ache often extends down the arm and the forearm, and sometimes focuses strongly over the lateral epicondyle of the elbow (Fig. 21.1). This epicondylar component distinguishes supraspinatus from infraspinatus TPs, which do not refer pain to the elbow.[29, 32] Rarely, pain is referred to the wrist from the supraspinatus. The tenderness and pain that it projects to the mid-deltoid region is easily mistaken for subdeltoid bursitis.

Other authors have described the pain referred from the supraspinatus as traveling toward, or into the shoulder,[10, 11, 14] to the outer side of the arm,[9, 10] and from the scapula to mid-humerus.[12]

Experimental injection of 6% hypertonic

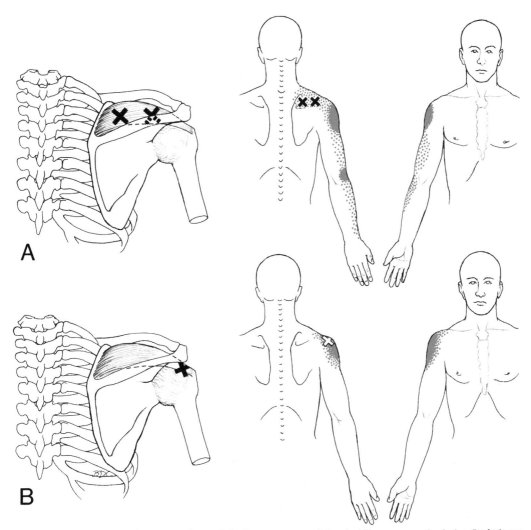

Figure 21.1. Referred pain patterns (essential reference zone *solid red*, spillover zone *stippled red*) of trigger points (×s) in the right supraspinatus muscle and tendon. *A*, medial and lateral trigger point areas located in the supraspinatus muscle. *B*, trigger point area located in the supraspinatus tendon.

saline into normal supraspinatus muscles caused referred pain to the shoulder (three subjects), to the upper back (two subjects) and to the elbow (one subject).[26]

2. ANATOMICAL ATTACHMENTS
(Fig. 21.2)

The supraspinatus muscle attaches *medially* to the supraspinatus fossa of the scapula and *laterally* to the upper part of the greater tubercle of the humerus[29] (Fig. 21.2).

Supplemental References

Other authors have clearly illustrated the supraspinatus muscle from be-

hind,[7, 16, 21, 25, 27] from above,[5] from in front,[28] in cross section,[3] and in sagittal section.[6, 17, 22]

3. INNERVATION

The supraspinatus muscle is innervated by the suprascapular nerve through the upper trunk, from the C_5 spinal nerve.

4. ACTIONS

The supraspinatus muscle abducts the arm, and pulls the head of the humerus inward toward the glenoid fossa,[2, 7, 13, 18] which prevents downward displacement of the head of the humerus when the arm is dependent at the side.[1, 4]

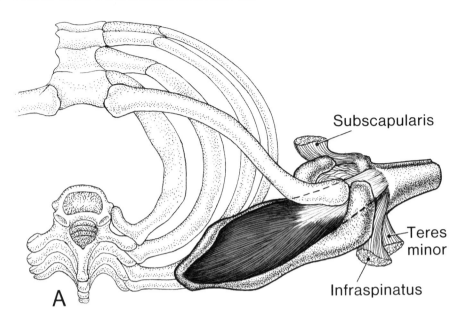

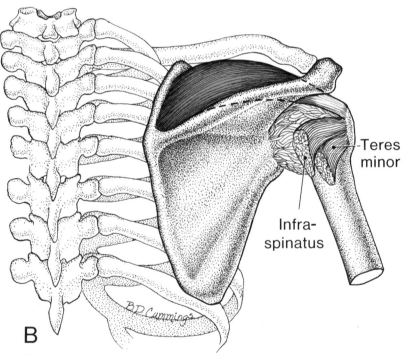

Figure 21.2.   Attachments of the supraspinatus muscle (*red*). The other rotator cuff muscles are cut and reflected to show their attachments more clearly. *A*, seen from above, including the relation of its humeral attachment to the other three rotator cuff muscles. *B*, seen from behind. It becomes obvious why such a long needle is required to reach the deep, lateral trigger point area through the overlying trapezius muscle if one envisions the trapezius attachments to the superficial surfaces of the three surrounding bones, the clavicle, acromion, and spine of the scapula.

Basmajian[1] showed electromyographically that supraspinatus activity alone, in the absence of other muscular activity at the shoulder, prevented downward displacement of the head of the humerus when the upper extremity, hanging at the side, was loaded to exhaustion with a 7-kg weight or was loaded with sudden downward jerks. The wedge action due to the angulation of the glenoid fossa and the cartilaginous labrium make this mechanism effective.[1,2]

The belief persists that the supraspinatus is more effective than the deltoid muscle for the initiation of abduction when the arm is at the side.[18] However, the clinical observations of Duchenne,[4] the electromyographic studies of Inman, et al.,[8] of Basmajian,[1] and the fact that experimental paralysis of the supraspinatus muscle simply reduces the force and endurance of abduction[1] establish the fact that this muscle and the deltoid work as a team throughout abduction of the arm at the shoulder.[1,2,13]

Stimulation of the supraspinatus muscle produced abduction, slight flexion, and slight internal rotation of the arm. However, this contraction of only the supraspinatus offered no resistance to passive external rotation of the arm; or to backward movement of the partially abducted arm.[4] Although Gray[7] attributes weak external rotation and flexion of the arm to this muscle, it appears that any such action is functionally insignificant. No electromyographic data were found to support a function of internal or external rotation.

The supraspinatus is active during walking, while the arm is swinging either forward or backward, but not at the ends of the swing. This activity apparently helps to prevent downward dislocation of the head of the humerus.

5. MYOTATIC UNIT

The middle deltoid and upper trapezius fibers are synergistic with the supraspinatus for abduction of the arm. The remaining three muscles of the rotator cuff, the infraspinatus, teres minor and subscapularis, assist the supraspinatus in stabilizing the head of the humerus in the glenoid fossa during abduction.[2] The serratus anterior is essential for stabilization of the scapula during abduction.[4]

The latissimus dorsi, teres major and teres minor muscles can act as antagonists to the supraspinatus.

6. SYMPTOMS

The chief complaint is referred pain, which is usually felt strongly during abduction of the arm at the shoulder and as a dull ache at rest. Supraspinatus TPs alone rarely cause severe, sleep-disturbing nocturnal pain. Other authors also have noted stiffness of the shoulder[12] and nighttime ache[10,12] due to involvement of the supraspinatus.

Some patients complain of snapping or clicking sounds around the shoulder joint, which may disappear when the supraspinatus TPs have been inactivated. Tautness of supraspinatus fibers due to TP activity probably interferes with the normal glide of the head of the humerus in the fossa, a mechanism which is well described by Cailliet.[2]

When the supraspinatus muscle on the dominant side is affected, the patient reports difficulty in reaching the head to comb the hair, brush the teeth or shave, and complains of restricted shoulder motion during sports activities, like a tennis serve. When TPs are located on the nondominant side, the patient may be unaware of the moderate restriction of motion, since the normal arm usually performs these arm-elevation activities.

7. ACTIVATION OF TRIGGER POINTS

Supraspinatus TPs can be activated by carrying heavy objects, such as a suitcase, briefcase, or package with the arm hanging down at the side, and by regularly walking a large dog pulling on a leash. The TPs of this muscle also may be activated by lifting an object to, or above, shoulder height with the arm outstretched.

8. PATIENT EXAMINATION

Sola and colleagues found the supraspinatus muscle to be one of the less frequently involved shoulder-girdle muscles, in both patients[23] and in young healthy adults.[24] We find it is seldom involved by itself, but often in association with the infraspinatus or the upper trapezius, which very commonly harbor TPs.

The Hand-to-shoulder Blade Test (see

PART 2

PART 2

Fig. 22.4) is restricted by supraspinatus TPs. Also, in the upright position, the patient is unable to fully abduct the arm because this shortens and loads the supraspinatus. The patient has less difficulty with this motion when lying supine because the muscle is not lifting the weight of the arm.

The lateral attachment of the supraspinatus tendon is most easily palpated if the hand of the upper extremity being examined is placed behind the back at waist level to internally rotate the arm and bring the tendon from beneath the acromion so it can be reached.

Palpation often reveals marked tenderness beneath the deltoid at the attachment of the supraspinatus tendon, which may show evidence of degeneration in elderly persons. The junior author has seen early calcific deposits at the insertion of the tendon resolve with inactivation of TPs in the supraspinatus muscle. Michelle, et al.[15] also noted this calcification in patients with tenderness deep in the region of this muscle. These deposits may be evidence of chronic tendon strain caused by TP tautness of the involved supraspinatus muscle fibers.

Differential Diagnosis

When evaluating a patient with pain referred from supraspinatus TPs, common differential diagnoses include cervical arthritis or spurs with nerve root irritation,[10] C_5 radiculopathy,[10, 19] and brachial plexus injuries. All of these neurogenic sources of pain are likely to exhibit, on electromyographic examination, spontaneous potentials in the muscles supplied by the compromised nerves; muscles with only myofascial TPs produce no spontaneous electromyographic activity.

The shoulder pain of the supraspinatus myofascial syndrome does not have the deep, aching quality of the infraspinatus TP pain, which is referred deep into the shoulder joint and is easily mistaken for arthritis of the glenohumeral joint.[19]

Subdeltoid bursitis, rotator cuff tears and supraspinatus TPs all may cause tenderness along the muscular attachments to the rotator cuff beneath the acromion. Only the TPs, however, cause spot tenderness within the supraspinatus muscle. When rotator cuff tears are present, these are likely to be associated with supraspinatus TPs, which add to the symptoms. In these cases, it may be preferable to inject rather than to stretch and spray the muscle.

Suprascapular nerve block has been recommended for relief of intractable shoulder pain that has no satisfactory explanation[31] and is associated with tenderness of the supraspinatus and infraspinatus mus-

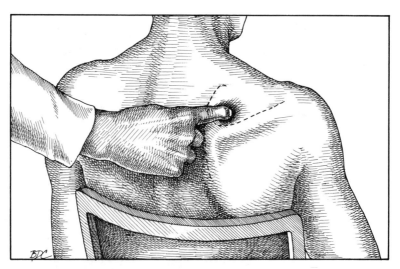

Figure 21.3. Application of digital pressure to the medial trigger point in the supraspinatus muscle. Sustained pressure evokes the pattern of referred pain when this medial trigger point is active, but rarely when the lateral trigger point is compressed.

cles to palpation.[20] These findings, in our experience, usually mean that active TPs are present in these two scapular muscles. It is not unreasonable to think that an effective block of the suprascapular nerve to the supraspinatus and infraspinatus muscles could temporarily interrupt the self-sustaining TP mechanism, permitting recovery of normal muscle function. However, direct injection of TPs responsible for the pain should be equally, if not more effective, and safer.

9. TRIGGER POINT EXAMINATION
(Fig. 21.3)

The patient sits comfortably, or lies on the opposite side, with the affected arm close to the body and relaxes. In the case of less active TPs, it may be desirable to place the arm in the stretch position, as for stretch and spray. The supraspinatus muscle must be palpated through the trapezius fibers; the locations of the medial and lateral TPs are shown in Fig. 21.1A. Other observers also have identified the lateral[30] and the medial[10] TP areas. Both TPs lie deep in the supraspinatus fossa of the scapula, underneath a relatively thick part of the trapezius muscle, so that a local twitch response of the supraspinatus is rarely perceived. The medial TP is located by flat palpation (Fig. 21.3) just above the spine of the scapula several centimeters (about 1 in) lateral to the vertebral border of the scapula. The lateral TP is palpated in the space between the scapula and the clavicle just medial to the acromion.

The severity and extent of the referred pain evoked by needling TPs in the lateral muscular area is usually out of proportion to the slight degree of tenderness to deep palpation reported by the patient. If an active supraspinatus TP is present, as shown by its characteristic pain pattern, and even though local tenderness seems minimal, the TP should be inactivated, usually by local anesthetic injection.

A third TP may lie in the tendon of the muscle at its lateral attachment to the joint capsule and greater tubercle under the acromial process (Fig. 21.1B). This tendinous TP acts and responds like the tendinous involvement of the long head of the biceps brachii, and may be associated with local calcification.

10. ENTRAPMENTS

No nerve entrapment is attributed to TP tension in the supraspinatus muscle.

11. ASSOCIATED TRIGGER POINTS

In our experience, the supraspinatus and infraspinatus muscles are frequently involved together, and also may involve the middle and upper trapezius as part of the myotatic unit.

Since the deltoid lies in the pain reference zone of the supraspinatus, it may develop satellite TPs.

If the latissimus dorsi muscle has become involved as an antagonist, inactivating its TPs will increase abduction of the arm by release of this adductor muscle tension.

12. STRETCH AND SPRAY
(Fig. 21.4)

The forearm of the seated patient is placed behind the back at waist level.

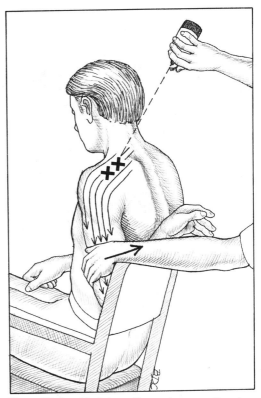

Figure 21.4.   Stretch position and spray pattern (*arrows*) for trigger points (×s) in the supraspinatus muscle. The *arrow on the operator's wrist* indicates pressure exerted by the operator toward the patient's hand.

PART 2

After a few preliminary sweeps of spray, the hand is raised as high toward the scapula as is tolerated. The patient is encouraged to relax in the stretch position by leaning back and pinning the arm against the chairback. The stream of vapocoolant spray is applied in unhurried parallel sweeps from medial to lateral in line with and over the supraspinatus muscle fibers, across the acromion and over the deltoid, down the arm to the elbow, and over the forearm (Fig. 21.4). By bending the head and neck toward the opposite side and spraying upward over the upper trapezius, obstructive tension in this muscle can be released, since it is often also involved. Hot packs are applied, followed by full range of active motion of the treated muscles.

If both the supraspinatus and infraspinatus TPs are extremely sensitive and the patient has difficulty in placing the hand behind the back, the arm may be brought, instead, across the front of the chest and stretched as illustrated for the posterior deltoid muscle (see Fig. 28.4B). Either way, the vapocoolant traces the pattern of Fig. 21.4, as described above.

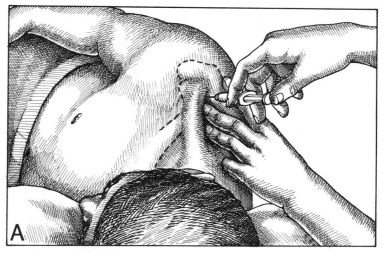

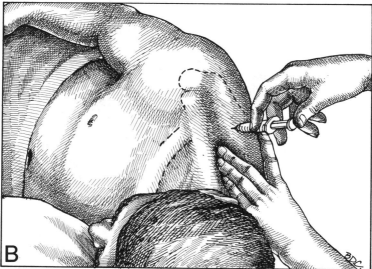

Figure 21.5.   Injection of trigger points in the right supraspinatus muscle and tendon with the patient lying on the left side. *A*, the lateral muscular trigger point, seen from above. *B*, the medial muscular trigger point, viewed from above. *C*, the tendinous trigger point, viewed from behind.

13. INJECTION AND STRETCH
(Fig. 21.5)

With the patient lying on the opposite side, the medial TP is located by palpation and injected, using a 3.2- to 3.8-cm (1¼- to 1½-in) needle, which is directed downward into the bony fossa of the scapula below and behind the edge of the upper trapezius (Fig. 21.5B). If one inserts the needle lateral to this TP in order to angle the needle medially, instead of vertically as in Figure 21.5B, the needle may encounter an active TP_2 in the upper trapezius (see Fig. 6.2). Penetration of this trapezius TP produces a visible local twitch response and elicits referred pain to the neck. Continued movement of the needle downward to the supraspinatus TP then elicits its referred pain pattern to the upper extremity. The operator should probe the region with the needle to locate any additional supraspinatus TPs.

If this injection, followed by stretch and spray and hot packs, does not fully restore shoulder motion, the operator should check for any tenderness just medial to the acromial process that would suggest a lateral supraspinatus TP. This other TP is difficult to detect by palpation because it lies deep in the supraspinatus and is covered by a roof of trapezius fibers. It announces its presence by a persistant referred pain pattern. The region of this lateral TP should be probed with the needle for TPs. In a large person, this may require a 5-cm (2-in) needle, which is directed caudally, deep into the supraclavicular fossa, parallel to, lateral to, and behind the rib cage (Fig. 21.5A). Contact with a TP there usually flashes referred pain to the deltoid and down the arm.

Injection is followed by passive stretch of the muscle during a few sweeps of the spray, and then by a hot pack. Occasionally, residual tenderness just beneath the tip of the acromial process is due to supraspinatus tendinitis, which may respond to injection of a local anesthetic and/or corticosteroid drug (Fig. 21.5C).

Other authors also have found that injection of the supraspinatus muscle effectively inactivates its TPs.[9, 10, 11]

14. CORRECTIVE ACTIONS

The patient should avoid overload by not carrying a heavy object, such as a briefcase, in the hand with the arm hanging down at the side, and by not lifting heavy things overhead. The patient also should avoid sustained contraction of the muscle, as when maintaining the arm in abduction or flexion, e.g. holding the arms up continuously for several minutes to put curlers in the hair, or to hang drapes.

The patient must learn to slowly, firmly stretch the supraspinatus muscle by pull-

PART 2

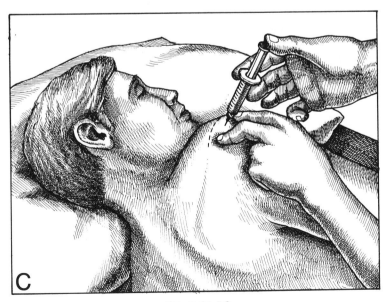

Figure 21.5C

ing the forearm across and upward behind the back, with the other hand to position the involved arm as in Fig. 21.4. This passive stretch may be done while the patient sits on a stool under a hot shower with the water beating on the muscle. The patient also may stretch the muscle by bringing the elbow of the involved side in front of the chest and, with the other hand, firmly pulling the elbow high across the chest (see Figs. 28.3B and 28.4A).

References

1. Basmajian JV: *Muscles Alive*, Ed. 4. Williams & Wilkins. Baltimore, 1978 (pp. 165, 186, 192, 193, 197, 199, 316).
2. Cailliet. R: *Soft Tissue Pain and Disability*. F.A. Davis, Philadelphia, 1977 (pp. 149–151, Fig. 122).
3. Carter BL, Morehead J, Wolpert SM, *et al.*: Cross-Sectional Anatomy. Appleton-Century-Crofts, New York, 1977 (Sects. 19, 20).
4. Duchenne GB: *Physiology of Motion*, translated by E.B. Kaplan. J.B. Lippincott, Philadelphia, 1949 (pp. 59–63).
5. Grant JCB: *An Atlas of Human Anatomy*, Ed. 7. Williams & Wilkins, Baltimore, 1978 (Fig. 6–33).
6. *Ibid.* (Fig. 6–48).
7. Gray H: *Anatomy of the Human Body*, edited by C.M. Goss, American Ed. 29. Lea & Febiger, Philadelphia, 1973 (p. 456, Fig. 6–37).
8. Inman VT, Saunders JB, Abbott LC: Observations on the function of the shoulder joint. *J Bone Joint Surg* 26:1–30. 1944 (pp. 18, 21).
9. Kellgren JH: A preliminary account of referred pains arising from muscle. *Br Med J* 1:325–327, 1938 (Case 3).
10. Kelly M: New light on the painful shoulder. *Med J Aust* 1:488–493, 1942 (Cases 2 and 8, Figs. 2B and 3C).
11. Kelly M: The nature of fibrositis. III. Multiple lesions and the neural hypothesis. *Ann Rheum Dis* 5:161–167, 1946 (Case 2).
12. Kelly M: Some rules for the employment of local analgesia in the treatment of somatic pain. *Med J Aust* 1:235–239, 1947 (Table 1 No. 4).
13. Kendall HO, Kendall FP, Wadsworth GE: *Muscles, Testing and Function*, Ed. 2. Williams & Wilkins, Baltimore, 1971 (p. 104).
14. Kraus H: *Clinical Treatment of Back and Neck Pain*. McGraw-Hill. New York, 1970 (p. 98).
15. Michele AA, Davies JJ, Krueger FJ, *et al.*: Scapulocostal syndrome (fatigue-postural paradox). *NY State J Med 50*:1353–1356, 1950 (p. 1355).
16. Pernkopf E: *Atlas of Topographical and Applied Human Anatomy*, Vol. 2. W.B. Saunders, Philadelphia, 1964 (Fig. 28).
17. *Ibid.* (Fig. 45).
18. Rasch PJ, Burke RK: *Kinesiology and Applied Anatomy*, Ed. 6. Lea & Febiger, Philadelphia, 1978 (pp. 163, 164).
19. Reynolds MD: Myofascial trigger point syndromes in the practice of rheumatology. *Arch Phys Med Rehabil 62*:111–114, 1981 (Tables 1 and 2).
20. Skillern PG: Suprascapular nerve syndrome as revealed by new (anterior) approach in induction of block. *Arch Neurol Psych 71*:185–188, 1954.
21. Sobotta J, Figge FHJ: *Atlas of Human Anatomy*, Ed. 9, Vol. 1. Hafner Division of Macmillan, New York, 1974 (p. 144).
22. *Ibid.* (p. 197).
23. Sola AE, Kuitert JH: Myofascial trigger point pain in the neck and shoulder girdle. *Northwest Med 54*:980–984, 1955.
24. Sola AE, Rodenberger ML, Gettys BB: Incidence of hypersensitive areas in posterior shoulder muscles. *Am J Phys Med 34*:585–590, 1955.
25. Spalteholz W: *Handatlas der Anatomie des Menschen*, Ed. 11, Vol. 2. S. Hirzel, Leipzig, 1922 (p. 324).
26. Steinbrocker O, Isenberg SA, Silver M, *et al.*: Observations on pain produced by injection of hypertonic saline into muscles and other supportive tissues. *J Clin Invest 32*:1045–1051, 1953 (Table 2).
27. Toldt C: *An Atlas of Human Anatomy*, translated by M.E. Paul, Ed. 2, Vol. 1. Macmillan, New York, 1919 (p. 312).
28. *Ibid.* (p. 313).
29. Travell J, Rinzler SH: The myofascial genesis of pain. *Postgrad Med 11*:425–434, 1952.
30. Webber TD: Diagnosis and modification of headache and shoulder-arm-hand syndrome. *JAOA 72*:697–710, 1973 (Fig. 28 Part 1, p. 10).
31. Wertheim HM, Rovenstine EA: Suprascapular nerve block. *Anesthesiology 2*:541–545, 1941.
32. Zohn DA. Mennell J McM: *Musculoskeletal Pain: Diagnosis and Physical Treatment*. Little, Brown & Company, Boston, 1976 (p. 192, Fig. 9–13).

CHAPTER 22
Infraspinatus Muscle
"Shoulder Joint Pain"

HIGHLIGHTS: **REFERRED PAIN** from the usual trigger point (TP) locations in the infraspinatus muscle concentrates deeply in the anterior deltoid region and in the shoulder joint, extending down the front and lateral aspect of the arm and forearm, and sometimes including the radial half of the hand. Pain also may be referred to the suboccipital and posterior cervical areas. An infrequent TP may refer pain over the adjacent rhomboid muscles. **ANATOMICAL ATTACHMENTS** are, medially, to the infraspinous fossa of the scapula and, laterally, to the greater tuberosity of the humerus. **ACTIONS** of this muscle include external rotation of the arm at the shoulder, and stabilization of the head of the humerus in the glenoid cavity during movement of the arm. **SYMPTOMS** are referred pain when sleeping on either side, inability to reach behind to a back pocket or to bra hooks and, in front, to comb the hair or brush the teeth. **ACTIVATION OF TRIGGER POINTS** usually results from overload while reaching backward and up. **PATIENT EXAMINATION** reveals restriction of internal and external rotation at the shoulder, demonstrated by the Mouth Wrap-around and the Hand-to-shoulder Blade Tests. **TRIGGER POINT EXAMINATION** locates active TPS a centimeter or two (½−1 in) below the spine of the scapula, occasionally more caudally. **ASSOCIATED TRIGGER POINTS** are commonly found in the supraspinatus, teres minor, anterior and posterior deltoid, biceps brachii, and pectoralis major muscles. **STRETCH AND SPRAY** of this muscle may be done by lifting the arm in front of, or behind, the chest, while directing the vapocoolant laterally over the muscle and down the arm over its referred pain pattern, including the hand. Separate sweeps are directed upward over the suboccipital area. **INJECTION AND STRETCH** are begun with the patient lying on the opposite side while the TP is localized between palpating fingers. Injection is followed by passive stretching, hot packs, and active range of motion. **CORRECTIVE ACTIONS** include elimination of recurrent overload on the muscle, proper positioning in bed at night, self-administered ischemic compression, and self-stretch exercises.

1. REFERRED PAIN
(Fig. 22.1)

We have found that when the patient feels referred pain from myofascial trigger points (TPs) intensely deep in the front of the shoulder, the infraspinatus muscle is the major source.[29]

Most reports of the referred pain pattern from this muscle identify the front of the shoulder as the major target area (Fig. 22.1).[8, 15, 20, 25, 28, 30, 32, 33, 34, 36] In 193 cases of infraspinatus referred pain, all patients identified the front of the shoulder as painful.[28] The shoulder pain is usually felt *deep* within the joint.[30] The pain is described as also projecting down the anterolateral aspect of the arm,[7, 8, 11, 14, 15, 20, 28, 30, 32, 34, 36] to the lateral forearm,[14, 15, 20, 25, 28, 30, 32, 34, 36] to the radial aspect of the hand,[14, 15, 20, 25, 30, 34, 36] and occasionally to the fingers.[14, 28] Patients usually identify the most painful area by covering the front of the shoulder with the hand.

A few authors located the pain in the back of the shoulder,[8, 11] which we find can be referred simultaneously from TPs that also are present in the adjacent teres minor muscle.

Much of the variation among these reports is probably due to the appearance of referred pain in the variable spillover zones. Among 193 subjects, 46% experienced pain in the deltoid and biceps brachii regions, none reported elbow pain, 21% reported pain in the radial forearm, 13% in the radial side of the hand, and 14% in the suboccipital posterior cervical area.[28] The medial TP of the two illustrated in Figure 22.1A is the most frequent. No distinction is made in the pain patterns arising from these two TPs.

An infrequent TP that lies more caudally, close to the vertebral border of the scapula (Fig. 22.1B), refers pain to the adjacent interscapular rhomboid muscles. This pain pattern is difficult to distinguish from that of the trapezius TP4 (see Fig. 6.3).

Among hundreds of patients seen with infraspinatus TPs, one aberrant pain pattern was observed; the pain was referred superficially to the front of the chest. After

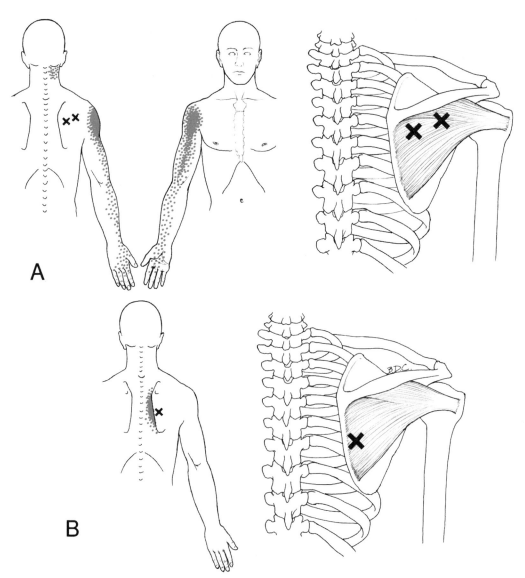

Figure 22.1. Referred pain patterns (*red*), and location of corresponding trigger points (✕s) in the right infraspinatus muscle. *Solid red* shows essential referred pain zones, *stippled red* areas show spillover zones. *A*, common location of trigger points. *B*, unusual trigger point location.

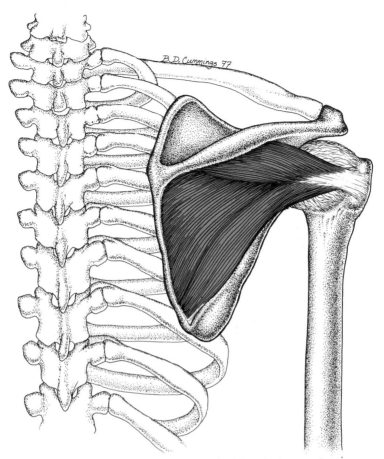

Figure 22.2. Attachments of the infraspinatus muscle.

the initial injection, the patient returned with the expected infraspinatus pain pattern, which, with additional injections of TPs, was resolved.[30]

Experimentally, increased alpha motor neuron excitability in the anterior deltoid muscle has been demonstrated by pressure stimulation of an active infraspinatus TP that referred pain to the anterior deltoid area. Motor unit activity appeared at rest in the deltoid during referred pain elicited by this application of pressure. The patient was unable to eliminate this motor unit activity by relaxation, although surrounding muscles, not within the pain reference zone, were electrically silent.[31]

Referred pain was experimentally induced from the infraspinatus by injecting the normal muscle with 6% hypertonic saline. Pain was felt deeply at the shoulder tip, in the posterior and lateral shoulder regions, and in the anterolateral aspect of the arm.[9]

2. ANATOMICAL ATTACHMENTS
(Fig. 22.2)

The infraspinatus attaches **medially** to the medial two-thirds of the infraspinous fossa below the spine of the scapula and to adjacent fascia. **Laterally** it fastens to the posterior aspect of the greater tuberosity of the humerus[6] (Fig. 22.2).

The upper medial portion of the muscle is covered by the lower trapezius.

Supplemental References

Other authors have illustrated the infraspinatus muscle in dorsal view without,[5, 6, 16, 21, 26, 27] and with its artery and nerve supply,[22] and in cross section.[3, 17]

3. INNERVATION

The infraspinatus muscle is supplied by the suprascapular nerve, through the upper trunk from spinal nerves C_5 and C_6.[6]

4. ACTIONS

The infraspinatus externally rotates the arm at the shoulder with the arm in any position,[4] and helps to stabilize the head of the humerus in the glenoid cavity during upward movement of the arm.[2, 12, 18] In addition, Gray[6] states that the upper fibers of this muscle help to abduct, and the lower fibers help to adduct the arm at the shoulder.

Inman et al.[7] demonstrated that, electromyographically, infraspinatus activity increased linearly with increasing abduction, with additional peaks of activity during flexion. Basmajian[1] clearly described how the angulation of the glenoid fossa, together with the activity of horizontal fibers in several muscles, provides a wedge action that prevents downward displacement of the head of the humerus. He showed that action of the supraspinatus and posterior fibers of the deltoid prevented downward displacement, even with considerable downward loading of the adducted arm. However, in other positions, additional protection of the joint by rotator cuff muscular activity, which includes contraction of the infraspinatus, becomes critical.[1] In abduction, many fibers contribute both to the abductive force and to stabilization of the humeral head in the glenoid fossa.

Electrical activity of the infraspinatus is not mentioned in conjunction with adduction of the shoulder, and Duchenne[4] denied an adduction component on stimulation.

5. MYOTATIC UNIT

The infraspinatus muscle functions in parallel with the teres minor and posterior deltoid for external rotation of the arm. The infraspinatus and teres minor have nearly identical actions, but different innervations. The infraspinatus also assists the supraspinatus and other rotator cuff muscles by stabilizing the head of the humerus in the glenoid cavity during abduction and extension of the arm.[1]

The subscapularis, pectoralis major and anterior deltoid muscles act as antagonists to the infraspinatus and posterior deltoid for rotation of the arm.

6. SYMPTOMS

We agree with other authors that when myofascial pain is referred to the shoulder joint, the infraspinatus, supraspinatus, and less frequently, the levator scapulae muscles are its most likely sources.[10, 23]

The patient with this TP commonly complains: "I can't reach into my back pants pocket; I can't fasten my bra behind my back; I can't zip up the back of my dress; I can't get my sore arm into my coat sleeve last, but must put it in first; or I can't reach back to the night stand beside my bed." Inability to internally rotate and to adduct the arm at the shoulder simultaneously is a revealing sign of infraspinatus TP activity. Tennis players complain that the shoulder pain limits the vigor of their strokes.

Sola and Williams[25] identified the symptoms of shoulder-girdle fatigue, weakness of grip, loss of mobility at the shoulder, and hyperhidrosis in the referred pain area as due to TP activity in the infraspinatus muscle.

Referred pain (Fig. 22.1) prevents the patient from lying on the same side (and sometimes on the back) at night, because the weight of the thorax compresses and stimulates the infraspinatus TPs.[30] When the patient lies on the other side for relief, the top-side arm is likely to fall forward and painfully stretch the affected infraspinatus muscle, again disturbing sleep. Thus, patients with very active infraspinatus TPs may find that they can sleep only by propping themselves up, seated in a chair or on a sofa for the night.

A major part of the shoulder-girdle pain associated with hemiplegia is commonly due to myofascial TPs in the trapezius, scalene, supraspinatus, infraspinatus and subscapularis muscles. In the absence of spasticity at rest, the TPs in these muscles usually respond well to local treatment.

7. ACTIVATION OF TRIGGER POINTS

Infraspinatus TPs are usually activated by multiple overload stresses, such as, frequently reaching out and back to a bedside stand, especially during an acute illness when muscles may be "below par;" grabbing backward for support to regain balance, e.g. grasping the railing when slip-

ping on steps; twisting the arm that holds
a ski pole during a fall; excessive poling
when skiing; delivering an especially hard
tennis serve when off balance, mishitting
the ball; or an experienced ice skater drag-
ging a novice skater around by the arm for
a long period of time. These patients can
usually identify the initiating trauma that
occurred within a few hours of the onset
of shoulder pain.

8. PATIENT EXAMINATION
(Figs. 22.3 and 22.4)

The Mouth Wrap-around and the Hand-
to-shoulder Blade Tests are valuable to
screen for involved shoulder-girdle muscles.

The Mouth Wrap-around Test requires
full abduction and external rotation of the
arm at the shoulder. The patient does this
test (Fig. 22.3) by bringing the hand and
forearm *behind* (not above) the head and
sliding the hand as far forward as possible
trying to cover the mouth. The head should
be turned no more than 45°, and not tilted.
Normally, the fingertips then cover the
mouth nearly to the midline in most persons, just to the corner of the mouth if the
patient has short upper arms, and over the
entire mouth with hypermobile joints.

Holding this position strongly contracts
the abductors and external rotators in the
shortened position. When involved, one of
these muscles slightly limits the range of
movement due to pain at the end point.
With only the infraspinatus involved, the
fingers are likely to reach as far as the ear
when the test is performed actively by the
patient, and a little further when tested
as passive movement; with additional
stretch-restriction by TPs in the subscapularis muscle, the fingers may not reach
the back of the neck. This limitation of
range due to restriction of subscapularis
stretch is as severe, or more so, when the
test is done passively.

Conversely, the Hand-to-shoulder-blade
Test requires full adduction and internal
rotation of the arm at the shoulder. The
patient does this test by placing the hand
behind the back (Fig. 22.4) and reaching as
far up the spinal column as possible. Normally, the fingertips should reach at least
to the spine of the scapula, farther than is

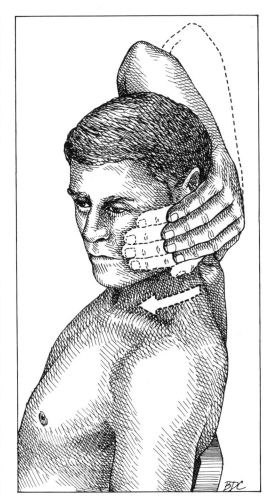

Figure 22.3.   Mouth Wrap-around Test of abduction
and external rotation of the arm. The *fully rendered
hand* shows slightly restricted range of motion. The
dotted white arrow and *dotted outline* show the additional normal reach for this subject with congenitally
short upper arms. Most persons can cover half the
mouth; individuals with hypermobile joints normally
cover the entire mouth with the hand.

shown in Figure 22.4. This stretches the
abductors and external rotators. When the
range of these muscles (e.g. the infraspinatus) is stretch limited because of TP
tautness and shortening of the fibers, the
fingers may barely reach to a hip pocket.
This limitation is similar when done actively or passively. On the other hand,
involvement of its antagonist, the subscapularis, may let the fingers reach the spinal
column, or farther, if done passively without contracting the muscle.

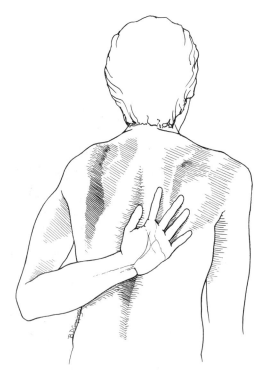

Figure 22.4. Hand-to-shoulder Blade Test of adduction and internal rotation of the arm at the shoulder, which places the infraspinatus muscle on stretch. This shows slight restriction of movement. In normal individuals, the fingertips usually reach the spine of the scapula.

Differential Diagnosis

Painfully restricted motion at the shoulder ("frozen shoulder") that is due to adhesive capsulitis (see Chapter 26) exhibits less pain and more rigidity than does restriction due to myofascial TPs. Adhesive capsulitis often requires short-term steroid therapy, which may be given orally.[33, 35]

The scapulohumeral syndrome, as defined by Long,[14] may be due to active infraspinatus TPs. This syndrome also might include pain referred from TPs in the pectoralis major and minor muscles and from the long head of the biceps brachii.

Infraspinatus TPs refer pain in the distributions of the C_5, C_6, and C_7 spinal nerves, which may cause diagnostic confusion with radiculopathy due to intervertebral disc disease,[19] unless neurological deficits and electromyographic findings are considered in addition to the distribution of pain.

Equally confusing is the fact that re-

ferred pain from TPs in the infraspinatus muscle closely mimics that arising in the glenohumeral joint itself.[19]

9. TRIGGER POINT EXAMINATION

The infraspinatus frequently harbors myofascial TPs. In 126 patients, referred pain to the shoulder region arose from the infraspinatus muscle in 31% of the cases, a frequency second only to that of the levator scapulae (55%).[23] Pace[15] made a similar observation. Among young, pain-free adults, the infraspinatus was third (18%) in the prevalence of latent TPs, fewer than the levator scapulae (20%) and the upper trapezius (35%).[24]

The muscle may be stretched gently for examination with the patient sitting, or lying on the opposite side as for a TP injection (see Fig. 22.6). When the patient is seated, the muscle is stretched by bringing the hand and arm across the front of the chest to grasp the far armrest of the chair (see TP_4, Fig. 6.8). Flat palpation discloses spot tenderness at the main TP, which is usually perpendicularly equidistant from the vertebral border and the spine of the scapula, caudal to the junction of the medial and second quarter of the length of the scapular spine (medial × in Fig. 22.1A).

The next most common TP (lateral × in Fig. 22.1A) is usually located caudal to the midpoint of the scapular spine, but may be as far lateral as the lateral border of the scapula. It, too, is found by flat palpation. Lange[13] illustrated the location of this infraspinatus trigger area.

The least common location for infraspinatus TPs (Fig. 22.1B) is about mid-muscle along the vertebral border of the scapula. This same location was described previously.[25, 35]

Firm bands in this muscle are readily palpable. Exquisite deep tenderness and local twitch responses are easily elicited by snapping palpation. Referred pain is usually evoked, or aggravated by sustained pressure on an active infraspinatus TP.

10. ENTRAPMENTS

No nerve entrapments are attributed to TPs in this muscle.

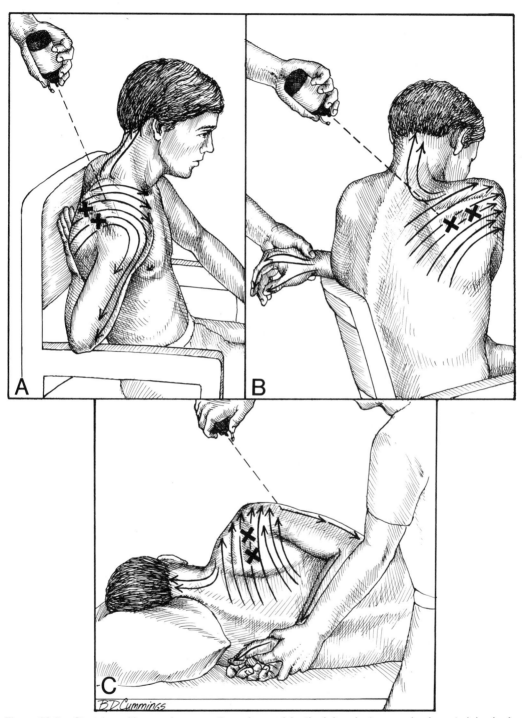

Figure 22.5. Stretch positions and spray patterns (*arrows*) for the infraspinatus muscle. *A*, seated, back-of-chest position. *B*, seated, front-of-chest position. *C*, recumbent, back-of-chest position.

11. ASSOCIATED TRIGGER POINTS

The teres minor lies in parallel, and is the chief synergist of the infraspinatus. In addition, three families of muscles develop active TPs in association with the infraspinatus, but any given patient usually exhibits involvement of only one of the three groups. The anterior deltoid muscle lies in the essential pain reference zone of the infraspinatus, and it often develops satellite TPs in response to prolonged activation of the infraspinatus TPs. Another family is the synergistic supraspinatus-infraspinatus team, which can be thought of as two traces of a wagon that raise the arm up and back, so that dual involvement is expected. The biceps brachii also may join this family. The third group includes the teres major and latissimus dorsi, which counter external rotation by the infraspinatus, and it sometimes involves the posterior deltoid, which assists them.

The antagonistic subscapularis and pectoralis major muscles also should be checked for associated TPs.

12. STRETCH AND SPRAY
(Fig. 22.5)

Three stretch positions may be employed effectively. (1) The position of the Hand-to-shoulder Blade Test may be used with the patient seated (Fig. 22.5A). (2) With the patient seated, the arm may be pulled across the chest in full horizontal adduction (Fig. 22.5B). (3) The upper extremity may be placed behind the back with the patient lying on the opposite side (Fig. 22.5C). In each position, slow parallel sweeps of the spray follow the muscle fibers in a medial to lateral direction, are then carried down the arm to the fingertips and over the thumb, and upward over the posterior cervical pain reference zone. Be-

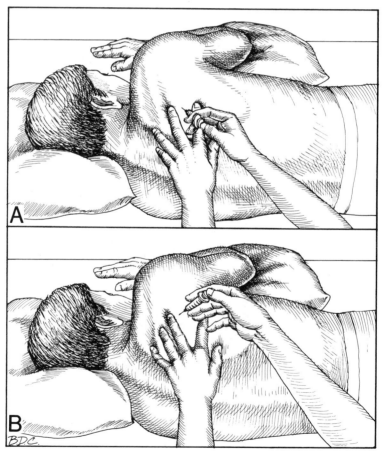

Figure 22.6. Technique for injecting the two common trigger points in the infraspinatus muscle. *A*, the medial trigger point. The left middle finger presses against the lower (caudal) border of the scapular spine. *B*, the lateral trigger point. The left ring finger presses against the lower border of the scapular spine.

fore finishing the treatment, stretch and spray are applied to the antagonistic anterior deltoid and pectoralis major muscles. These muscles are likely to experience shortening activation of latent TPs in response to the unaccustomed shortening associated with the release of infraspinatus tension. The treatment ends with application of a hot pack, and then active range of motion of the involved muscles.

If TP tenderness and local twitch responses remain in the infraspinatus muscle, ischemic compression may be helpful.

13. INJECTION AND STRETCH
(Fig. 22.6)

While the patient lies on the opposite side, the arm is abducted to about 90° and the elbow rests on a pillow that has been placed against the chest (Fig. 22.6A). The TP is located and pinned between the fingers against the scapula. The TP is probed with a 3.8-cm (1½-in) needle until the needle elicits a local twitch response, a local pain response, and usually, also, the referred pain pattern of the TP. As the procaine solution is injected, the needle peppers the area to reach any remaining TPs. Hemostasis is applied with the fingers of the palpating hand during and after injection. If residual tenderness and local twitch responses are still present, the remaining TPs are localized by palpation and probed with the needle. A full passive stretch is carried out during a few sweeps of vapocoolant spray, and then a hot pack is applied while the arm is supported in a comfortable neutral position.

Contrary to an early illustration,[28] the injection of TPs is never done in a seated patient; it is always performed in the recumbent position to minimize psychogenic syncope and the complications of falling, should the patient faint.

A physician described to the senior author his experience of producing a pneumothorax while injecting an infraspinatus TP. The needle penetrated the scapula through a fibrous membrane where he expected scapular bone. Portions of the infraspinous fossa can be paper thin. One must be aware of this possibility, and sensitive to the resistance encountered by the needle at that depth.

If, following injection therapy, the patient's range of motion in the Hand-to-shoulder Blade Test remains significantly restricted, the supinator muscle in the forearm should be checked for TPs, since they, too, can limit the movement in that test. This test can be restricted because the hand does not pronate fully.

14. CORRECTIVE ACTIONS
(Fig. 22.7)

The patient should avoid habitual sustained or repetitive motions that overload the infraspinatus, such as regularly rolling the hair up on night curlers, and reaching backward to objects on a bedside table. The table should be moved toward the foot of the bed, or the opposite arm used to reach across. On retiring, application of a hot pack to the muscle for 15–20 min can markedly reduce the irritability of its TPs.

When the patient lies on the uninvolved side, sleep is improved by supporting the uppermost elbow and forearm on a bed pillow (Fig. 22.7A) to avoid overstretching the affected infraspinatus muscle that can

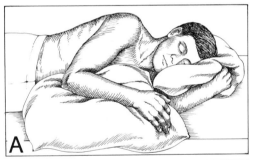

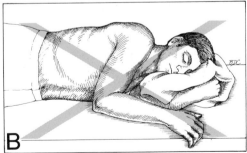

Figure 22.7. Pain-relieving and pain-producing sleep positions when right infraspinatus trigger points are active. *A*, mid-position of relief, with the affected arm supported by a pillow. *B*, poor position (*red* ✕) with the arm strongly adducted at the shoulder. This position places the infraspinatus on a pain-producing stretch.

cause referred pain (Fig. 22.7B); a neutral position (mid-muscle-length) is best.

The patient may "press out" an infraspinatus TP by lying on a tennis ball placed directly under a tender spot in the muscle; body weight is used to maintain increasing pressure at the discomfort level for 1 or 2 min. The tennis ball pressure treatment may be repeated daily or every second day, until TP tenderness disappears.

The patient learns to stretch the muscle daily, while seated under a hot shower. The arm is pulled across the body, first in the front to achieve the arm position in Fig. 22.5B, and then to the rear (Fig. 22.5A). The hot water is directed on the involved infraspinatus and associated muscles.

Supplemental References, Case Reports

The senior author has presented the management of patients with infraspinatus TPs.[28, 33]

References

1. Basmajian JV: *Muscles Alive*, Ed. 4. Williams & Wilkins, Baltimore, 1978 (pp. 194, 196–200).
2. Cailliet, R: *Soft Tissue Pain and Disability*. F.A. Davis, Philadelphia, 1977 (pp. 149–152).
3. Carter BL, Morehead J, Wolpert SM, et al.: *Cross-Sectional Anatomy*. Appleton-Century-Crofts, New York, 1977 (Sects. 20–23).
4. Duchenne GB: *Physiology of Motion*, translated by E.B. Kaplan, J.B. Lippincott, Philadelphia, 1949 (p. 64).
5. Grant JCB: *An Atlas of Human Anatomy*, Ed. 7. Williams & Wilkins, Baltimore, 1978 (Figs. 6-39, 6-40).
6. Gray H: *Anatomy of the Human Body*, edited by C.M. Goss, American Ed. 29. Lea & Febiger, Philadelphia, 1973 (pp. 456, 457, Fig. 6-37).
7. Inman VT, Saunders JB, Abbott LC: Observations on the function of the shoulder joint. *J Bone Joint Surg* 26:1–30, 1944 (Fig. 25, p. 23).
8. Judovich B, Bates W: *Pain Syndromes: Treatment by Paavertebral Nerve Block*. Ed. 3. F.A. Davis, Philadelphia, 1949 (Fig. 6, pp. 127, 128).
9. Kellgren JH: Observations on referred pain arising from muscle. *Clin Sci* 3:175–190, 1938 (pp. 179, 184, Fig. 7).
10. Kelly M: The nature of fibrositis 1. The myalgic lesion and its secondary effects: a reflex theory. *Ann Rheum Dis* 5:1–7, 1945.
11. Kelly M: Some rules for the employment of local analgesia in the treatment of somatic pain. *Med J Aust* 1:235–239, 1947 (Table 1).
12. Kendall HO, Kendall FP, Wadsworth GE: *Muscles, Testing and Function*, Ed. 2. Williams & Wilkins, Baltimore, 1971 (p. 120).
13. Lange M: *Die Muskelhärten (Myogelosen)*. J.F. Lehmanns, München, 1931 (Fig. 40b, p. 129).
14. Long C, II: Myofascial Pain Syndromes: Part II—Syndromes of the head, neck and shoulder girdle. *Henry Ford Hosp Med Bull* 4:22–28, 1956 (p. 26).
15. Pace JB: Commonly overlooked pain syndromes responsive to simple therapy. *Postgrad Med* 58:107–113, 1975 (Fig. 3, p. 110).
16. Pernkopf E: *Atlas of Topographical and Applied Human Anatomy*, Vol. 2. W.B. Saunders, Philadelphia, 1964 (Fig. 28).
17. *Ibid*. (Figs. 44, 60).
18. Rasch PJ, Burke RK: *Kinesiology and Applied Anatomy*, Ed. 6. Lea & Febiger, Philadelphia, 1978 (p. 168).
19. Reynolds MD: Myofascial trigger point syndromes in the practice of rheumatology. *Arch Phys Med Rehabil* 62:111–114, 1981 (Tables 1 and 2).
20. Rubin D: An approach to the management of myofascial trigger point syndromes. *Arch Phys Med Rehabil* 62:107–110, 1981.
21. Sobotta J, Figge FHJ: *Atlas of Human Anatomy*, Ed. 9, Vol. 1. Hafner Division of Macmillan, New York, 1974 (pp. 142, 144, 191).
22. Sobotta J, Figge FHJ: *Atlas of Human Anatomy*, Ed. 9, Vol. 3. Hafner Division of Macmillan, New York, 1974 (p. 283).
23. Sola AE, Kuitert JH: Myofascial trigger point pain in the neck and shoulder girdle. *Northwest Med* 54:980–984, 1955.
24. Sola AE, Rodenberger ML, Gettys BB: Incidence of hypersensitive areas in posterior shoulder muscles. *Am J Phys Med* 34:585–590, 1955 (Fig. 4, p. 983).
25. Sola AE, Williams RL: Myofascial pain syndromes. *Neurol* 6:91–95, 1956 (pp. 93, 94, Fig. 2).
26. Spalteholz W: *Handatlas der Anatomie des Menschen*, Ed. 11, Vol. 2. S. Hirzel, Leipzig, 1922 (p. 323).
27. Toldt C: *An Atlas of Human Anatomy*, translated by M.E. Paul, Ed. 2, Vol. 1. Macmillan, New York, 1919 (p. 312).
28. Travell J: Basis for the multiple uses of local block of somatic trigger areas (procaine infiltration and ethyl chloride spray). *Miss Valley Med J* 71:13–22, 1949 (Figs. 2 and 3, Case 3, pp. 17 and 18).
29. Travell J: Ethyl chloride spray for painful muscle spasm. *Arch Phys Med Rehabil* 33:291–298, 1952 (p. 293).
30. Travell J: Pain mechanisms in connective tissue. In *Connective Tissues, Transactions of the Second Conference, 1951*, edited by C. Ragan. Josiah Macy, Jr. Foundation, New York, 1952 (pp. 90, 91, 93).
31. Travell J, Berry C, Bigelow N: Effects of referred somatic pain on structures in the reference zone. *Fed Proc* 3:49, 1944.
32. Travell J, Rinzler S, Herman M: Pain and disability of the shoulder and arm: treatment by intramuscular infiltration with procaine hydrochloride. *JAMA* 120:417–422, 1942 (Fig. 2B).
33. Travell J, Rinzler SH: Pain syndromes of the chest muscles: Resemblance to effort angina and myocardial infarction, and relief by local block. *Can Med Assoc J* 59:333–338, 1948 (Fig. 1, Cases 1 and 3).
34. Travell J, Rinzler SH: The myofascial genesis of pain. *Postgrad Med* 11:425–434, 1952.
35. Webber TD: Diagnosis and modification of headache and shoulder-arm-hand syndrome. *JAOA* 72:697–710, 1973 (Fig. 28).
36. Zohn DA, Mennell J McM: *Musculoskeletal Pain: Diagnosis and Physical Treatment*. Little, Brown & Company, Boston, 1976 (Fig. 9-13, p. 192).

CHAPTER 23
Teres Minor Muscle
"Silver-dollar Pain"

HIGHLIGHTS: The teres minor functions as a "little brother" to the infraspinatus muscle. **REFERRED PAIN** from trigger points (TPs) in the teres minor is usually encountered as residual pain following inactivation of TPs in the infraspinatus muscle. The pain focuses on an area about the size of a silver dollar, sharply localized to the lower posterior deltoid region. **ANATOMICAL ATTACHMENTS** of this muscle are immediately adjacent to, and just below those of the infraspinatus muscle. **INNERVATION** of the teres minor is through the axillary nerve, whereas that of the infraspinatus is by the suprascapular nerve. **ACTIONS** of this muscle are nearly identical to those of the infraspinatus: external rotation of the arm at the shoulder and assistance in stabilization of the head of the humerus in the glenoid cavity during movement of the arm. **SYMPTOMS** are chiefly posterior shoulder pain. **ACTIVATION OF TRIGGER POINTS** results from overload on the muscle while reaching out and behind the shoulder. **PATIENT EXAMINATION** reveals slight restriction of internal rotation at the shoulder on performance of the Hand-to-shoulder Blade Test. **STRETCH AND SPRAY** are done by having the patient lie on the opposite side and by bringing the involved arm over and behind the head, while applying vapocoolant from below upward over the muscle and its referred pain pattern. **INJECTION AND STRETCH** of this muscle start, with the patient recumbent, by localization of the TP between the fingers, and then by injection. This is followed by passive stretch of the muscle. **CORRECTIVE ACTIONS** include elimination of mechanical stress on the muscle, attention to the sleeping position in bed, self-administration of ischemic compression, and self-stretch exercises.

1. REFERRED PAIN
(Fig. 23.1)

A patient with active teres minor trigger points (TPs) complains of a "painful bursa" about the size of a silver dollar deep in the posterior deltoid muscle (Fig. 23.1), just proximal to the deltoid's attachment at the deltoid tubercle of the humerus. The spot of pain appears well below the subacromial bursa, but feels like "bursitis" to the patient because of its sharp localization and deep quality. If the patient complains of a broadly distributed aching pain in the arm and shoulder posteriorly, it is rarely due to TPs in the teres minor alone.

2. ANATOMICAL ATTACHMENTS
(Fig. 23.2)

The teres minor muscle attaches **medially** to the dorsal surface of the scapula near its axillary border and to the aponeuroses which separate it from the infraspinatus and teres major muscles, and **laterally** to the lowermost impression on the greater tubercle of the humerus[6] (Fig. 23.2).

Supplemental References

Other authors have clearly illustrated the teres minor muscle as seen from behind,[4, 6, 10, 13, 17, 19] from the side,[14, 18] in cross section,[2, 11] and in sagittal section.[5]

PART 2

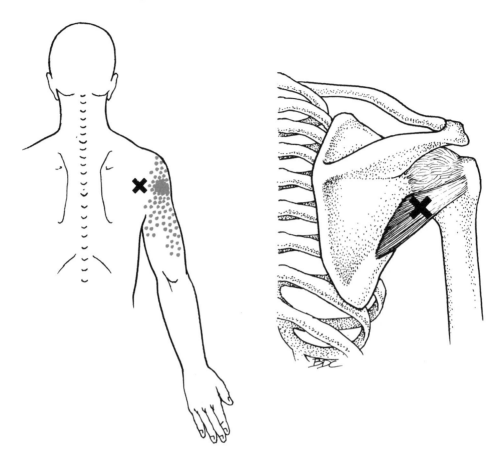

Figure 23.1.   Referred pain pattern (essential zone *solid red*, spillover zone *stippled red*) of a trigger point (×) in the right teres minor muscle.

3. INNERVATION

The teres minor muscle is innervated by the axillary nerve through the posterior cord from the C_5 and C_6 spinal nerves.

4. ACTIONS

Many of the sources reviewed[1, 3, 7, 9, 12] equated the actions of the teres minor and the infraspinatus. Both muscles externally rotate the arm at the shoulder regardless of whether the arm is abducted, flexed, or extended,[3] and help to stabilize the head of the humerus in the glenoid cavity during movement of the arm (see Section 4 in Chapter 22). Supporting this concept, the two muscles showed remarkably similar, almost linearly, increasing electrical activity as the arm was abducted at the shoulder and during flexion; the activity reached a peak at about 120° of flexion.[8] The same authors[8] confirmed electro-myographically the contribution of the teres major to external rotation of the arm.

Although Gray[6] identified weak adduction as one action of the teres minor muscle, Basmajian[1] makes no mention of electromyographic evidence that adduction is a function of this muscle.

5. MYOTATIC UNIT

The teres minor muscle functions in parallel with the infraspinatus, to which it is a "little brother," having similar attachments, but a different nerve supply. These muscles assist the other rotator cuff muscles, the supraspinatus and subscapularis, to stabilize the head of the humerus in the glenoid cavity during abduction and extension of the arm. The teres minor is also synergistic with the posterior fibers of the deltoid.

The teres minor may act as an antagonist to the subscapularis, pectoralis major and anterior deltoid muscles.

6. SYMPTOMS

Patients complain more of the pain (Fig. 23.1) than of restricted motion. When the patient presents with pain deep in the *front* of the shoulder, the symptom is likely to be due to active TPs in the infraspinatus. After treatment, with relief of the anterior shoulder pain and restoration of the normal length of the infraspinatus, the patient then becomes aware of the teres minor pain that is referred to the back of the shoulder. The infraspinatus-referred pain apparently dominates, and release of the infraspinatus tension uncovers the pain pattern of the next-tightest line of parallel muscle fibers, the teres minor.

7. ACTIVATION OF TRIGGER POINTS

The teres minor muscle is rarely involved alone. Its TPs are activated by the same overload stress, reaching out and behind the shoulder, that activates TPs in the infraspinatus muscle (see Chapter 22).

8. PATIENT EXAMINATION

This is one of the less commonly involved muscles. About 7% of patients with myofascial pain complaints in the shoulder region were found to have TPs in the teres minor.[15] Only 3% of healthy young adults had what we would call latent TPs in the teres major or minor muscles.[16]

Usually, the patient with obvious active TPs in the teres minor muscle has had the TPs in the infraspinatus inactivated by

PART 2

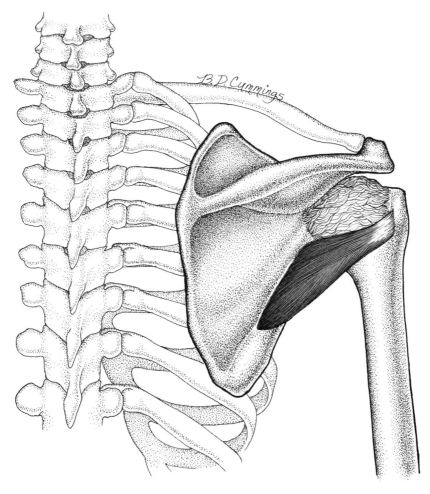

Figure 23.2. Attachments of the teres minor muscle.

treatment, but still shows restricted range of motion in the Hand-to-shoulder Blade Test. The Mouth Wrap-around Test also may be restricted. The pain has shifted from the front to the back of the shoulder, and palpation reveals evidence of TP activity in the teres minor muscle.

9. TRIGGER POINT EXAMINATION
(Fig. 23.3)

The patient lies on the opposite side with the uppermost arm resting on a pillow against the chest. The operator palpates along the lateral edge of the scapula, between the infraspinatus, above, and the teres major muscle, below, to locate active TPs in the parallel fibers of the teres minor muscle. Fig. 23.3 illustrates these anatomical relationships; see also Figure 25.3 which shows the palpation of the teres major. The teres minor lies immediately above the major, but attaches directly to the back of the humerus, rather than joining the latissimus dorsi to attach on the front of the humerus, as the teres major does (Fig. 23.3).

10. ENTRAPMENTS

No nerve entrapments are attributed to TP tension in this muscle.

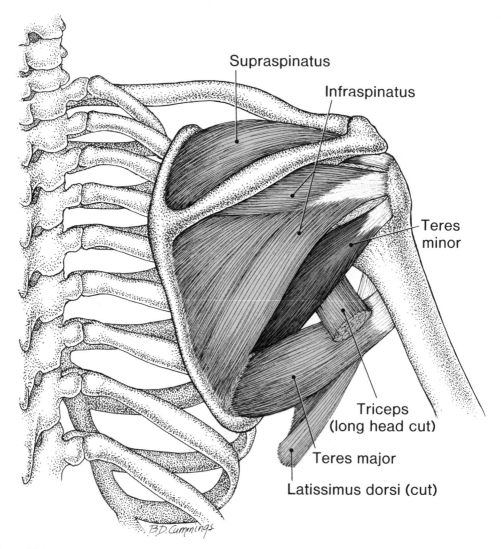

Figure 23.3.   Anatomical relations of the teres minor (*dark red*) to the dorsal scapular muscles (*light red*). The lateral border of the scapula is usually palpable as an orienting landmark in the space between the teres minor and the teres major muscles when using pincer palpation.

11. ASSOCIATED TRIGGER POINTS

The infraspinatus is the primary synergist of the teres minor, and in our experience has almost always become involved when there are TPs in the teres minor. Additional muscles likely to be involved are those presented in Section 11 of Chapter 22.

12. STRETCH AND SPRAY
(Fig. 23.4)

The patient lies on the opposite side and the operator first runs a few sweeps of spray over the muscle while flexing the arm to bring it over, and as far behind, the head as it will reach. While continuing to apply spray, the operator gradually stretches the muscle further by drawing the arm down toward the other side of the body *behind* the head and holding the arm internally rotated at the shoulder (Fig. 23.4). Parallel sweeps of the vapocoolant spray are applied along the line of the muscle fibers and over the pain reference zone. The treatment is followed by hot packs over the muscle.

Instead of, or in addition to this treatment, a member of the patient's family can be taught to apply ischemic compression by hand to the TP, or the patient can lie on a tennis ball for pressure, as recommended for the infraspinatus muscle (see Chapter 22).

13. INJECTION AND STRETCH
(Fig. 23.5)

The patient lies on the opposite side, with the involved arm in front, resting on

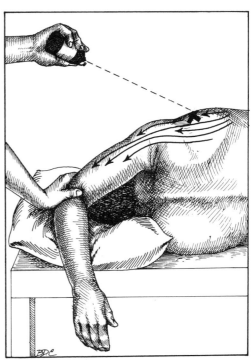

Figure 23.4.   Stretch position and spray pattern (*arrows*) for a trigger point (✗) in the teres minor muscle. The arm is held in internal rotation at the shoulder as it is brought up to and behind the head.

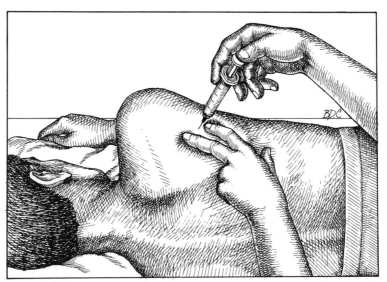

Figure 23.5.   Technique for injection of a trigger point in the teres minor muscle. The patient lies on the opposite side. The tip of the operator's index finger marks the lateral border of the scapula between the teres major and minor muscles.

a pillow. Alternatively, the patient may lie prone with the arm internally rotated (palm up) and abducted to approximately 45°, or less, to establish a tolerable stretch of the muscle. The TPs in the teres minor usually lie near the surface of the muscle and are located between the teres major and infraspinatus near the lateral border of the scapula. For injection, a TP is fixed between the index and middle fingers (Fig. 23.5), using a technique analogous to that described for the infraspinatus muscle (see Chapter 22). The needle is directed toward the scapula. Following injection, the patient makes the movement of the Hand-to-shoulder Blade Test to stretch the muscle while a few sweeps of vapocoolant are applied over it. A hot pack completes this treatment.

14. CORRECTIVE ACTIONS

Corrective actions for the teres minor are essentially those described in detail in Section 14 of Chapter 22. They include avoidance of excessive or repetitive load on the muscle, correct position of the arm to avoid full shortening during sleep, home application of hot packs and of ischemic compression, and self-stretch exercises.

References

1. Basmajian JV: *Muscles Alive*, Ed. 4. Williams & Wilkins, Baltimore, 1978 (p. 194).
2. Carter BL, Morehead J, Wolpert SM, *et al.*: *Cross-Sectional Anatomy*. Appleton-Century-Crofts, New York, 1977 (Sects. 21–23).
3. Duchenne GB: *Physiology of Motion*, translated by E.B. Kaplan. J.B. Lippincott, Philadelphia, 1949 (pp. 64, 66).
4. Grant JCB: *An Atlas of Human Anatomy*, Ed. 7. Williams & Wilkins, Baltimore, 1978 (Figs. 6-39, 6-40).
5. *Ibid.* (Fig. 6-48).
6. Gray H: *Anatomy of the Human Body*, edited by C.M. Goss, American Ed. 29. Lea & Febiger, Philadelphia, 1973 (p. 457, Fig. 6-37).
7. Hollinshead WH: *Functional Anatomy of the Limbs and Back*, Ed. 4. W.B. Saunders, Philadelphia, 1976 (p. 106).
8. Inman VT, Saunders JB, Abbott LC: Observations on the function of the shoulder joint. *J Bone Joint Surg* 26:1–30, 1944 (pp. 20, 22, 23, Figs. 26, 29).
9. Kendall HO, Kendall FP, Wadsworth GE: *Muscles, Testing and Function*, Ed. 2. Williams & Wilkins, Baltimore, 1971 (p. 120).
10. Pernkopf E: Atlas of Topographical and Applied Human Anatomy, Vol. 2. W.B. Saunders, Philadelphia, 1964 (Figs. 27, 28, 57).
11. *Ibid.* (Fig. 60).
12. Rasch PJ, Burke RK: *Kinesiology and Applied Anatomy*. Lea & Febiger, Philadelphia, 1967 (p. 168).
13. Sobotta J, Figge FHJ: *Atlas of Human Anatomy*, Ed. 9, Vol. 1. Hafner Division of Macmillan, New York, 1974 (pp. 142, 144, 191).
14. *Ibid.* (p. 192).
15. Sola AE, Kuitert JH: Myofascial trigger point pain in the neck and shoulder girdle. *Northwest Med* 54:980–984, 1955 (p. 983).
16. Sola AE, Rodenberger ML, Gettys BB: Incidence of hypersensitive areas in posterior shoulder muscles. *Am J Phys Med* 34:585–590, 1955.
17. Spalteholz W: *Handatlas der Anatomie des Menschen*, Ed. 11, Vol. 2. S. Hirzel, Leipzig, 1922 (p. 323).
18. Toldt C: *An Atlas of Human Anatomy*, translated by M.E. Paul, Ed. 2, Vol. 1. Macmillan, New York, 1919 (p. 311).
19. *Ibid.* (p. 312).

CHAPTER 24
Latissimus Dorsi Muscle
"Pernicious Mid-thoracic Backache"

HIGHLIGHTS: **REFERRED PAIN** from trigger points (TPs) in the latissimus dorsi is readily misjudged as resulting from enigmatic intrathoracic disease. Pain concentrates in the area of the inferior angle of the scapula and may extend to the back of the shoulder and down the medial arm and forearm to the ulnar aspect of the hand, including the ring and little fingers. **ANATOMICAL ATTACHMENTS** to the trunk present a fan shape that connects, below, to the spinous processes of the lower six thoracic and all the lumbar vertebrae, the sacrum, the crest of the ilium, and the last three or four ribs. Above, the muscle attaches jointly with the teres major to the humerus. **ACTIONS** include adduction and internal rotation of the arm at the shoulder and forceful depression of the scapula. **SYMPTOMS** are primarily pain which shows little aggravation or relief with activity or change of position. **ACTIVATION OF TRIGGER POINTS** results from repetitive reaching forward and upward, either to manipulate some awkwardly large object, or to pull something down. **PATIENT EXAMINATION** reveals minimal restriction of range of motion. **TRIGGER POINT EXAMINATION** requires pincer palpation of the posterior axillary fold at approximately the midscapular level to locate the source of pain. **ASSOCIATED TRIGGER POINTS** often appear in the teres major and triceps brachii muscles. **STRETCH AND SPRAY** of this muscle are often effective. The vapocoolant is applied upward over the entire muscle from the pelvis and is continued over the referred pain pattern. **INJECTION AND STRETCH** of TPs in this muscle are performed by grasping the muscle fibers within the posterior axillary fold in a pincer grip to inject them. Stretch is applied by flexing the arm at the shoulder and pulling the pelvis down. **CORRECTIVE ACTIONS** focus on teaching the patient to avoid overloading the muscle, to apply hot packs to the underarm area, and to perform stretching exercises regularly.

1. REFERRED PAIN
(Fig. 24.1)

The latissimus dorsi is a frequently overlooked myofascial cause of mid-back pain. The myofascial trigger points (TPs) responsible for that pain are usually located in the axillary portion of the muscle in the posterior axillary fold. A constant aching pain is referred to the inferior angle of the scapula and the surrounding mid-thoracic region (Fig. 24.1 *A* and *B*).[25] Referred pain also may extend to the back of the shoulder[17] and down the medial aspect of the arm, forearm and hand, including the ring and little fingers. In describing the center of this pain, the patient has difficulty reaching behind to the lower scapular region but, when asked, is apt to draw a solid circle centered on the inferior angle of the scapula to locate the pain.

Figure 24.1 *C* and *D* shows an unusual location of a latissimus dorsi TP, which refers pain to the front of the shoulder. This TP is located more caudally in the muscle, near where it attaches to the ribs. An intermediate TP refers pain locally over the lower end of the posterior axillary fold, lateral to the scapula, as previously illustrated.[36]

Injection of hypertonic saline into a normal latissimus dorsi within the posterior axillary fold induces referred pain in various parts of the pattern shown in Fig.

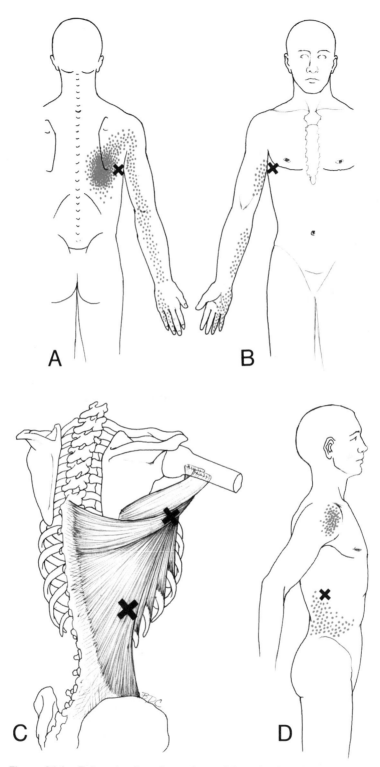

Figure 24.1   Referred pain patterns (essential portion is *solid red*, spillover portion is *stippled red*) referred from trigger points (✕s) in the right latissimus dorsi muscle. *A*, back view of the pain pattern from trigger points in their usual location within the axillary portion of the muscle. *B*, front view of same. *C*, usual location of trigger points (*upper* ✕) and unusual location (*lower* ✕). *D*, pain pattern of the unusual (*lower*) trigger point.

24.1A. Kellgren[15] reported that such an injection of 6% saline referred pain to the arm and forearm. Using 7.5% saline for injection, we found that the vertically oriented, deep fibers next to the teres major were likely to refer pain to the back in the scapular area, whereas the superficial, more horizontally oriented fibers were likely to refer pain to the upper extremity.[25]

Winter[37] attributed some cases of low back pain to TPs in the fascial attachments of the latissimus dorsi in the lumbosacral area.

2. ANATOMICAL ATTACHMENTS
(Fig. 24.2)

This muscle attaches **below** to the spinous processes of the lower six thoracic vertebrae and of all the lumbar vertebrae, to the sacrum *via* the lumbar aponeurosis, and to the crest of the ilium. The caudal ends of its most vertical fibers are anchored anteriorly to the last three or four ribs. **Above** the latissimus dorsi tendon fuses with that of the teres major, as they attach to the medial edge of the intertubercular groove of the humerus.

The teres major attachment ends distal and dorsal to that of the latissimus dorsi (Fig. 24.2). There the two tendons are covered by the pectoralis major, which all attach to the lateral edge of the same groove as they bridge the bicipital tendon. All latissimus fibers twist nearly 180° around the teres major muscle. The nearly vertical fibers of the latissimus dorsi, which attach to the ribs and crest of the ilium, hug the teres major in the axillary fold and attach proximally on the humerus. The nearly horizontal fibers, which overlap (and sometimes attach to) the tip of the scapula, form the free margin of the posterior axillary fold and attach distally on the humerus.

Rarely, a variant called the axillary arch muscle crosses the lower axillary fossa between the humeral end of the latissimus dorsi and the costal end of the pectoralis major muscle.[6, 11, 12]

Supplemental References

The latissimus dorsi has been well illustrated as seen from behind,[7, 11, 19, 22, 27, 32, 35] from the side,[6, 26] and from the front.[20, 30] Cross sections show the muscle at the tho-

racic level[9, 21] and at the lumbar level.[10, 29, 33] Details of the relationship between the latissimus dorsi and the teres major muscles in the axilla and their attachment to the humerus are shown from behind,[23, 28] from below,[34] and from in front.[8, 31]

3. INNERVATION

The muscle is supplied by the thoracodorsal (long subscapular) nerve through the posterior cord and spinal nerves C_6, C_7 and C_8.

4. ACTIONS

The latissimus dorsi primarily extends the arm at the shoulder, as when swimming the crawl or chopping wood. It adducts and assists internal rotation of the arm,[24] and depresses the humerus.[1] The combination of humeral depression and extension, acting through the glenohumeral joint, retracts the scapula and draws the shoulder downward and backward.[13] The vertical fibers of the latissimus dorsi, and to a lesser extent the lower fibers of the pectoralis major, support the body weight by depressing the scapula while "chinning" oneself and when crutch walking.

Stimulation studies[5] showed that the upper one-third (nearly horizontal fibers) of the latissimus dorsi adducted and extended the arm while strongly retracting the scapula. When the muscle contracted bilaterally, this retraction strongly extended the thoracic spine. Stimulation of the lowest third of the muscle strongly depressed the shoulder and extended the arm. Internal rotation was produced only when the arm had been placed in abduction. The tendency of strong contraction of the latissimus dorsi to subluxate the glenohumeral joint was countered by the long head of the tricep brachii and the coracobrachialis muscles.[5]

The latissimus dorsi showed minimal electromyographic activity during simulated automobile driving.[14] During 13 sport activities, both the lateral and medial parts of the muscle always showed slight to moderate motor unit activity bilaterally, with a few outstanding bursts of activity from just one part of one muscle.[2] As would be expected, typing and various sitting postures caused little, if any, activation of the latissimus dorsi.[18]

PART 2

PART 2

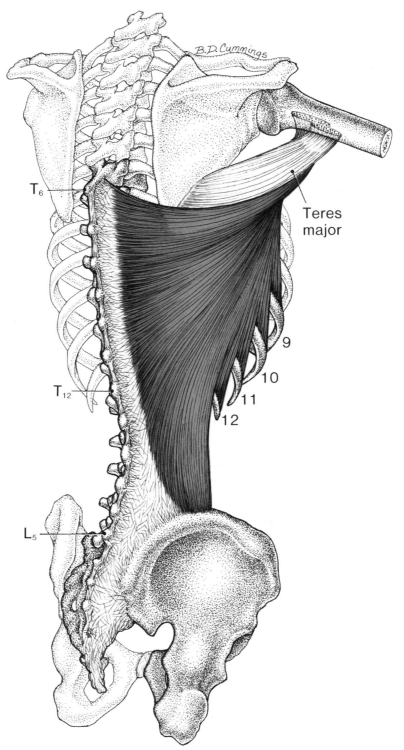

B.D. Cummings

T_6

Teres
major

T_{12}

9

10

11

12

L_5

Figure 24.2. Attachments of the latissimus dorsi (*red*), and its relation to the teres major muscle.

5. MYOTATIC UNIT

The functions of the teres major and the long head of the triceps brachii relate in a complex way to those of the latissimus dorsi; only the latissimus dorsi attaches to the trunk. Both the teres major and long head of the triceps connect the humerus and scapula, but in a crisscross fashion, with opposite leverage. With the arm at the side, the latissimus dorsi and long head of the triceps have antagonistic effects on displacement of the glenohumeral joint. In the abducted arm, their effect on this displacement is synergistic. The teres major and the latissimus dorsi, with the scapula stabilized, are strongly synergistic because of their common attachment to the humerus.

The thorax- and shoulder-elevation functions of the scalene and upper trapezius muscles are antagonistic to the depressor function of the latissimus dorsi.

Below, the anterior latissimus dorsi fibers interdigitate with the fibers of the abdominal external oblique to form a synergistic myotatic unit to depress the scapula with ribs fixed.

6. SYMPTOMS

The pernicious infrascapular mid-thoracic backache projected from the latissimus dorsi TPs is distressingly unresponsive to any kind of stretching movement or positioning by the patient in efforts to obtain relief. The latissimus dorsi is a long slack muscle and, therefore, rarely causes pain on movements that stretch it only partially, but does refer pain with depressor movements that load it. This occurs when the patient reaches up and far out in front to handle something bulky. The patient is likely to give a long history of negative diagnostic procedures, such as bronchoscopy, coronary angiogram, myelogram, or computerized tomography, and a history of unsuccessful therapy applied to the area of referred pain in the back.

Dittrich[4] attributed low back pain in many of his patients to tears and fibrous tissue pathology of the lumbodorsal and subfascial fat, which he illustrated. Based on operative findings, he surmised that the damage was done by excessive tension of the latissimus dorsi.[3] Certainly, tense TP bands would increase the tension unevenly on the muscle's attachments.

7. ACTIVATION OF TRIGGER POINTS

Aggravation of symptoms may result from repetitive reaching forward and upward, as when carrying an awkwardly large box or a bulky wicker armchair, when pulling heavy window drapes daily, or when working for several hours with a heavy chain saw at shoulder level. Other precipitating events have included: reaching overhead to exercise with a heavy weight in the hands, catching a high baseball, hanging from a swing or rope, and gardening (clipping, digging, twisting and pulling weeds).

8. PATIENT EXAMINATION

The patient is unaware of the slightly restricted range of motion that is demonstrated by the Mouth Wrap-around Test (see Fig. 22.3) and by the Triceps Brachii Test (see Fig. 32.4). To do the Triceps Test, the patient abducts the arm and, with the elbow held straight, brings the arm into firm contact with the ear and, if possible, behind the ear. Inability to hold the elbow straight in this test indicates additional involvement of the long head of the triceps.

Pain due to latissimus dorsi TPs may be elicited by reaching far forward and up (muscle stretched by arm flexion), or by having the patient press down hard on the iliac crests (muscle activated in the shortened position, performing its shoulder depressor function).

9. TRIGGER POINT EXAMINATION
(Fig. 24.3)

The examination position is similar to that for the subscapularis muscle. With the patient lying supine, the latissimus dorsi is put on half stretch by placing the hand under the head or under the pillow with the arm abducted to about 90°. The examiner grasps the latissimus dorsi muscle (Fig. 24.3) along the free border of the posterior axillary fold at the mid-scapular level where the teres major attaches, as also shown by Lange.[17] While lifting the muscle off the chest wall, the firm bands and their points of maximal tenderness (TPs) are rolled between the fingers and thumb to identify them. These TPs usually lie a few centimeters (about an inch) below the top of the arch of the posterior axillary fold. Snapping palpation of the bands elicits strong local twitch responses, which are readily seen along the scapular margin or over the lower thoracic and lumbar regions, depending on which fibers are involved. A large twitch response of several bands may cause the arm to jerk.

10. ENTRAPMENTS

No nerve entrapment has been identified as due to TP activity in this muscle.

11. ASSOCIATED TRIGGER POINTS

Eventually, the teres major usually develops active TPs in association with those in the latissimus dorsi, since these muscles are anatomically and functionally so closely related. The long head of the triceps brachii also tends to develop TPs because of synergistic or antagonistic overload, especially in chronic cases.

Diagnostically, one should consider the other muscles that may refer pain to the midback, including the upper rectus abdominus, subscapularis, iliocostalis, serratus anterior, and both the serratus posterior superior and inferior muscles.

12. STRETCH AND SPRAY
(Figs. 24.4 and 24.5)

Initially, the muscle may be stretched with the patient supine (Fig. 24.4). Before exerting tension, the vapocoolant spray is applied to the trunk in a cephalad direction, covering the length of the muscle and all of the posterior axillary fold, then down the posterior arm and forearm over the region of referred pain, including the fourth and fifth digits (Fig. 24.4). The full spray pattern is repeated as the muscle is passively stretched.

To ensure full stretch and complete coverage of the muscle posteriorly, the patient should next lie on the opposite side, and the painful arm should be slowly extended until it reaches tightly behind the ear (Fig. 24.5). While the muscle is stretched (Fig. 24.5), the sweeps of vapocoolant spray start in the area of the TPs and cover all the posterior thoracic zones of referred pain. Next the spray is directed from the TP area to the fingertips, covering the upper extremity part of the referred pain pattern.

When the nearly horizontal fibers contain TPs, they can be stretched by placing the patient's arm across the chest and pulling it into adduction, slowly and firmly to pain tolerance. The spray again follows the lines in Figures 24.4 and 24.5. The spray covers the muscle fibers and the pain reference pattern, first toward the spine, and then to the hand.

The vapocooling of this muscle is followed at once by hot packs, and then by active full range of motion.

13. INJECTION AND STRETCH
(Figs. 24.6 and 24.7)

The latissimus dorsi TPs within the posterior axillary fold are readily and effectively injected.[36] In the supine patient, they are located by pincer palpation, as described in Section 9. A TP is fixed between the digits for precise insertion of the needle and is then injected (Figs. 24.6 and 24.7); a strong local twitch response is usually both seen and felt when the needle penetrates a latissimus dorsi TP. Both the su-

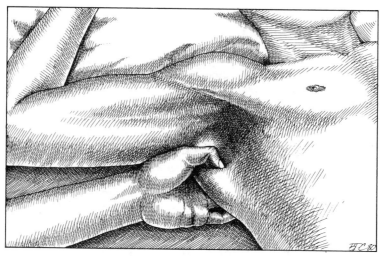

Figure 24.3. Pincer palpation of the right latissimus dorsi muscle to locate trigger points within the posterior axillary fold.

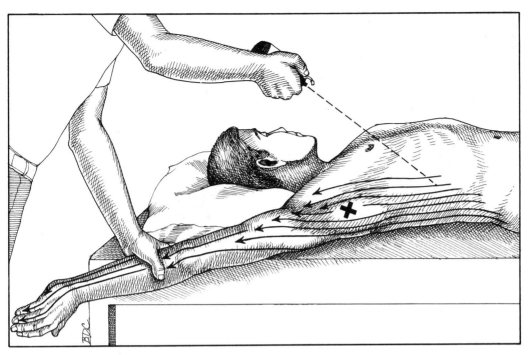

Figure 24.4. Supine stretch-position, usual location of trigger point (×), and vapocoolant spray pattern (*arrows*) for the latissimus dorsi muscle.

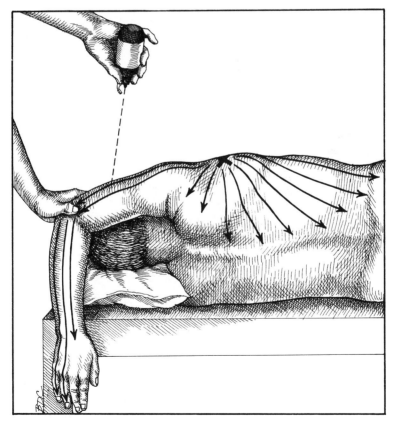

Figure 24.5. Side-lying stretch position, usual location of trigger point (×), and vapocoolant spray pattern (*arrows*) for the latissimus dorsi muscle.

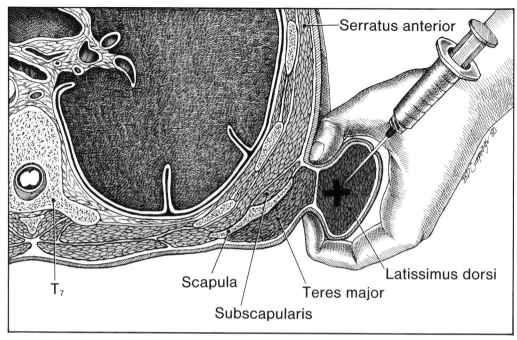

Figure 24.6.   Cross section view of injection technique for the right latissimus dorsi muscle, using pincer palpation. The "×" locates the trigger point to be injected at the level of the seventh thoracic vertebra.

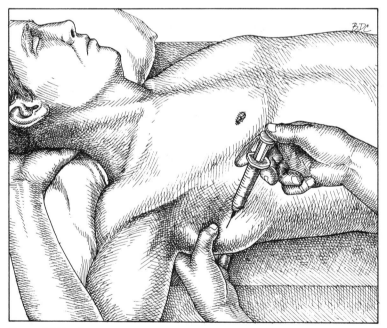

Figure 24.7.   Injection of trigger points at the usual location in the latissimus dorsi muscle.

perficial and deep axillary portions of the muscle should be probed for TPs, which tend to occur in clusters.

The teres major usually also harbors active TPs which can be injected through the same skin puncture by sliding the skin into position, with the tip of the needle held subcutaneously. The teres major TPs are injected within the pincer grasp as are those in the latissimus dorsi.

Immediate hemostasis is maintained by the palpating hand both during probing and after the injection.

Injections are followed again by stretch and spray. The treatment is completed, first with hot packs to the axillary region, and then with full acitve range of motion.

The referred pain from the fibrous tissue TPs described by Dittrich[3, 4] was relieved first by injection of the TPs with procaine and often followed by surgery.

14. CORRECTIVE ACTIONS

Following local treatment of the muscle, the patient is instructed, when pulling down on something, to keep the arm vertical (not forward of the abdomen) and the elbow beside the body; to step up on a stool so as not to reach high for a heavy object; and at night to keep a pillow in the axilla between the elbow and the chest to prevent prolonged shortening of the muscle at rest (see Fig. 30.8).

Home exercises to passively stretch the muscle include the Mouth Wrap-around Test (see Fig. 22.3) and the upper hand position of the In-doorway Stretch Exercise (see Fig. 42.10). To effectively stretch the latissimus dorsi while doing the latter, the low back must be arched (hyperextended) and the hips swung forward through the doorway; the patient should feel the tension in the latissimus dorsi muscle. Each stretch maneuver should be done smoothly, without jerking the muscle, for a few repetitions daily until relief is obtained. The effectiveness of the exercise is increased by following it with a hot pack, applied for 15–20 min, especially before retiring.

Effective self-treatment for latissimus dorsi TPs can be obtained through the home use of a tennis ball to apply pressure, as ischemic compression (see Section 14 in Chapter 22).

Supplemental References, Case Reports

The senior author[36] has reported the management of a patient with latissimus dorsi TPs. Kellgren[16] describes a patient with involvement of the latissimus dorsi and other shoulder-girdle muscles.

References

1. Basmajian JV: *Muscles Alive*, Ed. 4. Williams & Wilkins, Baltimore, 1978 (pp. 195, 356).
2. Broer MR, Houtz SJ: *Patterns of Muscular Activity in Selected Sports Skill.* Charles C Thomas, Springfield, Ill., 1967.
3. Dittrich, RJ: Low back pain—referred pain from deep somatic structure of the back. *Lancet* 73:63–68, 1953.
4. Dittrich RJ: Soft tissue lesions as cause of low back pain: anatomic study. *Am. J. Surg* 91:80–85, 1956.
5. Duchenne GB: *Physiology of Motion*, translated by E.B. Kaplan. J.B. Lippincott, Philadelphia, 1949 (pp. 38–39, 68–70).
6. Eisler P: *Die Muskeln des Stammes.* Gustav Fischer, Jena, 1912 (pp. 357–368, Fig. 48).
7. Grant JCB: *An Atlas of Human Anatomy*, Ed. 7. Williams & Wilkins, Baltimore, 1978 (Fig. 6-30).
8. *Ibid.* (Fig. 6-23).
9. *Ibid.* (Fig. 1-50).
10. *Ibid.* (Fig. 5-29).
11. Gray H: *Anatomy of the Human Body*, edited by C.M. Goss, American ed. 29. Lea & Febiger, Philadelphia, 1973 (pp. 446, 448–449, Fig. 6-33).
12. Hollinshead WH: *Anatomy for Surgeons*, Ed. 2, Vol. 3, *The Back and Limbs.* Harper & Row, New York, 1969 (pp. 280, 287, Fig. 4-19).
13. Hollinshead WH: *Functional Anatomy of the Limbs and Back*, Ed. 4. W.B. Saunders, Philadelphia, 1976 (p. 105).
14. Jonsson S, Jonsson B: Function of the muscles of the upper limb in car driving, IV. *Ergonomics* 18:643–649, 1975.
15. Kellgren JH: Observations on referred pain arising from muscle. *Clin. Sci.* 3:175–190, 1938 (p. 184, Fig. 7).
16. Kellgren JH: A preliminary account of referred pains arising from muscle. *Br Med J* 1:325–327, 1938 (Case 3).
17. Lange M: *Die Muskelhärten (Myogelosen).* J.F. Lehmanns, München, 1931 (p. 93 Case 3, p. 129 Fig. 40).
18. Lundervold AJS: Electromyographic investigations of position and manner of working in typewriting. *Acta Physiol Scand* 24:Supp. 84, 1951 (pp. 66–68, 126).
19. McMinn RMH, Hutchings RT: *Color Atlas of Human Anatomy.* Year Book Medical Publishers, Chicago, 1977 (pp. 87, 111, 112).
20. *Ibid.* (p. 118).
21. Pernkopf E: *Atlas of Topographical and Applied Human Anatomy*, Vol. 2. W.B. Saunders, Philadelphia, 1964 (Fig. 8).
22. *Ibid.* (Fig. 27).
23. *Ibid.* (Fig. 57).
24. Rasch PJ, Burke RK: *Kinesiology and Applied Anatomy.* Lea & Febiger, Philadelphia, 1967 (pp. 166–167).
25. Simons DG, Travell JG: The latissimus dorsi syndrome: a source of mid-back pain. *Arch Phys Med Rehabil* 57:561, 1976.
26. Sobotta J, Figge FHJ: *Atlas of Human Anatomy*, Ed. 9, Vol. 1, Hafner Division of Macmillan, New York, 1974 (p. 141).
27. *Ibid.* (p. 142).
28. *Ibid.* (p. 144).

29. *Ibid.* (p. 153).
30. *Ibid.* (p. 162).
31. *Ibid.* (p. 198).
32. Spalteholz W: *Handatlas der Anatomie des Menschen*, Ed. 11, Vol. 2. S. Hirzel, Leipzig, 1922 (p. 302).
33. *Ibid.* (p. 306).
34. *Ibid.* (p. 316).
35. Toldt C: *An Atlas of Human Anatomy*, translated by M.E. Paul, Ed. 2, Vol. 1. Macmillan, New York, 1919 (p. 266).
36. Travell J, Rinzler SH: Pain syndromes of the chest muscles: resemblance to effort angina and myocardial infarction, and relief by local block. *Can Med Assoc J* 59:333–338, 1948 (pp. 333, 334, Case 1, Fig. 2).
37. Winter Z: Referred pain in fibrositis. *Med. Rec* 157:34–37, 1944 (pp. 4, 5).

PART 2

CHAPTER 25
Teres Major Muscle
"Twin to Latissimus Dorsi"

HIGHLIGHTS: **REFERRED PAIN** from trigger points (TPs) in either the axillary or posterior portions of the teres major muscle penetrates deeply into the posterior deltoid region. **ANATOMICAL ATTACHMENT**, above, on the humerus merges with that of the latissimus dorsi muscle, which twists around the teres major to help it form the posterior axilliary fold. Below, the teres major attaches to the scapula while the latissimus dorsi attaches to the chest wall. **ACTIONS** of the teres major assist adduction, internal rotation, and extension of the arm from the flexed position, but only when these motions are resisted. **SYMPTOMS** are primarily pain when reaching forward and up, with little restriction of motion. **ACTIVATION OF TRIGGER POINTS** is likely to occur when driving a car that is hard to steer. **TRIGGER POINT EXAMINATION** of the axillary TP is performed by pincer palpation that surrounds the latissimus dorsi. Examination of the posterior TP is done with flat palpation against the scapula. **STRETCH AND SPRAY** may completely resolve acute symptoms. **INJECTION AND STRETCH** are often required. They should eliminate TPs in both areas of the muscle. **CORRECTIVE ACTIONS** include avoidance of overload, self-stretch exercises, and pillow positioning to prevent muscle shortening at night. All corrections may be essential for sustained relief.

1. REFERRED PAIN
(Fig. 25.1)

Trigger points (TPs) occur in the teres major muscle[24] in two locations (Fig. 25.1C): one medially overlying the posterior surface of the scapula (Fig. 25.1A) and the other more lateral in the posterior axillary fold, where the latissimus dorsi muscle wraps around the teres major (Fig. 25.1B). Both TP areas refer pain to the posterior deltoid region and over the long head of the triceps brachii, as also observed by Kelly.[8] Teres major TPs may refer pain into the shoulder joint posteriorly and occasionally to the dorsal forearm, but rarely, if ever, to the scapula or elbow.

2. ANATOMICAL ATTACHMENTS
(Fig. 25.2)

The teres major muscle attaches **medially** to an oval area on the dorsum of the scapula near its inferior angle, and to the fibrous septa shared with the teres minor

and infraspinatus muscles (see Fig. 23.3); **laterally** it attaches by a short tendon to the crest of the lesser tubercle of the humerus (Fig. 25.2). The borders of the teres major and latissimus dorsi tendons are fused at their humeral attachment (see Fig. 24.2).

Supplemental References

Other authors illustrate the teres major muscle from in front,[3, 12, 19, 23] from behind,[4, 5, 11, 13, 15, 18, 22] and in cross section.[14]

3. INNERVATION

The teres major muscle is innervated from spinal roots C_5 and C_6 *via* the posterior cord through the lower scapular nerve.

4. ACTIONS

This muscle assists internal rotation and is active during resisted adduction, and extension of the arm from the flexed position[1, 6]; it assists the latissimus dorsi in

403

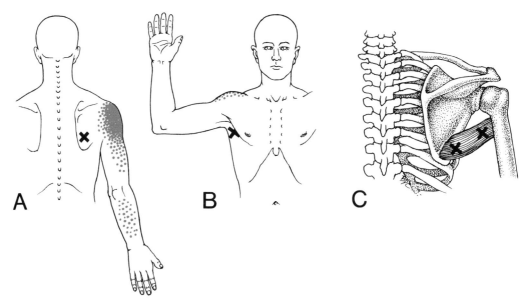

Figure 25.1.   Medial and lateral (posterior and axillary) trigger points (**X**s) in the right teres major muscle and their referred pain pattern. *Solid red* shows the essential portion; *stippled red* areas show the spillover portion of the pattern. *A*, rear view of pain pattern showing medial trigger point. *B*, front view showing lateral trigger point. *C*, location of both trigger points on the muscle.

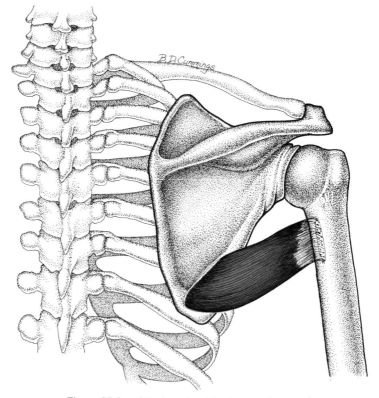

Figure 25.2.   Attachments of the teres major muscle.

the wood-chopping movement. Stimulation studies[2] showed that, alone, the teres major only weakly adducted the arm to the side. However, when the scapula was stabilized by the levator scapulae and rhomboidei to fix the inferior angle, teres major activity then strongly adducted the arm.

An early report[7] categorically stated that the muscle never exhibited activity during movement of the arm, but came into action only when necessary to maintain a static position. This was accepted as fact[16] until Basmajian[1] demonstrated that the muscle is electromyographically active when the arm is internally rotated or extended, but only against resistance. The teres major also is activated during the backward swing of the arm in walking.[1]

In an electromyographic study of typing, Lundervold[9] reported that writing long-hand caused moderate teres major activity; that striking a single typewriter key caused moderate activity of the muscle in most subjects; and that, with fatigue, activity increased markedly in amplitude. Elevation of the typewriter keyboard had little influence on teres major motor unit activity.[9]

5. MYOTATIC UNIT

The latissimus dorsi and the long head of the triceps brachii form a myotatic unit with the teres major for extension and internal rotation of the arm. These muscles commonly develop TPs together. The teres major and latissimus dorsi entwine so as to end in a common attachment on the humerus. The teres major and long head of the triceps attach to the same bones with reciprocal (spurt/shunt) leverage. The teres major attaches proximally on the humerus, whereas the long head of the triceps attaches distally on the humerus beyond the teres major.

6. SYMPTOMS

Pain (Section 1) on motion is the chief complaint, particularly while driving a heavy car without power steering. Occasionally pain occurs on reaching overhead, as in serving at tennis. Pain at rest is usually mild. Patients compensate for the slight restriction in the overhead range of arm motion without being aware of it.

7. ACTIVATION OF TRIGGER POINTS

A source of strain that repeatedly has been seen to activate teres major TPs is driving a heavy car without power steering. Apparently, force exerted across the top of the steering wheel when turning

toward the opposite side is most likely to activate these TPs on the weaker non-dominant side. For example, one lady drove a large car without power steering for several years without shoulder trouble until, by error, over-sized steel-belted radial tires were placed on the front wheels. This made the car much harder to steer and the added stress activated left teres major TPs, which resolved only with return to normal-sized front tires and local injection of the TPs.

8. PATIENT EXAMINATION

The patient has difficulty abducting the involved arm fully and cannot place it tightly against the homolateral ear (see Triceps Test, Fig. 32.4). The Mouth Wrap-around Test (see Fig. 22.3) is restricted by 3–5 cm (an inch or two) when only the teres major muscle is involved. Stretching the muscle by passively flexing and externally rotating the arm causes pain, as does loading the muscle by actively resisting extension and internal rotation of the arm at the shoulder.[10] Involvement of the teres major does not "freeze" the shoulder, or seriously restrict its motion, but it does cause disabling pain near the full range.

9. TRIGGER POINT EXAMINATION (Fig. 25.3)

Involvement of this muscle is seen repeatedly. TP tenderness was located in this muscle for 3% of the 256 latent TPs found in shoulder-girdle muscles of 200 normal young adult subjects,[20] and for 7% of the 126 active TPs found in the shoulder-girdle musculature among 80 somewhat older patients treated for shoulder pain.[21]

The TPs in the axillary portion of the teres major lie slightly cephalad to the most common location for latissimus dorsi TPs, and may be palpated by having the patient lie supine with the arm at 90° from the side and partly externally rotated (Fig. 25.3B). First, the muscle mass of the latissimus dorsi is grasped between the thumb and fingers; this muscle forms the free border of the posterior axillary fold as it wraps around the teres major muscle (see Fig. 24.2). Deep pincer palpation of the axillary fold a few centimeters (about 1 in) below the arm locates the border of the scapula (Fig. 25.3B). Since this is above the

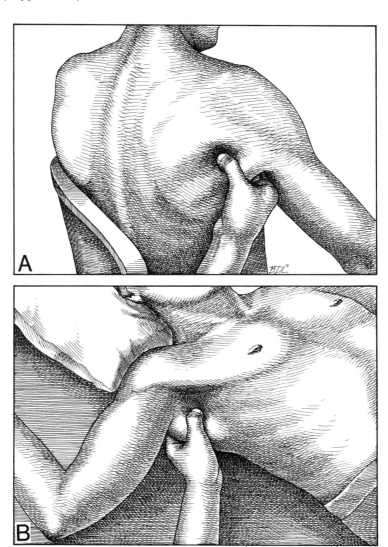

Figure 25.3. Examination of the teres major muscle. The examiner's digits must fully encompass the latissimus dorsi muscle to reach the teres major. *A,* patient seated; *B,* patient supine.

attachment of the teres major to the scapula, a groove is palpable anteriorly between the edge of the scapula and the teres major muscle. This groove lies just above the point where the teres major extends beyond the scapula and joins the latissimus dorsi. Axillary TPs of the teres major are found at the level of this groove. Below this, just above the inferior angle of the scapula, only the latissimus dorsi muscle forms the axillary fold; therefore, it is the only muscle within the pincer grasp when one palpates a groove between the lateral lower edge of the scapula and the axillary fold. At the level of the axillary TP in the

teres major, the axillary fold is formed by both muscles, which are separated by another palpable groove located between them (Fig. 25.3A). The teres major is the deeper (medial) one of the two muscles. Taut bands, when present in the muscle, can be readily located and their local twitch responses felt and seen in all but the most obese patients.

The posterior scapular TP area is best examined with the patient lying on the opposite side and the uppermost arm resting on a pillow against the chest to ensure relaxation. The teres major is located in the axillary fold as described above; the

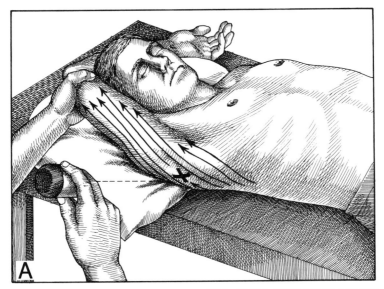

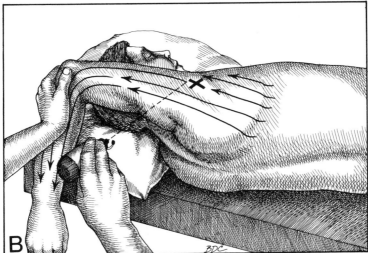

Figure 25.4.   Stretch position and spray pattern (*arrows*) for a trigger point (**X**) in the teres major muscle. *A*, patient supine; *B*, patient on opposite side.

borders of the teres major fibers are followed onto the scapula. Examination of the muscle by flat palpation reveals TPs close to the lateral border of the scapula at about mid-scapular level.

10. ENTRAPMENTS

No nerve entrapments by this muscle have been observed.

11. ASSOCIATED TRIGGER POINTS

The long head of the triceps brachii and the latissimus dorsi muscles commonly become involved with the teres major mus-

cle. Eventually, the posterior deltoid, teres minor and subscapularis also tend to develop associated TPs, causing greatly impaired function and much pain, a condition often diagnosed as "frozen shoulder".

12. STRETCH AND SPRAY
(Fig. 25.4)

The muscle may be stretched in the supine position (Fig. 25.4*A*), or with the patient lying on the opposite side (Fig. 25.4*B*); the arm is placed in full abduction at the shoulder with the elbow bent to permit controlled internal and external rotation.

PART 2

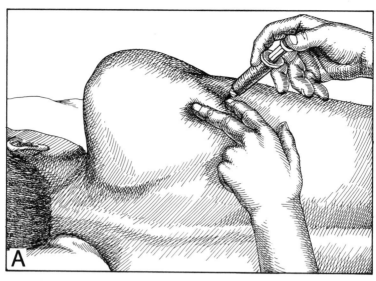

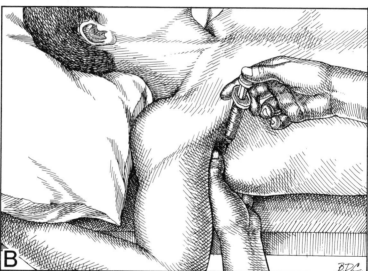

Figure 25.5.   Injection of trigger points in the teres major. *A,* posterior scapular (medial) trigger point, which is located over the lower scapula and is approached from behind with the patient lying on the opposite side. *B,* axillary (lateral) trigger point, located within the posterior axillary fold, and approached from the front with the patient supine.

After initial vapocooling, stretch tension is exerted on the muscle; the patient's hand is brought behind the head, while the inferior angle of the scapula is stabilized by resting the body weight on it. Stabilization of the scapula is easier in the supine position, but reaching the scapular portion of the muscle with sweeps of the vapocoolant spray is more difficult.

The skin is rewarmed at once with hot packs, and then function is restored by active range of motion against gravity

only. The patient should avoid strenuous effort by that muscle for several days.

The medial TP area is well suited to treatment by ischemic compression by the operator, or by the patient, using the tennis ball technique (see Section 14, Chapter 22).

13. INJECTION AND STRETCH
(Fig. 25.5)

The medial TPs in the teres major are injected against the back of the scapula like TPs in the infraspinatus muscle, but more caudally (Fig. 25.5A).

The axillary-fold (lateral) TPs of this muscle are injected with the patient supine and the arm abducted to 90°; they are approached from the inside, or anterior face, of the posterior axillary fold (Fig. 25.5B). The TPs are identified within the axillary fold and localized between the thumb and fingers, by pincer grasp. Local twitch responses are clearly felt when the needle impales a TP. The area is peppered with the needle, since a cluster of TPs is usually present. It is possible also to inject TPs in the overlying latissimus dorsi through the same skin puncture by sliding the skin and needle laterally.

14. CORRECTIVE ACTIONS

The patient should revise any activity that repeatedly stresses the teres major muscle, e.g. driving a car or truck without power steering, or lifting weights overhead.

The patient learns to stretch the muscle gently but firmly, first by placing the painful arm behind the head (start of Mouth Wrap-around Test), and then by pulling the arm with the other hand to stretch the teres major. The patient should do this seated under a hot shower, while the water beats on the skin overlying the region of the teres major muscle.

At night, to prevent full shortening of this muscle during sleep, a small pillow is placed between the elbow and side of the body; this prop maintains a slight stretch on the muscle (see Fig. 22.7).

Supplemental Reference, Case Report

The senior author has reported the management of a patient with teres major TPs.[17]

References

1. Basmajian JV: *Muscles Alive,* Ed. 4. Williams & Wilkins, Baltimore, 1978 (pp. 194, 195, 316).
2. Duchenne GB: *Physiology of Motion,* translated by E.B. Kaplan. J.B. Lippincott, Philadelphia, 1949 (pp. 81–83).
3. Grant JCB: *An Atlas of Human Anatomy,* Ed. 7. Williams & Wilkins, Baltimore, 1978 (Fig. 6-23).
4. *Ibid.* (Figs. 6-39, 6-40).
5. Gray H: *Anatomy of the Human Body,* edited by C.M. Goss, American Ed. 29. Lea & Febiger, Philadelphia, 1973 (pp. 456, 457).
6. Hollinshead WH: *Functional Anatomy of the Limbs and Back,* Ed. 4. W.B. Saunders, Philadelphia, 1976 (pp. 107–108).
7. Inman VT, Saunders JB, Abbott LC: Observations on the function of the shoulder joint. *J Bone Joint Surg* 26:1–30, 1944 (p. 24–26, Fig. 30).
8. Kelly M: Some rules for the employment of local analgaesics in the treatment of somatic pain. *Med J Aust* 1:235–239, 1947 (p. 236).
9. Lundervold AJS: Electromyographic investigations of position and manner of working in typewriting. *Acta Physiol Scand* 24:(Suppl 84), 1951. (pp. 66–68, 80–81, 94–95, 101, 157).
10. Macdonald AJR: Abnormally tender muscle regions and associated painful movements. *Pain* 8:197–205, 1980.
11. McMinn RMH, Hutchings RT: *Color Atlas of Human Anatomy.* Year Book Medical Publishers, Chicago, 1977 (pp. 111, 112).
12. *Ibid.* (p. 118).
13. Pernkopf E: *Atlas of Topographical and Applied Human Anatomy,* Vol. 2. W.B. Saunders, Philadelphia, 1964 (Fig. 28).
14. *Ibid.* (Figs. 44, 45).
15. *Ibid.* (Fig. 57).
16. Rasch PJ, Burke RK: *Kinesiology and Applied Anatomy,* Ed. 6. Lea & Febiger, Philadelphia, 1978 (p. 167).
17. Rinzler SH, Travell J: Therapy directed at the somatic component of cardiac pain. *Am Heart J* 35:248–268, 1948 (pp. 261–263, Case 3).
18. Sobotta J, Figge FHJ: *Atlas of Human Anatomy,* Ed. 9, Vol. 1. Hafner Division of Macmillan, New York, 1974 (pp. 142, 144, 191).
19. *Ibid.* (p. 196, 198).
20. Sola AE, Rodenberger ML, Gettys BB: Incidence of hypersensitive areas in posterior shoulder muscles. *Am J Phys Med* 34:585–590, 1955.
21. Sola AE, Kuitert JH: Myofascial trigger point pain in the neck and shoulder girdle. *Northwest Med* 54:980–984, 1955.
22. Toldt C: *An Atlas of Human Anatomy,* translated by M.E. Paul, Ed. 2, Vol. 1. Macmillan, New York, 1919 (pp. 266, 312).
23. *Ibid.* (p. 313).
24. Winter Z: Referred pain in fibrositis. *Med Rec* 157:34–37, 1944 (p. 4).

PART 2

CHAPTER 26
Subscapularis Muscle
"Frozen Shoulder"

HIGHLIGHTS: **REFERRED PAIN** from trigger points (TPs) in the subscapularis concentrates in the posterior deltoid area and may extend medially over the scapula, down the posterior aspect of the arm, and then skips to a band around the wrist. **ANATOMICAL ATTACHMENTS** of the subscapularis are, medially, to the inner surface of the scapula and, laterally, to the lesser tubercle on the anterior aspect of the humerus. **ACTIONS** of the subscapularis are chiefly internal rotation and adduction of the arm at the shoulder. It also helps to secure the head of the humerus in the glenoid fossa and, in this way, assists abduction of the arm. The **SYMPTOMS** of progressive painful restriction of abduction and external rotation of the arm due to subscapularis trigger points (TPs) are often diagnosed as a "frozen shoulder." **ACTIVATION OF TRIGGER POINTS** in this muscle is often caused by chronic muscular strain or sudden trauma to the shoulder. **PATIENT EXAMINATION** identifies involvement of this muscle by the marked reciprocal limitation of abduction and external rotation of the arm at the shoulder. The humeral attachment of the muscle is tender to palpation. The differential diagnosis of "frozen shoulder" includes myofascial TPs of the subscapularis and other shoulder-girdle muscles, adhesive capsulitis, and adhesions of subacromial structures. **TRIGGER POINT EXAMINATION** is exacting in its technique, but rewarding. Abduction of the scapula is necessary to reach many of the TPs in this muscle. **STRETCH AND SPRAY** of this muscle require that the patient's arm be gradually abducted and externally rotated while the vapocoolant is applied over the lateral chest wall, over the scapula, and over the pain pattern on the back of the arm and wrist. **INJECTION AND STRETCH** require identification of the TPs for injection by palpation of the subscapularis fibers against the scapula and a longer needle than usual. With proper positioning of the patient, careful technique, and follow-up stretch, injection of the TPs is safe and effective. **CORRECTIVE ACTIONS** include avoidance of prolonged shortening of the muscle both at night and during the daytime, and regular use of the In-doorway Stretch Exercise at home.

1. REFERRED PAIN
(Fig. 26.1)

Subscapularis trigger points (TPs) cause severe pain both at rest and on motion. The essential zone of the referred pain pattern lies over the posterior aspect of the shoulder (Fig. 26.1). Spillover reference zones cover the scapula and extend down the posterior aspect of the arm to the elbow. A diagnostically useful accent, when present, is a strap-like area of referred pain and tenderness around the wrist[36, 38]; the dorsum of the wrist is usually more painful and tender than the volar surface.

2. ANATOMICAL ATTACHMENTS
(Fig. 26.2)

The connection of the subscapularis to the humerus is the most anterior attachment of the four muscles that form the rotator cuff; the others are the supraspinatus, infraspinatus and teres minor muscles.[2]

Medially the subscapularis attaches to

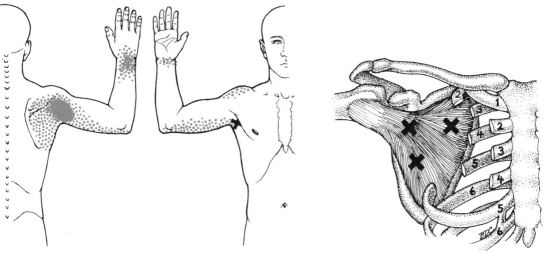

Figure 26.1.   Referred pain pattern projected from trigger points (×s) in the right subscapularis muscle. The essential referred pain zone is *solid red*; the spillover zone is *stippled red*. Portions of the second through the fifth ribs have been removed for clarity.

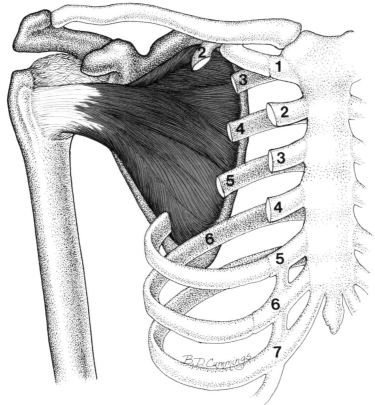

Figure 26.2.   Attachments of the right subscapularis muscle, as seen from the front with the arm externally rotated. Parts of ribs two through five are resected.

most of the inner (anterior) surface of the scapula, filling the subscapular fossa from the vertebral to the axillary border of the scapula (Fig. 26.2). **Laterally** it passes across the front of the shoulder joint *via* a tendon, which attaches to the lesser tubercle on the anterior (ventral) aspect of the humerus and the lower half of the capsule of the shoulder joint. A large bursa, which usually communicates with the cavity of the shoulder joint, separates the neck of the scapula from the muscle.[11]

Supplemental References

Other authors illustrate the subscapularis muscle as seen from in front, partially covered by overlying structures;[9, 21, 29, 35] from in front, with an unobstructed view;[30, 34] from below;[8] from the side;[33] and in cross section.[10, 25]

3. INNERVATION

The muscle is innervated by the upper and lower subscapular nerves, through the posterior cord of the brachial plexus from spinal nerves C_5 and C_6.[11, 13]

4. ACTIONS

Acting alone, the subscapularis internally rotates and adducts the arm, and helps to hold the head of the humerus in the glenoid fossa.[11] Because the deltoid muscle attaches proximal to the midpoint of the humerus, during abduction it tends to pull the head of the humerus upward, out of the glenoid fossa and against the acromion. During abduction, the depressor action of the subscapularis contributes a major force to counteract this upward displacement caused by the deltoid.[14] This stabilization function of the subscapularis was substantiated by electromyographic activity of the subscapularis during abduction that increases from 0°–90°, plateaus from 90°–130°, and rapidly diminishes from there to 180° as the deltoid no longer exerts an upward displacement force.[14]

The subscapularis is active during forward swing of the arm when walking.[2]

Electrical stimulation of the subscapularis elicits a strong internal rotation of the arm at the shoulder.[6] When a strongly shortened subscapularis maintains internal rotation of the arm, it is not possible to fully supinate the hand of the outstretched upper extremity because of the restricted external rotation at the shoulder.[6] In this way, subscapularis TPs can impair function at the hand.

5. MYOTATIC UNIT

The teres major most nearly matches the functions of the subscapularis muscle and is strongly synergistic with it. Both the latissimus dorsi and pectoralis major also adduct and internally rotate the arm, and thus can act synergistically with the subscapularis, but these muscles attach to the trunk rather than the scapula.

The arm-rotation function of the subscapularis is opposed primarily by the infraspinatus and teres minor muscles.

However, these three muscles are synergistic during arm flexion and abduction at the shoulder to prevent upward displacement of the humeral head. Thus, these three muscles form a myotatic unit with the deltoid and supraspinatus muscles for abduction and flexion of the arm at the shoulder.

6. SYMPTOMS

In the early stage of myofascial involvement of the subscapularis, patients can reach up and forward, but are unable to reach backward with the arm held at shoulder level, as when starting to throw a ball. With progression of TP hyperactivity, abduction at the shoulder becomes severely restricted to 45° or less. These patients complain of pain both at rest and on motion, and of inability to reach across to the opposite armpit. The patient has often been told that he or she has a "frozen shoulder," adhesive capsulitis or "pitcher's arm." When asked about the wrist, the patient often says that it is sore and painful in a strap-like area, especially on the dorsum. Because of this referred tenderness, the patient may move the wristwatch to the opposite wrist.

Active TPs are a major source of the pain and limited shoulder motion of hemiplegic patients, especially abduction and external rotation. The TP shortening also contributes to subluxation of the head of the humerus.

7. ACTIVATION OF TRIGGER POINTS

Subscapularis TPs are activated: (1) by unusual repetitive exertion requiring forceful internal rotation when the subject is out of condition, as in the overhead stroke of the crawl during swimming, or pitching a baseball; (2) due to repeated forceful overhead lifting while exerting strong adduction, as when swinging a small child back and forth, from between an adult's legs, up overhead, and down again; (3) by the sudden stress overload of reaching back at the shoulder level to arrest a fall; (4) when the muscles are stressed by dislocation of the shoulder joint; (5) at the time of fracture of the proximal humerus, or tear of the shoulder joint capsule; and (6) by prolonged immobilization of the shoulder joint in the adducted and internally rotated position.

8. PATIENT EXAMINATION

When examining a shoulder with restricted abduction, one of the first questions to be answered is the freedom of scapular mobility as distinguished from glenohumeral movement. Placing the hand on the scapula to note its movement as the arm is abducted answers the question. Involvement of only the subscapularis restricts glenohumeral movement, but not scapular movement on the chest. Restriction also of scapular mobility makes one think of TPs in the pectoralis minor, serratus anterior, trapezius, and rhomboid muscles.

When only the subscapularis muscle is shortened and taut, abduction and external rotation at the shoulder are reciprocally limited; one movement can trade for the other, which is easily demonstrated. If the patient has moderately active subscapularis TPs, abduction of the arm at the shoulder is limited to about 90° when the forearm hangs down, which fully internally rotates the arm. No external rotation of the arm at the shoulder is possible in this position. However, with the arm adducted by placing the elbow at the side and with the elbow bent at 90° to show shoulder joint rotation, close to 90° of external rotation is possible. The arm is internally rotated when the hand touches the abdomen and performs 90° of external rotation of the arm at the shoulder when the hand points forward. Involvement of the teres major, anterior deltoid and lower fibers of the pectoralis major also can produce this same response, but not as severely or consistently as the subscapularis.

A lesser degree of subscapularis involvement can be detected if the muscle refers pain in its characteristic pattern to the back when the arm is fully flexed in external rotation at the shoulder. This referred pain may be encountered when using this position to stretch and spray the long head of the triceps.[26]

The humeral attachment of the subscapularis (Fig. 26.2) is usually very tender to palpation when there is chronic TP involvement of the muscle. To examine this attachment, the arm is placed by the side and externally rotated as the patient extends the arm by trying to bring the elbow behind the plane of the back. This rotates the humeral attachment from the cover of the coracoid process to the front of the shoulder, where it can be palpated.

"Frozen Shoulder"

"Frozen shoulder" is a descriptive term that, in our opinion, should not be considered a diagnosis because so many authors use it to identify so many different conditions. First, a summary of current clinical usage of this term will be presented; the summary is organized under three categories of "frozen shoulder": idiopathic capsulitis, adhesive capsulitis, and subacromial fibrosis. Finally, these categories are reconsidered in terms of myofascial TPs.

Names. Synonyms for "frozen shoulder," or conditions reputed to cause it, include: adhesive capsulitis,[1, 4, 5] (adhesive) periarthritis or periarticular arthritis,[3, 4, 5, 15] pericapsulitis,[4, 5] scapulocostal syndrome,[15] calcific tendinitis of the rotator cuff,[3, 24, 32] degenerative tendinitis of the rotator cuff,[3, 4] and acromioclavicular arthritis.[3, 24]

Etiology. A "frozen shoulder" is considered by some writers to be the final stage of various disorders affecting the shoulder,[3] while others regard it as an independent, idiopathic condition.[19, 24, 37] The mechanisms proposed to account for it are often unconvincing. Cailliet[5] indicates that the "frozen shoulder" should be a clinical, not a pathological diagnosis.

Idiopathic "frozen shoulder" is considered a progressive, painful limitation of arm movement[3] that is supposed to start with pain, which then causes vasospasm and restricted movement. This, in turn, leads to a fibrotic reaction that causes more pain and more immobilization.[5, 19] What caused the pain in the first place? Further, Bateman[3] argues that a "frozen shoulder" cannot be caused by disuse alone, since it fails to develop in disuse caused by paralysis or by degenerative tendinitis of the rotator cuff.

Adhesive capsulitis is described as capsular fibrosis with the specific pathology[3] of a thickened, contracted, self-adherent synovial membrane associated with tightness and tenderness of muscles attributed to protective spasm,[3] and a thickened, shortened capsule.[23] What initiates the fibrosis?

Subacromial fibrosis is a transformation of the connective tissue within the subacromial space above the shoulder joint capsule. This space develops a thin, dry, brittle subacromial bursa and becomes laced with tough adhesions associated with thickened accessory ligaments.[3, 5, 15] Thompson and Kopell[32] also noted that increased irritability of the structures beneath the coracoacromial ligament appears to cause glenohumeral restriction and pain on motion. Again, what initiates the fibrotic changes?

Additional proposed etiologies of the "frozen shoulder" include acromioclavicular joint irritation,[3] entrapment of the suprascapular nerve[15, 32] (which can be verified by the nerve latency,[16]) prolonged immobilization of the upper extremity,[4, 24] cervical radiculopathy,[4, 20] muscle spasm,[24] myocardial infarction,[4, 20] and bicipital tendinitis.[3] Several authors hold that the bicipital tendinitis is not the cause, but the result of pathology in the shoulder joint.[4, 24]

There is no consensus in the literature concerning the etiology of "frozen shoulder."

Diagnosis. Pain has been variously described as occurring somewhere in the shoulder region,[3, 19, 31] specifically in the deltoid muscle,[4, 24, 37] worst at night,[3, 4, 15] and inceased by arm movement.[3]

Several authors apparently accepted any restriction of movement at the shoulder as diagnostic of a "frozen shoulder,"[4, 15, 24, 37] whereas some specifically designated decreased glenohumeral joint range,[3, 4] and others described restriction of both scapular glide and glenohumeral

movement as diagnostic.[5, 32] Impairment of abduction and rotation in general,[3, 19] and specifically external rotation,[20] were noted.

Cailliet identified muscle spasm as part of a pain-protective reaction in the "frozen shoulder."[5] He further noted that restricted abduction implicated the supraspinatus, that restricted external rotation implicated the subscapularis, and that impaired internal rotation implicated the infraspinatus and teres minor muscles. This was the only reference that we found in the "frozen-shoulder" literature which related restriction of particular movements to problems in specific muscles.

Patients with **idiopathic** "frozen shoulder" were most likely to be middle aged (40–50 years) and more likely to be female.[3, 4, 15, 20] Several authors reported that patients first complained chiefly of pain, then, as the pain subsided, restriction of movement developed.[5, 15, 19, 32] Two authors reported generalized shoulder tenderness in the "frozen shoulder" syndrome, without noting any localization.[3, 15]

Routine X-ray examination of the "frozen shoulder" may show that the humerus rides abnormally high in the glenoid fossa,[3] or may show calcification in the region of the rotator cuff insertions.[15, 20, 32]

In **adhesive capsulitis,** an abnormal arthrogram is reported to be diagnostic.[19, 22, 24] The arthrogram contrast medium shows that the normally rounded outline of the capsule is replaced by a squat, square contracted patch. The redundant fold at the inferior portion of the joint, which normally hangs down like a pleat, is obliterated.[3]

Adhesive capsulitis is reported as responding to manipulation under general anesthesia[37]; others express serious reservations about this form of treatment.[3, 5, 24]

Treatment. Some authors[5, 12, 19] consider the "frozen shoulder" to be self-limited; spontaneous recovery is expected in a year or two. Others emphasize that many patients never recover spontaneously.[3, 4, 31]

Oral steroids or phenylbutazone are commonly recommended for pain relief.[3, 4, 5, 20, 24] Local injection of steroid with local anesthetic also is used.[4, 24, 31, 37] Recommended sites of injection include subacromially,[5, 31, 37] into the joint capsule[20, 31] and into the bicipital tendon area.[31] Stein-brocker and Argyros[31] routinely injected these last three locations in every patient. In our opinion, much of the steroid is absorbed to produce a systemic effect that relieves pain on motion. They reported good results in combination with range of motion exercises. Marmor[19] advised against steroid injection.

Generally, a program of gradually increasing active range of motion at the shoulder joint under the guidance of a physical therapist is recommended in order to restore the normal daily use of that extremity.[3, 4, 5, 37] Many helpful exercises are well illustrated.[3] Rhythmic stabilization of the subscapularis is strongly recommended by one author,[5] but others recommend against active exercise because it aggravates pain in some patients.[19, 20] Refrigerant spray,[20] and ice packs with massage to the shoulder-girdle muscles[4] also have been recommended.

Surgery to release the restriction has been advised only for patients who had advanced adhesive capsulitis or severe subacromial fibrosis, and manipulation under anesthesia has been recommended only as part of a surgical procedure.[3, 24] Arthrography was reported to be helpful therapeutically at times when used diagnostically.[1, 20]

Myofascial Approach. When viewed in terms of myofascial TP phenomena, the etiology and natural history of most "frozen shoulders" is clear. The patient activates TPs in the subscapularis muscle which, in turn, causes associated TPs to develop in most of the remaining shoulder muscles. Also, the initiating trauma, in some cases, may activate primary TPs in several shoulder-girdle muscles. Connective tissue changes similar to those caused by TPs in other muscles (Chapters 37 and 40) combined with the marked limitation of motion due to active subscapularis TPs, may lead to adhesive capsulitis and subacromial fibrosis.

The **idiopathic "frozen shoulder,"** in our experience, usually starts with the activation of TPs in the subscapularis muscle. This restricts abduction at the shoulder, which sensitizes the pectoralis major and minor, latissimus dorsi, and triceps muscles to the development of TPs. The restriction of external rotation similarly sensitizes the anterior deltoid and teres major muscles. Referred pain from the subscapularis to the posterior deltoid region makes the latter muscle liable to satellite TPs. Involvement may continue to spread to other muscles through overload of antagonists and restriction of their range of motion. Eventually all of the shoulder-girdle muscles may become involved. Regardless of the name used, the important contribution by the muscles to this common condition remains the same. The peak age incidence of idiopathic "frozen shoulder" corresponds to that of the fibrositis syndrome (myofascial TPs) reported by Kraft et al. [17]

Diagnostically, the distribution of the referred pain and tenderness depends on which TPs are active in which muscles. The severely restricted range of motion is seldom missed, but the fact that the muscles are primarily responsible is only occasionally noted. That the subscapularis muscle is critically involved is usually overlooked.

Tenderness and calcification at the tendinous attachment of the supraspinatus muscle may develop as part of the "frozen shoulder" syndrome during prolonged TP activity and tension in that muscle.

Therapeutically, we find that stretch and spray of the specific muscles involved in an individual case is most helpful. Injection of 0.5% procaine solution in the deltoid and glenohumeral joint areas, which are zones of *referred* pain and tenderness, is much less effective than the same injection directed specifically to the parent TPs in the muscles that are referring the pain. As TP activity subsides with therapy, passive stretch, then rhythmic stabilization exercises, and finally strengthening exercises are instituted. Active exercise at first, when the TPs are still hyperirritable, can increase symptoms and thereby increase disability.

If the TPs are still in the neuromuscular dysfunction stage and have not yet progressed to the dystrophic phase (see Chapter 2), the injection of steroids and an oral course of phenylbutazone helps chiefly through temporary reduction of pain,[3] which facilitates stretching exercises and return to normal activity. In our experi-

PART 2

ence, TPs that are otherwise unresponsive to injection may respond well in conjunction with a week or two of intensive, diminishing-dose oral steroid therapy. When this is necessary, the TPs have probably progressed well into the dystrophic phase.

In time, TPs in the subscapularis muscle may subside spontaneously; or they may remain limited to just that muscle; or the TP involvement may spread to other shoulder-girdle muscles. If the patient manages to unload these muscles of excessive stress, if there are no significant perpetuating factors, and if the patient has a low tendency to develop fibrotic changes, spontaneous recovery may well occur. Responsiveness to treatment also is determined largely by these same considerations. Likely perpetuating factors are summarized in Chapter 4.

How does **adhesive capsulitis** relate to myofascial TPs in the "frozen shoulder?" The TP involvement of the subscapularis may facilitate the development of adhesive capsulitis which, in our experience, is seen in only a few percent of patients with symptoms of "frozen shoulder." Usually, the restricted range of motion initially is due entirely to TP activity in the shoulder-girdle muscles. In those patients whose muscles fail to respond to TP therapy and exercises, arthrography helps to identify a capsulitis component. To understand how subscapularis TPs could lead to capsulitis, it helps to remember that several muscles, including the trapezius, sternocleidomastoid, and infraspinatus are known to produce dramatic referred autonomic phenomena including vasoconstriction (see Chapters 6 and 7). The subscapularis also appears to exert a strong influence on reflex sympathetic vasomotor control. Fassbender[7] recently described mesenchymoid transformation, a focal proliferation of fibrous tissue, in connective tissue structures adjacent to muscles afflicted with non-articular rheumatism (myofascial TPs). The transformation was ascribed to hypoxia caused by vasoconstriction. The same process, initiated by TPs in the subscapularis, may induce fibrotic changes in the adjacent glenohumeral joint capsule that lead to adhesive capsulitis when combined with severely limited joint movement.

Diagnostically, it is not clear whether some of the arthrographic distortions of the lower bursal fold may not be caused by pressure from the taut, involved subscapularis fibers. The bursal fold lies between the subscapularis and the neck of the scapula.

How does **subacromial fibrosis** relate to myofascial TPs in "frozen shoulder?" Myofascial TPs in the remaining rotator cuff muscles (the supraspinatus, infraspinatus, and teres minor) are likely to develop as part of the total myofascial syndrome of the shoulder-girdle muscles. TPs in these muscles may induce pathologic changes in the adjacent subacromial connective tissue in a manner similar to that described for the subscapularis, above.

We know of no diagnostic test to determine how much of the limitation of motion is due to subacromial fibrosis and how much to myofascial TPs, except to inactivate the myofascial TPs in the adjacent muscles. Motion is sometimes more *painfully* limited by TP activity. Both fibrosis and TP activity may coexist; the latter is much more responsive to therapy.

9. TRIGGER POINT EXAMINATION
(Figs. 26.3 and 26.4)

The most common TPs in the subscapularis muscle lie within the subscapular fossa along the axillary border of the scapula (Fig. 26.1). Occasionally, TPs may lie more medially toward the superior angle of the scapula, where they are deeper and more difficult to palpate.

The examiner first abducts the arm of the supine patient away from the chest wall to 90°, if possible. In patients with marked shortening of the subscapularis muscle due to hyperactive TPs, it may not be possible to abduct the arm beyond 20° or 30°. Figure 26.3 shows the relationship of the subscapularis to the scapula, the latissimus dorsi, teres major and to other adjacent muscles. The arm is abducted to the 90° position for examination. Abduction (lateral displacement) of the scapula is necessary to adequately expose the ventral (inner) surface of the scapula and its subscapularis muscle for palpation.

Next, the examiner grasps the latissimus dorsi and teres major muscles (Fig. 26.3) in a pincer grip (Fig. 26.4 *A* and *B*) and locates the hard edge of the scapula with the tips

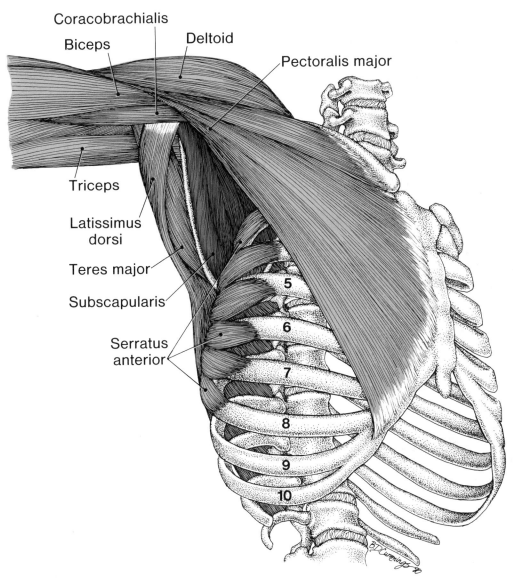

Figure 26.3.   Relation of the subscapularis muscle (*dark red*) to the surrounding muscles (*lighter red*) when the scapula (shown as a vertical white line) has been pulled away from the chest wall by the examiner (compare with Fig. 26.2).

of the digits. Traction must be maintained on the arm to abduct the scapula, (*arrow* in Fig. 26.4B shows direction of pull). The phantom finger "C" in Figure 26.4B locates the same portion of the subscapularis as is being palpated in Figure 26.4C, illustrating the increased accessibility of the subscapularis by abducting the scapula.

This is the most frequent location of TPs along the lateral margin of the muscle. The palpating finger slides into the space between the serratus anterior, which lies against the chest wall above the finger, and the subscapularis muscle, beneath the finger. The pressure is directed cephalad and toward the spine of the scapula to locate firm bands of muscle fibers in the TP area. Sustained, light-to-moderate pressure on an active subscapularis TP in a band is likely to reproduce the patient's posterior shoulder and scapular pain, occasionally with a referred twinge in the wrist. Local twitch responses are sometimes seen and are often felt.

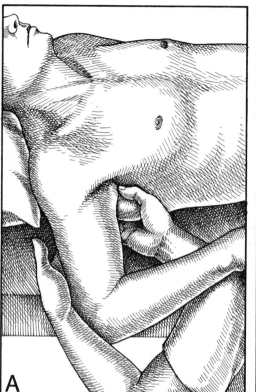

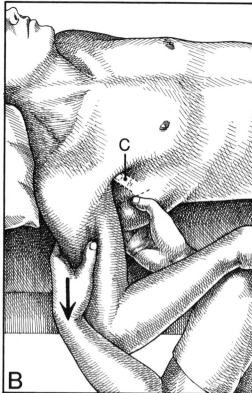

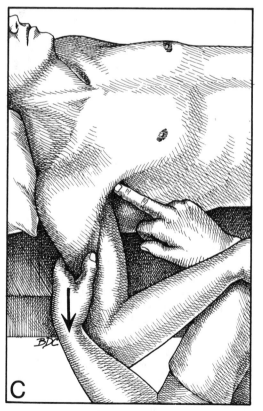

Figure 26.4. Examination of the subscapularis muscle. *A*, pincer grasp of the latissimus dorsi and teres major muscles demonstrates the inaccessibility of the subscapularis with the scapula in its usual resting position. *B*, same grasp as in Part *A*, with the scapula pulled away from the chest wall (*arrow*) to make the subscapularis muscle more accessible for palpation. The *dashed line* indicates where the thumb is pressed against the bony edge of the scapula. The phantom finger, ''*C*'', shows how far the actual finger position in Part *C* extends beyond the edge of the scapula. *C*, location of the finger to palpate the most cephalad trigger point area along the axillary border of the scapula.

In thin supple patients, more direct control of the scapula is obtained if the examiner hooks the fingers of the non-palpating hand directly on the vertebral border of the scapula and pulls it laterally, away from the midline of the body.

In patients with severe subscapularis involvement, deep tenderness in the muscle is usually so exquisite that they can tolerate only very light digital pressure on the muscle. Normal subscapularis muscles palpated in this way are non-tender.

The second most common TP area in this muscle is found more caudally, just inside the axillary border of the scapula (Fig. 26.1), and is readily palpated when the scapula is abducted. In our experience, it is nearly as common as the site described above. Lange[18] identified only this lower site, which is the most readily located, especially if the scapula is not abducted.

Palpation of the third, least common, TP area in the subscapularis is described in Section 13. One should not stimulate TPs by examination unless one is prepared to treat them immediately. Both the examination and injection of this TP area requires more skill than that of most beginners.

10. ENTRAPMENTS

No nerve entrapments have been attributed to this muscle.

11. ASSOCIATED TRIGGER POINTS

When there is moderate TP involvement of the subscapularis muscle, the patient's arm movement may be restricted by this muscle alone without associated TP activity in other shoulder-girdle muscles. When the subscapularis TPs become sufficiently active, the restriction of motion at the shoulder due to pain becomes severe. Then, myotatically related muscles quickly become involved (Section 5), so that many, or most, of these muscles develop active TPs. Motion at the shoulder is then "frozen." Autonomic trophic changes are likely to follow soon.

The pectoralis major tends to develop TPs early, probably due to the restriction of its normal range of motion. The teres major, latissimus dorsi and long head of the triceps brachii are often next to develop secondary TPs. The anterior and posterior parts of the deltoid soon become involved. No longer can any of these muscles be stretched to their full length; this severely limits all movement at the shoulder.

12. STRETCH AND SPRAY
(Fig. 26.5)

With the patient supine, the operator first applies a few initial sweeps of spray and then abducts the arm to the limit of tolerance, holding it in the neutral position between internal and external rotation. As the operator then starts to externally rotate the arm from the position of Figure 26.5A to the position of Figure 26.5B, the vapocoolant spray is again swept upward over the fold of the axilla (Fig. 26.5B). The patient's body weight helps to fix the scapula. Passive stretch on the subscapularis is gradually increased by placing the patient's hand successively under the head, then under the pillow, and finally over the edge of the bed, as the range of arm motion increases with respect to both abduction and external rotation (Fig. 26.5C). To achieve the full effectiveness of the spray, the patient's body is turned sufficiently to sweep the vapocoolant over the dorsal surface of the scapula, including its vertebral border.

When other shoulder muscles also are involved, the full range of abduction and external rotation at the shoulder may be blocked until these other muscles are released, especially the teres major, latissimus dorsi, pectoralis major and anterior deltoid. When full external rotation is approached during abduction, the unaccustomed shortening may cause shortening activation of an antagonist of the subscapularis, the supraspinatus muscle. This activation of its latent TPs may cause sudden, severe pain referred to the shoulder, but can be prevented or relieved if the supraspinatus muscle is promptly stretched and sprayed.

One may think of the release of these successively activated muscles as unravelling the history of the condition, much as one unwinds layers of a bandage, with the subscapularis as the original layer.

In hemiplegic patients, stretch and spray

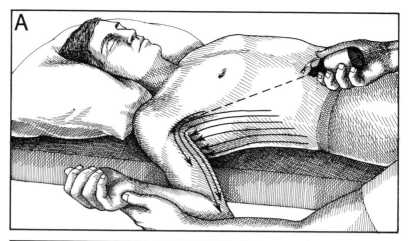

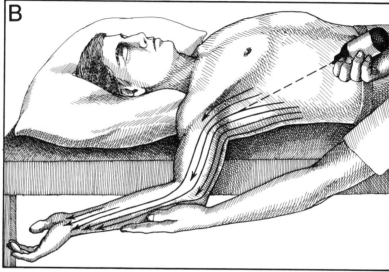

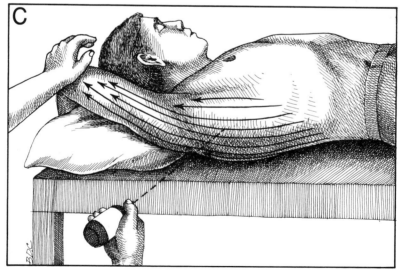

Figure 26.5. Stretch position and spray pattern (*arrows*) for trigger points in the subscapularis muscle. *A,* initial stretch position. *B,* intermediate stretch position that is reached as the tautness of the muscle partially releases. *C,* full stretch of the subscapularis muscle. The involved side of the chest is rolled up, away from the table, sufficiently for the spray to cover *all* of the skin that overlies the subscapularis posteriorly.

420

are likely to provide only temporary benefit in the acute phase, or if there is resting spasticity. There is no contraindication to the application of stretch and spray several times a day, and it can provide much relief of pain. After several months, with no resting spasticity, stretch and spray may lead to lasting relief of pain and to permanent improvement in the range of shoulder motion.

Stretch and spray are followed at once by hot packs, then by active range of motion exercises, and finally by the middle hand-position of the In-doorway Stretch Exercise (see Chapter 42).

13. INJECTION AND STRETCH
(Figs. 26.6 and 26.7)

If TP tenderness, pain and restriction of movement remain after non-invasive treatment by stretch and spray, precise injection of the active TPs may be effective. The patient lies supine in the same position as that used for vapocooling, with the arm abducted, if possible, to 90°. The patient's hand is placed under the pillow, or with the wrist at shoulder level (Fig. 26.5A), if that is as high as it will go. The patient's body weight holds the scapula in position after it is pulled laterally (Fig. 26.4 B and C). Active TPs are located in the two most common areas and are fixed between the fingers. A 6- or 7.5-cm (2½- or

3-inch), 22-gauge needle is inserted between the examiner's fingers into the depth of the axillary fossa; the needle is directed parallel to the rib cage and cephalad, toward the face of the scapula, into the TPs identified by palpation (Fig. 26.6). The needle is always inserted caudal to the TPs being injected, which avoids directing it toward the rib cage.

After the lateral TPs have been inactivated, if pain remains, the high medial TP area shown in Figure 26.1 may be responsible. These TPs lie in the thick band of fibers arching across the middle of the muscle and attaching to the scapula apparently between the posterior cut ends of ribs four and five, as shown in Figure 26.2.

To palpate these deep TPs located toward the superior angle of the scapula, one should first turn the patient on the opposite side and grasp the scapula with the non-palpating hand, placing the index finger just beneath the spine of the scapula as illustrated in Figure 26.7A, to be used as a target. While exerting counter pressure laterally with the hand holding the scapula, the palpating finger is pressed deep into the axilla, directly toward the tip of the target index finger. In this way, one locates precisely the TP tenderness as the patient lies supine, relaxes and rests the hand on the examiner's shoulder (Fig. 26.7B). The operator keeps clearly in mind

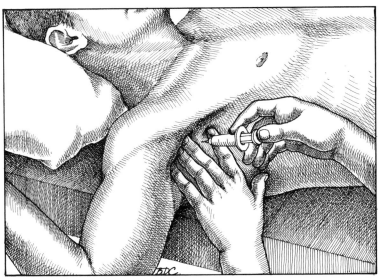

Figure 26.6.   Injection of trigger points in the subscapularis muscle along the axillary border of the scapula.

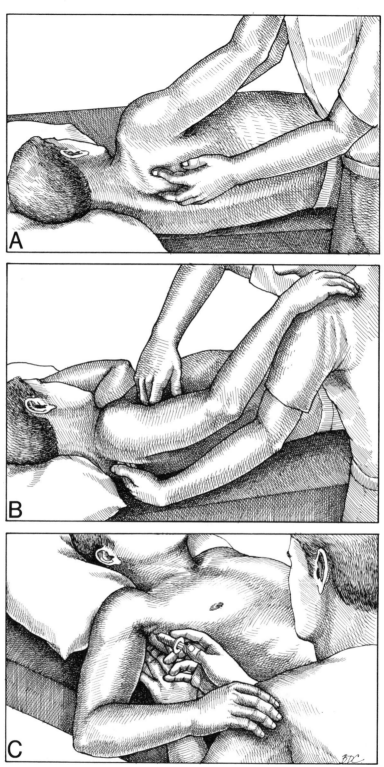

Figure 26.7. Injection of deep trigger points located high in the subscapularis, toward the superior angle of the scapula. *A,* the trigger point area is located approximately under the index finger of the left hand (see text). The patient has been turned to show this location. *B,* the patient is positioned for palpation of this trigger point area. The middle finger of the right hand probes the depth of the muscle, using the index finger of the left hand (placed as in Part *A*) as its target. *C,* injection of this medial trigger point area after it has been located.

the orientation of the TPs as the needle is directed precisely in the direction of the deep TP tenderness on the face of the scapula (Fig. 26.7C), while the examiner keeps one finger against the chest wall. To avoid the possibility of causing a pneumothorax, the needle is aimed away from, or, at most, tangent to, the rib cage, *toward* the scapula (Fig. 26.7C). Referred pain, and/or a local twitch response, signal contact with the TP.

The TP injection is followed immediately by stretch and spray, and then a hot pack to warm the skin over the subscapularis.

Use of steroid (see Section 13, Chapter 3) should be considered for inclusion in the injected solution, or for systemic administration in conjunction with procaine injections if subscapularis TPs fail to respond to this injection and no uncorrected perpetuating factors (see Chapter 4) can be found.

14. CORRECTIVE ACTIONS
(Fig. 26.8)

Sleep Position

When sleeping on the painful side or back, the patient should keep a small pillow between the elbow and side of the chest (Fig. 26.8), thus maintaining some arm abduction and preventing prolonged positioning of the subscapularis muscle in the fully shortened position. When sleeping on the pain-free side, the pillow is moved to support the painful arm in front of the body (see Fig. 22.7). This prevents folding the arm across the chest in the

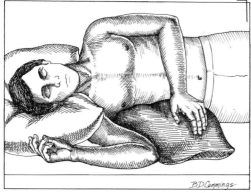

Figure 26.8. Use of a pillow at night to prevent sustained shortening of the right subscapularis muscle when lying on the affected side.

fully adducted and internally rotated position.

Posture Stress

The patient should hook the thumb in the belt or on the hip when standing for a period of time to prevent the arm from remaining close to the side. Also, when sitting, the patient should move the arm to stretch the muscle frequently. When driving a car, this stretching is done by resting the right arm across the back of the passenger's front seat, or by opening the window in warm weather and holding on to the roof of the car with the left hand. In cold weather, the armrest on the door may be used for the left arm. When driving long distances, the subscapularis muscle generates much referred pain if it remains in the shortened position without movement; a non-dominant left subscapularis is the more vulnerable, since a dominant right arm is more active.

Home Exercise

The patient learns to passively lengthen the muscle by using the middle and lower hand-positions of the In-doorway Stretch Exercise (Fig. 42.10). Three cycles of each of these hand positions should be performed at least twice daily, preferably after a hot pack, hot shower, or hot bath.

Circumduction, or an arm-swinging exercise, with the person leaning over and the arm hanging down (Codman's exercise) is very helpful. A weight may be hung from the fingers or wrist to increase the traction on the rotator cuff muscles. The circular movement should be clockwise for the left, and counter-clockwise for the right arm.

Rhythmic stabilization[28] of the subscapularis muscle (cyclic resisted abduction and external rotation at the shoulder to the limit of pain) increases the tolerance of the muscle to stretch by reflex reciprocal inhibition, thus improving its range of motion.

Supplemental Reference, Case Reports

The senior author described the management of a patient with TPs in multiple muscles, including the subscapularis.[27]

References

1. Annexton M: Arthrography can help free "frozen shoulder." *JAMA* 241:875–876, 1979.

PART 2

2. Basmajian JV: *Muscles Alive*, Ed. 4. Williams & Wilkins, Baltimore, 1978 (p. 316).
3. Bateman JE: *The Shoulder and Neck*. W.B. Saunders, Philadelphia, 1972 (pp. 134, 145–146, 149, 284–290).
4. Cailliet, R.: *Soft Tissue Pain and Disability*, F.A. Davis, Philadelphia, 1977 (pp. 161, 162).
5. Cailliet R: *Shoulder Pain*. F.A. Davis, Philadelphia, 1966 (Figs. 41, 42, pp. 64–70).
6. Duchenne GB: *Physiology of Motion*, translated by E.B. Kaplan. J.B. Lippincott, Philadelphia, 1949 (pp. 64, 66).
7. Fassbender HG: *Pathology of Rheumatic Diseases*. Springer-Verlag, New York, 1975 (pp. 94–98, 309, 314).
8. Grant JCB: *An Atlas of Human Anatomy*, Ed. 7. Williams & Wilkins, Baltimore, 1978 (Fig. 6–18).
9. *Ibid.* (Fig. 6–23).
10. *Ibid.* (Fig. 6–27).
11. Gray H: *Anatomy of the Human Body*, edited by C.M. Goss, American Ed. 29. Lea & Febiger, Philadelphia, 1973 (pp. 455–456).
12. Grey RG: The natural history of "Idiopathic" frozen shoulder. *J Bone Joint Surg* 60-A:564, 1978.
13. Hollinshead WH: *Functional Anatomy of the Limbs and Back*, Ed. 4. W.B. Saunders, Philadelphia, 1976 (p. 87).
14. Inman VT, Saunders JB, Abbott LC: Observations on the function of the shoulder joint. *J Bone Joint Surg* 26:1–30, 1944 (pp. 14, 15, 21–24).
15. Kopell HP, Thompson WAL: Pain and the frozen shoulder. *Surg Gynecol Obstet* 109:92–96, 1959.
16. Kraft GH: Axillary, musculocutaneous and suprascapular nerve latency studies. *Arch Phys Med Rehabil* 53:383–387, 1972.
17. Kraft GH, Johnson EW, LeBan MM: The fibrositis syndrome. *Arch Phys Med* 49:155–162, 1968.
18. Lange M: *Die Muskelhärten (Myogelosen)*. J.F. Lehmanns, München, 1931 (p. 129, Fig. 40A).
19. Marmor LC: The painful shoulder. *Am Fam Physician* 1:75–82, 1970 (pp. 78–79).
20. Mattingly S: The painful shoulder, Chapter 20. In *Progress in Clinical Rheumatology*, edited by A.ST.J. Dixon. J. & A. Churchill, London, 1965 (pp. 334–336).
21. McMinn RMH, Hutchings RT: *Color Atlas of Human Anatomy*. Year Book Medical Publishers, Chicago, 1977 (p. 118).
22. Mikasa M: Subacromial bursography. *J Jap Orthop Assoc* 53:225–231, 1979.
23. Neviaser JS: Adhesive capsulitis of shoulder: study of pathological findings in periarthritis of shoulder. *J Bone Joint Surg* 27:211–222, 1945.
24. Neviaser JS: Musculoskeletal disorders of the shoulder region causing cervicobrachial pain; differential diagnosis and treatment. *Surg Clin North Am* 43:1703–1714, 1963 (pp. 1708–1713).
25. Pernkopf E: *Atlas of Topographical and Applied Human Anatomy*, Vol. 2. W.B. Saunders, Philadelphia, 1964 (Fig. 60).
26. Reynolds MD: Personal communication, 1980.
27. Rinzler SH, Travell J: Therapy directed at the somatic component of cardiac pain. *Am Heart J* 35:248–268, 1948 (Case 3, pp. 261–263).
28. Rubin D: An approach to the management of myofascial trigger point syndromes. *Arch Phys Med Rehabil* 62:107–110, 1981.
29. Sobotta J, Figge FHJ: *Atlas of Human Anatomy*, Ed. 9, Vol. 1. Hafner Division of Macmillan, New York, 1974 (pp. 162, 191, 198).
30. Spalteholz W: *Handatlas der Anatomie des Menschen*, Ed. 11, Vol. 2. S. Hirzel, Leipzig, 1922 (p. 318).
31. Steinbrocker O, Argyros TG: Frozen shoulder: treatment by local injections of depot corticosteroids. *Arch Phys Med Rehabil* 55:209–213, 1974.
32. Thompson WAL, Kopell HP: The components of the frozen shoulder. *Bull NY Acad Med* 36:501–509, 1960.
33. Toldt C: *An Atlas of Human Anatomy*, translated by M.E. Paul, Ed. 2, Vol. 1. Macmillan, New York, 1919 (p. 277).
34. *Ibid.* (pp. 313).
35. *Ibid.* (pp. 315, 316).
36. Travell J, Rinzler SH: The myofascial genesis of pain. *Postgrad Med* 11:425–434, 1952.
37. Weiser HI: Painful primary frozen shoulder mobilization under local anesthesia. *Arch Phys Med Rehabil* 58:406–408, 1977.
38. Zohn DA, Mennell J McM: *Musculoskeletal Pain: Diagnosis and Physical Treatment*. Little, Brown & Company, Boston, 1976 (Fig. 9-13, p. 192).

CHAPTER 27
Rhomboideus Major and Minor Muscles
"Superficial Backache and Round Shoulders"

HIGHLIGHTS: Both of the rhomboid muscles often "complain" because of latent trigger points (TPs) in the powerful pectoralis major muscles, which shorten and pull the shoulders forward. This overloads the weaker interscapular muscles. **REFERRED PAIN** from the rhomboid muscles concentrates medially to the vertebral border of the scapula and extends over the supraspinous area of the scapula. **ANATOMICAL ATTACHMENTS** are to the spinous processes of vertebrae C_7 to T_5 medially, and laterally to the vertebral border of the scapula. **ACTIONS** are primarily to retract the scapula and rotate it, turning the glenoid fossa down. The **MYOTATIC UNIT** includes the trapezius muscle as the chief synergist, and the pectoral muscles as antagonists. **ACTIVATION OF TRIGGER POINTS** is usually caused by poor posture, which is often due to latent TPs in the pectoral muscles. **PATIENT EXAMINATION** reveals little, or no, restriction in the range of motion of the arm at the shoulder. **TRIGGER POINT EXAMINATION** by palpation usually discloses multiple TPs close to, and medial to, the vertebral border of the scapula. **STRETCH AND SPRAY** require, for full stretch, protraction of the scapula with upward rotation of the glenoid fossa. The spray is applied in a caudal direction, parallel to the muscle fibers. **INJECTION AND STRETCH** demand persistence and patience to inactivate all of the TPs. **CORRECTIVE ACTIONS** include inactivation of pectoral muscle TPs, correction of functional scoliosis, self-administration of ischemic compression, and home use of the Middle-trapezius and In-doorway Stretch Exercises.

1. REFERRED PAIN
(Fig. 27.1)

Pain referred from trigger points (TPs) in the rhomboid muscles concentrates along the vertebral border of the scapula between the scapula and the paraspinal muscles.[12] It may spread upward over the supraspinous portion of the scapula (Fig. 27.1). The pain pattern somewhat resembles that of the levator scapulae, but without the neck component and restriction of neck rotation. Referred pain has not been reported as extending to the arm.

Experimental injection of hypertonic saline into normal rhomboid muscle caused referred pain felt over the upper lateral part of the scapula and extending over the acromion.[10]

2. ANATOMICAL ATTACHMENTS
(Fig. 27.2)

The more cephalad and smaller of the two rhomboid muscles, the rhomboideus minor, attaches *above* to the ligamentum nuchae and to the spinous processes of the C_7 and T_1 vertebrae, and *below* to the medial border of the scapula at the root of its spine (Fig. 27.2). The rhomboideus major attaches *above* to the spinous processes of the T_2 through T_5 vertebrae, and *below* to the medial border of the scapula between its spine and inferior angle.

Supplemental References

Other authors have illustrated these muscles from behind,[3, 6, 7, 13, 14, 17, 20, 21] from the side,[4] and in cross section.[2, 5, 15]

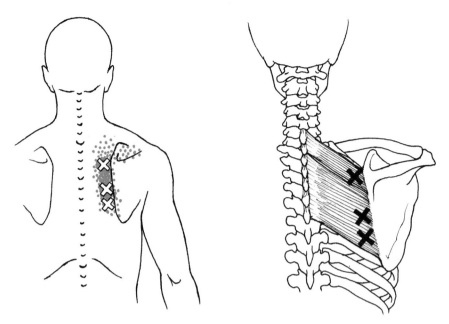

Figure 27.1. Composite referred pain pattern (essential zone *solid red*, spillover zone *stippled red*) of trigger points (×s) in the right rhomboid muscles.

3. INNERVATION

The rhomboid muscles are innervated by the dorsal scapular nerve *via* the upper trunk from the C_5 (occasionally also the C_4) root.

4. ACTIONS

Based on anatomical considerations, the rhomboid muscles adduct (draw medially) and elevate the scapula.[7, 8] The attachment of the rhomboideus major fibers to the lower vertebral border of the scapula tends to rotate the scapula, turning the glenoid fossa down (caudally).[1, 7, 8, 11, 16] These muscles, therefore, assist forceful adduction and extension of the arm by stabilizing the scapula in the retracted position.[16] The rhomboid muscles hold the lower angle of the scapula close to the ribs, preventing winging (protrusion of the inferior angle) of the scapula when the upper extremity is pushing forward against resistance, as when leaning forward against a wall.[16] With the scapula fixed, the two rhomboid muscles on one side rotate the spine, turning the face to the opposite side. Bilaterally, they extend the thoracic spine.[11]

Electromyographically, these muscles were reported to be more active during abduction than during flexion of the arm at the shoulder, like the fibers of the middle trapezius.[1] The electrical activity of the rhomboidei rapidly increased in intensity between 160° and 180° of either movement.[9] This activity is not predicted by any of the anatomically-based actions listed above. The stabilization function during lightly loaded abduction is apparently an additional action that fixes the scapula firmly against the paraspinal soft tissues. The rhomboid muscles are active during both forward and backward swings of the arm while walking,[1] probably also to stabilize the scapula.

No distinction was drawn between the functions of the rhomboideus major and rhomboideus minor by the authors quoted above. Because of the differences in attachments of these two muscles to the scapula, the rotator effect of the major may be much greater than that of the minor.

5. MYOTATIC UNIT

The rhomboid muscles act synergistically with the levator scapulae and with the upper trapezius for elevation of the scapula. They are synergistic with the levator scapulae[8] and latissimus dorsi,[16] but oppose the upper trapezius in rotation of

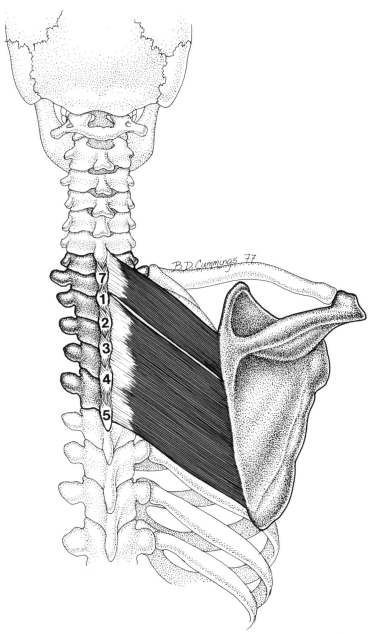

Figure 27.2. Attachments of the rhomboideus major and rhomboideus minor muscles to the vertebral spinous processes and to the medial border of the scapula.

the scapula. Basmajian[1] considers the rhomboidei synergistic with the middle trapezius for assisting abduction of the arm to 90° and in early flexion of the arm at the shoulder.

Scapular retraction by the rhomboid and middle trapezius muscles is opposed by the pectoralis major and minor, which protract the scapula.

6. SYMPTOMS

The rhomboid pair is infrequently involved among shoulder-girdle muscles.[18, 19]

Pain (Section 1) is rarely identified as originating in this muscle until TPs in neighboring involved muscles, such as the levator scapulae, trapezius and infraspinatus, have been inactivated. The complaint is of superficial, aching pain at rest, not influenced by ordinary movement.

Patients reach for, and try to rub, the painful area, whereas the pain referred from TPs in the underlying serratus posterior superior feels as though it were too deep to be reached by surface pressure.

Snapping and crunching noises during movement of the scapula may be due to TPs in the rhomboid muscles.

7. ACTIVATION OF TRIGGER POINTS

The TPs in the rhomboid muscles are activated by prolonged leaning forward and working in the round-shouldered position (as when writing or sewing); by overload due to prominence of the scapula on the convex side in upper thoracic scoliosis (due to idiopathic scoliosis, chest surgery, or a short leg); by prolonged holding of the arm in abduction at 90°; and by overload due to TPs in the pectoralis major.

8. PATIENT EXAMINATION

No obvious restriction of motion is caused by TPs in the rhomboid muscles. The patients tend to have a round-shouldered posture.

9. TRIGGER POINT EXAMINATION

The rhomboidei are best examined with the patient seated and the arms hanging forward to protract and spread the scapulae apart. Palpation reveals TPs just medial to, and along the vertebral border of, the scapula, as illustrated in Figure 27.1 and by Sola and Kuitert.[18] All but the caudal ends of the lowermost fibers of the rhomboideus major must be palpated through the trapezius. Local twitch responses are difficult to perceive, but the referred pain from active TPs may be induced by deep palpation.

If the precise borders of these muscles are in doubt, the patient to be examined should lie prone with his or her hand in the small of the back. The examiner tries to place a finger (reinforced with the opposite hand, if necessary) deep to the me-

dial border of the scapula. When the patient lifts the hand up off the back, the rhomboid muscles contract vigorously, pushing the examiner's finger out from under the scapula. Once the rhomboidei have been outlined, deep palpation across the muscle fibers with the patient in any convenient position should identify the firm "ropy" bands that contain TPs.

10. ENTRAPMENTS

No nerve entrapments have been attributed to these muscles.

11. ASSOCIATED TRIGGER POINTS

Active rhomboid TPs usually become obvious only after elimination of TPs in the levator scapulae, trapezius and infraspinatus muscles. Patients with rhomboid TPs complain of upper back and scapular pain. They are frequently stooped and round-shouldered, appear flat-chested, and are unable to stand up straight because of TP-induced tautness in either or both the pectoralis major and minor. The rhomboid and middle trapezius muscles on both sides are then overloaded by having to oppose the stronger, shortened pectoral muscles. The pectoralis TPs may be latent and not signaling trouble by pain, but they are nevertheless overloading their dorsal antagonists, which do the complaining.

12. STRETCH AND SPRAY
(Fig. 27.3)

Treatment should start with inactivation of any pectoral TPs and restoration of normal resting length to the pectoralis major and minor muscles. Stretch and spray are then applied to the rhomboid TPs, with the patient seated and relaxed, the upper thoracic spine flexed, and the arms hanging between the knees (Fig. 27.3A), or crossed in front of the chest (Fig. 27.3B). The patient should "hump" the back (flex the thoracic spine) and let the weight of the arms pull the shoulder blades forward and laterally. The operator may push forward and down on the acromial process to assist protraction of the scapula (Fig. 27.3C). The patient inhales deeply while the spray is applied downward in slow parallel sweeps over the rhomboid muscles, in the direction of their muscle fibers

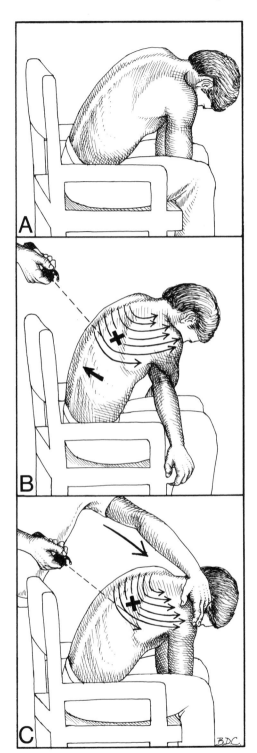

Figure 27.3. Stretch position and spray pattern (*thin arrows*) for a trigger point (✕) in the right rhomboideus major muscle. *A*, position for optimum stretch of the rhomboideus minor. *B*, position for optimum stretch of the rhomboideus major and spray pattern for both muscles. *C*, the operator increases the stretch on the

(Fig. 27.3*B*). The uppermost sweeps are continued across the scapula to cover the lateral extension of the referred pain pattern.

An alternate method provides more direct stretch, but the patient has more difficulty in relaxing completely: with the patient seated and well supported by the chair, the operator grasps the elbow on the involved side and pulls the shoulder forward and down by pulling the elbow across the front of the body toward the patient's opposite knee. Again, the patient humps the back and takes a deep breath, fully expanding the chest while the vapocoolant spray is applied in the pattern described above (Fig. 27*B*). Flexing the arm upward across the chest not only protracts but also rotates the scapula, glenoid fossa up. This places maximum stretch on the lowest rhomboid fibers. A maximum stretch on the rhomboideus minor may be obtained by having the patient hang the arms down between the knees.

Stretch and spray are followed by hot packs and active range of motion, as for the Middle-trapezius Stretch Exercise (see Fig. 6.11).

13. INJECTION AND STRETCH

The TP is localized and fixed against the chest wall between the fingers of the palpating hand. For injection of the TP, a 3.8-cm (1½-in) needle is directed almost tangential to the surface. The needle is aimed toward a rib to avoid penetrating an intercostal space. The rhomboid muscles often harbor multiple TPs, each of which should be injected individually by locating all the tender spots in the muscle.

Stretch and spray are then applied, as above. A hot pack follows to reduce postinjection soreness, and then active range of motion is performed to maintain normal muscle length.

14. CORRECTIVE ACTIONS

The patient should be taught how to apply ischemic compression to the rhomboid TPs by lying on a tennis ball placed

rhomboid muscles by pressing forward (*long single arrow*) and down on the acromion.

on the floor, or on a large thin book on the bed (see Section 14, Chapter 22). The patient can "press out" the spot tenderness due to each rhomboid TP by rolling the tennis ball along the inner border of the scapula and holding it centered against a tender spot until the pain gradually fades, usually in 20 or 30 sec, sometimes as long as a minute. One patient had learned by herself that placing a warm iron upside down in the bed and lying on it could relieve the TP pain and soreness.

The patient also should learn to do the Middle-trapezius Stretch Exercise (see Fig. 6.11), which also stretches the rhomboid muscles.

If the patient has involvement of the pectoral muscles, daily use of the In-doorway Stretch (see Fig. 42.10) is more effective if it is done after a hot shower, bath, or pack.

The use of a lumbar pillow, which maintains the normal lumbar curve when sitting, helps greatly to correct the round-shouldered posture, especially while working at a desk or driving a car. A chair with a vertical, flat backrest should be avoided; it pushes the upper torso and shoulders forward. Some backward slope of the backrest, with lumbar support, is needed for a comfortable seated posture.

For a patient who becomes preoccupied at a desk and forgets to change position and thus relieve the strain on the muscles from time to time, an interval timer can be set to ring across the room. Then, the patient must get up at regular intervals of 20–30 min to turn it off and reset it. This need not interrupt the train of thought.

Any protrusion of the scapula due to *functional* scoliosis that is caused by a short leg or small hemipelvis can be corrected by leveling the pelvis and straightening the spine with appropriate lifts (see Section 14, Chapter 48).

References

1. Basmajian JV: *Muscles Alive*, Ed. 4. Williams & Wilkins, Baltimore, 1978 (pp. 192, 316, Fig. 10.1).
2. Carter BL, Morehead J, Wolpert SM, et al.: *Cross-Sectional Anatomy*. Appleton-Century-Crofts, New York, 1977 (Sects. 19–23).
3. Eisler P: *Die Muskeln des Stammes*. Gustav Fischer, Jena, 1912 (Fig. 51).
4. *Ibid.* (Fig. 52).
5. *Ibid.* (Fig. 68).
6. Grant JCB: *An Atlas of Human Anatomy*, Ed. 7. Williams & Wilkins, Baltimore, 1978 (Figs. 5-26, 6-30).
7. Gray H: *Anatomy of the Human Body*, edited by C.M. Goss, American Ed. 29. Lea & Febiger, Philadelphia, 1973 (p. 449, Fig. 6-33).
8. Hollinshead WH: *Functional Anatomy of the Limbs and Back*, Ed. 4. W.B. Saunders, Philadelphia, 1976 (pp. 103, 104).
9. Inman VT, Saunders JB, Abbott LC: Observations on the function of the shoulder joint. *J Bone Joint Surg* 26:1–30, 1944 (p. 27, Fig. 33).
10. Kellgren JH: Observations on referred pain arising from muscle. *Clin Sci* 3:175–190, 1938 (p. 183).
11. Kendall HO, Kendall FP, Wadsworth GE: *Muscles, Testing and Function*, Ed. 2. Williams & Wilkins, Baltimore, 1971 (p. 122).
12. Kraus H: *Clinical Treatment of Back and Neck Pain*. McGraw-Hill, New York, 1970 (p. 98).
13. McMinn RMH, Hutchings RT: *Color Atlas of Human Anatomy*. Year Book Medical Publishers, Chicago, 1977 (p. 112).
14. Pernkopf E: *Atlas of Topographical and Applied Human Anatomy*, Vol. 2. W.B. Saunders, Philadelphia, 1964 (Fig. 28).
15. *Ibid.* (Fig. 44).
16. Rasch PJ, Burke RK: *Kinesiology and Applied Anatomy*. Lea & Febiger, Philadelphia, 1967 (p. 151).
17. Sobotta J, Figge FHJ: *Atlas of Human Anatomy*, Ed. 9, Vol. 1. Hafner Division of Macmillan, New York, 1974 (p. 142).
18. Sola AE, Kuitert JH: Myofascial trigger point pain in the neck and shoulder girdle. *Northwest Med* 54:980–984, 1955 (p. 983).
19. Sola AE, Rodenberger ML, Gettys BB: Incidence of hypersensitive areas in posterior shoulder muscles. *Am J Phys Med* 34:585–590, 1955.
20. Spalteholz W: *Handatlas der Anatomie des Menschen*, Ed. 11, Vol. 2. S. Hirzel, Leipzig, 1922 (p. 303).
21. Toldt C: *An Atlas of Human Anatomy*, translated by M.E. Paul, Ed. 2, Vol. 1. Macmillan, New York, 1919 (p. 267).

CHAPTER 28
Deltoid Muscle
"A Dull Actor"

HIGHLIGHTS: **REFERRED PAIN** from active trigger points (TPs) in the deltoid muscle is not projected to a distance as for most muscles, but only locally to the region of the affected (anterior or posterior) part of the muscle. **ANATOMICAL ATTACHMENTS** are, above, to the clavicle, acromion and spine of the scapula and, below, to the deltoid prominence of the humerus. **ACTIONS** of the anterior part of this superficial muscle, which covers the head of the humerus, are antagonistic to its posterior part in horizontal flexion and extension. Together with the middle fibers, the anterior and posterior fibers help the supraspinatus muscle abduct the arm at the shoulder. The **MYOTATIC UNIT** of the anterior part, synergistically, is the clavicular section of the pectoralis major, the biceps brachii (long head), and the coracobrachialis muscles. The posterior part acts synergistically with the latissimus dorsi, teres major, and the triceps brachii (long head) muscles. **ACTIVATION OF TRIGGER POINTS** may result from impact trauma in sports, from over-exertion, or from the hypodermic injection of irritant medication where latent TPs are located. They also may develop as satellite TPs lying within the pain reference zone of another muscle, especially the infraspinatus. **PATIENT EXAMINATION,** when TPs are active in the anterior deltoid, reveals painful restriction of the Mouth Wrap-around Test and painfully weakened abduction of the externally rotated arm. Posterior deltoid TPs painfully weaken abduction of the internally rotated arm. **STRETCH AND SPRAY** of anterior and posterior deltoid TPs employ a proximal-to-distal spray pattern. **INJECTION AND STRETCH** are technically simple and usually effective. **CORRECTIVE ACTIONS** include the elimination of perpetuating mechanical stresses, and a program of daily stretching exercises to prevent reactivation of TPs.

1. REFERRED PAIN
(Fig. 28.1)

The deltoid is one of the muscles that most often develops myofascial trigger points (TPs).[16] When these hyperirritable foci appear in the anterior part of the deltoid, they (Fig. 28.1A) refer pain to the anterior and middle deltoid regions.[21, 43, 46, 49] Active TPs in the posterior part of the deltoid (Fig. 28.1B) refer pain over the middle and posterior deltoid regions, sometimes spilling into adjacent areas of the arm. Like its corresponding pelvic-girdle muscle, the gluteus maximus, the deltoid lacks any distant projection of referred pain. Referred pain from this muscle was demonstrated experimentally by the injection of hypertonic saline.[39]

2. ANATOMICAL ATTACHMENTS
(Fig. 28.2)

Proximally the anterior third of the deltoid muscle attaches to the lateral one-third of the clavicle (Fig. 28.2); the middle part, to the acromion; and the posterior part, to the lateral portion of the spine of the scapula. *Distally* all fibers converge near the mid-point of the lateral aspect of the humerus and attach to its deltoid prominence. This point appears, in most patients, as a dimple in the skin at the base of the "v" formed by the belly of the muscle.

The anterior and posterior parts of the deltoid comprise long fiber-bundles which travel directly between attachments. The middle part is bipenniform. Its fibers travel

431

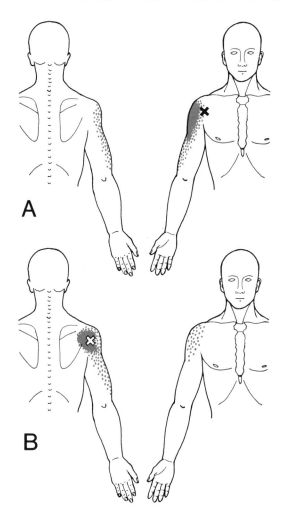
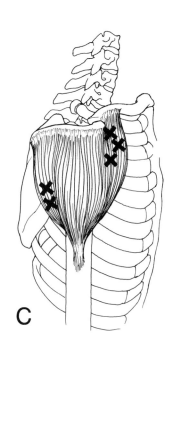

Figure 28.1.   Referred pain patterns (*red*) from trigger points (✕s) in the right deltoid muscle. *A*, pain pattern from trigger points in anterior part of the muscle; *B*, pain patterns from the posterior part; *C*, usual location of trigger points in the muscle, lateral view.

obliquely between tendons (usually four) that extend downward from the acromion, into the substance of the muscle, and three interdigitating tendons that extend upward from the deltoid prominence, as previously described[1, 15] and clearly drawn schematically.[14] Thus, the middle part of the muscle, by design, produces more force through a shorter distance than do the anterior and posterior parts.

Supplemental References

The deltoid muscle has been well illustrated from the anterior view,[10, 26, 29, 36, 40] the side view,[11, 27, 34, 37, 41] the posterior view,[12, 28, 30, 35, 38, 42] and in cross section.[13, 31]

3. INNERVATION

This muscle is supplied through the C_5 and C_6 spinal roots *via* the posterior cord and its terminal branch, the axillary nerve.[15]

4. ACTIONS

At one time, it was thought that the deltoid initiates abduction at the shoulder and that the supraspinatus completes it; however, the electrical activity of both the deltoid and supraspinatus muscles increases progressively throughout abduction. It is greatest in both muscles when the arm is elevated between 90° and 180°.[19]

Abduction of the arm at the shoulder

PART 2

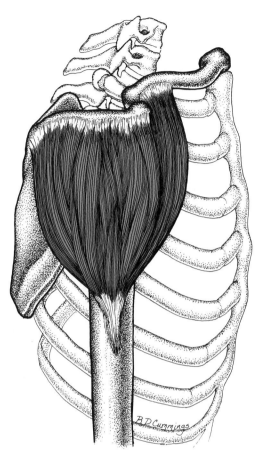

Figure 28.2. Attachments of the right deltoid muscle. Compare the complexly interwoven fibers in the middle part with the fusiform arrangement in the anterior and posterior parts.

progresses with smooth coordination of the glenohumeral joint movement and scapular rotation in a constant 2:1 ratio.[19] This mechanism is called the scapulohumeral rhythm.[6, 7] Paralysis of either the supraspinatus or deltoid muscle simply reduces the force and endurance of abduction.[8, 9] Patients with deltoid TPs, however, may show serious impairment of strength, or total inability to reach 90° of abduction in positions of the arm that load the affected part of the muscle.

Simultaneous contraction of the anterior, middle and posterior parts abduct the arm.[2, 15] Only the lowest fibers of both the anterior and posterior parts adduct the arm.[18] Otherwise, the anterior and posterior parts oppose each other.

The anterior part of the deltoid forward flexes the arm,[15, 18, 32] as confirmed by elec-

tromyographic[2] and electrical stimulation[9] studies; it also horizontally flexes the arm across the chest.[32] The attachments look as if this part of the muscle should internally rotate the arm,[15, 18] but this action is questioned by electromyographers.[2] Movement of the hand to the face requires adequate function of the anterior deltoid and serratus anterior muscles,[9] both of which contribute to the scapulohumeral rhythm.

The middle part of the deltoid muscle is designed structurally for abduction, during which it responds strongly electromyographically.[2]

The posterior part extends the arm[2, 15, 18, 32]; this function is essential in order to reach behind the body to the gluteal area and beyond.[9] Anatomically, this part should assist external rotation,[15, 18] but that function has not been substantiated electromyographically.[2] When the dependent upper extremity was carrying weight, marked increase in the electrical activity of the more horizontal, posterior marginal fibers of the deltoid confirmed its important role in securing the head of the humerus in the vertically oriented, capsule-rimmed glenoid cavity. Contraction of the deltoid and supraspinatus muscles helps to wedge the head of the humerus upward against the slope of the lower glenoid labrium to prevent downward dislocation of the humerus at the glenohumeral joint.[2, 5]

During sports activities that require underhand, overhand and sidearm movements, the amplitude of motor unit activity in the anterior part of the deltoid was consistently greater than in the other parts of the muscle, with one exception: during the tennis serve, the middle part of the muscle showed a strong double peak of maximum activity.[4]

Raising the typewriter keyboard clearly increased the continuous electrical activity (strain) present in the deltoid muscle.[25] In a subsequent methodological study Hagberg and Jonsson[17] showed that the activity load on the deltoid is increased if the work height is either too low or too high, and that amplitude distribution analysis is a useful method to clearly demonstrate this effect.

Driving a car with the hands on top of the steering wheel activated chiefly the anterior, and to a lesser extent the middle, part of the muscle. Activation occurred when the driver pushed the steering wheel toward the opposite side, a movement of horizontal flexion. The posterior deltoid was rarely activated.[20]

5. MYOTATIC UNIT

The anterior deltoid, coracobrachialis, clavicular section of the pectoralis major, and the long head of the biceps brachii are commonly involved together as a myotatic unit. The pectoralis minor muscle also may develop active TPs in association with those in the anterior deltoid.

The posterior deltoid forms a myotatic unit with the long head of the triceps brachii, the latissimus dorsi and teres *major* muscles. The teres *minor* fibers, which are aligned with the posterior deltoid only in full abduction, are less likely to develop associated TPs.

Since, as noted in Section 4, the anterior and posterior deltoid fibers commonly function as antagonists, they may develop active TPs together.

6. SYMPTOMS

The history may reveal onset of symptoms after impact trauma to the anterior deltoid muscle during sports activities.

The patient complains of pain on shoulder motion and to a lesser degree, of pain at rest, deep in the deltoid area (Fig. 28.1). The patient with active anterior deltoid TPs has difficulty in raising the arm to the horizontal, as in bringing the hand to the mouth, and in reaching back at shoulder level.

7. ACTIVATION OF TRIGGER POINTS

Anterior Part of Deltoid

Few other muscles are so likely to receive forceful impacts directly against underlying bone. Impact trauma may occur from a hit by a tennis or golf ball, or the repeated recoil of a gun when shooting. Trauma by sudden overload often occurs during a loss of balance when going down steps and reaching out to a bannister or railing to "catch the fall." Overload repetitive strain develops during prolonged lifting (holding a power tool at shoulder height), or episodic overexertion (unaccustomed deep sea fishing).

Posterior Part of Deltoid

Intramuscular injection of locally irritant solutions (e.g. B vitamins, penicillin, tetanus toxoid, diphtheria or influenza vaccine) into a latent TP is likely to activate it and to cause a persistently painful shoulder.[44] This disability can be avoided (1) by preliminary palpation of the injection site for tender points (latent TPs) so as to avoid them; (2) by adding enough 2% procaine solution in the syringe before injection to bring it to a 0.5% solution of procaine; (3) by peppering the site with 1 ml of 0.5% (or stronger) procaine solution immediately after the injection, if continuing pain at the injection site indicates that a TP was activated; (4) by routine stretch and spray of the muscle following any intramuscular injection; or (5) by selecting another site, such as, the lateral thigh.

Overexercise may activate TPs in the posterior deltoid e.g. by excessive poling when skiing. This part rarely develops TPs alone as the result of activity, but usually in association with TPs in other muscles.

8. PATIENT EXAMINATION

The patient straightens the elbow and tries to abduct the arm to 90°, first with the thumb up (palm forward) and then with the thumb down (palm backward). The thumb-up position is painful when fibers in the anterior part of the deltoid muscle harbor active TPs; the thumb-down position is painful when it loads TPs in the posterior part of the muscle.

Involvement of the anterior deltoid impairs performance of the Back-rub Test (see Fig. 29.3). When the patient with active TPs in the posterior deltoid attempts the Mouth Wrap-around Test (see Fig. 22.3), the arm can reach over the head, but not behind it, because of pain induced by forceful contraction of the affected posterior deltoid fibers in the shortened position.

Differential Diagnosis

Referred pain from the deltoid may mimic pain arising in the glenohumeral joint,[33] and thus, be misdiagnosed as arthritis of that joint.

Rotator cuff tears and tendinitis, and subdeltoid bursitis, may cause deep shoulder pain and tenderness similar to deltoid

TP-referred pain, but lack the specific physical signs of palpable bands and local twitch responses in the muscle.

The acromioclavicular joint underlies the proximal attachment of the anterior deltoid muscle. Pain due to sprain, subluxation, or complete dislocation of this joint mimics the pain pattern of anterior deltoid TPs, or *vice versa*. A sprain of the acromioclavicular joint produces localized tenderness over the joint, rather than TP tenderness in the deltoid muscle, and causes pain on passive mobilization of the joint by arm motion which rotates or elevates the scapula. Acromioclavicular subluxation and dislocation are identified by increasing loss of mobility.[3] In the latter two conditions, bilateral standing X-ray examination with a weight held in each hand for comparison, or physical examination of the joint under local anesthesia, help to identify the depression and forward displacement of the clavicle in relation to the acromion.[7] For this joint problem, either conservative[7] or surgical[3] treatment is recommended. Both the acromioclavicular joint and the deltoid muscle may be in trouble simultaneously.

9. TRIGGER POINT EXAMINATION

The deltoid is a superficial muscle, which simplifies detection of its palpable bands and vigorous local twitch responses. The relaxed muscle is examined by snapping palpation across the TPs, while the fibers are under moderate tension, which occurs when the arm has been abducted to about 30°. If the muscle is slackened by abducting the arm to 90° or more, as sometimes recommended,[22, 37] the taut bands and their twitch responses are less evident, if detectable at all.

Anterior deltoid TPs (Fig. 28.1C) and their palpable bands[22] are usually located high in the anterior margin of the muscle, in front of the glenohumeral joint.[47] Occasionally, middle deltoid fibers also may develop TPs, usually just below the acromion and distal to the attachment of the supraspinatus tendon. The supraspinatus attachment to the rotator cuff frequently becomes tender in response to the chronic tension caused by TPs in the supraspinatus muscle. When the arm is abducted to 90° at the shoulder, the supra-

spinatus attachment is protected from pressure, beneath the acromion; the deltoid TPs remain tender to palpation.

The posterior deltoid TPs (Fig. 28.1C) are usually located more distally along the posterior margin of the muscle.[24, 48]

One rarely finds TP involvement of the deltoid muscle alone.

10. ENTRAPMENTS

Entrapment of the axillary nerve due to TPs in this muscle has not been observed.

11. ASSOCIATED TRIGGER POINTS

Active TPs in the anterior part of the deltoid muscle are often associated with TPs: (1) in the clavicular section of the pectoralis major (adjacent to the anterior deltoid); (2) in the biceps brachii; and (3) in the antagonistic, posterior part of the deltoid.

When an active TP is found in the posterior deltoid, one should check the proximal one-third of the long head of the triceps brachii, the latissimus dorsi, and the teres major muscles for associated TPs. The posterior deltoid is unlikely to be the only muscle affected with active TPs, unless latent TPs were activated by local injection of an irritant solution into the muscle, after which the TP activity tends to be self-sustaining.

Because the deltoid lies in the essential pain reference zones of both the infraspinatus and supraspinatus muscles, it rarely escapes for long the development of satellite TPs when these two scapular muscles harbor active TPs. The increased irritability of motor units in the reference zone was demonstrated experimentally by motor unit activity in the anterior deltoid in response to pressure on an active TP in the infraspinatus muscle that caused referred pain over the front of the shoulder. At the same time, recording needles in the biceps and triceps brachii showed electrical silence.[45]

If inactivation of deltoid TPs restores abduction of the arm at the shoulder only to about 90°, then any active supraspinatus TPs should be located and eliminated. This usually restores the full range of arm motion in the overhead position, unless antagonists to abduction are also involved.

PART 2

12. STRETCH AND SPRAY
(Figs. 28.3 and 28.4)

With the patient seated, the *anterior* deltoid may be stretched by abducting the arm to 90°, externally rotating it at the shoulder, and bringing it backward (Fig. 28.3*A*). The vapocoolant spray pattern slowly traces the course of the muscle fibers distally and then covers the area of referred pain before and while applying stretch tension.

The *posterior* deltoid is stretched by internally rotating the arm and pulling it up across the chest of the seated patient (Fig. 28.3*B*). Sweeps of the spray are directed over the posterior deltoid fibers from above downward to cover the muscle and include the pain reference zone. This position also stretches the supraspinatus and infraspinatus muscles. Both should be included in the spray pattern, particularly if they are tender, or if a full range of shoulder motion is not achieved after release of the posterior part of the deltoid muscle by the stretch-and-spray procedure.

Two stretch positions and the spray pattern for the *middle* deltoid are shown in Figure 28.4*A* and *B*.

Deep massage, as described by Lange,[22] and ischemic compression also may be effective for inactivation of deltoid TPs.

13. INJECTION AND STRETCH
(Fig. 28.5)

The TPs in the anterior, middle, and posterior parts of the deltoid muscle are readily identified by flat palpation, and then localized between the fingers and injected as in Fig. 28.5. Active deltoid TPs give readily visible, strong local twitch responses and evoke nearby referred pain when impaled by the needle.

Myofascial TPs in the anterior deltoid lie close to the anterior border of the muscle where the cephalic vein passes between the deltoid and pectoralis major muscles. When injecting these TPs (Fig. 28.5*A*), the vein can be avoided by placing one finger of the palpating hand on it.

The pain and tenderness over the glenohumeral joint, which are referred from anterior deltoid TPs, may easily lead to the erroneous assumption that the joint is the

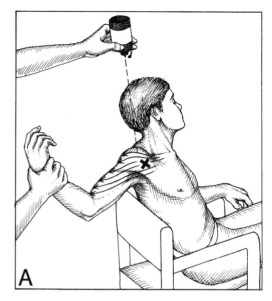

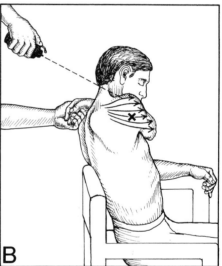

Figure 28.3. Seated stretch positions and spray patterns (*arrows*) for the deltoid muscle with active trigger points (×s). *A*, anterior part of the muscle. *B*, posterior part of the muscle. During the latter stretch, the arm is pulled high across the chest.

source of pain and needs to be injected instead. Since TPs in the anterior part of the deltoid lie in the path of the anterior approach to the joint, these TPs may be penetrated unintentionally, and thereby unknowingly inactivated, during the joint injection. The relief of pain thus obtained would further reinforce the incorrect conclusion that inflammation of the joint had been responsible for the pain. Any myo-

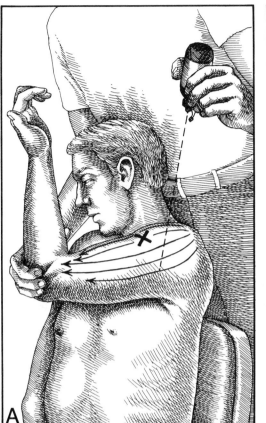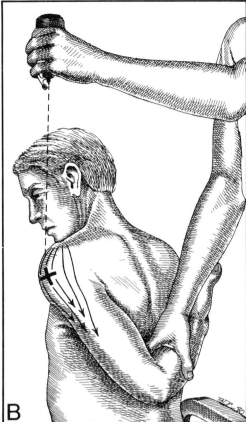

Figure 28.4.   Stretch positions and spray pattern (*arrows*) for trigger point (×) in the middle part of the deltoid muscle. *A*, anterior arm position. *B*, posterior arm position.

fascial TPs in the deltoid muscle should be inactivated and the response observed before deciding to inject the shoulder joint.

When attention is directed only to the subacromial area of referred pain and tenderness, and active TPs in the anterior and posterior borders of the deltoid are overlooked, a diagnosis of "subdeltoid bursitis" is often rendered. An innocent bursa is then injected, to the neglect of the guilty deltoid TPs, and a poor therapeutic result obtained.

14. CORRECTIVE ACTIONS

Any TPs should be eliminated that refer pain to the deltoid region and are therefore likely to activate satellite TPs in the deltoid muscle. The muscles most likely to do this are noted in Section 11.

At the same time, mechanical stress factors should be corrected. The patient should learn to lift heavy objects with the arm rotated so that the thumb is turned in the direction that unloads the affected part of the deltoid muscle (Section 8).

Activation of latent TPs by intramuscular injection into the posterior deltoid may be avoided as outlined in Section 7.

The patient is warned to watch the steps, to hold onto railings, and not to trip.

Shooting enthusiasts should place a pad in front of the shoulder to minimize direct trauma by the gun recoil.

For continuing relief, daily passive stretching of the affected part of the muscle may be necessary. To stretch the anterior part of the deltoid, the patient is taught to do the middle- and lower-hand positions of the In-doorway Stretch Exercise (Fig. 42.10), and the Against-doorjamb Exercise (Fig. 30.7). To self-stretch the posterior deltoid, the patient places the arm in the position of Figure 28.3B, grasps the

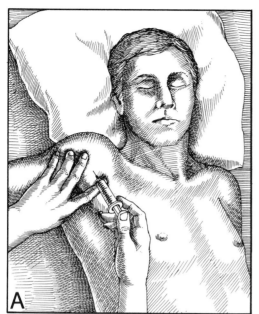

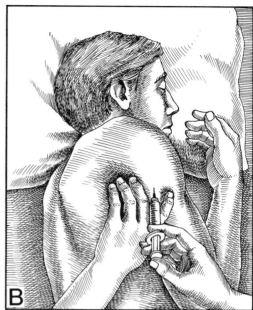

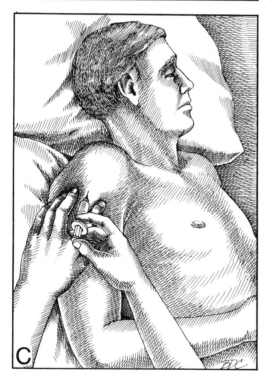

Figure 28.5. Injection of trigger points in the right deltoid muscle. A, anterior deltoid, with the patient supine. B, posterior deltoid, with the patient lying on the opposite side. C, middle deltoid, with the patient partially supine.

elbow of the affected arm with the other hand and pulls it across the chest, while sitting under a hot shower with the water directed over the muscle.

Supplemental Case Reports

The management of patients with deltoid TPs is reported by Kellgren[21] and Lange.[23]

References

1. Bardeen CR: The Musculature, Sect. 5. In *Morris's Human Anatomy*, edited by C.M. Jackson, Ed. 6. Blakiston's Son & Co., Philadelphia, 1921 (p. 399).
2. Basmajian JV: *Muscles Alive*, Ed. 4. Williams & Wilkins, Baltimore, 1978 (pp. 193–197).
3. Bateman JE: *The Shoulder and Neck*. W.B. Saunders, Philadelphia, 1972 (pp. 347–350, 424–433).
4. Broer MR, Houtz SJ: *Patterns of Muscular Activity in Selected Sports Skill*. Charles C Thomas,

Springfield, Ill. 1967.

5. Caillet R: *The Shoulder in Hemiplegia.* F.A. Davis, Philadelphia, 1980 (p. 23).
6. Cailliet, R: *Soft Tissue Pain and Disability,* F.A. Davis, Philadelphia, 1977 (p. 152).
7. Caillet R: *Shoulder Pain.* F.A. Davis, Philadelphia, 1966 (Fig. 19, pp. 82–85).
8. Dehne E, Hall RM: Active shoulder motion in complete deltoid paralysis. *J Bone Joint Surg 41-A:*745–748, 1959.
9. Duchenne GB: *Physiology of Motion,* translated by E.B. Kaplan. J.B. Lippincott, Philadelphia, 1949 (pp. 45–55).
10. Grant JCB: *An Atlas of Human Anatomy,* Ed. 7. Williams & Wilkins, Baltimore, 1978 (Fig. 6-14).
11. *Ibid.* (Fig. 6-37).
12. *Ibid.* (Fig. 6-30).
13. *Ibid.* (Fig. 6-33).
14. *Ibid.* (Fig. 6-38).
15. Gray H: *Anatomy of the Human Body,* edited by C.M. Goss, American Ed. 29. Lea & Febiger, Philadelphia, 1973 (p. 455).
16. Gutstein M: Common rheumatism and physiotherapy. *Br J Phys Med 3:*46–50, 1940 (p. 47).
17. Hagberg M, Jonsson B: The amplitude distribution of the myoelectric signal in an ergonomic study of the deltoid muscle. *Ergonomics 18:*311–319, 1975.
18. Hollinshead WH: *Functional Anatomy of the Limbs and Back,* Ed. 4. W.B. Saunders, Philadelphia, 1976 (p. 106).
19. Inman VT, Saunders JB, Abbott LC: Observations on the function of the shoulder joint. *J Bone Joint Surg 26:*1–30, 1944.
20. Jonsson S, Jonsson B: Function of the muscles of the upper limb in car driving. *Ergonomics 18:*375–388, 1975 (pp. 377–380).
21. Kellgren JH: A preliminary account of referred pains arising from muscle. *Br Med J 1:*325–327, 1938 (Cases 2 and 3).
22. Lange M: *Die Muskelhaerten (Myogelosen):* J.F. Lehmanns, Muenchen, 1931 (pp. 49, 66, Figs. 10, 27, 40b).
23. *Ibid.* (Cases 14, 15, 18, 20–22).
24. Llewellyn LJ, Jones AB: *Fibrositis.* Rebman, New York, 1915 (Fig. 35 facing p. 226).
25. Lundervold A: Occupation myalgia. Electromyographic investigations. *Acta Psychiatr Neurol Scand 26:*359–369, 1951 (p. 365, Fig. 5).
26. McMinn RMH, Hutchings RT: *Color Atlas of Human Anatomy.* Year Book Medical Publishers, Chicago, 1977 (p. 108).
27. *Ibid.* (p. 113A).
28. *Ibid.* (p. 111).
29. Pernkopf E: *Atlas of Topographical and Applied Human Anatomy,* Vol. 2. W.B. Saunders, Philadelphia, 1964 (p. 11).
30. *Ibid.* (p. 33).
31. *Ibid.* (pp. 54, 72).
32. Rasch PJ, Burke RK: *Kinesiology and Applied Anatomy,* Ed. 6. Lea & Febiger, Philadelphia, 1978 (pp. 161, 163).
33. Reynolds MD: Myofascial trigger point syndromes in the practice of rheumatology. *Arch Phys Med Rehabil 62:*111–114, 1981 (Table 1).
34. Sobotta. J, Figge FHJ: *Atlas of Human Anatomy,* Ed. 9, Vol. 1. Hafner Division of Macmillan, New York, 1974 (p. 192).
35. *Ibid.* (p. 142).
36. Spalteholz W: *Handatlas der Anatomie des Menschen,* Ed. 11, Vol. 2. S. Hirzel, Leipzig, 1922 (pp. 280, 282, 320).
37. *Ibid.* (p. 315).
38. *Ibid.* (pp. 303, 322).
39. Steinbrocker O, Isenberg SA, Silver, M et al.: Observations on pain produced by injection of hypertonic saline into muscles and other supportive tissues. *J Clin Invest 32:*1045–1051, 1953 (p. 1046).
40. Toldt C: *An Atlas of Human Anatomy,* translated by M.E. Paul, Ed. 2, Vol. 1. Macmillan, New York, 1919 (p. 274).
41. *Ibid.* (p. 310).
42. *Ibid.* (p. 266).
43. Travell J: Ethyl chloride spray for painful muscle spasm. *Arch Phys Med Rehabil 33:*291–298, 1952 (p. 293).
44. Travell J: Factors affecting pain of injection. *JAMA 158:*368–371, 1955.
45. Travell J, Berry C, Bigelow N: Effects of referred somatic pain on structures in the reference zone. *Fed Proc 3:*49, 1944.
46. Travell J, Rinzler SH: The myofascial genesis of pain. *Postgrad Med 11:*425–434, 1952 (p. 428).
47. Webber TD: Diagnosis and modification of headache and shoulder-arm-hand syndrome. *JAOA 72:*697–710, 1973.
48. Winter Z: Referred pain in fibrositis. *Med Rec 157:*34–37, 1944 (p. 4).
49. Zohn DA, Mennel J McM: *Musculoskeletal Pain: Diagnosis and Physical Treatment.* Little, Brown & Company, Boston, 1976 (p. 192, Fig. 9–13).

PART 2

CHAPTER 29
Coracobrachialis Muscle
"Hide-and-go-seek"

HIGHLIGHTS: Involvement of the coracobrachialis muscle usually is not apparent until trigger point (TP) activity has been resolved in associated muscles, such as, the anterior deltoid, biceps brachii (short head) and the triceps brachii (long head). **REFERRED PAIN** from TPs in this muscle appears in the front of the shoulder and in a line down the back of the arm and dorsum of the forearm to the back of the hand, but skips the elbow and wrist. **ANATOMICAL ATTACHMENTS** of the coracobrachialis are to the coracoid process, above, and to the middle of the humerus, below. **ACTIONS** are to assist flexion and adduction of the arm at the shoulder. **SYMPTOMS** are disabling pain with little restriction in the range of motion. **ACTIVITY OF TRIGGER POINTS** in the coracobrachialis usually develops secondary to the involvement of associated muscles. **PATIENT EXAMINATION** reveals a positive Back-rub Test and pain when the patient raises the straightened elbow above the head. **TRIGGER POINT EXAMINATION** is by direct palpation of the coracobrachialis muscle medial to the short head of the biceps brachii. **ENTRAPMENTS** by this muscle have not been observed, but theoretically compression of the musculocutaneous nerve by the taut coracobrachialis could occur. **STRETCH AND SPRAY** are performed with a technique similar to that for TPs in the anterior deltoid. **INJECTION AND STRETCH** of TPs in this muscle involve an anterior approach through the deltoid muscle with tactile guidance of the needle from the palpating hand. **CORRECTIVE ACTIONS** include relief of excessive stress from lifting, and home use of the In-doorway Stretch Exercise.

1. REFERRED PAIN
(Fig. 29.1)

Pain is referred over the anterior deltoid area, in a broken line down the posterior aspect of the arm over the triceps brachii, and over the dorsum of the forearm and again over the dorsum of the hand; the line of pain may extend to the tip of the middle finger (Fig. 29.1). Pain tends to skip the elbow and wrist, emphasizing the arm and forearm segments. The extent of referred pain is greater, and the pain is more intense, when the trigger points (TPs) are more active.

2. ANATOMICAL ATTACHMENTS
(Fig. 29.2)

The coracobrachialis joins the tendon of the short head of the biceps brachii, which, together, attach *above* to the apex of the coracoid process (Fig. 29.2). *Below* the coracobrachialis fastens to the medial surface of the humerus just proximal to the middle of the shaft of the bone, between the triceps and brachialis muscles.[7]

The brachial neurovascular bundle passes beneath the tendinous attachment of the pectoralis minor at the coracoid process and continues down the arm next to the coracobrachialis muscle.

Variations include total absence of the muscle, and extension of its humeral attachment to the medial epicondyle.[1]

Supplemental References

Other authors have illustrated the coracobrachialis as seen from the front,[8, 11, 13, 17, 19, 22] from the medial aspect,[4, 21] including the muscle's relation to the brachial neu-

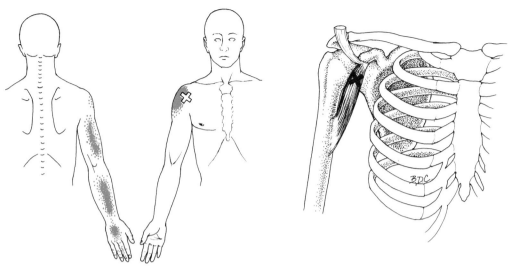

Figure 29.1. Pain pattern (*red*) referred from a trigger point (✗) in the right coracobrachialis muscle. Trigger points may be found as far distally as the middle of the muscle. In some cases, the pain may extend only to the elbow.

PART 2

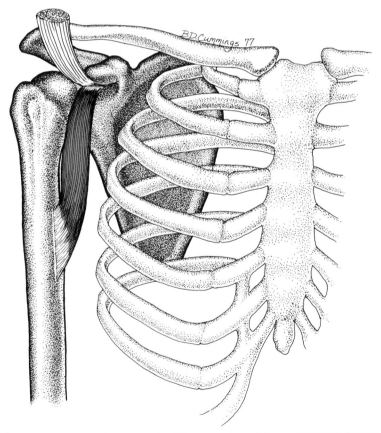

Figure 29.2. Usual attachments of the coracobrachialis muscle (*red*): above to the tip of the coracoid process, and below to a line along the humerus extending almost to midshaft. The short head of the biceps brachii has been cut and turned up.

rovascular structures,[5, 14, 20] and in cross section.[2, 15] Grant[6] illustrates a variation of the muscle.

3. INNERVATION

The coracobrachialis muscle is innervated from roots C_6 and C_7, through the upper and middle trunks, *via* the lateral cord of the brachial plexus and, finally, by a branch of the musculocutaneous nerve that separates before the nerve trunk penetrates the muscle.[7] As it passes through the muscle at its midpoint, the musculocutaneous nerve may divide the coracobrachialis into clearly defined superficial and deep portions.[1]

4. ACTIONS

The coracobrachialis helps to flex and adduct the arm at the shoulder,[1, 7, 9, 10, 16] and to hold the head of the humerus in the glenoid fossa.[1, 16] When contracted by faradic stimulation while the arm was held in the abducted position, the muscle forcefully drew the humerus toward the glenoid cavity.[3]

It assists in returning the arm to the neutral position from external[1, 16] or internal rotation.[16] Although considered by some to be a primary mover in horizontal flexion,[16] when contracted by faradic stimulation, it was able only to move the arm weakly forward and inward.[3]

The coracobrachialis can help to increase extreme abduction.[1]

5. MYOTATIC UNIT

The coracobrachialis acts synergistically with the anterior deltoid and short head of the biceps brachii in forward and horizontal flexion. In adduction, it assists the pectoralis major, subscapularis, infraspinatus, teres major and minor, and the long head of the triceps brachii. It may assist the middle deltoid and supraspinatus in extreme abduction.

6. SYMPTOMS

For coracobrachialis TPs, the primary complaint is upper extremity pain, particularly in the front of the shoulder and in the arm posteriorly. The patient experiences pain when reaching behind the body, across the low back, as in the Back-

rub Test (see Fig. 29.3). When only the coracobrachialis muscle is involved, reaching up to do the hair, or serving in tennis with the elbow bent, is not painful. However, reaching up in abduction and flexion at the shoulder may cause a painful contraction of the coracobrachialis in the shortened position.

7. ACTIVATION OF TRIGGER POINTS

Active TPs in this muscle develop secondarily to active TPs in related muscles of its myotatic unit, as listed above.

8. PATIENT EXAMINATION
(Fig. 29.3)

The Back-rub Test (Fig. 29.3) reveals a restriction in the range of shoulder motion due to pain caused by use of the involved coracobrachialis muscle.

The arm can be flexed as far as the ear, but not behind it.

Flexion at the shoulder may be slightly weak. To test the strength of the coracobrachialis, the patient first elevates the arm to about 45° of flexion and abduction. The elbow should be partially flexed and the hand fully pronated to minimize biceps

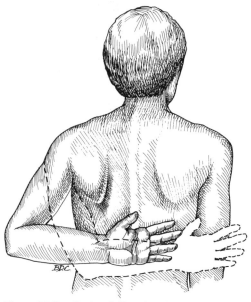

Figure 29.3. Back-rub Test for trigger points in the left coracobrachialis muscle. Before treatment of the coracobrachialis, the patient usually can reach only to the small of the back, but following successful inactivation of trigger points, the wrist can reach across the full width of the back (*dotted outline*).

PART 2

activity. Then the operator presses at the elbow, pushing the arm downward and slightly posteriorly.[10] Inability to resist such pressure indicates weakness of the coracobrachialis. Maximal resistance by the patient is likely to elicit pain if the coracobrachialis muscle harbors active TPs.

Stretching the involved coracobrachialis by passively extending the arm at the shoulder causes pain, as does loading the muscle by actively resisting flexion of the arm at the shoulder.[12]

9. TRIGGER POINT EXAMINATION (Fig. 29.4)

Involvement of the coracobrachialis is usually discovered when the patient returns following successful inactivation of

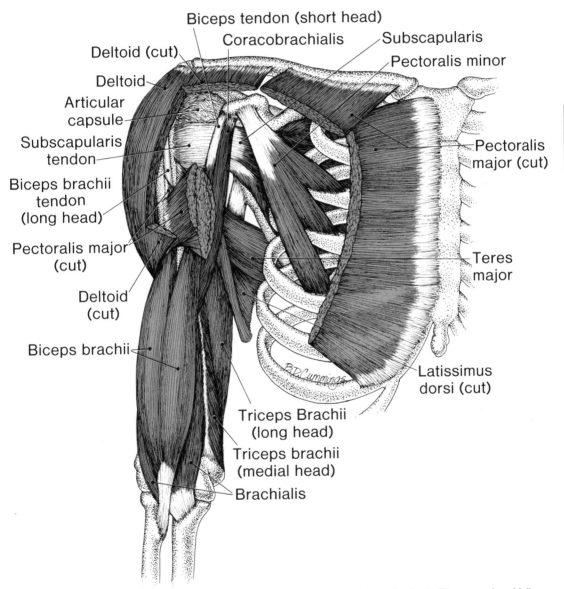

Figure 29.4. Muscular regional anatomy of the right shoulder, seen from the front. The coracobrachialis muscle (*dark red*) crosses superficial to the attachments of the subscapularis, latissimus dorsi, and teres major muscles, but lies deep to the pectoralis major muscle. For clarity, the serratus anterior muscle is not shown. The coracobrachialis lies medial to the short head of the biceps, and is palpated for trigger points against the humerus in the anterior axillary fossa, deep to the pectoralis major muscle.

multiple TPs in the shoulder muscles, especially the anterior deltoid. Although there is no recurrence of tenderness or detectable local twitch responses in the muscles previously treated, the patient complains of severe pain, and deep tenderness remains in the region of the anterior deltoid muscle. Careful examination reveals another tender spot, lying deeper than the deltoid, which may respond with a palpable, but not visible, local twitch response.

This coracobrachialis TP is found when palpating it against the humerus by sliding the finger into the axilla beneath the deltoid and pectoralis major (Fig. 29.4). The tip of the digit encounters the adjacent bellies of the short head of the biceps brachii and, more posteriorly, the coracobrachialis at a level where about half of the biceps fibers have become attached to their common tendon. The axillary neurovascular bundle passes along the coracobrachialis[5] and must be displaced posteriorly to permit the digit to explore the fibers of the coracobrachialis by rolling them against the humerus. The bundle lies posterior to the attachment of the muscle on the humerus. TPs may be found along the proximal half of the muscle, usually near the location indicated in Figure 29.1.

10. ENTRAPMENTS

One would expect that TPs in the coracobrachialis muscle could cause entrapment of the musculocutaneous nerve as it passes through that muscle to the biceps brachialis.[7, 18, 20] Clinical symptoms of this entrapment have not been noted to date, but nerve compression should be evidenced by a marked reduction in the force of elbow flexion (motor supply to the biceps brachii and most of the brachialis muscles) accompanied by disturbed sensation of the skin on the radial side of the forearm.[7]

11. ASSOCIATED TRIGGER POINTS

Since patients do not present themselves with symptoms of TPs in this muscle alone, it appears that coracobrachialis TPs develop in association with TPs in functionally related muscles, such as the anterior or posterior deltoid, the biceps brachii (short head), the supraspinatus, and the triceps brachii (long head).

12. STRETCH AND SPRAY

Stretch and spray are applied in a manner similar to that used for TPs in the anterior deltoid (see Fig. 28.3A). The same stretch position is used. For the coracobrachialis muscle, the spray pattern for the anterior deltoid is carried closer to the axilla, extended over the back of the arm and forearm, and over the dorsum of the hand to the tip of the middle finger.

13. INJECTION AND STRETCH
(Fig. 29.5)

With the patient supine and with the arm by the side placed in external rotation at the shoulder, the tender coracobrachialis TPs may be palpated deep in the axilla by reaching beneath the pectoralis major muscle and pressing against the humerus on the dorsal aspect of the combined bundle of the short head of the biceps and coracobrachialis muscles (Fig. 29.4). The pulsating brachial artery is felt in the neuromuscular bundle that lies dorsal and medial to the coracobrachialis, between the coracobrachialis and the attachment of the lateral head of the triceps to the humerus. The needle is inserted through the pectoralis major or anterior deltoid, directed toward the tender area that is localized with the operator's other hand (Fig. 29.5). The patient feels a brilliant flash of referred pain when the needle strikes the TP. Infiltration of the local anesthetic may cause temporary weakness and anesthesia in the distribution of the musculocutaneous nerve with prompt recovery in 15 or 20 min if 0.5% procaine solution was used for injection.

Spray and stretch are repeated and a hot pack applied.

14. CORRECTIVE ACTIONS

The patient must not lift heavy objects with the arms outstretched in front, but must keep the elbows close to the body; in lifting, the hands should be supinated and the shoulders externally rotated so that the weak coracobrachialis is not forced to substitute for the stronger biceps brachii muscle.

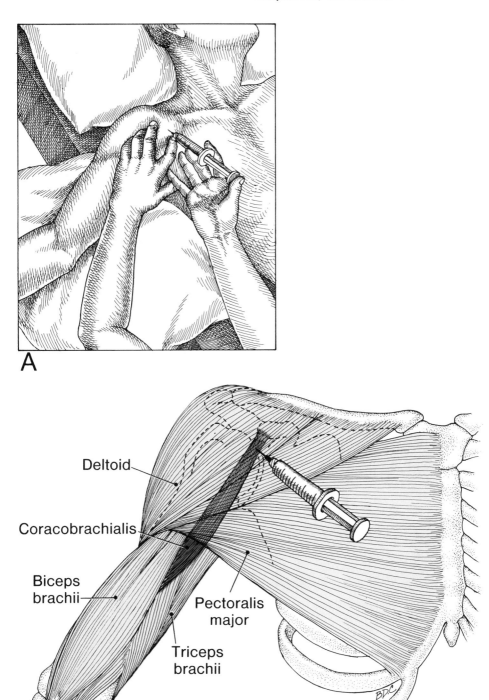

A

Deltoid

Coracobrachialis

Biceps
brachii

Pectoralis
major

Triceps
brachii

B

Figure 29.5.   The upper trigger point in the coracobrachialis muscle is injected through the anterior deltoid muscle at the level of the greater tuberosity of the humerus. *A*, injection technique. *B*, schematic diagram of injection showing the coracobrachialis muscle (*dark red*) through the deltoid and pectoralis major muscles.

The patient should do the Against-door-jamb Exercise (see Fig. 30.7) daily. As an additional means of restoring the normal full length of the coracobrachialis muscle, daily use of the In-doorway Stretch Exercise, lower hand-position, is helpful (see Fig. 42.10).

Local application of moist heat to the muscle just before, or after, the passive stretch exercises reduces postexercise soreness. If this occurs, an alternate-day program is wise, and may obviate this reaction.

References

1. Bardeen CR: The musculature. Sect. 5. In *Morris's Human Anatomy*, edited by C.M. Jackson, Ed. 6. Blakiston's Son & Co., Philadelphia, 1921 (pp. 413, 414).
2. Carter BL, Morehead J, Wolpert SM, *et al.*: *Cross-Sectional Anatomy.* Appleton-Century-Crofts, New York, 1977 (Sects. 21, 22, 49).
3. Duchenne GB: *Physiology of Motion*, translated by E.B. Kaplan. J.B. Lippincott, Philadelphia, 1949 (p. 87).
4. Grant JCB: *An Atlas of Human Anatomy*, Ed. 7. Williams & Wilkins. Baltimore, 1978 (Figs. 6-18, 6-20, 6-23).
5. *Ibid.* (Figs. 6-18, 6-25).
6. *Ibid.* (Fig. 6-121).
7. Gray H: *Anatomy of the Human Body*, edited by C.M. Goss, American Ed. 29. Lea & Febiger, Philadelphia, 1973 (pp. 459, 969).
8. *Ibid.* (p. 452).
9. Hollinshead WH: *Functional Anatomy of the Limbs and Back*, Ed. 4. W.B. Saunders, Philadelphia, 1976 (p. 133).
10. Kendall HO, Kendall FP, Wadsworth GE: *Muscles, Testing and Function*, Ed. 2. Williams & Wilkins, Baltimore, 1971 (pp. 108, 109).
11. Lockhart RD, Hamilton GF, Fyfe FW: *Anatomy of the Human Body*, Ed. 2. J.B. Lippincott, Philadelphia, 1969 (p. 206).
12. Macdonald AJR: Abnormally tender muscle regions and associated painful movements. *Pain* 8:197–205, 1980 (pp. 202, 203).
13. McMinn RMH, Hutchings RT: *Color Atlas of Human Anatomy.* Year Book Medical Publishers, Chicago, 1977 (p. 118).
14. *Ibid.* (p. 119).
15. Pernkopf E: *Atlas of Topographical and Applied Human Anatomy*, Vol. 2. W.B. Saunders, Philadelphia, 1964 (Figs. 44, 61).
16. Rasch PJ, Burke RK: *Kinesiology and Applied Anatomy*, Ed. 6. Lea & Febiger, Philadelphia, 1978 (pp. 165, 166).
17. Sobotta J, Figge FHJ: *Atlas of Human Anatomy*, Ed. 9, Vol. 1. Hafner Division of Macmillan, New York, 1974 (pp. 192, 196, 198).
18. Sobotta J, Figge FHJ: *Atlas of Human Anatomy*, Ed. 9, Vol. 3. Hafner Division of Macmillan, New York, 1974 (p. 291).
19. Spalteholz W: *Handatlas der Antomie des Menschen*, Ed. 11, Vol. 2. S. Hirzel, Leipzig, 1922 (p. 320).
20. *Ibid.* (p. 753).
21. Toldt C: *An Atlas of Human Anatomy*, translated by M.E. Paul, Ed. 2, Vol. 1. Macmillan, New York, 1919 (p. 314).
22. *Ibid.* (pp. 316, 317).

PART 2

CHAPTER 30
Biceps Brachii Muscle
"A Three-joint Motor"

HIGHLIGHTS: **REFERRED PAIN** from trigger points (TPs) in the biceps brachii is projected mainly upward, over the muscle to the front of the shoulder with a spillover pain pattern in the suprascapular region. **ANATOMICAL ATTACHMENTS** are, above, to the glenoid labrium (long head) and to the coracoid process (short head) of the scapula; and, below, to the tuberosity of the radius. **ACTIONS** of both heads of this muscle are complex, since the muscle crosses three joints: the glenohumeral, humeroulnar and radioulnar. The muscle flexes the forearm at the elbow, assists flexion of the arm at the shoulder and may assist abduction at the shoulder; it powerfully assists supination of the hand when the forearm is not fully extended at the elbow. **SYMPTOMS** are restricted motion and aching pain, and sometimes soreness to pressure over the bicipital tendon. **ACTIVATION OF TRIGGER POINTS** occurs as the result of acute or chronic strain of the muscle; the TPs are usually located a few centimeters above the elbow. Tenosynovitis of the bicipital tendon may develop secondary to TPs in the belly of the long head. **PA-TIENT EXAMINATION** for range-of-motion testing is misleading if the muscle is not stretched simultaneously across the three joints that it crosses. **TRIGGER POINT EXAMINATION** is done by both flat and pincer palpation, especially of the distal third of the muscle. **ASSOCIATED TRIGGER POINTS** are likely to develop in the brachialis, supinator, and triceps brachii muscles secondary to TPs in the biceps. **STRETCH AND SPRAY** require that the biceps brachii be passively stretched by abducting the arm to 90°, by extending it posteriorly with the arm externally rotated at the shoulder, and by extending the forearm at the elbow while pronating the hand. At the same time, the vapocoolant spray is applied cephalad over the muscle and its pain pattern. **INJECTION AND STRETCH** may inactivate the biceps brachii TPs, but true bicipital tenosynovitis may persist. Injection of the tendon area may then relieve the symptoms. **CORRECTIVE ACTIONS** include lifting objects with the hands in pronation to unload the biceps brachii muscle. The Against-door-jamb Exercise stretches it passively.

1. REFERRED PAIN
(Fig. 30.1)

Trigger points (TPs) in the biceps brachii are usually found in the distal part of the muscle.[27] They refer pain upward over the muscle and over the anterior deltoid region of the shoulder[9]; occasionally the pain skips to the suprascapular region (Fig. 30.1). These TPs also may initiate another additional pattern of milder pain downward in the antecubital space. Deep tenderness to palpation of the bicipital tendon in the area of pain referred from TPs in the biceps muscle may be mistaken for bicipital tendinitis or subdeltoid bursitis.

Experimental injection of 6% sodium chloride solution into the biceps tendon at the antecubital space in 10 normal subjects caused pain that was referred locally and also proximally over the biceps muscle (including the acromion in one case). Other phenomena that were referred distally to some part of the volar forearm and hand

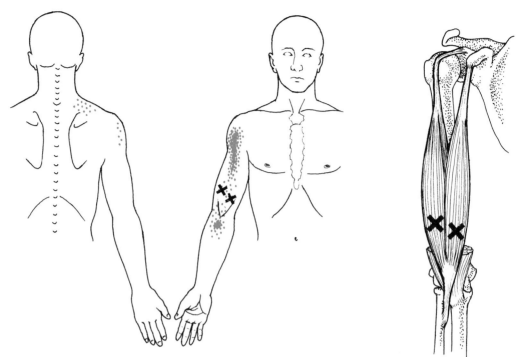

Figure 30.1.   Referred pain pattern (essential zone is *solid red*, spillover zone *stippled red*) of trigger points (×s) in the distal portion of the right biceps brachii muscle.

included deep tenderness, erythema, paresthesia, pallor, and a feeling of weakness.[22]

2. ANATOMICAL ATTACHMENTS
(Fig. 30.2)

Proximally the long head of the biceps brachii attaches to the superior margin of the glenoid cavity of the scapula (Fig. 30.2). Its tendon lies in the intertubercular groove and passes through the glenohumeral joint space over the head of the humerus. The short head attaches **proximally** to the coracoid process of the scapula, remaining free of the glenohumeral joint capsule.

Distally the common tendon of both heads attaches to the tuberosity of the radius. The attachment faces the ulna when the hand is supinated,[7] but in pronation the tendon wraps more than halfway around the radius.[17]

Supplemental References

Additional illustrations of the biceps brachii show the relation of the two heads to each other at the shoulder,[19, 21, 25] details of its tendinous relations at the shoulder

and of its tendinous attachment to the radius,[6, 19] and the relation of the biceps brachii to the brachialis.[19]

3. INNERVATION

The biceps brachii muscle is innervated by the musculocutaneous nerve, *via* the lateral cord and by spinal roots C_5, and C_6.[7]

4. ACTIONS

In summary, the biceps brachii (1) assists flexion of the arm at the shoulder; (2) assists abduction at the shoulder when the arm is externally rotated; (3) flexes the arm at the elbow most vigorously when the hand is supinated; (4) strongly supinates the hand from the pronated position when the elbow is at least partly bent, but not when the elbow is straight; and (5) the long head of the muscle helps to seat the head of the humerus in the glenoid fossa when a heavy weight is carried in the hand with the arm dependent.

Anatomically, the biceps brachii acts at the shoulder, elbow and radioulnar joints. It flexes the arm at the shoulder,[7] flexes the forearm at the elbow,[1, 4, 7, 10, 17] and assists forceful supination of the hand more

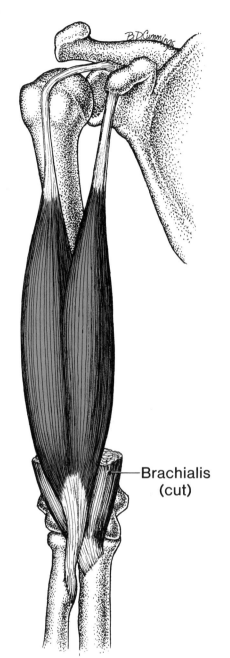

Figure 30.2. Attachments of the biceps brachii muscle (*red*), which covers most of the brachialis muscle. The brachialis has been cut for clarity.

vigorously when the elbow is flexed to 90° than when it is straight.[26] The long head draws the head of the humerus upward into the glenoid fossa.[7, 10, 17] The biceps is in a position to assist flexion at the shoulder when the arm is internally rotated, and to assist abduction of the arm when externally rotated.[10]

Electrical stimulation of the entire biceps strongly supinated and flexed the forearm. Supination was markedly weaker if the elbow was fully extended, or if only the long head was stimulated.[4] The effect of the loss of biceps function was demonstrated in patients who had selective atrophy of this muscle. Forceful flexion of the forearm at the elbow was achieved by the brachialis and brachioradialis muscles. However, this effort in lifting a heavy weight caused a painful partial dislocation of the humeral head from the glenoid fossa when the additional support of the biceps was absent[4]; the muscle is needed to keep the head of the humerus seated in the glenoid cavity.

The two heads of the biceps brachii, the brachialis, and the brachioradialis muscles distribute a sustained forearm-flexion load among themselves in an irregular and unpredictable manner.[1] With the elbow bent, motor unit activity in the biceps brachii appears during resistance to supination, but usually disappears when the forearm is then fully extended at the elbow.[1] Electrical activity is vigorous in the muscle during flexion at the elbow when the hand is supinated, but is markedly inhibited when the hand is pronated.[1, 24] The biceps is the auxiliary which reinforces fast supination, or forceful supination, against resistance.[26] Motor units are active in the long head during abduction at the shoulder,[17] but only when the arm is held in external rotation with the hand supinated.[1] During flexion at the shoulder, the long head is electrically more active than the short head.[1] The short head assists flexion, abduction, and internal rotation at the shoulder and movement of the arm horizontally across the chest.[17]

Sports requiring throwing with the arm strongly activate this muscle. An unusually vigorous motor-unit response of the biceps brachii appears near the end of the tennis serve, and also during the basketball spike (a one-leg jump made to block the ball), and during lay-up (a jumping one-handed shot in basketball made off the backboard from close under the basket). Minimal motor unit activity develops during the tennis forehand drive, batting a baseball and the golf drive.[2]

The biceps is moderately activated by longhand writing and by typing; the latter causes a marked increase in amplitude of biceps electrical activity as the speed of typing increases.[14]

During simulated driving of a car on a country road, electrical activity occurred in the right biceps chiefly when making left turns, and in the left biceps when making right turns. Occasional short bursts of electrical activity were observed in the biceps brachii during simulated driving on a main road.[11]

5. MYOTATIC UNIT

The biceps functions synergistically with the brachialis and brachioradialis muscles to flex the forearm at the elbow, with the supinator to supinate the pronated hand, and with the anterior deltoid and supraspinatus to abduct the arm at the shoulder. The coracobrachialis assists the short head in adduction at the shoulder.

The triceps brachii is its chief antagonist.

6. SYMPTOMS

When active TPs are present in the biceps brachii, the chief complaint is superficial anterior shoulder pain, but NOT deep pain in the shoulder joint, nor pain in the mid-deltoid region. Pain occurs during elevation of the arm above the shoulder level during flexion and abduction.[8] Other symptoms are tenderness over the bicipital tendon; diffuse aching over the anterior surface of the arm, but rarely in the antecubital space; weakness, as well as pain, on raising the hand above the head; snapping or grating sounds from the taut long-head tendon, on abduction of the arm; and frequently an associated ache and soreness in the upper trapezius region. This biceps-shoulder pain is often evoked by overstress during activities like a strong backhand tennis stroke executed with the elbow straight and the hand supinated to put top-spin on the ball.

In contrast to patients with TP involvement of the infraspinatus muscle, the patient with biceps TPs can lie comfortably on the affected side and can reach behind the waistline without pain.

7. ACTIVATION OF TRIGGER POINTS

Lifting heavy objects with the hand supinated may overload the biceps brachii.

Other activating stresses include sudden lifting with the arm extended (lifting the hood of a car, or boxes at arm's length); a sustained elbow-flexion load (playing the violin or guitar, using an electric hedge clipper); unaccustomed vigorous or repeated supination (turning a stiff doorknob, using a screwdriver); over-exertion (hard serving in competitive tennis, shovelling snow); and sudden over-stretching of the muscle (catching a fall with the arm by reaching behind to a railing with the elbow extended).

8. PATIENT EXAMINATION
(Fig. 30.3)

Restriction of shoulder or elbow motion due to TPs in the biceps is not obvious because the muscle crosses three joints and the muscle must be stretched across all of them at the same time to reveal the abnormal tension of its fibers. Limitation of stretch of the long head is tested using the Biceps-extension Test (Fig. 30.3): with the patient seated in a low-backed chair and leaning back to stabilize the scapula against the backrest, the patient's elbow is extended fully to stretch the muscle across this joint. Then the muscle is passively stretched across the shoulder joint by *externally* rotating and abducting the arm to 45°. Finally, the hand is pronated without letting the arm rotate at the shoulder as the arm is moved backward and upward (Fig. 30.3A). Normally, the arm will extend to the position drawn in black (Fig. 30.3B). If the muscle is shortened by TPs, as the stretch increases across the shoulder joint, the elbow flexes to relieve the abnormal tension, assuming the position outlined in red (Fig. 30.3B). This compensatory flexion of the elbow indicates a shortened biceps muscle. We find, as Macdonald[15] has reported, that stretching the involved biceps by passively extending the forearm causes pain, as does loading the muscle by actively resisting flexion of the forearm at the elbow.

Misinterpretations

Referred pain in the forearm that is experienced when the forearm has been flexed at the elbow with the hand supinated, but not with the hand pronated, is commonly attributed to bursitis of the bicipital bursa located at the radial attach-

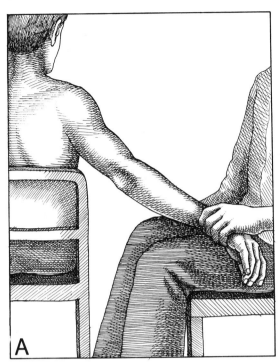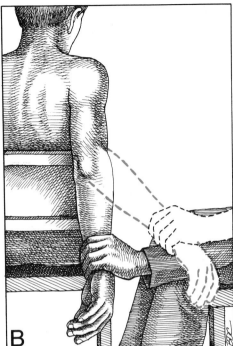

Figure 30.3. Extension test for muscle shortening due to myofascial trigger points in the biceps brachii muscle. *A*, initial test position. *B*, normal test position is black. *Red dashed lines* show abnormal flexion of the elbow as the arm approaches full extension at the shoulder while in abduction of about 45°.

ment of the biceps.[13] In our experience, this kind of pain is much more likely to be caused by active TPs in the biceps brachii or supinator muscles. Occasionally, the patient also may have the bursitis.

Because TPs in the biceps brachii may refer pain and tenderness to the region of the glenohumeral joint, these symptoms are easily misinterpreted as rheumatic disease of the joint unless the biceps is examined for TPs.[18] Both conditions may coexist.

9. TRIGGER POINT EXAMINATION
(Fig. 30.4)

The patient lies supine with the shoulder flat on the examining table, or seated with the elbow supported on a well padded surface. To slacken the biceps muscle slightly, the elbow is flexed about 15° and the hand supinated. Flat palpation is used to screen each head of the biceps for the tense bands that harbor TPs, especially in the distal third of the muscle (Fig. 30.4*A*). Deeper palpation may reveal additional TPs in the underlying brachialis muscle; they refer pain to the thumb.

For pincer palpation, the elbow is flexed another 15° to further slacken the biceps muscle. The entire muscle belly (both heads) is lifted away from the underlying brachialis; then the fibers are rolled between the fingers and thumb to accurately localize the firm bands and spot tenderness (TPs). Application of pincer palpation (Fig. 30.4*B*) with a snapping movement across the bands is likely to elicit local twitch responses of the tense bands. These responses and referred pain elicited by steady pressure confirm the sites of active TPs. The precise location of the TP is obtained by squeezing along the length of a band to pinpoint the spot of greatest tenderness. The tension on the muscle can be adjusted by lessening, or increasing elbow flexion to maximize the sensitivity of the TPs to digital compression.

10. ENTRAPMENTS

No entrapments of the musculocutaneous, median or radial nerves have been observed due to TPs in the biceps brachii muscle.

PART 2

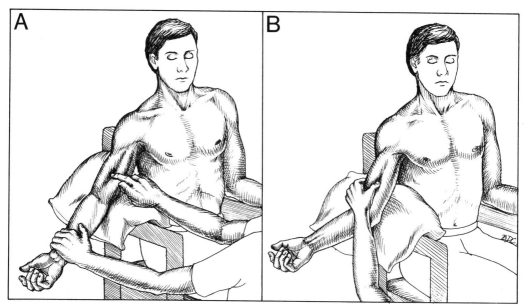

Figure 30.4.   Examination of the biceps brachii muscle for trigger points, patient seated: *A*, flat palpation. The tip of the finger rubs across the fibers. *B*, pincer palpation, which is facilitated by this position that increases elbow flexion and slackens the muscle.

11. ASSOCIATED TRIGGER POINTS

Secondary TPs commonly develop in the synergistic brachialis and supinator muscles, and also in the antagonistic triceps brachii muscle. Eventually, usually within a matter of weeks, the anterior deltoid, supraspinatus and upper trapezius muscles succumb to the added stress on these remaining muscles of the biceps brachii's myotatic unit. Finally, the coracobrachialis may develop TPs.

12. STRETCH AND SPRAY
(Fig. 30.5)

With the patient seated and leaning back in a relaxed position to stabilize the shoulders against the backrest of the chair (Fig. 30.5*A*), the patient's forearm is extended at the elbow. After external rotation of the arm at the shoulder and abduction to 90°, the hand is pronated. This position fully stretches both the long and short heads of the biceps. However, it is difficult to hold the position because pronation of the hand tends to release external rotation at the shoulder. It is, therefore, necessary to stabilize the patient's elbow with the operator's hand (Fig. 30.5*A* and *B*). After a few initial sweeps of spray, the muscle is

stretched by extending the elbow and by swinging the arm backward to extend it at the shoulder. Meanwhile, the jet stream of vapocoolant spray covers the muscle from the elbow cephalad over the front of the shoulder, and then continues over the upper trapezius to include all of the pain reference zone. Additional downsweeps of the spray should start above the TPs to cover the front of the elbow and upper part of the forearm, if that spillover reference region is painful. During vapocooling, full stretch is maintained on the biceps muscle.

To stretch and spray the biceps with the patient supine, the externally rotated arm hangs over the padded edge of the treatment table; the hand is pronated. The forearm and arm are extended together, while the spray is applied in parallel sweeps from the elbow upward over the muscle and over the front of the shoulder, as in Figure 30.5*A* and *B*. Again, the difficulty of keeping the arm externally rotated at the shoulder while pronating the hand requires stabilization of the elbow against the operator's knee or the table.

Before ending the treatment, the synergistic brachialis muscle is stretched and sprayed by insuring full extension at the elbow while covering the muscle and the

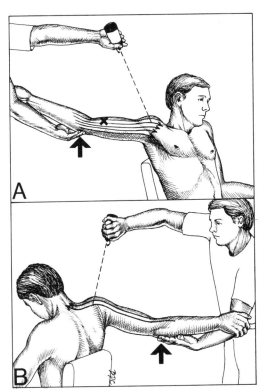

volar forearm with downsweeps of vapo-coolant (see Chapter 31). Reactive cramping of the opposing triceps brachii muscle should be prevented, especially if it has tender TPs on palpation, by likewise stretching and spraying it (see Chapter 32).

Hot packs are applied promptly to rewarm the cooled skin. Immediately after the packs, the patient is asked to move the shoulder, elbow and radioulnar joints actively through their combined ranges of motion. This fully stretches the biceps and triceps muscles.

Figure 30.5.   The stretch position and spray pattern (*thin arrows*) using cephalad sweeps for a trigger point (x) in the biceps brachii muscle. The arm is abducted to 90° and swung backward with the arm externally rotated, the elbow hyperextended, and the hand pronated. The operator must grasp the elbow firmly to hold this difficult position; the *bold arrows* indicate pressure exerted by the operator. *A*, front view; *B*, rear view.

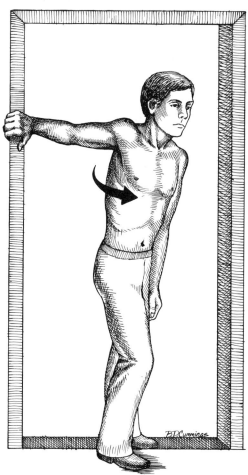

Figure 30.7.   Against-doorjamb Exercise for passive stretching of the biceps brachii, anterior deltoid, and coracobrachialis muscles. The patient gradually rotates the torso (*arrow*) to passively stretch these muscles. To stretch the biceps fully, the arm must be externally rotated at the shoulder, the forearm extended and the hand pronated with the thumb pointed down so that the antecubital space faces forward and as far upward as possible.

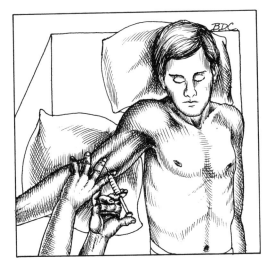

Figure 30.6.   Injection of trigger points in the biceps brachii muscle, with the patient supine.

13. INJECTION AND STRETCH
(Fig. 30.6)

If stretch and spray and/or ischemic compression have not fully inactivated these biceps TPs as evidenced by spots in the muscle that remain tender and hyper-irritable, procaine injection of the remaining active TPs in the muscle is frequently effective.

For injection, the elbow of the supine patient is flexed to about 45°, and the TPs located and held firmly in a pincer grasp. The TPs are precisely injected with 0.5% procaine solution, and the region within the pincer grasp is probed to ensure penetration of all TPs, which tend to form clusters in this muscle. Needle penetrations may be almost tangential to the humerus, or may be directed perpendicularly toward it.

Alternatively, the TPs may be located for injection, using flat palpation, by straddling them with two fingers of the free hand. The TPs are held against the underlying brachialis, as in Figure 30.6. Deeper injection may be required to reach associated TPs in the brachialis muscle (see Chapter 31). During injection, the median

and radial nerves,[16, 20] which lie, respectively, along the medial and lateral borders of both the distal biceps and brachialis muscles, should be avoided.

The injections are followed by full *passive* stretching during application of vapocoolant and then by a hot pack. Treatment is concluded with *active* alternate lengthening and shortening of the biceps.

Additional symptoms, often diagnosed as bicipital tendinitis (tenosynovitis), may be partly due to myofascial pain and tenderness referred primarily from the muscular TPs, and partly due to tension tenosynovitis caused secondarily by these TPs, which continuously tense some of the biceps brachii muscle fibers attached to the tendon. Connective tissue structures associated with muscles showing symptoms of nonarticular rheumatism (in this case equivalent to myofascial TPs) histologically exhibited degenerative changes.[5]

A coincidental, primary bicipital tendinitis may be encountered. It is diagnosed by tenderness of the tendon on palpation[23] and by a positive Yergason's test, in which pain is felt over the bicipital groove when the forearm is forcibly supinated against resistance with the elbow flexed.[3, 23] When

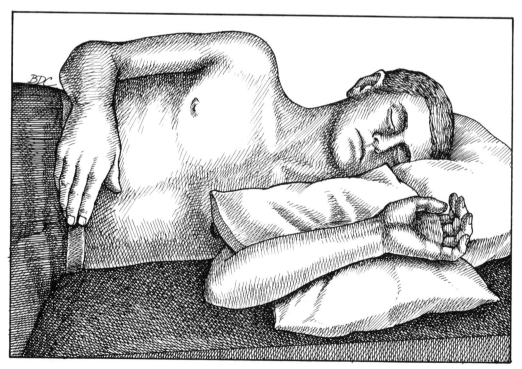

Figure 30.8.   The correct sleeping position for a patient with active trigger points in the left biceps brachii muscle. The pillow is positioned to prevent tight flexion at the elbow.

PART 2

signs of tendinitis persist after inactivation of the biceps brachii TPs, the synovial space around the tendon may be injected with a short-acting corticosteroid, using the fan-wise method of Steinbrocker and Neustadt.[23]

14. CORRECTIVE ACTIONS
(Figs. 30.7 and 30.8)

Following treatment for inactivation of TPs in the biceps brachii, the patient should passively and gently stretch both heads of the muscle daily by doing the Against-doorjamb Exercise (Fig. 30.7). To do this, the patient externally rotates the arm at the shoulder and pronates the hand to hook the fingers, thumb down, against the doorjamb. With the hand slightly above shoulder level, the patient leans forward and, keeping the elbow straight, gradually rotates the torso as shown in Figure 30.7. This is done to produce a steady passive stretching of the muscle, without jerking, for six slow repetitions. It is important to release the tension on the muscle by pausing to breathe between each stretch. This reminds the patient to relax.

The patient should learn to lift and carry objects with the hands pronated in order to transfer some of the load from the biceps to the brachioradialis and supinator muscles (see Fig. 36.3C).

At night, the patient should avoid sleeping with the elbow tightly flexed by placing a small pillow in the crook of the elbow (Fig. 30.8). This prevents prolonged shortening of the muscle.

Supplemental Case Report

The treatment of a patient with somewhat atypical involvement of the biceps brachii is described by Kelly.[12]

References

1. Basmajian JV: *Muscles Alive*, Ed. 4. Williams & Wilkins, Baltimore, 1978 (pp. 193, 194, 201–203).
2. Broer MR, Houtz SJ: *Patterns of Muscular Activity in Selected Sport Skills*. Charles C Thomas, Springfield, Ill. 1967.
3. Calliet R: *Shoulder Pain*. F.A. Davis, Philadelphia, 1966 (p. 73).
4. Duchenne GB: *Physiology of Motion*, translated by E.B. Kaplan. J.B. Lippincott, Philadelphia, 1949 (pp. 88, 98, 106).
5. Fassbender HG: Non-articular rheumatism, Chapter 13. In *Pathology of Rheumatic Diseases*, translated by G. Loewi. Springer-Verlag, New York, 1975 (pp. 307–310).
6. Grant JCB: *An Atlas of Human Anatomy*, Ed. 7. Williams & Wilkins, Baltimore, 1978 (p. 57).
7. Gray H; *Anatomy of the Human Body*, edited by C.M. Goss, American Ed. 29. Lea & Febiger, Philadelphia, 1973 (pp. 459, 460).
8. Gutstein M: Common rheumatism and physiotherapy. *Br J Phys Med* 3:46–50, 1940 (Case 1, p. 49).
9. Gutstein M: Diagnosis and treatment of muscular rheumatism. *Br J Phys Med* 1:302–321, 1938 (Cases 1 and 2; Figs. 1, 2; p. 308).
10. Hollinshead WH: *Functional Anatomy of the Limbs and Back*, Ed. 4. W.B. Saunders, Philadelphia, 1976 (p. 131).
11. Jonsson S, Jonsson B: Function of the muscles of the upper limb in car driving, I–III. *Ergonomics* 18:375–388, 1975 (pp. 383–387).
12. Kelly M: Interstitial neuritis and the neural theory of fibrositis. *Ann Rheum Dis* 7:89–96, 1948 (Case 10, p. 94).
13. Llewellyn LJ, Jones AB: *Fibrositis*. Rebman, New York, 1915 (p. 228).
14. Lundervold AJS: Electromyographic investigations of position and manner of working in typewriting. *Acta Physiol Scand* 24:(Suppl. 84), 1951 (pp. 66–67, 80–81, 94).
15. Macdonald AJR: Abnormally tender muscle regions and associated painful movements. *Pain* 8:197–205, 1980 (pp. 202, 203).
16. Pernkopf E: *Atlas of Topographical and Applied Human Anatomy*, Vol. 2. W.B. Saunders, Philadelphia, 1964 (Fig. 72, p. 83).
17. Rasch PJ, Burke RK: *Kinesiology and Applied Anatomy*. Lea & Febiger, Philadelphia, 1967 (pp. 188, 189).
18. Reynolds MD: Myofascial trigger point syndromes in the practice of rheumatology. *Arch Phys Med Rehabil* 62:111–114, 1981 (Table 1).
19. Sobotta J, Figge FHJ: *Atlas of Human Anatomy*, Ed. 9, Vol. 1. Hafner Division of Macmillan, New York, 1974 (pp. 109, 111, 192, 196, 198).
20. Sobotta J, Figge FHJ: *Atlas of Human Anatomy*, Ed. 9, Vol. 3. Hafner Division of Macmillan, New York, 1974 (p. 294).
21. Spalteholz W: *Handatlas der Anatomie des Menschen*, Ed. 11, Vol. 2. S. Hirzel, Leipzig, 1922 (p. 319).
22. Steinbrocker O, Isenberg SA, Silver M, et al.: Observations on pain produced by injection of hypertonic saline into muscles and other supportive tissues. *J Clin Invest* 32:1045–1051, 1953 (Fig. 3, p. 1049).
23. Steinbrocker O, Neustadt DH: *Aspiration and Injection Therapy in Arthritis and Musculoskeletal Disorders*. Harper & Row, Hagerstown, 1972 (pp. 44, 46; Fig. 5-6).
24. Sullivan WE, Mortensen OA, Miles M, Greene LS: Electromyographic studies of m. biceps brachii during normal voluntary movement at the elbow. *Anat Rec* 107:243–251, 1950.
25. Toldt C: *An Atlas of Human Anatomy*, translated by M.E. Paul, Ed. 2, Vol. 1. Macmillan, New York, 1919 (p. 315).
26. Travill A, Basmajian JV: Electromyography of the supinators of the forearm. *Anat Rec* 139:557–560, 1961.
27. Winter Z: Referred pain in fibrositis. *Med Rec* 157:34–37, 1944 (p. 4).

PART 2

CHAPTER 31

Brachialis Muscle

"Workhorse Elbow Flexor"

HIGHLIGHTS: **REFERRED PAIN** from trigger points (TPs) in the brachialis muscle is projected to the base of the thumb. **ANATOMICAL ATTACHMENTS** are to the humerus above, and to the ulna below. Its **ACTION**, therefore, is flexion of the forearm at the elbow. **ACTIVATION OF TRIGGER POINTS** is caused chiefly by stress overload. **PATIENT EXAMINATION** reveals aggravation of thumb pain by passive full extension at the elbow. **TRIGGER POINT EXAMINATION** of the brachialis requires that the bulk of the biceps brachii muscle be pushed aside. **ENTRAPMENT** of the sensory branch of the radial nerve may be due to TP activity of this muscle. **ASSOCIATED TRIGGER POINTS** are found in the brachioradialis, supinator and biceps brachii muscles. **STRETCH AND SPRAY** are performed by extending the forearm at the elbow while applying the spray with a down-pattern. **INJECTION AND STRETCH**, to be successful, require an appreciation of the unexpected thickness of this muscle. **CORRECTIVE ACTION** calls for relieving overload of the muscle.

1. REFERRED PAIN
(Fig. 31.1)

Pain is referred from brachialis trigger points (TPs) chiefly to the dorsum of the carpometacarpal joint at the base of the thumb and to the dorsal web of the thumb (Fig. 31.1), as also noted by Kelly.[10] The most common, distal TPs in the brachialis are located a few centimeters above the antecubital space. Spillover pain from them may cover the antecubital space. The pain that occasionally extends upward over the deltoid muscle arises from TPs lying more proximal in the brachialis.

Experimental injection of hypertonic saline into this muscle produced referred pain in the region of the elbow and over the radial aspect of the forearm. The pain was associated with referred tenderness that matched the pain in distribution, duration and severity.[11]

2. ANATOMICAL ATTACHMENTS
(Fig. 31.2)

The brachialis attaches *above* to the distal half of the shaft of the humerus ante-riorly and to the medial and lateral intermuscular septa. It attaches *below* to the coronoid process on the proximal end of the ulna (Fig. 31.2).

The overlying biceps brachii attaches distally to the radius.[7]

Supplemental References

Other authors have illustrated the brachialis muscle as it is seen from in front,[6, 19, 22, 23] from the medial aspect,[20] from the medial aspect with associated neurovascular structures,[13, 16, 21] from the lateral aspect,[4, 12, 15, 18] and as seen in cross section.[2, 5, 14]

3. INNERVATION

The brachialis muscle is supplied by the musculocutaneous nerve *via* the lateral cord from the C_5 and C_6 roots.[7]

4. ACTIONS

Due to its ulnar, rather than radial attachment, the brachialis performs only one motion, flexion of the forearm at the elbow.[1, 3, 8, 17] It is the "workhorse" of the

PART 2

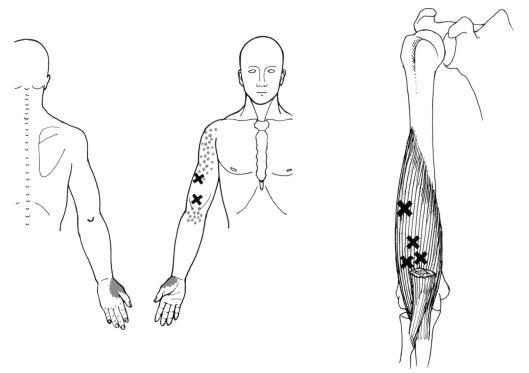

Figure 31.1.   The pain pattern (essential portion, *solid red*, spillover portion, *stippled red*) that is referred from trigger points (×s) in the right brachialis muscle. The uppermost trigger point may cause entrapment of the radial nerve.

elbow flexors. Like the deltoid, it shows no activity when the dependent arm is heavily loaded with weights.[1] There is fine interplay between the biceps brachii, the brachialis and the brachioradialis muscles during resisted forearm flexion. The interplay shows striking variability on repeated trials.[1]

During the act of driving a car, the brachialis generally showed a low level of electrical activity that was relatively constant, and only occasionally showed short bursts of more intense activity.[9]

5. MYOTATIC UNIT

The brachialis is synergistic with the biceps brachii, brachioradialis, and that part of the supinator that functions as an elbow flexor.

The brachialis functions as an antagonist to the triceps brachii.

6. SYMPTOMS

Symptoms may be due to referred pain and tenderness from brachialis TPs, or secondary to radial nerve entrapment. Re-ferred pain is felt in the base of the thumb at rest and often also with use of the thumb. Diffuse soreness of the thumb may represent referred tenderness. Pain referred over the anterior deltoid region from the upper brachialis TPs alone does not lead to impairment of shoulder motion.

Symptoms caused by brachialis entrapment of the superficial sensory (cutaneous) branch of the radial nerve are dysesthesia, tingling, and numbness on the dorsum of the thumb. The aching of referred pain and these symptoms of entrapment, which are also experienced in the thumb, may each arise from TPs located in different parts of the muscle.

7. ACTIVATION OF TRIGGER POINTS

Brachialis TPs are activated by stress overload of forearm flexion during heavy lifting. Examples are holding a power tool, carrying groceries, meticulous ironing, and playing a violin or guitar. Another cause is unaccustomed weight bearing on forearm crutches, as for a leg injury. In "tennis elbow," brachialis involvement tends to develop together with that of the biceps

PART 2

PART 2

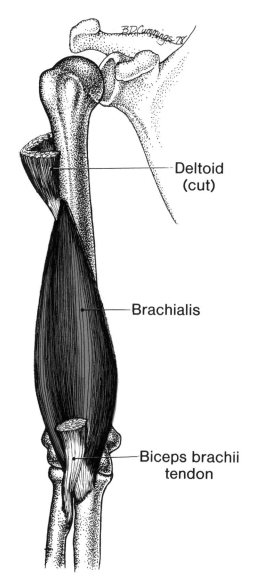

Figure 31.2. Attachments of the right brachialis muscle to the humerus above, and ulna below. The cut end of the overlying biceps brachii muscle appears below. The deltoid, above, also has been cut for clarity.

brachii after initial activation of TPs in the supinator (see Chapter 36).

8. PATIENT EXAMINATION

Pain referred from TPs is increased by passively extending the elbow fully, although limitation of motion is not a complaint. The range of elbow extension is restricted by only a few degrees, and often is detectable only on comparison with the other arm, or by improvement after treatment. Surprisingly, active motion of the

thumb in the pain reference zone usually hurts, but active movement of the elbow does not.

Radial nerve compression is indicated when a tingling in the thumb results from pressure exerted on the region where the nerve exits through the lateral intermuscular septum (see Fig. 32.3). The place to apply pressure is about mid arm, just below the dimple that marks the apex (distal end) of the triangular bulge which represents the deltoid muscle.

9. TRIGGER POINT EXAMINATION
(Fig. 31.3)

The patient's elbow is flexed between 30 and 45°, and the bulk of the biceps brachii pushed aside, medially, to palpate the underlying brachialis TPs (Fig. 31.3). The most frequent brachialis TPs are located in the distal part of the muscle (Fig. 31.1) and refer pain to the thumb, and sometimes to the front of the elbow. One of these TPs is often located beneath the lateral edge of the undisplaced biceps brachii, but others may be found toward the radial side of the muscle. The more proximal TPs, which refer pain up the arm, are likely to be centered under the biceps muscle.

The TP that causes entrapment of the radial nerve usually lies in the lateral border of the brachialis muscle just above the level where the nerve penetrates the intermuscular septum, and possibly passes through some of the brachialis fibers.

10. ENTRAPMENT

The symptoms of nerve entrapment include "numbness," hypoesthesia or hyperesthesia, and dysesthesia (as distinguished from the deep ache of referred pain). These symptoms, like the referred pain, appear over the dorsum of the thumb and its adjacent web space. This entrapment of the sensory branch of the radial nerve is apparently caused by TP tension of brachialis fibers at the level of the origin of the brachioradialis muscle, as the radial nerve exits the musculospiral groove from beneath the triceps brachii through the lateral intermuscular septum (see Fig. 32.3).

These symptoms of entrapment are relieved by injection of the brachialis TP, which feels like an almond in the lateral

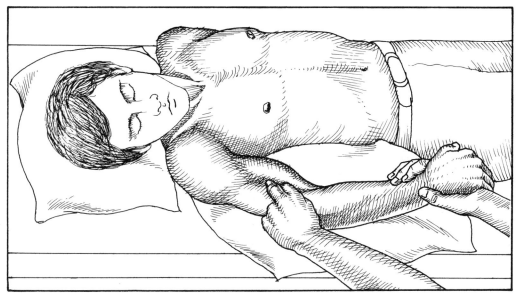

Figure 31.3. Examination of the brachialis muscle for trigger points while pushing the biceps brachii medially in order to reach under it.

border of the muscle, just proximal to the nerve. The resultant resolution of the taut band and the relief of nerve-entrapment signs and symptoms strongly suggest that muscle shortening associated with the TPs produced the nerve compression and should be confirmable by sensory nerve conduction velocities before and after relief by treatment.

11. ASSOCIATED TRIGGER POINTS

The brachialis is likely to be involved when the biceps brachii, brachioradialis or supinator muscles harbor active TPs.

Pain at the base of the thumb also may be referred from TPs in the supinator, brachioradialis and adductor pollicis muscles.

12. STRETCH AND SPRAY
(Fig. 31.4)

The operator rests the end of the humerus at, or just above, the olecranon on a firm support (operator's knee, or armrest of the chair covered by a pillow), as in Figure 31.4. The elbow is gradually extended while the vapocoolant spray is applied over the brachialis downward, in the direction of its chief zone of referred pain and on to the end of the thumb. The spray also is applied upward to cover the brachialis again and the anterior deltoid region, if pain also is felt there.

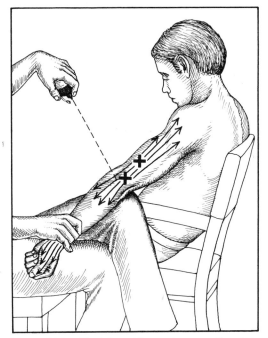

Figure 31.4. Stretch position and spray pattern (*arrows*) for trigger points (×s) in the brachialis muscle. The elbow is hyperextended by applying counter pressure at, or just above, the olecranon process with the wrist supinated, while the vapocoolant spray is applied over the muscle and over the hand.

13. INJECTION AND STRETCH
(Fig. 31.5)

The arm is flexed approximately 45° less than full extension to slacken the biceps

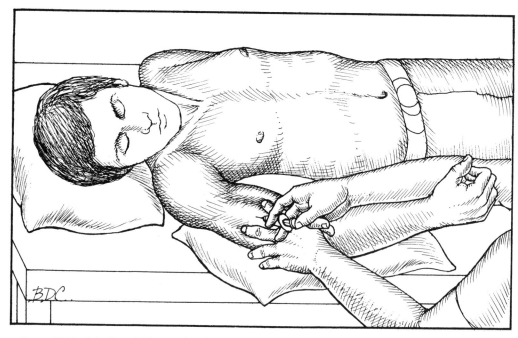

Figure 31.5.   Injection of trigger points in the brachialis muscle, with the biceps brachii pushed medially.

brachii, which is pressed aside, medially. For injection, the needle should be at least 3.8 cm (1½ in) long. The brachialis is a surprisingly thick muscle; its TPs lie deep, next to the humerus. Approaching the muscle from the lateral side of the arm (Fig. 31.5), the needle is directed medially and upward, probing widely to explore the lateral and middle portions of the muscle for TPs to infiltrate. The needle may lightly contact the humerus, which insures reaching the full depth of the muscle.

After injection, the brachialis is stretched passively to its full range of motion as the vapocoolant is applied to the skin, followed by a hot pack.

14. CORRECTIVE ACTIONS
(Fig. 31.6)

Stress overload of forearm flexion is avoided by lifting only light or moderate loads, with the hands supinated. This brings the biceps brachii into play, avoiding additional load on the brachialis (see Chapter 30).

The patient learns to place a pillow in the angle of the elbow at night to avoid sleeping with the arm tightly folded (see Fig. 30.8), a position which immobilizes the brachialis in a very shortened position. Likewise, the elbow should not be held sharply flexed during a long telephone call.

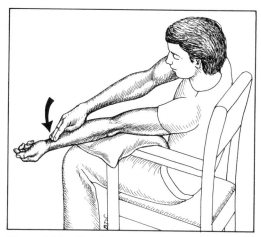

Figure 31.6.   Passive self-stretch of the brachialis muscle.

A purse strap should not hang on the forearm with the elbow bent; the purse may be held in the fingers with the elbow straight, or hung over the opposite shoulder or on a belt.

When playing a musical instrument, like a violin, the bent elbow should be straightened at every opportunity.

The patient learns to passively stretch the brachialis, by supporting the humerus just above the elbow, while pushing the supinated wrist down with the other hand (Fig. 31.6). The patient should do several such stretches once or twice daily after soaking the arm and forearm in hot water, or after application of a hot pack.

References

1. Basmajian JV: *Muscles Alive*, Ed. 4. Williams & Wilkins, Baltimore, 1978 (pp. 165, 187, 199, 201, 203).
2. Carter BL, Morehead J, Wolpert SM, *et al.*: *Cross-Sectional Anatomy*. Appleton-Century-Crofts, New York, 1977 (Sects. 50–54).
3. Duchenne GB: *Physiology of Motion*, translated by E.B. Kaplan. J.B. Lippincott, Philadelphia, 1949 (p. 98).
4. Grant JCB: *An Atlas of Human Anatomy*, Ed. 7. Williams & Wilkins, Baltimore, 1978 (Fig. 6-37).
5. *Ibid.* (Fig. 6-41).
6. *Ibid.* (Fig. 6-53, 6-55).
7. Gray H: *Anatomy of the Human Body*, edited by C.M. Goss, American Ed. 29. Lea & Febiger, Philadelphia, 1973 (p. 460).
8. Hollinshead WH: *Functional Anatomy of the Limbs and Back*, Ed. 4. W.B. Saunders, Philadelphia, 1976 (p. 133).
9. Jonsson S, Jonsson B: Function of the muscles of the upper limb in car driving. *Ergonomics* 18:375–388, 1975 (pp. 383–386).
10. Kellgren JH: Observations on referred pain arising from muscle. *Clin Sci* 3:175–190, 1938 (pp. 187, 188).
11. Kelly M: The nature of fibrositis. I. The myalgic lesion and its secondary effects: a reflex theory. *Ann Rheumatol Dis* 5:1–7, 1945 (Case 1).
12. McMinn RMH, Hutchings RT: *Color Atlas of Human Anatomy*. Year Book Medical Publishers, Chicago, 1977 (pp. 113, 128).
13. *Ibid.* (p. 119).
14. Pernkopf E: *Atlas of Topographical and Applied Human Anatomy*, Vol. 2. W.B. Saunders, Philadelphia, 1964 (pp. 61, 80).
15. *Ibid.* (p. 58).
16. *Ibid.* (p. 56).
17. Rasch PJ, Burke RK: *Kinesiology and Applied Anatomy*, Ed. 6. Lea & Febiger, Philadelphia, 1978 (p. 185).
18. Sobotta J, Figge FHJ: *Atlas of Human Anatomy*, Ed. 9, Vol. 1. Hafner Division of Macmillan, New York, 1974 (p. 192).
19. *Ibid.* (pp. 196, 204).
20. *Ibid.* (p. 198).
21. Sobotta J, Figge FHJ: *Atlas of Human Anatomy*, Ed. 9, Vol. 3. Hafner Division of Macmillan, New York, 1974 (pp. 291, 296).
22. Spalteholz W: *Handatlas der Anatomie des Menschen*, Ed. 11, Vol. 2. S. Hirzel, Leipzig, 1922 (pp. 320, 321, 327).
23. Toldt C: *An Atlas of Human Anatomy*, translated by M.E. Paul, Ed. 2, Vol 1. Macmillan, New York, 1919 (pp. 315, 316, 321).

PART 2

CHAPTER 32
Triceps Brachii Muscle (Anconeus)
"The Three-headed Monster"

HIGHLIGHTS: The three heads of the triceps brachii may develop trigger points (TPs) in five locations, each with its own referred pain pattern. **REFERRED PAIN** from the muscle's TPs is projected mostly up and down the posterior aspect of the arm and to the lateral, more often than to the medial, epicondyle with spillover into the fourth and fifth fingers. It may be projected also to the suprascapular region. The long head is commonly overlooked as a source of pain because it spans two joints. **ANATOMICAL ATTACHMENTS** of the medial and lateral heads are to the humerus and the adjacent olecranon process of the ulna, thus crossing one joint, unlike the long head, which spans two joints. Above, the triceps attaches to the scapula; below, it forms the common tendon of all three heads at the olecranon process. **ACTION** of all parts of the triceps brachii is extension of the forearm at the elbow. In addition, the long head adducts, and may extend the arm at the shoul- der. **ACTIVATION OF TRIGGER POINTS** is usu- ally due to overload stress. **PATIENT EXAMI- NATION** to identify restricted range of motion requires flexion of both the elbow and the shoul- der, an awkward unnatural position. **TRIGGER POINT EXAMINATION** of the long head requires deep pincer palpation of the muscle adjacent to the humerus. Flat palpation may be used for the other heads. **ENTRAPMENT** of the radial nerve may be caused by taut bands in the lateral head. **STRETCH AND SPRAY** of the triceps brachii requires simultaneous flexion of both the joints that the long head transverses with application of the vapocoolant mainly from the proximal to the distal direction. **INJECTION AND STRETCH** of this muscle may be needed to completely inactivate its TPs. **CORRECTIVE ACTIONS** call for modification of activities and mechanical fac- tors that stress this muscle, including the use of chairs with inadequate elbow support.

1. REFERRED PAIN
(Figs. 32.1 and 32.2)

The referred pain patterns of five trigger point (TP) areas in the three heads of the triceps brachii are shown in Figure 32.1. The TPs are numbered in order of decreas- ing prevalence, based on our experience.

TP$_1$, Long Head
(Fig. 32.1A)

Referred pain extends from the TP up- ward over the posterior arm to the back of the shoulder, occasionally to the base of the neck in the upper trapezius region, and sometimes down the dorsum of the fore- arm, skipping the elbow.

TP$_2$, Medial Head, Distal Lateral Border
(Fig. 32.1A)

This TP lies in the lateral border of the medial head. Referred pain and tenderness are projected to the *lateral* epicondyle, and are a common component of the "tennis elbow." Pain also may extend to the radial aspect of the forearm.

TP$_3$, Lateral Head, Mid-belly Lateral Border
(Fig. 32.1*B*)

From this TP, pain is referred over the arm posteriorly, sometimes to the dorsum of the forearm, and occasionally to the fourth and fifth digits. The taut muscle bands may entrap the radial nerve.

TP$_4$, Medial Head, Central Distal End
(Fig. 32.1*B*)

This TP refers pain and tenderness distally to the olecranon process.

TP$_5$, Medial Head, Distal Medial Border
(Fig. 32.1*C*)

Most easily located by an anterior approach, this TP refers pain and tenderness to the *medial* epicondyle. Pain may extend to the volar surface of the fourth and fifth digits and sometimes also to the adjacent palm and middle finger. Winter[34] also included pain along the inner side of the forearm.

Anconeus
(Fig. 32.2)

An active TP in the anconeus (pronounced anco'neus) muscle refers pain and tenderness locally to the *lateral* epicondyle (Fig. 32.2).

2. ANATOMICAL ATTACHMENTS
(Fig. 32.3)

The three heads of the triceps brachii muscle attach **distally** to the olecranon process of the ulna *via* a common tendon (Fig. 32.3). **Proximally** the **long head** attaches to the infraglenoid lip of the scapula; this head crosses two joints. The **medial head** attaches to the humerus **medial** and **distal** to the radial nerve. This head lies deep against the bone, and just above the elbow it extends across the humerus to both the medial and lateral sides of the arm. **Proximally** the **lateral head** attaches to the humerus **lateral** and **proximal** to the radial nerve. It bridges the radial nerve and covers much of the medial head (Fig. 32.3*C*). The medial and lateral heads cross only the elbow joint.[12]

The **anconeus** muscle appears as an extension of the triceps between the olecranon process and the lateral epicondyle (Fig. 32.3). It attaches **above** to the lateral epicondyle and **below** to the side of the olecranon process and to the dorsal surface of the ulna.[12]

Supplemental References

Other authors have illustrated the triceps brachii as viewed from the medial aspect,[6, 28, 31] from the lateral aspect,[7, 21, 26] from behind,[8, 19, 22, 27, 30, 32] from behind showing the lateral head reflected to reveal its relation to the radial nerve,[9, 29] and in cross section.[3, 11, 20] The anconeus was sometimes included.[10, 27]

3. INNERVATION

All heads of the muscle are innervated by branches of the radial nerve *via* the posterior cord from spinal roots C_7 and C_8.

4. ACTIONS

All parts of the triceps brachii extend the forearm at the elbow.[1, 5, 13, 23] However, the medial head is the workhorse that exhibits the earliest and greatest activity.[1, 33] The long head also adducts[1, 13, 23] and is said to extend[13, 23] the arm at the shoulder; on stimulation of the long head, adduction is the dominant action.[5]

The scapular attachment of the long head influences actions at the glenohumeral joint. Electrical stimulation studies[5] demonstrated that activation of the long head alone, with the arm hanging down, elevated the head of the humerus toward the acromion. Stimulation with the arm abducted to 90° forced the head of the humerus into the glenoid cavity. The long head of the triceps, the pectoralis major and latissimus dorsi all strongly adduct the arm, but the long head counteracts the strong tendency of the other two muscles to pull the head of the humerus down out of the glenoid fossa.[5] Stimulation of the long head adducted the arm at the glenohumeral joint by drawing the humerus to the scapula without rotating the scapula, whereas stimulating the teres major tended to draw the inferior angle of the scapula toward the humerus without moving the arm.[5] This is not surprising since these two muscles have reverse long and short lever arms across the glenohumeral joint.

The anconeus muscle assists the triceps

PART 2

PART 2

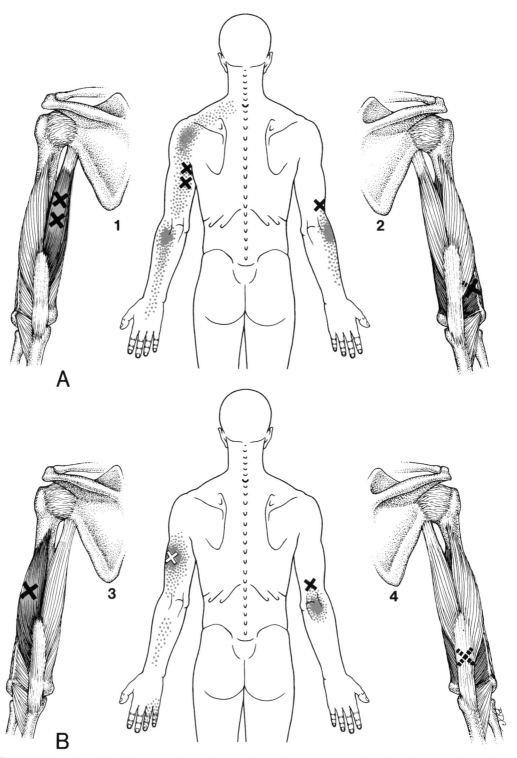

Figure 32.1 A–C. Referred pain patterns (*dark red*) from trigger points (×s) in the triceps brachii muscle (*medium red*). *A,* trigger point number 1 (TP$_1$), left long head; TP$_2$, lateral portion of the right medial head. *B,* TP$_3$, lateral border of the left lateral head; TP$_4$, deep in the distal right medial head, centrally. *C,* TP$_5$, deep in the medial border of the right medial head (*medium red*).

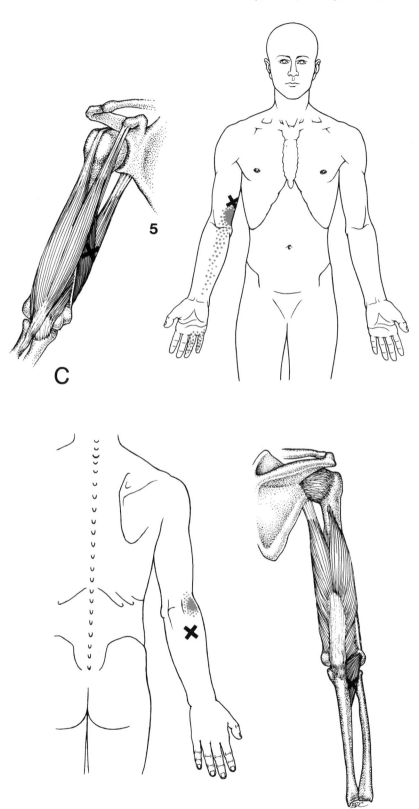

Figure 32.2.   Location of a trigger point (✗) in the anconeus muscle (*light red*) and its referred pain pattern (*dark red*).

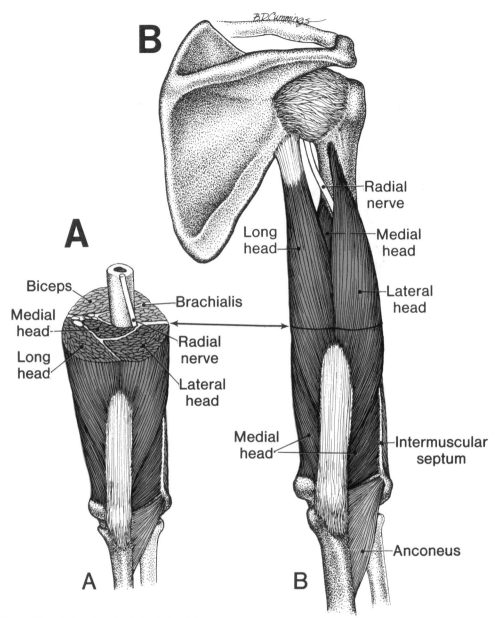

Figure 32.3 A–C. Attachments of the right triceps brachii muscle (*dark red*) seen from one view and three degrees of dissection. Other muscles are *light red*. *A*, cross section just proximal to the level where the radial nerve penetrates the lateral intermuscular septum. *B*, posterior view of the intact triceps brachii. *C*, posterior view with the lateral head reflected, showing the course of the radial nerve, which separates the humeral attachments of the medial and lateral heads. The medial head attaches to the humerus *medially* and *distally*; the lateral head attaches *laterally* and *proximally* to the nerve.

in extension of the forearm at the elbow.[1] The anconeus was thought by Duchenne[5] to contribute specifically to abduction of the ulna during pronation of the hand. It was observed electromyographically to be activated by all index finger movements and to contribute to stabilization of the humeroulnar joint.[25] Other electromyographic evaluations of anconeus activity concluded that the anconeus, supinator and medial head of the triceps brachii work together to stabilize the elbow joint during pronation and supination of the hand.[1, 33]

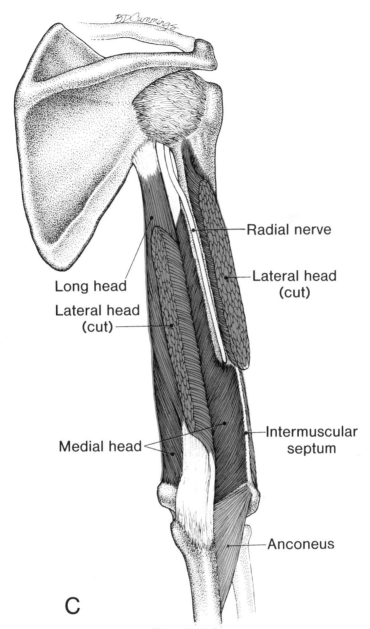

Figure 32.3 C.

Activities

Bilateral triceps brachii muscles were monitored electromyographically with surface electrodes during 13 sports activities that included overhand and underhand throws, tennis, golf, baseball hits and 1-ft jumps. Most of the records showed briefer, more intense contraction of the dominant than of the non-dominant triceps muscle. The more prolonged activity of the non-dominant triceps appeared to relate to rotational counterbalance. Two outstanding exceptions were batting a baseball and golf swings, in which the non-dominant triceps acted as a prime mover.[2]

Electromyographic monitoring during typewriting showed minimal activity in the triceps, and that only as the subject approached maximum typing speed.[16] Triceps activity during driving showed no meaningful correlation with deviation of the steering wheel.[14]

5. MYOTATIC UNIT

The triceps and anconeus muscles are synergistic extensors of the forearm at the elbow. The long head of the triceps is synergistic with the latissimus dorsi, teres major and teres minor muscles, all of which can act as adductors and extensors of the arm at the shoulder.

As antagonists to the triceps, the biceps and brachialis muscles are prone to develop TPs—often latent—during chronic TP involvement of the triceps.

6. SYMPTOMS

The patient is likely to complain of vague, hard-to-localize pain posteriorly in the shoulder and upper arm. Most patients are unaware of any restriction of arm or forearm motion because of the tendency to keep the elbow slightly flexed, out of the painful range, and to compensate for the slightly reduced reach by additional scapular or body movement. Because of tenderness referred to the medial epicondyle, the elbow may be held away from the side to avoid contact.

Pain occurs during activity which requires forceful extension at the elbow: in the dominant arm when playing tennis, and in the non-dominant arm (elbow held straight) when playing golf. Myofascial elbow pain interferes with either game. As the activity of TP$_2$ increases, it becomes an important source of pain in the chronic "tennis elbow" (see Chapter 36).

7. ACTIVATION OF TRIGGER POINTS

Activation of TPs in the triceps brachii may occur due to overload from overuse of forearm crutches; from the stress of a cane that is too long (used because of injury to the back or leg); from strain of the muscle in sports (backhand "mis-hit" in tennis); from overenthusiastic conditioning exercises (golf practice or push-ups); or from repetitively pressing tightly bound books on a photocopy machine. Surprisingly, the TPs in the long head are likely to be activated by sitting for long periods with the elbow held forward in front of the plane of the chest or abdomen and lacking elbow support, e.g. driving a car on a long trip, holding down a sheet of paper with the left hand while writing with the right, or doing needlepoint without elbow support.

8. PATIENT EXAMINATION
(Fig. 32.4)

When the long head is involved, the patient is unable to abduct the arm against the ear with the elbow held straight (Fig. 32.4); nor can he or she simultaneously fully flex the forearm at the elbow and fully flex the arm at the shoulder, as in the stretch position shown later in Figure 32.6. The patient is unable to fully straighten the elbow against a load when the medial, or lateral head is involved. Stretching the

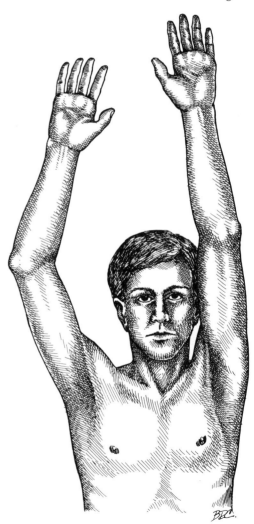

Figure 32.4. Positive Triceps Brachii Test. If the long head contains active trigger points, the patient cannot bring the involved right arm tight against the ear while the muscle holds the elbow straight.

PART 2

involved triceps by passively flexing the forearm causes pain, as does loading the muscle by actively resisting extension of the forearm at the elbow.[17]

An epicondyle that is painful because of TPs also is sensitive to tapping because of referred tenderness. Pain in the lateral epicondyle due to activity of triceps TP$_2$ often persists in patients with "tennis elbow" after their supinator, biceps brachii and brachioradialis TPs have been inactivated. Then, residual percussion tenderness of the posterior aspect of the epicondyle indicates that this triceps TP is probably active.

Differential Diagnosis

Pain referred from the triceps brachii to the vicinity of the elbow joint may be mistakenly attributed to arthritis.[24]

Since pain from this muscle may focus on the back of the arm and extend into the hand, it is sometimes erroneously thought to result from a C$_7$ radiculopathy.[24]

The cubital tunnel syndrome is more likely to cause hypoesthesia of the skin in the ulnar distribution of the hand, and weakness and clumsiness of the hand, than pain.[4] The entrapment syndrome is associated with slowing of ulnar nerve conduction through the cubital tunnel, whereas the pain from myofascial TPs is not.

9. TRIGGER POINT EXAMINATION (Fig. 32.5)

The muscle is slackened by bending the elbow 15° or 20°, with the arm comfortably supported. Active TPs in the triceps, especially in the long head, respond to palpation with visible local twitch responses and projection of referred pain in their predictable patterns.

TP$_1$

This TP area lies deep in the long head slightly proximal to mid-belly, a few centimeters distal to where the teres major crosses the long head (Fig. 32.1A). Pincer palpation is used to explore the long head by starting at the humerus and by encircling all of its fibers with the digits (right hand in Fig. 32.5). Clusters of TPs are often present and are identified by their multiple taut bands and local twitch responses.

TP$_2$

This common component of the "tennis elbow" lies in the distal lateral portion of

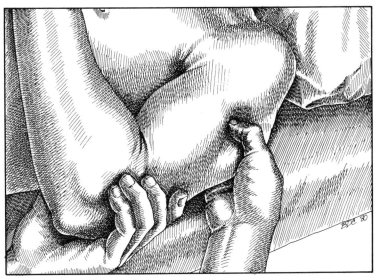

Figure 32.5.   Pincer palpation of a trigger point (TP$_1$) in the long head of the left triceps brachii muscle. The fingers encircle the long head in a pincer grasp, separating it from the humerus and the adjacent neurovascular bundle. Individual taut bands and their trigger points are located by rolling the muscle fibers between the digits. A taut band is examined by snapping it back and forth, to elicit local twitch responses.

the medial head, 4–6 cm (1½–2½ in) above the lateral epicondyle, to which it refers pain in association with other TPs contributing to a "tennis elbow" myofascial syndrome. The TP is found by flat palpation; a local twitch response is often seen in a band of muscle that extends down to the lateral epicondyle (Fig. 32.1A).

TP₃

This is a small superficial "button" located by flat palpation at mid-belly in the lateral border of the lateral head, just above the point where the radial nerve exits from the musculospiral groove (Figs. 32.1B and 32.3C). This TP₃ band may entrap the sensory fibers of the radial nerve. In this case, firm palpation along the lateral intermuscular septum, in the region where the radial nerve penetrates the septum, is likely to set off a tingle in the hand. The button-like ridge in the muscle at the TP lies just above this point of nerve hypersensitivity.

TP₄

TP₄ is found deep in the medial head, close to the mid-line of the muscle just above the olecranon, to which it refers pain (Figs. 32.1B and 32.3).

TP₅

This TP is located deep in the medial border of the medial head just above the medial epicondyle, where it projects its pain and tenderness (Fig. 32.1C). This TP is found by flat palpation, with the patient lying supine and the arm externally rotated at the shoulder.

10. ENTRAPMENT

The TP₃ "button" is found in the lateral border of the lateral head of the triceps brachii (Fig. 32.1B), just proximal to the exit of the radial nerve from the musculospiral groove (Fig. 32.3C). Activation of this TP is often associated with sensory signs and symptoms of compression of the radial nerve. The patient complains of tingling and numbness (dysesthesias) over the dorsum of the lower forearm, wrist, and hand to the base of the middle finger, which lies in the sensory distribution of the radial nerve. By comparison, the aching pain referred from TP₃ appears in the two "ulnar" (fourth and fifth) digits.

Symptoms of nerve compression may be relieved within minutes to days after an injection of the TP that relaxes the responsible taut band of muscle. The local anesthetic solution may temporarily block the radial nerve. This TP₃ responds poorly to stretch and spray.

Clinical and electromyographic evidence of radial nerve neuropraxia indicates that entrapment occurred along its passage beneath the triceps muscle. Careful dissection of cadavers revealed in almost every body an accessory part of the lateral head that originated below the spiral groove. The attachment of this slip of muscle to the humerus forms a fibrotic arch of variable snugness over the radial nerve. This arch is distinct from the opening of the lateral intermuscular septum.[15] A patient with a 3-year history of an atraumatic radial paresis progressing to paralysis was relieved by surgical release of lateral head fibers that attached near the radial nerve.[18] The TP₃ fibers may tense this arch, ensnaring the nerve.

11. ASSOCIATED TRIGGER POINTS

The synergistic latissimus dorsi, teres major and teres minor muscles often exhibit associated TPs.

If the elbow pain persists in the lateral epicondylar area after eliminating TPs in the triceps brachii, then the anconeus, supinator, brachioradialis and extensor carpi radialis longus muscles may be harboring TPs that also refer pain to that region.

12. STRETCH AND SPRAY
(Fig. 32.6)

With the patient seated and the forearm fully flexed at the elbow, the muscle is further stretched by passively flexing the arm at the shoulder (Fig. 32.6A). The operator stretches the triceps brachii by pulling back on the patient's elbow while pressing the patient's forearm forward (Fig. 32.6A). The spray is swept upward, starting at the latissimus dorsi in the posterior axillary fold and continuing over the triceps brachii, around the elbow, and down the forearm to include the fourth and fifth fingers (Fig. 32.6A). Full flexion at the shoulder may be limited also by latissimus dorsi TPs.

To obtain a similar stretch of the triceps

PART 2

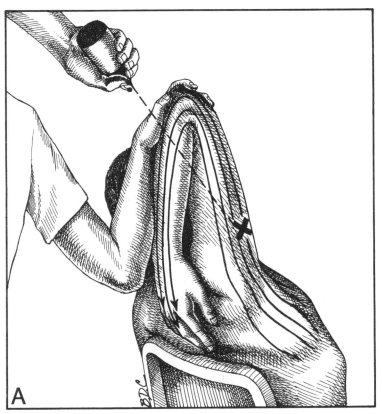

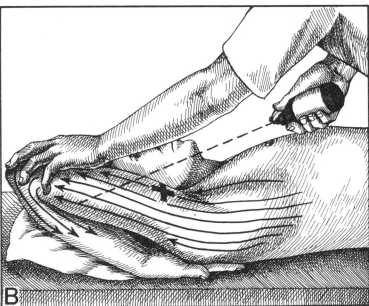

Figure 32.6. Stretch position and spray pattern (*arrows*) for a trigger point (×) in the long head of the triceps brachii. This technique is also effective for the other two heads. *A*, patient seated. *B*, patient supine; this position is likely to be more effective because the patient relaxes more completely.

brachii muscle in the supine patient, the forearm is flexed at the elbow and the arm flexed at the shoulder to place the supinated hand beneath the shoulder, as in Figure 32.6*B*. The vapocoolant spray is again applied in parallel sweeps, starting at the latissimus dorsi adjacent to the scapula, covering the triceps distally over the arm and around the elbow to the wrist. Meanwhile the operator presses down on the elbow to further flex the arm at the shoulder, stretching especially the long head of the muscle.

13. INJECTION AND STRETCH
(Figs. 32.7–32.10)

TP₁, Patient Supine or Side-lying
(Fig. 32.7)

To inject this TP by approaching the medial side of the long head of the triceps, the supine patient externally rotates the arm so that the antecubital space faces up

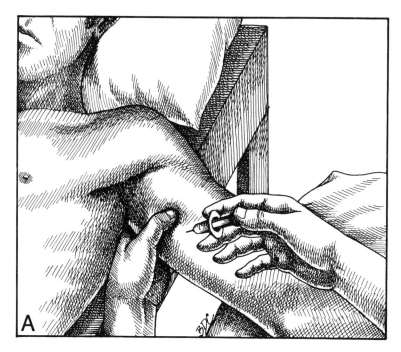

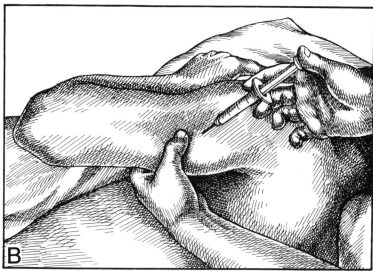

Figure 32.7. Injection of trigger points (TP₁ region) in the long head of the left triceps brachii. *A*, anterior approach, with the patient supine. *B*, posterior approach, with the patient lying on the opposite side.

and abducts the arm sufficiently to place the long head on a slight stretch (Fig. 32.7A). The operator encircles the long head of the muscle in a pincer grasp and lifts it away from the underlying bone, blood vessels and nerve trunks, and from the lateral head of the triceps, beneath which the radial nerve courses. A TP in a palpable band is fixed and injected between the tips of the digits. Penetration of these TPs by the needle produces local twitch responses that are easily seen and can be felt by the encompassing fingers and thumb.

If it is a more convenient position, or the TPs are in the lateral part of the long head, this TP area can be approached from the lateral aspect of the arm. To do so, the patient lies on the opposite side, facing away from the operator (Fig. 32.7B), permitting the operator to grasp the muscle and inject the TPs as described above. These TPs also can be injected through the muscle from the anterior approach.

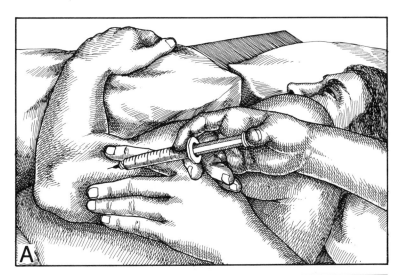

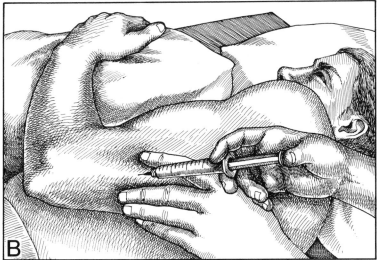

Figure 32.8.   Injection of trigger points (TP$_2$ and TP$_3$ regions) in the left triceps brachii with the patient lying on the right side and the uppermost arm resting on a pillow against the chest wall, elbow bent. A, TP$_2$ lies in the lateral border of the medial head distally; it refers pain and tenderness to the lateral epicondyle. This trigger point is located about three or four fingerbreadths proximal to the lateral epicondyle. B, TP$_3$ lies in the lateral border of the lateral head about mid-humerus; it refers pain locally over the muscle, to the dorsum of the forearm, and to the fourth and fifth digits.

TP₂, Patient Side-lying
(Fig. 32.8A)

The patient lies on the opposite side with the arm supported on a pillow (Fig. 32.8A). TP₂ is palpated distally in the lateral border of the medial head, adjacent to the attachments of the extensor carpi radialis longus and the brachioradialis muscles. For injection, the TP is fixed between the fingers by pressing it against the humerus (Fig. 32.8A).

TP₃, Patient Side-lying
(Fig. 32.8B)

For injection of TP₃, the patient is placed in the same position as described above for TP₂. TP₃ is located along the lateral border of the lateral head, just above the exit of the radial nerve, which courses beside the brachialis and then beneath the brachioradialis muscle. The needle is inserted tangentially into a thin layer of muscle (Fig. 32.8B) and may be directed either distally or proximally (whichever is more convenient), probing for TPs in a fan-like pattern.

It is not unusual for some procaine solution to infiltrate the radial nerve and cause a temporary nerve block. If the dilute 0.5% procaine solution is used for injection, the nerve recovers its function within 15–20 min.

TP₄, Patient Side-lying

The patient lies on the opposite side, facing away from the operator, as in Figure 32.8. This TP is located only by spot tenderness to deep palpation through the thick aponeurosis of all heads of the triceps brachii. This TP area is injected deeply, aiming toward the olecranon process. Penetration of the TP by the needle is confirmed primarily by the patient's report of a local pain response and of referred pain. Occasionally, the operator feels a local twitch of the muscle when the needle encounters TP₄.

TP₅, Patient Supine
(Fig. 32.9)

The patient's externally rotated and partially abducted arm lies on the padded lap of the operator (Fig. 32.9). TP₅ lies deep in the distal medial head of the muscle and is identified by its spot tenderness and local twitch response. The region of the TP is fixed between the fingers to inject it, with

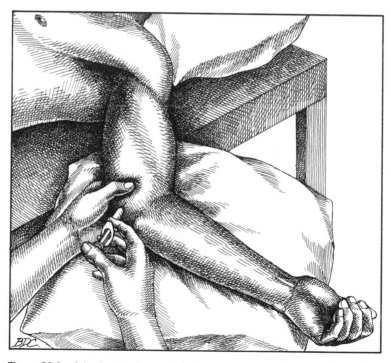

Figure 32.9. Injection of trigger points (TP₅ region) in the distal medial head of the left triceps brachii, with the patient supine. The arm is externally rotated, the forearm supinated, and the slightly flexed elbow is supported on a pillow.

PART 2

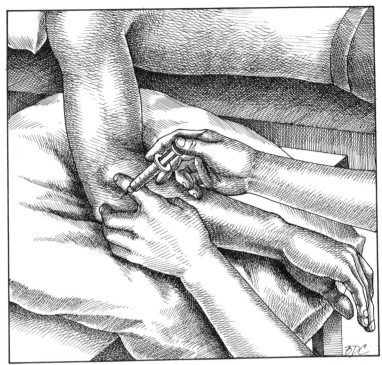

Figure 32.10. Injection of trigger point in the right anconeus muscle of a supine patient. The patient's elbow is flexed slightly and the hand pronated. The tender trigger point is localized by the fingers against the ulna, between the olecranon process and the lateral epicondyle.

the needle directed parallel to the muscle fibers and usually upward toward the shoulder.

This TP is not especially close to the neurovascular bundle, but, if one peppers and injects the area too widely, one can cause a temporary block of the median or ulnar nerve.

Anconeus
(Fig. 32.10)

The arm of the supine patient is supported on a padded surface with the forearm flexed about 45° at the elbow and the hand pronated (Fig. 32.10). For injection, the TP is fixed between the fingers of the palpating hand.

14. CORRECTIVE ACTIONS

When typing, writing, reading, etc., the patient should keep the upper arm vertical, with the elbow behind the plane of the chest and not projected forward. Whenever possible, an armrest of suitable height should support the elbow.

To correct for short upper arms in relation to the torso height, a writing-board

with padding glued underneath is used to raise the armrests, or the height of the armrests above the seat is increased directly.

If forearm crutches are necessary, their use should be started gradually to avoid sudden overload of the arm muscles, especially the triceps.

In tennis, the patient may change to a lighter weight racquet or to one not so heavy in the head. Also, it may be helpful to shorten the grip on the racquet handle, which reduces the leverage on this elbow extensor muscle.

Chinning on a bar and push-ups, which easily overload the arm muscles, should be avoided until after recovery.

The patient should be taught how to stretch the triceps brachii, by assuming the patient position in Figure 32.6A, while seated under a hot shower with the water streaming over the muscle.

References

1. Basmajian JV: *Muscles Alive*, Ed. 4. Williams & Wilkins, Baltimore, 1978 (pp. 164, 165, 186, 204, 205).

2. Broer MR, Houtz SJ: *Patterns of Muscular Activity in Selected Sports Skill.* Charles C Thomas, Springfield, Ill. 1967.
3. Carter BL, Morehead J, Wolpert SM, *et al.*: *Cross-Sectional Anatomy.* Appleton-Century-Crofts, New York, 1977 (Sects. 51, 52).
4. Craven PR, Green DP; Cubital tunnel syndrome. *J Bone Joint Surg 62-A*:986–989, 1980.
5. Duchenne GB: *Physiology of Motion,* translated by E.B. Kaplan. J.B. Lippincott, Philadelphia, 1949 (pp. 85, 86).
6. Grant JCB: *An Atlas of Human Anatomy,* Ed. 7. Williams & Wilkins, Baltimore, 1978 (Fig. 6-25).
7. *Ibid.* (Fig. 6-37).
8. *Ibid.* (Fig. 6-39).
9. *Ibid.* (Fig. 6-40).
10. *Ibid.* (Fig. 6-64).
11. *Ibid.* (Fig. 6-41).
12. Gray H: *Anatomy of the Human Body,* edited by C.M. Goss, American Ed. 29. Lea & Febiger, Philadelphia, 1973 (pp. 460, 461, 470).
13. Hollinshead WH: *Functional Anatomy of the Limbs and Back,* Ed. 4. W.B. Saunders, Philadelphia, 1976 (p. 33).
14. Jonsson S, Jonsson B: Function of the muscles of the upper limb in car driving. *Ergonomics 18*:375–388, 1975.
15. Lotem M, Fried A, Levy M, *et al.*: Radial palsy following muscular effort. *J Bone Joint Surg 53-B*:500–506, 1971.
16. Lundervold AJS: Electromyographic investigations of position and manner of working in typewriting. *Acta Phys Scand 24 Suppl. 84*:1–171, 1951 (pp. 66, 67, 94, 95, 97, 100).
17. Macdonald AJR: Abnormally tender muscle regions and associated painful movements. *Pain 8*:197–205, 1980.
18. Manske PR: Compression of the radial nerve by the triceps muscle. *J Bone Joint Surg 59A*:835–836, 1977.
19. McMinn RMH, Hutchings RT: *Color Atlas of Human Anatomy.* Year Book Medical Publishers, Chicago, 1977 (p. 120).
20. Pernkopf E: *Atlas of Topographical and Applied Human Anatomy,* Vol. 2. W.B. Saunders, Philadelphia, 1964 (Figs. 44, 61).
21. *Ibid* (Fig. 57).
22. *Ibid* (Fig. 59).
23. Rasch PJ, Burke RK: *Kinesiology and Applied Anatomy,* Ed. 6. Lea & Febiger, Philadelphia, 1978 (pp. 179, 180).
24. Reynolds MD: Myofascial trigger point syndromes in the practice of rheumatology. *Arch Phys Med Rehabil 62*:111–114, 1981 (Tables 1 and 2).
25. Sano S, Ando K, Katori I, *et al.*: Electromyographic studies on the forearm muscle activities during finger movement. *J Jap Orthop Assoc 51*:331–337, 1977.
26. Sobotta J, Figge FHJ: *Atlas of Human Anatomy,* Ed. 9, Vol. 1. Hafner Division of Macmillan, New York, 1974 (p. 192).
27. *Ibid.* (p. 194).
28. Sobotta J. Figge FHJ: *Atlas of Human Anatomy,* Ed. 9, Vol. 3, Hafner Division of Macmillan, New York, 1974 (p. 291).
29. *Ibid.* (p. 293).
30. Spalteholz W: *Handatlas der Anatomie des Menschen,* Ed. 11, Vol. 2. S. Hirzel, Leipzig, 1922 (p. 322).
31. Toldt C: *An Atlas of Human Anatomy,* translated by M.E. Paul, Ed. 2, Vol. 1. Macmillan, New York, 1919 (p. 314).
32. *Ibid.* (p. 318).
33. Travill AA: Electromyographic study of the extensor apparatus of the forearm. *Anat Rec 144*:373–376, 1962.
34. Winter SP: Referred pain in fibrositis. *Med Rec 157*:34–37, 1944, (p. 37).

PART 2

PART 3

CHAPTER 33
Elbow to Finger
Pain-and-Muscle Guide

INTRODUCTION TO PART 3

This third part of THE TRIGGER POINT MAN-UAL includes the forearm and hand muscles, and all those that cross the elbow joint, except the anconeus, biceps, brachialis and triceps.

PAIN GUIDE TO INVOLVED MUSCLES

This guide lists the muscles that may be responsible for pain in the areas shown in Figure 33.1 The muscles most likely to refer pain to each specific area are listed below under the name of that area. One uses this chart by locating the name of the area that hurts and then by looking under that heading for a listing of all the muscles that might cause the pain. Then, reference should be made to the individual muscle chapters; the number for each follows in parenthesis.

In a general way, the muscles are listed in the order of the liklihood that each may be the cause of pain in that area. This order is only an approximation; the selection process by which patients reach an examiner greatly influences which muscles are most likely to be involved. Bold-face type indicates that the muscle refers an essential pain pattern to that pain area. Normal type indicates that the muscle refers a spillover pattern to that pain area. TP stands for trigger point.

PAIN GUIDE

LATERAL EPICONDYLAR PAIN

Supinator (36)
Brachioradialis (34)
Extensor carpi radialis longus (34)
Triceps brachii (TP$_2$) (32)
Supraspinatus (21)
Fourth and fifth finger extensors (35)
Anconeus (32)

MEDIAL EPICONDYLAR PAIN

Triceps brachii (TP$_5$) (32)
Pectoralis major (42)
Pectoralis minor (43)

ANTECUBITAL PAIN

Brachialis (31)
Biceps brachii (30)

DORSAL FOREARM PAIN

Triceps brachii (TPs$_{1-3}$) (32)
Teres Major (25)
Extensores carpi radialis longus and brevis (38)
Coracobrachialis (29)
Scalenus minimus (20)

OLECRANON PAIN

Triceps brachii (TP$_4$) (32)
Serratus posterior superior (45)

RADIAL FOREARM PAIN

Infraspinatus (22)
Scaleni (20)
Brachioradialis (34)
Supraspinatus (21)
Subclavius (42)

VOLAR FOREARM PAIN

Palmaris longus (37)
Pronator teres (38)
Serratus anterior (46)
Triceps brachii (TP$_5$) (32)

ULNAR FOREARM PAIN

Latissimus dorsi (24)
Pectoralis major (42)
Pectoralis minor (43)
Serratus posterior superior (45)

VOLAR WRIST AND PALMAR PAIN

Flexor carpi radialis (38)
Flexor carpi ulnaris (38)

Opponens pollicis (39)
Pectoralis major (42)
Pectoralis minor (43)
Latissimus dorsi (24)
Palmaris longus (37)
Pronator teres (38)
Serratus anterior (46)

DORSAL WRIST AND HAND PAIN

Extensor carpi radialis brevis (34)
Extensor carpi radialis longus (34)
Index to little finger extensors (35)
Extensor indicis (35)
Extensor carpi ulnaris (34)
Subscapularis (26)
Coracobrachialis (29)
Scalenus minimus (20)
Latissimus dorsi (24)
Serratus posterior superior (45)
First dorsal interosseus (40)

BASE-OF-THUMB AND RADIAL HAND PAIN

Supinator (36)
Scaleni (20)
Brachialis (31)
Infraspinatus (22)
Extensor carpi radialis longus (34)
Brachioradialis (34)
Opponens pollicis (39)
Adductor pollicis (39)
First dorsal interosseus (40)
Flexor pollicis longus (38)

VOLAR FINGER PAIN

Flexores digitorum sublimis and profundus (38)
Interossei (40)
Latissimus dorsi (24)
Serratus anterior (46)
Abductor digiti minimi (40)
Subclavius (42)

DORSAL FINGER PAIN

Extensor digitorum (35)
Interossei (40)
Scaleni (20)
Abductor digiti minimi (40)
Pectoralis major (42)
Pectoralis minor (43)
Latissimus dorsi (24)
Subclavius (42)

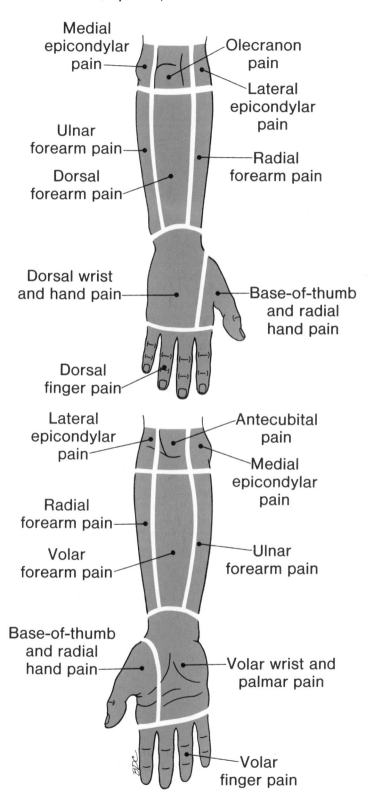

Figure 33.1. The designated areas within the elbow-to-finger region that may encompass pain referred there by myofascial trigger points.

PART 3

CHAPTER 34
Hand Extensor and Brachioradialis Muscles
"Painful Weak Grip"

HIGHLIGHTS: The extensor muscles of the hand at the wrist are the extensores carpi radialis longus and brevis, and the extensor carpi ulnaris. The "painful weak grip" muscles are primarily the extensores carpi radialis longus and brevis, and the extensor digitorum. The brachioradialis and supinator also may develop trigger points (TPs) in association with the radial hand extensors. The active TPs of these "extensor mass" muscles occur close together in the proximal forearm, distal to but near the lateral epicondyle. REFERRED PAIN from TPs in the extensores carpi radialis longus and brevis appears over the lateral epicondyle, lightly over the dorsum of the forearm, and it accents the dorsum of the hand. The extensor carpi ulnaris refers pain to the dorsal surface of the ulnar side of the wrist. The brachioradialis refers pain chiefly to the lateral epicondyle and down over the length of the muscle to the dorsal aspect of the web of the thumb. ANATOMICAL ATTACHMENTS of the hand extensors are to the region of the lateral epicondyle at the elbow, and to various carpal bones at the wrist. The brachioradialis attaches to the shaft of the humerus above the elbow, and to the radial side of the styloid process at the wrist. ACTION of the extensor carpi radialis longus is chiefly radial deviation of the hand; the brevis chiefly extends the hand; the extensor carpi ulnaris primarily deviates the hand toward the ulnar side; and the

brachioradialis assists flexion of the forearm at the elbow. SYMPTOMS are usually pain as described above—often diagnosed as a "tennis elbow" syndrome—and an unreliable or weak grip that lets objects fall from the patient's hand. ACTIVATION OF TRIGGER POINTS in these muscles arises from abuse of combined gripping and twisting motions, as in some sports, digging with a trowel in the garden, and using a screw driver. PATIENT EXAMINATION that reveals a painful and weak grip when the hand is ulnarly deviated indicates involvement of the extensores carpi radialis longus and brevis. TRIGGER POINT EXAMINATION localizes the active TPs in each muscle by pincer palpation for the brachioradialis and flat palpation for the others. ENTRAPMENT of either the motor, or sensory branch of the radial nerve may be caused by tension of the flexor carpi radialis brevis. STRETCH AND SPRAY require that the brachioradialis and extensores carpi radialis muscles be stretched across both the elbow and wrist joints. A proximal-to-distal spray pattern is used. INJECTION AND STRETCH of these muscles present no special difficulty when the TP is fixed between the fingers. CORRECTIVE ACTIONS include eliminating strain of the involved muscles, establishing a home program of stretch exercises, and the gradual resumption of normal activities.

1. REFERRED PAIN
(Figs. 34.1 and 34.2)

Radial Hand Extensors
(Fig. 34.1)

Trigger points (TPs) in the extensor carpi radialis longus refer pain and tender-

ness to the lateral epicondyle (Fig. 34.1C), and to the dorsum of the hand in the region of the anatomical snuff box, which is often described by the patient as "the thumb."[58, 60] Extensor carpi radialis brevis TPs project pain to the back of the hand and wrist (Fig. 34.1B), as originally deter-

480

PART 3

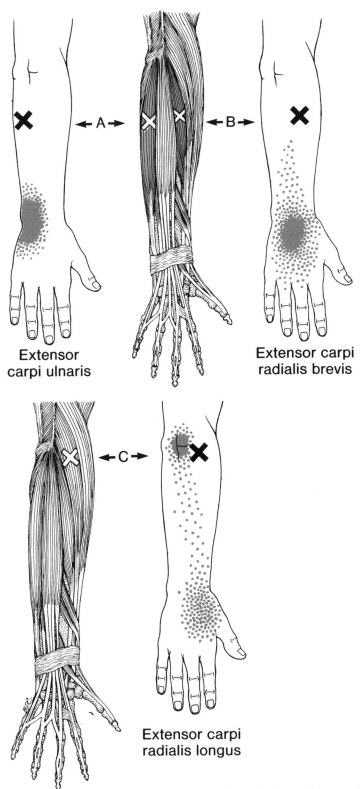

Figure 34.1.   Referred pain patterns (*dark red*) and location of trigger points (×s) in the three primary hand extensor muscles (*medium red*) on the right side. *A*, extensor carpi ulnaris. *B*, extensor carpi radialis brevis. *C*, extensor carpi radialis longus.

PART 3

mined in 45 patients.[58] This is one of the most common myofascial sources of pain in the back of the wrist.

Gutstein-Good,[23] who later wrote as Good,[15] reported a case of "idiopathic myalgia," or "muscular rheumatism," in which pain was projected deep in the upper arm with dysesthesia (numbness, pins-and-needles and painful vibratory sensations) along the forearm to the thumb and index finger. The pain was reproduced by pressure on tender spots in the extensor carpi radialis muscles. Kelly[27, 28] reported three cases of "fibrositis" with pain in the elbow, radiating down the dorsum of the forearm, or to the radial side of the wrist. The pain originated in a tender spot within the extensor muscle mass several centimeters (about 1 in) distal to the lateral epicondyle. This is where the authors find TPs in the extensor carpi radialis longus. Bates and Grunwaldt[6] reported a similar myofascial pain pattern for the extensor carpi radialis muscles in children.

Extensor Carpi Ulnaris
(Fig. 34.1A)

The extensor carpi ulnaris muscle harbors TPs less often than the extensores carpi radialis. The referred pain pattern of the extensor carpi ulnaris includes primarily the ulnar side of the back of the wrist (Fig. 34.1A). Gutstein[22, 23] identified this TP in a doctor.

Brachioradialis
(Fig. 34.2)

The brachioradialis projects its essential pain pattern to the wrist and base of the thumb in the web space between the thumb and index finger (Fig. 34.2). The brachioradialis, like the underlying supinator, refers pain also to the lateral epicondyle. For the supinator, this is an essential pain pattern, but an inconsistent spillover pattern for the brachioradialis. Pain referred to the lateral epicondyle from TPs in either muscle causes the epicondyle to become tender to light tapping on its distal face. Referred pain from the brachioradialis rarely extends to the olecranon process.

The brachioradialis is a thin muscle, which immediately overlies the extensor carpi radialis longus, and it is usually difficult to distinguish by flat palpation which of these muscles is giving rise to a

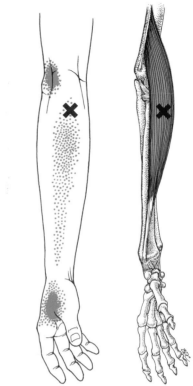

Figure 34.2.   Referred pain pattern (*dark red*) and location of trigger point (✕) in the right brachioradialis muscle (*medium red*).

particular referred pain. Kelly[27] ascribed to the brachioradialis muscle a pattern of pain and tenderness close to the elbow, and of diffuse referred pain and tenderness across the dorsum of the hand. However, in our experience, pain across the back of the hand arises chiefly from associated TPs in the extensor carpi radialis brevis or longus.

2. ANATOMICAL ATTACHMENTS
(Figs. 34.3 and 34.4)

Radial Hand Extensors
(Fig. 34.3)

The extensor carpi radialis longus attaches **proximally** to the distal third of the lateral supracondylar ridge of the humerus, between the lateral epicondyle and the attachment of the brachioradialis muscle. The longus attaches **distally** to the base of the second metacarpal bone on its dorso-radial aspect. The muscle extends one-third, and its tendon the remaining two-thirds, of the length of the forearm.

The **proximal** attachments of the exten-

PART 3

sor carpi radialis brevis (Fig. 34.3*B*), which lie beneath the belly of its companion, the longus, include the common extensor attachment to the lateral epicondyle, the radial ligament of the elbow, and intermuscular septa between it and adjacent muscles.[21] The belly of the extensor carpi radialis brevis expands to full thickness near the junction of the upper and middle thirds of the forearm, as the more lateral longus muscle dwindles to a tendon.[35, 38, 44] **Distally** the extensor carpi radialis brevis attaches to the base of the third metacarpal bone on its dorso-radial aspect (Fig. 34.3*B*).[21]

Not always clearly described is the fact that **proximally** the strong aponeurosis of the brevis forms a bridge of fascia, which stretches between the lateral epicondyle and the deep fascia of the dorsal forearm. It may become thickened,[14, 30] where the deep (motor) branch of the radial nerve passes beneath it to enter the supinator muscle (Fig. 34.3*C*). Usually, the superficial radial nerve has branched off before the deep radial nerve dips beneath the extensor carpi radialis brevis (Fig. 34.3*B*). In some cases, however, the nerve divides more distally (Fig. 34.3*C*), so that the superficial branch must penetrate the belly of the extensor carpi radialis brevis muscle to return to its course beneath the brachioradialis muscle.[30]

Extensor Carpi Ulnaris
(Fig. 34.3*A*)

The extensor carpi ulnaris muscle attaches **proximally** to the common extensor tendon of the lateral epicondyle; and **distally** to the ulnar side of the base of the fifth metacarpal bone (Fig. 34.3*A*).

Brachioradialis
(Fig. 34.4)

The brachioradialis attaches **proximally** to both the lateral supracondylar ridge of the humerus and to the lateral intermuscular septum, distal to where the radial nerve penetrates the septum at mid-arm level (Fig. 34.4). **Distally** the brachioradialis tendon expands laterally as it approaches the styloid process of the radius and connects with the neighboring ligaments.[2] It is then anchored by a tendinous attachment to the styloid process.[2, 21, 32, 47] A variable slip may attach distally to several carpal bones, and to the third metacarpal.[2, 21]

Supplemental References

The radial hand extensors are well illustrated by other authors from the dorsal view,[19, 36, 38, 53, 56] the lateral view,[16, 35, 44, 52] and in cross section.[10, 39] The distal attachments at the wrist are shown in detail.[20, 36, 40, 45]

The extensor carpi ulnaris is illustrated in the dorsal view,[19, 36, 38, 53, 56] the lateral view,[35] and in cross section.[9, 39] Its distal attachment is also shown in detail.[40, 45]

The brachioradialis muscle is depicted in the dorsal view,[19, 36, 38, 56] the lateral view,[16, 35, 44, 52] the volar view,[18, 48, 51, 57] and in cross section.[8, 39] Details of its distal attachment are shown.[36, 46] Other figures show the course of the superficial branch of the radial nerve lying beneath this muscle.[17, 37, 49]

3. INNERVATION

Hand Extensors

The radial nerve supplies the extensor carpi radialis longus and the brachioradialis muscles as it passes beneath them, proximal to the elbow joint. The nerve also usually divides into superficial and deep branches proximal to this joint. The deep branch of the radial nerve then supplies the extensor carpi radialis brevis and the supinator muscles, before entering the supinator muscle through the arcade of Frohse. This entrance is formed by the space between the superficial and deep layers of the supinator (see Fig. 36.2*B*).[21] The deep branch also gives off the recurrent (epicondylar) nerve, which exits by again passing beneath the archway formed between the proximal attachments of the extensor carpi radialis brevis muscle.[21]

The extensor carpi radialis muscles are supplied by fibers from spinal nerves C_6 and C_7, and the extensor carpi ulnaris muscle is supplied by fibers from C_6, C_7 and C_8. These muscles are supplied by the radial nerve, which receives fibers through all three posterior divisions and the posterior cord.[21]

Brachioradialis

The brachioradialis muscle is supplied by a branch of the radial nerve from the posterior cord, the upper trunk and spinal nerves C_5 and C_6.

PART 3

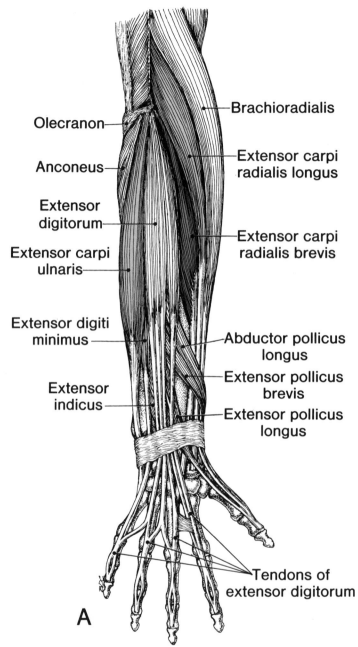

Olecranon

Anconeus

Extensor digitorum

Extensor carpi ulnaris

Extensor digiti minimus

Extensor indicus

Brachioradialis

Extensor carpi radialis longus

Extensor carpi radialis brevis

Abductor pollicus longus

Extensor pollicus brevis

Extensor pollicus longus

Tendons of extensor digitorum

A

Figure 34.3 A–C.   The relations of the hand extensor muscles and part of the radial nerve in the right forearm. *A*, dorsal view showing the attachments of the extensor carpi radialis longus and brevis, and extensor carpi ulnaris muscles. *B*, lateral view showing the deep branch of the radial nerve before it passes beneath the fibrous arch formed by the proximal attachments of the extensor carpi radialis brevis and the normal course of the superficial (sensory) branch. *C*, variant course of the superficial branch of the radial nerve *through* the extensor carpi radialis brevis muscle (adapted from Kopell and Thompson[30]).

4. ACTIONS

Hand Extensors

There is general agreement[1, 4, 12, 21, 24, 41] that both the extensores carpi radialis lon-gus and brevis participate in extension and abduction (radial deviation) of the hand, while the extensor carpi ulnaris extends and adducts the hand (ulnar deviation) at the wrist. Duchenne[12] emphasizes that the

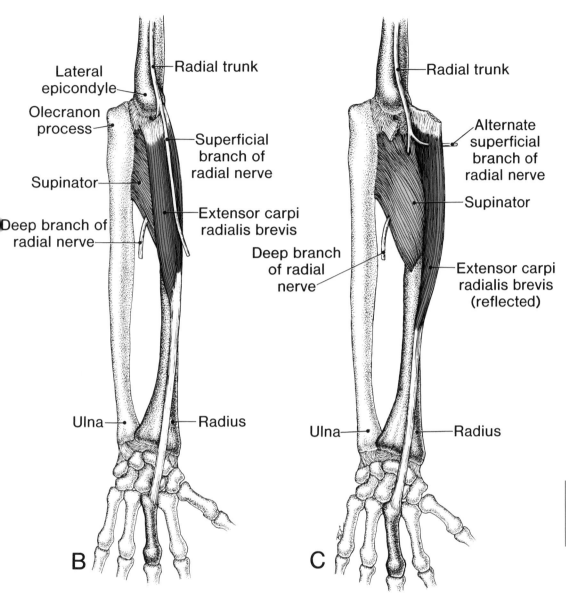

Lateral epicondyle

Radial trunk

Olecranon process

Supinator

Superficial branch of radial nerve

Deep branch of radial nerve

Extensor carpi radialis brevis

Ulna

Radius

B

Radial trunk

Alternate superficial branch of radial nerve

Supinator

Deep branch of radial nerve

Extensor carpi radialis brevis (reflected)

Ulna

Radius

C

Figure 34.3. *B* and *C*.

extensor carpi radialis longus, which attaches to the second metacarpal bone, mainly abducts the hand; the extensor carpi radialis brevis, which attaches to the third metacarpal, chiefly extends it; and the extensor carpi ulnaris, which attaches to the ulnar side of the fifth metacarpal, mainly adducts the hand. The extensor carpi radialis longus and the extensor carpi ulnaris muscles, acting together, can extend the hand at the wrist, but do so only to exert strong force.[12, 24]

Activation of the hand extensors is essential to the power grip.[41]

Electromyographic monitoring of subjects while they repeatedly pressed a typewriter key at a maximal rate, or wrote with a pencil, showed moderate activity of the finger and hand extensors. At slow rates of typing, the amplitude of this electrical activity dropped to less than one-tenth of that at very rapid rates.[33]

Bilateral electromyographic monitoring of the radial wrist and finger extensors as a group, and of the brachioradialis muscle separately, was performed with surface electrodes during 13 sports activities. They included overhand throws, underhand

PART 3

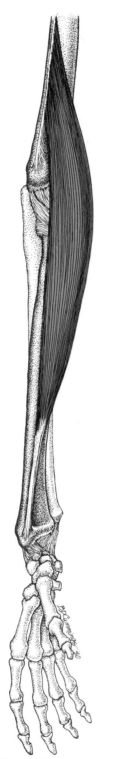

Figure 34.4. The attachments of the right brachioradialis muscle, from the radial view.

throws, tennis, golf, hitting a baseball and 1-ft jumps. The *extensor group* consistently showed slight to moderate activity,

bilaterally similar. The *brachioradialis* frequently showed an activity pattern similar to, but slightly stonger than, that of the hand and finger extensors, especially on the non-dominant side. The two exceptions to this relationship were batting a baseball and driving a golf ball, when the extensors on the non-dominant side showed more electrical activity than did the brachioradialis.[7]

Brachioradialis

Reports on the function of this muscle began with misunderstanding and confusion, some of which persist. Initially, this muscle was named the "supinator longus," on the assumption that its primary action was supination of the hand. Duchenne demonstrated clearly by stimulation studies that it functioned chiefly as a flexor at the elbow,[12] which led to its present name, brachioradialis. He also reported that its stimulation brought the forearm to a neutral position from either supination or pronation.

Authors agree that it flexes the forearm at the elbow.[2, 21, 29, 32, 47, 50] Electromyographically,[3] brachioradialis activity usually is reserved for speedy movement and the lifting of weight by flexing the elbow, especially if the hand is in the neutral position. However, none of the elbow flexors is used to counteract gravity when a weight is held in the dependent hand with the elbow straight.[3]

The brachioradialis is also the classic example of a "shunt muscle"; it is attached in such a manner that its contraction prevents separation of the elbow joint by centrifugal force during rapid elbow movement. In contrast, the biceps brachii and brachialis, "spurt muscles," accelerate movement at the elbow without counteracting distraction of the elbow joint.

In consonance with Duchenne,[12] textbooks generally state that the brachioradialis returns the forearm to mid-position from pronation or supination.[2, 29, 50] However, Gray[21] makes no mention of this function, and Lockhart[32] states that the brachioradialis is never a pronator or supinator of the forearm. In a 1957 study that employed bipolar needle electrodes inserted into the middle of the muscle, Basmajian[5] reported that the brachioradialis assisted both pronation and supination, but only when these motions were resisted.

In an electromyographic study of two subjects by the authors,[43] a monopolar needle electrode recorded electrical activity of the brachioradialis only during resisted pronation, and not during resisted supination. This agrees with Duchenne's early observation[12] that it acted more as a pronator than as a supinator, and with Hollinshead's conclusion[24] that it probably provides limited assistance in pronation, but little, if any assistance in supination. Its use for supination may vary among individuals because of variations in its distal attachment.

During typewriting (by subjects who demonstrated no resting electromyographic activity) there was no difference in brachioradialis electrical activity whether the elbow was bent at an acute angle, at a right angle, or at an obtuse angle.[33] Elevation of the typewriter does not create a problem for this muscle, as for the shoulder muscles.

During simulated driving, [26] the brachioradialis and brachialis muscles worked nearly synchronously when most subjects turned the steering wheel to the opposite side. A few subjects apparently did not use these muscles when driving.

The wrist-cocking local twitch response observed during examination of the brachioradialis for TPs, and the kinds of activities that cause TPs in this muscle, indicate that in some individuals the deepest layer may function to cock (radially deviate) the wrist. This movement may depend upon its variable attachment, occasionally, to the scaphoid, navicular, or third metacarpal bones.[1] This attachment also could make the corresponding muscle fibers more vulnerable than the rest of the muscle to overload. No reference to this action was found in the literature. It is not always possible to unambiguously distinguish by palpation the deep brachioradialis fibers from those of the underlying extensor carpi radialis longus, the primary source of this wrist-cocking movement.

5. MYOTATIC UNIT

Hand Extensors

For extension of the hand at the wrist, the extensor carpi radialis longus is synergistic with the brevis, the extensor carpi ulnaris, and the finger extensors.

For radial deviation of the hand, the extensores carpi radialis muscles are synergistic with the flexor carpi radialis. For ulnar deviation, the extensor and flexor carpi ulnaris muscles are similarly synergistic.

During flexion of the hand at the wrist, electromyographically, the extensor carpi ulnaris functioned as the primary antagonist.[5]

Brachioradialis

Kinesiologically, synergists with the brachioradialis muscle are the biceps brachii and brachialis muscles. However, in terms of TP phenomena, the brachioradialis is more closely associated with the extensores carpi radialis longus and brevis, the extensor digitorum, and supinator muscles. These muscles become a myotatic unit during grasp, or during hand rotation and grasp with the wrist cocked.

6. SYMPTOMS

It is difficult to sharply delineate which symptoms are caused by the radial hand extensors, and which by the brachioradialis, when both are involved.

Pain, as described in Section 1, is a major complaint. The pain is likely to appear first in the lateral epicondyle, and then spread to the wrist and hand. The epicondylar pain, often diagnosed as "tennis elbow," is frequently a composite pain that is referred in part from the supinator, the extensor carpi radialis longus,[11] and the extensor digitorum. With involvement of the latter two muscles, patients complain of pain when they attempt a firm grip with the hand in ulnar deviation, e.g. shaking hands. Pain is more likely to be felt if forceful supination or pronation are added to the movement, as when turning a doorknob, or using a screwdriver.[23]

Weakness of the grip during these movements may be pronounced, so that objects tend to slip out of the hand, particularly when the movement uncocks (ulnarly deviates) the wrist, futher weakening the grip. Examples include letting the head of the tennis racquet drop, loss of control when pouring milk or juice from a carton, or when drinking coffee—just as the cup reaches the lip and is tipped to drink. The muscles act as if the finger flexors are reflexly inhibited by TP activity in the simultaneously contracting extensors. An autoinhibition of the extensors also may occur, like that seen when TPs in the vastus medialis muscle cause buckling of the knee instead of pain. Weakness of the grip is aggravated when the patient grasps a large, rather than a small object. However, TPs in these extensor muscles cause no problem in using scissors, whereas TPs in the finger flexors do.

7. ACTIVATION OF TRIGGER POINTS

In the extensor carpi radialis longus and brevis and in the brachioradialis muscles, TPs are activated by repetitive forceful handgrip. The larger the object being gripped, and the greater the ulnar deviation of the hand, the more likely the muscles are to develop TPs.

The following examples illustrate how patients have activated TPs in these muscles: executing a one-hand backhand with the head of the tennis racquet dropped (see Fig. 36.6), weeding with a trowel, extensive handshaking, scraping ice off the windshield with a scraper, repeatedly lifting a *heavy* large paperweight to test for muscle soreness, meticulous ironing, pulling open a sticking drawer with the middle finger under the latch, and hours of frisbee-throwing.[13]

These activities cause referred elbow pain that is frequently called "tennis-elbow." The muscles around the elbow that cause this lateral epicondylar pain are likely to develop TPs in approximately the following sequence: (1) supinator, (2) brachioradialis, (3) extensor carpi radialis longus, (4) extensor digitorum, (5) triceps brachii, (6) the anconeus, and (7) the biceps and brachialis together.

The supinator muscle usually becomes involved with the brachioradialis, and *vice versa*. One patient, while paddling a canoe, developed lateral epicondylar pain due to TPs in the brachioradialis of the non-dominant forearm, with less severe involvement of the extensor carpi radialis muscles, but with *no* involvement of the supinator. This was an unusual combination.

Lange[31] observed that "writer's cramp" was more likely to involve the brachioradialis and forearm extensor muscles than the antagonistic flexors.

The extensor carpi ulnaris, which is seldom required to support a load against gravity, rarely develops TPs. Its involvement is usually secondary to gross trauma, such as fracture of the ulna, or as part of a "frozen-shoulder" syndrome in which most of the shoulder muscles and many of the elbow muscles harbor TPs. This latter condition may follow dislocation of the shoulder joint, its prolonged immobilization in a cast, or surgery on structures around the shoulder or elbow joint (see Section 8 in Chapter 26).

8. PATIENT EXAMINATION

Involvement of the extensor group of muscles in the forearm, which includes the radial and ulnar hand extensors, the finger extensors and the brachioradialis, is tested with the *Handgrip Test* by having the patient squeeze the examiner's hand cocked in radial deviation at the wrist in the normal hand-shake position, and then uncocked into ulnar deviation. A strong grip effort is likely to reproduce the spontaneous referred pain pattern and to reveal a weakened grip. The grip is further weakened when the patient drops the hand into the "uncocked" position at the wrist. If grip strength is tested with a dynamometer in the usual cocked position at the wrist, this weakness due to TPs is not as evident; in the dropped position, the weakness becomes clearly demonstrable.

The TP origin of the pain is confirmed by the *Compression Test*, strongly and widely compressing the extensor mass of muscles below the elbow in a pincer grasp, which is held during the Handgrip Test. This pressure often eliminates the pain response; release of pressure restores the pain during the handgrip. A similar effect may sometimes be obtained by firmly pinching the skin over the muscle mass.

Tapping the lateral epicondyle with the fingertip is likely to demonstrate referred tenderness over the *distal half* of the epicondyle, when the active TPs are in the forearm, in the extensor carpi radialis longus, brachioradialis or supinator muscles, which refer pain upward from TPs that are distal to the lateral epicondyle. Triceps TPs are located in the arm proximal to the lateral epicondyle, and when they refer pain and tenderness to it, they cause tenderness mainly of the *proximal half* of the lateral epicondyle.

Identification of the involved muscle is confirmed by eliciting referred pain when the muscle is passively stretched (Section

12, below) and when it is actively loaded in the shortened position. Macdonald[34] reported that passively stretching an involved extensor carpi ulnaris muscle by flexing and abducting the hand at the wrist caused pain, as did loading the muscle by actively resisting the patient's effort to extend and adduct the hand at the wrist. In addition, testing for the strongest local twitch response helps to identify which muscle harbors the most active TPs. The patient must be positioned so that the TP can be stimulated by snapping palpation and so a twitch response would be seen or felt.

Following inactivation of the TPs in each of these muscles by treatment, these tests no longer evoke referred pain, deep tenderness and local twitch responses.

Differential Diagnosis

The pain and tenderness that is referred from myofascial TPs to the dorsum of the hand and wrist, especially in the region of the base of the thumb, may easily be mistaken for tenosynovitis (de Quervain's disease), which presents similar symptoms.[55] In both conditions, the pain is aggravated by either loading or stretching the involved tendons and muscles. Palpation of the extensores carpi radialis and the brachioradialis muscles for TPs that reproduce the patient's pain largely establishes the myofascial TP diagnosis. However, this finding does not exclude the additional diagnosis of coexisting tenosynovitis until myofascial treatment has been successful.

The wrist pain and tenderness arising from the hand extensor muscles can be mistaken for arthritis.[42] On the other hand, arthritic wrist pain may be aggravated by referred myofascial pain from these muscles; the latter can be dealt with directly. The osteoarthritic wear-and-tear changes may be only coincidental, and not the immediate cause of the patient's pain.

9. TRIGGER POINT EXAMINATION
(Figs. 34.5 and 34.6)

Hand Extensors
(Fig. 34.5)

The TPs in the extensor carpi *radialis longus* are found in the forearm at nearly the same distance from the elbow as are the TPs in the brachioradialis muscle, but closer to the ulna. The relaxed, supported forearm is examined by deep pincer palpation, with the hand hanging down at the wrist and the elbow flexed about 30° (Fig. 34.5A). A local twitch response from the longus muscle produces strong radial abduction of the hand and some extension at the wrist. Active TPs are found more often in the longus than in the brevis.

TPs in the extensor carpi *radialis brevis* are located distal to those in the longus, located in the muscle mass on the ulnar side of the brachioradialis muscle (Fig. 34.5B). These brevis TPs lie 5 or 6 cm (a full 2 in) distal to the crease at the elbow. The muscle may be examined by flat palpation against the radius and snapped transversely to elicit its local twitch response, which produces hand extension with slight radial deviation at the wrist (Fig. 34.5B).

For palpation, the extensor carpi *ulnaris* stands out clearly from the other forearm muscles, if the patient vigorously spreads the fingers. The TP tenderness is found by flat palpation 7 or 8 cm (about 3 in) distal to the lateral epicondyle and 2 or 3 cm (about 1 in) from the sharp edge of the ulnar bone toward the dorsal surface of the forearm (Fig. 34.1A). A local twitch response causes ulnar deviation of the hand (Fig. 34.5C).

Brachioradialis Muscle
(Fig. 34.6)

For palpation of this muscle, the patient sits comfortably with the forearm resting on a padded armrest, and with the elbow slightly bent. The brachioradialis muscle is held in a pincer grasp between the thumb and fingers (Fig. 34.6). For injection purposes, it is useful to distinguish TPs that lie in the deepest brachioradialis fibers, which usually have no effect on wrist motion but may occasionally extend or cock the wrist, from those in the underlying extensor carpi radialis longus fibers, which always cock the wrist; the superficial (sensory) branch of the radial nerve passes between these two muscles. When the patient tries to forcefully flex the elbow held at 90° of flexion, the brachioradialis stands out and, using pincer palpation, can be encircled with the digits and separated from the underlying extensores carpi radialis longus and brevis. TPs are

PART 3

PART 3

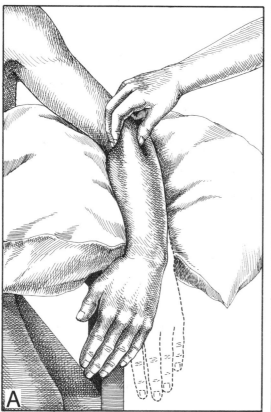

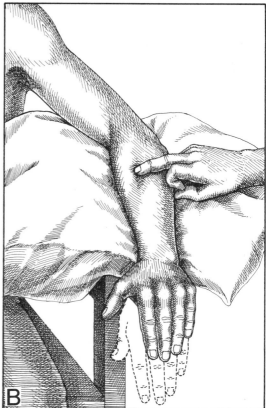

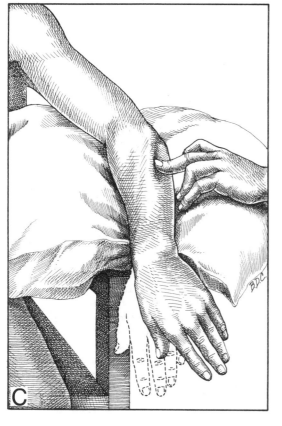

Figure 34.5.   Examination for trigger points in the hand extensor muscles, with their respective local twitch responses, which deviate the hand from its rest position (*dotted lines*). *A,* extensor carpi radialis longus, causing radial deviation of the hand. *B,* extensor carpi radialis brevis, producing extension of the hand at the wrist. *C,* extensor carpi ulnaris, evoking ulnar deviation of the hand.

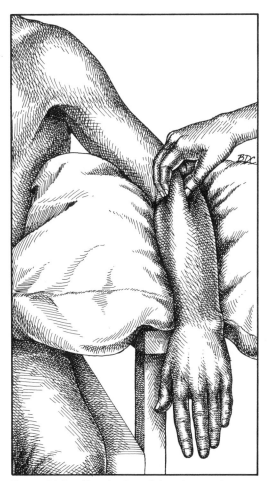

Figure 34.6. Examination of the trigger point area in the brachioradialis muscle. The muscle is held in a deep pincer grasp over the radius, approximately 2 cm (nearly 1 in) distal to the antecubital crease.

usually found only in the deep part of the brachioradialis muscle. Compression of these active TPs often evokes their characteristic referred pain pattern, primarily to the dorsal web between the thumb and index finger (Fig. 34.2).

10. ENTRAPMENTS

The extensor carpi radialis brevis muscle may entrap parts of the radial nerve in either of two ways (Fig. 34.3 B and C): (1) When the bridge of fascia between the proximal attachments of the muscle develops a thickened margin, this hard edge may impinge on the deep radial nerve (forcibly when the forearm is fully pronated),[54] where the nerve passes beneath it to penetrate the supinator muscle.[13, 14, 25, 30] (2) If, as sometimes happens, the sensory fibers branch from the motor

fibers *distal* to this bridge of fascia, the sensory branch must penetrate the substance of the extensor carpi radialis brevis to resume its normal course.

The first type of entrapment is less likely to be due to TP tautness of the extensor carpi radialis brevis than the second is. It also is more likely to cause symptoms during forceful pronation by exerting direct pressure on the deep radial nerve. Normally, this first entrapment produces only motor weakness of the muscles innervated by that nerve. These muscles include the following extensors: the indicis, pollicis longus, pollicis brevis, carpi ulnaris, digitorum, and digiti minimi; it also includes the abductor pollicis longus.

The second mechanism entraps only the superficial (sensory) branch of the radial nerve when it penetrates the belly of the extensor carpi radialis brevis muscle (Fig. 34.3 C).[30] In the presence of this anatomical variation, compression of the nerve by taut bands associated with active TPs in the extensor carpi radialis brevis can cause purely sensory neuropraxia with numbness and tingling over the dorsum of the thumb and hand, but no motor symptoms unless the first entrapment mechanism is also present. This sensory entrapment was confirmed surgically in four patients.[30]

Other mechanisms may cause entrapment symptoms of the radial nerve (see Section 10 in Chapter 36). Patients with entrapment of the deep radial nerve due to TP activity of the supinator muscle as the nerve penetrates the muscle can present with referred pain due to the TPs and with motor weakness due to the nerve compression. Both are relieved by procaine injection of the TPs.[28] Tumor entrapment of the deep radial nerve in this region is pain-free and the motor symptoms are relieved by surgical excision of the tumor.[14]

Parenthetically, entrapment of the recurrent (epicondylar) branch of the radial nerve between the brevis muscle and the head of the radius, which is sometimes blamed for the aching pain of "tennis elbow,"[30] would be more likely to produce numbness and parenthesias than aching pain and deep tenderness, which is characteristic of myofascial TP activity. In the patients seen by the authors, epicondylar pain is most frequently referred from TPs in the surrounding muscles, and is rarely of neuritic origin.

11. ASSOCIATED TRIGGER POINTS

Myofascial TPs frequently occur both in the extensores carpi radialis and brachioradialis muscles; involvement of either is likely to be associated with TPs in the extensor digitorum and supinator muscles. Myofascial TPs are rarely observed in the extensor carpi ulnaris without at least one TP in the neighboring parallel extensor digitorum muscle.

TPs in the brachioradialis often develop secondary to TPs in the supinator and extensor carpi radialis longus muscles. Involvement then spreads to the long finger extensors, especially to the middle and ring fingers. The distal lateral end of the medial head of the triceps brachii, proximal to the lateral epicondyle, also may develop associated TPs, which refer pain to the lateral epicondyle.

12. STRETCH AND SPRAY
(Figs. 34.7 and 34.8)

Hand Extensors
(Fig. 34.7)

Both the extensores carpi radialis longus and brevis muscles are stretched with the

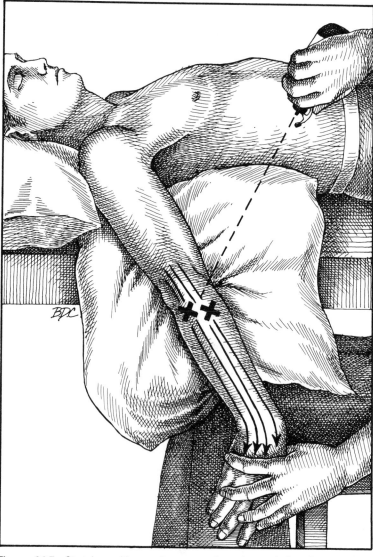

Figure 34.7 Stretch position and spray pattern (*arrows*) for trigger points (×s) in the hand extensor muscles. The more radial "×" identifies the region of the extensores carpi radialis longus and brevis trigger points. The ulnar "×" locates the extensor carpi ulnaris trigger point.

PART 3

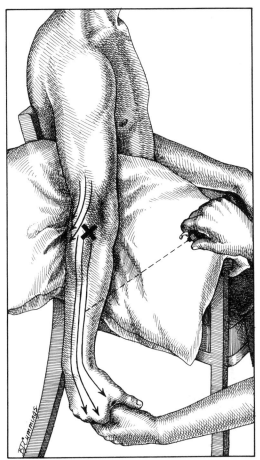

Figure 34.8.   Stretch position and spray pattern (*arrows*) for a trigger point (✕) in the brachioradialis muscle. With the arm supinated, the forearm is extended at the elbow. Maximum stretch may be obtained by placing the hand in ulnar deviation and pronation, while extending the elbow against a padded surface to avoid internal rotation at the shoulder. Sweeps of the vapocoolant cover the muscle in the forearm and its referred pain patterns: first, the lateral epicondyle, and second, the dorsum of the hand and the web space between the thumb and index finger.

patient either seated or supine, with the forearm extended at the elbow, and with the hand pronated and forcefully flexed at the wrist (Fig. 34.7). During this stretch, the vapocoolant spray is applied in parallel sweeps over the muscle from the humerus to the hand, covering the epicondyle and distal referred pain areas in the wrist. Muscles with associated TPs, the brachioradialis, finger extensors and supinator, also are stretched and sprayed.

The extensor carpi ulnaris is stretched by flexing the wrist and supinating the hand without particular concern for elbow

extension. Sweeps of the spray are applied in a distal direction, covering the muscle from the lateral epicondyle to the ulnar styloid process, including the reference zone at the wrist.

Brachioradialis
(Fig. 34.8)

The patient is seated comfortably in a relaxed position with the forearm extended at the elbow and the elbow resting on a padded support. Full pronation is used in order to stretch the brachioradialis as it crosses the forearm. The spray is applied as in Figure 34.8. After covering the TP area, the proximal-to-distal spray pattern detours to cover the lateral epicondyle, then sweeps over the forearm to cover the dorsum of the hand and dorsal web between the thumb and the index finger.

Hot packs follow promptly.

13. INJECTION AND STRETCH
(Figs. 34.9 and 34.10)

Hand Extensors
(Fig. 34.9)

The patient lies supine with the arm resting on a pillow, or other support. Since all three hand extensor muscles are relatively superficial, palpation can precisely localize their TPs for injection. The operator fixes the extensor carpi radialis longus TP between the index and middle fingers and injects it as shown in Fig. 34.9A. The brevis TP is 3 or 4 cm (about 1½ in) more distal (Fig. 34.9B). These TPs, when impaled by the needle, generally respond with obvious local twitch responses and clear referred pain patterns. After injection, stretch and spray are applied as above, followed by a hot pack, and then full range of active movement.

Cyriax[11] described a similar technique for injecting an extensor carpi radialis muscle with procaine.

Procaine injection of TPs in the extensor mass of the forearm restored the strength of handgrip in a patient with strong evidence of hysteria.[59]

Brachioradialis
(Fig. 34.10)

The forearm of the supine patient is supported slightly flexed at the elbow with the hand pronated. The muscle may be injected by holding the TP in a pincer

PART 3

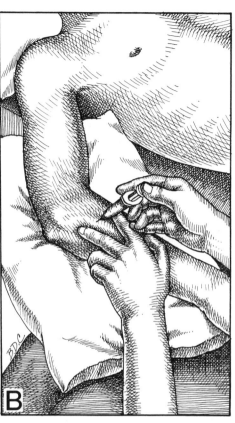

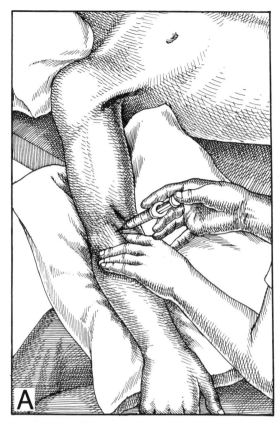

Figure 34.9.   Injection technique for two trigger points. *A*, in the extensor carpi radialis longus muscle. The brachioradialis muscle is displaced to the radial side by the index finger. *B*, in the extensor carpi radialis brevis.

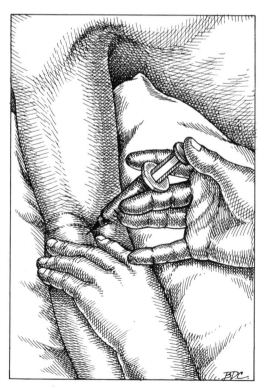

grasp between the finger and thumb, as in Figure 34.6, or by using flat palpation, as in Figure 34.10.

When referred pain is evoked in the base of the thumb by a deep injection in the proximal forearm, the TP may lie either in the brachioradialis or in the underlying supinator. The fact that during this procedure the sensory branch of the radial nerve may be temporarily blocked by the local anesthetic should be explained in advance to the patient.

14. CORRECTIVE ACTIONS
(Fig. 34.11)

Hand Extensors

The patient with active TPs in the radial hand extensors should avoid forceful activity with the hand flexed or in ulnar

Figure 34.10.   Injection of a trigger point in the right brachioradialis muscle. The needle must reach the deepest fibers of the muscle to penetrate the trigger point. Note the difference in the position of the operator's index finger, as compared with Figure 34.9*A*.

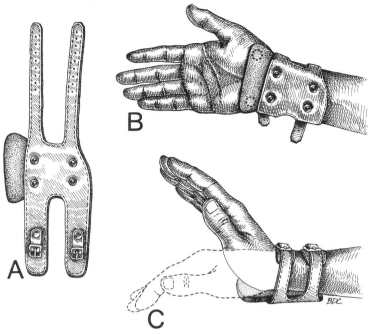

Figure 34.11. The design and application of a leather wrist brace that supports the bony thenar and hypothenar prominences to limit hand flexion at the wrist. This brace relieves the hand extensors of strain during forceful movements that combine grasp, pronation and/or supination by limiting flexion and, to some extent, ulnar deviation at the wrist. It does not limit extension. *A*, pattern of the brace. The outer strap portion is made of flexible leather. The inner piece is made of stiff material. *B*, volar view of the brace strapped into position. The *dotted circles* locate the pisiform bone and base of the first metacarpal, which must be covered to restrict hand flexion effectively. *C*, side view, demonstrating the limits of flexion and extension permitted by the wrist brace.

deviation at the wrist. Liquid should be poured from a container by rotating the arm at the shoulder, instead of deviating the hand at the wrist; the head of the tennis racquet should be angled up; in a receiving line, the hand should be offered with the palm facing upward, and the right and left hand alternated in shaking hands. If work requires stressful twisting motions, a strap wrist support that prevents hand flexion (Fig. 34.11) protects these extensor muscles from overload during the course of treatment and recovery.

Brachioradialis

The patient learns to avoid activities which aggravate brachioradialis TPs, such as digging with a trowel, prolonged shaking of hands, and playing tennis with too heavy a racquet. If the activity must be pursued, then the patient should be encouraged to maintain the wrist cocked in radial deviation. This is especially important when playing tennis (see Fig. 36.6).

The strap support for the wrist, mentioned above (Fig. 34.11) reminds the patient to rotate the hand from the shoulder and trunk, not at the wrist and elbow.

The patient may be taught to self-stretch the supinator by placing the affected elbow on a support, while seated as in Figure 34.8. The arm must be held externally rotated at the shoulder so that the antecubital space faces up. The other hand applies the external force to fully flex the pronated hand on the involved side and to stretch the muscles passively to reach the same position as Fig. 34.8, while water beats on it from a hot shower or vapocoolant spray is applied.

References

1. Bardeen CR: The musculature, Sect. 5. In *Morris's Human Anatomy*, edited by C.M. Jackson, Ed. 6. Blakiston's Son & Co., Philadelphia, 1921 (pp. 421–425).
2. *Ibid.* (pp. 421, 423).
3. Basmajian JV: *Muscles Alive*, Ed. 4. Williams & Wilkins, Baltimore, 1978 (pp. 152, 187, 204, 208).

PART 3

4. *Ibid.* (p. 213).
5. Basmajian JV, Latif A: Integrated actions and functions of the chief flexors of the elbow. *J Bone Joint Surg* 39A:1106–1118, 1957.
6. Bates T, Grunwaldt E: Myofascial pain in childhood. *J Pediatr* 53:198–209, 1958.
7. Broer MR, Houtz SJ: *Patterns of Muscular Activity in Selected Sports Skill.* Charles C Thomas, Springfield, Ill. 1967.
8. Carter BL, Morehead J, Wolpert SM, et al.: *Cross-Sectional Anatomy.* Appleton-Century-Crofts, New York, 1977 (Sections 51–57).
9. *Ibid.* (Sections 53–59).
10. *Ibid.* (Sections 51–59).
11. Cyriax J: *Textbook of Orthopaedic Medicine,* Ed. 5, Vol. 1. Williams & Wilkins, Baltimore, 1969 (pp. 315, 316).
12. Duchenne GB: *Physiology of Motion,* translated by E.B. Kaplan. J.B. Lippincott, Philadelphia, 1949 (pp. 99, 100, 114–116).
13. Fraim CJ: Unusual cause of nerve entrapment. *JAMA* 242:2557–2558, 1979.
14. Goldman S, Honet JC, Sobel R, Goldstein AS: Posterior interosseous nerve palsy in the absence of trauma. *Arch Neurol* 21:435–441, 1969 (p. 440).
15. Good MG, Acroparaesthesia—idiopathic myalgia of elbow. *Edinburgh Med J* 56:366–368, 1949.
16. Grant JCB: *An Atlas of Human Anatomy,* Ed. 7. Williams & Wilkins, Baltimore, 1978 (Fig. 6–37).
17. *Ibid.* (Figs. 6–55, 6–69).
18. *Ibid.* (Fig. 6–66).
19. *Ibid.* (Fig. 6–91).
20. *Ibid.* (Fig. 6–104).
21. Gray H: *Anatomy of the Human Body,* edited by C.M. Goss, American Ed. 29. Lea & Febiger, Philadelphia, 1973 (pp. 467–470, 961, 976, 978).
22. Gutstein M: Diagnosis and treatment of muscular rheumatism. *Br J Phys Med* 1:302–321, 1938 (Fig. 8, Case 8).
23. Gutstein-Good M: Idiopathic myalgia simulating visceral and other diseases. *Lancet* 2:326–328, 1940 (Fig. 6, Case 7).
24. Hollinshead WH: *Functional Anatomy of The Limbs and Back,* Ed. 4. W.B. Saunders, Philadelphia, 1976 (pp. 162–164).
25. Jackson FE, Fleming PM, Cook RC, et al.: Entrapment of deep branch of radial nerve by fibrous attachment of extensor carpi radialis brevis: case report with operative decompression and cure. *US Navy Med* 58:10–11, 1971.
26. Jonsson S, Jonsson B: Function of the muscles of the upper limb in car driving, I–III. *Ergonomics* 18:375–388, 1975 (pp. 383–387).
27. Kelly M: Pain in the forearm and hand due to muscular lesions. *Med J Aust* 2:185–188, 1944 (Figs. 1 and 3, Cases 1 and 5).
28. Kelly M: Interstitial neuritis and the neural theory of fibrositis. *Annals Rheum Dis* 7:89–96, 1948.
29. Kendall HO, Kendall FP, Wadsworth GE: *Muscles, Testing and Function,* Ed. 2. Williams & Wilkins, Baltimore, 1971 (pp. 98, 99).
30. Kopell HP, Thompson WAL: *Peripheral Entrapment Neuropathies,* Ed. 2. Williams & Wilkins, Baltimore, 1963 (Fig. 54, pp. 138–139).
31. Lange M: *Die Muskelhärten (Myogelosen).* J.F.
Lehmanns, München, 1931 (Fig. 38, p. 116).
32. Lockhart RD, Hamilton GF, Fyfe FW: *Anatomy of the Human Body,* Ed. 2. J.B. Lippincott, Philadelphia, 1969 (p. 215).
33. Lundervold AJS: Electromyographic investigations of position and manner of working in typewriting. *Acta Physiol Scand* 24:(Suppl. 84), 1951 (pp. 66, 67, 80, 131).
34. Macdonald AJR: Abnormally tender muscle regions and associated painful movements. *Pain* 8:197–205, 1980 (pp. 202, 203).
35. McMinn RMH, Hutchings RT: *Color Atlas of Human Anatomy.* Year Book Medical Publishers, Chicago, 1977 (p. 128).
36. *Ibid.* (pp. 127, 141).
37. *Ibid.* (p. 125).
38. Pernkopf E: *Atlas of Topographical and Applied Human Anatomy,* Vol. 2. W.B. Saunders, Philadelphia, 1964 (Figs. 78, 79).
39. *Ibid.* (Figs. 81, 82).
40. *Ibid.* (Fig. 90).
41. Rasch PJ, Burke RK: *Kinesiology and Applied Anatomy,* Ed. 3. Lea & Febiger, Philadelphia, 1967 (pp. 204, 206, 218).
42. Reynolds MD: Myofascial trigger point syndromes in the practice of rheumatology. *Arch Phys Med Rehabil* 62:111–114, 1981 (Table 1).
43. Simons DG, Travell J: Unpublished data, 1978.
44. Sobotta J, Figge FHJ: *Atlas of Human Anatomy,* Ed. 9, Vol. 1. Hafner Division of Macmillan, New York, 1974 (pp. 192, 206).
45. *Ibid.* (p. 208).·
46. *Ibid.* (p. 218).
47. *Ibid.* (p. 207).
48. *Ibid.* (pp. 199, 202).
49. Sobotta J, Figge FHJ: *Atlas of Human Anatomy,* Ed. 9, Vol. 3. Hafner Division of McMillan, New York, 1974 (pp. 294, 295).
50. Spalteholz W: *Handatlas der Anatomie des Menschen,* Ed. 11, Vol. 2. S. Hirzel, Leipzig, 1922 (p. 325).
51. *Ibid.* (p. 326).
52. *Ibid.* (p. 330).
53. *Ibid.* (p. 332).
54. Spinner M: *Injuries to the major branches of peripheral nerves of the forearm,* Ed. 2. W.B. Saunders, Philadelphia, 1978 (p. 94).
55. Strandness DE Jr.: Pain in the extremities, Chapter 10. In *Harrison's Principles of Internal Medicine,* edited by M.M. Wintrobe, et al., Ed. 7. McGraw-Hill Book Co., New York, 1974 (p. 44).
56. Toldt C: *An Atlas of Human Anatomy,* translated by M.E. Paul, Ed. 2, Vol. 1. Macmillan, New York, 1919 (p. 326).
57. *Ibid.* (p. 322).
58. Travell J: Pain mechanisms in connective tissue. In *Connective Tissues, Transactions of the 2nd Conference, 1951,* edited by C. Ragan. Josiah Macy, Jr. Foundation, New York, 1952 (pp. 98, 99, Fig. 33A).
59. Travell J, Bigelow NH: Role of somatic trigger areas in the patterns of hysteria. *Psychosom Med* 9:353–363, 1947 (p. 356).
60. Travell J, Rinzler SH: The myofascial genesis of pain. *Postgrad Med* 11:425–434, 1952 (p. 428).

CHAPTER 35
Finger Extensor Muscles
Extensor Digitorum and Extensor Indicis
"Stiff Fingers"

HIGHLIGHTS: **REFERRED PAIN** from the extensor digitorum is projected down the forearm to the back of the hand, and often to the fingers that are moved by the involved muscle fibers. Pain from the extensor indicis is felt most strongly at the junction of the wrist and the dorsum of the hand. Sometimes, pain distal to the lateral epicondyle of the elbow arises from trigger points (TPs) in the ring and little finger extensors. The thumb extensors, unlike the extensors of the other digits, seldom develop TPs. **ACTIONS** of the finger extensors are primarily extension of the fingers and of the hand at the wrist. They make an essential contribution to forceful finger flexion. **SYMPTOMS** may include, separately or in combination, pain, weakness, stiffness and tenderness of the proximal interphalangeal joints; symptoms appear in the finger that corresponds to the involved portion of the extensor muscle group. **ACTIVATION OF TRIGGER POINTS** commonly results from too forceful gripping activities, or repetitive finger movements. **PATIENT EXAMINATION** reveals pain and weakness when the patient attempts to grip an object strongly. **TRIGGER POINT EXAMINATION** demonstrates deep tenderness distal to the lateral epicondyle, in the extensor muscle mass. **ASSOCIATED TRIGGER POINTS** are likely to be found in the supinator, brachioradialis and extensor carpi radialis longus muscles. **STRETCH AND SPRAY** are most effective if the hand and finger extensors are treated as a group. Both the wrist and the fingers must be fully flexed, as the spray is applied in a proximal-to-distal pattern. **INJECTION AND STRETCH** of TPs in the extensor group should employ a needle technique that also reaches any TPs in the underlying supinator muscle. **CORRECTIVE ACTIONS** include avoidance of unnecessary muscular strain and the use of a home-exercise program to achieve and maintain a full range of motion.

1. REFERRED PAIN
(Fig. 35.1)

Trigger points (TPs) in the finger extensors project pain down the dorsum of the forearm to the back of the hand and often into the fingers dorsally. The pain consistently stops short of the ends of the fingers, leaving the last phalanx and nail bed pain-free. (In comparison, the long finger *flexors* project pain to, "and beyond," the finger tips.) Confirming our observations, Gutstein[11] noted tender spots in the forearm extensors distal to the lateral epicondyle that referred pain from the dorsum of the forearm to include the middle and ring fingers.

Extensor Digitorum
(Fig. 35.1 *A* and *B*)

Involvement of the middle finger extensor is extremely common.[11] The pain, which is felt most intensely in the hand, forms a line that extends onto the dorsum of the forearm, wrist and hand, including the metacarpophalangeal (MCP) and proximal interphalangeal joints of the middle finger. There also may occasionally be an area of pain on the volar side of the wrist (Fig. 35.1A). Patients complain of pain in the hand and finger, and of stiffness and soreness in the painful finger joints.[14, 38, 41] The original report of this pain pattern was based on 38 patients.[38]

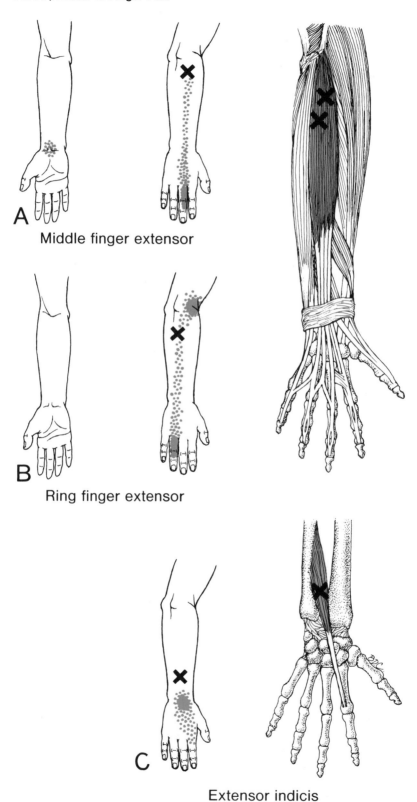

Figure 35.1.   Pain patterns (*dark red*) and location of TPs (✕s) in selected right finger extensor muscles (*medium red*). *A,* middle finger extensor. *B,* ring finger extensor. *C,* extensor indicis.

The ring finger extensor refers pain similarly to the ring finger.[41] However, unlike the middle finger extensor, TPs in the ring and little finger extensors are likely also to project pain and tenderness proximally into the region of the lateral epicondyle (Fig. 35.1B). When asked whether the pain is felt more on the top or the underside of the fingers, the patient may say he is not sure, but is likely to show the location by rubbing the dorsal surface of the fingers.

Other authors described the finger extensors as referring pain to the elbow or lateral epicondyle,[5, 13] to the forearm,[5, 13, 14] and to the hand.[13] "Tennis elbow" pain in the region of the lateral epicondyle was associated with signs of TPs in the finger extensors.[15, 16, 42]

Kellgren[12] injected 0.2 ml of 6% sodium chloride solution into the belly of a normal extensor digitorum muscle. Pain developed in the dorsal forearm and more severely over the back of the hand. During the pain, there was slight tenderness to deep pressure, definite tenderness to tapping, but no hypersensitivity of the skin in the painful area.

Extensor Indicis
(Fig. 35.1C)

Myofascial TPs are found in the more distal portion of this muscle. They refer pain toward the radial side of the dorsum of the wrist and hand, but not into the fingers (Fig. 35.1C).

2. ANATOMICAL ATTACHMENTS
(Fig. 35.2)

Extensor Digitorum
(Fig. 35.2A)

This muscle arises **proximally** from the lateral epicondyle of the humerus, from intermuscular septa, and from the antebrachial fascia. It occupies the space on the dorsal surface of the forearm between the extensor carpi radialis brevis and the extensor carpi ulnaris muscles. All three muscles arise from the common tendon at the lateral epicondyle.

The tendons of the extensor digitorum are united over the back of the hand by oblique bands that tend to limit independent movement (Fig. 35.2A). The tendinous slips to the index and little fingers are usually joined by heavier tendons from the separate extensor indicis and the ex-

tensor digiti minimi muscles, respectively. Many of the extensor digitorum fibers contribute to extension of the middle finger, directly or indirectly, through the oblique bands.[10]

Distally each tendinous slip of the extensor digitorum muscle is bound by fasciculi to the collateral ligaments of its metacarpophalangeal joint, as the tendon crosses the joint. The tendon spreads out to cover the dorsal surface of the proximal phalanx of each finger. Here, it is joined by tendons of the lumbrical and interosseous muscles.[21] This aponeurosis then divides into slips which insert on the base of the second phalanx and onto the dorsal surface of the distal phalanx of each finger.

Extensor Digiti Minimi
(Fig. 35.2)

The extensor digiti minimi is not considered separately in this chapter because its belly is adjacent to, and clinically indistinguishable from, the corresponding fibers of the extensor digitorum muscle to the fifth finger.[10]

Extensor Indicis
(Fig. 35.2B)

This muscle arises **proximally** from the dorsal and medial surface of the body of the ulna. It attaches **distally** to the ulnar side of the slip of the extensor digitorum muscle to the index finger, at the level of the head of the second metacarpal bone.

Supplemental References

The extensor digitorum muscle is illustrated by other authors from the dorsal view,[6, 10, 25, 34, 36] from the radial aspect,[7, 26, 32] and retracted to show its innervation and blood supply.[29] Also shown in detail is the arrangement of its tendons on the dorsum of the hand,[8, 10, 21, 27, 30, 33, 36] and its tendinous attachments to each finger.[9, 28] The extensor indicis is seen in the deepest layer of the dorsal forearm muscles.[22, 31, 35, 37]

3. INNERVATION

Both the extensor digitorum and extensor indicis muscles are supplied by the deep radial nerve and the posterior cord, which is formed from all three posterior divisions and all three trunks of the brachial plexus. Both muscles are innervated through spinal nerves C_6, C_7 and C_8. The

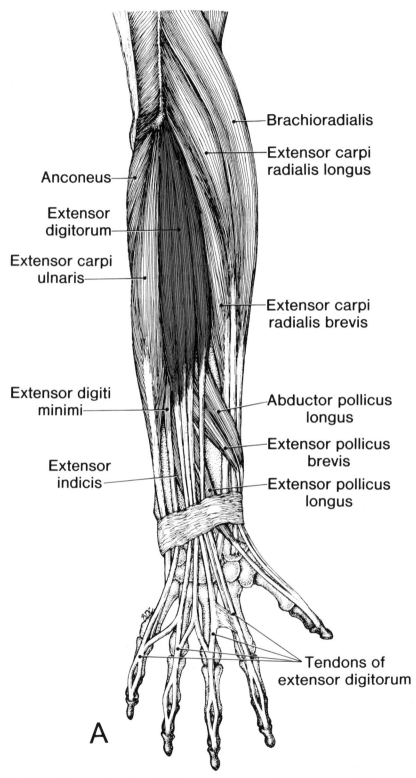

Figure 35.2 *A–B.* Attachments of the right finger extensor muscles. A, extensor digitorum (*red*), showing oblique bands that interconnect the distal tendons, and the attachment of the extensor indicis to the index finger tendon of the extensor digitorum muscle. *B,* extensor indicis (*red*), which passes beneath the extensor digitorum tendons.

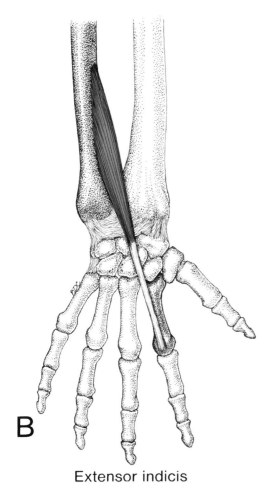

B

Extensor indicis

Figure 35.2 *B*

extensor indicis is the last muscle to be supplied by the radial nerve.

4. ACTIONS

The extensor digitorum muscle extends all phalanges of the fingers,[1, 10, 17] especially the proximal phalanges,[3] and assists extension of the hand at the wrist.[1, 10] All of the extrinsic hand muscles become involved in a power grip, in proportion to the strength of the grip.[1, 19] When the proximal phalanges are held in flexion, the extensor digitorum extends the more distal phalanges, but when the proximal phalanges and the hand are held in extension, then, its contraction has little additional effect on the last two phalanges.[23]

The extensor indicis, in addition to acting on the index finger in the same way that the extensor digitorum acts,[24] is said to adduct the index finger into ulnar de-

viation,[3, 23] because of the angulation of its tendon across the dorsum of the hand.

Electromyographic monitoring of the hand and finger extensors with surface electrodes was performed during 13 sports, including tennis, golf, baseball, overhand throws, and 1-ft jumps. All records showed similar motor unit activity bilaterally. The greatest activity appeared in the dominant right forearm during a right-handed golf swing.[2]

5. MYOTATIC UNIT

Strong agonist-antagonist interactions are needed between the flexors and extensors of the hand and fingers to produce forceful hand grip. Powerful *flexion* of the distal phalanges requires strong activity also of the *finger extensors*.

The ring and little finger extensors form a myotatic unit with the supinator for twisting motions, such as opening jar tops and door handles. Understandably, these three muscles often develop TPs together.

6. SYMPTOMS

Patients complain of pain, as described in Section 1. It may be identified with "tennis elbow," or arthritis of the fingers.[15, 16, 42] In the days of long skirts, when ladies suffered elbow pain from holding them up, the pain was called epicondylalgia, or brachialgia.[18] The pain may awaken patients at night.[14] If a firm grip, as when shaking hands, is distressingly painful, TPs in the extensor muscles of the ring and little fingers are likely to be responsible.

When the middle finger extensor alone is involved, the patient may still complain of weakness of the grip, without pain.[40] The finger extensors are essential to a powerful grip, and this weak grip presents another example of the fact that TPs can inhibit muscular contraction to the degree required to prevent pain.[40] Muscles learn.[39]

Symptoms of impaired finger *flexion* may be due to TPs in the finger *extensor* muscles. Stiffness and painful cramping of the fingers prevented one patient from milking his cows, until tender TPs in his extensor digitorum muscle had been inactivated.[14] Another patient of the senior author could not type because the ring and little fingers would "not work separately,"

PART 3

until the TPs were injected in the extensor fibers of those fingers.

7. ACTIVATION OF TRIGGER POINTS

Myofascial TPs in the finger extensors commonly occur due to such activities as overuse of forceful repetitive finger movements by professional pianists, carpenters, or mechanics; habitual fingering of worry beads; constantly stretching a rubber band with the finger extensors; and repeatedly pulling a sticking drawer with one finger in the handle. Local infection of the ring finger in a seamstress resulted in a stiff and painful ring finger that was relieved months later by injection, high in the forearm, of a TP in the muscle fibers that extended that finger. Activation of finger extensor TPs by fracture of the forearm has been observed by the authors and was reported by Kelly.[14]

When a finger extensor tendon loses its mooring over the metacarpophalangeal joint, the tendon may be said to "jump its trolley." This is a serious source of muscular strain due to the resultant ulnar deviation of the finger, and the tendon displacement must be surgically repaired for restoration of function.[4]

8. PATIENT EXAMINATION
(Fig. 35.3)

Limitation of the *range of motion* is tested by having the patient flex the interphalangeal joints to bring the tips of the fingers against the palmar pads, while extending the metacarpophalangeal joints (Fig. 35.3). Tightness (resistance to stretch) of an affected finger extensor muscle results in that finger standing out from the others, away from the palm, e.g., the middle finger extensor in Fig. 35.3. Passive flexion of the finger beyond this point is painful.

Weakness due to finger extensor TPs is detected in the grip during a handshake. Bilateral comparison is improved by testing both hands simultaneously. Dropping the hand into ulnar deviation and flexion at the wrist during handshake increases the sensitivity of the test beyond that obtainable with the hand held in an extended or neutral position. This test may reveal weakness without pain when the TPs are latent.

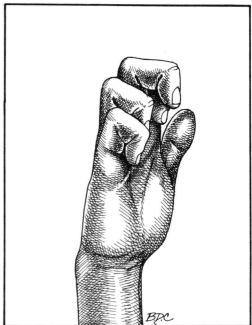

Figure 35.3. Positive finger test, illustrating involvement of only the middle finger extensor muscle. All of the other finger tips can be pressed firmly against the palmar pads while the metacarpophalangeal joints are held straight, not flexed.

Tenderness of the proximal interphalangeal joint is commonly associated with the finger stiffness and "soreness" due to finger extensor TPs, sometimes without referred *pain* in the joint.[40] This may be analogous to the tendinitis associated with TPs in the fibers of the long head of the biceps brachii (see Chapter 30). Both conditions may be completely relieved by inactivation of the myofascial TPs in the responsible muscle.

When an extensor pollicis longus muscle with evidence of TP activity was stretched by passively flexing the thumb, pain was experienced in the thumb and interphalangeal area. Loading the muscle by actively resisting extension of the thumb also caused pain.[20]

9. TRIGGER POINT EXAMINATION
(Fig. 35.4)

Palpation of a TP in the middle finger extensor produces one of the commonest and most easily elicited local twitch responses. This TP is located 3–4 cm (about 1¼ in) distal and slightly dorsal to the head

PART 3

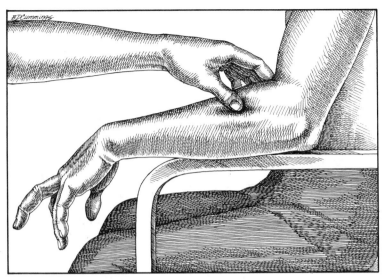

Figure 35.4. Demonstration of a local twitch response, the movement of the middle finger, produced by snapping palpation of a TP in its fibers of the extensor digitorum muscle. The response in many adults without symptoms is readily demonstrable and due to latent trigger points.

of the radius, which lies 2 cm (nearly 1 in) or more distal to the lateral epicondyle (Figs. 35.1A and 35.4). Often the TP is latent; only when the TP is active, does the patient also have spontaneous pain in the middle finger.

The TPs in the fibers of the extensor digitorum that supply the ring and little fingers are difficult to locate (Fig. 35.1B) because they are deep in the muscle mass beneath the aponeurosis of origin, part of which covers the surface of the muscle. They lie next to the extensor carpi ulnaris, which is the muscle mass lateral to the ulna, and close to the underlying supinator muscle. On palpation, they tend to refer pain distally to the wrist and hand, and sometimes proximally to the lateral epicondyle. Local twitch responses that extend the little and ring fingers confirm their location.

An active TP in the extensor indicis is found in the distal portion of the muscle (Fig. 35.1C) and, when stimulated by pressure, the TP projects pain to the wrist, not to the finger. This TP is rarely found by itself; when the activity of other TPs has been eliminated and wrist pain persists, an extensor indicis TP is likely to be the culprit.

Rarely do any of the thumb muscles in the forearm develop TPs, apparently be-cause the extensor pollicis longus and brevis are minimally involved in flexor activity, and control of the thumb involves only two, rather than three phalangeal joints.

10. ENTRAPMENTS

No entrapments have been observed due to TP activity in the finger extensor muscles.

11. ASSOCIATED TRIGGER POINTS

Unless TPs are activated by specific stress or injury of the extensor musculature, they are likely to appear in association with the "tennis elbow"; usually, the supinator becomes involved first, followed by the brachioradialis and extensor carpi radialis longus muscles. With the passage of time and spread of the involvement to the middle and ring finger extensors, gripping and hand-twisting motions become painful. At this point, the extensor carpi ulnaris also may develop TPs.

12. STRETCH AND SPRAY
(Fig. 35.5)

The patient sits in a chair with suitable armrests so that the elbow can be supported in extension and, simultaneously,

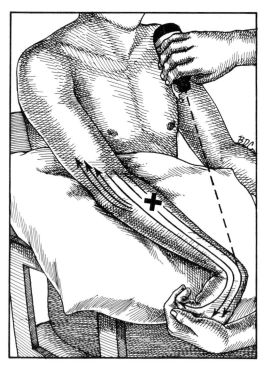

Figure 35.5. Stretch position and spray pattern (*arrows*) for the long finger extensor muscle. The "**x**" marks the approximate trigger point area. The downward spray pattern should swing around to include the lateral epicondyle, especially when that, too, exhibits referred pain and tenderness.

the hand and fingers can be fully flexed (Fig. 35.5). Curling only the fingers, or bending only the wrist, fails to stretch the long finger extensors sufficiently to eliminate their TPs during vapocooling. Stretching across all finger and wrist joints must be performed simultaneously, while parallel sweeps of the spray cover the muscle and its referred pain pattern. When TPs in the ring and little finger extensor muscles refer pain over the lateral epicondyle, an up-sweep (proximal) pattern is added to cover that region also. A hot pack is then applied over the forearm muscles.

Following treatment, the patient is encouraged to increase activities gradually, avoiding those that stress the involved muscle enough to make it hurt. Some patients are Spartan and determined to "exercise" and "strengthen" the weak muscle; they must be discouraged from purposely repeating painful activities, and thus aggravating their condition. Slow, passive stretch held briefly at the point of

pain is helpful, but painful active contraction tends to reactivate the TP mechanism.

13. INJECTION AND STRETCH
(Fig. 35.6)

Other authors have found, as we have, that injection into the site of TP tenderness in the finger extensors is effective in relieving the patient's myofascial signs and symptoms.[5, 13]

For injection, the patient lies supine with the arm placed so that the hand and fingers hang down limply, which stretches the finger extensors moderately.

After injection, the muscle is passively stretched to its full range of motion, usually during vapocooling, and a hot pack is applied.

Then, the same activity guidelines apply as after the stretch-and-spray treatment.

Extensor Digitorum

The TPs in the middle finger extensor are identified by flat palpation and injected with 0.5% procaine solution (Fig. 35.6A). Strong local twitch responses and clear pain patterns, as elicited by examination and needle penetration of the TPs, are characteristic of this muscle.

The TPs in the ring and little finger extensors are located between those in the middle finger extensor fibers and the extensor carpi ulnaris muscle. The needle is directed toward the point of deep tenderness (Fig. 35.6B). It is not always clear whether the TP, which is encountered by the needle at considerable depth and which refers pain to the lateral epicondyle, is actually in the finger extensor, or in the underlying supinator muscle. Normal grip strength may return immediately after elimination of these extensor TPs.[40]

Occasionally, a deep radial (dorsal interosseous) nerve block may inadvertently be produced during injection of these TPs. The patient should be warned, beforehand, of possible temporary extensor-muscle weakness, which resolves in 15 or 20 min when the dilute 0.5% procaine solution has been injected.

Extensor Indicis

This TP is found by flat palpation through, or between the extensor tendons. The TP lies in the belly of the muscle

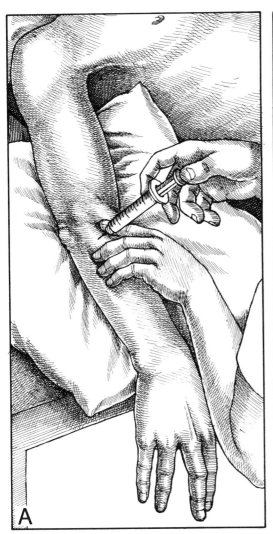

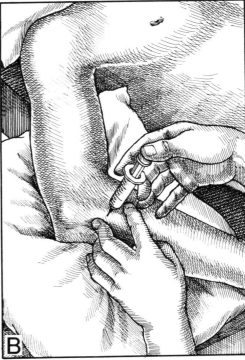

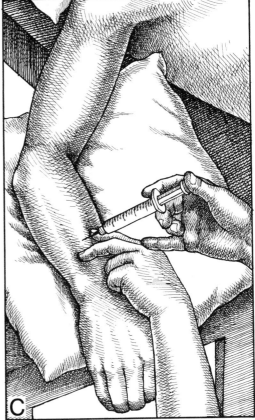

Figure 35.6.   Injection of the finger extensor muscles. *A*, middle finger extensor. *B*, ring and little finger extensors. Injection deep into the 4th and 5th finger extensors sometimes also reaches a trigger point in the underlying supinator muscle, which refers pain to the lateral epicondyle. *C*, extensor indicis muscle.

PART 3

approximately mid-way between the radius and ulna, as the muscle crosses the forearm to attach to the ulna (Fig. 35.6C).

14. CORRECTIVE ACTIONS
(Figs. 35.7–35.11).

Activity Stress

The patient learns to avoid overload of the finger extensors. When gripping or twisting with the hand, as in tennis, the patient should maintain the hand slightly extended and radially deviated (in a cock-up position of the wrist), rather than flexed and ulnarly deviated. The stress of shaking hands repeatedly can be reduced by offering the hand with the palm up and the hand slightly extended, so that the other person cannot squeeze tightly. The patient, thus, uses the biceps brachii instead of the forearm muscles to flex the elbow and, if standing in a receiving line, can gracefully alternate left and right hands between guests. External support for the wrist is provided by a leather strap, as illustrated before in Figure 34.11; it helps to maintain the wrist in the cocked position and to prevent excessive strain on the extensor

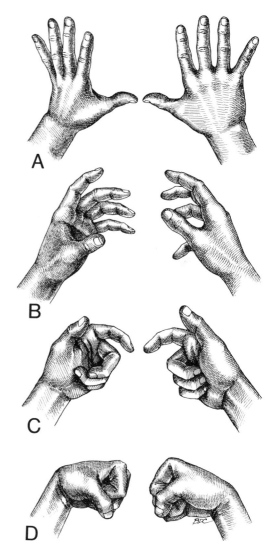

Figure 35.8.   Artisan's Finger-stretch Exercise. *A*, the exercise begins with the pronated hand open, and the wrist and fingers in forceful extension. *B* and *C*, the hand is supinated and the fingers closed in a smooth, continuous movement, starting with the little fingers. *D*, the hand is flexed and supinated as the fist is closed forcefully with the thumb overlapping the index finger.

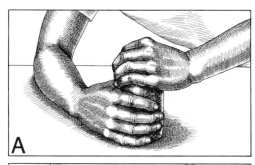

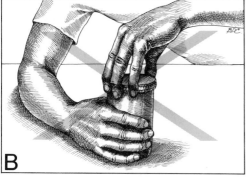

Figure 35.7.   Unscrewing a jar top. *A*, position of strength, with the wrist cocked. *B*, position of weakness of the grip, (*red* ✕). This position is likely to strain forearm extensor muscles.

muscles in the forearm. Unfortunately, such a support is not known to be commercially available, and elastic is not as effective as leather for this strap.

The patient should avoid testing painful motions, and permit the muscles to rest and recover, resuming only those activities that do not precipitate pain. A *variety* of activities is desirable, with gradual resumption of more kinds of movement and

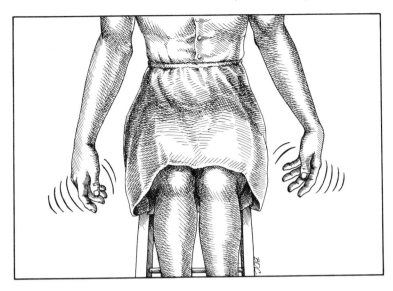

Figure 35.9.   The Finger-flutter Exercise for the long finger and hand extensors shakes the relaxed hand and fingers with the shoulder-girdle and arm muscles.

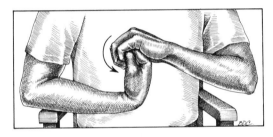

Figure 35.10.   Passive Self-stretch Exercise for the right extensor digitorum muscle. The right hand and fingers are fully and strongly flexed simultaneously.

an increased level of activity as function improves.

A common abuse of hand extensors is the grasping of jar lids in a manner that places this muscle at a mechanical disadvantage (Fig. 35.7*B*). By keeping the wrist cocked and by using the entire arm as a lever (Fig. 35.7*A*), stress on the hand extensors is greatly reduced.

Exercises

The Artisan's Finger-stretch Exercise (Fig. 35.8) and the Finger-flutter Exercise (Fig. 35.9) are especially useful for people who must hold their hands for long periods in tense positions with repetitive finger movements. Examples are those who do fine tool work, piano playing, or longhand writing.

The Artisan's Finger-stretch Exercise

begins by placing the hands pronated in front of the face with the fingers extended and spread apart (Fig. 35.8*A*). As the hand is slowly supinated, the fingers are flexed, little finger first (Figs. 35.8 *B* and *C*), to make a fist with the hand fully supinated and flexed at the wrist (Fig. 35.8*D*). The Finger-stretch Exercise has the advantage of stretching and activating both flexor and extensor muscles of the fingers, thumb, and hand, in addition to the intrinsic muscles of the hand.

The Finger-flutter Exercise (Fig. 35.9) is done by dropping the hands to the sides, completely relaxed, and shaking the hands and fingers from the shoulders and elbows.

The Passive Self-stretch, as illustrated in Figure 35.10, enables the patient to relieve the tension of the taut finger extensors. It is essential that both the wrist and finger joints crossed by the finger extensor muscles and tendons be fully flexed.

Positioning

Positioning at night is important if the patient tends to hold the hand and fingers in a fully flexed position (Fig. 35.11*B*). To avoid this, it may be necessary to have the patient affix a small pillow, or bath towel, to the volar surface of the hand and forearm at night, to maintain the mid-position and to avoid cramping pain (Fig. 35.11*A*).

PART 3

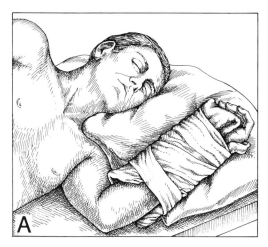

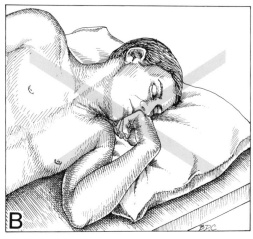

Figure 35.11. Sleep positions. A, use of a soft splint to maintain the correct, neutral positions of the elbow, wrist and fingers. B, an incorrect position (*red* ✕) that must be prevented, if assumed spontaneously in sleep.

References

1. Basmajian JV: *Muscles Alive*, Ed. 4. Williams & Wilkins, Baltimore, 1978 (pp. 213, 217).
2. Broer MR, Houtz SJ: *Patterns of Muscular Activity in Selected Sports Skill*. Charles C Thomas, Springfield, Ill., 1967.
3. Duchenne GB: *Physiology of Motion*, translated by E.B. Kaplan. J.B. Lippincott, Philadelphia, 1949 (p. 126).
4. Flatt AE: *The care of the rheumatoid hand*, Ed. 3. C.V. Mosby, St. Louis, 1974 (pp. 249–277).
5. Good MG: The role of skeletal muscles in the pathogenesis of diseases. *Acta Med Scand* 138:285–292, 1950 (p. 287).
6. Grant JCB: *An Atlas of Human Anatomy*, Ed. 7. Williams & Wilkins, Baltimore, 1978 (Fig. 6-91).
7. *Ibid*. (Fig. 6-93).
8. *Ibid*. (Figs. 6-102, 6-104).
9. *Ibid*. (Fig. 6-106).
10. Gray H: *Anatomy of the Human Body*, edited by C.M. Goss, American Ed. 29. Lea & Febiger, Philadelphia, 1973 (pp. 468, 469, 472).
11. Gutstein M: Common rheumatism and physiotherapy. *Br J Phys Med* 3:46–50, 1940 (p. 47).
12. Kellgren JH: Observations on referred pain arising from muscle. *Clin Sci* 3:175–190, 1938 (p. 187).
13. Kelly M: New light on the painful shoulder. *Med J Aust* 1:488–493, 1942 (Case 8, Figs. 3D and 3F).
14. Kelly M: Pain in the forearm and hand due to muscular lesions. *Med J Aust* 2:185–188, 1944 (Cases 2, 7, and 9; Fig. 4).
15. Kelly M: Some rules for the employment of local analgesia in the treatment of somatic pain. *Med J Aust* 1:235–239, 1947 (p. 236).
16. Kelly M: The relief of facial pain by procaine (Novocaine) injections. *J Am Geriatr Soc* 11:586–596, 1963 (Case 3, p. 589).
17. Kendall HO, Kendall FP, Wadsworth GE: *Muscles: Testing and Function*, Ed. 2. Williams & Wilkins, Baltimore, 1971 (p. 77).
18. Llewellyn LJ, Jones AB: *Fibrositis*. Rebman, New York, 1915 (Fig. 35 opposite p. 226; p. 227).
19. Long C, Conrad PW, Hall EA, *et al.*: Intrinsic-extrinsic muscle control of the hand in power grip and precision handling. *J Bone Joint Surg* 52-A:853–867, 1970.
20. Macdonald AJR: Abnormally tender muscle regions and associated painful movements. *Pain* 8:197–205, 1980 (pp. 202, 203).
21. McMinn RMH, Hutchings RT: *Color Atlas of Human Anatomy*. Year Book Medical Publishers, Chicago, 1977 (pp. 127, 141, 142, 145).
22. *Ibid*. (p. 127).
23. Rasch PJ, Burke RK: *Kinesiology and Applied Anatomy*, Ed. 6. Lea & Febiger, Philadelphia, 1978 (pp. 200, 203).
24. Sano S, Ando K, Katori I, *et al.*: Electromyographic studies on the forearm muscle activities during finger movements. *J Jap Orthop Assoc* 51:331–337, 1977.
25. Sobotta J, Figge FHJ: *Atlas of Human Anatomy*, Ed. 9, Vol. 1. Hafner Division of Macmillan, New York, 1974 (p. 206).
26. *Ibid*. (p. 192).
27. *Ibid*. (p. 212).
28. *Ibid*. (p. 222).
29. Sobotta J, Figge FHJ: *Atlas of Human Anatomy*, Ed. 9, Vol. 3. Hafner Division of Macmillan, New York, 1974 (p. 299).
30. *Ibid*. (p. 304).
31. Sobotta J, Figge FHJ: *Atlas of Human Anatomy*, Ed. 9, Vol. 1. Hafner Division of Macmillan, New York, 1974 (p 208).
32. Spalteholz W: *Handatlas der Anatomie des Menschen*, Ed. 11, Vol. 2. S. Hirzel, Leipzig, 1922 (p. 330).
33. *Ibid*. (p. 334).
34. *Ibid*. (p. 331).
35. *Ibid*. (p. 333).
36. Toldt C: *An Atlas of Human Anatomy*, translated by M.E. Paul, Ed. 2, Vol. 1. Macmillan, New York, 1919 (p. 326).
37. *Ibid*. (pp. 326, 328, 330).
38. Travell J: Pain mechanisms in connective tissue. In *Connective Tissues, Transactions of the Second Conference, 1951*, edited by C. Ragan. Josiah

Macy, Jr. Foundation, New York, 1952 (Fig. 33, pp. 98, 99).

39. Travell J: Myofascial trigger points: clinical view. *In Advances in Pain Research and Therapy,* edited by J.J. Bonica and D. Albe-Fessard, Vol. 1. Raven Press, New York, 1976 (pp. 919–926).

40. Travell J, Bigelow NH: Role of somatic trigger areas in the patterns of hysteria. *Psychosom Med* 9:353–363, 1947 (p. 356).

41. Travell J, Rinzler SH: The myofascial genesis of pain. *Postgrad Med* 11:425–434, 1952 (p. 428).

42. Winter Z: Referred pain in fibrositis. *Med Rec* 157:34–37, 1944 (pp. 37, 38).

PART 3

CHAPTER 36
Supinator Muscle
"Tennis Elbow"

HIGHLIGHTS: "Tennis Elbow" or "epicondylitis," as pain in the lateral epicondyle is often called, is frequently of myofascial origin, usually due to trigger points (TPs) in the supinator muscle. **REFERRED PAIN** from TPs in the supinator is projected chiefly to the lateral epicondyle, frequently to the dorsal aspect of the web and base of the thumb, and sometimes to the forearm dorsally. **ANATOMICAL ATTACHMENT** along the dorsal surface of the ulna at the elbow positions the supinator to wrap around the lateral surface of the radius lateral to its attachment on the volar surface of the radius. The radius acts like a windlass that winds up the supinator and the biceps brachii tendon when the hand is pronated. **ACTIONS** of the supinator are primarily to supinate the hand, and secondarily to assist flexion at the elbow. **SYMPTOMS** are mainly elbow pain, both at rest and when the arm is used. **ACTIVATION OF TRIGGER POINTS** in the supinator may occur due to stress overload, as when playing tennis, "flipping" a briefcase onto the desk, or wresting a stiff doorknob. **PATIENT EXAMINATION** reveals marked referred tenderness of the lateral epicondyle to tapping. **TRIGGER POINT EXAMINATION** proceeds by bending the elbow slightly, supinating the hand, pushing the brachioradialis muscle aside, and palpating the supinator against the head and shaft of the radius in the distal antecubital space. **ENTRAPMENT** of the deep radial nerve may occur as it enters the arcade of Frohse, or within the belly of the supinator muscle. **ASSOCIATED TRIGGER POINTS** in the "tennis elbow" syndrome are found in the nearby hand and finger extensors, the brachioradialis, the distal triceps and occasionally the anconeus muscles. The brachialis, biceps and palmaris longus muscles also may become involved, but do not contribute to the lateral epicondylar pain of the "tennis elbow." For **STRETCH AND SPRAY** of the supinator, the elbow is extended and the hand pronated, while the vapocoolant spray is applied upward and around the forearm over the muscle, and then down over the dorsal forearm and thumb. **INJECTION AND STRETCH** are begun by directing the needle into the tender spot overlying the head and neck of the radius in the distal antecubital space. Passive stretch of the supinator follows injection. **CORRECTIVE ACTIONS** include keeping the wrist dorsiflexed and the elbow slightly bent to prevent strain when playing tennis, applying ischemic pressure over the muscle, and carrying packages with the hands supinated to transfer the load from the supinator to the biceps brachii and brachialis muscles.

1. REFERRED PAIN
(Fig. 36.1)

Trigger points (TPs) in the supinator muscle refer pain primarily to the lateral epicondyle and the surrounding lateral aspect of the elbow.[40] They also project spillover pain to the dorsal aspect of the web of the thumb and, if sufficiently intense, the pain may include some of the dorsal forearm[42] (Fig. 36.1).

Kelly[20] reported a patient with tenderness in the region of the most common supinator TP and in the wrist and finger extensors, with numbness in the thumb and tingling in the index and ring fingers. These symptoms, and additional areas of tenderness in the lower brachialis and in the volar aspect of the wrist, disappeared when the tender spots in the finger extensor group and the supinator were injected with a local anesthetic. Two other pa-

510

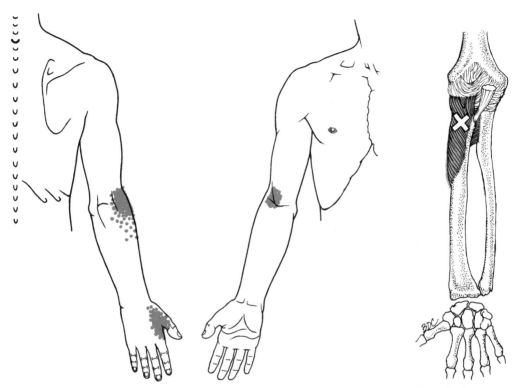

Figure 36.1.   Referred pain pattern (*dark red*) of a frequent trigger point (✕) in the right supinator muscle (*light red*).

tients[19] had the typical supinator pattern of referred pain to the thumb, with relief by injection in the area of the supinator TPs.

2. ANATOMICAL ATTACHMENTS
(Fig. 36.2)

The supinator is a flat muscle, the proximal part of which is divided into two layers. The muscle spirals around the lateral (outer) side of the radius to attach **proximally** to the dorsal surface of the ulna, the lateral epicondyle of the humerus, the lateral and ventral ligaments of the radioulnar joint, and the anterior capsule of the humeroulnar joint (Fig. 36.2B and C). **Ventrally** and **distally** the fibers form a "Y" shaped attachment to the volar surface of the radius just distal to the tendon of the biceps brachii (Fig. 36.2A). The bare bone between the arms of the "Y" (Fig. 36.2C) separates the proximal portion of the muscle into superficial and deep layers.[1, 36] Distally the muscle is undivided. When the hand pronates, the supinator muscle and the biceps tendon wrap around the radius into the space between the ra-

dius and the ulna. The deep radial (posterior interosseous) nerve enters between the superficial and deep layers of the muscle beneath the archway formed by the superficial layer, the arcade of Frohse.[36]

"Supinator longus" is an outmoded name for the brachioradialis, not the supinator muscle; the brachioradialis has very little, if any, supinator function.

Supplemental References

Anatomy books illustrate the supinator muscle from the medial aspect,[24] from in front without the radial nerve,[24, 39] with the radial nerve,[12] from the lateral side,[11, 23, 24] from the posterior (dorsal) view without the radial nerve,[13, 34, 38] with the deep radial nerve,[28, 35] from the medial view without the radial nerve,[37] and in cross section.[6, 29]

3. INNERVATION

This muscle is supplied primarily by the C_6 and partly by the C_5 spinal nerves, from the posterior cord, and the deep branch of the radial nerve.

PART 3

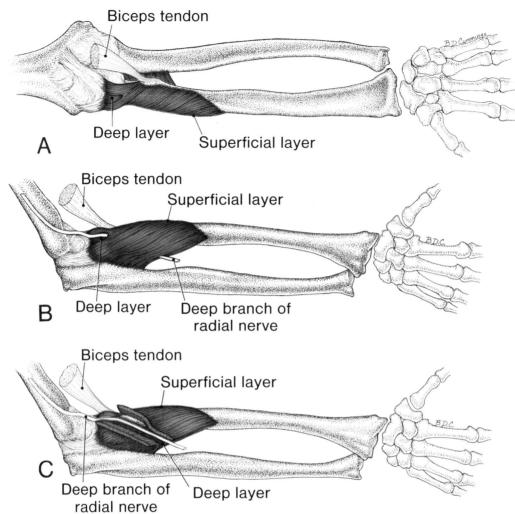

Figure 36.2.   Attachments of the right supinator muscle (*red*), and its relation to the deep radial nerve. *A*, ventral view of the forearm, hand supinated. In the foreground, the muscle attaches to the volar surface of the radius; in the background, it crosses the interosseous space to its dorsal ulnar attachment. A small part of the deep layer is seen through the arched opening in the superficial layer. *B*, lateral view of the forearm, hand in neutral position. The deep radial nerve enters the arched opening in the superficial layer and continues between the two layers of the muscle. *C*, same view as *Part B*, with the superficial layer of the muscle reflected to show the deep layer and the nerve. The area of the radius that is free of muscle fiber attachments is seen just above the nerve. This bare bone separates the two layers. The division of the muscle into two layers ceases in its distal half, where the nerve tunnels through the undivided muscle belly.

4. ACTIONS
(Fig. 36.3)

The supinator, as its name implies, is the primary supinator of the hand and forearm at the radioulnar joint of the forearm.[2, 9, 18, 31, 43] Supinator activity predominates over biceps activity during unresisted supination of the hand, and "holds" the hand in supination.[2, 43] The much stronger biceps assists supination when the forearm is at least slightly flexed at the elbow and when force is needed to overcome resistance to supination.[43] However, the biceps assists very little, if at all, when the elbow is straight. Strong supination, therefore, requires at least a slight degree of elbow flexion.

Based on electromyography, forceful elbow flexion with the hand pronated, as in Figure 36.3C, inhibits contraction of the biceps (which is a supinator) and, there-

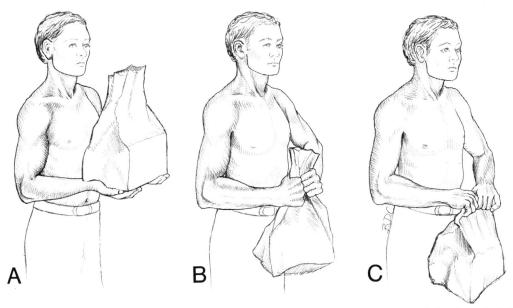

Figure 36.3.   Three hand positions for carrying a heavy object with the elbow flexed. *A*, hands supinated, which loads the biceps brachii and unloads the supinator. *B*, hands in the neutral position, which loads both muscles. *C*, hands pronated, which tends to unload the biceps and to load the brachialis, brachioradialis, and some fibers of the supinator for elbow flexion.

fore, tends to load the supinator, brachio-radialis and brachialis muscles. Forceful elbow flexion in the supinated position of Figure 36.3*A* tends to load the biceps and to unload the supinator. The supinator also assists flexion of the forearm at the elbow when the hand is held intermediate between supination and pronation,[33] as in Figure 36.3*B*.

The supinator fibers that attach to the anterior capsule of the humeroulnar joint contribute primarily to elbow flexion, rather than to supination; they pass between the deep radial nerve and the biceps tendon. The epicondylar fibers also may contribute to flexion.

5. MYOTATIC UNIT

Supination is augmented by the biceps brachii during increased effort. The supinator is synergistic with the forearm flexors, as described in Section 4, above.

The chief antagonist to the supinator is the prime pronator, the pronator quadratus; the secondary antagonist is the pronator teres.[2]

6. SYMPTOMS

Patients with active TPs in the supinator muscle complain of twinges of pain in either, or both, the lateral epicondyle and the dorsal surface of the web of the thumb. Pain is caused by activities like carrying a heavy briefcase with the elbow fully extended, playing tennis, and other movements listed under Section 7, below. These patients also are likely to experience continuing elbow pain at rest following such activities. In our experience, nearly every patient with lateral epicondylar pain and tenderness has an active supinator TP; the supinator is the muscle most frequently responsible for the pain of "tennis elbow."

7. ACTIVATION OF TRIGGER POINTS

Symptoms of "tennis elbow" may occur when the player mis-hits the ball "off-center," twisting the racquet with the elbow completely extended (more likely in backhand, than in forehand strokes). During full elbow extension, the biceps cannot assist the supinator to resist the added force. Supinator strain may occur when resisting unexpected pronation or when executing an extremely forceful supination.

At times, the commonly used term "tennis elbow" is really a "briefcase elbow," "door-handle elbow," or "dog-walker's elbow." Any excessively forceful, repetitive, or sustained supination of the hand, especially with the elbow straight, may initiate symptoms. So can forceful elbow flexion when the forearm is held in pronation (Fig. 36.3C). "Briefcase elbow" occurs when the briefcase is flipped with the carrying hand onto the top of a desk, ready to open, ending with the forearm in the position of Fig. 36.3C. Also traumatic is carrying a heavy briefcase with the elbow straight when it must be stabilized by the supinator with each step, especially if the leg bumps the back end of the briefcase while walking.

Additional initiating and perpetuating stresses include turning stiff doorknobs, wringing clothes when doing laundry, meticulous ironing, unscrewing a tight jar lid by movement only at the wrist, walking a large dog pulling on a leash, handshaking in long receiving lines at receptions (as by politicians), erasing chalk lines on a blackboard, washing walls by hand, and raking leaves.

8. PATIENT EXAMINATION

Tapping the lateral epicondyle elicits exquisite tenderness; referred tenderness also may be present in the web of the thumb when it is squeezed. The combination of epicondylar tenderness and pain at the base of the thumb strongly suggests an active supinator TP. Thumb motion is usually not restricted and often is not painful. The Hand-to-shoulder-blade Test (see Fig. 22.4) shows slight restriction, and causes pain as described in Section 1, above. A handshake with a firm grip becomes painful when extensor muscles of the wrist and fingers have secondarily developed active TPs.

Differential Diagnosis

The symptoms of "tennis elbow," or lateral epicondylitis of the elbow, appear in the literature as a confusing polyglot of conditions ascribed chiefly to overstrain of the hand extensors at the wrist.[21, 25] The multiplicity of conditions and treatments found in the literature is typified by a current textbook's coverage of "tennis elbow."[7] A common etiology emerges for the many patients who fit one of these varieties when the findings are related to myofascial TP phenomena.

Cyriax[7] identified four varieties of the "tennis elbow." The teno-periosteal variety was explained as a partial tear at the ligamentous attachment of the hand and finger extensor muscles to the lateral epicondyle, which produced a painful scar.[25] This was treated with local triamcinolone injection and complete rest of the upper extremity for a week. The muscular variety required injection of 0.5% procaine solution precisely into the tender point in the "extensor carpi radialis" belly. The tendinous variety was described as a lesion in the "body of the tendon," presumably the common extensor tendon, at the level of the head of the radius. Surgical exploration of this area with removal of tissue revealed microscopic rupture of the origin of the extensor carpi radialis brevis with abortive regeneration.[27] It was treated with four to eight sessions of massage. The supracondylar variety displayed a tender point along the supracondylar ridge above the lateral epicondyle at the origin of the extensor carpi radialis longus muscle. It, too, was relieved by deep massage.

We see myofascial TP syndromes that fit each of these four varieties of "tennis elbow" described by Cyriax.[7] The teno-periosteal variety fits the pain and tenderness that is referred by active TPs in the supinator muscle, upward to the distal edge of the lateral epicondyle. The location of the injection is illustrated by Cyriax[7] as distal to the head of the radius where the belly of the supinator muscle is located, not between the head of the radius and the epicondyle where the common extensor tendon lies. Injection is described as directed to the area of tenderness, which would locate TPs in the extensor muscle mass (the extensor carpi radialis longus and extensor digitorum). Supinator fibers, which develop TPs, also often attach to this area of the radius; deep injection here is likely to include these supinator fibers. The prescribed rest would avoid overload and reduce the irritability of TPs in the supinator and extensor mass muscles.

The muscular variety fits closely our description of extensor carpi radialis longus TPs, which refer pain and tenderness to the lateral epicondylar area (see Chapter 34). Since injection of the deep radial nerve with procaine was a concern in the treatment of this variety,[7] the needle must have penetrated the supinator muscle to reach the nerve. This is one approach that we use for injection of the lateral supinator TP area, which also refers pain to the lateral epicondyle (Section 13).

The tender point described for the *tendinous* variety includes one of the areas of attachment of the supinator muscle (Fig. 36.2A). The massage would include those supinator fibers.

The location of the tender point in the *supracondylar* variety, also treated by massage, corresponds closely to the location of Triceps TP_5, which refers pain and tenderness to the medial epicondyle (*see* Fig. 32.1C).

Gunn[15] attributed the "tennis elbow" symptoms in one group of patients to a reflex localization of pain from radiculopathy of the cervical spine. Cyriax[7] considered pain due to cervical radiculopathy as a separate and distinguishable disease. We find that cervical radiculopathy may be an initiating and perpetuating cause of myofascial TPs; thus, both authors could be correct in their analysis of individual cases.

Arthritis of either joint at the elbow is a possible, but unlikely, cause of pain localized to the lateral epicondyle. It should be diagnosed by radiologic examination.

9. TRIGGER POINT EXAMINATION

The most frequent location of supinator TPs is close to the attachment of the superficial layer of the supinator muscle on the ventral aspect of the radius, which, in turn, is just lateral and somewhat distal to the biceps tendon (Fig. 36.1). The brachioradialis is slackened by flexing the elbow slightly (15–30°) and this muscle is pushed aside laterally. The hand is fully supinated; otherwise the TPs are easily missed. In this position, these supinator TPs lie directly over the radius and immediately beneath the skin between the biceps tendon and the brachioradialis muscle. Both muscular landmarks are readily identified by asking the patient to flex the forearm against resistance. Snapping palpation may produce a supination twitch response of the hand in spite of the shortened position of the muscle.

A second, deeply situated, supinator TP also may be found by pressing on the outer side of the forearm as the muscle approaches its attachment where the lateral joint capsule meets the ulna. This TP is evidenced by tenderness to deep palpation through the mass of the hand extensor muscles, especially through the extensor carpi ulnaris longus, 4 or 5 cm (nearly 2 in) distal to the lateral epicondyle, and 1 or 2 cm (about ¾ in) distal to the head of the radius. This second TP is likely to be associated with deep radial nerve entrapment.

10. ENTRAPMENTS

A sharp distinction can be drawn between the painless weakness caused by tumorous encroachment on the deep radial nerve[10] and the painful "tennis elbow" with myofascial referred pain and sometimes weakness due to deep radial nerve entrapment by the supinator muscle, or as the nerve enters the arcade of Frohse.[17, 22] Myofascial TPs cause the pain of "tennis elbow," while entrapment of the deep radial nerve causes motor symptoms of weakness. Involvement of the supinator can cause both pain and the entrapment, but usually only pain.

Goldman *et al.*[10] reviewed 28 cases of deep radial nerve palsy without sensory symptoms. Of the 18 cases operated on in which the cause of entrapment was verified, 17 were due to a tumor compressing the nerve. In the other case, the thickened edge of the arched attachment of the extensor carpi radialis brevis compressed the nerve. Another patient, with painless palsy at operation, had a fibrous band that bound the deep radial nerve as it entered the supinator muscle.[4] These correlations of painless palsy with non-TP nerve entrapment, plus the fact that the deep radial nerve is primarily a motor, not a cutaneous sensory nerve, strongly suggests that the pain of "tennis elbow" is *not caused* by entrapment of the deep radial nerve. This also was the conclusion reached by Van Rossum, *et al.*[44]

Pain from myofascial TPs in muscles that refer to the elbow region readily account for the pain of "tennis elbow." How can TPs in the supinator also cause entrapment of the deep radial nerve? An entrapment of the deep radial (posterior interosseous) nerve can occur as it enters the supinator muscle beneath the arcade of Frohse. An anatomical study showed that the proximal edge of the superficial layer of muscle fibers had formed the arcade, as a tendinous thickened border, in 30% of 50 "normal" adult arms.[36] The nerve enters an arcade about 1 cm lateral to the biceps tendon. Here, the nerve lies against the anterior capsule of the radiohumeral joint, cushioned slightly by the fibers of the deep layer of the supinator muscle as they attach to the joint capsule.

Supinator TPs can cause entrapment of the deep radial nerve if those supinator fibers that are attached to an arcade with a thick tendinous edge are shortened by activity of the less common supinator TP described in the previous Section. That this TP lies close to the nerve is evidenced by occasional temporary local anesthetic block of the nerve when that TP is injected.

The deep radial nerve supplies motor branches to the extensor carpi ulnaris, extensor digiti minimi, extensor digitorum, abductor pollicis longus, extensor pollicis longus and brevis, and extensor indicis muscles. It carries deep sensory fibers from the wrist joints and from the muscles that it supplies. Entrapment of the deep radial nerve, therefore, weakens extension of the hand, fingers and thumb, and sometimes causes a disagreeable dysesthesia of the wrist and distal forearm without a clearly definable pain pattern.

This myofascial concept is supported by two groups of investigators who recently reported operative findings in patients who presented with *pain* in the lateral proximal forearm (extensor mass).[17, 22] In one group, pain was reported to be increased by use.[22] In the other group, patients were awakened by pain in the early hours of the morning (43 of 48) and complained of weakness (34 of 48). All of these symptoms are characteristic of myofascial TPs in the supinator.[17]

On examination, all patients of both groups[17] had tenderness to palpation 4–5 cm (nearly 2 in) distal to the lateral epicondyle (over the course of the radial nerve), which is also where one finds tenderness of the supinator TP that is associated with this nerve entrapment. Nearly every patient (43 of 50, and 19 of 20) experienced pain when resisting supination, a cardinal sign of supinator TP involvement. Many (29 of 50, and 20 of 20) experienced pain when resisting extension of the middle finger; this finger extensor is one of the muscles most often involved with supinator TPs. Half (26 of 50) of one group[17] exhibited weakness of hand and finger extension that seemed to be pain induced, again, a sign of myofascial TPs.

All patients were treated by surgical release of the arcade of Frohse with 87% excellent or good results for both groups.[17] A number of these operations may not have been necessary had the active TPs been identified and inactivated first.

The report of another group of authors[22] identified four potential sources of radial nerve entrapment in patients who failed to respond to conservative treatment for chronic "tennis elbow": (1) a fibrous band of the joint capsule in front of the radial head, (2) the "radial recurrent fan" of the blood vessels in the antecubital space, (3) the sharp tendinous margin of the extensor carpi radialis brevis, and (4) compression by the arcade of Frohse. At operation, these investigators observed convincing pressure on the nerve by a thickened arcade of Frohse in all 20 patients, and by the edge of the extensor carpi radialis brevis in 14 of the patients. The arcade of Frohse was released in all patients of both groups. The nerve was freed of recurrent vessels in 14 of the 20 cases. Only three nerves had fibrous bands to be released over the joint capsule. No entrapment was observed proximal to the arcade. Since multiple possible causes of entrapment were released in many patients, the contribution of each cause is speculative in this study.

Other investigators[17] found that the arcade of Frohse had caused an impression on the nerve in 34 of the 39 patients on whom surgery was performed to relieve elbow pain. It is clear that the arcade is a *common* source of entrapment in patients with elbow pain. This operation should relieve radial nerve entrapment by the muscle, but might not inactivate the supinator TPs, which would account for incomplete pain relief by the surgical procedure alone.

We find that inactivation of all local myofascial TPs relieves the pain, and inactivation of the supinator TP on the ulnar

PART 3

side of the nerve usually relieves the deep radial nerve entrapment, without surgical intervention. Patients with a well developed arcade may be more vulnerable to entrapment of the radial nerve by supinator TPs.

11. ASSOCIATED TRIGGER POINTS

With the "tennis elbow" symptoms of pain and tenderness in the region of the lateral epicondyle, TPs are often found also in the triceps brachii, in the lower end of the lateral margin of its medial head (TP$_2$), in the long finger extensors, the extensor carpi radialis longus and brevis, and the brachioradialis muscles. When all of these TPs have been eliminated, an anco-

neus TP may still cause lateral epicondylar pain and tenderness to tapping.

Additional muscles that may become involved as part of the supinator's myotatic unit, but which do not refer pain to the lateral epicondyle, are the brachialis, biceps brachii (TPs in the distal third of the muscle), and sometimes the palmaris longus.

12. STRETCH AND SPRAY
(Fig. 36.4)

The elbow rests on a padded armrest, or over the operator's knee. This support permits full elbow extension and, as the forearm is fully pronated, prevents internal rotation at the shoulder. After several initial

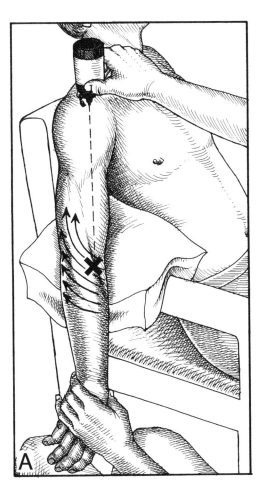
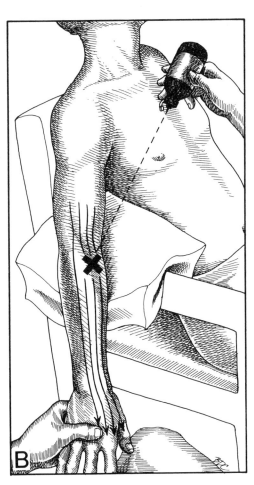

Figure 36.4.   Stretch position and spray pattern (*arrows*) for trigger points (✕s) in the supinator. *A,* the elbow must be supported to maintain effective elbow extension and pronation of the hand. The operator blocks internal rotation at the shoulder by locking the medial epicondyle against the elbow support. The up-sweep spray pattern covers the muscle and lateral epicondyle. *B,* the down-sweep spray pattern covers the muscle and its referred pain pattern on the forearm and at the base of the thumb, dorsally.

PART 3

sweeps of spray, passive stretch is applied as the vapocoolant spray is again swept upward and outward diagonally over the forearm following the muscle fibers from t̶ to the region of the lateral ....ig. 36.4A). Then, down- ...ied over the dorsum of the web of the thumb. (Fig.

part of the stretch-and-spray procedure, tension should be released in adjacent muscles likely to have developed associated TPs, and which are likely to protest painfully after release of the supinator; stretch and spray are applied to the biceps and brachialis, brachioradialis, extensor carpi radialis, and triceps muscles and to any associated TPs in the finger extensors.

Ischemic compression, applied by pressing TPs in the taut supinator muscle against the underlying radius, is most effective when combined with stretch and spray. Following successful treatment, the elbow should straighten to a degree of hyperextension not obtainable before, and the Hand-to-shoulder-blade Test (see Fig. 22.4) should show no restriction. All tenderness to tapping on the lateral epicondyle should be gone. If not, residual TPs may remain in the supinator, or in nearby muscles, especially the anconeus and triceps.

Hot packs are applied promptly to treated regions.

13. INJECTION AND STRETCH
(Fig. 36.5)

With the patient in the same position as for examination, the 22-gauge, 3.8-cm (1½-in) needle is directed proximally into the TP just lateral to the attachment of the biceps brachii tendon, where maximum tenderness is found on palpation (Fig. 36.5); it is difficult to see or feel a local twitch response. When the hand is supinated, the deep radial nerve passes through the muscle lateral to this TP area (Fig. 36.2 B and C) and, thus, is not usually encountered during TP injection.

An injection that misses the TP may aggravate referred pain instead of relieving it. Therefore, it is wise to probe the tender area thoroughly, searching for all TPs in this thin muscle. No tenderness should remain after the injection.

Injection is followed promptly by stretch and spray to restore full normal muscle length. The elbow area is then rewarmed with a hot pack. The injection and stretch are repeated in a few days, as necessary.

To assess the effect of the solution injected, 95 patients with "tennis elbow" were injected in the area of pain and tenderness (not specifically supinator TPs) in a double-blind experiment with one of three solutions. Ninety-two percent of those injected with 1 ml of methylprednisolone acetonide, 20% of those injected with 1% Xylocaine, and 24% of those injected with 0.9% saline were either cured or improved.[8] Thus, the corticosteroid was much more effective. In other studies, injection of the most tender point with corticosteroid and lidocaine together was effective in more than half of 202 cases of "tennis elbow"[3]; injection of triamcinolone acetate alone afforded relief in 66% of patients.[26]

Effective elimination of TP activity by injection with a local anesthetic or saline requires precise targeting of the TPs so that needle contact elicits a local twitch response or a clear pattern of referred pain. In agreement with the above studies, it has been the authors' experience that a corticosteroid can be helpful if the injection of TPs is imprecise. The steroid may relieve the pain because it is absorbed and produces systemic effects. With needle penetration of the TPs, we see no advantage in the use of the steroid in the injection solution, except for a few cases that are refractory to our usual therapeutic approach. These TPs may have progressed well into the dystrophic phase. If a more general steroid effect is desired, the medication may be given by mouth.

Surgery of varying extensiveness for "tennis elbow" is reported enthusiastically, including excision of the proximal attachment of the extensor carpi radialis brevis,[27] a medio-lateral incision to the bone in the tender area through a stab wound,[25] division of the deep fascia that covers the extensor group of muscles distal to the epicondyle,[30] surgical release of the common origin of the radial hand extensors,[32] and extensive removal of tendinous and joint tissue in the painful area.[5] The common denominator of these surgical ap-

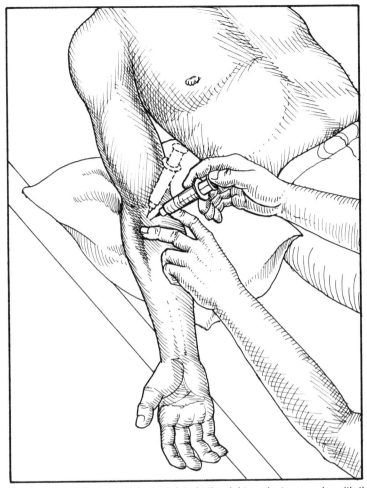

Figure 36.5.   Injection of trigger points in the right supinator muscle, with the brachioradialis pushed aside. The primary drawing shows the syringe position for injecting the usual trigger point in this muscle. The ghosted syringe (*dashed lines*) shows the approach for the more lateral and proximal trigger point location below the arcade of Frohse near the deep radial nerve.

PART 3

proaches is release of hand, and sometimes finger extensor tendons, which are described as showing structural changes characteristic of mechanical stress. In the opinion of the authors of this Manual, the taut bands caused by TPs in the forearm extensor muscles place a chronic strain on their tendinous attachments at the lateral epicondyle that could result in the structural changes described. Inactivation of the responsible TPs would seem to be a simpler initial approach than surgery, and is often effective.

"Tennis elbow" syndromes also have been treated with acupuncture at motor points.[16] To the extent that the acupuncture needles impale TPs, they should be

effective. Dry needling TPs is helpful, but probably less effective than needling them with 0.5% procaine solution and more painful to the patient.[41]

14. CORRECTIVE ACTIONS
(Figs. 36.6 and 36.7)

Tennis players should keep the wrist slightly dorsiflexed and the elbow slightly bent (Fig. 36.6A). Allowing the head of the racquet to drop (Fig. 36.6B) reduces grip strength. With slight dorsiflexion and no ulnar deviation of the hand at the wrist, the increase in strength protects the supinator from mis-hit overload and is easily demonstrated on a grip-strength meter.

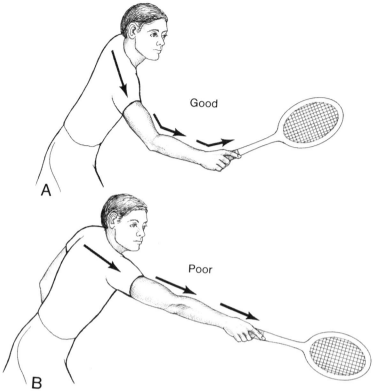

Figure 36.6.   Use and misuse of the tennis racquet (backhand stroke). *A*, good position. The elbow is slightly bent and the wrist cocked to raise the head of the racquet. *B*, poor position. The elbow is straight and the wrist dropped, which overloads the supinator muscle during supination at the end of the stroke and weakens the grip.

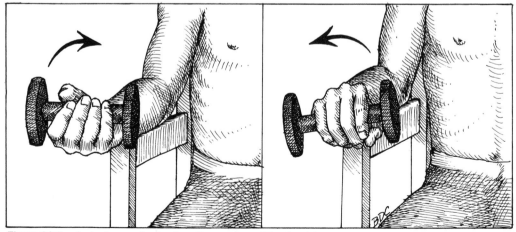

Figure 36.7.   Isotonic exercise to strengthen and condition the right supinator muscle. The hand is alternately supinated (*left*) and pronated (*right*) while holding a weight, which is increased progressively as strength improves.

Slight dorsiflexion places the forearm flexors at some mechanical advantage. Ulnar deviation places the ring and little finger flexors at a mechanical disadvantage. The bent elbow insures biceps assistance in supination and helps to prevent supinator overload.

If the player still has difficulty with the racket slipping in the hand because the grip is weak, the size of the racquet handle should be reduced so that the fingers wrap fully around it. Otherwise, the extensors, especially those of the ring and little fingers, which are essential for a strong grip, again function at a disadvantage. A weak grip permits the racquet to turn in the hand when the ball is mis-hit off-center, causing sudden muscle strain. The additional effort required to keep a tight grip on a large handle further strains the finger extensors.

Elbow pain often begins when a person gets a new racquet that is too heavy, that has a larger handle, or is unbalanced with too heavy a head. The position of the grip on the racquet may be shortened to reduce the length of the lever arm against which the forearm muscles must operate. The two-handed backhand stroke protects the supinator by preventing complete elbow extension during the stroke.

Tennis players with this elbow problem should not play on consecutive days, but should rest the supinator muscle until the postexercise soreness from overuse has worn off, usually in a day or two.

A snug figure-8 elastic support may be worn that encompasses the muscles just above and below the elbow, but leaves an opening for the olecranon process. It is sold in sporting goods and some drug stores, and may be worn during tennis, gardening, etc. This provides supporting counter pressure over the supinator and other vulnerable elbow muscles, and discourages full elbow extension.

A patient with "briefcase elbow" may find it better to carry the briefcase tucked under the arm with the elbow bent, and should avoid flipping the briefcase onto the desk; it should be placed there in two steps: (1) lift it on top of the desk and (2) with *two* hands, lay it flat for opening.

For some activities, wrist-rotation stress may be avoided temporarily by using the other hand or by using the affected hand differently. Instead of wringing washed clothes, they may be pressed against the bottom of the sink to drain the water from them. Raking leaves and walking a large dog pulling on a leash should be discontinued. If shaking hands in a receiving line is unavoidable, the right and left hands are alternated from person to person, reaching across with the opposite arm to the next guest in line; the hand is presented with the *palm up* to gracefully avoid a friendly crushing hand grip.

The patient with supinator TPs should learn to carry packages with the hands supinated (Fig. 36.3A), rather than pronated (36.3C); this substitutes the biceps for the supinator as an assistant to the brachialis to flex the elbow when lifting loads. The biceps is much stronger than the supinator for this purpose.

For a strengthening and conditioning isotonic exercise, the hand is alternately supinated and pronated, holding a weight (Fig. 36.7). A progressive program increases the weight of the object as strength improves. This exercise is started after the elbow pain and soreness have subsided. It increases the supinator's tolerance to activity.

References

1. Bardeen CR: The musculature, Sect. 5. In *Morris's Human Anatomy*, edited by C.M. Jackson, Ed. 6. Blakiston's Son & Co., Philadelphia, 1921 (p. 426).
2. Basmajian JV: *Muscles Alive*, Ed. 4. Williams & Wilkins, Baltimore, 1978 (pp. 207–210, 213, 217).
3. Bernhang AM: The many causes of tennis elbow. NY State J Med 79:1363–1366, 1979.
4. Blom S, Hele P, Parkman L: The supinator channel syndrome. *Scand J Plast Reconstr Surg* 5:71–73, 1971 (Case 2).
5. Bowden BW: Tennis elbow. *JAOA* 78:97–98, 101–102, 1978.
6. Carter BL, Morehead J, Wolpert SM, *et al.*: *Cross-Sectional Anatomy.* Appleton-Century-Crofts, New York, 1977 (Sects. 54, 55).
7. Cyriax J: *Textbook of Orthopaedic Medicine*, Ed. 5, Vol. 1. Williams & Wilkins, Baltimore, 1969 (pp. 312–316).
8. Day BH, Govindasamy N, Patnaik R: Corticosteroid injections in the treatment of tennis elbow. *Practitioner* 220:459–462, 1978.
9. Duchenne GB: *Physiology of Motion*, translated by E.B. Kaplan. J.B. Lippincott, Philadelphia, 1949 (pp. 99, 100).
10. Goldman S, Honet JC, Sobel R, *et al.*: Posterior interosseous nerve palsy in the absence of trauma. *Arch Neurol* 21:435–441, 1969.
11. Grant JCB: *An Atlas of Human Anatomy*, Ed. 7. Williams & Wilkins, Baltimore, 1978 (Fig. 6-93).
12. *Ibid.* (Fig. 6-70).

PART 3

13. Gray H: *Anatomy of the Human Body*, edited by C.M. Goss, American Ed. 29. Lea & Febiger, Philadelphia, 1973 (p. 471).

14. *Ibid.* (pp. 470, 471).

15. Gunn CC, Milbrandt WE: Tennis elbow and the cervical spine. *Can Med Assoc J* 114:803–809, 1976.

16. Gunn CC, Milbrandt WE: Tennis elbow and acupuncture. *Am J Acupunc* 5:61–66, 1977.

17. Hagert C-G, Lundborg G, Hansen T: Entrapment of the posterior interosseous nerve. *Scand J Plast Reconstr Surg* 11:205–212, 1977.

18. Hollinshead WH: *Functional Anatomy of the Limbs and Back*, Ed. 4. W.B. Saunders, Philadelphia, 1976 (p. 164).

19. Kelly M: Pain in the forearm and hand due to muscular lesions. *Med J Aust* 2:185–188, 1944 (Cases 1 and 4).

20. Kelly M: The nature of fibrositis. I. The myalgic lesion and its secondary effects: a reflex theory. *Ann Rheum Dis* 5:1–7, 1945 (p. 3, Case 1).

21. Lafreniere JG: "Tennis elbow" evaluation, treatment, and prevention. *Phys Ther* 59:742–746, 1979.

22. Lister GD, Belsole RB, Kleinert HE: The radial tunnel syndrome. *J Hand Surg* 4:52–59, 1979.

23. McMinn RMH, Hutchings RT: *Color Atlas of Human Anatomy*. Year Book Medical Publishers, Chicago, 1977 (p. 128).

24. *Ibid.* (p. 129).

25. Murtagh JE: Tennis elbow: description and treatment. *Aust Fam Physician* 7:1307–1310, 1978.

26. Nevelös AB: The treatment of tennis elbow with triamcinolone acetonide. *Curr Med Res Opin* 6:507–509, 1980.

27. Nirschl RP, Pettrone FA: Tennis elbow: the surgical treatment of lateral epicondylitis. *J Bone Joint Surg* 61-A:832–839, 1979.

28. Pernkopf E: *Atlas of Topographical and Applied Human Anatomy*, Vol. 2. W.B. Saunders, Philadelphia, 1964 (Fig. 79).

29. *Ibid.* (Fig. 81).

30. Posch JN, Goldberg VM, Larrey R: Extensor fasciotomy for tennis elbow: a long-term follow-up study. *Clin Orthop* 135:179–182, 1978.

31. Rasch PJ, Burke RK: *Kinesiology and Applied Anatomy*, Ed. 6. Lea & Febiger, Philadelphia, 1978 (p. 187).

32. Rosen MJ, Duffy FP, Miller EH, *et al.*: Tennis elbow syndrome: results of the "lateral release" procedure. *Ohio State Med J* 76:103–109, 1980.

33. Simons DG, Travell JG: Unpublished data, 1979.

34. Sobotta J, Figge FHJ: *Atlas of Human Anatomy*, Ed. 9, Vol. 1. Hafner Division of Macmillan, New York, 1974 (p. 208).

35. Sobotta J, Figge FHJ: *Atlas of Human Anatomy*, Ed. 9, Vol. 3. Hafner Division of Macmillan, New York, 1974 (p. 299).

36. Spinner M: *Injuries to the Major Branches of Peripheral Nerves of the Forearm*, Ed. 2. W.B. Saunders, Philadelphia, 1978 (pp. 80–94).

37. Toldt C: *An Atlas of Human Anatomy*, translated by M.E. Paul, Ed. 2, Vol. 1. Macmillan, New York, 1919 (p. 324).

38. *Ibid.* (p. 328).

39. *Ibid.* (pp. 321, 327).

40. Travell J: Basis for the multiple uses of local block of somatic trigger areas (procaine infiltration and ethyl chloride spray). *Miss Valley Med J* 71:12–21, 1949 (p. 18, Fig. 4).

41. Travell J: Pain mechanisms in connective tissue. In *Connective Tissues, Transactions of the Second Conference, 1951*, edited by C. Ragan. Josiah Macy, Jr. Foundation, New York, 1952 (p. 117).

42. Travell J, Rinzler SH: The myofascial genesis of pain. *Postgrad Med* 11:425–434, 1952 (p. 428, Fig. 6).

43. Travill A, Basmajian JV: Electromyography of the supinators of the forearm. *Anat Rec* 139:557–560, 1961.

44. Van Rossum J, Buruma OJS, Kamphuisen HAC, *et al.*: Tennis elbow—a radial tunnel syndrome? *J Bone Joint Surg* 60-B:197–198, 1978.

CHAPTER 37

Palmaris Longus Muscle

"Dupuytren's Contracture"

HIGHLIGHTS: **REFERRED PAIN** is felt as a distinctive, prickling, needle-like sensation over the palm. Tenderness of the palm and the progression of contracture are frequently relieved when trigger points (TPs) in the palmaris longus are inactivated. **ANATOMICAL ATTACHMENTS** of this muscle are the medial epicondyle of the humerus and the palmar fascia. **ACTIONS** are chiefly to cup the palm and assist flexion of the hand at the wrist. **SYMPTOMS** are pain and tenderness in the palm that interfere with the use of tools. Contracture of the palmar fascia also may be present. **ACTIVATION OF TRIGGER POINTS** is initiated by direct trauma to the palm, and excessive use of the grasping function of the hand. **ASSOCIATED TRIGGER POINTS** in the wrist and finger flexor muscles should be inactivated. **STRETCH AND SPRAY** of the muscle are accomplished by strongly extending the fingers and the hand at the wrist while applying the spray in a distal pattern. This treatment can be effectively supplemented with ischemic compression of the palmaris longus TPs. **INJECTION AND STRETCH** are relatively simple, when using flat palpation to localize the TPs. **CORRECTIVE ACTIONS** entail the avoidance of activities that overload the palmar cupping function, or that traumatize the palm.

---

1. REFERRED PAIN
(Fig. 37.1)

Like another muscle, the platysma, which also acts primarily on cutaneous tissue, the trigger points (TPs) in the palmaris longus refer a superficial, needle-like prickling pain, rather than the deep aching pain of most other muscles. The referred pain pattern (Fig. 37.1) centers in the palm. It extends to the base of the thumb and to the distal crease of the palm, but not into the digits. The prickling sensation feels as if produced by many fine needles. The spillover pattern may extend to the distal volar forearm.

2. ANATOMICAL ATTACHMENTS
(Fig. 37.2)

The palmaris longus arises **above** chiefly from the medial epicondyle of the humerus, and inserts **below** into the triangular palmar aponeurosis and the transverse carpal ligament (Fig. 37.2). At the wrist, its tendon passes superficial to the flexor retinaculum; the tendon stands out clearly when the hand is actively flexed and the palm cupped.

Normally, the palmaris longus is a slender fusiform muscle with its belly located in the proximal third of the forearm between the flexor carpi radialis and the flexor carpi ulnaris muscles. It overlies the flexor digitorum sublimis.

However, it is anatomically highly variable. Variations include congenital absence (often bilateral), a distally placed muscle belly, a double-bellied muscle, and a distally placed anomalous muscle that shows a variety of attachments.[10, 22] The incidence of total absence ranges from 12.7%–20.4% in studies of occidental and black persons, but only from 2.2%–3.4% in Orientals. Bilateral absence is nearly twice as common as the absence of just one muscle. Either the right or left muscle is equally likely to be missing.[22] Absence is slightly more common in females than

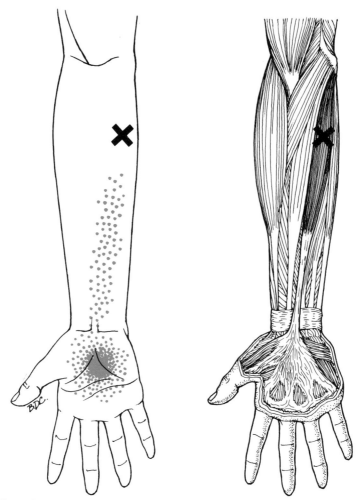

Figure 37.1.   Referred sensation pattern (*dark red*) arising from a trigger point (×) in the right palmaris longus muscle (*light red*). The referred sensation is described as a superficial painful prickle, rather than an aching pain. The belly of this variable muscle, and therefore its trigger points, may lie higher or lower in the forearm.

males and in whites than blacks. It may be inherited as a sex-linked dominant trait.[22] Anomalies other than absence occur in approximately 9% of individuals.

The palmar aponeurosis comprises two layers. A superficial layer of longitudinal fibers extends directly from the palmaris longus tendon at the wrist to the fingers. There, the fibers fan out in bundles to cover the flexor tendons of each finger and often of the thumb. Some of the superficial fibers attach to the skin of the flexor crease at the base of the fingers. Others continue into the digits to merge with the digital sheaths. The rest of the distal superficial fibers arch as bands between each metacarpal bone and the overlying transverse

metacarpal ligament to form a tunnel over the head of each metacarpal bone.[10] The deep layer, which consists mainly of transverse fibers, blends with the transverse metacarpal and transverse palmar ligaments. The fibers of the two layers of aponeurosis intertwine.

Two cases of what appeared to be carpal tunnel syndrome were found to have a variation of the palmaris longus in which the tendon passed beneath, rather than above, the volar carpal ligament.[4] Three other cases proved to have anomalous distal bellies of the palmaris longus which compressed the median nerve against the underlying tendons.[1] All were relieved by surgical decompression.

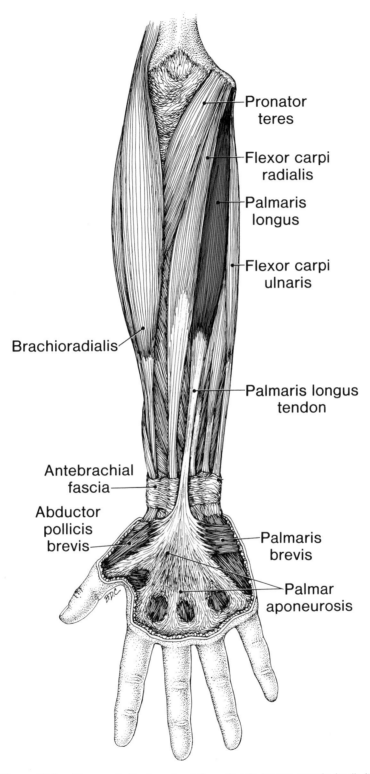

Figure 37.2. The usual attachments of the palmaris longus muscle (*red*). It originates at the medial epicondyle, and attaches distally to the palmar aponeurosis. The superficial layer of the palmar aponeurosis has fibrous bands that extend into the fingers and often to the thumb.

PART 3

Supplemental References

A number of authors have illustrated the palmaris longus muscle from the volar view,[8, 14, 16, 18, 24, 26, 28] and others in cross section.[5, 7, 20] Some have detailed its palmar fascial attachments,[17, 19, 25, 27] and many of its variations.[9, 22]

3. INNERVATION

The palmaris longus muscle is supplied by a branch of the median nerve from the lateral cord, through the anterior secondary divisions, the upper and middle trunks of the brachial plexus, and either spinal roots C_6 and C_7,[10, 21] roots C_7 and C_8 (the usual arrangement),[11, 13] or C_7, C_8 and T_1.[26] The nerve to the palmaris longus muscle also is variable; it may penetrate the flexor carpi radialis muscle,[11] or the superficial fibers of the flexor digitorum sublimis muscle.[2]

4. ACTIONS

This muscle functions to flex the hand at the wrist and to tense the palmar fascia. It probably assists pronation of the hand against resistance, and may assist flexion of the forearm at the elbow.

Duchenne,[6] upon stimulation of the palmaris longus, observed only hand flexion without pronation or deviation of the hand to either side. Authors have consistently noted this flexor function.[2, 3, 10–13, 21]

Two authors[13, 21] reported that the muscle tensed the fascia of the palm, which, anatomically, should be its primary function.

Beevor[3] observed that the palmaris longus contracted with the flexor carpi radialis as the hand was pronated against resistance; others agreed with this pronator function.[2, 12, 13] Because of the muscle's attachment to the medial epicondyle of the humerus, some authors propose a possible weak, flexor action at the elbow.[2, 13]

5. MYOTATIC UNIT

The palmaris longus has no antagonistic muscle. The thenar and hypothenar muscles are synergistic with it by helping to cup the hand but, of these, only the palmaris brevis also attaches to the subcutaneous palmar fascia.

6. SYMPTOMS

In addition to pain, as described in Section 1, patients complain of difficulty in handling tools because of soreness and tenderness in the palm; they frequently call attention to tender nodules there. The pressure of working with the handle of a screwdriver or trowel in the palm becomes intolerably painful. For instance, a sculptor was unable to pound his chisel with his palm to chip marble.

Advanced cases may exhibit palmar contracture. In 2278 cases of Dupuytren's contracture, over half had contractures in both hands, 29% in the right hand only, and 16% in the left hand only. The male:female prevalence was reported as 6:1[23] and 8:1.[15]

7. ACTIVATION OF TRIGGER POINTS

Myofascial TPs in the palmaris longus muscle tend to develop as satellites of primary TPs in the distal medial head of the triceps brachii muscle, which refer pain to the region of the palmaris longus (see TP_5, Fig. 32.1C).

Myofascial TPs in the palmaris longus also may be activated by direct trauma, as by a fall on the hand. Use of a tool forcibly pressed or held firmly in the cupped palm can aggravate, and may initiate, TP activity in the palmaris longus muscle. Examples are gardening and using a screwdriver or other carpenter's tool. Holding a tennis racquet with the end of the handle against the palm, and leaning on a cane with an angular, rather than a round, handle pressing into the palm also may activate or perpetuate TPs in this muscle.

Dupuytren's Contracture

In our experience, patients with Dupuytren's contracture consistently have one or more active TPs in the fibers of the palmaris longus muscle.

Authors agree that heredity is a factor in the development of the contracture,[15, 23] but have become increasingly negative toward repeated trauma as a primary cause.[15, 23] Patients, on the other hand, tend to make the latter association because of the referred palmar tenderness. Contracture is more likely to be encountered in those who do not perform regular manual labor than in those who do.[15] The novice worker is apt to maintain the palm in the tightly cupped position for longer periods while holding a tool; the skilled craftsman does not.

The prevalence of Dupuytren's contracture is reported to rise sharply in the 4th decade; it is higher in patients with alcoholism, epilepsy and diabetes mellitus. The condition may be associated with increased sympathetic tone, and frequently also with the reflex sympathetic dystrophy of the shoulder-hand syndrome.[23]

Initially, tender nodular thickenings usually appear on the ulnar side of the palm, short of the distal palmar crease. The nodules develop within the fibrofatty tissue superficial to the palmar aponeurosis.[23] Next, fibrous bands extend centrifugally from these nodules.[15, 23] Finally, the palmar aponeurosis develops non-tender, contracted, dense fibrous bands which hold the fingers flexed, crippling the hand. These stages usually overlap, and progression may stop at any point.[23]

8. PATIENT EXAMINATION

The patient cups the hand (as in Fig. 37.3 in Section 9) to make the tendon stand out at the wrist, superficial to the transverse carpal ligament. To the examiner, this verifies the existence of the palmaris longus muscle, and helps the patient to see and feel the relationship between the fibrotic palmar fascia and the palmaris longus muscle.

A TP in the superficial palmaris longus is located in the proximal half of the muscle belly (Fig. 37.1). Palpation of the palm that is developing Dupuytren's contracture reveals discretely tender nodules with a background of diffuse referred palmar tenderness, which is the usual "soreness" in response to pressure; only the TP-referred sensation has a prickling quality.

9. TRIGGER POINT EXAMINATION
(Fig. 37.3)

An active TP in this muscle is located in a palpable band that can be rolled back and forth between two fingers, as shown in Figure 37.3. The tender TP usually responds with a local twitch response. Stimulation of this TP by pressure often elicits

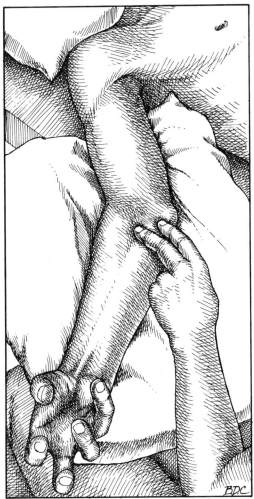

Figure 37.3. The strongly cupped hand illustrates a major function of the palmaris longus muscle. The active contraction makes its superficial tendon stand out at the wrist. The region of the muscle belly that is likely to contain an active trigger point lies between the two examining fingers.

the projection of referred pain in the pattern described in Section 1. However, if intense *spontaneous* pain is present due to maximal hyperactivity of this TP, its further stimulation by digital pressure cannot increase the already maximum referred pain. In this case, the examiner may erroneously assume that the tender spot in the palmaris longus is not related to the pain.

10. ENTRAPMENTS

No nerve entrapments have been observed due to TPs in this muscle.

PART 3

11. ASSOCIATED TRIGGER POINTS

Active TPs in the palmaris longus are frequently associated with TPs in the hand and finger flexors. However, the palmaris TPs are rarely associated with TPs in the muscles that refer pain to the elbow, as in "tennis elbow," or with the carpal tunnel syndrome.

12. STRETCH AND SPRAY
(Fig. 37.4)

The patient is seated with the forearm of the affected side supported on a padded surface. The fingers and hand are extended (Fig. 37.4), while parallel sweeps of the vapocoolant spray are applied in a distal direction over the muscle and palm. Extending the forearm at the elbow may add to the passive stretch.

Applications of the stretch-and-spray technique may be alternated with ischemic compression to inactivate palmaris longus TPs; these TPs generally respond well to ischemic compression.

After this muscle is stretched and sprayed, or its TPs injected, the entire group of forearm flexor muscles, particularly the hand and finger flexors, is then stretched and sprayed to eliminate any associated TP involvement of parallel muscles. After inactivation of the palmaris longus TPs, mild to moderate contractures of the palmar fascia may be stretched by firmly and regularly extending the fingers and palm under hot water, or while applying 2–3 watts/cm^2 of ultrasound.[23]

With inactivation of TPs in the palmaris longus muscle, the referred tenderness of the nodules and palm usually disappears immediately. The further the fibrotic contracture has progressed, the greater the likelihood that local tenderness will persist after TP inactivation.

13. INJECTION AND STRETCH
(Fig. 37.5)

The patient lies supine with the elbow extended on the affected side. After locating any TPs in the palmaris longus by palpation (Fig. 37.3), the area of each TP is probed and injected with 0.5% procaine solution (Fig. 37.5). Immediately after the TP injection, passive stretching of the muscles is carried out, usually again with vapocooling, and a hot pack is then applied. Restoration of full muscle length relieves the prickling palmar pain and releases the sustained tension that the taut muscle fibers placed on the palmar aponeurosis.

Troublesome palmar nodules that remain after inactivation of palmaris longus

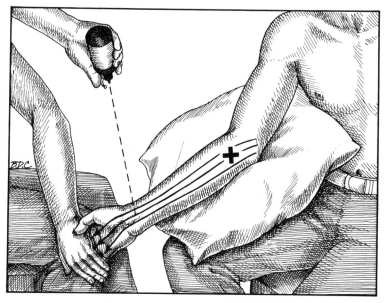

Figure 37.4. Stretch position and spray pattern (*arrows*) for the palmaris longus muscle. To fully stretch the muscle, the operator simultaneously extends both the patient's fingers and the hand at the wrist as far as tolerable.

Any TPs in the triceps brachii muscle should be inactivated, particularly if they refer pain to the medial epicondylar region of the palmaris longus muscle, where they can establish and perpetuate satellite TPs.

The patient should self-stretch the palmar fascia and palmaris longus muscle in a hot bath or shower, using the stretch position shown (Fig. 37.4).

References

1. Backhouse KM, Churchill-Davidson D: Anomalous palmaris longus muscle producing carpal tunnel-like compression. *Hand* 7:22–24, 1975.
2. Bardeen CR: The musculature, Sect. 5. In *Morris's Human Anatomy*, edited by C.M. Jackson, Ed. 6. Blakiston's Son & Co., Philadelphia, 1921 (p. 432).
3. Beevor CE: Muscular movements and their representation in the central nervous system. *Lancet* 1:1715–1724, 1903 (pp. 1718, 1719).
4. Brones MF, Wilgis EFS: Anatomical variations of the *palmaris longus*, causing carpal tunnel syndrome. *Plast Reconstr Surg* 62:798–800, 1978.
5. Carter BL, Morehead J, Wolpert SM, *et al.: Cross-Sectional Anatomy.* Appleton-Century-Crofts, New York, 1977 (Sects. 53–59).
6. Duchenne GB: *Physiology of Motion*, translated by E.B. Kaplan. J.B. Lippincott, Philadelphia, 1949 (p. 120).
7. Grant JCB: *An Atlas of Human Anatomy*, Ed. 7. Williams & Wilkins, Baltimore, 1978 (Fig. 6-72).
8. *Ibid.* (Fig. 6-67).
9. *Ibid.* (Figs. 6-66, 6-124).
10. Gray H: *Anatomy of the Human Body*, edited by C.M. Goss, American Ed. 29. Lea & Febiger, Philadelphia, 1973 (pp. 463, 476).
11. Hollinshead WH: *Anatomy for Surgeons*, Ed. 2, Vol. 3, *The Back and Limbs*. Harper & Row, New York, 1969 (p. 403).
12. Hollinshead WH: *Functional Anatomy of the Limbs and Back*, Ed. 4. W.B. Saunders, Philadelphia, 1976 (p. 151).
13. Kendall HO, Kendall FP, Wadsworth GE: *Muscles, Testing and Function*, Ed. 2. Williams & Wilkins, Baltimore, 1971 (p. 85).
14. Langman J, Woerdeman MW: *Atlas of Medical Anatomy*. W.B. Saunders, Philadelphia, 1978 (p. 241).
15. Larsen RD, Posch JL: Dupuytren's contracture with special reference to pathology. *J Bone Joint Surg* 40-A:773–793, 1958 (pp. 773, 774).
16. McMinn RMH, Hutchings RT: *Color Atlas of Human Anatomy*. Year Book Medical Publishers, Chicago, 1977 (p. 124).
17. *Ibid.* (pp. 131, 132).
18. Pernkopf E: *Atlas of Topographical and Applied Human Anatomy*, Vol. 2. W.B. Saunders, Philadelphia, 1964 (Fig. 75).
19. *Ibid.* (Fig. 84).
20. *Ibid.* (Figs. 82, 83).
21. Rasch PJ, Burke RK: *Kinesiology and Applied Anatomy*, Ed. 6. Lea & Febiger, Philadelphia, 1978 (pp. 197, 199).
22. Reimann AF, Daseler EH, Anson BJ, Beaton LE: The palmaris longus muscle and tendon. A study

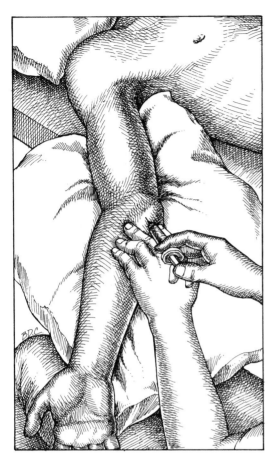

Figure 37.5. Injection of a trigger point in the palmaris longus muscle with the patient supine, the forearm extended and well supported.

TPs are likely to resolve more rapidly if each is injected with about 0.3 ml of a soluble steroid, such as dexamethasone sodium phosphate, solution mixed with sufficient 2% procaine solution to make its concentration 0.5%. Sigler[23] recommended the injection of a steroid only in the early stages of the nodules.

This treatment may stop the progression of fibrosis, but cannot reverse advanced palmar contracture. Surgical recommendations range from simple cutaneous fasciotomy and nodule excision to limited fasciotomy; radical fasciotomy is rarely, if ever, indicated.[23]

14. CORRECTIVE ACTIONS

The patient must avoid such activities as those listed in Section 7, which activate TPs in the palmaris longus muscle.

of 1600 extremities. *Anat Rec* 89:495–505, 1944.

23. Sigler JW: Dupuytren's contracture, Chapter 81. In *Arthritis and Allied Conditions*, edited by J.E. Hollander, D.J. McCarty, Jr., Ed. 8. Lea & Febiger, Philadelphia, 1972 (pp. 1503–1510).

24. Sobotta J, Figge FHJ: *Atlas of Human Anatomy*, Ed. 9. Vol. 1. Hafner Division of Macmillan, New York, 1974 (pp. 199, 202).

25. *Ibid.* (pp. 213, 223).

26. Spalteholz W: *Handatlas der Anatomie des Menschen*, Ed. 11, Vol. 2. S. Hirzel, Leipzig, 1922 (p. 325).

27. *Ibid.* (p. 335).

28. Toldt C: *An Atlas of Human Anatomy*, translated by M.E. Paul, Ed. 2, Vol. 1. Macmillan, New York, 1919 (p. 322).

CHAPTER 38

Hand and Finger Flexors in the Forearm

Flexores Carpi Radialis and Ulnaris, Flexores Digitorum Superficialis and Profundus, Flexor Pollicis Longus (Pronator Teres)

"Lightning Pain" and "Trigger Finger"

HIGHLIGHTS: **REFERRED PAIN** from each finger flexor is experienced throughout the length of the digit which it flexes. Pain may be projected "beyond" the tip of the digit like a bolt of lightning. Trigger points (TPs) in the hand flexors refer pain that centers on the volar wrist crease. A trigger finger is an annoying, but painless dysfunction that appears to be caused by restriction of the flexor tendon and is relieved by procaine injection into the tender point beneath the tendon just proximal to the corresponding metacarpal head. **ANATOMICAL ATTACHMENTS** of the finger flexors are to the medial epicondyle and to the middle and terminal phalanges of each finger. The flexors of the hand also arise from the medial epicondyle. The flexor carpi ulnaris inserts on the pisiform bone, and the flexor carpi radialis inserts on the bases of the second and third metacarpal bones. **ACTION** of the hand flexors is to flex the hand at the wrist; the finger flexors flex the hand and both the distal and middle phalanges. The **MYOTATIC UNIT** of the finger flexors includes the finger extensors, contraction of which is required for effective grasp. **SYMPTOMS** include

pain on forceful use of scissors and when cupping and supinating the hand to receive coins scooped into it. **ACTIVATION OF TRIGGER POINTS** results from repetitive or prolonged strong gripping, or repeated strenuous twisting and pulling movements with the fingers. **PATIENT EXAMINATION** causes pain to be projected to the end of the finger tips when the finger and hand flexors are passively stretched simultaneously. **ENTRAPMENT** of the ulnar nerve near the elbow may be aggravated by TPs in the proximal end of the flexor digitorum superficialis. **STRETCH AND SPRAY** are accomplished by fully extending the hand and fingers while applying the vapocoolant in a distal pattern. **INJECTION AND STRETCH** are often not required for TPs in the hand and finger flexor muscles, but are required to relieve a trigger finger or thumb. **CORRECTIVE ACTIONS** call for avoidance of prolonged, tight gripping, and the establishment of self-stretch habits by regular use of the Artisan's Finger-stretch, the Finger-extension, the Finger-spreading, or the Finger-flutter Exercises.

1. REFERRED PAIN
(Fig. 38.1)

The pain patterns presented in this chapter are based on a local twitch response to identify the muscle being in-

jected and the patient's report of the distribution of pain induced by needle penetration of the trigger point (TP).

Winter[54] described TPs in the flexors of the hand and fingers near their common attachment to the medial epicondyle as a

531

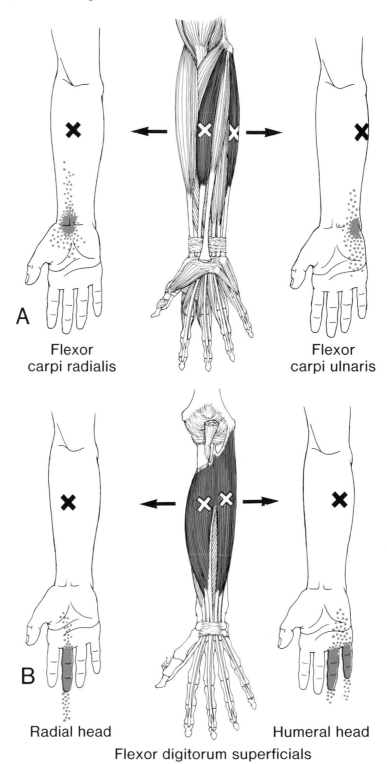

Figure 38.1 *A–D*. Composit referred pain patterns (*dark red*) and location of trigger points (×s) in the right hand and finger flexors (*medium red*). *A*, flexor carpi radialis and flexor carpi ulnaris. *B*, flexor digitorum superficialis and profundus: *left*—middle finger pattern; *right*—4th and 5th finger patterns. The index finger pattern, not shown, is comparable. *C*, flexor pollicis longus. *D*, pronator teres.

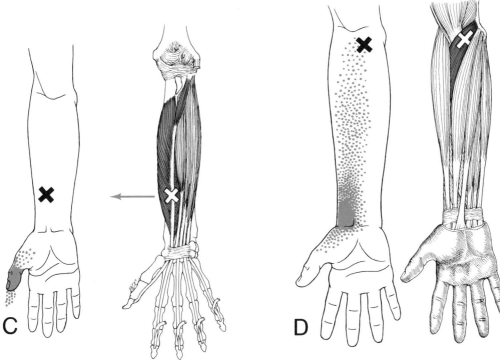

C Flexor pollicis longus   **D** Pronator teres

Figure 38.1 C and D.

frequent source of referred pain. Good[9] depicted the pain as projecting to the volar aspect of the wrist, or to the corresponding digit. Good[11] also attributed idiopathic myalgia of the elbow (comparable to myofascial pain) to referred pain from localized myalgic areas, some of which were in the flexors of the wrist and fingers. He relieved the symptoms by procaine injection of the myalgic spots (comparable to TPs).

Hand Flexors
(Fig. 38.1A)

An active TP in the flexor carpi radialis refers pain and tenderness that center in the radial aspect of the volar crease of the wrist, with some spillover into the adjacent forearm and palm (Fig. 38.1A, left).

An active TP in the flexor carpi ulnaris refers pain and tenderness to the ulnar side of the volar aspect of the wrist with similar spillover (Fig. 38.1A, right).

Finger Flexors
(Fig. 38.1B)

No distinction is made between the referred pain patterns of the flexores digitorum superficialis and profundus. A TP in these fibers refers pain to the same digit that the fibers activate. For example, a TP in the fibers of the middle finger flexor projects pain through the length of the middle finger (Fig. 38.1B, left); similarly, TPs in fibers that flex the ring and little fingers project pain throughout those digits (Fig. 38.1B, right). Pain is frequently described as an explosive pain that "shoots right out the end of the finger, like lightning." This pattern differs from the pain referred from the finger extensors, which stops short of the end of the digit. When patients with active TPs in the flexors are asked whether the pain is more on the top or underside of the finger, they are likely to rub the volar aspect and reply, "I don't know"; the movement reveals their answer.

Kellegren[23] reported that injection of 6% salt solution into the flexor digitorum profundus muscle produced metacarpophalangeal (MCP) joint pain that was indistinguishable from the pain caused by injecting 0.3 ml of the same solution directly into the same joint space of the opposite hand. The similar nature of the joint pain due to these two sources causes confusion between the pain of articular disease and that referred from myofascial TPs in the finger muscles.

Pain referred to the hypothenar eminence and the 5th knuckle (MCP joint), induced by injection of 0.2 ml of 6% salt solution into the flexor digitorum profundus muscle, persisted despite *total anesthesia* of the painful structures by local anesthetic block of the ulnar nerve at the wrist.[23] This observation is compatible with the convergence-projection mechanism of referred pain.[37] The referred pain in this experiment was not dependent on impulses arising in the pain reference zone; a significant part of the afferent nerve discharges caused by the irritant saline solution in the muscle, and of those perceived as pain from the reference area, must have followed a common pathway in the central nervous system. One might describe this as a phantom pain. (The pain referred to the hypothenar eminence may have been due to inadvertent saline infiltration of the flexor carpi ulnaris muscle as well.)

Long Thumb Flexor
(Fig. 38.1*C*)

When the flexor pollicis longus (Fig. 38.1*C*) harbors an active TP, it projects pain throughout the volar aspect of the thumb to its tip.

Pronator Teres
(Fig. 38.1*D*)

The pronator teres TPs refer pain deep in the volar radial region of the wrist and also of the forearm (Fig. 38.1*D*).

Trigger Finger

The painless phenomenon of a trigger finger, a "trick" or "locking" finger, consists of the finger sticking in the flexed position until it is extended by an external force. This condition responds to injection of a tendor spot deep in the fascial sheath, which is apparently responsible for the constriction of the flexor tendon at the MCP joint. The constriction may ensnare a knot-like enlargement of the tendon itself. Such a fascial band that might anchor the tendon is described just short of the end of the distal palmar synovial sheath for digits two, three and four[17]. The long

thumb flexor also may suffer this locking phenomenon (see Chapter 39).

2. ANATOMICAL ATTACHMENTS
(Fig. 38.2)

Hand Flexors
(Fig. 38.2A)

The **flexor carpi radialis** muscle is subcutaneous and nearly centered on the volar side of the forearm between the pronator teres, which crosses the forearm above it on the radial side and the palmaris longus, which tends to overlap it on the ulnar side (Fig. 38.2A). This radial hand flexor attaches *above* to the medial epicondyle *via* the common tendon and to intermuscular septa. The muscle belly extends only to the mid-forearm. Its tendon attaches *below* mainly onto the base of the second metacarpal bone, with a slip extending to the base of the third metacarpal bone.

The **flexor carpi ulnaris** muscle lies superficially along the volar side of the sharp edge of the ulna. *Proximally* it attaches by two heads: the humeral head attaches to the medial epicondyle of the humerus *via* the common tendon; the ulnar head fastens to the medial margin of the olecranon and to the proximal two-thirds of the dorsal border of the ulna through an aponeurosis shared in common with the extensor carpi ulnaris and flexor carpi profundus, and to intermuscular septa. *Distally* its tendon attaches to the pisiform bone.[17]

Finger Flexors
(Fig. 38.2 B and C)

Proximally the **flexor digitorum superficialis** (sublimis) comprises three heads: humeral, ulnar and radial (Fig. 38.2B). The humeral head attaches to the medial epicondyle of the humerus *via* the common tendon and to intermuscular septa; the ulnar head attaches to the medial side of the coronoid process of the ulna, proximal to the attachment of the pronator teres, beneath the humeral head; and the radial head attaches to the oblique line of the radius, between the attachments of the biceps brachii and pronator teres muscles. The median nerve passes beneath the fibrous archway between the attachments of the ulnar and radial heads.[42] This muscle covers most of the volar forearm, beneath the palmaris longus muscles and flexores carpi muscles (Fig. 38.2B).[17]

The tendons at the wrist, and to some extent the fibers of the flexor digitorum superficialis, lie in a deep and superficial plane. The superficial plane carries tendons to the middle and ring fingers, and the deep plane to the index and little fingers.

Distally at the first phalanx, each tendon of the **flexor digitorum superficialis** divides to pass around the deep tendon of the flexor profundus, as each superficialis tendon attaches to the sides of a middle phalanx.

The fibers of the **flexor digitorum profundus** (Fig. 38.2C) extend through the proximal half, on the ulnar side of the forearm. The muscle attaches *above* to the proximal three-fourths of the volar, medial and dorsal surfaces of the ulna; to an aponeurosis shared by the flexor and extensor carpi ulnaris; to the medial side of the coronoid process of the ulna; and to the ulnar half of the interosseous membrane. Each tendon fastens *below* onto the base of the terminal phalanx of the respective finger.[17]

The **flexor pollicis longus** (Fig. 38.2C) extends throughout most of the forearm, chiefly on the radial side. It attaches *proximally* to the radius and the adjacent interosseous membrane, and *distally* to the base of the distal phalanx of the thumb.[17] The belly of the flexor digitorum superficialis covers both the deep finger flexor and the long thumb flexor muscles.

The **pronator teres** attaches *above* and *medially* by two heads. The humeral head fastens proximal to the medial epicondyle and to adjacent fascia. The ulnar head fastens to the medial side of the coronoid process of the ulna, and the median nerve enters the forearm between these two heads. The muscle attaches *below* and *laterally* to the lateral surface of the radius at its midpoint in the forearm.

Supplemental References

The flexor carpi radialis has been well illustrated in the volar view,[12, 19, 28, 32, 40, 45, 50] and in cross section.[5, 15, 20, 33] The flexor carpi ulnaris has been shown in the volar view,[12, 13, 19, 28, 32, 39, 40, 45, 50] in the lateral view,[41] and in cross section.[6, 15, 20, 33]

The flexor digitorum sublimis has been clearly illustrated in the volar view,[13, 16, 18, 30, 32, 35, 39, 40, 42, 46, 49, 50, 53] and in cross section.[7, 15, 20, 33] The flexor digitorum profundus has been drawn in the volar view,[14, 16, 18, 21, 29, 30, 35, 39, 47, 53] and in cross section.[7, 15, 20, 33] The fibrous loop that restrains the flexor tendons at the point of constriction in the trigger finger also has been depicted.[31, 34, 43, 44, 51]

Other authors have illustrated the flexor pollicis longus in the volar view,[14, 18, 21, 28, 29, 32, 39, 40, 46, 47, 50, 52] and in cross section.[8, 15, 20]

The pronator teres is portrayed in volar view[12, 19, 28, 32, 40, 45, 47, 50] in relation to the median nerve,[42] and in cross section.[15, 33]

3. INNERVATION

Hand and Finger Flexors

Most of the flexor muscles in the forearm, including the flexor carpi radialis, flexor digitorum sublimis and flexor pollicis longus muscles, are supplied by the median nerve. However, the flexor carpi ulnaris and half of the flexor digitorum profundus are supplied by the ulnar nerve, and the other half, by the median nerve.

The flexor carpi radialis derives its innervation from spinal nerves C_6 and C_7; the flexor digitorum sublimis from C_7 and C_8; and the flexor carpi ulnaris, flexor digitorum profundus and flexor pollicis longus from C_8 and T_1.[17] Thus the lowest of these spinal segments innervate the deepest flexor muscles and those on the ulnar side of the forearm.

Pronator Teres

The pronator teres is supplied by a branch of the median nerve through spinal nerves C_6 and C_7.

4. ACTIONS

Hand Flexors

The flexor carpi radialis flexes the hand[17, 36] and assists abduction of the hand at the wrist.[36] The flexor carpi ulnaris flexes and strongly adducts the hand,[17, 36] and participates in finger-flexion movements.[38]

Finger Flexors

The flexor digitorum superficialis primarily flexes the middle phalanx of each

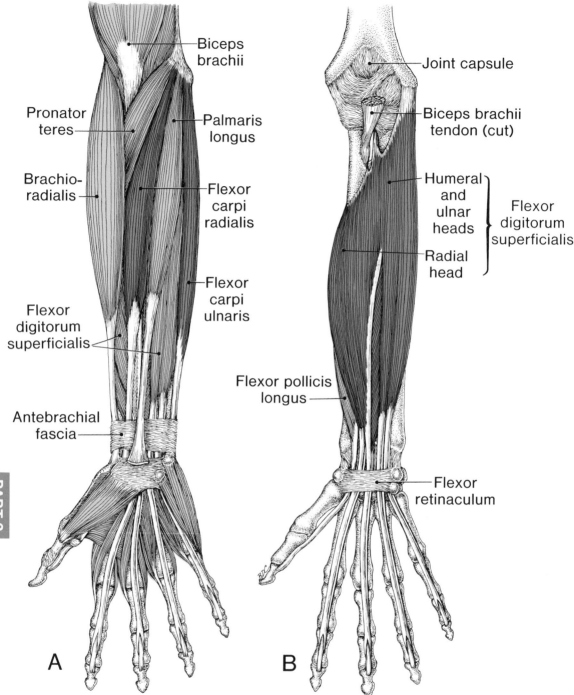

Figure 38.2 A–C. Volar view of the right upper extremity showing the attachments of the hand and finger flexors in the forearm. *A,* flexor carpi radialis and flexor carpi ulnaris are *dark red,* other muscles including the pronator teres are *medium red. B,* flexor digitorum superficialis (*dark red*). The ulnar head lies unseen beneath the humeral head. *C,* flexor digitorum profundus and flexor pollicis longus (*dark red*) and cut ends of flexor digitorum superficialis (light red).

finger, but also flexes the proximal phalanx, as well as the hand at the wrist.[17, 36]
The flexor digitorum profundus primar-

ily flexes the terminal phalanx of each
finger, and also all the other phalanges and
the hand.[17, 36] It is used not so much for

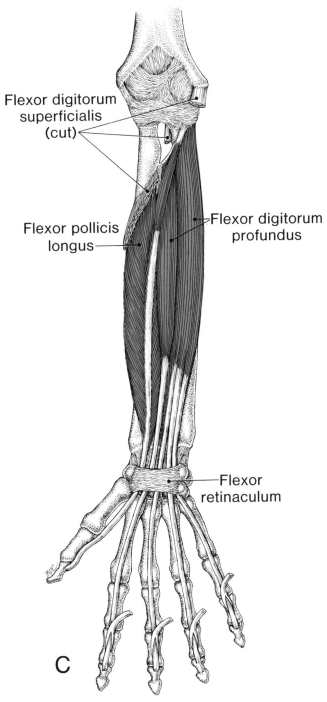

Flexor digitorum
superficialis
(cut)

Flexor pollicis
longus

Flexor digitorum
profundus

Flexor
retinaculum

C

Figure 38.2 C.

PART 3

wrist flexion, as for gross closure of the fist at all joints simultaneously.[1]

Long Thumb Flexor

The flexor pollicis longus initially flexes the terminal phalanx of the thumb, then the proximal phalanx with adduction of the metacarpal bone,[17] and eventually assists in flexion and abduction of the hand at the wrist.[36]

Pronator Teres

The pronator teres assists the pronator quadratus, the primary pronator, in fast movements and to overcome resistance. The pronator teres also assists flexion at the elbow, but only when resistance is offered.[2]

Activities

Motor unit activity of the hand and finger flexor muscles was monitored bilaterally with surface electrodes during 13 sports activities that included overhand throws, underhand throws, tennis, golf, hitting a baseball, and 1-ft jumps in basketball. Examination of the records showed moderate to strong activity, which was bilaterally similar in pattern, but of higher amplitude on the dominant right side, especially when the hand was gripping a handle.[3]

Lundervold[27] studied the electrical activity in the muscles of 135 subjects, 63 of whom had "occupational myalgia" (signs and symptoms including pain and muscle tenderness that strongly suggested TPs). He found that the symptomatic subjects were much more likely than pain-free subjects to show continuous, larger amplitude motor unit activity when striking a typewriter key repetitively with one finger. When muscular tenderness and pain involved the flexors in the forearm on one side only, typing with the *asymptomatic* arm greatly increased the sustained motor unit activity of these flexor muscles on the symptomatic side, which were "at rest." Subjects with symptoms also were more likely than normal subjects to respond to needle electrode insertion in the muscle with marked motor unit activity (muscle tension) that slowly subsided over a minute or more; normal subjects usually showed little or no such muscle-tension response. Symptomatic subjects were more likely than were pain-free subjects to respond to psychic stress (gruff commands), insufficient light, a cold draft, and to loud noise with increased and sustained motor unit activity. The motor units in the involved forearm flexor muscles were clearly more excitable, which would aggravate myofascial TP activity in those muscles.

5. MYOTATIC UNIT

Hand and Finger Flexors

All flexion movements of the fingers involve some activity of the extensor digi-

torum. When the fingers are held in extension at the interphalangeal joints, only the interossei and the lumbricales produce MCP flexion.[1]

During hand flexion at the wrist, the palmaris longus assists the finger and hand flexors.

For thumb flexion, the flexor pollicis brevis assists the flexor pollicis longus.

During flexion of the hand at the wrist, electromyographic records showed that only the extensor carpi radialis was an active antagonist.[1] In general, the hand and finger extensors function as described in Chapter 34.

Pronator Teres

The pronator teres assists the pronator quadratus. The brachioradialis may assist pronation from full supination (see Chapter 34).

6. SYMPTOMS

Hand and Finger Flexors

Patients with TPs in the flexor muscles of the forearm report difficulty in using scissors for cutting heavy cloth or for gardening, or in using tin shears. In contrast, patients with active TPs in the extensor forearm muscles and "tennis elbow" report no problem with the use of scissors.

Active TPs in the finger flexors interfere with the placement of curlers in the hair and with the insertion of bobby-pins into a bun at the back of the head.

Patients with active TPs in the pronator teres are likely to be unable to cup and supinate the hand when coins are scooped into it from a bureau. The combined motion of full supination, slight extension and cupping of the hand becomes prohibitively painful. These patients usually compensate by rotating the arm at the shoulder, thus overloading the shoulder muscles.

Active TPs in the finger extensors compromise finger flexion. Stiffness and painful cramping of the fingers prevented one patient from milking his cows, until the tender extensor digitorum muscle had been treated for its TPs.[24]

Trigger Finger

This phenomenon, also called "locking finger," is a painless but very annoying locking of the digit in the flexed position, despite a maximum active effort to extend the finger; the digit must be extended passively by an external force.

7. ACTIVATION OF TRIGGER POINTS

TPs in these hand and finger flexors are not aggravated by the fine pincer movements that tend to activate TPs in the intrinsic hand muscles, but rather by abuse of gross gripping movements. The skier who grips ski poles hard for long periods, and the carpenter who tightly grips small-handled tools are likely to activate these TPs.

The finger flexor muscles may develop active TPs as a result of driving a car with the fingers tightly gripping the steering wheel, especially when the hand grasps the top of the wheel so that the hand is flexed at the wrist. Symptoms are especially likely to occur after long, hard driving.

The passive-stretch position for treatment of the finger extensors, placing the fingers and hand in full flexion, can cause sudden shortening activation of latent TPs in the hand and finger flexors.

Activation of the flexor pollicis longus TP causes symptoms that may be termed "weeder's thumb." This results from forceful rocking, twisting and then pulling motions, all of which can strain this and other thumb muscles.

The pronator teres TP can be activated as the result of a fracture at the wrist or elbow.

The locking of a trigger finger appears to be due to a nodule in the tendon being caught by the constriction of the annular band that anchors the tendon sheath.[4] The precise mechanism that causes the nodule in the tendon is not clear. It may be a TP in the lumbrical muscle. One patient reactivated a trigger finger (middle digit) by the continuing use of a cane, the angled head of which pressed on the trigger-finger sore spot just proximal to the head of the third metacarpal bone.

8. PATIENT EXAMINATION
(Fig. 38.3)

When asked to fully supinate the hand with the fingers and hand extended, the patient may be unable to turn it beyond the mid-position if the finger flexors, the flexor carpi radialis, or the pronator teres are involved.

The patient does the Finger-extension Test by first placing the finger tips of the right and left hands together (Fig. 38.3 A), and then pushing the palms tightly against each other while bringing the forearms into as straight a line as possible (Fig. 38.3 B). Active TPs in the flexor muscles then are revealed by tightness and pain in the pain reference areas specific to the involved muscles (Section 1). Involvement of individual finger flexors can be tested by passive hyperextension of each digit in turn.

9. TRIGGER POINT EXAMINATION

The TPs in these flexor muscles are located in the proximal portions of the muscle bellies,[26] as shown in Figure 38.1. Both the flexor carpi radialis and ulnaris muscles are sufficiently superficial for their TPs to be identifiable by local twitch responses and by referred pain patterns evoked by palpation of tender spots in the muscle. To elicit the local twitch responses, the forearm is supinated and the hand must hang limply in the extended position. However, the finger and long thumb flexors are so deeply placed that the examiner may be able to identify only a region of deep tenderness which may, or may not, respond to pressure with the characteristic referred pain pattern.

10. ENTRAPMENTS
(Fig. 38.4)

Entrapment neuropathy of the ulnar nerve at the elbow is well known as the "cubital tunnel syndrome." When neuropathic symptoms develop as the late consequence of a known or presumed injury, they are sometimes known as "tardy ulnar palsy." Symptoms begin with disturbed sensation in the 4th and 5th digits, including dysesthesia, burning pain and a feeling of numbness. Hypoesthesia may be present. Motor involvement leads to clumsiness and weakness of the grip.

The ulnar nerve exits the upper arm through the medial intermuscular septum, to pass through a groove behind the medial epicondyle (Fig. 38.4 A). The nerve is held in this groove by a fibrous expansion of the common flexor tendon, which forms the roof of the cubital tunnel. From there,

PART 3

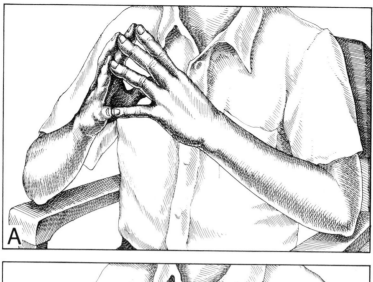

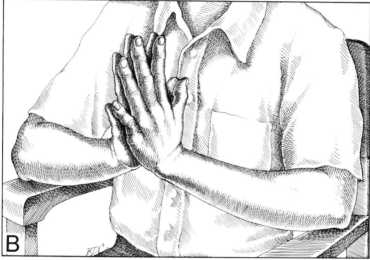

Figure 38.3. The Finger-extension Test showing some tightness of the hand and finger flexors. *A*, starting position. *B*, nearly normal extension. The final position must have the palms together and both forearms in a horizontal line for a completely negative, normal test.

it enters the forearm beneath an arch formed by the humeral and ulnar heads of the flexor carpi ulnaris muscle.[17] The ulnar nerve next occupies the triangular space bounded by three flexor muscles: the flexor carpi ulnaris covers the space superficially toward the medial (ulnar) side of the forearm; the flexor digitorum superficialis lies superficial and lateral; and the flexor digitorum profundus lies beneath, deep to the nerve.[5] The ulnar nerve continues through the proximal half of the forearm sandwiched between the flexor carpi ulnaris and the flexor digitorum profundus (Fig. 38.4*B*).

Kopell and Thompson[25] attributed entrapment syndromes to combined stretching of, and trauma to, the nerve through the cubital tunnel by the following mechanisms: (1) tethering of the nerve, where it penetrates the intermuscular septum both as it enters the tunnel and as it exists beneath the two heads of the flexor carpi ulnaris; (2) entrapment between the fibrous roof and bone within the cubital tunnel; and (3) external pressure forcing the nerve against the underlying bone that causes trauma within the tunnel.

A fourth, myofascial, source of entrapment can be the predominant cause of symptoms. This is seen in patients with TPs in the region of the flexor digitorum superficialis or profundus near the medial epicondyle. Symptoms due to this entrapment are relieved by injection of all active TPs in the flexor muscles that lie beneath the flexor carpi ulnaris, which is the muscle that, anatomically, one would expect to be responsible. Anatomically, just how TPs in one of the other flexor muscles cause this entrapment is not clear. In some patients with this entrapment syndrome, their only pain complaint is characteristic of TPs in the flexor carpi ulnaris (pain in the wrist), rather than of TPs in the flexores digitorum (pain in the fingers). Different entrapment mechanisms may operate for each muscle.

Harrelson and Newman[22] reported a case with compression of the ulnar nerve in the distal part of the forearm due to hypertrophy of the fibers of the flexor carpi ulnaris muscle, which attached to the deep side of the distal 7 cm (2¾ inches) of the tendon, before the tendon attached to the pisiform bone. Clinically, a visible and palpable mass overlying the ulnar nerve was tender to palpation throughout this distance. Electrodiagnostically, sensory and motor ulnar deficits were present distal to the wrist. At operation, the hypertrophic muscle fibers were excised, which relieved the patient's symptoms and neurological deficits. It is not clear if the entrapment was caused merely by the excessive space required by the muscle fibers, or included a myofascial TP component.

11. ASSOCIATED TRIGGER POINTS

TPs in the parallel flexores digitorum and flexores carpi muscles tend to develop together. However, TPs may appear in the flexor carpi radialis alone following an elbow fracture, or comparable discrete trauma.

Active TPs in the finger flexors may develop as satellites to TPs in muscles of the shoulder and neck that refer pain into the volar forearm, especially when TPs in these upper muscles tend also to cause nerve entrapment, e.g. the scalene or pectoralis minor muscles.

Myofascial TPs in the flexor pollicis longus tend to develop independently of active TPs in the other forearm flexor muscles.

12. STRETCH AND SPRAY
(Fig. 38.5)

For treatment of involved flexores digitorum and flexores carpi radialis and ulnaris muscles, the patient lies comfortably with the elbow resting on a padded surface and the hand supinated. The hand hangs over the edge of the support, so that the hand and fingers can be passively extended simultaneously, as the hand is pressed into full supination (Fig. 38.5A). Unless all three postures are established together, full stretch of the flexors is not obtained. Immediately before and while the muscles are being stretched, the vapocoolant spray is applied in parallel sweeps from the medial epicondyle to the finger tips over the involved muscles and their referred pain patterns (Fig. 38.5A).

To stretch and spray the flexor pollicis longus muscle, the hand and the thumb are extended similarly, while the sweeps of spray travel from the medial epicondyle down over the radial side of the forearm and the thumb (Fig. 38.5B). A hot pack to the volar forearm is applied promptly.

These patients are deeply concerned, and sometimes misinformed, about the cause of their pain. Reproduction of their pain during examination by pressure on a TP demonstrates that the pain is primarily muscular in origin, and is therefore reassuring. After treatment, the demonstration of freedom from pain during a repeat of the Hand-grip Test (see Section 8 in Chapter 34) and the normalization of measured grip strength reassures the patient that the pain has a myofascial source that is amenable to treatment.

13. INJECTION AND STRETCH
(Fig. 38.6)

Usually, hand and finger flexor muscles respond well to stretch and spray. Their TPs often do not require injection, except TPs that aggravate an ulnar nerve entrapment at the elbow, and those responsible for trigger fingers. Following TP injection, stretch and spray are immediately employed, as above, and a hot pack applied to the treated region.

Hand Flexors

Injection of TPs in these muscles also has been found effective by others.[10, 38]

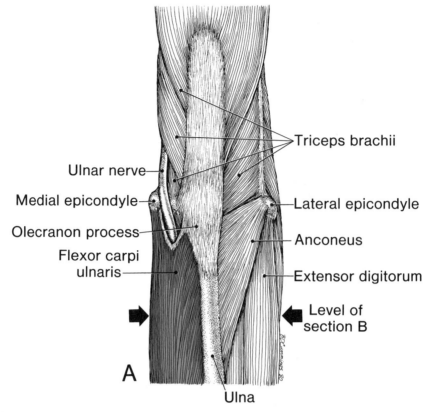

Figure 38.4. Dorsal view of the normal relation between the right ulnar nerve and the flexor carpi ulnaris muscle (*dark red*) A, tendinous arch between the muscle's humeral and ulnar heads, through which the ulnar nerve passes. B, cross section showing the relation of the ulnar nerve to the flexor carpi ulnaris (*dark red*), flexores digitorum superficialis and profundus muscles (*light red*), several centimeters below the elbow in the region of the trigger points that may cause the nerve entrapment.

To inject a TP in the **flexor carpi radialis**, the elbow of the supine patient is extended and the hand supinated. When the active TP has been located by flat palpation, it is injected with 0.5% procaine solution (Fig. 38.6A), and then passively stretched before the hot pack is applied.

To inject an active TP in the **flexor carpi ulnaris** muscle, the supine patient is asked to flex the elbow and externally rotate the arm (Fig. 38.6B). Since this TP is quite superficial, it, too, is located by flat palpation and injected under direct tactile control. A local twitch response is often observed when the needle encounters the TP.

Finger Flexors

Tender spots in the superficial flexors are located by flat palpation and the area of focal tenderness is injected. The TPs in

the deep finger flexor muscles are usually located approximately 3 cm (about 1½ in) distal to the medial epicondyle. These deep TPs are sometimes reponsible for entrapment of the ulnar nerve, and are injected as illustrated for the flexor carpi ulnaris (Fig. 38.6B), except that they lie deeper, requiring penetration to at least 2 cm (nearly 1 in); this depth reaches beyond the flexor carpi ulnaris, into the flexor digitorum sublimis or profundus. One obtains the impression that there may be a family of TPs in several muscles. In ridding this muscular region of TP activity, it is not uncommon to cause a temporary block of the ulnar nerve; the local anesthesia disappears in 15–20 min when 0.5% procaine solution is used.

Every muscle that was injected should be passively stretched at once, usually during vapocooling. A hot pack is applied promptly.

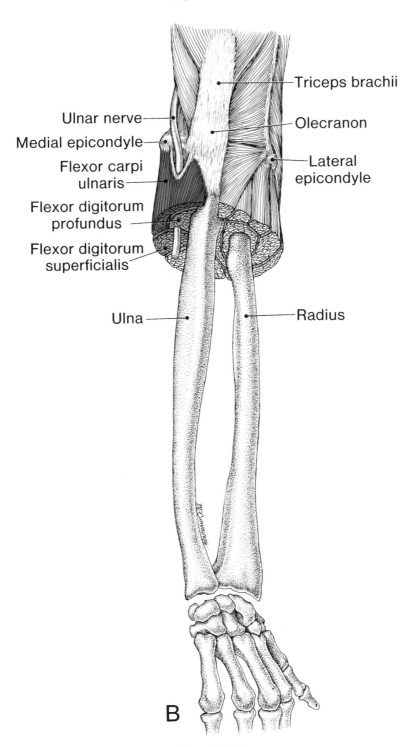

Triceps brachii

Ulnar nerve

Olecranon

Medial epicondyle

Flexor carpi
ulnaris

Lateral
epicondyle

Flexor digitorum
profundus

Flexor digitorum
superficialis

Ulna

Radius

B

Figure 38.4 B.

PART 3

Trigger Finger

A trigger finger may be promptly and permanently relieved by injection, but the return of full function is likely to require a few days after the treatment. The needle tip is aligned with the midline of the finger and is inserted in the center of the tender point, apparently deep in the restricting fibrous ring around the flexor tendon, in

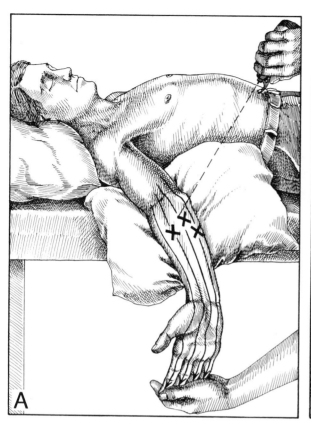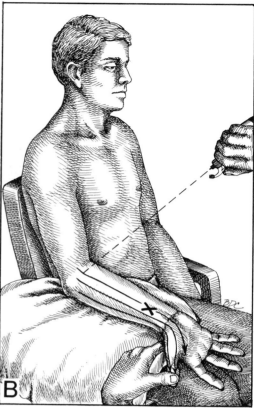

Figure 38.5.   Stretch position and spray pattern (*arrows*) for trigger points (**Xs**) in muscles of the hand, thumb and finger flexors in the forearm. *A*, flexores carpi radialis and ulnaris, and flexores digitorum muscles. The patient's hand is supinated, elbow extended, and both the hand and fingers are fully extended. The patient's fingers are included in the downsweep spray pattern. *B*, flexor pollicis longus muscle.

the midline, just proximal to the head of the metacarpal bone (Fig. 38.6C). Injection of 1–1.5 ml of 0.5% procaine solution precisely into the tender spot sufficies. No local twitch response is observed. This TP may be purely fascial, and not located within muscular tissue.

A trigger thumb, present in one patient for 10 years following trauma to the upper extremity, was immediately and permanently unlocked by a single injection. The result is representative of the senior author's experience.

An alternate treatment applies a flexible splint around the proximal interphalangeal joint to restrict flexor action of that finger for a period long enough to significantly reduce the frequency of triggering. This approach also restricts function.[48]

14. CORRECTIVE ACTIONS

When prolonged gripping, such as tightly holding a ski pole or a steering

wheel, activates TPs in the flexor muscles, the patient should learn consciously to relax the grip frequently, to pronate the hand rather than holding it supinated, and to stretch the muscles at frequent intervals. Relaxation is aided by doing the Artisan's Finger-stretch Exercise (see Fig. 35.8). Grasping the sides of the steering wheel halfway between the top and bottom places the wrist in a more neutral position. If the patient rows on a crew or paddles a canoe, he should fully open the fingers on the return stroke while holding the oar or paddle between the thumb and palm, in order to relieve tension and to stretch the flexor muscles. For those playing racquet games, the wrist should be held in the "cock-up" position and not allowed to droop, in order to strengthen the grip. A patient with latent TPs in the flexor muscles should learn to keep the hand, as well as the forearm, supported on the armrest when sitting and not to let the hand dangle

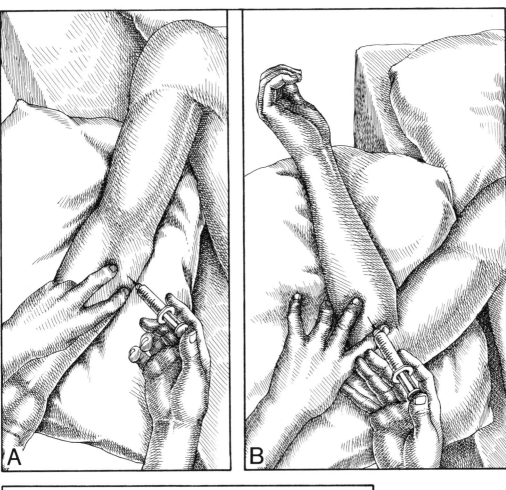

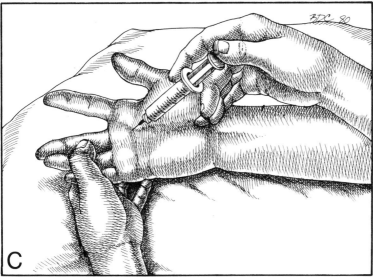

Figure 38.6.   Injection technique for trigger points in the hand and finger flexors, and for a trigger finger. *A,* flexor carpi radialis, with the elbow straight. *B,* flexor carpi ulnaris, with the forearm flexed and the arm externally rotated to provide convenient access to this muscle. *C,* injection to relieve a trigger finger. The injection apparently releases a fibrous ring that ensnares the flexor tendon of the middle finger.

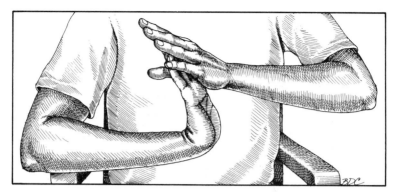

Figure 38.7.   The Finger-extension Exercise is a self-stretch passive movement for inactivating trigger points and relieving tension in the hand and finger flexor muscles. The right forearm under stretch is well supported and relaxed.

over the end, thus shortening the hand flexors.

When treating the hand and finger extensors by stretch and spray, a shortening reactivation of the flexor muscles can be avoided by routinely applying stretch and spray to them also.

In general, TP activity in the hand and finger flexors can be avoided, or treated, by daily use of four hand exercises: the Finger-extension Exercise (Fig. 38.7), the Artisan's Finger-stretch Exercise (see Fig. 35.8), the Finger-flutter Exercise (see Fig. 35.9), and the Interosseous-stretch Exercise (see Fig. 40.6).

The trigger finger is apparently a fascial entrapment which seems not to be influenced by muscle-stretch exercises. Recurrent heavy pressure on the tender spot against the metacarpal head, as by a cane or the handle of a tool, should be avoided.

References

1. Basmajian JV: *Muscles Alive,* Ed. 4. Williams & Wilkins, Baltimore, 1978 (pp. 213, 217).
2. *Ibid.* (pp. 204, 205).
3. Broer MR, Houtz SJ: *Patterns of Muscular Activity in Selected Sports Skill.* Charles C Thomas, Springfield, Ill., 1967.
4. Cailliet, R: *Soft Tissue Pain and Disability,* F.A. Davis, Philadelphia, 1977 (p. 188, Fig. 155).
5. Carter BL, Morehead J, Wolpert SM, *et al.: Cross-Sectional Anatomy.* Appleton-Century-Crofts, New York, 1977 (Sects. 53–58).
6. *Ibid.* (Sects. 53–59).
7. *Ibid.* (Sects. 53, 54, 56–63).
8. *Ibid.* (Sects. 56–61).
9. Good MG: What is "fibrositis"? *Rheumatism* 5:117–123, 1949 (pp. 120, 121; Fig. 3).
10. Good MG: Acroparaesthesia—an idiopathic myalgia of elbow. *Edinburgh Med J* 56:366–368, 1949 (Case 1).
11. Good MG: The role of skeletal muscles in the pathogenesis of diseases. *Acta Med Scand* 138:285–292, 1950 (p. 287).
12. Grant JCB: *An Atlas of Human Anatomy,* Ed. 7. Williams & Wilkins, Baltimore, 1978 (Fig. 6–66).
13. *Ibid.* (Fig. 6–68).
14. *Ibid.* (Figs. 6–69, 6–70).
15. *Ibid.* (Fig. 6–71).
16. *Ibid.* (Fig. 6–85).
17. Gray H: *Anatomy of the Human Body,* edited by C.M. Goss, American Ed. 29. Lea & Febiger, Philadelphia, 1973 (pp. 463–466).
18. *Ibid.* (p. 466, Fig. 6–42).
19. *Ibid.* (p. 462, Fig. 6–40).
20. *Ibid.* (p. 467, Fig. 6–43).
21. *Ibid.* (p. 465, Fig. 6–41).
22. Harrelson JM, Newman M: Hypertrophy of the flexor carpi ulnaris as a cause of ulnar-nerve compression in the distal part of the forearm. *J Bone Joint Surg* 57A:554–555, 1975.
23. Kellgren JH: Observations on referred pain arising from muscle. *Clin Sci* 3:175–190, 1938 (pp. 179, 188, 189).
24. Kelly M: Pain in the forearm and hand due to muscular lesions. *Med J Aust* 2:185–188, 1944 (Cases 2, 7, and 9; Fig. 4).
25. Kopell HP, Thompson WAL: *Peripheral Entrapment Neuropathies.* Williams & Wilkins, Baltimore, 1963 (pp. 113, 114, 116).
26. Lange M: *Die Muskelhärten (Myogelosen).* J.F. Lehmanns, München, 1931 (p. 116, Fig. 38).
27. Lundervold AJS: Electromyographic investigations of position and manner of working in typewriting. *Acta Physiol Scand* 24:(Suppl. 84), 1951.
28. McMinn RMH, Hutchings RT: *Color Atlas of Human Anatomy.* Year Book Medical Publishers, Chicago, 1977 (p. 124C).
29. *Ibid.* (p. 126A).
30. *Ibid.* (pp. 132A, 134A, 139).
31. *Ibid.* (p. 135C).
32. Pernkopf E: *Atlas of Topographical and Applied Human Anatomy,* Vol. 2. W.B. Saunders, Philadelphia, 1964 (Figs. 75, 76).
33. *Ibid.* (Figs. 81, 82).
34. *Ibid.* (Figs. 86, 87).
35. *Ibid.* (Fig. 85).
36. Rasch PJ, Burke RK: *Kinesiology and Applied Anatomy,* Ed. 6. Lea & Febiger, Phildelphia, 1978 (pp. 185, 197, 199, 200, 206).

37. Ruch TC, Patton HD: *Physiology and Biophysics*, Ed. 19. W.B. Saunders, Philadelphia, 1965 (pp. 375, 378).

38. Sano S, Ando K, Katori I, *et al*.: Electromyographic studies on the forearm muscle activities during finger movements. *J Jpn Orthop Assoc* 51:331–337, 1977.

39. Sobotta J, Figge FHJ: *Atlas of Human Anatomy*, Ed. 9, Vol. 1. Hafner Division of Macmillan, New York, 1974 (p. 204).

40. *Ibid*. (pp. 199, 202).

41. *Ibid*. (p. 206).

42. Sobotta J, Figge FHJ: *Atlas of Human Anatomy*, Ed. 9, Vol. 3. Hafner Division of Macmillan, New York, 1974 (p. 295).

43. Sobotta J, Figge FHJ: *Atlas of Human Anatomy*, Ed. 9, Vol. 1. Hafner Division of Macmillan, New York, 1974 (p. 220).

44. *Ibid*. (p. 216).

45. Spalteholz W: *Handatlas der Anatomie des Menschen*, Ed. 11, Vol. 2. S. Hirzel, Leipzig, 1922 (p. 326).

46. *Ibid*. (p. 327).

47. *Ibid*. (pp. 328, 329).

48. Swezey RL: *Arthritis; Rational Therapy and Rehabilitation*. W.B. Saunders, Philadelphia, 1978 (Fig. 57, p. 86).

49. Toldt C: *An Atlas of Human Anatomy*, translated by M.E. Paul, Ed. 2, Vol. 1. Macmillan, New York, 1919 (pp. 321, 323).

50. *Ibid*. (p. 322).

51. *Ibid*. (p. 333).

52. *Ibid*. (p. 324).

53. *Ibid*. (pp. 331, 335, 336).

54. Winter Z: Referred pain in fibrositis. *Med Rec* 157:34–37, 1944 (p. 4).

CHAPTER 39
Adductor and Opponens Pollicis Muscles; Trigger Thumb
"Weeder's Thumb"

HIGHLIGHTS: "Weeder's thumb" is a painful disability of the thumb that is primarily due to active trigger points (TPs) in the adductor and opponens pollicis muscles. The pain patterns and treatment approach for the opponens pollicis are applicable to the abductor and flexor pollicis brevis muscles. The latter two muscles lie directly over the opponens and are difficult to distinguish from it by palpation. **REFERRED PAIN** from both the adductor and opponens pollicis muscles projects to the radial and palmar aspects of the thumb; the opponens pollicis also may refer pain to the radial side of the palmar aspect of the wrist. **ANATOMICAL ATTACHMENT**, medially, of the transverse head of the *adductor pollicis* is to the carpometacarpal region of the index and middle fingers. Medially, the oblique head attaches to the shaft of the third metacarpal bone. Laterally, both heads fasten to the base of the proximal phalanx of the thumb. The *opponens pollicis* extends from the trapezoid bone of the wrist and the flexor retinaculum in the heel of the hand to wrap partially around and attach to the first metacarpal bone. The **ACTION** of the adductor pollicis is to adduct the thumb toward the index finger, while the opponens pollicis is essential in bringing the thumb pad across the palm to touch the pads of the ring and little fingers (opposition). **SYMPTOMS** due to active TPs in these muscles are referred thumb pain at rest and on motion, with awkwardness of pincer grip between the thumb and fingers. **ACTIVATION of TRIGGER POINTS** in these muscles may be caused by strong, prolonged pincer gripping, as when sewing, weeding, writing longhand, and opening jar tops. **PATIENT EXAMINATION** should include a check for a Heberden's node on the ulnar side of the interphalangeal joint of the thumb, a node that is often associated with TPs in the adductor pollicis. "Trigger thumb" is usually caused by a TP located beside, and radial to, the flexor pollicis longus tendon, just proximal to the first metacarpophalangeal (MCP) joint. **ASSOCIATED TRIGGER POINTS** are likely to occur in the first dorsal interosseous. **STRETCH AND SPRAY** require maximal spread of the thumb away from the index finger while bending the thumb backward. Vapocoolant spray is swept radially over the thenar eminence and thumb, and proximally over the wrist. Ischemic compression of TPs in the opponens pollicis can be helpful. **INJECTION AND STRETCH** are usually effective and, in the long run, less painful than the combination of stretch and spray with ischemic compression of the TPs. "Trigger thumb" is relieved by injection of the tender point just radial to a point of possible ensnarement of the flexor pollicis longus tendon by the flexor sheath at the distal end of the first metacarpal bone. **CORRECTIVE ACTIONS** include home exercises, such as, the Adductor Pollicis-stretch, the Opponens Pollicis-stretch, the Finger-flutter and the Finger-extension Exercises. These movements provide important intermittent relief during activities that require sustained or vigorous contraction of the thumb muscles.

PART 3

1. REFERRED PAIN
(Fig. 39.1)

Adductor Pollicis

An active trigger point (TP) in the adductor pollicis muscle causes aching pain along the outside of the thumb and hand at the base of the thumb distal to the wrist crease (Fig. 39.1A). The spillover pain area hits the palmar surface of the first metacarpophalangeal (MCP) joint, and may include most of the thumb, thenar eminence, and dorsal web space.[30, 31]

Opponens Pollicis

Pain is referred from TPs in this muscle to the palmar surface of most of the thumb and also to a spot on the radial side of the palmar aspect of the wrist, where the patient is likely to place a finger to locate the pain (Fig. 39.1B).

2. ANATOMICAL ATTACHMENTS
(Fig. 39.2)

Adductor Pollicis

The adductor pollicis spans the web space between the thumb and index finger. Both the oblique and transverse heads lie beneath (volar to) the tendon of the flexor pollicis longus and attach *laterally* to the ulnar side of the base of the proximal phalanx of the thumb (Fig. 39.2A), in common with the flexor pollicis and abductor pollicis brevis muscles (Fig. 39.2B). *Medially* the oblique head of the adductor pollicis attaches to the bases of the second and third metacarpals and to the capitate bone. The transverse head attaches *medially* to the distal two-thirds of the palmar surface of the third metacarpal bone (Fig. 39.2A).[11]

Opponens Pollicis

The opponens pollicis attaches *medially* to a ridge on the trapezoid bone of the wrist and to the flexor retinaculum, and *laterally* and *distally* along the whole length of the radial side of the first metacarpal bone (Fig. 39.2A).[11]

This muscle lies beneath the abductor pollicis brevis, and between the superficial and deep heads of the flexor pollicis brevis muscle (Fig. 39.2B).[11] By palpation it is indistinguishable from the two overlying muscles, which may well contain TPs that

are attributed in this manual to the opponens pollicis.

Trigger Thumb

Apparently, a bulbous enlargement of the flexor pollicis longus tendon becomes ensnared by a restricted flexor sheath at the head of the first metacarpal bone, where the tendon is firmly attached to the thumb after it has passed over the adductor pollicis and between the two heads of the flexor pollicis brevis muscle (Fig. 39.2B).[12] This triggering phenomenon is similar to that described for the tendons of the finger flexors (see Chapter 38).

Supplemental References

Other authors have pictured the adductor pollicis from the palmar view[7, 8, 11, 16, 22, 27, 28] including nerves and arteries,[12] from the medial (radial) aspect,[9, 17, 21] from the dorsal view including related arteries,[26] and in cross section.[3, 6, 19, 23]

They also have shown the opponens pollicis from the palmar view,[8, 10, 11, 22, 27, 29] from the medial aspect,[17, 25] and in cross section.[4, 19, 23]

Others have portrayed the region of the flexor pollicis longus tendon where the trigger thumb phenomenon occurs.[7, 13, 18, 24]

3. INNERVATION

Adductor Pollicis

This muscle is supplied by the deep palmar branch of the ulnar nerve from the medial cord and lower trunk through spinal nerves C_8 and T_1.

Opponens Pollicis

The opponens pollicis is supplied by a branch of the median nerve from the lateral cord and upper and middle trunks through spinal nerves C_6 and C_7.

4. ACTIONS

Contrary to what one might expect, flexion-extension of the thumb is defined as occurring in the plane of the palm, and adduction-abduction is defined as occurring in a plane perpendicular to the palm.[1, 11, 14, 15]

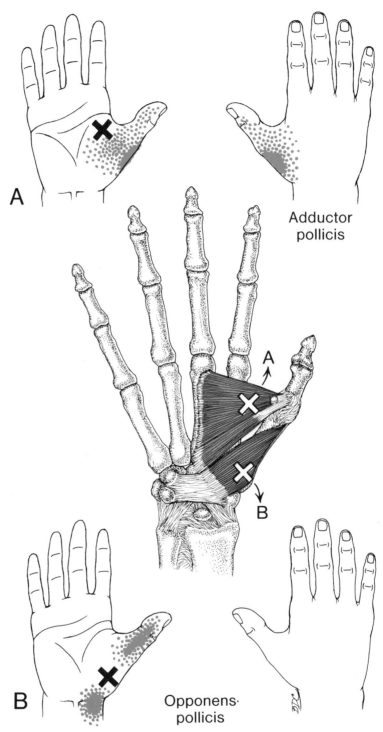

Figure 39.1.   Referred pain patterns (*dark red*) and location of trigger points (**X**s) for two thumb muscles (*medium red*), right hand. *A*, adductor pollicis. *B*, opponens pollicis.

PART 3

Adductor Pollicis

This muscle adducts the thumb. It also assists in flexion at the MCP joint of the thumb.

The adductor pollicis is activated electromyographically during any adduction, and also during forceful opposition of the thumb, which rotates the thumb to face the other fingers.[1]

Opponens Pollicis

The opponens muscle of the thumb abducts,[1, 16] flexes,[1, 14, 16] and rotates the metacarpal bone of the thumb into a position of opposition.[1, 5, 14, 15, 16]

Electromyographically, the opponens was consistently active during opposition of the thumb and, surprisingly, was moderately active during extension, and markedly active during abduction, of the thumb.[2]

5. MYOTATIC UNIT

The adductor pollicis brevis, flexor pollicis brevis, and the opponens pollicis generally act together synergistically. The abductors and extensors of the thumb are their antagonists. Functionally, this group of adductors and their opposers act in conjunction with the first dorsal interosseous and extrinsic finger muscles for forceful index-finger pinch, and with the opponens digiti quinti for forceful finger opposition.

6. SYMPTOMS

In addition to pain (Section 1), patients with active TPs in these thumb muscles may complain that their thumb is "clumsy." Their handwriting often has become illegible because they "can hardly hold a pen." They have trouble with the fine manipulations necessary for buttoning clothing, sewing, drafting and painting that require the prehensile pincer grip provided by the thumb.

7. ACTIVATION OF TRIGGER POINTS

A common syndrome, "weeder's thumb," is caused by activation of TPs in these muscles when the patient pulls well-rooted weeds, like dock or plantain. The trouble arises when the patient repeatedly firmly grasps the base of the weed in a strong pincer grip, twists the weed to loosen the root, and then exerts an even stronger pincer grip to pull it. Sustained, unrelieved tension will activate these TPs when using a fine paintbrush, sewing, or writing longhand—especially if writing requires pressing firmly with a ball-point pen that is held perpendicular to the paper.

When TPs result from the stresses on muscle that are imposed during the fracture of a bone in the hand, patients may say, "Of course it hurts, I had a fracture there years ago." They do not realize that the hand should be pain-free when the bone has healed. They are unaware that the continuing pain is probably due to residual myofascial TPs in the hand muscles.

8. PATIENT EXAMINATION
(Fig. 39.3)

Since deep tenderness in the web space of the thumb may be referred from the scalene, brachialis, supinator, extensor carpi radialis longus, or brachioradialis muscles, these should be checked first for active TPs. If these muscles are involved, they should be treated *before* attempting to inactivate TPs in the thumb muscles; the tenderness in the region of the thumb, if referred, may disappear following inactivation of TPs in the distant forearm and arm muscles. In the "weeder's thumb" syndrome, the first interosseous usually responds to treatment immediately, leaving the more complex thumb muscles still causing symptoms.

Flexion, adduction, and abduction movements of the thumb are weaker on the affected side when one of these muscles is involved, taking into account differences due to right and left hand dominance. The strength of the adductor pollicis is easily tested by the ability to hold a piece of paper tightly between the thumb and the second metacarpal bone. Abduction, and especially extension, of the thumb are often painful.

Pain and tenderness referred to the first MCP joint from TPs in the adductor pollicis muscle are easily mistaken for evidence of joint disease, if their myofascial origin is not recognized.[20]

Heberden's nodes have been observed on the ulnar (inner) side of the thumb. When a node is present there, an associ-

PART 3

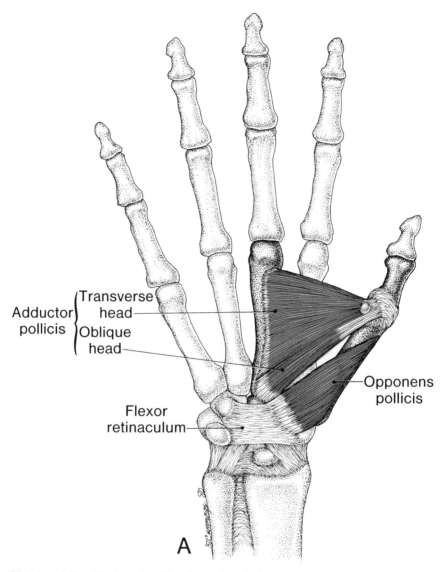

Figure 39.2 A and B.   Attachments of thumb muscles. *A*, the adductor pollicis and opponens pollicis (*dark red*) after removal of the flexor and abductor pollicis brevis muscles. *B*, course of the tendon of the flexor pollicis longus muscle with restraining fascial sheath at the base of the first phalanx just distal to the metacarpophalangeal joint, and the cut attachments of the overlying (*light red*) flexor pollicis brevis and abductor pollicis brevis muscles.

ated TP is nearly always found in the adductor pollicis muscle. This muscle adducts the thumb, much as the palmar interossei adduct the fingers, and the association with the Heberden's node probably has a similar basis (see Chapter 40).

Trigger Thumb
(Fig. 39.3)

The phenomenon of "trigger thumb" is identified by the patient's inability to ex-

tend the thumb without external assistance after flexing it; the thumb "locks" in flexion.

The cause of the problem is associated with a tender spot located lateral to the tendon of the flexor pollicis longus, possibly in the flexor pollicis brevis. To locate this TP, the patient supinates the hand, fully extends the MCP joint of the thumb, and then alternately flexes and extends the distal phalanx, while the examiner identifies the tendon (Fig. 39.3). To identify

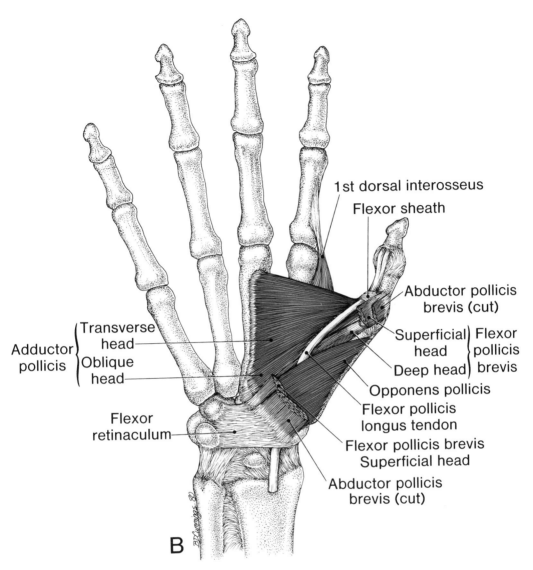

1st dorsal interosseus

Flexor sheath

Abductor pollicis
brevis (cut)

Transverse
head

Adductor
pollicis

Oblique
head

Superficial
head

Flexor
pollicis
brevis

Deep head

Opponens pollicis

Flexor pollicis
longus tendon

Flexor pollicis brevis
Superficial head

Abductor pollicis
brevis (cut)

Flexor
retinaculum

B

Figure 39.2 *B.*

PART 3

the tendon of the flexor pollicis longus, the examiner places a finger against the bulge of the MCP joint, pressing on the space between the flexor pollicis brevis and the adductor pollicis muscles where the tendon of the flexor pollicis longus enters the flexor sheath of the thumb (Fig. 39.2B). As the patient moves the distal phalanx back and forth, the cord of the subcutaneous tendon is located proximal to where it enters the anchoring arch of fibers at the head of the first metacarpal bone in the region of the "trigger" phenomenon. The TP tenderness is located several millimeters *lateral (radial)* to the tendon, just

proximal to the bony bulge of the MCP joint.

9. TRIGGER POINT EXAMINATION

Adductor Pollicis

With the patient seated comfortably and the hand pronated and relaxed, the web space of the thumb is examined by pincer palpation, through the dorsal approach. The first dorsal interosseous muscle, which lies superficial to the transversely oriented adductor fibers, is pushed aside. Exquisite spot tenderness, referred pain, and local twitch responses are, in most

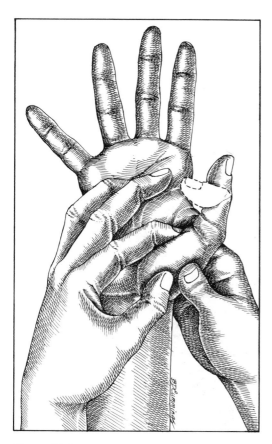

Figure 39.3. Technique for palpating the trigger point of a "trigger thumb." The distal phalanx is wiggled back and forth (as indicated by "ghosting" of it) to help identify the flexor pollicis longus tendon. Pressure against the head of the metacarpal bone, radial (lateral) to the tendon, elicits spot tenderness. Needle in Fig. 39.5C points to tender spot.

cases, easily elicited from active TPs in the adductor pollicis muscle.

Opponens Pollicis

Active TPs in this muscle are identified by flat, snapping palpation across the direction of the muscle fibers over the thenar eminence (Fig. 39.2A). When the TP is deeply located, a local twitch response is more difficult to elicit than when the TP lies in the superficial abductor or flexor pollicis brevis muscle fibers (Fig. 39.2B).

10. ENTRAPMENTS

No nerve entrapments are attributed to active TPs in these muscles.

11. ASSOCIATED TRIGGER POINTS

Active TPs are nearly always found in the first dorsal interosseous muscle when they are present in the adductor and opponens pollicis. One gains the impression that the thumb muscles are involved primarily, and the first interosseous is affected secondarily, due to its synergistic function.

The flexor pollicis brevis and abductor pollicis brevis muscles are eventually also likely to become involved.

12. STRETCH AND SPRAY
(Fig. 39.4)

For TP involvement in the adductor and opponens pollicis muscles, the hand is supinated while resting on a supporting sur-

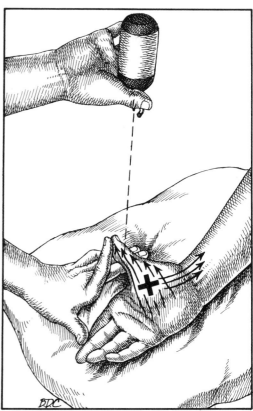

Figure 39.4. Stretch position and spray pattern (*arrows*) for a trigger point in either the adductor or opponens pollicis muscles. The "**X**" locates the adductor pollicis trigger point. The spray sweeps across the palm and thenar eminence to the end of the thumb. The up-pattern of spray across the wrist is added when the opponens pollicis is involved.

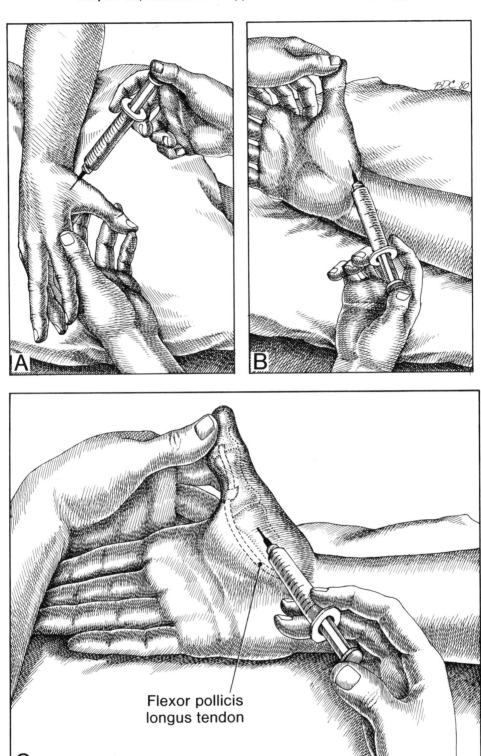

PART 3

Figure 39.5.   Techniques of trigger point injection. *A*, dorsal approach for the adductor pollicis muscle. *B*, palmar approach for the opponens pollicis. *C*, injection for "trigger thumb."

face that permits full extension (Fig. 39.4) and then hyperabduction of the thumb. The vapocoolant spray is applied in parallel sweeps across the palm, toward and over the radial surface of the thumb, while the adductor and opponens pollicis muscles are stretched. A proximal spray pattern is added across the radial side of the wrist to cover the pain pattern of the opponens pollicis. Ischemic compression can be helpful. A hot pack follows this treatment.

Stretch and spray of these muscles often are not as effective as TP injection.

Trigger thumb is not released by stretch and spray alone.

13. INJECTION AND STRETCH
(Fig. 39.5)

Adductor Pollicis

The patient's pronated hand is palpated for TPs in the adductor pollicis, as described in Section 9. When a TP has been located by its spot tenderness and local twitch response, the operator's finger presses against it from the palmar side to fix it and provide guidance (Fig. 39.5A). As the needle is directed toward this guiding

finger, it should pass to the radial side of, or perhaps penetrate, the first dorsal interosseous muscle. Following the injection, the muscle is passively stretched while release of the muscle is aided by sweeps of vapocoolant, followed by application of a hot pack.

Opponens Pollicis

When a TP in this muscle has been located by flat palpation (Section 9), it may be injected as illustrated in Figure 39.5B. The muscle is then passively stretched during vapocoolant application (Fig. 39.4), and the skin rewarmed by a hot pack.

Trigger Thumb

When the flexor pollicis longus tendon, and the tender area apparently responsible for its ensnarement, have been located by palpation with the thumb fully extended as described in Section 8, the tender spot is injected as illustrated in Fig. 39.5C. The needle probes widely down to the head of the first metacarpal bone, lateral and deep to the tendon, which need *not* be injected to eliminate the locking mechanism in the thumb.

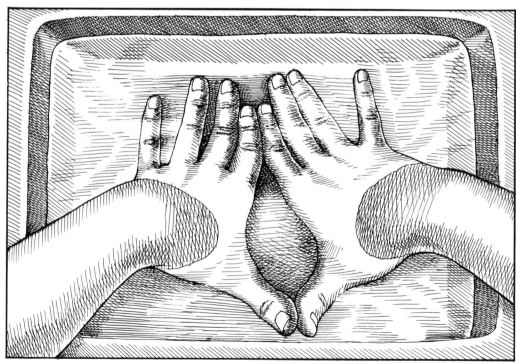

Figure 39.6.   The Adductor Pollicis-stretch Exercise is performed by pressing the thumb and index finger apart on each hand, in a basin of hot water.

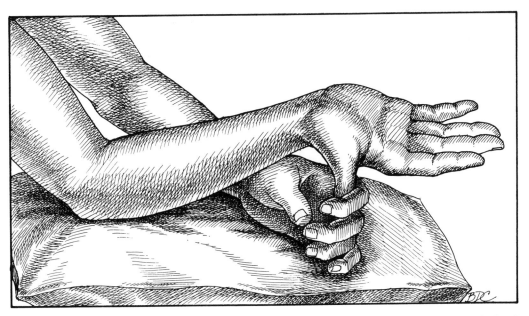

Figure 39.7.   The Opponens Pollicis-stretch Exercise is accomplished with the fingers of the opposite hand by passively hyperadducting the extended thumb.

14. CORRECTIVE ACTIONS
(Figs. 39.6 and 39.7)

The patient avoids persistent, vigorous weeding by limiting the time spent, by alternating hands in this activity, or by loosening the dirt with a spading fork before pulling the weeds out. He or she learns to use a soft felt-tip pen, which requires much less pressure on the paper than does a ball-point pen, especially when the latter is held in the up-ended position. The hours spent doing needlepoint continuously should be limited.

Reactivation of "weeder's thumb" can be avoided by having the patient frequently interrupt the gardening activity with the Artisan's Finger-stretch Exercise (see Fig. 35.8). Artisans who use tools that require sustained muscular tension for fine finger control are taught to pause and break the sustained activity every 10 or 15 min by a stretch exercise, such as the Finger-extension Exercise (see Fig. 38.7). In the Finger-flutter Exercise (see Fig. 35.9), the patient drops the hands at the side with elbows straight and shakes the fingers loosely in a limp fluttery motion. This should relax the muscles and increase their circulation.

The patient is taught also to do the Adductor Pollicis-stretch Exercise (Fig. 39.6) by placing the hands in a basin of hot water, while pressing the thumbs and index fingers of both hands against each other, to achieve full passive abduction and extension of the thumbs.

The Opponens Pollicis-stretch Exercise is performed by passively hyperadducting after fully extending the thumb, with the fingers of the opposite hand providing the external force (Fig. 39.7). The first metacarpal bone of the opposite hand is used as a fulcrum to provide leverage. A different line of muscle fibers (specifically, the opponens) is stretched if less extension is applied during the hyperadduction stretch. This stretch is more effective if done under a hot shower or with the hands in hot water.

References

1. Basmajian JV: *Muscles Alive*, Ed. 4. Williams & Wilkins, Baltimore, 1978 (pp. 220, 230).
2. Ibid. *(pp. 222, 223)*.
3. Carter BL, Morehead J, Wolpert SM, *et al.*: Cross-Sectional Anatomy. Appleton-Century-Crofts, New York, 1977 (Sect. 60).
4. *Ibid.* (Sects. 59, 60).
5. Forrest WJ, Basmajian JV: Functions of human thenar and hypothenar muscles. *J Bone Joint Surg* 47A:1585–1594, 1965.
6. Grant JCB: *An Atlas of Human Anatomy*, Ed. 7. Williams & Wilkins, Baltimore, 1978 (Fig. 6–73).
7. *Ibid.* (Fig. 6–78).
8. *Ibid.* (Fig. 6–83).
9. *Ibid.* (Figs. 6–87, 6–88).
10. *Ibid.* (Figs. 6–69, 6–70, 6–79).

PART 3

11. Gray H: *Anatomy of the Human Body*, edited by C.M. Goss, American Ed. 29. Lea & Febiger, Philadelphia, 1973 (pp. 482, 484; Fig. 6–52).

12. *Ibid.* (Fig. 12–48).

13. *Ibid.* (Fig. 6–53).

14. Hollinshead WH: *Functional Anatomy of the Limbs and Back*, Ed. 4. W.B. Saunders, Philadelphia, 1976 (p. 188).

15. Kendall HO, Kendall FP, Wadsworth GE: *Muscles, Testing and Function*, Ed. 2. Williams & Wilkins, Baltimore, 1971 (pp. 69, 70).

16. McMinn RMH, Hutchings RT: *Color Atlas of Human Anatomy*. Year Book Medical Publishers, Chicago, 1977 (pp. 132A, 136).

17. *Ibid.* (p. 142B).

18. *Ibid.* (p. 132A).

19. Pernkopf E. *Atlas of Topographical and Applied Human Anatomy*, Vol. 2. W.B. Saunders, Philadelphia, 1964 (Fig. 92).

20. Reynolds MD: Myofascial trigger point syndromes in the practice of rheumatology. *Arch Phys Med Rehabil* 62:111–114, 1981 (Table 1).

21. Sobotta J, Figge FHJ: *Atlas of Human Anatomy*, Ed. 9, Vol. 1. Hafner Division of Macmillan, New York, 1974 (p. 192).

22. *Ibid.* (pp. 215, 218, 220).

23. *Ibid.* (p. 223).

24. *Ibid.* (p. 218).

25. Sobotta J, Figge FHJ: *Atlas of Human Anatomy*, Ed. 9, Vol. 3. Hafner Division of Macmillan, New York, 1974 (p. 300).

26. *Ibid.* (p. 305).

27. Spalteholz W: *Handatlas der Anatomie des Menschen*, Ed. 11, Vol. 2. S. Hirzel, Leipzig, 1922 (p. 338).

28. Toldt C: *An Atlas of Human Anatomy*, translated by M.E. Paul, Ed. 2, Vol. 1. Macmillan, New York, 1919 (p. 334).

29. *Ibid.* (p. 335).

30. Travell J, Rinzler SH: The myofascial genesis of pain. *Postgrad Med* 11:425–434, 1952 (p. 428).

31. Zohn DA, Mennell J McM: *Musculoskeletal Pain: Diagnosis and Physical Treatment*. Little, Brown & Company, Boston, 1976 (p. 192, Fig. 9–13).

CHAPTER 40
Interosseous Muscles of the Hand
"Associates of Heberden's Nodes"

HIGHLIGHTS: Heberden's nodes are regularly associated with trigger points (TPs) in the interosseous musculature of the hand. **REFERRED PAIN** from either the dorsal or palmar interosseous muscles extends along the side of the finger to which that interosseous muscle attaches and, in the case of the first dorsal interosseous, may include the dorsum of the hand and ulnar side of the little finger. Pain from the lumbrical muscles is not distinguished from that referred by the interossei. The **ACTION** of each dorsal interosseous is to move a finger away from the midline of the middle finger (abduction). The abductor digiti minimi abducts the little finger. The palmar interossei adduct each of the other fingers toward the middle finger. **SYMPTOMS** caused by active TPs in the interossei include pain, finger stiffness, and awkwardness and are often associated with a tender nodule on the distal interphalangeal joint. This nodule is a Heberden's node, generally equated with osteoarthritis of the distal interphalangeal joint. **ACTIVATION OF TRIGGER POINTS** in the interossei is caused by prolonged or repetitive pincer grasp. **TRIGGER POINT EXAMINATION** reveals spot tenderness in the involved muscle; referred pain is rarely elicited and local twitch responses are not evident. **ENTRAPMENTS** of digital nerves by the interossei are seen occasionally. **INJECTION AND STRETCH** are more effective than stretch and spray, or ischemic compression, in eliminating these TPs. **CORRECTIVE ACTIONS** entail a change in daily activities and the interruption of sustained muscular contraction by the Finger-flutter, Finger-extension, Adductor Pollicis-stretch, and the Interosseous-stretch Exercises, as appropriate.

1. REFERRED PAIN
(Fig. 40.1)

The first dorsal interosseous trigger points (TPs) refer pain (Fig. 40.1A) strongly down the same (radial) side of the index finger and deeply in the dorsum and through the palm of the hand; the referred pain also may extend along the dorsal and ulnar sides of the little finger.[54, 56] Generally, patients experience the most intense pain at the distal interphalangeal joint where a Heberden's node would appear. No distinction is made between the patterns of pain referred from the dorsal and the palmar interossei.

The first dorsal interosseous TPs are the second most frequent source of referred pain in the palm, exceeded only by TPs in the palmaris longus. Some patients have difficulty in deciding whether the pain referred from first dorsal interosseous TPs is more severe on the palmar or on the dorsal aspect of the hand.

Myofascial TPs in the remaining dorsal and palmar interossei refer pain along the side of the finger to which that interosseous muscle attaches (Fig. 40.1C). Pain extends as far as the distal interphalangeal joint. The exact pain pattern varies somewhat, depending on the location of the TP in the interosseous muscle. An active TP

559

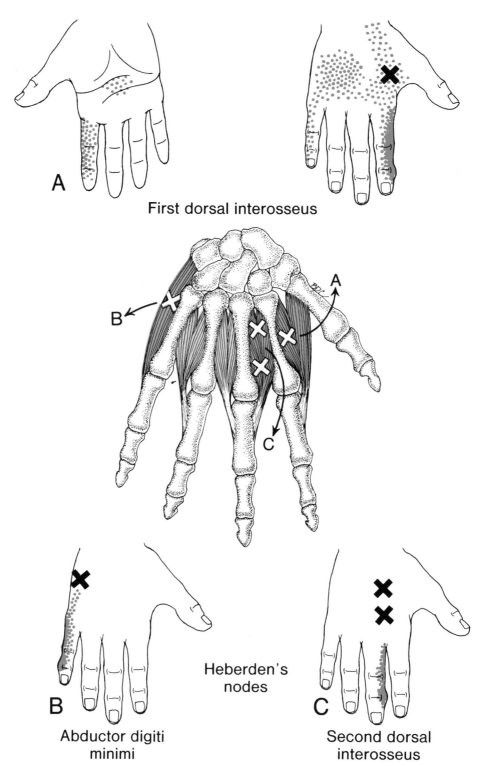

First dorsal interosseus

**Abductor digiti
minimi**

**Heberden's
nodes**

**Second dorsal
interosseus**

Figure 40.1.   Referred pain patterns (*dark red*) and location of trigger points (**X**s) for selected intrinsic muscles of the right hand. Essential zones are *solid red*, spillover zones are *stippled red. A*, the first dorsal interosseous *medium red. B*, the abductor digiti minimi (*medium red*). *C*, the second dorsal interosseous (*medium red*). *Light red*, third and fourth dorsal interossei. Trigger points may be found anywhere in the interossei, proximally or distally. Note the small Heberden's nodes in the essential pain reference zones.

in an interosseous muscle is often associated with a Heberden's node located within the TP's zone of referred pain and tenderness.

Experimental injection of hypertonic saline solution into the third dorsal interosseous of one subject referred pain to the ulnar aspect of both the dorsal and palmar surfaces of the hand, but apparently not to the fingers.[19]

The abductor digiti minimi similarly refers pain along the outer aspect of the little finger to which it attaches (Fig. 40.1B).

Heberden's Nodes

Heberden's nodes, which develop on the dorsolateral or dorsomedial aspect of the terminal phalanx at its joint, may be annoyingly tender, especially soon after they appear. With the passage of time, they tend to become pain-free.

The nodes are frequently associated with TPs in the interossei; the TPs may have been latent for years. Heberden described the nodes as "little hard knobs, about the size of a small pea, which are frequently seen upon the fingers particularly a little below the top, near the joint. They have no connection with the gout; ...they continue for life; and being hardly ever attended with pain, are rather unsightly than inconvenient, though they must be some little hindrance to the free use of the fingers."[17]

2. ANATOMICAL ATTACHMENTS
(Fig. 40.2)

As the name denotes, the interossei lie between adjacent metacarpal bones. Each dorsal interosseous muscle arises *proximally* by two heads (Fig. 40.2A), which form a bipenniform fish-bone pattern, as these heads attach to adjacent metacarpal bones. Each muscle attaches *distally* at the base of the proximal phalanx of the related finger and to that finger's extensor aponeurosis. Each muscle attaches on the side of the phalanx away from the midline of the hand.[11]

As the abductor of the index finger, the first dorsal interosseous is larger than the other interossei, but follows the same attachment pattern (Fig. 40.2A). One head arises *proximally* from the ulnar border of the metacarpal bone of the thumb, and the other head from almost the entire length of the radial border of the second metacarpal bone. Both heads attach *distally* to the extensor aponeurosis of the index finger on the radial side. This muscle fills the dorsal web space of the thumb.

Each of the three palmar interossei arises *proximally* from the palmar interosseous surface of one metacarpal bone (Fig. 40.2B) and lies palmar to the related dorsal interosseous muscle (Fig. 40.2C). Each then attaches *distally* to that finger's extensor aponeurosis at the base of the proximal phalanx on the side closest to the midline of the hand (center of the middle finger).

The four lumbricals attach *proximally* to the four tendons of the flexor digitorum profundus in mid-palm, and *distally* to the radial side of the extensor aponeurosis on each of the four fingers. Strictly speaking, the lumbricals are not interosseous muscles, but they function similarly. In terms of locating and inactivating their TPs, the first and second lumbricales lie palmar to the first and second dorsal interossei, but with the transverse head of the adductor pollicis interposed between these two lumbricales and the dorsal interossei. The third and fourth lumbricales lie palmar and adjacent to the second and third palmar interossei (Fig. 40.2C).

Abductor Digiti Minimi

This muscle provides half of what would be the next dorsal interosseous muscle, were there a 6th digit. It abducts the 5th digit (*light red*, Fig. 40.2A and B). The muscle arises *proximally* from the pisiform bone, and attaches *distally* to the ulnar side of the base of the first phalanx of the little finger and to its associated extensor aponeurosis.

Supplemental References

Other authors have illustrated the interossei of the hand from the dorsal view,[8, 13, 21, 24, 28, 32, 37, 41, 43, 48, 53] and in relation to arteries,[45] from the palmar view,[7, 11, 21, 24, 30, 34, 43, 47, 51, 52] from the lateral view,[12, 31, 44] and in cross section.[3, 6, 36, 40]

The abductor digiti minimi has been similarly portrayed from the dorsal view,[32, 49] from the palmar view,[14, 29, 35, 42, 52] from the lateral view,[10, 22] and in cross section.[4, 36, 40]

The lumbricales are shown in palmar

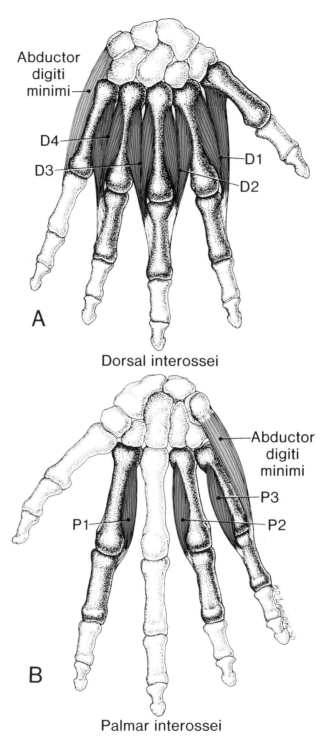

Abductor
digiti
minimi

D4

D3

D1

D2

A

Dorsal interossei

Abductor
digiti
minimi

P3

P1

P2

B

Palmar interossei

Figure 40.2. Attachments of the right interossei. *A,* dorsal view of the dorsal interosseous muscles (*dark red*), which move the fingers away from the mid-line of the middle finger, and of the abductor digiti minimi (*light red*). *B,* palmar view of all (the first, second and third) palmar interossei (*dark red*), which deviate the 2nd, 4th and 5th digits, respectively, toward the middle finger. Abductor digiti minimi, (*light red*). *C,* cross-sectional view through the metacarpal bones showing the relationship between the dorsal (D1, D2, D3, and D4, *dark red*) and the palmar (P1, P2 and P3, *medium red*) interossei. The lumbricales are the *light red* muscle masses on the radial side of the four flexor digitorum profundus tendons. *D,* appearance of Heberden's nodes on the sides of the distal interphalangeal joints.

view without[14] and with adjacent nerves,[9] and in cross section.[16]

Heberden's Nodes

Heberden's nodes are often identified with osteoarthritis,[33, 46] particularly with the primary idiopathic form, rather than the traumatic secondary form.[2] The node is an enlargement of soft tissue, sometimes partly bony, on the dorsal surface on either side of the terminal phalanx at the distal interphalangeal joint (Fig. 40.2D). The patient may eventually develop a flexion deformity with lateral or medial deviation of the distal phalanx.[33] Similar nodes located at the proximal interphalangeal joints are called Bouchard's nodes, but they are seen in only 25% of individuals with Heberden's nodes.[26]

3. INNERVATION

All of the interosseous and the abductor digiti minimi muscles are supplied by branches of the ulnar nerve, through the medial cord and lower trunk from spinal nerves C_8 and T_1.[15]

4. ACTIONS

Interossei and Lumbricales

To understand the actions of these intrinsic hand muscles, it is important to remember that the extensor digitorum strongly extends the first (proximal) pha-

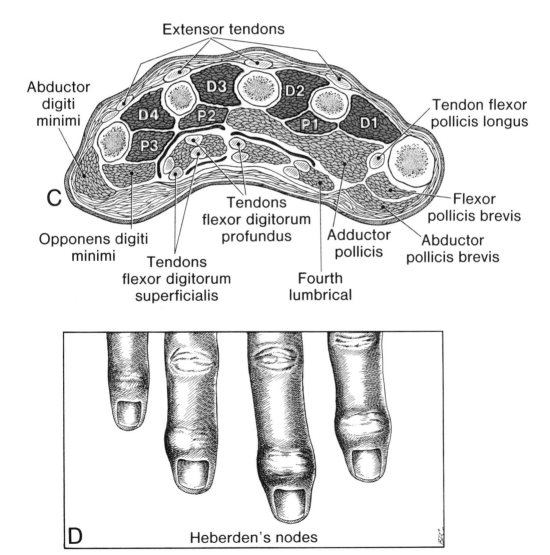

Figure 40.2C–D.

lanx of each finger, but only weakly extends the two distal phalanges. The flexor digitorum superficialis attaches to the middle of the second phalanx, flexing the proximal and middle phalanges. The flexor digitorum profundus attaches to the distal phalanx, flexing it and the more proximal phalanges.

The four dorsal and three palmar interossei have opposing actions in abduction, adduction and rotation, but both groups of interossei plus the lumbricales flex the fingers at the metacarpophalangeal (MCP) joints and extend the distal phalanges.[1, 5, 11, 18, 21] It is the interossei and lumbricales that extend the distal two phalanges when any degree of flexion of the proximal phalanx is present. The flexion or extension of the latter is controlled by the flexor digitorum superficialis and the extensor digitorum working as antagonists. The *d*orsal interossei *ab*duct (mnemonic—DAB), and the *p*almar interossei *ad*duct (mnemonic—PAD) with reference to the midline of the middle finger.[1, 5, 11, 18, 21] Electromyographic studies have shown that the interosseous hand muscles act as flexors of the MCP joints only when this function does *not* conflict with their extensor function at the interphalangeal joints.[1]

The flexion-extension function of the interosseous muscles requires considerably less force than the lateral motions of abduction and adduction. Therefore, in disease, the lateral motions are lost earlier, and recover more slowly than flexion-extension. The abduction-adduction functions of the interossei must be tested with the fingers extended at the MCP joints. Spreading the fingers apart is normally severely limited when the fingers are flexed at the MCP joint.[5]

The first *dorsal* interosseous rotates the proximal phalanx to make the index finger pad face toward the ulnar side of the hand whereas the first *palmar* interosseous rotates it in the opposite direction. The first dorsal and first palmar interossei counterbalance their rotational movements while combining their flexion-extension actions. In precision handling of objects, the interossei function mainly as abductors and adductors of the fingers. In spherical grip, their rotational forces were found to position the proximal phalanges for best finger pad contact.[25]

The lumbricales are unusual in that they anchor not to bone but to the tendons of other muscles. Thus, the lumbricales function as the equivalent of an adjustable physiological tendon transplant. Contraction of these muscles converts the distal phalanx-flexion action of the flexor digitorum profundus to extension of the distal phalanges. The lumbricales specifically permit the flexor digitorum superficialis to strongly grip with the proximal two phalanges, yet release the distal phalanx grip in the presence of flexor digitorum profundus activity. The usual test of the intrinsic muscles' flexion-extension function, by resisting interphalangeal joint extension with the MCP joint flexed, tests both the interossei and the lumbricales.[21] The lumbricales should be most useful when a strong grip is required in the absence of fingertip pressure.

5. MYOTATIC UNIT

As noted above, the dorsal and palmar interossei are synergistic for flexion at the metacarpophalangeal joint and extension of the two most distal phalanges; they are antagonistic for adduction-abduction and for rotation of the proximal phalanges.

The interossei and the lumbricales are synergistic. Full effectiveness of these intrinsic muscles for holding and grasping objects also requires the assistance of the thumb muscles in the thenar eminence.

6. SYMPTOMS

Patients with myofascial TPs in an interosseous muscle characteristically complain of "arthritis pain in my finger." They have finger stiffness that produces impairment of hand functions, such as, buttoning a shirt, writing, and grasping. One would not expect numbness and paresthesia to be associated with activity of this TP unless the muscle also entrapped the digital nerve. Some patients will complain of the Heberden's node as a "sore joint that is swollen." Careful examination shows a tender Heberden's node but, as a rule, no true synovial or bony swelling. The tenderness may be *referred* to the joint. In time, the Heberden's node becomes less tender. Again, clinically it appears that myofascial TPs in muscles can contribute to joint disease.[39]

The arthritis literature dealing with Heberden's nodes describes symptoms of brief morning stiffness[26, 33, 55] due to increased viscosity of periarticular structures.[55] Subsequent loss of range of motion was ascribed to muscle spasm and contracture,[33] which are often simulated by the muscle shortening due to myofascial TP activity. Heberden's nodes are sometimes, but not always, associated with local pain and tenderness.[26, 33] A relationship of Heberden's nodes to osteoarthritis in other parts of the body is seriously questioned by some,[2, 50] and claimed by others.[20, 27]

7. ACTIVATION OF TRIGGER POINTS

Myofascial TPs in the interossei are activated by sustained or repetitive pincergrasp, as performed by a seamstress, painter, sculptor, mechanic, or a modelmaker who holds small pieces firmly in place while the glue sets. A nervous habit like fiddling with the cap of a pen while writing with the other hand can be the cause. Activities requiring sustained forceful finger movements, such as pulling weeds, manipulation of foot muscles by a physical therapist, or the retraction of nail cuticles by a manicurist, have initiated interosseous TPs. "Golf hands" have been found to be due to a constant tight grip on the handle of the golf club, especially when the handle has a very small diameter. Playing the piano, or batting a baseball, seem not to activate these TPs.

The distal interphalangeal joints of the fingers preferentially develop Heberden's nodes. This evidence of an osteoarthritic process is most common in the finger joint that has by far the highest load per unit area of joint surface and in those individuals who commonly do activities that particularly load that joint.[38] The increased strain on the interosseous muscles caused by the abnormal hand mechanics associated with the distorted joint function of arthritis can activate and perpetuate these TPs. *Vice versa*, it appears that the myofascial TPs (fibrositis) also can contribute to the arthritis.[39] Inactivating the related myofascial TPs and the *elimination of their perpetuating factors* appears to be an important part of early therapy to delay or abort the progression of some kinds of osteoarthritis.

8. PATIENT EXAMINATION

Patients with active TPs in the interossei have difficulty flexing their fingers, which may "stick out" due to a degree of uncontrolled extension, preventing full closure of the finger tips to the palm. Myofascial TPs in the dorsal interossei produce uncontrolled separation between fingers. Most noticeable is abduction of the index or the little finger. The patient finds it difficult, if not impossible, to bring all four fingers tightly together.

Involvement of the palmar interossei restricts voluntary separation of adjacent fingers.

Heberden's Nodes

The presence of Heberden's nodes is a common finding in patients with TPs in the interossei. A node is palpable as an excrescence on the dorsal margin of the distal phalanx, or the distal end of the middle phalanx on either side, always near the distal interphalangeal joint (Fig. 40.2D). A Heberden's node also may appear on the thumb, usually on its ulnar side in conjunction with TPs in the adductor pollicis muscle. Idiopathic Heberden's nodes are most commonly seen on the index and middle fingers.[18] They appear on the side of the finger to which the involved interosseous muscle attaches. Also, Heberden's nodes are associated with irritation and increased sensitivity of the connective tissue similar to that seen in the biceps brachii tendon due to active TPs in the biceps muscle.

The prevalence of idiopathic Heberden's nodes among 220 white women increased from an insignificant 0.4% during the 4th decade to an impressive 30% by the 9th decade of life. Onset usually was in the 5th and 6th decades, at an average age of 48½ years.[50] In a hospital-based practice, the number of female patients with a myofascial TP syndrome (fibrositis) was significantly greater than the number of male patients, and the greatest number were in the 5th or 6th decades of life.[23] This is consistent with our impression of a significant relation between Heberden's nodes and myofascial TPs.

The mechanism by which TPs in the interossei may lead to Herberden's nodes is speculative. Myofascial TPs produce bands of taut muscle fibers, which could cause a sustained increase of tension on the tendon. The question also arises as to why, if trauma is a significant factor, distal joints of the fingers are involved, but not of the toes.[2] One possible answer is that fine manipulation with the digits overloads the hand interossei, but not those of the toes. The idiopathic form may be genetically governed. Early cases of idiopathic Heberden's nodes, radiographically, may show small islands of calcium deposit in the extensor tendons near the distal phalanx before the condition is apparent clinically.[50]

Idiopathic Heberden's nodes have sometimes, but not generally, been considered an inherited, autosomal, sex-influenced trait that is dominant in women and recessive in men, with a prevalence 10 times greater in women than in men.[33] The nodes require a normal nerve supply to develop.[50] Idiopathic Heberden's nodes have been closely related to menopause; nodes were first noted within 3 years of the last menstrual period in one-half of 99 cases.[50]

Heberden's nodes may be secondary to trophic changes induced by nerve entrapment (Section 10) or, more likely, may be due to an autonomic component within the reference zone of a TP in the corresponding interosseous muscle.

9. TRIGGER POINT EXAMINATION

Heberden's nodes serve as guides to TPs in the interossei. They are identified as nodules located over the distal interphalangeal joints, as seen in Figures 40.1 and 40.2D.[26] Nodes develop dorsally on that side of the finger to which the interosseous muscle attaches.

Usually only one or two interosseous muscles contain active TPs at one time; others may harbor latent TPs. Myofascial TPs in these muscles are difficult to palpate. Separating the fingers widely, which moves the metacarpal bones apart, permits pincer palpation between the bones. Meanwhile, counter-pressure is produced with a finger against the palm, beneath the muscle to be palpated. One may elicit deep tenderness in the interossei and lumbricals but, except for the first dorsal interosseous, referred pain and local twitch responses are rarely induced until a needle impales the TP.

10. ENTRAPMENTS

One may observe cutaneous hypoesthesia along one side of a finger where the patient reports a sensation of numbness when an active TP lies in the corresponding interosseous muscle. This neurological deficit disappears following inactivation of the TP, suggesting that a digital nerve had been entrapped by the increased tension of the involved interosseous muscle.

On their way through the palm to the digits, the median and ulnar nerves lie next to the lumbrical and palmar interosseous muscles. The deep (motor) branch of the ulnar nerve pierces the opponens digiti minimi before supplying all interossei, the third and fourth lumbricales, the adductor pollicis, and the deep head of the flexor pollicis brevis.[15] Active TPs in the opponens digiti minimi can be responsible for weakness of these ulnar-innervated muscles and, if weakness is present, the opponens should be examined for TPs.

11. ASSOCIATED TRIGGER POINTS

When the interosseous muscles are involved, one should look for associated TPs in the intrinsic thumb muscles. Other muscles that may refer myofascial pain into the fingers include the long finger flexors and extensors, the latissimus dorsi, the pectoralis major, scalene muscles, and either the lateral or the medial head of the triceps brachii.

Finger pain and numbness also may be due to nerve entrapment of the brachial plexus by taut scalene muscles, or as it passes beneath the scapular attachment of a taut pectoralis minor.

12. STRETCH AND SPRAY
(Fig. 40.3)

With the exception of the first dorsal interosseous, stretch and spray is not generally effective for the management of interosseous TPs, since it is difficult to adequately stretch these muscles. Their TPs are often inaccessible to ischemic compression, so that TP injection usually provides the most rapid and sustained relief.

The first dorsal interosseous is stretched and sprayed by the operator's forcefully abducting the thumb and adducting the index finger after initiating the down-

PART 3

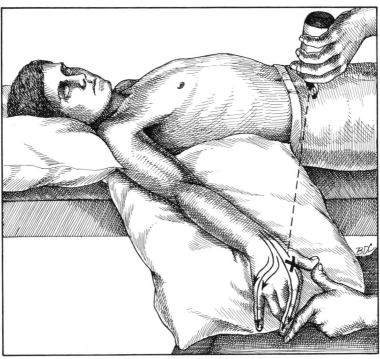

Figure 40.3.   Stretch position and direction of the sweeps of spray (*arrows*) for a trigger point (**X**) in the first dorsal interosseous muscle.

sweep pattern of the vapocoolant (Fig. 40.3).

Stretch and spray is more likely to be effective if the TPs are superficial (dorsal interossei), if the fingers and their metacarpal bones can be separated widely, and if the down-sweep spray pattern is used over both the involved musculature and its pain pattern (Fig. 40.1A). Stretch and spray also is applied to these muscles immediately following injection of TPs.

13. INJECTION AND STRETCH
(Figs. 40.4 and 40.5)

Since the precise location of TPs in the dorsal and palmar interossei and in the lumbricals is difficult to palpate, adequate exploration of the area with a 2.5-cm (1-in), 25-gauge needle is important.

Interossei

When the first dorsal interosseous harbors an active TP, the patient's index finger is held between the operator's thumb and middle finger (Fig. 40.4A), with the operator's middle finger pressed firmly into the web space beneath the first dorsal

interosseous, so that the muscle is held firmly in a pincer grasp; this permits identification and fixation of the TP for injection (Fig. 40.4A).

The dorsal interossei have a bipenniform structure with attachments to both adjacent metacarpal bones, and both halves must be explored with the needle for TPs. For example, to inject the second dorsal interosseus, the needle is aligned with the side of the third metacarpal bone in the second interosseus space and is inserted into the center of the tender area (Fig. 40.5). If any tenderness remains, the needle is aligned with the second metacarpal bone on the other side of the space and the other penna of the muscle probed for TPs.

To inject the first palmar interosseous (Fig. 40.5A), the needle is directed away from the third metacarpal bone to reach the muscle, which lies beneath the ulnar side of the second metacarpal (Fig. 40.5B).

Following inactivation of TPs in an interosseous muscle, soreness in the related distal interphalangeal joint and joint stiffness disappear. Tenderness of the Heberden's node usually disappears at once,

PART 3

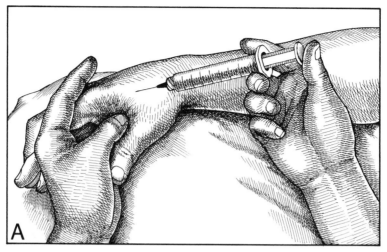

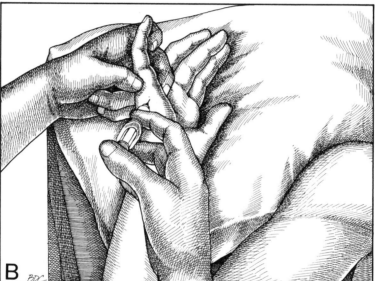

Figure 40.4.   Injection technique for trigger points in the intrinsic hand muscles. *A*, first dorsal interosseous muscle, approached from the dorsal aspect. *B*, the abductor digiti minimi, approached from the ulnar aspect of the hand.

whereas it diminishes in size with the passage of time.

Lumbricales

The four lumbricales, unlike the interossei, are injected from the palmar side of the hand because no major structure lies between them and the palmar skin. Each lumbrical muscle is found at the radial side of its corresponding metacarpal bone, in close association with a flexor digitorum profundus tendon (Fig. 40.2C).

Abductor Digiti Minimi

Either flat or pincer palpation may be used to locate TPs in the abductor digiti minimi. To inject a TP in this muscle, the patient turns the hand ulnar side up and rests it on a pillow (Fig. 40.4B). The palpable band and TP are located and precisely injected, using a pincer grasp.

Heberden's Nodes

After injection of the related TPs in the interosseous musculature, the nodes may eventually disappear completely without direct treatment of the nodes themselves.

14. CORRECTIVE ACTIONS
(Fig. 40.6)

The patient should learn to reduce the force and duration of pincer grip activities

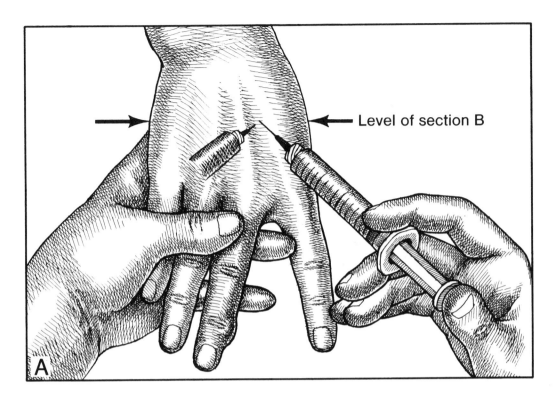

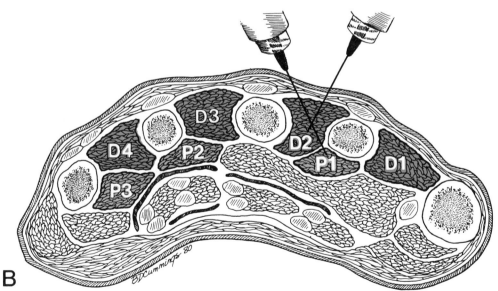

Figure 40.5.   Injection technique for the interossei. *A*, the *complete syringe* is injecting a trigger point in the more ulnar penna of the second dorsal interosseous muscle; its corresponding Heberden's node is shown. The *incomplete syringe* is injecting the first palmar interosseous, which is reached as the needle penetrates deep to the second metacarpal bone. A frequently related node on the index finger is not shown. *B*, cross section showing relation of the needles to the muscles being injected (see also Figure 40.2C). *Dark red*, dorsal interossei; *light red*, palmar interossei.

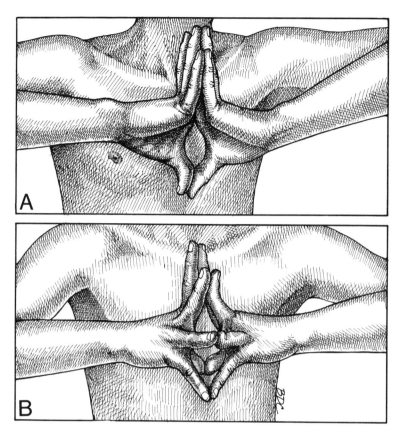

Figure 40.6.   Two views of the Interosseous-stretch Exercise. Both hand positions are effective. The forearms are held in a straight line, and an effort is made to firmly oppose the palmar aspects the metacarpal heads, while the fingers and thumbs are spread apart and hyperextended at all joints. *A*, hands fully pronated at the forearm. *B*, hands in the neutral position.

in order to lessen strain on the interosseous muscles. Patients who use ballpoint pens should, if their work permits, write with a more freely flowing felt-tip pen that needs a much lighter touch. A manual typewriter should be replaced by an electric one because it places less strain on the intrinsic hand muscles.

The patient should interrupt prolonged fine manual activity with the Finger-flutter Exercise (see Fig. 35.9), the Finger-extension Exercise (see Fig. 38.7), or the Artisan's Finger-stretch Exercise (see Fig. 35.8) to lessen tension of the intrinsic muscles of the hand.

In addition at home, daily, the patient should perform the Interosseous-stretch Exercise, illustrated in Figure 40.6. In doing this exercise, it is important that the forearms form a straight line. When active TPs are present in the first dorsal interosseous muscle, regular use of the Adductor Polli-

cis-stretch Exercise (see Fig. 39.6) also may be necessary to ensure continued recovery.

References

1. Basmajian JV: *Muscles Alive*, Ed. 4. Williams & Wilkins, Baltimore, 1978 (pp. 215–216).
2. Boyle JA, Buchanan WW: *Clinical Rheumatology*. F.A. Davis, Philadelphia, 1971 (pp. 5, 27, 32–34).
3. Carter BL, Morehead J, Wolpert SM, *et al.: Cross-Sectional Anatomy*. Appleton-Century-Crofts, New York, 1977 (Sects. 60–63).
4. *Ibid.* (Sects. 59–62).
5. Duchenne GB: *Physiology of Motion*, translated by E.B. Kaplan. J.B. Lippincott, Philadelphia, 1949 (Fig. 25; pp. 128–130, 134–136, 153–154).
6. Grant JCB: *An Atlas of Human Anatomy*, Ed. 7. Williams & Wilkins, Baltimore, 1978 (Fig. 6–73).
7. *Ibid.* (Fig. 6–85).
8. *Ibid.* (Fig. 6–104).
9. *Ibid.* (Fig. 6–79).
10. *Ibid.* (Fig. 6–95).
11. Gray H: *Anatomy of the Human Body*, edited by C.M. Goss, American Ed. 29. Lea & Febiger, Philadelphia, 1973 (pp. 485–487, Fig. 6–55).
12. *Ibid.* (p. 466, Fig. 6–42).

13. *Ibid.* (p. 471, Figs. 6–46, 6–54).
14. *Ibid.* (p. 484, Fig. 6–53).
15. *Ibid.* (pp. 971–975).
16. *Ibid.* (Fig. 6–51).
17. Heberden W: Digitorum nodi, Chapter 28. In *Commentaries on the History and Cure of Diseases*, facsimile of the London 1802 edition. Hafner, New York, 1962 (pp. 148–149).
18. Hollinshead WH: *Functional Anatomy of the Limbs and Back*, Ed. 4. W.B. Saunders, Philadelphia, 1976 (pp. 190, 191).
19. Kellgren JH: Observations on referred pain arising from muscle. *Clin Sci* 3:175–190, 1938 (p. 183).
20. Kellgren JH, Moore R: Generalized osteoarthritis and Heberden's nodes. *Br Med J* 1:181–187, 1952.
21. Kendall HO, Kendall FP, Wadsworth GE: *Muscles, Testing and Function*, Ed. 2. Williams & Wilkins, Baltimore, 1971 (pp. 80, 81, 82).
22. *Ibid.* (p. 76).
23. Kraft GH, Johnson EW, LeBan MM: The fibrositis syndrome. *Arch Phys Med Rehabil* 49:155–162, 1968.
24. Langman J, Woerdeman MW: *Atlas of Medical Anatomy*. W.B. Saunders, Philadelphia, 1978 (p. 253).
25. Long C, Conrad PW, Hall EW, et al.: Intrinsic-extrinsic muscle control of the hand in power grip and precision handling. *J Bone Joint Surg* 52-A:853–867, 1970.
26. Mannik M, Gilliland BC: Degenerative joint disease, Chapter 361. In *Harrison's Principles of Internal Medicine*, edited by M.M. Wintrobe, et al., Ed. 7. McGraw-Hill Book Co., New York, 1974 (p. 2006).
27. Marks JS, Stuart IM, Hardinge K: Primary osteoarthrosis of the hip and Heberden's nodes. *Ann Rheum Dis* 38:107–111, 1979.
28. McMinn RMH, Hutchings RT: *Color Atlas of Human Anatomy*. Year Book Medical Publishers, Chicago, 1977 (pp. 127B, 141).
29. *Ibid.* (pp. 132A, 135B).
30. *Ibid.* (pp. 136, 138).
31. *Ibid.* (p. 142B).
32. *Ibid.* (p. 143).
33. Moskowitz RW: Clinical and laboratory findings in osteoarthritis, Chapter 56. In *Arthritis and Allied Conditions*, edited by J.L. Hollander, D.J. McCarty, Ed. 8. Lea & Febiger, Philadelphia, 1972 (pp. 1034, 1037, 1045).
34. Pernkopf E: *Atlas of Topographical and Applied Human Anatomy*, Vol. 2. W.B. Saunders, Philadelphia, 1964 (p. 85).
35. *Ibid.* (p. 87).
36. *Ibid.* (p. 92).
37. *Ibid.* (p. 90).
38. Radin EL, Parker HG, Paul IL: Pattern of degenerative arthritis, preferential involvement of distal finger-joints. *Lancet* 1:377–379, 1971.
39. Reynolds MD: Myofascial trigger point syndromes in the practice of rheumatology. *Arch Phys Med Rehabil* 62:111–114, 1981.
40. Sobotta J, Figge FHJ: *Atlas of Human Anatomy*, Ed. 9, Vol. 1. Hafner Division of Macmillan, New York, 1974 (p. 223).
41. *Ibid.* (pp. 208, 214).
42. *Ibid.* (pp. 215, 216).
43. *Ibid.* (p. 222).
44. Sobotta J, Figge FHJ: *Atlas of Human Anatomy*, Ed. 9, Vol. 3. Hafner Division of Macmillan, New York, 1974 (p. 300).
45. *Ibid.* (p. 304).
46. Sokoloff L: The pathology and pathogenesis of osteoarthritis, Chapter 55. In *Arthritis and Allied Conditions*, edited by J.L. Hollander, D.J. McCarty, Ed. 8. Lea & Febiger, Philadelphia, 1972 (pp. 1018, 1019).
47. Spalteholz W: *Handatlas der Anatomie des Menschen*, Ed. 11, Vol. 2. S. Hirzel, Leipzig, 1922 (p. 340).
48. *Ibid.* (p. 341).
49. *Ibid.* (p. 334).
50. Stecher RM, Hersh AH, Hauser H: Heberden's nodes. *Am J Hum Genet* 5:46–60, 1953.
51. Toldt C: *An Atlas of Human Anatomy*, translated by M.E. Paul, Ed. 2, Vol. 1. Macmillan, New York, 1919 (pp. 335, 336).
52. *Ibid.* (p. 334).
53. *Ibid.* (pp. 330, 331).
54. Travell J. Rinzler SH: The myofascial genesis of pain. *Postgrad Med* 11:425–434, 1952 (p. 428).
55. Wright V, Goddard R, Dawson D and Longfield MD: Articular gelling in osteoarthrosis—a bioengineering study. *Ann Rheum Dis* 29:339, 1970.
56. Zohn DA, Mennell J McM: *Musculoskeletal Pain: Diagnosis and Physical Treatment*. Little, Brown & Company, Boston, 1976 (p. 192, Fig. 9–13).

PART 3

PART 4

CHAPTER 41
Torso Pain-and-Muscle Guide

INTRODUCTION TO PART 4

This fourth part of the TRIGGER POINT MAN-UAL includes those muscles of the front of the chest, abdomen, and back that were not previously covered. Excluded are the muscles that attach to the scapula and those that cross the glenohumeral joint. Muscles that give rise to buttock pain, including the quadratus lumborum, intrapelvic muscles, and muscles that cross the hip joint will be covered in a subsequent volume.

PAIN GUIDE TO INVOLVED MUSCLES

This guide lists the muscles that may be responsible for pain in the areas shown in Figure 41.1. The muscles most likely to refer pain to a given area are listed below under the name of that area. One uses this chart by locating the name of the area that hurts and then by looking under that heading for all the muscles that are likely to cause the pain. Then, reference should be made to the individual muscle chapters; the number for each follows in parenthesis.

In a general way, the muscles are listed in the order of the frequency in which they are likely to cause pain in that area. This order is only an approximation; the selection process by which patients reach an examiner greatly influences which of their muscles are most likely to be involved. Boldface type indicates that the muscle refers an essential pain pattern to that pain area. Regular type indicates that the muscle refers a spillover pattern to that pain area.

PAIN GUIDE

LOW THORACIC BACK PAIN

Iliocostalis thoracis (48)
Multifidi (48)
Serratus posterior inferior (47)
Rectus abdominis (49)
Latissimus dorsi (24)

LUMBAR PAIN

Longissimus thoracis (48)
Iliocostalis lumborum (48)
Iliocostalis thoracis (48)
Multifidi (48)
Rectus abdominis (49)

SACRAL AND GLUTEAL PAIN

Longissimus thoracis (48)
Iliocostalis lumborum (48)
Multifidi (48)

SIDE-OF-CHEST PAIN

Serratus Anterior (46)
Latissimus dorsi (24)

FRONT-OF-CHEST PAIN

Pectoralis major (42)
Pectoralis minor (43)
Scaleni (20)
Sternocleidomastoid (sternal) (7)
Sternalis (44)
Iliocostalis cervicis (48)
Subclavius (42)
External abdominal oblique (49)

ABDOMINAL PAIN

Rectus abdominis (49)
Abdominal obliques (49)
Transversus abdominis (49)
Iliocostalis thoracis (48)
Multifidi (48)
Pyramidalis (49)

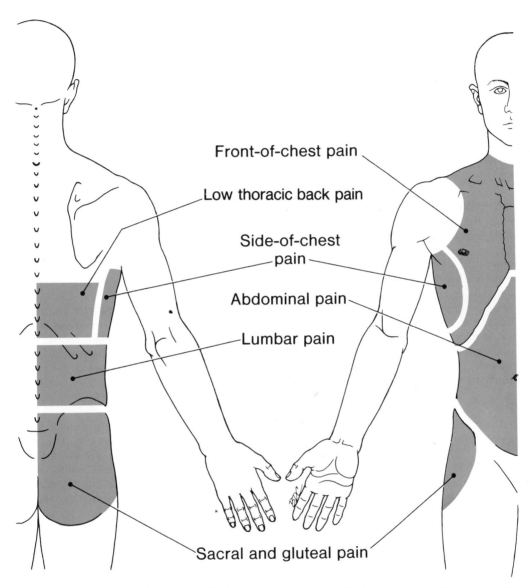

Front-of-chest pain

Low thoracic back pain

Side-of-chest pain

Abdominal pain

Lumbar pain

Sacral and gluteal pain

Figure 41.1.   The designated areas within the torso region where the patient may describe pain referred there by myofascial trigger points.

CHAPTER 42
Pectoralis Major Muscle (Subclavius Muscle)
"Poor Posture" and "Heart Attack"

HIGHLIGHTS: **REFERRED PAIN** from pectoralis major trigger points (TPs) may localize substernally, may include the anterior chest and breast, and may extend down the ulnar aspect of the arm to the 4th and 5th fingers. The pectoralis major muscle can harbor a somatovisceral TP in its costal section medially on the *right* side. The extinction of this TP terminates episodes of cardiac arrhythmia. When on the *left* side, pectoralis major TPs refer pain in patterns that are easily mistaken for the pain of ischemic heart disease. **ANATOMICAL ATTACHMENTS** are complex. It is rarely mentioned that this muscle consists of multiple overlapping laminae in a playing-card arrangement. The muscle is divided into clavicular, sternal, costal, and abdominal sections. Several caudal laminae wrap around the lateral border of the muscle. **ACTIVATION OF TRIGGER POINTS** may be caused by stress overload on the muscle or by referred phenomena associated with a myocardial infarction. **PATIENT EXAMINATION** reveals shortening of the pectoralis major muscle by active or latent TPs, which pulls the shoulders forward to produce a stooped, round-shouldered posture. **TRIGGER POINT EXAMINATION** is performed by palpating the clavicular, sternal and costal sections of the muscle for tender TPs within firm bands, which react with strong local twitch responses. **STRETCH AND SPRAY** are done by abducting and flexing the arm at the shoulder while applying the vapocoolant cephalad over the stretched muscle fibers and distally over the arm. **INJECTION AND STRETCH** usually require the injection of multiple TPs to be effective. **CORRECTIVE ACTIONS** start with convincing the patient (when true) that the myofascial chest pain is a treatable pain of skeletal muscle, rather than of cardiac origin. Correction of poor standing and sitting posture, avoidance of mechanical overload of this muscle, and the In-doorway Stretch Exercise help to insure continued freedom from this myofascial pain.

1. REFERRED PAIN
(Figs. 42.1 and 42.2)

Edeiken and Wolferth,[11] in 1936, identified the "trigger zone" as a hypersensitive spot in the skeletal musculature of the chest. The "trigger zone" was responsible for referred chest pain that persisted following an acute myocardial infarction.[11, 35] Subsequent authors noted that tender spots in the left pectoralis major muscle ("pectoral myalgia")[19] referred pain to the chest in a manner that confusingly simulated the pain of coronary insufficiency in persons with no history or evidence of cardiac disease.[20, 25, 34, 52, 70] Other authors recognized the non-cardiac nature of this pain, but were unaware of its trigger point (TP) origin.[6, 13, 47] Lange[37] emphasized the shoulder and arm components of pain arising from the pectoralis major muscle.

This muscle is likely to develop TPs in five areas, each with a distinctive pain reference pattern. Pain and tenderness are referred unilaterally.

The TPs located in the *clavicular section*

PART 4

(Fig. 42.1A) refer pain over the anterior deltoid muscle and locally to the clavicular section of the pectoralis major itself.

Active TPs in the *intermediate sternal section* of the pectoralis major (Fig. 42.1B) are likely to refer intense pain to the anterior chest[33, 34, 41, 72] (to the precordium, if on the left side) and down the inner aspect of the arm. The arm pain accents the medial epicondyle. If sufficiently active, these TPs refer pain also to the volar aspect of the forearm and ulnar side of the hand. The hand pain includes the last two, or two and one half, digits (more than the one and one half digits usually innervated by the sensory fibers of the ulnar nerve).[69] The uppermost of these sternal-section TPs (Fig. 42.1B) lies at the three-way confluence of the clavicular and manubrial sections of the pectoralis major and the underlying pectoralis minor muscle. Active TPs occur frequently in all three of these layers.

Active TPs located in the *medial sternal section* of the pectoralis major refer pain locally and over the sternum without crossing the midline[33, 41, 66] (Fig. 42.2A). At times, when injecting TPs located over the sternum in the area of a sternalis muscle (see Chapter 44), one may encounter TPs in a second, deeper layer of muscle, 1.5–2 cm (½–¾ in) beneath the surface. These TPs are probably located in pectoralis major fibers close to their musculotendinous junctions, beneath a sternalis muscle.

In the *costal and abdominal section* of the pectoralis major, TPs develop in two regions. One of these regions lies along the lateral border of the muscle. These TPs (Fig. 42.1C) cause breast tenderness with hypersensitivity of the nipple, intolerance to clothing, and often breast pain.[63] Complaints of this distressing syndrome are made by both women and men, but more often by women.

More medially, a TP associated with somatovisceral cardiac arrhythmias[64] is located on the right side between the fifth and sixth ribs, just below the point where the lower border of the fifth rib crosses a vertical line that lies midway between the margin of the sternum and the nipple (Fig. 42.2B). This TP has been observed only on the right side, except in *situs inversus*. The spot tenderness of this TP is associated with ectopic cardiac rhythms, but not with

any pain complaint. There may be nearby tender points over or between adjacent ribs, but they are not pertinent to cardiac arrhythmia.

When active TPs occur in the left pectoralis major muscle, the referred pain is easily confused with that due to coronary insufficiency.[13, 36, 68] Chest pain that persists long after an acute myocardial infarction is often due to myofascial TPs.[26, 51, 52, 67]

Subclavius
(Fig. 42.3)

The subclavius muscle can develop active TPs that refer pain into the upper extremity on the same side (Fig. 42.3). The pain travels across the front of the shoulder, and down the front of the arm and along the radial side of the forearm, but skips the elbow and wrist to reappear on the radial half of the hand. The dorsal and volar aspects of the thumb, index and middle fingers also may hurt.

2. ANATOMICAL ATTACHMENTS
(Figs. 42.4 and 42.5)

Anatomy books contradict each other in their descriptions of the arrangement of the lowest fibers of the pectoralis major muscle. They generally agree that the fibers of the entire muscle attach **medially** as four separate sections (Fig. 42.4): (1) clavicular fibers to the clavicle, (2) sternal fibers to the sternum, (3) costal fibers to the cartilages of the second to sixth or seventh ribs, and (4) abdominal fibers (Fig. 42.5) to the superficial aponeuroses of the obliquus externus abdominis and rectus abdominis muscles.[2, 12, 23, 28, 29, 40, 41, 54, 56] These are also the components of the muscle that authors illustrate in very nearly all anatomical atlases.[12, 22, 28, 29, 40, 48, 54, 56, 59] The abdominal section of the pectoralis major is more likely to be omitted and occasionally fails to develop.[2, 7, 22]

Anatomists, except Eisler[12] who identified three layers, agree that the **lateral** termination of the muscle on the humerus comprises two layers, a ventral and a dorsal. All are attached to the crest of the greater tubercle of the humerus (along the lateral lip of the groove for the bicipital tendon).[2, 23, 28, 29, 40, 46, 49, 54, 56, 59]

In 1912, Eisler[12] described the bulk of the muscle as strips of fibers that overlap each other like the shingles on a roof or the

PART 4

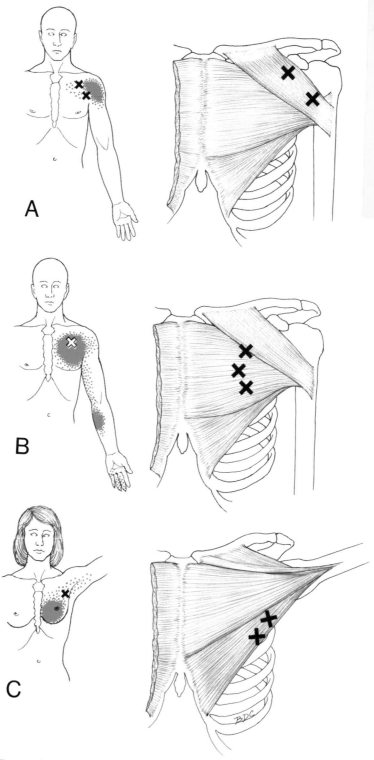

Figure 42.1. Referred pain patterns (*red*) and trigger points (×s) in the left pectoralis major muscle. *Solid red* shows essential areas of referred pain, and *stippled red* shows the spillover pain areas. *A*, the clavicular section. *B*, the intermediate sternal section. *C*, the lateral free margin of the muscle, which includes fibers of the costal and abdominal sections that form the anterior axillary fold.

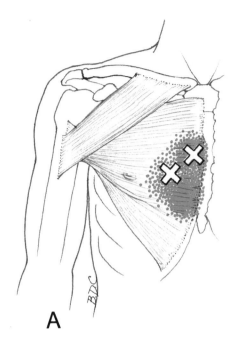

A

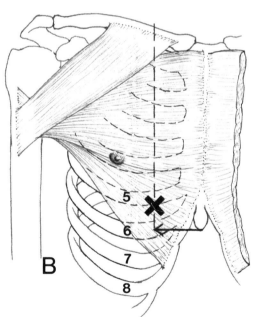

B

Figure 42.2.   Right pectoralis major muscle trigger-point phenomena. *A*, overlapping referred pain patterns (*red*) of two parasternal trigger points (×s) located in the medial sternal section of the muscle. *B*, location of the "cardiac arrhythmia" trigger point (×) below the lower border of the fifth rib in the vertical line that lies midway between the sternal margin and the nipple line. On this line, the sixth rib is found at the level of the tip of the xiphoid process (*arrow*).

leaves of a fan. Hollinshead[28] clearly described this relationship between the clavicular and sternocostal sections. A few other authors recognized the overlap of these sections.[2, 23, 28, 40, 49, 56] Many illustrations of the muscle show a variable degree of this overlap,[2, 22, 28, 40, 45, 48, 56, 59] while others do not.[22, 23, 54]

Eisler[12] described the lower sternocostal fibers and the abdominal section as folding upward beneath the rest of the muscle at its lateral end; because of this folding, the lowermost fibers had the most proximal attachment to the humerus. Hollinshead[28] also described this folding process and illustrated it diagrammatically.[28] Some illustrations of the muscle also portray this feature,[12, 22, 23, 28, 40, 45, 54, 56, 59] but others do not.[2, 22, 48] Drawings of the muscle with and without this fold sometimes appear in the same volume.

Frustrated by these inconsistencies, Ashley[1] dissected 60 adults and 8 fetuses to establish the facts. He reported clear schematic drawings of his findings. The arrangement of most of the pectoralis major fibers can be seen clearly ONLY from the dorsal (under) side of the muscle, a view not found in anatomy texts. Ashley's drawings[1] were followed closely in the preparation of Figure 42.5, which is a semischematic presentation of the muscle's fiber arrangement. However, his terminology has been modified to clarify the description.

Ashley[1] found (Fig. 42.5) that the tendinous pectoralis major attachment **laterally** to the humerus has two layers, each of which is made up of laminae. The ventral layer at the humerus, as previously described by Eisler,[12] is composed of six or more overlapping laminae splayed in the manner of playing cards. These six laminae attach **medially** to the clavicle, sternum, and ribs. The lower sternal and costal laminae of this ventral (superficial) layer at the humerus attach **medially** as underlying, but unfolded, *deep* fibers of this superficial layer.

As seen from the usual ventral view, however, these deep lower laminae are hidden by a more superficial lamina of lower sternal, costal, and abdominal fibers that wrap or fold around the caudal end of the pectoralis major to attach on the humerus as most, if not all, of the dorsal

PART 4

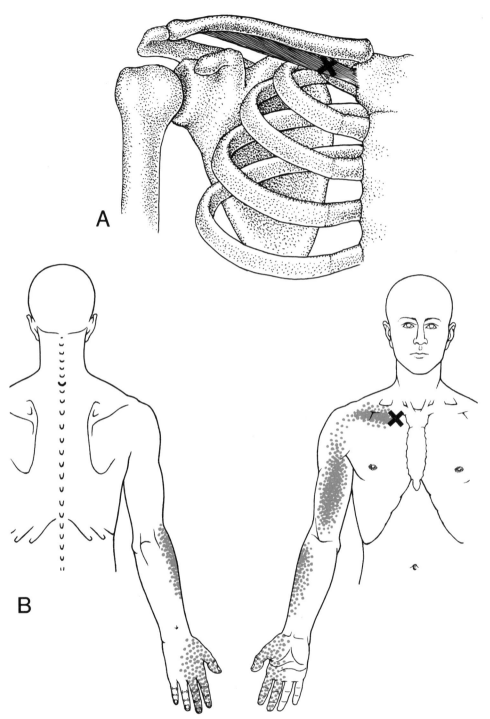

Figure 42.3. Subclavius muscle. *A*, attachments, and location (×) of trigger points in this muscle (*medium red*). *B*, Referred pain pattern (*dark red*) of the trigger point (×).

(deep) layer at that location. The folded arrangement reverses the order of attachment of these fibers. They wrap around an unfolded lamina that usually attaches to

the sixth rib, sometimes to the fifth and seventh ribs. This pivotal costal lamina joins the folded lamina to complete the dorsal layer in approximately 9 of 10 bod-

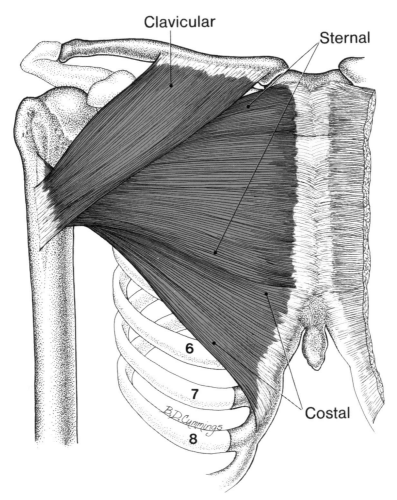

Figure 42.4.   Attachments of the pectoralis major muscle (*red*), anterior (ventral) view. Fibers of the uppermost clavicular section overlap fibers of the sternal section to form part of the ventral layer at the humeral attachment. Costal fibers curl around the lateral border (anterior axillary fold) to form most of the dorsal layer at the humerus. The variable abdominal fibers are not shown (see Fig. 42.5).

ies. In the rest, the costal lamina joins the ventral layer, leaving the folded lamina to form all of the dorsal layer.[1]

The semischematic version of the usual anterior view of the undisturbed pectoralis major muscle (Fig. 42.5*A*) clearly shows the first two overlapping laminae of the ventral layer, which are the fibers of the clavicular section and the manubrial portion of the sternal section. The remaining sternal, costal, and abdominal fibers visible in Fig. 42.5*A* are superficial at their medial attachments, but fold under the ventral layer fibers to form the bulk of the dorsal layer at the humerus.

A glimpse of the remaining laminae of the ventral layer at the humerus is revealed in Figure 42.5*B* by retraction of the folded lamina. These remaining laminae are clearly seen in the reflected dorsal view of the fibers in Figure 42.5*C*. These ventral layer fibers attach **medially** to the sternum and ribs, deep to the more superficial folded lamina.

Knowledge of this arrangement is important in order to interpret accurately the direction of the fibers palpated for TPs and the direction of contraction when a local twitch response is elicited.

Rarely, all or a portion of the pectoralis

PART 4

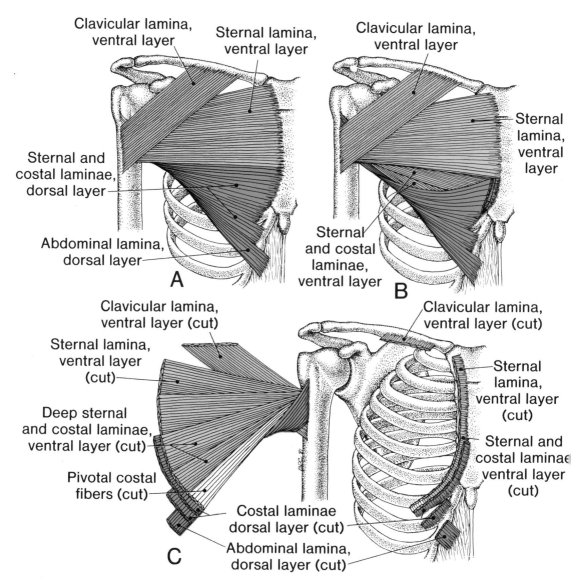

Clavicular lamina,
ventral layer

Sternal lamina,
ventral layer

Clavicular lamina,
ventral layer

Sternal
lamina,
ventral
layer

Sternal and
costal laminae,
dorsal layer

Abdominal lamina,
dorsal layer

Sternal
and costal
laminae,
ventral layer

A

B

Clavicular lamina,
ventral layer (cut)

Clavicular lamina,
ventral layer (cut)

Sternal lamina,
ventral layer
(cut)

Sternal
lamina,
ventral layer
(cut)

Deep sternal
and costal laminae,
ventral layer (cut)

Sternal and
costal laminae
ventral layer
(cut)

Pivotal costal
fibers (cut)

Costal laminae
dorsal layer (cut)

Abdominal lamina,
dorsal layer (cut)

C

Figure 42.5.   Semischematic drawings of the fiber arrangement in the pectoralis major muscle, adapted from Ashley.[1] *A*, usual ventral view. *B*, ventral view with the superficial dorsal-layer fibers retracted to show the deep lamina of the ventral layer (*light red*) when it attaches to the humerus. *C*, muscle reflected laterally to show the dorsal aspect of the seldom seen playing card arrangement of the deep lamina of the ventral layer. The dorsal layer (*dark red*) swings around the other fibers to attach on the humerus dorsal to them.

major muscle may be congenitally absent; the sternocostal sections are more likely to be absent than the clavicular section.[42] An axillary arch variant of the pectoralis major has been illustrated.[28] This and other variations have been well described.[2, 12]

Subclavius Muscle

The subclavius muscle (Fig. 42.3*A*) lies beneath the clavicle over the first rib and attaches **medially** by a short thick tendon

to the junction of the first rib with its cartilage. The muscle attaches **laterally** in a groove on the under side of the clavicle.[24] A number of authors have clearly illustrated its attachments.[24, 46, 55]

3. INNERVATION

The pectoralis major muscle is innervated by the medial and lateral pectoral nerves.

Spinal nerves C_5 through C_7 supply the

lateral pectoral nerve.[29] This nerve branches from, or just above, the lateral cord of the brachial plexus to supply the clavicular and sternal sections of the pectoralis major muscle.[23]

The *medial* pectoral nerve arises from spinal nerves C_8 and T_1 and passes *via* the medial cord of the brachial plexus to supply the caudal third, the costal and abdominal sections, of the muscle. This nerve may skirt the lateral border of, but usually pierces, the pectoralis minor muscle, which it supplies en route.[29]

The innervation of the pectoralis major fibers progresses segmentally from above downward. The clavicular section is supplied chiefly by spinal segments C_5 and C_6. The sternal section is innervated mainly by segments C_6 and C_7. The costal section innervation is usually a transition zone between the two nerves by segments C_7 and C_8. The costal and abdominal sections are supplied by segments C_8 and T_1 through the medial pectoral nerve.[12]

4. ACTIONS

When passively stretching this muscle, it is important to remember that it crosses three joints, namely, the sternoclavicular, acromioclavicular, and glenohumeral. It also spans an area that functions like a joint to provide the gliding movement of the scapula over the ribs.

Electrical stimulation of the entire pectoralis major muscle internally rotates the arm.[9] Stimulation of only the clavicular section moves the shoulder obliquely upward and forward. This stimulation also moves the arm obliquely upward, forward and inward, so as to press it against the thorax. Stimulation of the sternocostal section lowers the shoulder and extends the flexed arm, and strongly adducts it.[9]

All fibers contribute to three movements of the arm at the shoulder: (1) adduction[23, 29] (electromyographically only the sternocostal fibers are reported as active[3]), (2) movement across the chest,[29, 49] and (3) internal rotation.[23, 29, 49] Electromyographically, the muscle was active during internal rotation only against resistance. All fibers assist forced protraction of the scapula.[3]

The *clavicular section* assists flexion at the shoulder when the movement is started with the arm at the side,[31, 49] draws the arm upward across the chest toward the opposite ear,[23, 29] and assists abduction at the shoulder above the horizontal.[49] Electromyographically, throughout flexion, chiefly the clavicular fibers were active,[3, 31] with some assistance from the sternal fibers.[31]

The *sternal, costal* and *abdominal* fibers extend,[23, 29, 49] but do not hyperextend[29] the arm; they depress the arm and shoulder.[23, 42] The unassisted pectoralis major could not bring the arm far enough across the chest for the hand to touch the opposite ear, but only to reach the opposite side of the chest; the unassisted anterior deltoid, however, can complete the former movement.[3, 9]

Bilateral, surface-electrode electromyographic activity in the clavicular and sternal sections of the pectoralis major muscles was reported for the right-handed execution of sport skills in four underhand patterns, three overhand patterns, four sidearm patterns and two kinds of 1-ft jumps.[4] Generally, both right and left muscles were slightly-to-moderately active. They were most active when the subject batted a baseball. Generally, the left clavicular section responded most vigorously and showed a prolonged or double burst of activity. The bursts of activity seen in the left pectoralis major muscle appeared to counterbalance rotary movement imparted to the body by acceleration of the right hand; this effect was noteworthy in all but the underhand throwing patterns.[4]

The subclavius muscle assists protraction of the shoulder by drawing it in a ventral and caudal direction.[24]

5. MYOTATIC UNIT

All sections of the pectoralis major muscle contract together during strong adduction of the arm, assisted by the teres major and minor, the anterior and posterior deltoid, the subscapularis, and the long head of the triceps muscles. For protraction of the scapula, the serratus anterior, pectoralis minor, and subclavius assist the pectoralis major below its clavicular section.

Agonist muscles in parallel and in series, which may assist the *clavicular* section of the pectoralis major, include the anterior deltoid, coracobrachialis, subclavius, scalenus anterior and sternocleidomastoid muscles on the same side. The clavicular

PART 4

section and the anterior deltoid work very closely together. They lie side-by-side with adjacent attachments and are separated only by the groove of the cephalic vein.

The more vertical, lower fibers of the *costal* and *abdominal sections* of the pectoralis major depress the shoulder with the help of corresponding fibers of the latissimus dorsi, lower trapezius, and lower serratus anterior. These lower pectoralis major fibers are also assisted by the subclavius and the pectoralis minor muscles. The pectoralis major muscle contracts bilaterally during forceful adduction of both arms together.

The major antagonists to the sternal section of the pectoralis major are the rhomboidei and middle trapezius muscles. For adduction of the arm at the shoulder, antagonists are the supraspinatus and deltoid muscles.

6. SYMPTOMS

In addition to pain in the front of the shoulder and in the subclavicular region (Fig. 42.1A), patients with active TPs in the clavicular section of the pectoralis major muscle may be aware of restricted abduction at the shoulder.

Active TPs in the central part of the pectoralis major refer pain widely over the precordium (if on the left side) and down the ulnar aspect of the arm to the 4th and 5th fingers (Fig. 42.1B), and also may cause a sense of chest constriction that is readily confused with angina pectoris. The patient with TPs in the intermediate fibers of the left sternal section is likely to complain of intermittent, intense chest pain (Fig. 42.2A) that appears in the precordial region at rest and/or on effort. Nocturnally this pain often disturbs sleep.

Breast pain and diffuse soreness are a feature of TPs in the free margin of the costal section, laterally (Fig. 42.1C). The nipple may be hypersensitive.

Differential Diagnosis

The intensity, quality and distribution of true cardiac pain can be reproduced in every detail by the pain referred from active TPs in the anterior chest muscles.[36, 50, 68] Although these patterns strongly mimic cardiac pain, myofascial TP pain shows a much wider variability in its response to activity from day-to-day than does the more consistent limit imposed by angina pectoris.

A definite diagnosis of active myofascial TPs based on their characteristic signs and symptoms, and a dramatic response to local treatment, does NOT exclude cardiac disease. Adding to this diagnostic challenge is the fact that non-cardiac pain may induce transient T-wave changes in the electrocardiogram.[17] A disorder of the heart may coexist and must be ruled out by appropriate tests of cardiac function.[60]

Complaints of circumscribed areas of unilateral parasternal pain should arouse suspicion of parasternal TPs in the pectoralis major muscle (Fig. 42.2A). However, one should be aware that pain clearly of cardiac origin can be abolished temporarily or permanently by the application of a vapocoolant spray to,[52, 60, 67] or by infiltration of procaine subcutaneously into, the area of referred cardiac pain[21, 39]; these measures also eliminate pain solely of myofascial origin. Hence, relief of pain by a vapocoolant spray or by local injection cannot be used diagnostically to exclude myocardial ischemia as a cause of the pain.[50]

On the other hand, relief of pain by nitrites does not ensure that the pain is due to coronary artery insufficiency, because a placebo sometimes is equally effective in angina pectoris.[18] Furthermore, nitrites dilate the peripheral, as well as the coronary arteries; nitrites occasionally have relieved skeletal muscle pain.[8, 21, 36] Foley and colleagues[14, 15] showed that, in the patient with Raynaud's disease or who had an absent radial pulse due to vasospasm, sublingual nitroglycerin promptly restored the pulsation of the radial artery.

The pectoralis minor muscle (see Chapter 43) has a similar referred pain pattern and a close anatomical relationship to the pectoralis major. Active TPs in the scaleni, (see Chapter 20) also refer pain to the pectoral region.[69] Tender spots in the deep paraspinal muscles to the left of the second to the sixth thoracic vertebrae,[73] and in the region of the left upper rectus abdominis muscle, induce chest pain that strongly mimics cardiac disease.[33] Experimentally,

Lewis and Kellgren[38] accurately reproduced the pain of effort angina by injecting hypertonic saline to the left of the interspinous ligaments below both the C_7 and T_1 spinous processes.

Other sources of chest pain to be considered include intercostal neuritis or radiculopathy; irritation of the bronchi, pleura or esophagus; hiatal hernia with reflux; distension of the stomach by gas, mediastinal emphysema;[53] gasseous distension of the splenic flexure of the colon;[10] and lung cancer.

Some of the less common non-cardiac skeletal syndromes that cause pain and tenderness in the chest include the chest wall syndrome.[13] Tietze's syndrome,[32, 58] costochondritis, the hypersensitive xiphoid, the precordial catch syndrome,[5] the slipping rib syndrome,[27] and the rib-tip syndrome.[43] Each patient should be carefully examined to determine if the symptoms are partially or entirely due to myofascial referred pain and tenderness, especially from TPs in the pectoralis major muscle. Of the above conditions, each has been reported as sometimes relieved by injection of the tender area with a local anesthetic. Relief by injection is characteristic of TPs.

The patient who presents with a painful or tender breast, often with hypersensitivity of the nipple to light contact, may harbor responsible TPs in the lateral margin of the pectoralis major muscle[63, 69] (Fig. 42.1C). Cancer may be a serious, but *unexpressed* fear in patients who express enormous relief when they realize that the pain has a benign treatable myofascial cause.

Somatovisceral Effects

A common example of a somatovisceral response is found in the patient who experiences episodes of supraventricular tachycardia, supraventricular premature contractions, or ventricular premature contractions without other evidence of heart disease. The patient with such an ectopic rhythm should be checked for an active TP in the right pectoralis major muscle between the fifth and sixth ribs at the specific site[64] (Fig. 42.2B). Although this TP is tender to palpation, it is not a source of spontaneous pain. Inactivation of the TP promptly restores normal sinus rhythm when an ectopic supraventricular rhythm is present, and often eliminates recurrences of the paroxysmal arrhythmia or frequent premature contractions for a long period of time.

A comparable somatovisceral effect is the well known onset of angina pectoris appearing when an anginal patient suddenly breathes cold air through the nose.[16] Another is the slowing of the heart rate that occurs when the face is placed in cold water, known as the diving reflex.

The somatic area of referred pain exerts a strong influence on the perceived pain originating in an ischemic myocardium. The pain of angina pectoris was relieved in three patients by infiltrating the painful area subcutaneously with 2% procaine.[71] Even the application of only vapocoolant spray to the area of chest pain referred from a myocardial infarct relieved the pain at once.[44, 64] Chest pain that persisted in 12 patients following a myocardial infarct, or angina pectoris that developed shortly after a myocardial infarct, was relieved by procaine injection or vapocoolant spray of the TPs in the chest wall muscles.[52]

Another example of somatic modulation of visceral cardiac pain was observed using the intravenous ergonovine test, which induces sufficient myocardial ischemia to cause anginal pain and depression of the S-T segment in the normal resting electrocardiograms of patients subject to effort angina, but not in pain-free controls. This pain and electrocardiographic response to intravenous ergonovine is quickly reversed by sublingual nitroglycerin, but persists for more than 10 min when untreated.

Patients who responded to the ergonovine test in this manner were sprayed with vapocoolant over the somatic areas of anginal pain that developed on effort and after intravenous ergonovine injection.[64] In no case did the vapocoolant delay or modify the electrocardiographic ischemic response. However, 10 of 12 patients whose pain areas were sprayed immediately following injection obtained complete relief of pain, and two patients obtained partial relief. More surprisingly, when the spray was applied just *before* the ergonovine injection to the areas that were known to become painful in response to the myocardial ischemia caused by this test and by their effort angina, 9 of 15 patients experienced no pain at all, although the electrocardiographic effects of coronary ischemia developed as before. The other six patients had a delayed onset or attenuation of anginal pain after intravenous ergonovine.

Viscerosomatic Effects

An example of a myofascial viscerosomatic interaction begins with coronary artery insufficiency, or other intrathoracic disease, that refers pain from these visceral structures to the anterior chest wall. As a result, satellite TPs develop in the somatic pectoral muscles. Kennard and Haugen[35] related the presence of palpably tender TPs in the chest muscles to chest and arm pain, and to the disease process responsible for the pain. They found that 61% of 72 patients with cardiac disease, 48% of 35 patients with other visceral chest disease, and only 20% of 46 patients with pelvic and lower extremity disease, had tender TPs in the chest muscles. In the patients with chest and arm pain due to cardiac and other unilateral intrathoracic disease, tender TPs were strongly lateralized to the affected side.

Additional examples of somatovisceral and viscerosomatic effects in relation to the abdominal viscera[57] are presented in Section 6 of Chapter 49, where the neurophysiology of referred visceral pain is summarized.

7. ACTIVATION OF TRIGGER POINTS

Pectoralis major TPs may be initiated or re-activated in many ways: by heavy lifting (especially when reaching out in front), by overuse of arm adduction (use of manual hedge clippers), by sustained lifting in a fixed position (use of a power saw), by immobilization of the arm in the adducted position (arm in a sling or cast), by sustained high levels of anxiety, or by exposure of fatigued muscles to cold air (while sitting in the shade in a wet suit after a swim, or when exposed to the draft from an air conditioner).

Pectoralis major TPs are activated by a round-shouldered posture, because it produces sustained shortening of the pectoral muscles. This is likely to occur during prolonged sitting, when reading and writing, and when standing with a slouched, flat-chested posture.

In acute myocardial infarction, pain is commonly referred from the heart to the mid-region of the pectoralis major and minor muscles. The injury to heart muscle initiates a viscerosomatic process that activates TPs in the pectoral muscles. Following recovery from the acute infarction, these self-perpetuating TPs tend to persist in the chest wall unless wiped away like dust from a shelf.

8. PATIENT EXAMINATION

The TPs in the pectoralis major, when it is involved alone, cause minimal restriction of motion at the shoulder, as shown by the Hand-to-shoulder-blade Test (see Fig. 22.4). Pectoralis TPs do not cause restriction of the Finger-flexion Test (see Fig. 20.6) as is the case when the similar upper extremity pain pattern is caused by TPs in the scalene muscles. The patient with chest pain due to pectoralis major TPs is likely to suffer additional referred pain and restriction of movement at the shoulder due to associated myofascial TPs in functionally related shoulder-girdle muscles.

The diagnosis of angina pectoris sometimes is made clinically when there is no definite evidence that the chest pain is due to myocardial ischemia. In many such patients, one can demonstrate that the pain is referred from TPs in the pectoralis major muscle.[13] The patient with the diagnosis of angina pectoris is naturally *fearful* of any activity that produces the pain. This fear inhibits full movement, which accelerates both physical and psychological deterioration and perpetuates the myofascial TPs.

When a patient complains of breast soreness (referred tenderness), she or he also may describe a feeling of congestion in that breast. When compared with the other side, the breast may be slightly enlarged and feel doughy. These signs of impaired lymph drainage, possibly due to entrapment or reflex inhibition of peristalsis, soon disappear after inactivation of the responsible TPs in the lateral border of the taut pectoralis major muscle (Fig. 42.1C).

Sudden pain in the muscle during strenuous effort may be due to rupture of the muscle belly. The tear is easily recognized by the visible and palpable discontinuity of the muscle belly when compared with the normal side.[42]

9. TRIGGER POINT EXAMINATION
(Fig. 42.6)

Most of the TPs found in the clavicular section, and all of the TPs in the parasternal section of the muscle are identified by flat palpation. The TPs in the intermediate and lateral parts of the sternal and costal sections are best located by pincer palpation (Fig. 42.6). The muscle is placed on moderate tension by abducting the arm to approximately 90° in order to maximize the spot tenderness and local twitch responses of the taut bands.

To find the "cardiac arrhythmia" TP (Fig. 42.2B), the tip of the xiphoid process is first located. Then, at this level on the right side, in a vertical line midway between the sternal border and the nipple line, the hollow between the fifth and sixth ribs is examined for a tender spot. This TP is found by pressing upward against the inferior edge of the fifth rib and exploring the muscle for spot tenderness.

10. ENTRAPMENTS

Lymphatic drainage from the breast usually travels in front of, and around, the pectoralis major muscle to the axillary lymph nodes. A lymph vessel from the cephalad portion of the breast may pierce the pectoralis major muscle and terminate in the subclavicular lymph nodes.[23] Entrapment of this lymph duct by passage between tense fibers of an involved pec-

toralis major muscle, may cause edema of the breast. These signs of entrapped lymphatic drainage and breast tenderness are relieved by extinction of the related pectoralis major TPs.

No nerve entrapments by this muscle have been observed.

11. ASSOCIATED TRIGGER POINTS

Parallel myotatic muscles, the anterior deltoid and coracobrachialis, are agonists that substitute in part for impaired function of the pectoralis major. The anterior deltoid is especially likely to develop satellite TPs because it also lies within the pain reference zone of the pectoralis major. Before long, the sternalis, sternocleidomastoid and scalene muscles, which are also part of the agonist myotatic unit, may develop active TPs.

Involvement of the serratus anterior and the rhomboid and middle trapezius antagonists often follows, especially in the patient with round-shouldered posture. The subscapularis, teres minor and posterior deltoid antagonistic muscles also may develop active TPs, with the end result of a "frozen" shoulder.

12. STRETCH AND SPRAY
(Fig. 42.7)

All sections of the pectoralis major are usually more effectively stretched with the patient seated than supine. The former

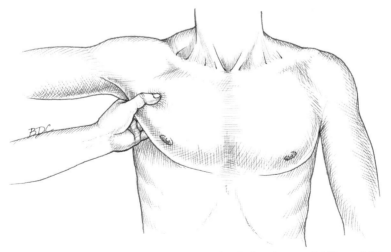

Figure 42.6.   Pincer palpation of trigger points in the sternocostal fibers of the pectoralis major muscle. Local twitch responses are best elicited when the muscle is placed on a moderate stretch by abducting the arm.

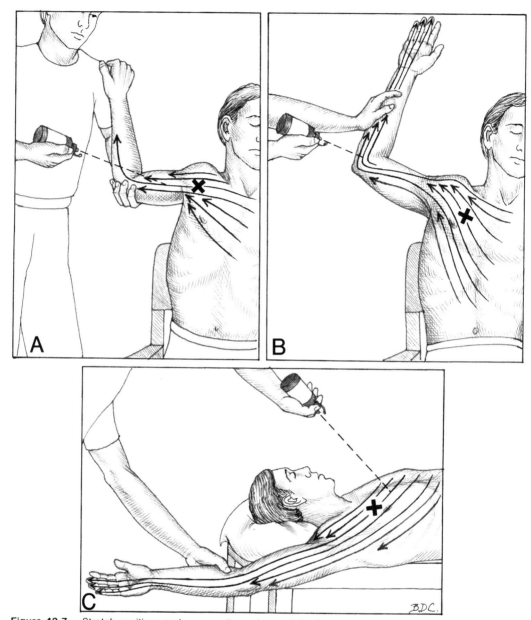

Figure 42.7. Stretch positions and spray patterns (*arrows*) for the pectoralis major muscle and location of the corresponding trigger points (×s). *A*, clavicular section with the patient seated. *B*, sternocostal sections, with the patient seated. *C*, sternocostal sections, with the patient supine. The patient lies with the shoulder slightly over the edge of the examining table. This provides freedom of movement for the arm and scapula to respond to traction on the arm with full stretch of the muscle.

position permits freer motion of both the scapula and arm. The freedom is important because this muscle must effectively be stretched across three joints (Section 4). Therefore, traction is applied to the arm as part of the stretch. The object is not only to increase the range of motion at the glenohumeral joint, but also to glide the

scapula over the chest wall to induce additional stretch of the muscle.

In any of the three stretch positions described below, but particularly when stretching the most caudal fibers, tightness of the subscapularis due to TPs can limit stretch of the pectoralis major. If the subscapularis is also involved, its spray pattern (see Fig. 26.5C) must be included alternately with the pectoralis pattern to release both muscles together.

For passive stretch of the *clavicular section* (Fig. 42.7A), the arm is externally rotated and horizontally extended at the shoulder so as to place maximal stretch on the clavicular fibers. The vapocoolant spray is swept laterally from the clavicle across the muscle and then over the shoulder and upper extremity to cover the referred pain pattern before and while stretching force is applied.

To stretch the *intermediate sternal fibers*, the arm is placed at about 90° of abduction, then externally rotated and pressed backward into maximum tolerated extension. Just before and while this position is achieved, parallel sweeps of the vapocoolant are directed laterally and upward across the sternal portion of the muscle, starting at the sternum and continuing over the upper extremity to cover all of its referred pain patterns, including the fingers (Figs. 42.1B and 42.7B). TPs in the anterior deltoid muscle will also restrict this movement, but their spray pattern is already included in that of the pectoralis major.

When inactivating *parasternal* TPs, the stretch position of Fig. 42.7B is used. The spray is swept medially across the sternal section of the muscle from its lateral border, over the TPs and pain reference zone, to the midline.

The pectoralis major muscle can be stretched and sprayed with the patient in the supine position, if care is taken not to fix the scapula against the table. Figure 42.7C shows the supine technique for the *lower sternal and costal sections*.

For stretch of the *lowest costal section*, with the patient either seated or supine, the arm is flexed at the shoulder while held in external rotation (like the stretch used for the pectoralis minor muscle). As much force is applied as the patient can tolerate without loss of relaxation. Meanwhile, the path of the spray courses *downward* and medially from the humerus over the passively stretched fibers, also covering the tender breast.

Hot packs follow each stretch-and-spray treatment at once. Afterward any residual TPs usually can be inactivated by ischemic compression or by injection with 0.5% pro-

caine solution, followed again by brief stretch and spray and then a hot pack.

The antagonistic posterior shoulder-girdle muscles, the rhomboidei and middle trapezius, are likely to develop shortening activation and pain after the tension in the pectoralis major has been released. Latent TPs in the antagonist muscles are apparently activated by the unaccustomed shortening during stretch of the pectoralis major. Therefore, as a routine procedure, stretch and spray should be applied to both anterior and posterior groups of chest muscles.

Vapocooling the skin over the pectoralis major muscle in the pattern shown (Fig. 42.7 A and B) may relieve the pain of true cardiac ischemia, as well as pain arising from active myofascial TPs.[61, 69] Thus, the cardiac status should be known in every patient who experiences relief of chest pain by these simple measures.

With proper technique, many pectoralis major TPs respond to stretch-and-spray therapy. However, the arrhythmia TP and the parasternal TPs may require repeated ischemic compression, or local anesthetic injection. It is important to teach the patient with arrhythmias the self-application of ischemic compression. With the thumb of one hand on top of the finger of the other hand to reinforce it, increasing pressure is directed onto the tender TP against the rib for a minute or more. The patient may thus learn to abort a paroxysmal ectopic tachycardia as soon as the attack is recognized.

13. INJECTION AND STRETCH
(Fig. 42.8)

The patient lies supine for all injections of TPs in the pectoralis major muscle.

Clavicular Section

Flat palpation localizes these TPs between the fingers for injection, in the manner shown in Fig. 42.8A; the needle is aimed cephalad and nearly tangent with the chest wall to avoid penetrating an intercostal space.[51]

Mid-sternal Section

Figure 42.8A also applies to the similar technique for injecting the frequent TPs in the mid-sternal section, where the clavic-

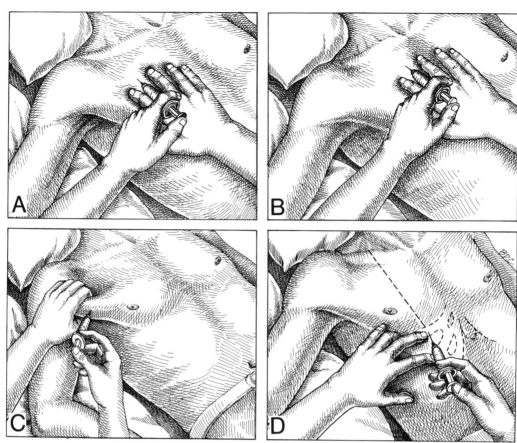

Figure 42.8.   Injection of trigger points in the pectoralis major muscle. *A*, the trigger points are localized and fixed by flat palpation for injection where the clavicular and sternal sections overlap. If the needle is not directed nearly tangent to the chest wall; beware of entering the pleura. *B*, similar technique for injection of parasternal trigger points. *C*, pincer grasp for injection of fibers in the lateral "roll" of the costal and abdominal sections. *D*, flat palpation for injection of the cardiac arrhythmia trigger point, while directing the needle upward toward the lower margin of the fifth rib, into the spot of maximal tenderness.

ular and sternal portions of the pectoralis major overlap the pectoralis minor muscle (uppermost × in Fig. 42.1*B*). These TPs can strongly induce all parts of the pectoralis major pain pattern. The TPs in this region are injected by directing the needle upward toward the coracoid process, away from the thoracic cage. Which of these three layers of muscle contains the TPs may be inferred by the depth of the needle on contact with a TP and the direction of the local twitch response.

Intermediate Sternal Section

In patients with mobile subcutaneous tissue, active TPs in the intermediate sternal section may be held for injection in a pincer grasp, as in Figure 42.8*C*, but with more of the muscle between the fingers.

To do this, the muscle must be slackened by bringing the arm closer to the patient's side. This permits the operator's fingers to slip between the thoracic cage and the underside of the pectoral musculature.

Medial Sternal Section

Parasternal TPs in the medial part of the sternal section are localized for injection between the fingers by flat palpation (Fig. 42.8*B*).

When the patient has pain and tenderness along the border of the anterior axillary fold, as in Figure 42.1*B*, these referred phenomena due to TP activity in that part of the pectoralis major may be secondary to a primary TP located among the lowest fibers of the sternal section close to the border of the sternum. If one first injects the latter TP, the other, secondary, TPs and referred phenomena along the lateral margin of the muscle may disappear.

Costal Section

To inject any remaining active TPs in the lateral margin of the costal section of the pectoralis major, the muscle is grasped between the thumb and fingers of one hand, as in Figure 42.8C. For this TP, however, adequate muscle tension is provided by abducting the arm to approximately 90°. The TPs in palpable bands are readily identified by the vigorous local twitch responses. For TPs in the most superficial fibers, the needle should enter at an acute angle to the fibers; for deep TPs, using pincer palpation, the needle may be directed perpendicularly to the skin in order to locate a cluster of TPs in the middle of, or on the far side of, the fold. Skin mobility permits multiple TP injections through one skin penetration.

Hemostasis is maintained by constant counterpressure during and after each injection.[63]

Subclavius Muscle

If, after injection of TPs in the clavicular section, tenderness to deep subclavicular pressure persists, and particularly if this pressure elicits pain in the referred pattern of the subclavius muscle (Fig. 42.3), the TPs in that muscle should be injected. For this, the needle is directed toward the point of maximum tenderness beneath the clavicle, usually close to the junction of its medial and middle thirds. Strong referred pain patterns are likely to be elicited by needle penetration of these TPs.

Arrhythmia Trigger Point

After locating the precise spot tenderness of the arrhythmia TP by flat palpation, the needle is directed cephalad toward the fifth rib (Fig. 42.8D). The needle is aimed nearly tangential to the skin, since the TP lies no deeper than the anterior surface of the lower border of the rib. This TP is not located as deep as the intercostal muscles. During and after treatment, the patient breathes so as to keep the chest diameter small, using normal, coordinated respiration and *not* the surprisingly common paradoxical breathing (see Fig. 20.13). Resolution of this TP has been difficult in

patients with an emphysematous, large-diameter chest.

For all parts of the pectoralis major muscle, the TP injection is followed by brief stretch and spray, and then a hot pack. Any residual TPs may be inactivated by ischemic compression or by repeated stretch and spray after rewarming. Both procedures seem to be more effective during, rather than before or after, local procaine analgesia. The patient should make active, full-range movements of the shoulder and arm after removal of the hot packs. This activity "re-educates" the muscle in its normal range of motion.[65]

14. CORRECTIVE ACTIONS
(Figs. 42.9 and 42.10)

Patient Education

For patients who have *no* demonstrable evidence of heart disease, but who suffer from chest pain that is assumed to be cardiac in origin, identification of TPs in the pectoralis major muscle as the cause of the pain completely changes the management and prognosis. By demonstrating to these patients that the kind and distribution of their pain is reproduced by pressure on the TPs, and by demonstrating local twitch responses, the patients are convinced that the pain is indeed myofascial, not cardiac, in origin. A normal, active life again becomes possible. Relief of pain by treatment of the afflicted muscles reassures the patient that it is safe to follow instructions and to perform the reconditioning exercise program, which is often critical for restoring normal function of the skeletal musculature and the quality of life.

When coronary artery disease and pectoralis major TPs coexist, relief of the TP-induced pain is important for more than comfort. Pain itself may reflexly diminish the caliber of the coronary arteries and thereby even further increase myocardial ischemia.[17, 39, 44]

Standing Posture

An important mechanical factor that perpetuates TPs in the pectoralis major muscle is poor standing and sitting posture. When the standing posture of the patient is slouched, with the shoulders and head projected forward, the center of the

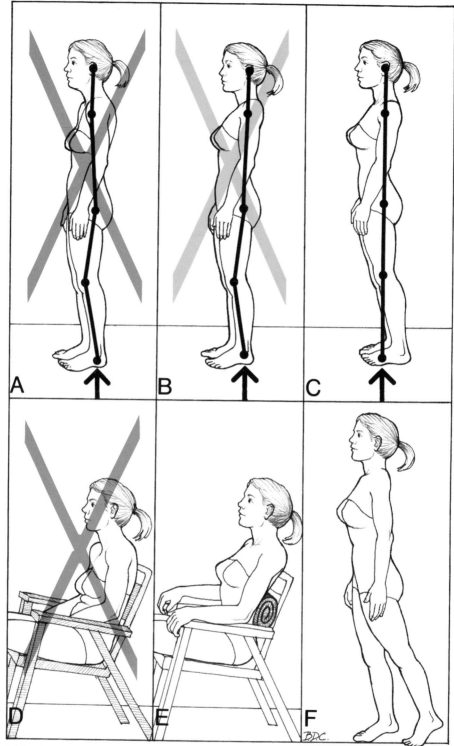

Figure 42.9. Improvement of standing and seated posture. *A*, this stooped, round-shouldered standing posture is aggravated by the increased tension that is caused by trigger points in the pectoralis major muscles. *B*, slight improvement in posture by having the patient "Stand up straight and hold the shoulders back!". *C*, marked improvement when the patient shifts the body weight from the heels onto the balls of the feet, which moves the head backward over the shoulders as a counterweight and straightens the lines of weight bearing. The *arrows* mark the shift in the *center-of-gravity line*, through the feet. *D*, the stooped, round-shouldered seated posture that often results from pectoralis major trigger points and poorly designed chairs. *E*, addition of a lumbar pillow or roll maintains the normal lumbar curve (lordosis) and moves the head backward, in balance. *F*, forward-leaning posture of the Indian Lope, which exaggerates the weight shift in panel *C* and greatly improves walking posture.

body weight rests solidly on the back of the heels (Fig. 42.9A). With instructions to "Stand up straight!," posture improves slightly, but the center of gravity remains on the heels (Fig. 42.9B). Maintaining this straightened position requires constant muscular effort by the patient, who soon becomes tired and discouraged.

If, instead, the body weight is rocked forward onto the balls of the feet (Fig. 42.9C), the head shifts backward over the shoulders as a counterweight and becomes more erect. The center of gravity through the feet moves forward, restoring the normal cervical and lumbar curves. The chest automatically expands. The patient now finds that the normal upright, balanced posture is easily maintained without muscular strain. Seeing the improvement *in a mirror*, the patient enjoys the straightened posture and feeling of comfort. Reminders from others are welcomed to help incorporate this "new look" into the day.

The Indian Lope (Fig. 42.9F) exaggerates the shift of weight to the balls of the feet, ensuring an erect, balanced, head-back posture. The person leans forward, on the verge of losing the balance, and walks very rapidly (too rapidly to swing the arms) to keep from falling forward. Each step receives a vigorous push-off with the toes (from the calf muscles). The feet actually follow the body. The pace is about twice the minimum energy rate of walking, just short of running. The American Indians used it to cover very long distances quickly.

Sitting Posture

Poor sitting posture arises largely from the much too common practice of constructing chairs with inadequate lumbar support.[62] This historic practice was reinforced by early research that established the model for seating design.[30] This study erroneously concluded that there was no need to shape the backrest to fit the lumbar curve because the spine could straighten and conform to a flat backrest. Neither comfort, normal posture, nor resultant muscular strain were considered in the study.

Recently, a comprehensive approach has provided more realistic data for the design of comfortable physiologic seating.[7]

Selection of a pain-relieving chair requires that serious consideration be given to the needs of the muscles.[62] Fig. 42.9D shows the result of sitting in a chair without lumbar support; the shoulders are "rounded," the head is projected forward, and the lumbar curve is flattened in a stooped posture.

These faults are corrected by fitting a small roll behind the lumbar spine about where a belt would go around the waist (Fig. 42.9E). The roll should comfortably support the normal lumbar curve. Foam rubber is usually too soft, but an old bath towel, tightly rolled, provides the desirable combination of firmness and resilience. The towel can be folded about 30 cm (12 in) wide, and enough of it rolled up to provide the needed lumbar support (usually 7.5 to 10 cm, or 3 to 4 in, in diameter) when used with a particular chair or auto seat. The towel can be slipped into an attractive cover with ties around the backrest to hold the roll in place. The roll also may be supported by two straps thrown over the top of the backrest, with enough lead weight sewn into the end of each strap to counterweight the roll and hold it in place.

The chair seat must also be designed with sufficient hollow or backward slope at the bottom of the backrest so that the buttocks are not pushed forward.

For comfort in reading, talking and watching TV (but not for eating), the chairback should slope 25–30° from the vertical. If it slopes 20° or less, for relaxation the person must slide the hips forward on the seat to obtain adequate slope for the torso; this requires a larger lumbar roll. Inadequate lumbar support is a major contributory factor in most patients for whom riding in an automobile aggravates back, chest, or neck pain.

When sitting, crossing the arms in front of the chest swings the scapulae forward and shortens the pectoralis major. Instead, the elbows should be placed on armrests, if they are of suitable height. For prolonged sitting, the patient should avoid a chair without armrests, or with armrests too low to support the elbows.

Unnecessary muscular tension should be reduced. To achieve relaxation, the patient should focus attention on *consciously*

PART 4

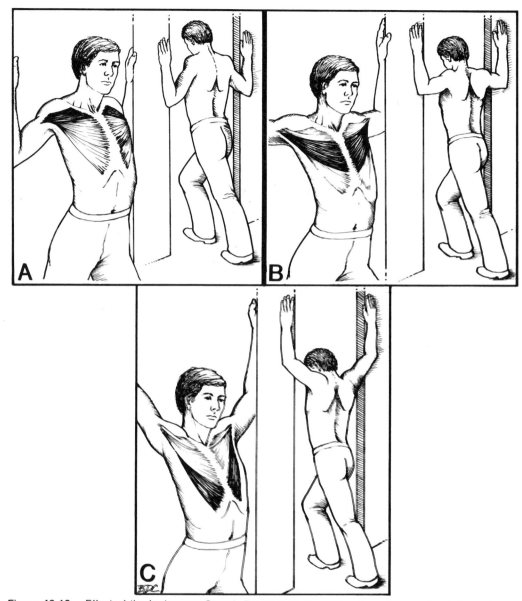

Figure 42.10.   Effect of the In-doorway Stretch Exercise on the pectoralis major muscle. *A*, lower hand-position to stretch the clavicular section bilaterally. *B*, middle hand-position to stretch the sternal section bilaterally. *C*, upper hand-position to stretch the fibers of the costal and abdominal sections. Hyperextension of the low back is optional for additional stretch of the latissimus dorsi and iliopsoas muscles.

feeling the support provided by various parts of the chair (armrests, seat, backrest and perhaps headrest). The same method of relaxation applies in bed at night; the patient concentrates on detecting the texture of the sheet and mattress wherever it supports the body.

Activities that overload flexion and adduction movements of the arm (especially if unaccustomed) should be identified and then modified, or avoided, such as heavy lifting (especially while reaching out in front); working forcefully with large, scissor-type hand tools (hedge clippers); and sustained-position strain for long periods (pulling the rope in a tug-of-war, holding ropes when sailing a boat, or holding a chain saw high and away from the body).

Sleeping Posture

At night, the patient must avoid shortening of the pectoralis major muscle, as occurs when the arms are folded across the chest. The corner of the pillow should be tucked between the head and shoulder to drop the shoulder backward, *not* tucked under the shoulder (see Fig. 7.7A). When lying on the pain-free side, the patient should support the uppermost forearm on a pillow; this prevents the arm from dropping forward to the bed and thus shortening the affected pectoralis major (see Fig. 22.7A). When the patient lies on the affected side, the pillow fits in the axilla, between the arm and the chest to maintain some degree of pectoralis major stretch (see Fig. 26.8).

Stretch Exercises

The In-doorway Stretch Exercise is useful to stretch all of the adductors and internal rotators at the shoulders. To do it, the patient stands in a narrow doorway with the forearms against the doorjambs (Fig. 42.10). One foot is placed in front of the other, and the forward knee is bent. The patient holds the head erect looking straight ahead, neither craning the neck forward, nor looking down at the floor. As the forward knee bends and the patient leans through the doorway, a slow, gentle, passive stretch is exerted bilaterally on the pectoralis major muscle and on its synergistic muscles. The stretch is held briefly, for only a few seconds. The patient pauses, relaxes, and breathes between each cycle. The hand position against the doorjamb is adjusted to vary the stretch on different sections of the muscle. Fibers of the clavicular section are stretched best in the low hand-position (Fig. 42.10A). By raising the hands to the middle hand-position with the upper arms horizontal (Fig. 42.10B), the sternal section is stretched. Moving the hands as high as possible, while keeping the forearms against the doorjambs (Fig. 42.10C), stretches the costal and more vertical abdominal fibers that form the lateral margin of the muscle.

When doing this exercise, the patient is encouraged to distinguish the different feeling of stretch for each section of the muscle.

If desired, the patient may be told also to swing the hips forward through the doorway to hyperextend the low back. This option stretches the iliopsoas and the more vertical fibers of the latissimus dorsi muscles on the side of the rear leg.

Supplemental References, Case Reports

The senior author has presented case reports of patients with myofascial pain and myocardial infarction or effort angina,[52, 60] with pseudoangina,[68] and with breast pain and soreness due to TPs in the lateral border of the pectoralis major.[63]

References

1. Ashley GT: The manner of insertion of the pectoralis major muscle in man. *Anat Rec* 113:301–307, 1952.
2. Bardeen CR: The musculature. Sect. 5. In *Morris's Human Anatomy*, edited by C.M. Jackson. Ed. 6. Blakiston's Son & Co., Philadelphia, 1921 (pp. 405, 406).
3. Basmajian JV: *Muscles Alive*, Ed. 2. Williams & Wilkins, Baltimore, 1967 (pp. 162, 163).
4. Broer MR, Houtz SJ: *Patterns of Muscular Activity in Selected Sports Skills*. Charles C Thomas, Springfield, Ill., 1967.
5. Calabro JJ, Jeghers H, Miller KA, et al.: Classification of anterior chest wall syndromes. *JAMA* 243:1420–1421, 1980.
6. DeMaria AN, Lee G, Amsterdam EA, et al.: The anginal syndrome with normal coronary arteries. *JAMA* 244:826–828, 1980.
7. Diffrient N, Tilley AR, Bardagjy JC: *Humanscale 1/2/3*. The MIT Press, Cambridge, Mass., 1974.
8. Dixon RH: Cure or relief of cases misdiagnosed "angina of effort." *Br Med J* 2:891, 1938.
9. Duchenne GB: *Physiology of Motion*, translated by E.B. Kaplan. J.B. Lippincott, Philadelphia, 1949 (pp. 71–74).
10. Dworken HJ, Fructuoso JB, Machella TE: Supradiaphragmatic reference of pain from the colon. *Gastroenterology* 22:222–228, 1952.
11. Edeiken J, Wolferth CC: Persistent pain in the shoulder region following myocardial infarction. *Am J Med Sci* 191:201–210, 1936.
12. Eisler P: *Die Muskeln des Stammes*. Gustav Fischer, Jena, 1912 (pp. 456–464).
13. Epstein SE, Gerber LH, Borer JS: Chest wall syndrome, a common cause of unexplained cardiac pain. *JAMA* 241:2793–2797, 1979.
14. Foley WT, McDevitt E, Tulloch JA, Tunis M, Wright IS: Studies of vasopasm: 1, The use of glyceryl trinitrite as a diagnostic test of peripheral pulses. *Circulation* 7:847–854, 1953.
15. Foley WT, Wright IS: *Color Atlas and Management of Vascular Disease*. Appleton-Century-Crofts, New York, 1959 (p. 86).
16. Gilbert NC: Influence of extrinsic factors on the coronary flow and clinical course of heart disease. *Bull NY Acad Med* 18:83–92, 1942.
17. Gold H, Kwit NT, Modell W: The effect of extracardiac pain on the heart. *Proc A Res Nerv Ment Dis* 23:345–357, 1943.

18. Gold H, Kwit NT, Otto H: The xanthines (theobromine and aminophylline) in the treatment of cardiac pain. *JAMA* 108:2173–2179, 1937.

19. Good MG: What is "fibrositis"? *Rheumatism* 5:117–123, 1949 (p. 121, Fig. 7).

20. Good MG: The role of skeletal muscles in the pathogenesis of diseases. *Acta Med Scand* 138:285–292, 1950 (pp. 286, 287).

21. Gorrell RL: Local anesthetics in precordial pain. *Clin Med Surg* 46:441–442, 1939.

22. Grant JCB: *An Atlas of Human Anatomy*, Ed. 7. Williams & Wilkins, Baltimore, 1978 (Figs. 2–5, 2–6, 6–14).

23. Gray H: *Anatomy of the Human Body*, edited by C.M. Goss, American Ed. 29. Lea & Febiger, Philadelphia, 1973 (pp. 453, 750, 751).

24. *Ibid.* (pp. 452, 454; Fig. 6–36).

25. Gutstein M: Diagnosis and treatment of muscular rheumatism. *Br J Phys Med* 1:302–321, 1938 (p. 309, Case IX; p. 311, Case 52).

26. Gutstein-Good M: Idiopathic myalgia simulating visceral and other diseases. *Lancet* 2:326–328, 1940.

27. Heinz GJ, Zavala DC: Slipping rib syndrome; diagnosis using the "hooking maneuver." *JAMA* 237:794–795, 1977.

28. Hollinshead WH: *Anatomy for Surgeons*, Ed. 2, Vol. 3, *The Back and Limbs.* Harper & Row, New York, 1969 (pp. 285–287, Figs. 4–18, 4–19).

29. Hollinshead WH: *Functional Anatomy of the Limbs and Back*, Ed. 4. W.B. Saunders, Philadelphia, 1976 (pp. 94, 95).

30. Hooten, EA: *A Survey in Seating.* Heywood-Wakefield Co., Gardner, Mass., 1945. Reprinted by Greenwood Press, Westport, Conn., 1970.

31. Inman VT, Saunders JB, Abbott LC: Observations of the function on the shoulder joint. *J Bone Joint Surg* 26:1–30, 1944.

32. Jelenko C III: Tietze's syndrome at the xiphisternal joint. *South Med J* 67:818–819, 1974.

33. Kelly M: The treatment of fibrositis and allied disorders by local anaesthesia. *Med J Aust* 1:294–298, 1941. (p. 296).

34. Kelly M: Pain in the Chest: Observations on the use of local anaesthesia in its investigation and treatment. *Med J Aust* 1:4–7, 1944. (pp. 5, 6; Cases V, VII, IX).

35. Kennard MA, Haugen FP: The relation of subcutaneous focal sensitivity to referred pain of cardiac origin. *J Am Soc Anesthesiologists* 16:297–311, 1955.

36. Landmann HR: "Trigger areas" as cause of persistent chest and shoulder pain in myocardial infarction or angina pectoris. *J Kans Med Soc* 50:69–71, 1949.

37. Lange M: *Die Muskelhaerten (Myogelosen); Ihre Entstehung und Heilung.* J.F. Lehmanns, München, 1931 (pp. 118–135, Fig. 40A, Examples 14, 20, 21, 22).

38. Lewis T, Kellgren JH: Observations relating to referred pain, viscero-motor reflexes and other associated phenomena. *Clin Sci* 4:47–71, 1939 (p. 48).

39. Lindgren I: Cutaneous precordial anaesthesia in angina pectoris and coronary occlusion (an experimental study). *Nord Med Cardiologia* 11:207–218, 1946.

40. Lockhart RD, Hamilton GF, Fyfe FW: *Anatomy of the Human Body*, Ed. 2. J.B. Lippincott, Philadelphia, 1969 (pp. 200–203, Fig. 322).

41. Long C II: Myofascial pain syndromes, part III—some syndromes of the trunk and thigh. *Henry Ford Hosp Med Bull* 4:102–106, 1956.

42. Marmor L, Bechtol CO, Hall CB: Pectoralis major muscle: function of sternal portion and mechanism of rupture of normal muscle: case reports. *J Bone Joint Surg* 43A:81–87, 1961.

43. McBeath AA, Keene JS: The rib-tip syndrome. *J Bone Surg* 57A:795–797, 1975.

44. McEachern CG, Manning GW, Hall GE: Sudden occlusion of coronary arteries following removal of cardiosensory pathways. *Arch Intern Med* 65:661–670, 1940.

45. McMinn RMH, Hutchings RT: *Color Atlas of Human Anatomy.* Year Book Medical Publishers, Chicago, 1977 (p. 108).

46. *Ibid.* (p. 109).

47. Pasternak RC, Thibault GE, Savoia M, et al.: Chest pain with angiographically insignificant coronary arterial obstruction. *Am J Med* 68:813–817, 1980.

48. Pernkopf E: *Atlas of Topographical and Applied Human Anatomy*, Vol. 2. W.B. Saunders, Philadelphia, 1964 (p. 47, Fig. 38).

49. Rasch PJ, Burke RK: *Kinesiology and Applied Anatomy.* Ed. 6. Lea & Febiger, Philadelphia, 1978 (pp. 164, 165).

50. Reeves TJ, Harrison TR: Diagnostic and therapeutic value of the reproduction of chest pain. *Arch Intern Med* 91:8–25, 1953 (p. 15).

51. Rinzler SH: *Cardiac Pain.* Charles C Thomas, Springfield, Ill., 1951 (pp. 82, 84).

52. Rinzler SH, Travell J: Therapy directed at the somatic component of cardiac pain. *Am Heart J* 35:248–268, 1948 (pp. 249, 256; Cases 1 and 3).

53. Smith JR: Thoracic pain. *Clinics* 2:1427–1459, 1944.

54. Sobotta J, Figge FHJ: *Atlas of Human Anatomy*, Ed. 9, Vol. 1. Hafner Division of Macmillan, New York, 1974 (pp. 154, 155).

55. *Ibid.* (pp. 162, 174).

56. Spalteholz W: *Handatlas der Anatomie des Menschen*, Ed. 11, Vol. 2. S. Hirzel, Leipzig, 1922 (pp. 280, 281).

57. Theobald GW: The relief and prevention of referred pain. *J Obstet Gynaecol Br Com* 56:447–460, 1949 (pp. 451–452).

58. Tietze A: Ueber eine eigenartige Häufung von Fällen mit Dystrophie der Rippenknorpel. *Berl Klin Wochenschr* 58:829–831, 1921.

59. Toldt C: *An Atlas of Human Anatomy*, translated by M.E. Paul, Ed. 2, Vol. 1. Macmillan, New York, 1919 (p. 274).

60. Travell J: Early relief of chest pain by ethyl chloride spray in acute coronary thrombosis, case report. *Circulation* 3:120–124, 1951.

61. Travell J: Introductory remarks. In *Connective Tissues, Transactions of the Fifth Conference, 1954*, edited by C. Ragan. Josiah Macy, Jr. Foundation, New York, 1954 (p. 18).

62. Travell J: Chairs are a personal thing. *House Beautiful*, Oct. 1955 (pp. 190–193).

63. Travell J: Referred pain from skeletal muscle: the pectoralis major syndrome of breast pain and

soreness, and the sternomastoid syndrome of headache and dizziness. *NY State J Med* 55:331–339, 1955 (p. 332, Fig. 1*A*, Cases 1 and 2).

64. Travell J: *Office Hours: Day and Night.* The World Publishing Company, New York, 1968 (pp. 261, 263, 264).

65. Travell J: Myofascial trigger points: clinical view. In *Advances in Pain Research and Therapy,* edited by J.J. Bonica and D. Albe-Fessard, Vol. 1. Raven Press, New York, 1976 (pp. 919–926).

66. Travell J, Bigelow NH: Role of somatic trigger areas in the patterns of hysteria. *Psychosom Med* 9:353–363, 1947.

67. Travell J, Rinzler SH: Relief of cardiac pain by local block of somatic trigger areas. *Proc Soc Exp Biol Med,* 63:480–482, 1946.

68. Travell J, Rinzler SH: Pain syndromes of the chest muscles: resemblance to effort angina and myocardial infarction, and relief by local block. *Can Med Assoc J 59:*333–338, 1948 (Case 1).

69. Travell J, Rinzler SH: The myofascial genesis of pain. *Postgrad Med 11:*425–434, 1952.

70. Webber TD: Diagnosis and modification of headache and shoulder-arm-hand syndrome. *JAOA* 72:697–710, 1973.

71. Weiss S, Davis D: The significance of the afferent impulses from the skin in the mechanism of visceral pain. Skin infiltration as a useful therapeutic measure. *Am J Med Sci* 176:517–536, 1928.

72. Winter Z: Referred pain in fibrositis. *Med Rec* 157:34–37, 1944 (pp. 4, 5).

73. Young D: The effects of novocain injections on simulated visceral pain. *Ann Intern Med,* 19:749–756, 1943 (pp. 751, Cases 1 and 2).

CHAPTER 43
Pectoralis Minor Muscle
"Neurovascular Entrapper"

HIGHLIGHTS: When the pectoralis minor muscle harbors trigger points (TPs), its taut fibers are likely to entrap the axillary artery and the brachial plexus. **REFERRED PAIN** from a left-sided muscle, pectoralis major or minor, may refer pain to the precordium that mimics the angina of myocardial ischemia. The pectoralis minor refers pain over the front of the chest, primarily to the front of the shoulder, and sometimes down the ulnar side of the arm, forearm and fingers. **ANATOMICAL ATTACHMENTS** of this muscle differ from the pectoralis major by connecting the anterior rib cage to the coracoid process, rather than to the humerus. **ACTIONS** of the pectoralis minor, therefore, are to pull the scapula and shoulder down and forward, and to assist the upper chest muscles in forced inspiration. **PATIENT EXAMINATION** discloses a round-shouldered posture. Shoulder motion is somewhat restricted when reaching forward and upward, and more restricted when reaching backward at shoulder level. **TRIGGER POINT EXAMINATION** proceeds by palpating the pectoralis minor indirectly through the pectoralis major, or directly by grasping it from beneath and through the pectoralis major, using pincer palpation. **ENTRAPMENT** symptoms due to compression of the brachial plexus (medial and lateral cord) and of the axillary artery by an abnormally taut pectoralis minor muscle are accentuated when the arm is hyperabducted. **STRETCH AND SPRAY** are executed by extending the arm and sweeping lines of spray upward over the muscle and shoulder, and continuing down the length of the upper extremity to cover its pain pattern as well. **INJECTION AND STRETCH** are performed by directing the needle upward toward the coracoid process, not toward the ribs. **CORRECTIVE ACTIONS** for long-term relief require that a stooped posture, or other stress overload on the muscle, be eliminated.

1. REFERRED PAIN
(Fig. 43.1)

The trigger points (TPs) in the pectoralis minor muscle refer pain most strongly over the anterior deltoid area. With very active TPs, the pain may extend upward over the subclavicular area, and sometimes covers the entire pectoral region on the same side. Spillover referred pain extends along the ulnar side of the arm, elbow, forearm, and palmar hand to include the last three fingers (Fig. 43.1). No distinction is drawn between the pain originating from an upper or lower TP in the pectoralis minor.

Essentially the same pattern also is referred from adjacent TPs in the pectoralis major.[34]

Pain from either pectoral muscle[19, 26] and specifically the pectoralis minor,[21] can closely mimic the pain of cardiac ischemia.

2. ANATOMICAL ATTACHMENTS
(Fig. 43.2)

The pectoralis minor muscle attaches *above* to the medial aspect of the tip of the coracoid process of the scapula; and *below* to the third, fourth and fifth ribs near their costal cartilages[15] (Fig. 43.2). It also may attach as low as the sixth rib, or as high as the first rib.[1]

PART 4

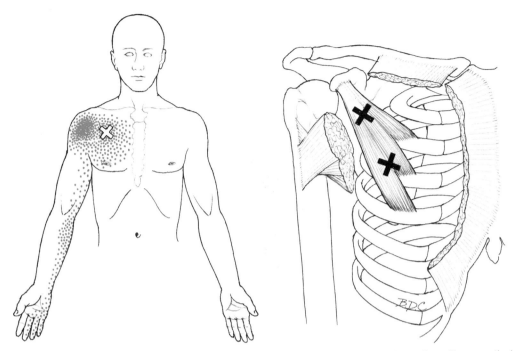

Figure 43.1.   Referred pain pattern (*solid red* is the essential portion, *stippled red* shows the spillover portion), and trigger point locations (×s) in the right pectoralis minor muscle.

The tip of the coracoid process also provides attachment for the tendons of the coracobrachialis and the short head of the biceps brachii muscles.

A slip of the pectoralis minor may extend beyond the coracoid process in about 15% of bodies to attach to tendons of adjacent muscles, or to the greater tuberosity of the humerus.[1, 14]

Two other, relatively infrequent, anatomical variations are described.[10] The pectoralis *minimus* connects the first rib cartilage to the coracoid process, effectively extending the pectoralis minor muscle cephalad.[25] The pectoralis *intermedius* may attach more medially than the pectoralis minor onto the third, fourth and fifth rib cartilages and attach above to the fascia covering the coracobrachialis and biceps brachii muscles. This arrangement sandwiches the intermedius between the pectoralis major and minor muscles.[10]

Supplemental References

Other authors have clearly illustrated the pectoralis minor muscle as seen from the front,[9, 11, 16, 20, 25, 30, 32] from in front with neurovascular structures,[12] from the side,[22] from the side with neurovascular struc-

tures,[29] from below with neurovascular structures,[23] and in cross section.[5, 8] In a common variation, fibers extend over the coracoid process to reinforce the coracohumeral ligament.[14]

3. INNERVATION

The pectoralis minor is innervated by the medial pectoral nerve from the medial cord, and by fibers of roots C_8 and T_1.[15]

4. ACTIONS

The pectoralis minor draws the scapula forward, downward and inward at nearly equal angles.[25] Depression of the shoulder by this muscle[7, 15, 17] stabilizes the scapula when the arm exerts downward pressure against resistance.[25] Since, when this muscle contracts, the inward force component is blocked by the clavicle, the resultant force draws the glenoid fossa of the scapula obliquely down and forward.[7] At the same time, this tends to lift its medial border and inferior angle away from the ribs (winging of the scapula).[25]

The scapular protraction by this muscle is used to pull the shoulders forward. The muscle stabilizes the scapula for down-

PART 4

Cut pectoralis major

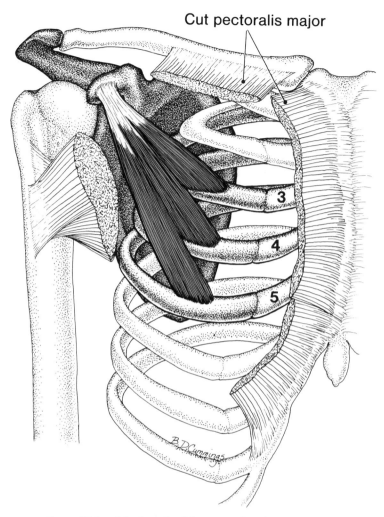

Figure 43.2.   Attachments of the pectoralis minor muscle (*red*).

ward thrust (crutch walking and driving a stake into the ground).[31]

When the scapula is fixed in elevation by the upper trapezius and levator scapulae muscles, the pectoralis minor becomes active during strong inspiratory efforts that involve the upper chest.[7] It thus can serve as an accessory respiratory muscle during forced inspiration.[2, 15, 25]

5. MYOTATIC UNIT

The pectoralis minor forms a synergistic myotatic unit for vigorous inspiration with the levator scapulae, upper trapezius, sternocleidomastoid and scalene muscles. Electromyographically, the pectoralis minor is active in forced inspiration, but not

in quiet breathing.[2] The pectoralis minor assists the pectoralis major in depression of the shoulder, protrusion of the scapula, and downward rotation of its lateral angle (glenoid fossa). It also assists the latissimus dorsi in depression of the shoulder.

The rhomboid and lower trapezius muscles act as antagonists to the pectoralis minor in scapular rotation and protraction.

6. SYMPTOMS

The patient's chief complaint is pain; no sharp distinction is made between the pain referred from TPs in the pectoralis minor and from TPs in the overlying and adjacent portions of the pectoralis major. The intensity and quality, as well as the distribution, of cardiac pain may be reproduced by this pectoral muscle's referred pain.[26]

The patient may be aware of difficulty in reaching forward and up, or reaching backward with the arm at shoulder level.

The shortened pectoralis minor may cause distinctive neurovascular symptoms through entrapment of the neurovascular bundle to the upper extremity[28] (see Section 10, Fig. 43.4).

7. ACTIVATION OF TRIGGER POINTS

Pectoralis minor TPs may be activated: as satellite TPs due to their presence within the zone of pain induced by myocardial ischemia, or their presence within the reference zone of scalene TPs; by trauma (a gunshot wound through the upper chest, or fracture of upper ribs); by strain through overuse as a shoulder depressor (unaccustomed crutch-walking); by strain as an accessory muscle of inspiration (during paroxysms of severe coughing, or to assist paradoxical breathing); by poor seated posture (keeping the muscle chronically shortened because of a poorly designed chair or work space); or by prolonged compression of the muscle (knapsack with a tight strap over the front of the shoulder).

8. PATIENT EXAMINATION

The increased tension due to TPs in the pectoralis minor prevents the patient from reaching fully behind the back at shoulder level. The protraction of the scapula and downward rotation of the glenoid fossa that are caused by the taut pectoralis minor limits full flexion at the shoulder.[18] Arm extension may show some weakness because power in this movement depends on fixation of the scapula in part by the pectoralis minor.

When they are shortened by TPs, both the pectoralis minor and subscapularis muscles restrict the combined movement of abduction and external rotation at the shoulder. However, subscapularis TPs restrict only glenohumeral motion, whereas pectoralis minor TPs restrict only scapular mobility on the chest wall. The movement of the scapula is palpable and sometimes visible. With the arm abducted to 90°, external rotation is restricted markedly by both muscles; with the arm at the side, only the subscapularis seriously restricts external rotation. Also, when abduction of the arm at the shoulder is restricted by pectoralis minor tautness, the patient may be aware of pulling on the ribs at the limit of abduction. These observations are of confirmatory value; the subscapularis and pectoralis minor muscles have different referred pain patterns, which are not likely to be confused.

9. TRIGGER POINT EXAMINATION (Fig. 43.3)

First, the pectoralis major should be examined for active TPs which might obscure and confuse the localization of TPs in the underlying pectoralis minor.

The examiner, if unsure of the position of the pectoralis minor muscle under the pectoralis major, can locate the muscle by having the patient tense the pectoralis minor. To do this, the supine patient raises the shoulder away from the examining table, while relaxing the arm and carefully avoiding downward pressure against the table with the hand, which would also tense the pectoralis major.[18] In the sitting position, the patient holds the arm close to the side, a little to the rear to inhibit the pectoralis major, strongly protracts the shoulder, and then inhales deeply with the chest.[25] Both maneuvers activate only the pectoralis minor so that it can be located for examination.

In both the supine and seated positions, pectoralis minor TPs can be localized either by flat palpation through the pectoralis major against the chest wall (Fig. 43.3A), as also illustrated by Webber,[35] or by pincer palpation (Fig. 43.3B). With either approach, the pectoralis major is slackened by keeping the patient's arm toward the front of the body and the forearm on the abdomen; the pectoralis minor may be placed on the desired degree of stretch by retracting the shoulder toward the military-brace position. The two pectoral muscles may be distinguished by noting the muscle fiber direction of palpable bands and of local twitch responses.

Although the patient achieves better relaxation in the supine than in the seated position, it is often convenient and inform-

PART 4

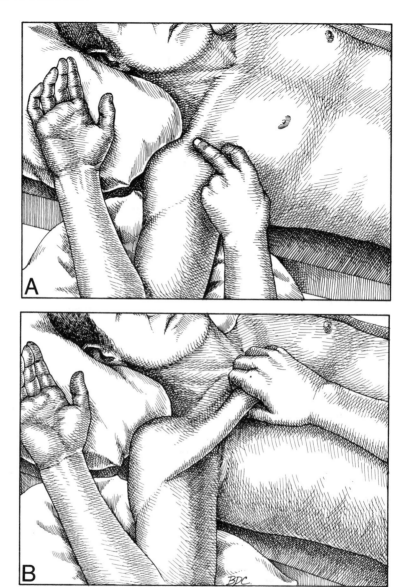

Figure 43.3. Palpation of trigger points in the pectoralis minor muscle. The overlying pectoralis major is slackened by elevating the arm as shown, or by placing the forearm on the abdomen. *A,* flat palpation of the pectoralis minor through the pectoralis major. *B,* pincer palpation around the pectoralis major. The thumb contacts the pectoralis minor, through only the skin. The fingers grasp it through the pectoralis major. The pectoralis minor may be tautened for better identification of its trigger points by elevating the shoulder.

ative to screen both pectoral muscles for TPs using flat palpation with the patient seated. The seated position simplifies range-of-motion testing and the Irving S. Wright hyperabduction maneuver.[36]

In the supine position, and in non-obese patients with relatively loose skin, the pectoralis minor can usually be palpated di- rectly by pincer palpation (Fig. 43.3*B*). The pectoralis major is slackened by placing the arm in the position described above, and, if additional relief is necessary, the shoulder is protracted by padding placed under it. The operator places a digit in the apex of the axilla and slides it along the chest wall beneath the pectoralis major toward the midline, until it encounters the muscle mass of the pectoralis minor. That muscle, and the pectoralis major above it, are then encompassed by a pincer grasp between the thumb and fingers (Fig. 43.3B). The fibers of the pectoralis minor can then be palpated directly through the skin for taut bands and spots of TP tenderness. Identification of TPs in the pectoralis minor may be enhanced by elevating the shoulder cephalad to tauten the pectoralis minor, which increases the sensitivity of its TPs without tightening the pectoralis major.

10. ENTRAPMENTS
(Fig. 43.4)

The pectoralis minor is the landmark for anatomically dividing the axillary artery into three parts; the second part of the artery lies beneath the muscle. Likewise, the distal portion of the brachial plexus passes deep to the pectoralis minor muscle where the muscle attaches to the coracoid process. When the arm is abducted and externally rotated at the shoulder, the artery, vein, and nerves are bent and stretched around the pectoralis minor muscle close to its attachment, and are likely to be compressed if the muscle is firm and tautened by myofascial TPs (Fig. 43.4B).

The entrapment of the axillary artery is demonstrated by the Wright maneuver,[36] which places the arm in external rotation and abduction at the shoulder (Fig. 43.4A) while the radial pulse is palpated. The test is more effective if the patient is not allowed to elevate the shoulder and relieve tension on the neurovascular structures. This position can produce compression of the neurovascular structures by the pectoralis minor,[3, 4] and by closure of the costoclavicular space if the scapula also is retracted. Entrapment symptoms and obliteration of the radial pulse by abduction of the arm to only 90° at the shoulder demonstrates the effect of severe pectoralis minor shortening due to TP involvement. Further hyperabduction (Fig. 43.4) increases tension on both the pectoralis minor muscle and the neurovascular structures, which may produce demonstrable compression in some normal subjects.[36]

Arterial entrapment is detected by loss of the radial pulse at the wrist or by a reduction of arterial blood flow, which is more precisely detected by Doppler ultrasound.[24] If arterial compression in abduction or hyperabduction is primarily due to TP activity of the pectoralis minor, the radial pulse may be restored in the test position by eliminating hyperirritability of the TPs. When patients with active pectoralis minor TPs were placed in the hyperabducted position to the point of just obliterating the radial pulse, pulsation returned immediately while vapocooling the skin over the stretched pectoralis minor muscle, without changing the arm position.

Symptoms of neurological entrapment are similar to those described for the scalene muscles in Chapter 20. When the Wright maneuver (above) is used to detect nerve entrapment beneath the pectoralis minor, the test is more effective if the patient is not allowed to elevate the shoulder to relieve tension on the brachial plexus. Entrapment of the medial cord (Fig. 43.4B), which connects the lower trunk to the ulnar nerve,[6, 13] causes numbness and paraesthesias of the 4th and 5th digits, usually not of the thumb and other fingers. Entrapment of the lateral cord, which connects with the upper and middle trunks proximally, and the musculocutaneous and median nerves distally,[6, 13] disturbs sensation over the dorsum and radial aspects of the forearm and over the palmar side of the first three and one-half digits.[15] Compression of both cords disturbs much of the sensation below the elbow.

Entrapment by the taut pectoralis minor does not produce the hand edema and stiffness of the fingers so characteristic of entrapment by the scalenus anterior. Scalenus anterior entrapment is more likely to impair venous, than arterial, circulation by compression of the subclavian vein between the clavicle and first rib. This occurs because the first rib is elevated by shortening of the scalenus anterior muscle.

Entrapment due to the costoclavicular syndrome is caused by compression of either, or both, the axillary artery and the distal brachial plexus between the clavicle and the first rib. The effects of this compression are demonstrated by having the patient assume the military brace position (chest elevated and shoulders retracted).

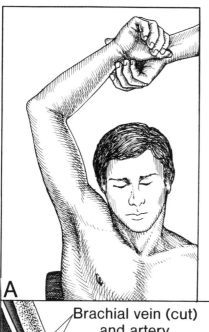

Figure 43.4. Entrapment of the lower brachial plexus and axillary artery by the right pectoralis minor during the Wright hyperabduction test. *A,* hyperabduction test position. *B,* stretch and torsion of the brachial plexus and axillary artery can occur as they hook beneath the pectoralis minor muscle where it attaches to the coracoid process. The clavicle also may compress these neurovascular structures directly against the first rib as the scapula is retracted (pulled backward), in the military stance.

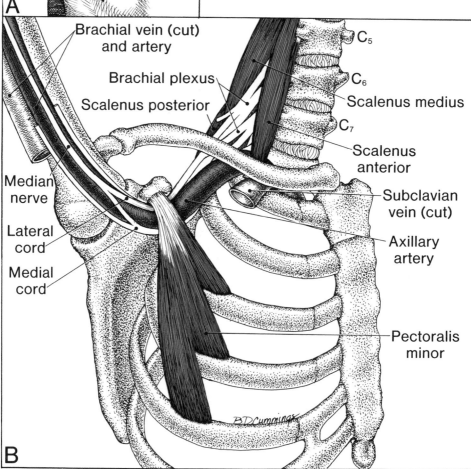

11. ASSOCIATED TRIGGER POINTS

One rarely, if ever, finds active TPs in the pectoralis minor without active TPs in the pectoralis major. Therefore, the same muscles that are commonly associated with pectoralis major involvement are likely to harbor active TPs when the pectoralis minor is involved: the anterior deltoid, scalene, sternocleidomastoid, and sternalis muscles.

On the other hand, one may find TPs in the pectoralis major without involvement of the pectoralis minor, especially when the TPs are located in the parasternal section and lower lateral border of the costal section of the pectoralis major muscle.

Connective tissue TPs have been found in post-traumatic scar tissue in the region of the coracoid attachment of the pectoralis minor. These TPs have referred tenderness, hot burning pain, prickling, and lightening-like jabs to the pectoral region and olecranon process on the same side. Injection of these connective tissue TPs caused brilliant momentary flashes of local and referred pain, followed by relief.

12. STRETCH AND SPRAY
(Fig. 43.5)

The patient sits in a relaxed position with the low back well supported. The arm is grasped firmly so that the shoulder can be pulled backward to retract the scapula and place the pectoralis minor muscle on stretch. Abducting and horizontally extending the arm also stretches the pectoralis major. Before and during the application of stretching force, vapocoolant spray is applied in parallel sweeps from below, upward across the muscle, and is

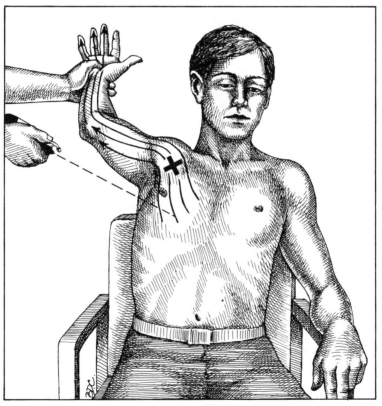

Figure 43.5. Stretch position and spray pattern (*arrows*) for a trigger point (✗) in the pectoralis minor muscle. The arm is abducted and shoulder pulled back to elevate and retract the scapula. Up-sweeps of the spray cover the pectoralis minor muscle and its pain pattern. By thus hyperabducting and externally rotating the arm, the pectoralis major also is stretched and should be sprayed at the same time. Frequently the two pectoral muscles are involved together.

PART 4

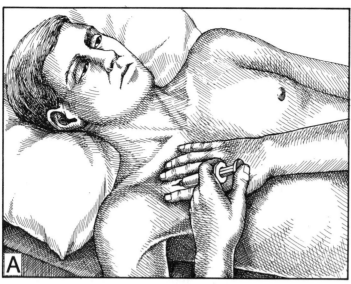

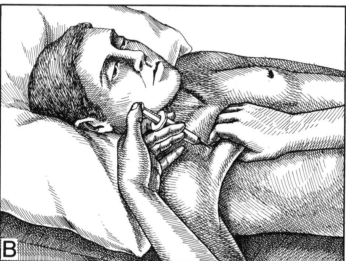

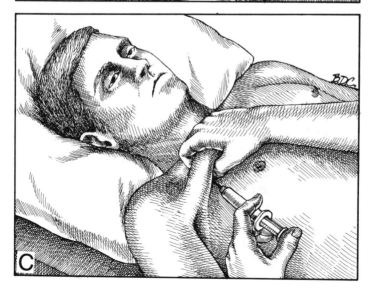

Figure 43.6. Injection of the pectoralis minor muscle by a left handed operator. *A,* injection of the upper trigger point after its localization by flat palpation. *B,* injection of the lower trigger point from above with the trigger point localized between the digits by pincer palpation. *C,* injection of the upper trigger point from below with the trigger point localized between the digits in a pincer grasp.

extended over the referred pain distribution to the fingertips (Fig. 43.5).

The stretch position illustrated in Fig. 43.5 combines a position that stretches the pectoralis major muscle across the glenohumeral joint and at the same time uses the arm as a convenient lever to force the scapula back and down to stretch the pectoralis minor muscle. If the pectoralis major muscle is also involved, which it usually is, it is important to extend the spray pattern to cover that of the pectoralis major muscle (see Fig. 42.7 B or C).

13. INJECTION AND STRETCH
(Fig. 43.6)

Injection of pectoralis minor TPs should be done with the patient supine, *not* seated, to avoid psychologically induced syncope and only after TPs in the pectoralis major have been inactivated to avoid recurrence. The upper TPs are close to the musculotendinous junction at the coracoid process and are reached by directing the needle toward the coracoid process,[26] as illustrated in Fig. 43.6 A and C. Whenever possible, the hand of the operator locates the pectoralis minor underneath the pectoralis major. This uses pincer palpation as described in Section 9, with the fingers (or thumb) contacting the pectoralis minor directly (Fig. 43.6 B and C). The needle is preferably directed away from the chest wall and toward the coracoid process.

The lower TPs in the pectoralis minor lie close to the ribs. When necessary, they are approached with the needle directed caudad, as tangential to the plane of the chest wall as possible (Fig. 43.6B), so as to preclude the needle's entering an intercostal space.

After injection of TPs, passive stretch during vapocooling is applied, as above, followed by a hot pack over the pectoral region.

14. CORRECTIVE ACTIONS

TPs should be inactivated in any muscles, such as the scalene group and pectoralis major, that refer pain to the region of the pectoralis minor and thus may induce satellite TPs in it.

Activity stress due to overuse must be avoided by identifying and limiting the offending activity, such as gardening, working at a desk, and crutch walking.

Paradoxical breathing (see Fig. 20.13A) needs correction, as described in Chapter 20.

Standing and seated posture (see Fig. 42.9) should be improved, as described in Chapter 42.

A strap that compresses the pectoralis minor should be avoided; it may be placed on the acromion to relieve pressure on the muscle, or may be padded to distribute the load more widely.

The patient learns to maintain full pectoral muscle length by using the In-doorway Stretch Exercise (see Fig. 42.10).

To minimize aggravation of pectoralis minor TPs when the muscle is placed in the shortened position at night, the patient avoids sleeping "curled up" on the side with the shoulder forced strongly forward.[28]

Supplemental References, Case Reports

Examples of the diagnosis and management of patients with active pectoralis minor TPs are presented by the senior author.[27,33]

References

1. Bardeen CR: The musculature, Sect. 5. In *Morris's Human Anatomy*, edited by C.M. Jackson, Ed. 6. Blakiston's Son & Co., Philadelphia, 1921 (pp. 406, 407).
2. Basmajian JV: *Muscles Alive*. Ed. 4. Williams & Wilkins, Baltimore, 1978 (p. 160).
3. Cailliet, R: *Soft Tissue Pain and Disability*, F.A. Davis, Philadelphia, 1977 (pp. 144–146, Fig. 116).
4. Cailliet R: *Neck and Arm Pain*. F.A. Davis, Philadelphia, 1964 (pp. 95, 96).
5. Carter BL, Morehead J, Wolpert SM, *et al.*: *Cross-Sectional Anatomy*. Appleton-Century-Crofts, New York, 1977 (Sects. 21–25).
6. Clemente CD: *Anatomy*. Lea & Febiger, Philadelphia, 1975 (Fig. 14).
7. Duchenne GB: *Physiology of Motion*, translated by E.B. Kaplan. J.B. Lippincott, Philadelphia, 1949 (pp. 19, 479, 481).
8. Eisler P: *Die Muskeln des Stammes*. Gustav Fischer, Jena, 1912 (Fig. 68).
9. *Ibid*. (Fig. 69).
10. *Ibid*. (Fig. 73, pp. 477–479).
11. Grant JCB: *An Atlas of Human Anatomy*, Ed. 7. Williams & Wilkins, Baltimore, 1978 (Fig. 1–15).
12. *Ibid*. (Fig. 6-20).
13. *Ibid*. (Fig. 6-24).
14. *Ibid*. (Fig. 6-120).
15. Gray H: *Anatomy of the Human Body*, edited by C.M. Goss, American Ed. 29. Lea & Febiger, Philadelphia, 1973 (p. 454).
16. *Ibid*. (Fig. 6-36).
17. Hollinshead WH: *Functional Anatomy of the Limbs and Back*, Ed. 4. W.B. Saunders, Philadelphia, 1976 (p. 96).

PART 4

18. Kendall HO, Kendall FP, Wadsworth GE: *Muscles, Testing and Function*, Ed. 2. Williams & Wilkins, Baltimore, 1971 (p. 113).

19. Kraus H: *Clinical Treatment of Back and Neck Pain*. McGraw-Hill, New York, 1970 (p. 98).

20. McMinn RMH, Hutchings RT: *Color Atlas of Human Anatomy*. Year Book Medical Publishers, Chicago, 1977 (p. 109).

21. Mendlowitz M: Strain of the pectoralis minor, an important cause of precordial pain in soldiers. *Am Heart J* 30:123–125, 1945.

22. Pernkopf E: *Atlas of Topographical and Applied Human Anatomy*, Vol. 2. W.B. Saunders, Philadelphia, 1964 (Fig. 38).

23. *Ibid.* (Fig. 39).

24. Pisko-Dubienski ZA, Hollingsworth J: Clinical application of doppler ultrasonography in the thoracic outlet syndrome. *Can J Surg* 21:145–150, 1978.

25. Rasch PJ, Burke RK: *Kinesiology and Applied Anatomy*, Ed. 6. Lea & Febiger, Philadelphia, 1978 (pp. 154, 155, 164).

26. Rinzler SH: *Cardiac Pain*. Charles C Thomas, Springfield, Ill. 1951 (pp. 37, 85).

27. Rinzler SH, Travell J: Therapy directed at the somatic component of cardiac pain. *Am Heart J* 35:248–268, 1948 (pp. 261–263, Case 3).

28. Rubin D: An approach to the management of myofascial trigger point syndromes. *Arch Phys Med Rehabil* 62:107–110, 1981.

29. Sobotta J, Figge FHJ: *Atlas of Human Anatomy*, Ed. 9, Vol. 3. Hafner Division of Macmillan, New York, 1974 (p. 281).

30. Spalteholz W: *Handatlas der Anatomie des Menschen*, Ed. 11, Vol. 2. S. Hirzel, Leipzig, 1922 (p. 282).

31. Steindler A: *Kinesiology of the Human Body*. Charles C Thomas, Springfield, Ill., 1955 (pp. 468, 469).

32. Toldt C: *An Atlas of Human Anatomy*, translated by M.E. Paul, Ed. 2, Vol. 1. Macmillan, New York, 1919 (p. 274).

33. Travell J, Rinzler SH: Pain syndromes of the chest muscles: Resemblence to effort angina and myocardial infarction, and relief by local block. *Can Med Assoc J* 59:333–338, 1948 (pp. 333, 334; Case 1).

34. Travell J, Rinzler SH: The myofascial genesis of pain. *Postgrad Med* 11:425–434, 1952.

35. Webber TD: Diagnosis and modification of headache and shoulder-arm-hand syndrome. *JAOA* 72:697–710, 1973 (pp. 10, 11; Fig. 29).

36. Wright IS: The neurovascular syndrome produced by hyperabduction of the arms. *Am Heart J* 29:1–19, 1945.

CHAPTER 44
Sternalis Muscle
"Anomalous Substernal Ache"

HIGHLIGHTS: **REFERRED PAIN** from active trigger points (TPs) in the anomalous sternalis muscle produces a deep substernal ache which is unrelated to movement. **ANATOMICAL ATTACHMENTS** of the sternalis muscle are highly variable. The fibers are superficial and generally lie parallel with the margins of the sternum. The muscle may be located on one or both sides, running at right angles to, and overlying, the sternal end of the pectoralis major muscle. It is reported to be present in approximately 1 of 20 adults. **ACTIVATION OF TRIGGER POINTS** in this muscle occurs when pain is referred to the sternum from the heart during myocardial ischemia or from the lower end of the sternocleidomastoid muscle. **TRIGGER POINT EXAMINATION** for sternalis TPs is by flat palpation of the muscle against underlying bone to locate exquisite spot tenderness at a TP and to elicit referred pain. **INJECTION** is directed precisely into the TPs, which overlie bone. The TPs also are readily accessible to ischemic compression. **CORRECTIVE ACTIONS** include primarily self-application of ischemic compression by the patient to ensure sustained relief.

1. REFERRED PAIN
(Fig. 44.1)

The referred pain pattern of the sternalis usually includes the entire sternal and substernal region, and may extend on the same side across the upper pectoral area and front of the shoulder to the underarm and to the ulnar aspect of the elbow (Fig. 44.1).[15, 17] This pattern closely mimics the substernal ache of myocardial infarction or angina pectoris. The chest pain referred from this muscle has a terrifying quality that is remarkably independent of body movement. Its left-sided pattern differs from the referred pain of the left pectoralis major muscle in that the latter is more likely to extend beyond the elbow into the ulnar aspect of the left forearm and hand. Both muscles may contribute simultaneously to the pain reported by the patient; this is illustrated in case reports.[12, 14, 15]

Trigger points (TPs) may be located anywhere within the sternalis muscle: as high as the manubrium, as low as the xiphoid process, and on either or both sides, including the midline of the sternum when the muscle fuses across the sternum. Sternalis TPs usually occur over the upper two-thirds of the sternum and are most likely to be found slightly to the left of the midline at the mid-sternal level. Anatomically, a unilateral muscle is as common on the right as on the left, but active TPs are more common on the left side, probably because of their activation as satellite TPs within the locus of referred pain from the heart.

Albeit the sternalis may be only a small remnant of muscle, the intensity of pain arising from its TPs is not related to the size of the muscle, but to the degree of hyperirritability of these abnormal foci.

At times, a TP located at the confluence of the sternalis, pectoralis major and sternal division of the sternocleidomastoid muscles can be the source of a dry, hacking cough. Penetration of this TP with a

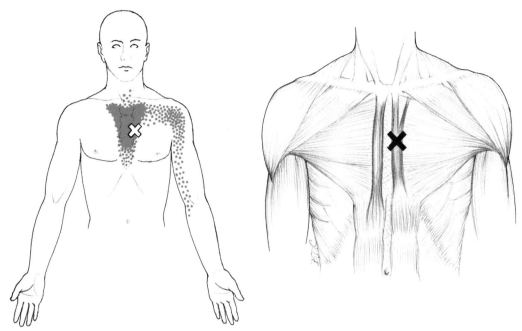

Figure 44.1.   A trigger point (×) in the left sternalis muscle gives rise to the referred pain pattern shown in *red*.

needle, in whichever muscle it lies, activates the cough momentarily, and then relieves it.

2. ANATOMICAL ATTACHMENTS
(Fig. 44.2)

The anomalous sternalis muscle is highly variable in presence, laterality, length, bulk, attachments and innervation. It may occur bilaterally (Fig. 44.2), or more often unilaterally, on either side of the sternum or, rarely, the two muscles may fuse across the sternum. It may attach **above** to the sternum, to the fascia over either the pectoralis major or sternocleidomastoid muscle, or it may form a continuation of those muscles. **Below** it may attach to the third through seventh costal cartilages, the fascia covering the pectoralis major, and/or to the sheath of the rectus abdominis muscle.

The sternalis was found in 1.7% to 14.3% (median 4.4%) of cases in 13 studies of at least 10,200 bodies;[3] at most, in 48% of anencephalic monsters;[3] in 4.3% of 2062 cadavers as summarized by Christian;[2] and in 6% of 535 cadavers according to Barlow.[1] Eisler,[3] Hollinshead,[7] Grant[6] and Toldt[10] each have illustrated the sternalis muscle. Christian[2] illustrated two bilateral

muscles. Barlow[1] reported no significant difference in the incidence of the sternalis muscle in white and black Americans. The muscle may be as thick as 2 cm (¾ in) over the sternum, a depth at which it is difficult to distinguish the sternalis from the pectoralis major muscle.

3. INNERVATION

Based on the innervation of 26 muscles in 20 cadavers,[2] the sternalis muscle was considered a variant of either the pectoralis major or the rectus abdominis muscle. Sixteen of 26 sternalis muscles (62%) received their innervation from intercostal nerves (anterior primary divisions of thoracic spinal nerves), and were considered homologous to the rectus abdominis. The remaining 38% received their innervation from the cervical plexus, usually *via* the medial pectoral nerve, which is derived from spinal nerves C_8 and T_1, so that these muscles were considered homologous with the sternal portion of the pectoralis major. Two muscles received a dual innervation.[2] Whether the sternalis muscle has an exact analogue in other species has been the subject of unresolved controversy. Its diverse innervation suggests that it may represent variable remnants of several muscles.

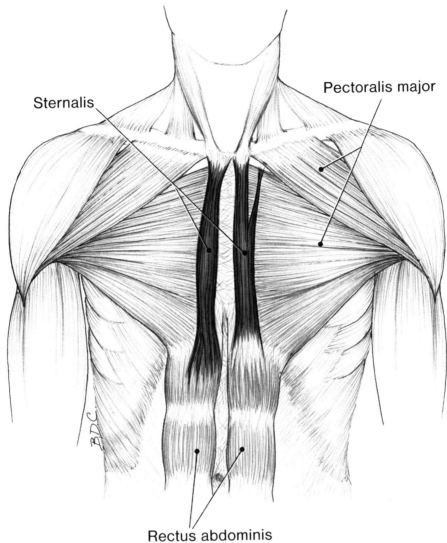

Figure 44.2.   Common attachments of the anatomically variable sternalis muscle (*red*). It is twice as likely to be unilateral as bilateral and equally likely to occur on the right or left sides.

4. ACTIONS

No skeletal movement is attributed to this muscle. No electromyographic data or clinical reports of muscular contraction of the sternalis were located; thus, when or why it contracts is unknown.

5. MYOTATIC UNIT

The functional relation of the sternalis to other muscles must await determination of its function.

6. SYMPTOMS

The symptoms associated with TPs in this muscle are intense deep substernal pain and occasionally, soreness over the sternum. Since the pain arising from this muscle is not aggravated by movement, its musculoskeletal origin is easily overlooked.

7. ACTIVATION OF TRIGGER POINTS

It is important to realize that patients with either acute myocardial infarction or angina pectoris are likely to develop active TPs in both the sternalis and left pectoralis major muscles. A sternalis TP that was activated by an episode of myocardial ischemia, as in acute infarction, is likely to persist long after this initiating event.

Right or left sternalis muscles may de-

PART 4

velop satellite TPs when the sternalis lies within the zone of pain referred downward from the lower portion of the sternal division of the sternocleidomastoid muscle.

Activation of TPs also may result from direct trauma to the costosternal area.

8. PATIENT EXAMINATION

Range-of-motion tests are negative, since the pain is neither relieved nor aggravated by any musculoskeletal activity, such as, movement of the shoulder girdle, deep breathing, or stooping.

9. TRIGGER POINT EXAMINATION

Sternalis TPs are found by systematic palpation against the underlying sternum and costal cartilages; firm pressure elicits focal deep tenderness at the TP and projection of referred pain, but rarely local twitch responses. On examination, the patient has difficulty in distinguishing between the local and the referred pain that is elicited from this muscle, unless the pain radiates not only beneath the sternum, but also to the shoulder or arm. Referred pain responses due to needle penetration of the TP are more clearly distinguishable. The TPs may appear anywhere in the muscle, including in the midline, but they are most likely to occur to the left of the midline at the mid-sternal level.[15, 16]

When multiple areas of spot tenderness are found over the costochondral junctions without the referred pain feature of sternalis TPs, the examiner should consider costochondritis or Tietze's syndrome.[8] This syndrome is identified by upper anterior chest pain with tender, non-suppurative swelling in the area of the costal cartilages or the sternoclavicular junctions. Multiple lesions are more frequent than single lesions, and usually involve adjacent articulations. Also, in Tietze's syndrome, systemic manifestations are absent; radiographic and laboratory studies are normal, except for occasional reports of increased calcification at affected sites.[8] The importance of distinguishing between chest pain of cardiac origin and that of chest wall origin has recently been emphasized.[4]

10. ENTRAPMENTS

None are attributed to this muscle.

11. ASSOCIATED TRIGGER POINTS

One rarely observes sternalis TPs alone, without the presence of active TPs in the pectoralis major muscle. The possibility that a sternalis TP represents a satellite of a distant primary TP makes it important to examine the lower portion of the sternal division of the sternocleidomastoid muscle, which may refer pain downward over the sternum.

12. STRETCH AND SPRAY

Application of vapocoolant spray is only occasionally effective in the treatment of these myofascial TPs, since stretch of the sternalis muscle is not possible. Application in a crisscross pattern while the patient holds a deep breath[14] has been the most successful spray technique for TPs in this muscle. The sternalis TPs are responsive, however, to ischemic compression against the underlying bone, and the TPs may be easily injected. Deep friction massage applied to the muscle fibers in the region of the TP is also beneficial.

Local treatment of the sternalis myofacial pain syndrome is not complete until active TPs in the pectoralis major, or in the lower end of the sternal division of the sternocleidomastoid muscle, have been inactivated, often by stretch and spray (see Chapters 7 and 42). The patient is less likely to experience recurrence of pain due to TPs in the sternalis muscle if these other two muscles are stretched and sprayed prophylactically, even though they contain only latent TPs which are clinically silent with respect to pain.

Relief of sternal pain by the spray does not rule out a cardiac etiology of the pain.[11]

13. INJECTION AND STRETCH

A TP in the sternalis is identified by flat palpation; it is then fixed between two fingers, probed, and precisely infiltrated. When a sternalis TP is encountered by the tip of the needle, the patient reports projection of pain under the sternum, and sometimes across the upper pectoral region and down the ulnar aspect of the arm as far as the elbow. Injection has not been observed to induce a local twitch response.

Both sides of the sternum must be checked for sternalis TPs. During injection, TPs on the front of the sternum may be found as deep as 2 cm (¾ in) beneath the skin surface. These deep TPs may lie in the pectoralis major, rather than in sternalis fibers. This possibility is strengthened by the sensation that the needle sometimes penetrates two layers of muscle, a superficial and then a deeper one, either or both of which may contain TPs.

A hot pack is applied promptly after injection of TPs. This muscle can not be stretched.

14. CORRECTIVE ACTIONS

The patient should learn to perform ischemic compression on his or her own sternalis TPs, followed by moist heat. The patient selects a tender spot and presses on it steadily with one finger, reinforced by pressure from the other hand. Pressure is gradually increased to maintain a sense of discomfort, but not severe pain, until strong pressure on that spot no longer hurts. Sustained pressure for about 30 sec, sometimes for as long as 2 min, obliterates the tenderness at the TP. With release of pressure, the compressed skin is blanched, but quickly turns pink. This reddening represents reactive hyperemia that may last a long time, even hours.

It is likely that the underlying muscle which contains the TP, as well as the skin, is flushed by reactive hyperemia. The pressure is sufficiently firm and should be held long enough to produce also a significant degree of ischemic nerve block,[5] as indicated by the disappearance of spot tenderness; this may require a minute longer. When the previously tender spot of muscle at the TP becomes normo-sensitive, it is no longer a source of referred pain. It may remain quiescent indefinitely, unless the TP is reactivated, as by the recurring pain due to the coronary insufficiency of angina pectoris.[13]

References

1. Barlow RN: The sternalis muscle in American whites and Negroes. *Anat Rec* 61:413–426, 1935.
2. Christian HA: Two instances in which the musculus sternalis existed—one associated with other anomalies. *Bull Johns Hopkins Hosp* 9:235–240, 1898.
3. Eisler P: *Die Muskeln des Stammes.* Gustav Fischer Verlag, Jena, 1912 (pp. 470–475, Figs. 70, 72).
4. Epstein SE, Gerber LH, Borer JS: Chest wall syndrome, a common cause of unexplained cardiac pain. *JAMA* 241:2793–2797, 1979.
5. Gasser HS, Erlanger J: The role of fiber size in the establishment of a nerve block by pressure or cocaine. *Am J Physiol* 88:581–591, 1929.
6. Grant JCB: *An Atlas of Human Anatomy,* edited by J.E. Anderson, Ed. 7. Williams & Wilkins, Baltimore, 1978 (Fig. 6-120B).
7. Hollinshead, WH: *Anatomy for Surgeons.* Ed. 2, Vol. 3, *The Back and Lungs,* Harper & Row, New York, 1969 (p. 287 Fig. 4-19).
8. Levey GS, Calabro JJ: Tietze's Syndrome: Report of two cases and review of the literature. *Arthritis Rheum* 5:261–269, 1962.
9. Rinzler SH: *Cardiac Pain.* Charles C Thomas, Springfield, Ill., 1951 (pp. 80, 81).
10. Toldt C: *An Atlas of Human Anatomy.* Translated by M.E. Paul, Vol. 1. Macmillan Company, New York, 1919 (p. 282).
11. Travell J: Early relief of chest pain by ethyl chloride spray in acute coronary thrombosis. *Circulation* 111:120–124, 1951.
12. Travell J: Pain mechanisms in connective tissue. In *Connective Tissues, Transactions of the Second Conference, 1951.* Josiah Macy, Jr. Foundation, New York, 1952 (pp. 86–125).
13. Travell J, Rinzler SH: Therapy directed at the somatic component of cardiac pain. *Am Heart J* 35:248–268, 1958.
14. Travell J, Rinzler SH: Pain syndromes of the chest muscles: Resemblance to effort angina and myocardial infarction, and relief by local block. *Can Med Assoc J* 59:333–338, 1948 (Cases 2 and 3).
15. Travell J, Rinzler SH: The myofascial genesis of pain. *Postgrad Med* 11:425–434, 1952 (p. 429).
16. Webber TD: Diagnosis and modification of headache and shoulder-arm-hand syndrome. *JAOA* 72:697–710, 1973 (pp. 10, 12; Fig. 32).
17. Zohn DA, Mennell J McM: *Musculoskeletal Pain: Diagnosis and Physical Treatment.* Little, Brown & Co., Boston, 1976 (p. 193, Fig. 9-14).

CHAPTER 45
Serratus Posterior Superior Muscle
"Cryptic, Deep, Upper-back Pain"

HIGHLIGHTS: Referred pain from trigger points (TPs) in the serratus posterior superior is a frequent source of scapular pain. **REFERRED PAIN** from this muscle is strongly felt deep under the upper portion of the scapula, often with extension to the back of the shoulder, the upper triceps area, the elbow, ulnar side of the forearm and hand, and to the entire little finger. **ANATOMICAL ATTACHMENTS** are to the dorsal midline fascia from C_7 through T_3, above, and to the second through fifth ribs, below and laterally. The **ACTION** established for this muscle is to assist inspiration. The **SYMPTOM** of pain may be increased by reaching out forward with the hands. **ACTIVATION OF TRIGGER POINTS** is likely to occur from overloading of thoracic respiratory effort, as by coughing or paradoxical breathing. **TRIGGER POINT EXAMINATION** requires strong protraction and abduction of the scapula to uncover the TPs and make them accessible to palpation against the ribs. **STRETCH AND SPRAY** require the seated patient to lean forward and drop the head, hump the back, and exhale deeply as the vapocoolant spray is directed caudally along the muscle fibers. Ischemic compression is helpful. For **INJECTION AND STRETCH** the needle is directed into the TP, which is pinned down against a rib. **CORRECTIVE ACTIONS** include learning abdominal breathing and the home application of ischemic compression.

1. REFERRED PAIN
(Fig. 45.1)

Trigger points (TPs) in the serratus posterior superior frequently cause scapular and shoulder pain. Among 76 painful shoulders in 58 patients, this muscle was a cause of pain in 98%, and the single source of pain in 10%.[15]

The essential pain reference of this muscle is a *deep ache* under the upper portion of the scapula (Fig. 45.1). When asked to point to the painful area, patients usually reach back with the opposite arm, but are unable to touch the sore area because the shoulder blade covers it. This pain is perceived as deeper than the similar upper-back pain that arises from TP_5 in the middle trapezius. Pain is also usually felt in-tensely over the posterior border of the deltoid and the long head of the triceps brachii muscles.[14, 15, 16] It often covers the entire triceps region, with an accent on the medial epicondyle of the elbow, and occasionally includes the ulnar side of the forearm, hand, and all of the little finger. Anteriorly, the pectoral region may occasionally be painful.

2. ANATOMICAL ATTACHMENTS
(Figs. 45.2 and 45.3)

The serratus posterior superior muscle attaches *above* to the dorsal midline fascia, from C_7 through T_2 or T_3, and *below* and *laterally* by four digitations, to the cranial borders of the second through the fifth

PART 4

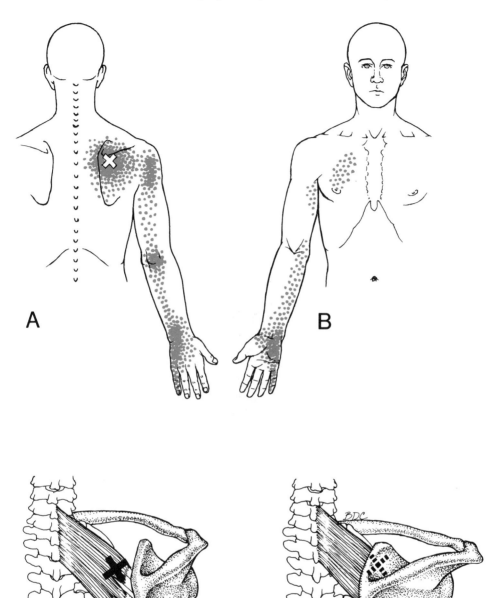

Figure 45.1. Referred pain pattern of a trigger point (✕) in the right serratus posterior superior muscle. Essential pain is *solid red*, spillover pain is *stippled red*. *A*, back view of pain pattern. *B*, front view of pain pattern. *C*, scapula abducted, making the trigger point (✕) accessible to palpation and injection. *D*, scapula in the normal rest position, and the trigger point (*dashed* ✕) *inaccessible*.

A

B

C

**Trigger point
palpable**

D

**Trigger point
not palpable**

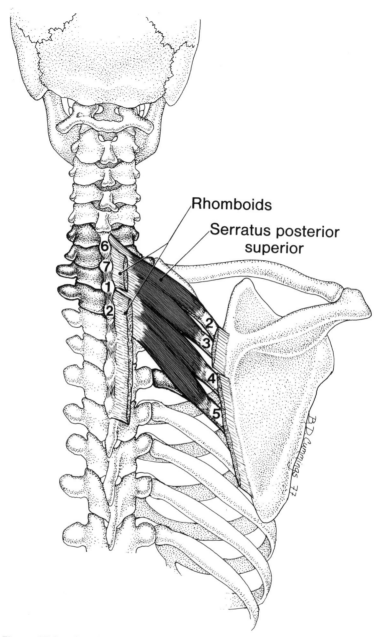

Figure 45.2.   Attachments of the serratus posterior superior muscle (*red*) to numbered vertebrae and ribs.

ribs[5] (Fig. 45.2). The number of digitations is variable.[5]

The fibers of the serratus superior are inclined at approximately 45°, and lie immediately beneath the fibers of the rhomboid muscles, which nearly parallel them (Fig. 45.3). Both of these muscles lie beneath the fibers of the trapezius muscle, which are aligned nearly horizontally.

Paraspinally, the longissimus thoracis and iliocostalis muscles lie deep to the serratus posterior superior.

Supplemental References

Anatomy atlases present the serratus posterior superior as seen from behind,[3, 4, 8, 11-13] and in cross section.[2]

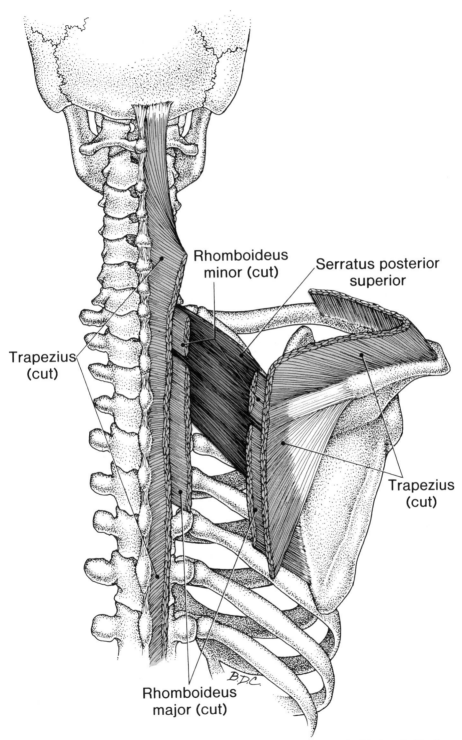

Figure 45.3.   Anatomical relations of the serratus posterior superior muscle (*dark red*). The trapezius and rhomboid muscles (*light red*) lie over all of it, and the iliocostalis and longissimus thoracis muscles (not shown) lie beneath part of this muscle.

3. INNERVATION

The serratus posterior superior muscle is innervated by the anterior primary divisions of spinal nerves T_1 through T_4.[5]

4. ACTIONS

The serratus posterior superior muscle raises the ribs to which it is attached, thereby expanding the chest and aiding inspiration.[1, 5, 6, 9] No electromyographic or stimulation studies are known.

5. MYOTATIC UNIT

Presumably, the intercostal and the scalene muscles act synergistically with the serratus posterior superior for inspiration.

6. SYMPTOMS

The patient complains of a steady deep ache at rest, as described in Section 1. Little or no change in the intensity of pain occurs with movement or activity. Pain may be increased by lifting objects with outstretched hands, or by other activities which cause the scapula to press against active TPs in the serratus posterior superior muscle.

7. ACTIVATION OF TRIGGER POINTS

Like the scalene muscles, TPs in the serratus posterior superior muscle are activated by overload of the thoracic respiratory effort because of coughing, as in pneumonia, asthma or chronic emphysema, and by paradoxical breathing (use of the diaphragm and abdominal muscles out of phase), which reduces rather than augments tidal volume (see Fig. 20.13A).

Movements and postures that force the scapula against the serratus posterior superior also appear to activate its TPs. Those causes include sitting for long periods writing at a high desk or table, when the shoulders are elevated and rotated forward to permit the arms to reach the high surface; repeatedly reaching to the rear of a high work surface, as by laboratory technicians; and protrusion of the thorax against the scapula by scoliosis (see Chapter 27).

8. PATIENT EXAMINATION

Patients with intrathoracic disease that compromises ventilation, such as emphysema, are in double trouble if they also develop TPs in this serratus muscle. These people are generally *not* round-shouldered (as compared with those who suffer from rhomboid and pectoral muscle involvement), and they have little or no restriction of movement. They often have scoliosis, especially the functional type due to a short leg and small hemipelvis, observed when the patient stands with the feet together (see Fig. 48.9B), or sits straight on a flat wood seat (see Fig. 48.10B).

The referred pain pattern of this muscle mimics the distribution of pain caused by eighth cervical root compression;[10] both diagnoses must be considered. The serratus myofascial syndrome causes no neurological deficit. The radiculopathy *per se* causes no TP tenderness, palpable bands, or referred pain evoked from the muscle.

9. TRIGGER POINT EXAMINATION (Fig. 45.4)

The patient sits and leans forward slightly, with the arm hanging down on the side to be examined (Fig. 45.4), or with the homolateral hand placed in the opposite axilla, to fully abduct the scapula.[15] The scapula **must** be protracted and pulled laterally to uncover the serratus TPs beneath the scapula (Figs. 45.1C and 45.4). The serratus posterior superior is palpated through the trapezius and rhomboid muscles (Fig. 45.3), as also illustrated by Michele *et al.*[7] Snapping palpation elicits local twitch responses of the overlying trapezius fibers, which can be identified because of the nearly horizontal orientation of those superficial fibers. However, local twitch responses in the deeper, obliquely oriented rhomboid and serratus fibers are not usually perceived.

A serratus TP is identified as a spot of exquisite deep tenderness in a palpable band when the muscle is pressed against the underlying rib. Pressure on the active TP readily induces the characteristic serratus referred pain pattern and convincingly demonstrates to the patient the relationship between this myofascial TP and the pain suffered.

10. ENTRAPMENTS

No nerve entrapment has been attributed to this muscle.

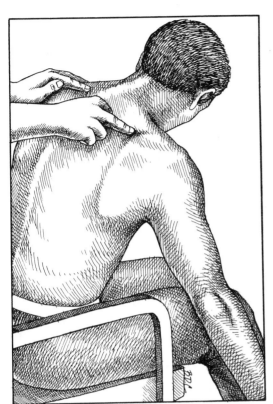

Figure 45.4. Digital examination of the right serratus posterior superior muscle. The scapula *must* be abducted to uncover the trigger point area (Fig. 45.1 *C* and *D*).

11. ASSOCIATED TRIGGER POINTS

The TPs in the serratus posterior superior lie within the pain reference zone of the synergistic scalene muscles, and may appear as satellites of scalene involvement. The scalene TPs may mimic, in part, the pain pattern of the serratus posterior superior. The neck should always be examined for scalene TPs, if a TP is found in the serratus posterior superior.

The overlying rhomboid and nearby iliocostalis, longissimus thoracis, and multifidus muscles also may develop associated TPs.

12. STRETCH AND SPRAY
(Fig. 45.5)

The seated patient hooks the fingers on the side to be treated under the chair seat (Fig. 45.5) to anchor the chest. The patient drops the head forward so that the operator can press the base of the neck forward and to the opposite side in order to stretch

the muscle. Meanwhile, vapocoolant spray is applied in slow parallel sweeps laterally and downward over the course of the muscle fibers and then outward over the shoulder and down the arm. Lines of spray should cover the referred pain pattern, which includes the 5th digit (Figs. 45.1A and 45.5). While the spray is being applied, the patient "humps the back" (flexes the

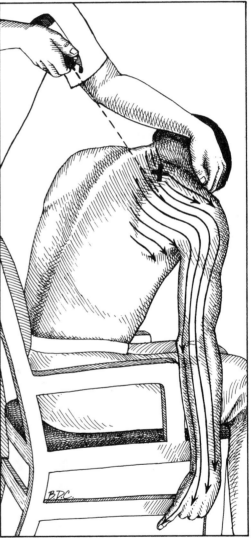

Figure 45.5. Stretch position and spray pattern (*arrows*) for a trigger point (×) in the serratus posterior superior muscle. The seated patient hooks the fingers of one hand under the chair seat, fully flexes the upper thoracic spine, then exhales deeply and holds the breath. Meanwhile, the operator presses the base of the neck forward and to the opposite side, while applying the spray over the muscle and its referred pain pattern.

thoracic spine) and exhales deeply to increase the stretch on the serratus muscle.

When the patient is in the above stretch-and-spray position, ischemic compression is easily applied to these TPs, which lie directly over the ribs. This finger pressure therapy is often helpful; it is most effective if the muscle is on stretch while pressure is applied.

The position of placing the arm across the chest and the hand under the opposite axilla, while useful for examination of the muscle, should not be used for stretch and spray. Abduction of the scapula is not essential for stretch and spray, as it is for examination. This position tends to elevate, rather than to lower, the rib cage and makes it difficult for the patient to achieve full relaxation of this chest muscle.

13. INJECTION AND STRETCH
(Fig. 45.6]

If stretch and spray or ischemic compression are not effective, injection of the TPs usually succeeds, but this carries a significant hazard of pneumothorax, if performed without precautions.

With the patient lying on the opposite side and the scapula fully abducted (Fig. 45.6), a TP is localized and fixed against the underlying rib. The needle is directed nearly tangent to the skin and is pointed toward a rib at all times, not toward an intercostal space; the operator, or the patient, might sneeze or unexpectedly startle and jump. The possibility of causing a pneumothorax must be kept in mind.

Following TP injection, stretch and spray are repeated, as above, and a hot pack applied over the muscle.

14. CORRECTIVE ACTIONS

It is most important that the patient uses coordinated chest and abdominal breathing (see Fig. 20.13B and C) and not paradoxical breathing, so as to avoid overload of the upper-chest accessory muscles of inspiration.

The patient should maintain normal lumbar lordosis, both standing and sitting. When seated, this is facilitated by placing an appropriate-sized lumbar pillow in the small of the back, then relaxing and leaning against the back of the chair so that the pillow maintains both the normal lumbar and thoracic curves without muscle strain (see Fig. 42.9E).

While supine, the patient may find it possible to apply ischemic compression by lying on a tennis ball placed under the interscapular region (see Chapters 22 and 27), if, for this muscle, the scapula is abducted sufficiently. Alternatively, a friend may be taught to apply ischemic compression to this TP for the patient, as part of the home program.

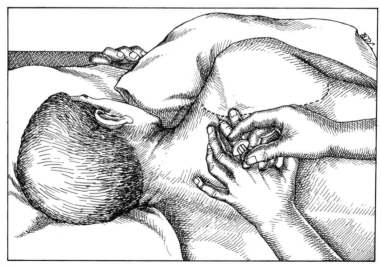

Figure 45.6. Injection of a trigger point in the serratus posterior superior muscle. The scapula must be abducted to reach the trigger points in most of this muscle. The needle is directed nearly tangent to the chest wall and toward a rib to avoid penetrating an intercostal space and causing a pneumothorax.

References

1. Campbell EJM: Accessory muscles, Chapter 9. In *The Respiratory Muscles*, edited by E.J.M. Campbell, E. Agostoni, J.N. Davis, Ed. 2. W.B. Saunders, Philadelphia, 1970 (pp. 181–195).
2. Carter BL, Morehead J, Wolpert SM, *et al.*: *Cross-Sectional Anatomy*. Appleton-Century-Crofts, New York, 1977 (Sections 19–21).
3. Eisler P: *Die Muskeln des Stammes*. Gustav Fischer, Jena, 1912 (Figs. 50, 53, 55).
4. Grant JCB: *An Atlas of Human Anatomy*, Ed. 7. Williams & Wilkins, Baltimore, 1978 (Fig. 5-26).
5. Gray H: *Anatomy of the Human Body*, edited by C.M. Goss, American Ed. 29. Lea & Febiger, Philadelphia, 1973 (p. 411).
6. Hollinshead WH: *Functional Anatomy of the Limbs and Back*, Ed. 4. W.B. Saunders, Philadelphia, 1976 (p. 226).
7. Michele AA, Davies JJ, Krueger FJ, *et al.*: Scapulocostal syndrome (fatigue-postural paradox). *NY State J Med* 50:1353–1356, 1950 (Fig. 2).
8. Pernkopf E: *Atlas of Topographical and Applied Human Anatomy*, Vol. 2. W.B. Saunders, Philadelphia, 1964 (Fig. 29).
9. Rasch PJ, Burke RK: *Kinesiology and Applied Anatomy*. Lea & Febiger, Philadelphia, 1967 (p. 256).
10. Reynolds MD: Myofascial trigger point syndromes in the practice of rheumatology. *Arch. Phys Med Rehabil* 62:111–114, 1981 (Table 2).
11. Sobotta J, Figge FHJ: *Atlas of Human Anatomy*, Ed. 9, Vol. 1. Hafner Division of Macmillan, New York, 1974 (Fig. 144).
12. Spalteholz W: *Handatlas der Anatomie des Menschen*, Ed. 11, Vol. 2. S. Hirzel, Leipzig, 1922 (p. 307).
13. Toldt C: *An Atlas of Human Anatomy*, translated by M.E. Paul, Ed. 2, Vol. 1. Macmillan, New York, 1919 (pp. 267, 269).
14. Travell J: Basis for the multiple uses of local block of somatic trigger areas (procaine infiltration and ethyl chloride spray). *Miss Valley Med J* 71:12–21, 1949 (p. 18, Fig. 4).
15. Travell J, Rinzler S, Herman M: Pain and disability of the shoulder and arm: treatment by intramuscular infiltration with procaine hydrochloride. *JAMA* 120:417–422, 1942 (p. 418, Fig. 2).
16. Travell J, Rinzler SH: Pain syndromes of the chest muscles: Resemblance to effort angina and myocardial infarction, and relief by local block. *Can Med Assoc J* 59:333–338, 1948 (p. 336, Fig. 5).

CHAPTER 46
Serratus Anterior Muscle
"Stitch-in-the-Side"

HIGHLIGHTS: **REFERRED PAIN** from the serratus anterior muscle is projected to the side and back of the chest and sometimes down the ulnar aspect of the arm. **ANATOMICAL ATTACHMENTS** of the muscle are in three fiber arrangements all of which run between the ribs in front and the vertebral border of the scapula behind. **INNERVATION** of the serratus anterior muscle is by the long thoracic nerve. **ACTIONS** of the muscle include rotation of the scapula to turn the glenoid fossa upward, protraction and elevation of the scapula, and prevention of winging of the scapula. **SYMPTOMS** of trigger points (TPs) in this muscle are pain and sometimes a sense of air hunger with short panting respiration. **ACTIVATION OF TRIGGER POINTS** is caused by stressful running, coughing, and by psychogenic factors, which may lead to disturbed respiration. **PATIENT EXAMINATION** may reveal reduced chest expansion, winging of the scapula, but little, if any, restriction of shoulder motion. **TRIGGER POINT EXAMINATION** locates the TPs along the mid-axillary line at about the fifth or sixth rib. **STRETCH AND SPRAY** require forceful retraction of the scapula with the spray directed first posteriorly, then anteriorly, to cover the muscle and all of its pain pattern. **INJECTION AND STRETCH** are directed at a TP fixed between the fingers against a rib. **CORRECTIVE ACTIONS** include modification of patient activities to reduce and eliminate overuse of the muscle, as by coughing, paradoxical breathing, push-ups, and body-lift exercises. Appropriate self-stretch exercises include the Serratus Anterior and the In-doorway Stretch Exercises.

1. REFERRED PAIN
(Fig. 46.1)

Referred pain from trigger points (TPs) concentrates anterolaterally at mid-chest level,[22] and in a separate posterior area medial to the inferior angle of the scapula (Fig. 46.1). Pain may also be projected down the arm, extending to the palm and ring finger.[28, 38, 39, 40] Respiratory symptoms[36] are described under Section 6.

In some patients, TPs in the serratus anterior contribute to abnormal breast sensitivity, in addition to the TPs in the pectoralis major muscle[35] (Fig. 42.1C) that are usually responsible for this breast symptom.[36]

2. ANATOMICAL ATTACHMENTS
(Fig. 46.2)

The serratus anterior muscle is composed structurally of three groups of fibers. The serration which attaches **anteriorly** to the first (and sometimes the second) rib connects **posteriorly** to the superior angle of the scapula.[1] This bundle of fibers lies nearly parallel to the underlying ribs (Fig. 46.2).

The next two serrations connect **anteriorly** to the second and third ribs to form a flat sheet, which attaches **posteriorly** to the length of the vertebral border of the scapula. These fibers lie snugly against the ribs, angling across them at nearly 45°.

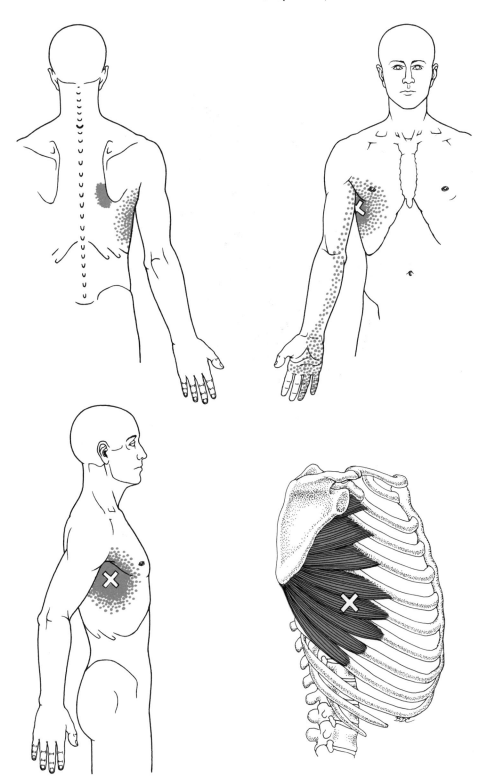

Figure 46.1.   Referred pain pattern (essential areas *solid dark red*, spillover areas *stippled dark red*) from a trigger point (**X**) in the right serratus anterior muscle (*medium red*), as seen from the back, front, and side view.

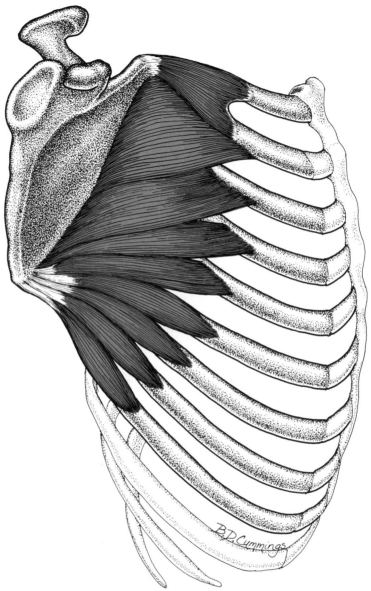

Figure 46.2.   Attachments of the right serratus anterior muscle (*red*). The clavicle has been removed and the scapula rotated forcibly backward. The fibers of the muscle are divided into three groups (see Section 2 of text).

The serrations attached **anteriorly** to the next five or six ribs, the third group, are the strongest part of the muscle and form a quarter-circle fan, which converges **posteriorly** on the inferior angle of the scapula[17] (Fig. 46.2). These lowest serrations develop TPs along the mid-axillary line.

The fibers attached to the lower ribs interdigitate anteriorly with the costal attachments of the external oblique muscle of the abdomen.

Supplemental References

Other authors illustrate this muscle as seen from the side,[6, 10, 14, 34] from in front,[7, 18, 30, 32] from behind,[11, 25] and in cross section.[4, 9, 12, 24] The serratus anterior also is shown in relation to the long thoracic nerve, which supplies it.[13, 15, 26, 31] A drawing of a variation of the muscle shows a group of interior fibers attaching posteriorly to superficial fascia instead of to the scapula.[8]

3. INNERVATION

The serratus anterior is supplied by the long thoracic nerve of Bell, directly from the anterior rami of the C_5, C_6, C_7 and sometimes C_8 spinal nerves. The fibers of the upper portion of the muscle derive their innervation mainly from C_5; the middle portion is innervated from C_5 and C_6, and the lower portion mainly from C_6 and C_7.[17]

The nerve of Bell lies superficial to the serratus anterior muscle, in the line of the anterior axillary fold, anterior to the usual location of TPs in the muscle.

4. ACTIONS

Stimulation of the long thoracic nerve to the entire serratus anterior muscle causes the scapula to move upward, laterally and forward.[5]

Trauma to the long thoracic nerve may cause paralysis of this muscle, which results in winging of the scapula.

Five of eight reported functions of the serratus anterior have been substantiated by electromyography:

1. It supports flexion and abduction of the arm. Contraction of the most caudal fibers of the muscle rotates the scapula so that it turns the glenoid fossa to face upward.[2, 17, 19, 23, 27] These fibers, when stimulated, initially rotate the inferior angle of the scapula forward around the medial (superior) angle.[5]

The serratus anterior is not active during unloaded elevation of the arm until it reaches about 30°. The middle trapezius, rhomboid, and upper third of the pectoralis major muscles provide the initial force.[5, 27] The lower, triangular group of serratus anterior fibers are electromyographically more active than the middle trapezius fibers during flexion of the arm, and *vice versa* during abduction of the arm.[2]

2. It protracts the scapula, as when the individual exerts effort to push an object forward;[17, 19, 23, 27] this also is described as an oblique lateral motion.[33]

3. It elevates the scapula. Prolonged stimulation of the *lowest* fibers eventually produces powerful elevation of the entire scapula, but not until the rhomboid and levator scapulae muscles have first been stretched by the serratus anterior as it rotates the inferior angle forward and outward. Stimulation of only the *middle* portion elevates the acromion.[5] The middle portion contributes to elevation of the scapula and is increasingly activated as the arm is elevated.[20]

4. It holds the medial border of the scapula firmly against the thorax.[19, 23]

5. It carries the thorax during a push-up.[23]

6. The lowest fibers are said to depress the scapula,[19, 23, 33] although neither direct stimulation[5] nor electromyography[2] support this contention. This function is questionable.

7. The original stimulation studies and observations were made in severely abnormal muscular situations and indicated that the serratus anterior functioned to support forceful inspiration;[5] this conclusion was perpetuated by others.[1, 23] However, an inspiratory function has been strongly refuted by multiple electromyographic studies in normal subjects.[2]

8. Electrical activity of the serratus anterior is *not* needed to support the shoulder girdle against gravity,[2] as first reported.[20]

Electromyographic monitoring of the serratus anterior during simulated auto driving showed activity in almost all cases when the top of the steering wheel was rotated contralaterally.[21]

Electromyographic monitoring of serratus anterior activity during 13 sports activities showed slight to moderate motor unit activity of nearly equal intensity bilaterally.[3]

5. MYOTATIC UNIT

Synergistic muscles, which also act to protract the scapula, include the pectoralis minor and upper fibers of the pectoralis major. The serratus anterior assists the upper trapezius in elevation of the glenoid fossa.

Protraction is antagonized by the more horizontal fibers of the latissimus dorsi, rhomboidei and middle trapezius muscles. Glenoid elevation is antagonized by the more vertical fibers of the latissimus dorsi and pectoralis major muscles.

PART 4

6. SYMPTOMS

Chest pain from serratus anterior TPs may be present at rest in severe cases. When the TPs are less hyperirritable, pain may be precipitated by deep breathing, *i.e.* a "stitch-in-the-side" while running. Similar pain also may arise from TPs in the abdominal oblique muscles. The runner may press against, or squeeze, the painful area for relief in order to keep going. Patients have difficulty finding a comfortable position at night and often are unable to lie on the affected muscle. See Section 1 for the referred pain distribution.

Patients with this myofascial syndrome may report that they are "short of breath," or that they "can't take a deep breath, it hurts." They frequently are unable to finish an ordinary sentence without stopping to breathe;[36] patients find this especially bothersome when talking on the telephone. Although these patients are likely to receive a cardiopulmonary work-up for dyspnea, the cause is reduced tidal volume due to restricted chest expansion.

Serratus anterior TPs can contribute to the pain associated with myocardial infarction. The pain has been relieved by inactivating pectoral muscle and serratus anterior TPs on the left side.[29]

Pain is rarely aggravated by the usual tests for range of motion at the shoulder, but may result from a strong effort to protract the scapula.

7. ACTIVATION OF TRIGGER POINTS

Serratus anterior TPs may be activated by muscle strain during excessively fast or prolonged running, push-ups, lifting heavy weights overhead, or severe coughing due to respiratory disease. High levels of anxiety, and of hysteria, apparently increase the likelihood of serratus anterior TPs.[36]

Patients with emphysema do not seem to be especially prone to develop these TPs, but this finding is not surprising in view of the usually over-expanded barrel chest in these patients, which would tend to stretch the serratus anterior muscle.

8. PATIENT EXAMINATION

Round-shouldered posture and prominence of the superior border and spine of the scapula on the affected side result from protraction and rotation of the scapula by the taut serratus anterior fibers. Viewed from the back, the protracted scapula stands out. From the front, the patient has a unilateral round-shouldered posture similar to that seen when the pectoralis major muscle develops active TPs, but the latter muscle tends to be affected nearly equally on both sides of the body.

The feeling of air hunger may be associated with rapid shallow respirations, which usually revert to normal depth when all active serratus anterior TPs have been inactivated.[36]

Active TPs in the serratus anterior muscle inhibit expansion of the lower chest. On inspiration, the patient can expand the upper thoracic cage, but measurement of chest expansion around the lower margin of the rib cage is likely to show marked restriction. After inactivation of TPs in this muscle, there is a smaller minimum and a larger maximum lower chest circumference. The resultant marked increase in volume of tidal air is associated with immediate relief of the respiratory pain and dyspnea.

Before treatment, the patient is likely to overuse the accessory muscles of respiration in the neck, and also to make poor use of the diaphragm. The diaphragmatic dysfunction and the reduced lower chest expansion appear to represent reflex inhibitory influences on respiration since the serratus anterior is not considered a respiratory muscle.

9. TRIGGER POINT EXAMINATION
(Fig. 46.3)

The TPs in the serratus anterior muscle are usually located in the subcutaneous portion of the muscle in the mid-axillary line at approximately the level of the nipple, over the fifth or sixth ribs,[37] but occasionally they are located higher or lower, as also illustrated by Webber.[39] For examination, the recumbent patient lies turned half-way toward the opposite side with the ipsilateral arm partly extended (Fig. 46.3). When the operator pushes the shoulder backward to retract the scapula for palpation and injection of the TPs, the mid-axillary line of the chest appears to be aligned with the anterior axillary fold of

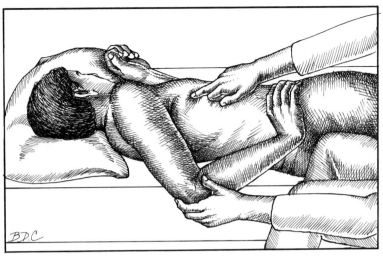

Figure 46.3.   Palpation of a trigger point in the serratus anterior muscle at the level of the sixth rib just anterior to the mid-axillary line. Retraction of the shoulder displaces the anterior axillary fold toward the mid-axillary line.

the shoulder. Flat palpation against the ribs in this area reveals spot tenderness in palpable bands within the muscle, just under the skin. At these points of exquisite tenderness, the palpable bands may respond to snapping palpation with local twitch responses.

10. ENTRAPMENTS

No nerve entrapments by the serratus anterior muscle have been observed. However, two of the three cervical roots that form the long thoracic nerve pass through the scalenus medius muscle[16, 17] and are potentially vulnerable to entrapment by TP activity in that scalene muscle. Thus, the nerve supply to the serratus anterior muscle may suffer entrapment due to TPs in the scalenus medius.

11. ASSOCIATED TRIGGER POINTS

Patients with active TPs in the serratus anterior muscle often have involvement of only this muscle. They may show no clinical involvement of other muscles in its myotatic unit.

The other muscles that may become overloaded due to shortening and reduced function of the serratus anterior include its main antagonist, the latissimus dorsi, and surprisingly, accessory muscles of inspiration in the neck, namely, the scalene and sternocleidomastoid muscles. These associated muscles may develop TPs that remain latent for a long period of time.

12. STRETCH AND SPRAY
(Fig. 46.4)

The patient lies on the opposite side with the back toward the operator and the uppermost arm drawn backward (Fig. 46.4A) to initiate passive stretch of the serratus anterior. Before and during forceful stretching, the vapocoolant is sprayed anteroposteriorly over the muscle. With continued backward and downward pressure on the arm, the patient assumes the position shown in Figure 46.4B. The patient's pelvis is blocked from rotation by the operator's hip so as to place controlled stretch on the serratus anterior. During this stretch, the patient takes a deep breath and holds it to enlarge the lower rib cage. This further stretches the muscle, while the vapocoolant spray is first applied in slow parallel sweeps as in Figure 46.4A, from the TP area backward along the line of the muscle fibers, then over the posterior pain reference zone, and finally over the anterior pain reference zone (Fig. 46.4B). Sweeps are extended down the arm to the palm of the hand in the patient who experiences this referred pain pattern.

In place of stretch-and-spray treatment, application of ischemic compression initially to the TPs in this muscle may be quite effective. Finger pressure also is useful to "clean up" any residual TPs following stretch and spray or injection. The results of treatment are checked by carefully palpating for residual TP tenderness.

13. INJECTION AND STRETCH
(Fig. 46.5)

With the patient lying on the opposite side, as for stretch and spray, a serratus anterior TP is located by flat palpation and pinned against a rib, between the fingers of one hand. The needle is directed toward the rib, at a shallow angle *nearly* tangential with the chest wall, until the needle tip encounters the TP, which lies in the thin layer of muscle between the rib and the skin (Fig. 46.5). The pain reaction on needle contact with a TP in this muscle is usually less intense than the response from TPs in many other muscles.

One should be scrupulously careful to replace immediately any needle that has developed a burr on its tip due to contact with bone.

The long thoracic nerve usually passes anterior to the region of the TPs. The nerve

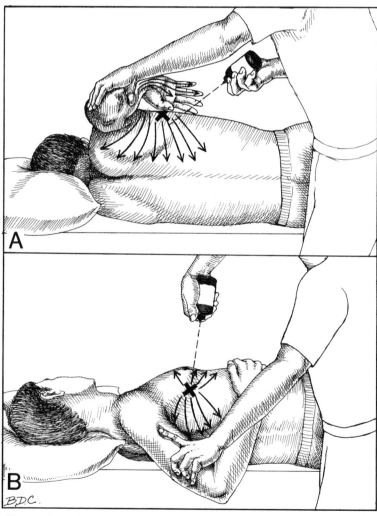

Figure 46.4. Stretch positions and spray patterns (*arrows*) for a trigger point (**X**) of the right serratus anterior muscle in the mid-axillary line. A, initial side-lying position. *B*, full retraction of the right scapula, which effectively stretches the serratus anterior if the operator's hip prevents the patient's pelvis from rotating backward.

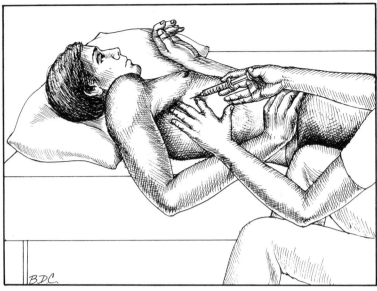

Figure 46.5.   Injection of a trigger point in the serratus anterior muscle over the sixth rib in the mid-axillary line. The patient is lying partially on the opposite side. Retraction of the scapula and the position of the arm moves the landmark of the anterior axillary fold backward. The needle is directed toward an underlying rib, avoiding intercostal spaces.

might be temporarily anesthetized if the procaine solution were infiltrated anterior to the usual TP locations, or if the nerve had a deviant path. In our experience, no patient has reported effects suggesting that a nerve block had resulted from the injection.

14. CORRECTIVE ACTIONS

Patients must avoid or modify activities that are likely to reactivate TPs in the serratus anterior muscle, particularly the activity that precipitated the initial TPs. They should learn to clear the throat rather than to cough, to use synchronized (not paradoxical) breathing (see Section 14 in Chapter 20), to avoid push-ups and heavy overhead lifting, and to avoid hanging from, or chinning themselves on, a bar.

Patients with very irritable TPs in the serratus anterior often are unable to sleep on the affected side because of pressure on the TPs, nor are they able to sleep on the other side if the arm of the affected side falls forward onto the bed and places the muscle in a cramped, shortened position. The latter problem is remedied by use of a pillow to support the arm, and to keep it and the scapula from falling forward, as illustrated in Figure 22.7B.

The seated patient should do the Serratus Anterior Self-stretch Exercise by leaning forward slightly and grasping the wrist on the involved side from behind the body at waist level and then pulling the affected arm toward the opposite side, which forces the scapula backward. The patient also should do the In-doorway Stretch Exercise in the lower and middle hand-positions (See Fig. 42.10).

Supplemental References, Case Reports

The management of a patient with serratus anterior TPs, including injection of procaine, is presented by the senior author.[30]

References

1. Bardeen CR: The musculature, Sect. 5. In *Morris's Human Anatomy*, edited by C.M. Jackson, Ed. 6. Blakiston's Son & Co., Philadelphia, 1921 (p. 394).
2. Basmajian JV: *Muscles Alive*, Ed. 4. Williams & Wilkins, Baltimore, 1978 (pp. 186, 191, 192, 356; Fig. 101).
3. Broer MR, Houtz SJ: *Patterns of Muscular Activity in Selected Sports Skill*. Charles C Thomas, Springfield, Ill., 1967.
4. Carter BL, Morehead J, Wolpert SM, *et al.: Cross-Sectional Anatomy*. Appleton-Century-Crofts, New York, 1977 (Sects 20–29).
5. Duchenne GB: *Physiology of Motion*, translated by E.B. Kaplan. J.B. Lippincott, Philadelphia, 1949

(pp. 24–36, 45).

6. Eisler P: *Die Muskeln des Stammes.* Gustav Fischer, Jena, 1912 (Fig. 52).
7. *Ibid.* (Fig. 76).
8. *Ibid.* (Fig. 77).
9. *Ibid.* (Fig. 68).
10. *Ibid.* (Fig. 52).
11. Grant JCB: *An Atlas of Human Anatomy,* Ed. 7. Williams & Wilkins, Baltimore, 1978 (Fig. 5–26).
12. *Ibid.* (Fig. 6–27).
13. *Ibid.* (Fig. 6–28).
14. *Ibid.* (Fig. 2–5).
15. *Ibid.* (Figs. 6–22, 6–23).
16. *Ibid.* (Fig. 9–5).
17. Gray H: *Anatomy of the Human Body,* Edited by C.M. Goss, American Ed. 29. Lea & Febiger, Philadelphia, 1973 (pp. 454, 963).
18. *Ibid.* (Fig. 6–36).
19. Hollinshead WH: *Functional Anatomy of the Limbs and Back,* Ed. 4. W.B. Saunders, Philadelphia, 1976 (p. 105).
20. Inman VT, Saunders JB, Abbott LC: Observations on the function of the shoulder joint. *J Bone Joint Surg* 26:1–30, 1944 (p. 26).
21. Jonsson S, Jonsson B: Function of the muscles of the upper limb in car driving, Part IV. *Ergonomics* 18:643–649, 1975 (p. 646).
22. Kelly M: Pain in the Chest: Observations on the use of local anaesthesia in its investigation and treatment. *Med J Aust* 1:4–7, 1944 (Case 2, p. 5).
23. Kendall HO, Kendall FP, Wadsworth GE: *Muscles, Testing and Function,* Ed. 2. Williams & Wilkins, Baltimore, 1971 (pp. 130, 131).
24. Pernkopf E: *Atlas of Topographical and Applied Human Anatomy,* Vol. 2. W.B. Saunders, Philadelphia, 1964 (Fig. 8).
25. *Ibid.* (Fig. 28).
26. *Ibid.* (Fig. 39).
27. Rasch PJ, Burke RK: *Kinesiology and Applied Anatomy,* Ed. 6. Lea & Febiger, Philadelphia, 1978 (pp. 153, 154).
28. Rinzler SH: *Cardiac Pain.* Charles C Thomas, Springfield, Ill., 1951 (pp. 79, 80, 82).
29. Rinzler SH, Travell J: Therapy directed at the somatic component of cardiac pain. *Am Heart J* 35:248–268, 1948 (pp. 255–257, Case 1).
30. Sobotta J, Figge FHJ: *Atlas of Human Anatomy,* Ed. 9, Vol. 1. Hafner Division of Macmillan, New York, 1974 (pp. 154, 162).
31. Sobotta J, Figge FHJ: *Atlas of Human Anatomy,* Ed. 9, Vol. 3. Hafner Division of Macmillan, New York, 1974 (pp. 280, 281).
32. Spalteholz W: *Handatlas der Anatomie des Menschen,* Ed. 11, Vol. 2. S. Hirzel, Leipzig, 1922 (p. 283).
33. Steindler A: *Kinesiology of the Human Body.* Charles C Thomas, Springfield, Ill., 1955 (pp. 468, 469).
34. Toldt C: *An Atlas of Human Anatomy,* translated by M.E. Paul, Ed. 2, Vol. 1. Macmillan, New York, 1919 (p. 277).
35. Travell J: Referred pain from skeletal muscle: the pectoralis major syndrome of breast pain and soreness and the sternomastoid syndrome of headache and dizziness. *NY State J Med* 55:331–339, 1955 (p. 333).
36. Travell J, Bigelow NH: Role of somatic trigger areas in the patterns of hysteria. *Psychosom Med* 9:353–363, 1947 (pp. 354, 355).
37. Travell J, Rinzler SH: Pain syndromes of the chest muscles: Resemblence to effort angina and myocardial infarction, and relief by local block. *Can Med Assoc J* 59:333–338, 1948 (Case 1, p. 256).
38. Travell J, Rinzler SH: The myofascial genesis of pain. *Postgrad Med* 11:425–434, 1952 (p. 429, Fig. 3).
39. Webber TD: Diagnosis and modification of headache and shoulder-arm-hand syndrome. *JAOA* 72:697–710, 1973 (p. 10, Fig. 31).
40. Zohn DA, Mennell J McM: *Musculoskeletal Pain: Diagnosis and Physical Treatment.* Little, Brown & Company, Boston, 1976 (p. 193, Fig. 9–14).

PART 4

CHAPTER 47
Serratus Posterior Inferior Muscle
"Nuisance Residual Backache"

HIGHLIGHTS: **REFERRED PAIN** from this muscle is relatively uncommon and is usually identified as an annoying ache that remains after the pain from associated paraspinal trigger points (TPs) has been relieved. The serratus pain radiates over and around the muscle. **ANATOMICAL ATTACHMENTS** of this muscle anchor, above and laterally, to the lowest four ribs. Below and medially, it attaches by an aponeurosis to the spinous processes of four vertebrae. **ACTIONS** of this muscle are to depress the lower ribs, and probably to rotate or extend the thoracolumbar spine when acting on one, or on both sides, respectively. **ACTIVATION OF TRIGGER POINTS** usually results from an acute back strain, which may also activate TPs in the nearby major back muscles at the same time.

TRIGGER POINT EXAMINATION is made by flat palpation across the muscle fibers. **ASSOCIATED TRIGGER POINTS** often are found in the adjacent iliocostalis and longissimus thoracis muscles. **STRETCH AND SPRAY** employ flexion of the back and forward rotation of the ipsilateral shoulder, while the stream of spray is directed upward and laterally over the muscle. Ischemic compression is helpful. For **INJECTION AND STRETCH** of these TPs, the needle is directed toward a rib, not between ribs. **CORRECTIVE ACTIONS** include relief of chronic stresses on the muscle by correcting a small hemipelvis or short leg, by adding a lumbar support to the straight backrest of a chair, by sleeping on a non-sagging mattress, and by the normalization of paradoxical breathing.

1. REFERRED PAIN
(Fig. 47.1)

An active trigger point (TP) in the serratus posterior inferior muscle produces aching discomfort over and around the muscle (Fig. 47.1). The pain extends across the back and over the lower ribs. Patients are likely to identify this annoying ache as muscular in origin.

2. ANATOMICAL ATTACHMENTS

The serratus posterior inferior muscle attaches **medially** to the thin aponeurosis from the spinous processes of the last two thoracic and the first two lumbar vertebrae. **Laterally** its four digitations attach to the last four ribs just medial to their an-

gles[6] (Fig. 47.2). The digitations to one or more ribs, especially to the ninth and twelfth ribs, are sometimes missing; rarely, the entire muscle is absent.[3]

Supplemental References

Other authors have illustrated the muscle clearly as seen from behind,[5, 8, 9, 11, 14, 15] from the side,[3, 4, 12] and in cross section.[2] A variation of the muscle is viewed from behind.[13]

3. INNERVATION

The serratus posterior inferior is supplied by branches of the anterior primary divisions of thoracic spinal nerves 9 through 12.[6] It is not supplied by the pos-

PART 4

terior divisions, as are the paraspinal muscles.

4. ACTIONS

This muscle attaches to the lower ribs and is generally considered a muscle of exhalation[10] that stabilizes the lower ribs against the upward pull of the diaphragm.[6, 7] However, an electromyographic study found no respiratory activity attributable to the muscle.[1] Unilateral contraction probably contributes to rotation, and bilateral contraction to extension of the spine.

5. MYOTATIC UNIT

The serratus posterior inferior muscle appears to act synergistically with the iliocostalis and longissimus thoracis muscles of the same side, unilaterally for rotation and bilaterally for extension of the spine. As a muscle of exhalation, it would act synergistically with the quadratus lumborum muscle, which bilaterally also can assist in extension of the spine.

6. SYMPTOMS

After symptoms due to active TPs in associated major muscles of the back have been eliminated, the patient may be left with a nagging ache in the lower thoracic region. The ache is annoying, but not a severely threatening pain.

Patients may report that squirming and stretching provide some relief.

Maximal deep inhalation and coughing do not evoke pain from the serratus posterior inferior, as they may from active TPs in the serratus anterior and in the quadratus lumborum muscles.

7. ACTIVATION OF TRIGGER POINTS

This is one of the many back muscles which are susceptible to strain during the combined movement of lifting, turning and reaching. Active TPs in the serratus posterior inferior develop due to overload strain at the same time as TPs in associated muscles. Standing on a ladder with the back hyperextended to reach up and work overhead has activated TPs in this muscle;

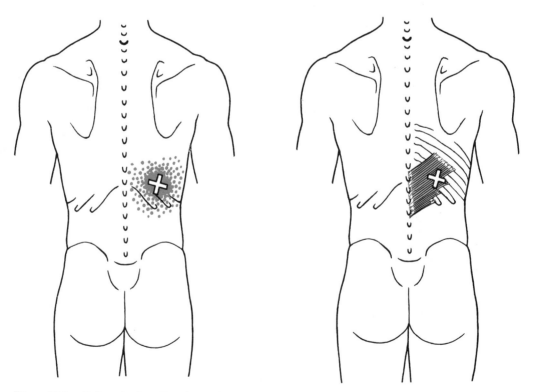

Figure 47.1. Referred pain pattern (essential zone is *solid dark red*, spillover zone is *stippled dark red*) of an active trigger point (**X**) in the right serratus posterior inferior muscle (*light red*).

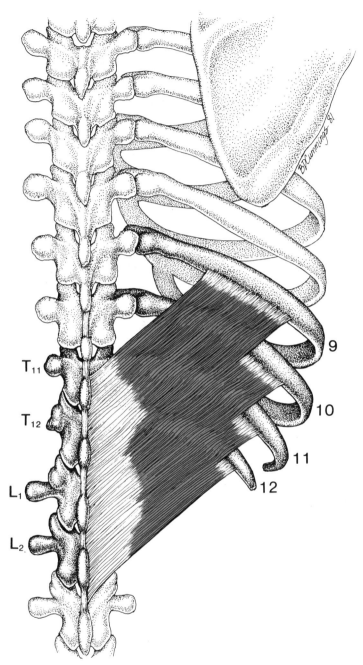

Figure 47.2.   Attachments of the serratus posterior inferior muscle laterally to the lowest four ribs and medially to the aponeurosis extending from the spinous processes of the T_{11} to L_2 vertebrae.

paradoxical breathing and unequal leg lengths are likely to perpetuate them.

8. PATIENT EXAMINATION

Patients may have slight restriction of thoracolumbar flexion, of spinal exten-

sion, and of rotation of the torso away from the painful side.

9. TRIGGER POINT EXAMINATION

As in the serratus posterior superior muscle, TP tenderness in this inferior muscle is found by flat palpation against an underlying rib at the lateral end of the muscle close to its rib attachment. Local twitch responses are not usually seen, or felt, in response to snapping palpation, but may be felt during TP injection.

10. ENTRAPMENTS

No entrapment of a peripheral nerve is attributed to this muscle.

11. ASSOCIATED TRIGGER POINTS

Like the pain evoked by TPs in the coracobrachialis muscle, this patch of discomfort is likely to be noticed only after successful treatment of myofascial symptoms arising from TPs in associated muscles. In this case, the associated muscles are the adjacent iliocostalis and longissimus thoracis.

12. STRETCH AND SPRAY

Stretch and spray is usually most useful as a follow-up to injection of this muscle. Before applying pressure to stretch the muscle, it is covered with a few preliminary sweeps of spray. With the patient seated, leaning forward, and the feet resting comfortably on the floor, the operator presses the shoulder of the involved side forward to flex and rotate the thoracolumbar spine. Meanwhile, the operator directs a stream of vapocoolant spray in parallel sweeps upward and outward from the spine to cover the muscle and its referred pain pattern. The skin is then rewarmed with a hot pack.

Ischemic compression followed by stretch and spray is more likely to be effective in this muscle than stretch and spray alone. The skin is again rewarmed with a hot pack.

13. INJECTION AND STRETCH
(Fig. 47.3)

To inject the serratus posterior inferior muscle, the patient lies on the opposite side and the active TPs are located by palpation. The needle is angled (Fig. 47.3) for injection of the TP so that its point is aimed toward the ninth, tenth, eleventh, or twelfth rib, depending on which digitations are involved. Penetration between the ribs must be avoided. Injection of the

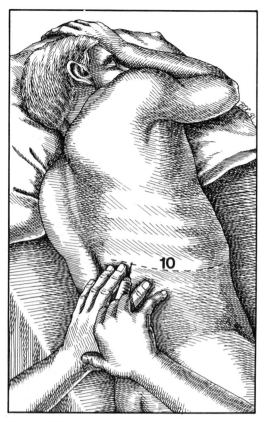

Figure 47.3. Injection of an active TP in a digitation of the serratus posterior inferior muscle that attaches to the ninth or tenth rib. The needle is directed toward a rib, not between ribs.

TPs in this muscle characteristically elicits palpable local twitch responses, and affords prompt relief of the nagging discomfort.

After injection, the muscle is stretched and sprayed, as above, and a hot pack applied.

14. CORRECTIVE ACTIONS

Many of the corrective actions to be considered are covered in other chapters. These include use of a "butt lift" to correct the compensatory scoliosis caused by a small hemipelvis when sitting, or by a short leg when standing (see Chapters 4 and 48); normalization of paradoxical breathing (see Fig. 20.13); sitting in chairs that fit, with adequate lumbar support (see Fig. 42.9E); standing with a normal lordotic lumbar curve (see Fig. 42.9C); and sleeping on a firm mattress that does NOT sag.

References

1. Campbell EJM: Accessory muscles, Chapter 9. In *The Respiratory Muscles*, edited by E.J.M. Campbell, E. Agostoni, and J.N. Davis, Ed. 2. W.B. Saunders, Philadelphia, 1970 (p. 188).
2. Carter BL, Morehead J, Wolpert SM, *et al.*: *Cross-Sectional Anatomy*. Appleton-Century-Crofts, New York, 1977 (Sects. 27–29).
3. Eisler P: *Die Muskeln des Stammes*. Gustav Fischer, Jena, 1912 (Fig. 52).
4. Grant JCB: *An Atlas of Human Anatomy*, Ed. 7. Williams & Wilkins, Baltimore, 1978 (Figs. 2–122, 2–123).
5. *Ibid.* (Fig. 5–26).
6. Gray H: *Anatomy of the Human Body*, edited by C.M. Goss, American Ed. 29. Lea & Febiger, Philadelphia, 1973 (p. 412).
7. Hollinshead WH: *Functional Anatomy of the Limbs and Back*, Ed. 4. W.B. Saunders, Philadel-phia, 1976 (p. 226).
8. McMinn RMH, Hutchings RT: *Color Atlas of Human Anatomy*. Year Book Medical Publishers, Chicago, 1977 (p. 157).
9. Pernkopf E: *Atlas of Topographical and Applied Human Anatomy*, Vol. 2. W.B. Saunders, Philadelphia, 1964 (Fig. 29).
10. Rasch PJ, Burke RK: *Kinesiology and Applied Anatomy*, Ed. 6. Lea & Febiger, Philadelphia, 1978 (p. 256).
11. Sobotta J, Figge FHJ: *Atlas of Human Anatomy*, Ed. 9, Vol. 1. Hafner Division of Macmillan, New York, 1974 (p. 144).
12. Spalteholz H: *Handatlas der Anatomie des Menschen*, Ed. 11, Vol. 2. S. Hirzel, Leipzig, 1922 (Fig. 53).
13. *Ibid.* (Fig. 54).
14. *Ibid.* (p. 307).
15. Toldt C: *An Atlas of Human Anatomy*, translated by M.E. Paul, Ed. 2, Vol. 1. Macmillan, New York, 1919 (pp. 267, 269).

CHAPTER 48

Thoracolumbar Paraspinal Muscles

"Lumbago"

HIGHLIGHTS: The paraspinal musculature consists of a superficial group of long-fibered longitudinal muscles, and a deep group of short diagonal muscles. In the superficial (erector spinae) group, the longissimus thoracis, iliocostalis thoracis, and iliocostalis lumborum are most likely to develop active trigger points (TPs). The deep paraspinal group includes the semispinalis, multifidus and rotatores, at successively deeper levels. **REFERRED PAIN** from TPs in the iliocostalis thoracis is projected laterally across the back of the chest. It may spill over anteriorly in the abdomen and up toward the back of the shoulder. The lumbar iliocostalis TPs refer pain to the mid-buttock. Active TPs in the longissimus thoracis muscle at the low thoracic and high lumbar levels also refer pain downward to the sacroiliac region and the buttock. Pain from the multifidus and rotatores muscles centers on the spinous processes at the segmental level of the TP or, in the lumbar region, it may be referred a few segments caudal to the TP. **ACTIONS** of the paraspinal muscles are to extend and rotate the spine. The superficial fibers are extensors. The successively deeper, shorter and more diagonal fibers supply an increasing rotational component. **ACTIVATION OF TRIGGER POINTS** in the paraspinal muscles is caused by either sudden overload, as when lifting objects with the back twisted and flexed, or by sustained overload during stooping, or when these back muscles are maintained in a fully shortened (hyperlordotic) position. **PATIENT EXAMINATION** reveals restricted range of back motion. Tightness of the more superficial group of muscles can be felt best when the patient is positioned between side-lying and prone. **TRIGGER POINT EXAMINATION** assists identification of the deeper TPs by focal deep tenderness and sometimes by eliciting their characteristic referred pain patterns. **ENTRAPMENT** of the posterior primary rami of both thoracic and lumbar spinal nerves may be due to TPs and their tense bands in the paraspinal muscles. **STRETCH AND SPRAY** of the long-fibered erector spinae muscles are accomplished by flexing the spine of the seated patient, while a jet stream of vapocoolant is applied in downward parallel sweeps. Successively deeper muscle layers require progressively more spinal rotation, with the patient's face turning toward the affected side. **INJECTION AND STRETCH** of the deep paraspinal TPs may require needle penetration to the depth of the laminae of the vertebrae, followed by strong rotary stretch. **CORRECTIVE ACTIONS** include compensation for body asymmetries, modification of the patient's daily activities to reduce stress on the back muscles, self-administered ischemic compression of TPs by use of a tennis ball, and graduated stretch and strengthening exercises.

1. REFERRED PAIN
(Figs. 48.1 and 48.2)

The referred pain patterns illustrated for these back muscles at specific segmental levels are common examples, but trigger points (TPs) may develop at any segmental level. Determining the precise depth of the TP and identifying its exact muscular layer is often difficult.

Pain patterns similar to these observed in adults were reported from the longissimus and multifidus muscles of children.[8]

Superficial Paraspinal (Erector Spinae) Muscles
(Fig. 48.1)

In the mid-back and low back, the two muscles of this group that are most likely to develop TPs are the longissimus thoracis and the iliocostalis thoracis. The iliocostalis thoracis refers pain chiefly upward, while the iliocostalis lumborum and the longissimus thoracis refer pain mainly downward.[112]

The pattern of referred pain from TPs in the iliocostalis at the mid-thoracic level (Fig. 48.1A), is upward toward the shoulder, and laterally to the chest wall which, on the left side, is easily misdiagnosed as cardiac angina,[34, 78] or as pleurisy on either side.[56] At the low thoracic level (Fig. 48.1B), iliocostalis TPs may refer pain upward across the scapula, around to the abdomen, and downward over the lumbar area.[112, 116] This pain referred to the abdomen from a back muscle may be mistaken for visceral pain.[45, 78, 115]

From iliocostalis TPs at the upper lumbar level (Fig. 48.1C), pain is referred strongly downward, concentrating on the mid-buttock,[110, 112, 116] and is a frequent source of unilateral posterior hip pain. "Fibrositis" of the iliocostalis muscles (we regard this term in these papers to mean TPs) is one common cause for the pain described as "lumbago."[65, 84] The patient usually draws an up-and-down pattern to represent the pain referred from ilicostalis TPs, but a crosswise pattern in the same region of the back to demonstrate the pain referred from TPs in the lower rectus abdominis muscle.

Myofascial TPs at the low thoracic level in the longissimus thoracis muscle (Fig. 48.1D, right side) refer pain strongly low in the buttock.[112, 116] This remote source of buttock pain is easily overlooked. Longissimus TPs toward the caudal end of the muscle fibers in the upper lumbar area usually refer pain several segments caudally, but still within the lumbar region[112, 116] (Fig. 48.1D, left side). This is another muscular source of "lumbago."

Lange,[60] in 1931, identified myogelosis of the erector spinae muscles (probably myofascial TPs) at the lumbar level as a frequent cause of "lumbago" and sacral pain. Gutstein[44] reported numerous patients with referred pain from myalgic spots or muscular rheumatism in the erector spinae muscles.

Kellgren[54] mapped the referred pain patterns of the erector spinae experimentally by injecting hypertonic salt solution into normal muscles. He reported that the superficial erector spinae muscles at the mid-lumbar level referred pain to the upper part of the buttock. In a similar study, hypertonic saline injection of the structures along the edge of the interspinous ligament at the L_1 level[55] referred pain characteristic of renal colic to the loin, inguinal, and scrotal areas, causing retraction of the testicle. At the T_9 level, the hypertonic saline injection caused palpable rigidity and deep tenderness of the lowest part of the abdominal wall.[61]

Deep Paraspinal Muscles
(Fig. 48.2)

Although the semispinalis thoracis is classified anatomically as the outermost of the deep paraspinal muscles, we have the impression that its pain patterns correspond to those of the longissimus fibers at the same segmental level.

The severe aching "bone" pain from TPs in this deep group of muscles is persistent, worrisome and disabling.

The next layer of the deep group of paraspinal muscles, the multifidi, refer pain primarily to the region around the spinous process of the vertebra adjacent to the TP (Fig. 48.2A). Multifidus TPs located from L_1 to L_5 may also refer pain anteriorly to the abdomen, which is easily misjudged as visceral in origin (Fig. 48.2B).[112, 116] Multifidus TPs at the S_1 level project pain downward to the coccyx (Fig. 48.2B), and render the coccyx hypersensitive to pressure (referred tenderness). The combination is often identified as coccygodynia.

Involvement of the deepest paraspinal muscles, the rotatores, throughout the length of the thoracolumbar spine produces midline pain and referred tenderness to tapping on the spinous process adjacent to the TP. Only deep palpation of the muscles can determine from which side the midline pain arises.

When Kellgren[54] injected hypertonic saline experimentally into normal deep paraspinal muscles, he concluded that these

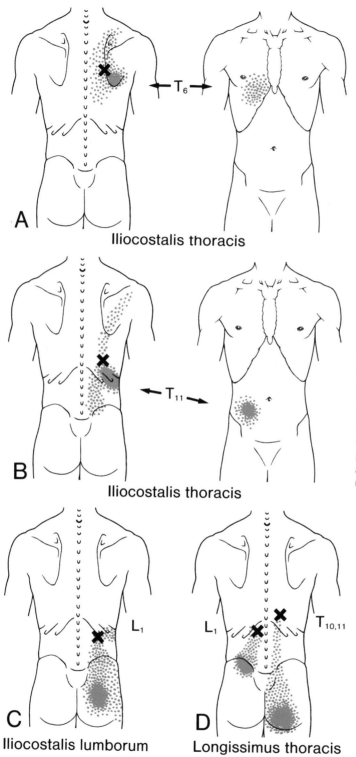

A
Iliocostalis thoracis

B
Iliocostalis thoracis

C
Iliocostalis lumborum

D
Longissimus thoracis

Figure 48.1. Examples of referred pain patterns (essential reference zones are *solid red*, spillover areas are *stippled red*) with their corresponding trigger points (**X**s), at several levels in the erector spinae (superficial paraspinal) muscles. *A*, the mid-level of the right iliocostalis thoracis. *B*, the caudal portion of the right iliocostalis thoracis. *C*, the upper end of the right iliocostalis lumborum. *D*, the lower thoracic (*right*) and upper lumbar (*left*) longissimus thoracis. Longissimus fibers often reach the upper lumbar region.

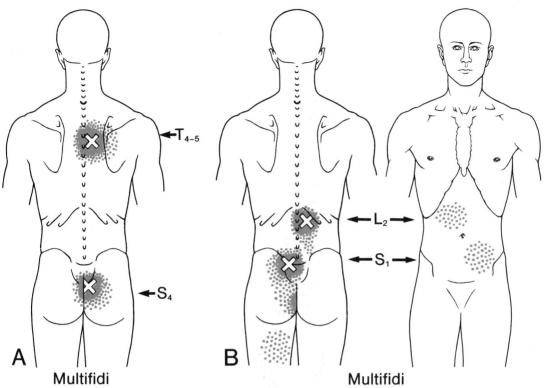

Figure 48.2.   Referred pain patterns (*red*), and their corresponding trigger points (**X**s) in the deep paraspinal muscles (multifidi and rotatores). *A*, examples of local patterns characteristic of trigger points at the midthoracic and low sacral levels; *B*, local and projected pain patterns of trigger points in these muscles at the intermediate L_2 and S_1 levels.

deep muscles were more likely than the superficial group to refer pain anteriorly to the abdomen. At the L_5 level, hypertonic saline injected in the deep muscles also referred pain down the posterolateral aspect of the thigh and leg.

Fascial and Fat Trigger Points

Dittrich[25] identified fibrosis of the subcutaneous lumbosacral fascia, presumably in response to tears caused by muscular strain, as a cause of low back pain. In 109 patients, these lesions with TP characteristics referred pain from either the midsacral, mid-lumbar, or the low cervical areas, as judged by the relief afforded for days, weeks, or months, by the injection of procaine.[24] Local surgical intervention relieved 14 of 19 patients.[23] Pain localized at the posterior portion of one iliac crest (iliolumbar syndrome) was frequently relieved by injections of a local anesthetic that penetrated sometimes the iliolumbar ligament, sometimes the quadratus lumborum muscle, and sometimes both.[47]

Fat lobules and herniations of fat through the subcutaneous fascia in the lumbosacral area were identified as the source of referred backache[19] and were considered the cause of coccygodynia when they were located at the mid-sacral level, lateral to the midline.[22] As reported, the possibility had not been excluded that the connective tissue associated with this fat harbored TPs responsible for the pain.

2. ANATOMICAL ATTACHMENTS
(Figs. 48.3 and 48.4)

The bewildering complexity of the paraspinal muscles is simplified by thinking of them as two layers, a superficial layer of long-fibered extensors (erector spinae or sacrospinalis muscles), and a deep layer of shorter, more diagonal extensor rotators (transversospinal muscles).

Superficial Group (Erector Spinae)
(Fig. 48.3)

As a source of TP pain, the two important muscles of the superficial group are

PART 4

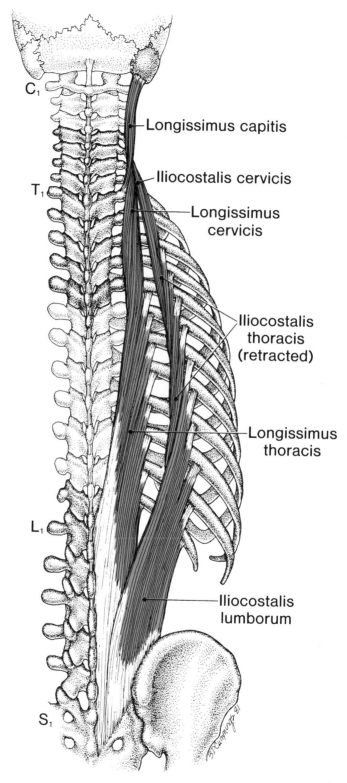

Figure 48.3.   Attachments of the two most important of the superficial (erector spinae) group of paraspinal muscles (*red*): *medially* the longissimus thoracis, and *laterally* the iliocostalis thoracis and iliocostalis lumborum.

the more medial longissimus thoracis and the laterally placed iliocostalis thoracis. Both of these muscles span the thoracic spine, but only the iliocostalis extends to the sacrum across the lumbar spine. The third superficial muscle, the spinalis, is usually small and has not been identified separately as a source of TP pain.

The medial-lying longissimus thoracis has the longest fibers of the paraspinal muscles (Fig. 48.3). **Above** it attaches primarily to the transverse processes of all the thoracic vertebrae and to the adjacent first to ninth or tenth ribs; **below** it attaches to the lumbar transverse processes, and to the anterior layer of the lumbocostal aponeurosis. Caudally, it blends with the iliocostalis and spinalis muscles.[41]

The more lateral iliocostalis thoracis (Fig. 48.3) is a continuation of the iliocostalis cervicis. It connects **above** to the transverse process of the seventh cervical vertebra and to the angles of the *upper* six ribs; **below** it attaches to the angles of the *lower* six ribs.[41]

The iliocostalis lumborum extends **below** to the sacrum and **above** from the angles of the lowest six ribs.

Deep Paraspinal Muscles
(Fig. 48.4)

As the fibers of the deeper muscles of this group become progressively more horizontal, they increasingly also rotate the spine, rather than solely extending it.[41] Among the deep group of paraspinal muscles, the semispinalis thoracis extends caudally as far as T_{10}, overlying the multifidi (Fig. 48.4). The multifidi and rotatores continue beyond the lumbosacral junction where they fill the multifidus triangle of the sacrum[64] and are covered by the tendinous extensions of the superficial longissimus and iliocostalis muscles.

The deeper multifidi and rotatores muscles attach **medially** and **above** near the base of a vertebral spinous process. **Laterally** and **below** they attach to a transverse process (Fig. 48.4), spaced as follows: the semispinalis thoracis fibers cross at least five vertebrae and extend caudally to the tenth thoracic vertebra (Fig. 48.4). Multifidus fibers cross two-to-four segments throughout the thoracic and lumbar spine, and sometimes extend to S_4. The short rotatores attach to adjacent vertebrae; the

long rotatores span one segment throughout the spine.[41]

Supplemental References

Other authors have clearly illustrated the longissimus thoracis, and the iliocostalis thoracis and lumborum as seen from behind,[30, 38, 68, 69, 80, 92, 96, 105, 106] from the side,[109] and in cross section.[17, 52, 53]

The semispinalis thoracis has been presented as seen from behind,[31, 38, 80, 93, 94, 97, 106] and in cross section.[18]

The multifidus has been illustrated from behind,[31, 80, 81, 93, 95, 98, 106, 107] from the side,[32] and in cross section.[39, 52, 53]

The rotatores have been shown from behind[40, 69, 80, 81, 94, 99] and from the oblique rear view.[108]

3. INNERVATION

All the paraspinal muscles are supplied by branches of the dorsal primary divisions of the spinal nerves.[41] Each dorsal primary division in the thoracic and lumbar spine has a medial and a lateral branch. The medial branch innervates the *deepest* spinal muscles at the level of exit of the spinal nerve, so that in the lower thoracic and lumbar regions, the nerve, the rotator muscle, and the tip of the spinous process, which has the same number as the nerve, are at the same level. The lateral branch innervates the longer, more superficial, muscles by running obliquely in a lateral-caudal-dorsal direction.[51] It may cross one or two segments before terminating in muscle fibers.[36, 55]

4. ACTIONS

Superficial Paraspinal (Erector Spinae) Muscles

Electrical stimulation of the superficial paraspinal lumbar muscles produced extension and lateral bending of the spine to the same side.[27]

Some authorities[49, 53] identify three functions for both major components of the erector spinae muscles: acting unilaterally, the iliocostalis and longissimus produce lateral flexion and rotation to the opposite side; acting bilaterally, they extend the spine. Their contribution to rotation appears to be minor. Hollinshead[49] states that these muscles function in a checkrein fashion to resist gravity in the stooping-for-

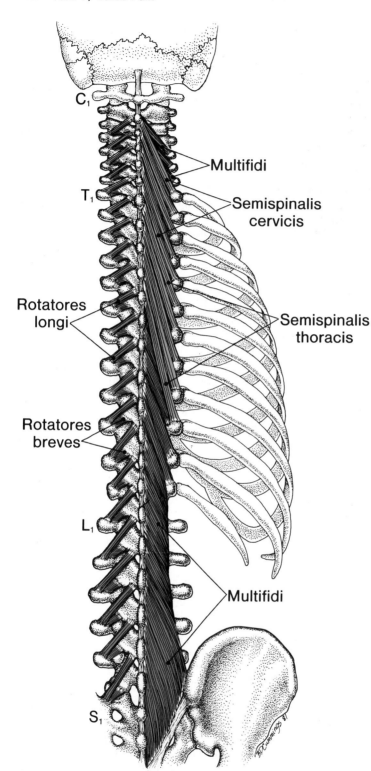

C₁

Multifidi

T₁

Semispinalis
cervicis

Rotatores
longi

Semispinalis
thoracis

Rotatores
breves

L₁

Multifidi

S₁

Figure 48.4. Attachments of the deep group of paraspinal muscles. **Right,** The more superficial of this group are the semispinalis thoracis at the thoracic level (*light red*), which overlies the multifidi, and the multifidi at the thoracic, lumbar and sacral levels (*dark red*). **Left,** The rotatores form the deepest layer at both the thoracic and lumbar levels.

ward position. Electromyographic studies support a major role for this "paying out" action during spinal flexion and side-bending.[7]

Electromyographic studies have shown, further, that, in persons on their feet, the erector spinae can achieve complete relaxation: when standing erect, when bending forward with the spine fully flexed,[7] and when side bending if all traces of spinal flexion or extension are eliminated.[79] The erector spinae muscles contract vigorously during coughing and straining to have a bowel movement.[7] When bending forward, their contraction is increased in proportion to the amount of flexion[4] down to an angle of 45°. Beyond that angle, increasing ligamentous tension unloads the erector spinae.

Surface electrodes over the lumbar sacrospinalis muscles consistently showed bilateral activity during 13 sport activities; the muscles on the left side were clearly more active than those on the right when the right hand was used.[12]

In a study of seated subjects, the paraspinal muscles were more active at the thoracic than at the lumbar level.[3] Backward inclination of the chair back reduced the activity of these muscles more effectively than did contouring of the chair to provide lumbar or thoracic support.[2, 3] However, a radiographic study showed that only a lumbar support, not the inclination of the backrest, significantly influenced the lumbar lordosis.[1]

As muscles of respiration, the bilateral iliocostalis lumborum usually become active at the end of inhalation, and also during exhalation, if the ventilation rate is close to its maximum.[16]

In patients with low back pain and with tenderness to palpation of the paraspinal muscles, the superficial layer tended to show less than a normal amount of electromyographic activity until the test movement became painful. Then these muscles showed increased motor unit activity, or "splinting".[82] During 6 min of standing, the root mean square amplitude of electrical activity of the L_4 and L_5 paraspinal muscles, recorded from surface electrodes, increased in seven patients with recent onset of low back pain, and decreased in four pain-free controls.[50] This observation fits the concept of normal muscles "taking over" (protective spasm) to unload and protect a parallel muscle that is the site of significant TP activity.

Deep Paraspinal Muscles

Acting bilaterally, the semispinalis thoracis, the thoracic and lumbar multifidi, and the rotatores extend the vertebral column. Acting unilaterally, they rotate the homolateral shoulder forward.[7, 53, 79, 82]

The deep group of muscles is believed to function primarily for fine adjustments between vertebrae, rather than for gross spinal movements.[26] The abdominal muscles are the primary flexors and rotators of the lumbar spine, and the quadratus lumborum is the most important for side-bending.

Electromyographically, the deep paraspinal muscles were activated by rotation to the opposite side, and were activated in complex patterns by flexion, extension and rotation of the spine.[7] Responses recorded by fine wire electrodes were illustrated for each of these movements.[71]

5. MYOTATIC UNIT

Spinal extension by the thoracic and lumbar paraspinal muscles is assisted by the serratus posterior inferior and the quadratus lumborum muscles, and is opposed by the rectus abdominis and abdominal oblique muscles.

Rotation of the lumbar spine is provided primarily by the oblique abdominal muscles, and is assisted by the deep paraspinal muscles. Rotation also may be assisted in the thoracolumbar region by the serratus posterior inferior and one group of diagonal deep fibers of the quadratus lumborum.

6. SYMPTOMS

The chief complaint caused by active TPs in the thoracolumbar paraspinal muscles is pain in the back and sometimes in the buttock and abdomen, as described in Section 1. This pain markedly restricts spinal motion and the patient's activity. When the longissimus muscles are involved bilaterally, often at the L_1 level, the patient has difficulty rising from a chair and climbing stairs, if he or she faces forward in the usual manner.

When the initial complaint of "lumbago" is due to TPs in the deep lumbar paraspinal muscles, it usually is a unilateral, extremely disagreeable, steady ache deep in the spine. It becomes bilateral as the muscles on both sides become involved. The patient may point to a one-sided bulging of the long muscles of the low back. The

PART 4

patient finds little relief by changing position, and is often convinced by the way it feels that the pain originates in the bony spine, not in the muscles.

7. ACTIVATION OF TRIGGER POINTS

In these back muscles, TPs may be activated by sudden overload (a grossly traumatic event), or by sustained muscular contraction over a period of time (obscure microtrauma).

A quick awkward movement that combines bending and twisting of the back, especially when the muscles are fatigued or chilled, is likely to activate TPs in the iliocostalis, even though no additional loading (lifting) is involved; this may be caused by disproportionate loading of one group of muscle fibers as the result of poor coordination.

Lange[60] and Lindstedt[62, 63] both thought that flat feet caused muscular strain which activated myogelosis or muscular rheumatic symptoms (described in terms indicative of TPs) in many back, hip, and thigh muscles and produced pain patterns commonly identified as "sciatica" or "lumbago." The authors of this manual find that structural disproportions, such as leg and pelvic asymmetry, can overload specific muscles and tend to perpetuate, rather than to initiate, the pain-producing TPs.

The whiplash type of accident caused by sudden acceleration or deceleration, then impact of the body parts is likely to rapidly stretch the stiffened spinal muscles which, in turn, is likely to activate TPs in them.

Prolonged immobility, as when sitting for hours in an aircraft or automobile with the seat belt fastened, may activate TPs in the paraspinal muscles. Substantiating this, an electromyographic study of the thoracic and lumbar erector spinae showed that typists who remained immobile in their optimally relaxed position (initial electrical silence) developed muscular activity in about ½ hr or sooner; repositioning temporarily quieted this motor unit activity at rest.[66] It is noteworthy that immobility built up muscle tension in every-one tested, in some much sooner than in others.

8. PATIENT EXAMINATION

Superficial Paraspinal (Erector Spinae) Muscles

When standing, the patient with involvement of the erector spinae may be unable to flex the torso more than a few degrees. Palpation of specific paraspinal muscles is less effective with the patient standing because of postural muscle tension and protective splinting by normal muscles. The examiner must obtain relaxation of the patient's back muscles so that abnormally taut muscle fibers are distinguishable. When the seated patient leans forward, dangles the arms between the legs, and relaxes, an involved lumbar longissimus on one side is evident like a hard rope. For greatest sensitivity to palpation, the patient lies on one side and brings the knees toward the chest far enough to take up the slack in the long erector spinae.

After the erector spinae on the painful side have been passively stretched during vapocooling, and the muscles on that side have relaxed, mirror-image pain and muscular tension may appear, so that the opposite lumbar longissimus now stands out and feels tense. The two sides function together as a unit.

Deep Paraspinal Muscles

Active TPs in the deep paraspinal muscles cause guarded movements and restrict side bending, rotation, and hyperextension of the trunk. Deep lumbar paraspinal TPs are likely to occur in patients with either an excessive or absent lumbar lordosis; deep thoracic paraspinal TPs tend to occur in patients with marked thoracic kyphosis.

Active TPs in the deep group of paraspinal muscles impair movement between two vertebrae during flexion or side bending of the spine. During flexion, a hollow or a flat area develops in the smooth curve formed by the spinous processes. The flattening usually spans one to three vertebrae. Involvement of a multifidus or a rotator muscle on either side produces midline tenderness over the adjacent spinous process. This tenderness is easily located by tapping each spinous process in succession; it disappears after inactivation of the responsible TPs, which may be located on either or both sides.

Local reduction of skin resistance to direct current was identified as characteristic of the musculoskeletal and myofascial symptoms of backache with limitation of spinal motion.[57, 58]

Differential Diagnosis

Radiculopathy, strain of spinal ligaments, and myofascial TPs in the paraspinal muscles may cause similar pain complaints. Radiculopathy may be caused by pressure from a ruptured disc, by encroachment within the spinal foramen, as from osteoarthritis, or by a tumor.

The rupture of an intervertebral disc, ligamentous strain, and paraspinal muscular overload that activates myofascial TPs are all likely to be caused by similar strains when lifting with the back twisted and flexed, instead of erect and straight.[74]

When the sacrospinal muscles are heavily loaded in flexion, compressive forces on the lumbar intervertebral discs increase. At 20° of trunk flexion with a 10-kg weight hanging in each hand, intra-discal pressure can reach 280 kg.[73] Twisting the trunk adds torsional forces on the discs, and greatly increases the likelihood of a disproportionate load on the deeper diagonal paraspinal muscles; it increases both intra-discal pressure and muscular load.[5]

Lumbar radiculopathy usually causes pain that radiates into the lower extremity; paraspinal TPs alone do not. However, when active TPs in the back muscles induce satellite TPs in the gluteal muscles, the latter TPs often refer myofascial pain down the lateral or posterior aspect of the thigh or leg, sometimes extending to the foot.[91, 110, 111, 112] Radiculopathy is characterized by neurological deficits: decreased tendon reflexes, impaired cutaneous sensation, and motor weakness with atrophy. Myofascial TPs per se do not cause such neurological deficits unless the TP tautness of the muscle fibers entraps a peripheral nerve. The number of these specific muscle-nerve entrapment syndromes is limited, and the degree of nerve damage is rarely more than neuropraxia.

Electrodiagnostic studies,[35] computerized axial tomography, thermography,[83] and, if surgery is seriously contemplated, myelography may be required to establish

that the clinical signs are due to intervertebral disc disease. A helpful sign of another source of root compression, spinal stenosis, (the cauda equina syndrome) is a positive Stoop Test,[28] in which the patient assumes a progressively stooped posture to relieve the increasing pain experienced during upright ambulation. Radiograms are useful to demonstrate abnormalities of the spinal column that contribute to radiculopathy[29] and to identify hip disease which can mimic some low back pain disorders,[101] but radiography and electromyography fail to reveal any soft tissue changes that identify myofascial TPs.

Most important, radiographic signs of degenerative joint disease correlate poorly with the occurrence of pain.[100] In the absence of intervertebral disc degeneration, about one-third of a group of industrial cases with low back pain were labeled simply "low back strain." On the other hand, over one-third of 50 asymptomatic control subjects had radiographic evidence of minor degenerative changes; one had slight narrowing of the lumbosacral disc space.[42] Thus, it can not be assumed that these degenerative changes cause back pain. In another study, only 40% of 936 symptom-free Air Force Academy or Air Cadet applicants between 17 and 27 years of age were free of congenital variations and other abnormalities of the spine.[20] Many patients with these abnormalities are completely relieved of their pain when the responsible TPs are inactivated.

The muscles supplied by a compressed nerve root are likely to develop TPs.[42] The pain caused by these myofascial TPs may be identified by their specific referred pain patterns, by reproduction of the patient's pain in response to pressure on the TP, by the physical findings of spot tenderness in palpable bands, and by a local twitch response of the band. Myofascial TP pain develops for many reasons other than radiculopathy, but when radiculopathy activates TPs, they are likely to persist long after the nerve root compression has been relieved; these TPs produce symptoms of stiffness and pain similar in distribution to the radicular pain, and may explain the complication known as the postlumbar-laminectomy pain syndrome.[87]

Another, less common source of low back pain is herniation of fat lobules

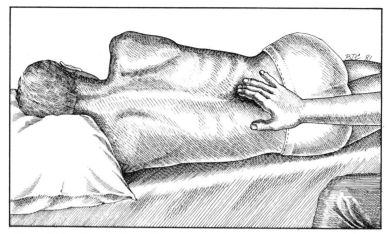

Figure 48.5.   Examination of the right erector spinae muscles. The back muscles are relaxed by placing the patient on the side, and the slack in the muscles is taken up by bringing the knees toward the chest.

through subcutaneous fascia.[19, 22] Similar paraspinal fibrolipomatous nodules at the T_{12} through L_2 levels referred pain to the back, abdomen, groin and testicle; the pain was temporarily relieved by local injection of 2% procaine solution and permanently relieved by surgical excision.[76]

The skin overlying involved lumbar paraspinal muscles often exhibits superficial tenderness and resistance to skin rolling (panniculosis),[6] or trophedema,[43] which disappears after inactivation of the underlying myofascial TPs.

Some additional causes of *acute* back pain that should be considered are systemic infectious illness; myositis; tumors, including metastases from the breast, ovaries and prostate; retrocecal appendicitis; dissecting aortic aneurysm or saddle thrombus; biliary, renal or ureteral stones; torsion of the kidney; pelvic inflammatory disease; and endometriosis.

Causes of *chronic* backache include many of the above, as well as ankylosing spondylitis, Paget's disease, osteoporosis with vertebral compression fracture, leukemia with enlarged retroperitoneal nodes, Hodgkin's disease, primary psychogenic backache, tumors of the kidney, prostatitis and seminal vesiculitis,[90] ligamentous and apophyseal joint sprains, sacroiliitis, and osteitis condensans ilii.

Back pain referred from TPs in the abdominal wall musculature is discussed in Chapter 49.

9. TRIGGER POINT EXAMINATION (Fig. 48.5)

Superficial Paraspinal (Erector Spinae) Muscles

The patient lies on the uninvolved side in a comfortable, relaxed position with a pillow under the side of the abdomen for semiprone support. The full prone position often strains the patient's neck and tends to over-slacken the paraspinal muscles for examination. The back muscles must have an intermediate degree of stretch, so that the taut bands containing the TPs can be distinguished from the adjacent normal, slackened muscle fibers. The degree of stretch is regulated by bringing the patient's knees toward the chest (Fig. 48.5). Flat palpation of the muscles then elicits spot tenderness and often referred pain.

Deep Paraspinal Muscles

With the patient recumbent as above, or seated and leaning forward to flex the spine slightly, a flattened region or slight hollow that extends over one to three vertebrae indicates the probable TP source of trouble. The examiner taps or presses on the tips of successive spinous processes to elicit tenderness. When a spinous process in the flat area is hypersensitive, the deep musculature on each side of it is palpated by firm pressure in the groove between the process and the longissimus muscle. Finger pressure is directed medially toward the body of the vertebra to elicit maximum spot tenderness. If two or three spinous processes are tender, one expects to find adjacent TPs on at least one side at each level of tenderness.

10. ENTRAPMENTS

The dorsal primary divisions (rami) of the spinal nerves supply skin sensation to the back. Since these dorsal rami pass through the paraspinal muscles to reach the skin, it is not surprising that many patients with active TPs in these muscles, in addition to pain, complain of nerve-entrapment symptoms. In the presence of entrapment, these symptoms include hyperesthesia, dysesthesia or hypoesthesia of the skin of the back. The medial branches of these rami supply afferent fibers to the skin for most of the thoracic segments above T_8, where they pass through the semispinalis thoracis and longissimus thoracis muscles. The lateral branches supply most of the skin below T_8, including the lumbar region, and are likely to be entrapped by the more lateral iliocostalis muscle.[42, 48]

Richter[86] reported 500 patients with these symptoms of nerve entrapment in whom focal TP tenderness was found. Nearly half of the patients were successfully treated solely by injection of the tender area with a local anesthetic. He[85] reported permanent relief in 144 patients by surgically excising the entrapped nerve or releasing herniated fat. Symptoms in the high lumbar region were usually due to compression of the low thoracic dorsal rami by bands of tense fibers in the iliocostalis lumborum muscle.[86]

11. ASSOCIATED TRIGGER POINTS

The deep paraspinal group is more likely to show isolated muscle involvement, whereas the more superficial paraspinal muscles are likely to accumulate associated TPs in functionally related muscles, especially the contralateral superficial muscles.

When TPs are active in the longissimus and iliocostalis muscles, the latissimus dorsi and quadratus lumborum also are often involved, either secondarily, or by the same initiating event that activated the

paraspinal group. The serratus posterior inferior, and sometimes the serratus posterior superior, also may develop associated TPs.

12. STRETCH AND SPRAY
(Figs. 48.6 and 48.7)

Superficial Paraspinal (Erector Spinae) Muscles
(Fig. 48.6)

Either of two seated stretch positions can be used. The less strenuous seated position stretches chiefly the long thoracic paraspinal muscles. The more strenuous long-sitting position, in addition to strongly stretching the thoracic paraspinal muscles, also stretches the lumbosacral, gluteal and hamstring muscles.

For a less strenuous technique, the patient sits in a chair with the feet placed comfortably on the floor and the legs apart. The patient leans forward, lets the head hang forward, and lets the arms drop between the knees (Fig. 48.6A). After a few initial sweeps of spray, the operator gradually increases pressure on the back of the head and neck as the vapocoolant spray is directed over the paraspinal muscles bilaterally in long downward parallel sweeps, on both sides. At the same time, in order to hyperflex the thoracic spine, the patient is told to take a deep breath and to "Hump the back!" The instruction, "Arch your back!" usually causes the patient to extend, rather than to flex the spine. Vapocooling is followed promptly by application of moist heat to rewarm the skin, in the recumbent position, and then by active range of motion.

To obtain greater stretch of the low paraspinal muscles, the patient assumes the long-sitting position on a flat surface with the legs extended and knees straight (Fig. 48.6B). The paraspinal and gluteal muscles are then sprayed in parallel down sweeps, as above for the seated position, but extending over the buttocks (Fig. 48.6B). This position places a strong stretch on the gluteus maximus and hamstring muscles, which, if tight, should first be released by stretch and spray during straight-leg raising to permit the full range of flexion at the hips. A proximal-to-distal

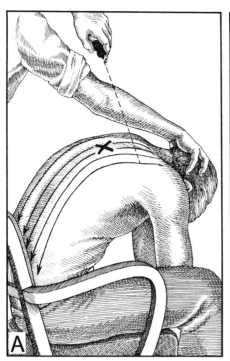
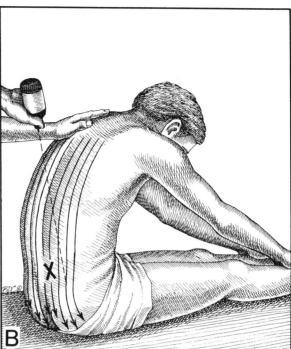

Figure 48.6.   Stretch positions and spray pattern (*arrows*) for the right erector spinae muscles. Typical locations of trigger points are indicated by "**X**s". *A,* stretch of chiefly the thoracic segments when the patient is seated in a chair with the knees bent. *B,* stretch of the low thoracic and lumbar paraspinal muscles, plus the gluteals and hamstrings, with the patient in the long-sitting position with the knees straight. The posterior spinal musculature is stretched bilaterally, and must be vapocooled *bilaterally.*

spray pattern is applied over the gluteal and hamstring muscles.[91]

Deep Paraspinal Muscles
(Fig. 48.7)

To stretch the multifidus and rotatores muscles, the seated patient's spine is flexed and simultaneously rotated, turning the face to the same side. Before the operator applies pressure to the opposite shoulder to assist this movement (Fig. 48.7), an initial set of sweeps is completed. Then, as pressure is exerted, the vapocoolant spray is simultaneously applied in a downward, diagonal pattern over these muscles.

If this procedure fails to eliminate tenderness in the paraspinal TPs, and to restore normal spinal contour on flexion, ischemic compression of the remaining tender spots may be effective. Local, deep kneading massage (pétrissage) also may be helpful.[45] If the treatment was effective, the depressed spinous processes will have returned to their normal contour on full flexion of the thoracic spine.

Manipulative techniques to mobilize the

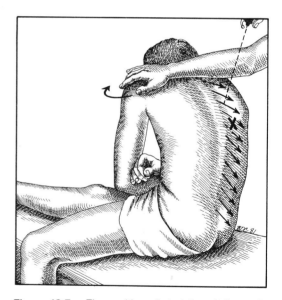

Figure 48.7.   The position of stretch and diagonal spray pattern (*arrows*) for the right deep paraspinal muscles. To stretch these muscles requires both flexion and rotation of the torso. The **X** is an example of a trigger point location in this layer. A tight left iliocostalis thoracis may need to be released by adding lines of spray over that muscle before full stretch can be realized.

PART 4

small joints of the spine are another approach that can relieve back pain and release taut paraspinal muscles.[11, 21, 67, 70, 113] Joint manipulation may inactivate TPs by restoration of normal joint play or by stretch of the muscles while inhibiting protective spasm mediated by the central nervous system.

13. INJECTION AND STRETCH
(Fig. 48.8)

The practice of needling tender spots in lumbar muscles for the treatment of low back pain is not new. In 1912 Osler[77] wrote, "For lumbago, acupuncture is, in acute cases, the most efficient treatment. Needles of from three to four inches in length (ordinary bonnet-needles, sterilized, will do) are thrust into the lumbar muscles at the seat of pain, and withdrawn after five or ten minutes. In many instances the relief is immediate, and I can corroborate fully the statements of Ringer, who taught me this practice, as to its extraordinary and prompt efficacy in many instances."

When multiple TPs are spread throughout the paraspinal musculature, it is usually desirable to start with stretch and spray. When only a few refractory TPs remain, or they lie deep in the paraspinal musculature, we find that injection is best. Injection of TPs in the paraspinal musculature has previously been reported very extensively.[9, 10, 13, 33, 46, 59, 64, 88, 115]

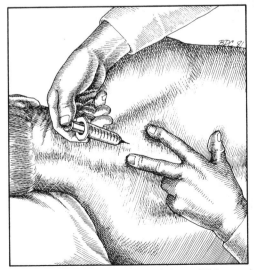

Figure 48.8. Injection of the right multifidus and rotatores muscles at the upper thoracic level. The needle is aimed slightly caudad to avoid penetrating between the vertebral laminae.

The TP injection is followed at once by a repetition of stretch and spray, and then by hot packs and active range of motion.

Superficial Paraspinal (Erector Spinae) Muscles

The longissimus and iliocostalis TPs are clearly palpable and readily located for injection in all but very obese patients. When injecting the iliocostalis thoracis muscle, the needle must be directed tangent to, and not between, the ribs, to avoid pericardial penetration if at the cardiac level on the left side, and to avoid pleural insertion with pneumothorax if elsewhere.

When injecting TPs in the superficial group of muscles at the mid- to low-thoracic level, needle-penetration of TPs located more medially in the longissimus thoracis muscle refers pain caudally. The patient sometimes expresses surprise when injection of another TP located 1–2 cm (about ¾ in) more laterally in the iliocostalis thoracis muscle refers pain upward toward the shoulder, instead of downward.

Deep Paraspinal Muscles

The TPs in the deep paraspinal thoracic muscles are injected by directing the needle caudally (not upward) and slightly medially (Fig. 48.8). When it is necessary to inject the deepest muscles (rotatores), which lie against the laminae of the vertebrae and attach at the base of each spinous process, a needle that is at least 5 cm (2 in) long is used. It is directed somewhat caudally and medially, nearly parallel to the long axis of the spine and toward the base of the spinous process, but not *between* the spinous processes.

This angle of the needle, while reaching the tender spots in the deepest paraspinal muscles, eliminates the possibility of introducing the needle between the ribs, or between the vertebrae into the epidural space. The caudal slant of the needle is indicated because of the shingle-like overlap of the laminae. Penetration to a depth greater than the laminae is unnecessary and undesirable.

14. CORRECTIVE ACTIONS
(Figs. 48.9–48.14)

The patient can reduce the hyperirritability of TPs in the paraspinal muscles in several ways: self-application of ischemic

PART 4

compression; reduction of the total load on the muscles by correcting structural inadequacies (body asymmetry and short upper arms); revision of daily activities; modification of the environment, especially chair design; by performance of passive stretch exercises for the paraspinal muscles; and with graded active strengthening exercises for the abdominal muscles.

Acutely and severely involved back muscles may be partially relieved of stress without incapacitating most patients by temporary application of a corset or brace for low back support, as described by Cailliet.[14]

Ischemic Compression

The patient can apply this compression therapy to TPs in the superficial back muscles by lying supine on a tennis ball, either on the floor, or on a bed with a large, thin book placed under the ball. The patient moves around until the ball presses directly on the sensitive TP; body weight is used to apply gradually increasing pressure for a minute or more, until the spot loses its deep tenderness. This technique is especially useful where back muscles overlie the ribs, such as the iliocostalis and longissimus thoracis and both serrati posterior muscles. A hot pack applied afterward enhances the beneficial effect and reduces soreness the next day.

Correction of Structural Inadequacies
(Figs. 48.9 and 48.10)

This subject is presented in more detail in Chapter 4. The following summarizes the essential facts.

A functional scoliosis develops in order to compensate for lateral tilting of the pelvis that is caused by a short leg when standing, or by a small hemipelvis when sitting. Such body asymmetry imposes

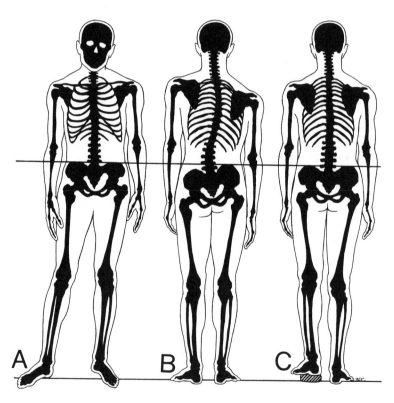

Figure 48.9.   Skeletal asymmetry due to a short left leg. *A*, to compensate, the patient stands on the short leg, placing the long leg forward and slightly to the side. This levels the pelvis. *B*, tilted pelvis, functional scoliosis, and tilted shoulder-girdle axis when the patient stands with the feet nearly together. *C*, the discrepancy in leg length is corrected by adding the precise heel lift under the short (left) leg. This levels the pelvis with the feet nearly together.

persistent muscle strain that perpetuates TPs in the paraspinal and associated musculature, and must be corrected.

Short Leg. Nichols[75] recognized a short leg, when present, as making a critical contribution to musculoskeletal pain. Ordinarily, a difference of as much as 1.3 cm (½ in) in leg length alone does not activate TPs and cause pain. It is usually a perpetuating, not an activating, factor. When an injury or muscular strain activates TPs in the paraspinal or quadratus lumborum muscles, the body asymmetry then perpetuates the TPs. The persistent TP activity causes chronic referred pain. In addition, focal reduction of skin resistance over the tender spots in the muscles demonstrates an autonomic effect of these TPs.[58] The functional scoliosis (Fig. 48.9B) due to the short leg and tilted pelvis requires, when the person is upright, continuous compensatory muscular activity, which overloads the paraspinal muscles.

The scoliotic spine also tilts the shoulder-girdle axis. Usually, the shoulder sags on the side of the long leg (Fig. 48.9B); but if the disparity in leg length is about 1.3 cm (½ in) or more, the shoulder is likely to be lower on the short side. The patient often stands on the short leg with the long leg in front or to the side (Fig. 48.9A).

To ensure lasting relief from the myofascial pain, it is important to correct a leg length discrepancy of as little as 0.3 cm (⅛ in) in a short person. The correction must be worn at *all* times that these patients are on their feet, including the use of bedroom slippers. The patient should avoid walking, or jogging, on slanted ground or a slanted beach.

To make a functional determination of the leg length difference, the patient stands with the feet together, or at most 7.6 cm (3 in) apart, and is observed from behind. To identify a short leg, the patient is examined: (1) for asymmetry of the body silhouette between the ribs and the pelvis; (2) for lateral tilt of the lumbar spine as it leaves the sacrum; (3) for the ensuing lateral scoliosis; (4) for a tilted shoulder-girdle axis (the symmetry of the scapular bulges are more reliable than the line of the shoulders, which is easily modified by trapezius muscle involvement); (5) for a low posterior superior iliac spine, by palpation or by eye for one low dimple; and (6) by palpation for a low iliac crest on one side.

A sufficient lift (pages of a pad or magazine) is placed under the heel of the side on which the pelvis is low in order to level the pelvis and straighten the spine. This usually corrects the other signs of asymmetry. The necessity for the correction is convincingly demonstrated to the patient by calling attention to the asymmetry seen in a full-length mirror, especially when the heel lift is briefly transferred under the heel of the long leg, doubling the existing difference. The patient feels uncomfortable with the correction on the wrong side, and the resulting marked aggravation of the indicators of asymmetry confirms the shortness of the other leg. A difference of 0.5 cm (³⁄₁₆ in) is often a significant source of muscle strain that requires correction.

The difference in leg length is corrected temporarily by inserting the correct thickness of firm felt inside the heel of the shoe, or permanently by building up the thickness of the heel outside, on the short side if a low heel (Fig. 48.9C), or by cutting down the heel on the long side, if a high heel. With large corrections of about 1.3 cm (½ in) or more, it is wise to divide the difference by removing half of the correction from the heel on the long side and by adding half to the other heel.

Correcting the leg length discrepancy alone may be sufficient to relieve the pain of muscular origin.[89] The active TPs causing the pain may spontaneously revert to latent TPs in a few days or weeks.

Small hemipelvis. Usually, the vertical dimension of the pelvis is smaller on the side of the short leg. This tilts the pelvis when sitting, just as the short leg tilts it when standing, and with the same musculoskeletal effects (Fig. 48.10B).

While the patient sits on a flat level wood seat, pelvic tilt is estimated and corrected by placing enough pages or sheets of paper under the ischial tuberosity on the short side to level the pelvis exactly (Fig. 48.10C). A hard surface requires less correction than a well padded seat, since the softness of the seat allows the body to tilt to the short side. This shifts more weight to that side, and increases the pelvic tilt (Fig. 48.10D). The patient's muscles become very discriminating as to the size of the "butt" lift needed, in relation to each chair seat. Some seats are domed and others are scooped, as in the bucket seat.

A pelvic tilt also may be produced un-

PART 4

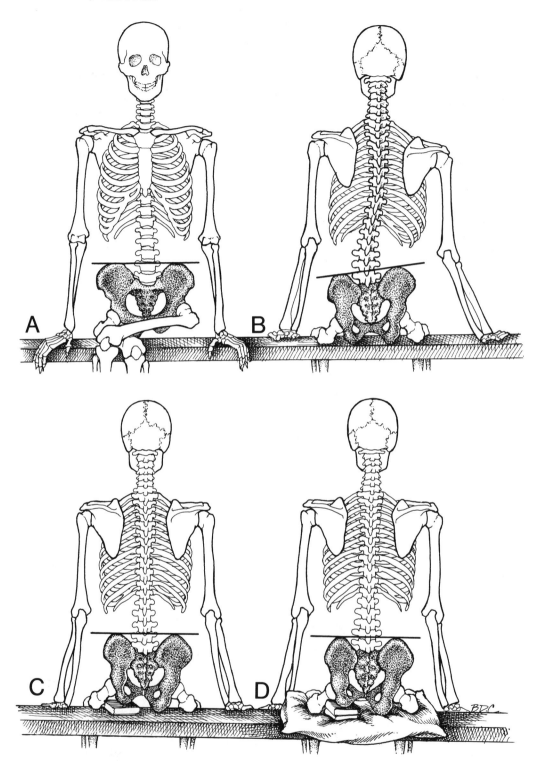

Figure 48.10. Effects of skeletal asymmetry due to a small hemipelvis on the left side are demonstrated by sitting on a flat level wood bench. *A*, crossing the leg on the short side over the opposite knee helps to level the pelvis. *B*, the tilted pelvis causes compensatory scoliosis, which tilts the shoulder-girdle axis. *C*, a small butt lift levels the pelvis on a hard surface. *D*, on a soft cushioned surface, a thicker butt lift is required to provide the same correction as that obtained on a hard surface.

wittingly by sitting on a wallet in the back pocket, causing "back-pocket sciatica,"[37] or by sitting regularly in a tilted office chair, or on a piano bench that has two rubber feet missing at one end or is placed on a slanted stage.

The patient often tries to compensate for a small hemipelvis by crossing one knee over the other to cantilever up the low side (Fig. 48.10A).

Modification of Activities

The patient should modify those activities which induce stress when bending over forward. The patient must learn to pick up *any* low object by bending the knees while keeping the back upright, thus transferring the load from the back muscles to the hip and knee extensors. Tichauer[102, 104] graphically illustrated the mechanical advantage to, and the reduction of electrical activity in, the back muscles when this method of lifting is used. During

lifting, as shown in Figure 48.11, a heavy object must be *held close to the body* with the pelvis "tucked in" under a somewhat flattened lordotic curve of the lumbar spine, thus maintaining the center of gravity through the hip joints, rather than in front of the body.[15, 103] Contracting the abdominal muscles to increase intra-abdominal pressure acts as a thoracic lifting force and relieves some of the compressive forces on the lumbar intervertebral discs.

By learning the "Sit-to-stand" and "Stand-to-sit" Technique (Fig. 48.12B), the patient avoids the usual "bent-over-the-sink" posture (Fig. 48.12A) when getting into, and out of, a chair. To rise from the chair, the hips are moved forward to the front of the chair seat before starting to rise; the body is turned somewhat sideways, and one foot is placed beneath the front edge of the chair; finally, the torso is held erect while the knees and hips are straightened, lifting the body.

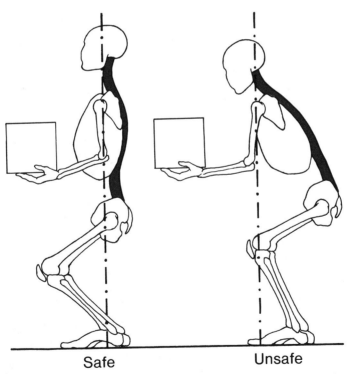

Safe   Unsafe

Figure 48.11.   Safe, and unsafe ways of lifting. *A,* safe position, keeping the object close to the body and lifting with the hip and knee extensors. The center of gravity falls through the pelvis. *B,* unsafe way, with the object held out in front of the body. Here, the trunk leans forward, which forces the paraspinal muscles to lift like a crane, overloading them and increasing compressive forces on the lumbar intevertebral discs.

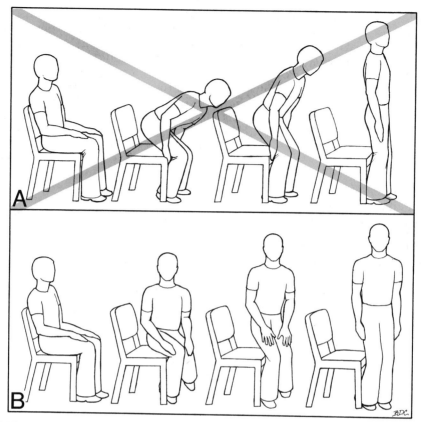

Figure 48.12.   The Sit-to-stand and Stand-to-sit Technique is a method for minimizing strain on the low back muscles and the intervertebral fibrocartilaginous discs while getting up from, or sitting down in a chair. *A*, poor, usual method of rising from a chair which places the back in a strained "leaning-over" posture. *B*, the better Sit-to-stand Technique (reading from left to right) keeps the spine erect throughout, from sitting to standing. This movement loads the hip and knee extensors instead of the thoracolumbar back muscles. The reverse Stand-to-sit technique is illustrated by reading from right to left.

The process is reversed in Stand-to-sit by turning sideways and placing one foot under the front edge of the chair, keeping the torso erect, and aiming the buttocks at the *front* edge of the chair seat rather than at the *rear* of the seat. The person then slides backward on the seat to meet the backrest. This procedure again maintains the back in an erect position and transfers the load from the paraspinal to the hip and thigh muscles.

The patient with myofascial back pain has difficulty going upstairs or climbing a ladder while facing the steps or rungs because of the tendency to lean forward and flex the spine. The pain can be avoided by turning the entire body at an angle with the steps, to face about 45° toward one side. It may be slower climbing, and the feet must travel around each other, but

this position automatically straightens the patient's posture, lightens the load on the paraspinal muscles, and may enable the patient to go up and down steps without pain.

Correction of faulty body posture when standing and sitting, as described in Chapter 42 and by Cailliet,[14] reduces muscle strain and, therefore, the likelihood of recurrence of myofascial pain.

Modification of Environment

The paraspinal musculature can be relieved of much unnecessary stress by modifying the seating to fit the person and the task. The backrest of a chair should provide enough lumbar support to maintain the normal lumbar lordotic curve when the muscles relax. The chair, not the muscles, should do the work of maintaining correct posture. Simply reclining the back-rest does not affect lumbar lordosis.[1, 2] If the seat has a straight back with no forward curvature at waist level (a fault of many chairs), support for the normal lumbar lordosis should be supplied by a pad, such as a small pillow or a roll of folded bath towel (see Fig. 42.9E). It is placed at belt level against the back of the chair, or auto seat, and adjusted up or down for comfort. Seated posture which completely eliminates lumbar lordosis[114] may be helpful for brief periods as a postural variation but can, by itself, cause muscle strain if maintained for a prolonged time, as when driving a car. To relieve tension during prolonged sitting, the paraspinal muscles should be stretched regularly by changing position.

In an extensive study to determine what chair design causes minimum muscular stress, as measured electromyographically when typing, Lundervold[66] found that the chair should have: a backrest with a backward slope, a seat which is slightly hollowed out, no casters, and firm upholstery. Seat height should be low enough so that the feet rest flat on the floor without compression of the thigh by the front edge of the seat. A footrest may be used, if necessary, to avoid underthigh compression. The lower edge of the backrest is positioned to support that part of the lumbar spine which flexes the most when bending forward, and the upper edge of the backrest should reach high enough to cover and support at least the inferior angles of the scapulae. The under surface of the typing table should fit just above the typist's knees, keeping the typewriter close to lap-level. Lundervold[66] did not recommend armrests for typists, but short armrests can be helpful, if they are the correct height for that person's body structure and work set-up. An electric, as compared to a manual, typewriter markedly reduces stress on the muscles.

A bed that is too soft and sags in the middle like a hammock aggravates tension in the back muscles. This is remedied by placing a plywood bed board, nearly as large as the mattress, between the mattress and the bed spring. Alternatively, several separate boards 1.3 cm (½ in) thick and 15–20 cm (6–8 inches) wide, cut three-quarters of the length of the mattress, may be placed lengthwise. The separate boards are more readily installed under the mattress, and also may be transported on a trip. Boards or slats placed crosswise underneath the mattress do not correct the hammock-like longitutinal sag of the bed.

When sleeping on the side rather than supine in a firm flat bed, the patient with myofascial back pain is usually more comfortable with a pillow placed under the uppermost knee. This prevents the rotary torsion of the lumbar spine that occurs when the knee drops forward onto the bed.

Exercises

The In-bathtub Stretch Exercise (Fig. 48.13) should be performed in comfortably hot water (provided there is no medical contraindication to the increased cardiovascular load caused by the heat). The patient leans forward with the knees straight, and assists relaxation by letting the head hang forward. The patient then walks the fingers down the shins until a pull is felt on the stretched paraspinal muscles, and then a little further to slight discomfort. After holding this degree of stretch for several seconds, tautness usually slackens. The patient leans back, relaxes, and breathes deeply with abdominal respiration. Then another step of the fingers "takes up the slack" to re-establish the previous degree of tension on the slightly longer paraspinal muscles. This slow, step-wise passive stretch helps to recapture the lost range of motion of the long back muscles. At the same time, the hamstring muscles are passively stretched as the pelvis rotates.

The Pelvic Tilt Exercise (see Fig. 49.10) stretches the paraspinal muscles while strengthening the muscles of the abdomen. Further strengthening of the abdominals is achieved by using the Sit-back, Abdominal-curl, and Sit-up Exercises (see Fig. 49.11 A–C). Strong abdominal muscles can provide 30% to 50% additional weight-carrying support to the thoracolumbar spine.[33, 72]

The Low-back Stretching Exercise in the supine position begins by drawing one knee to the chest with the hands clasped around the thigh behind the knee. This stretches the hip extensors (Fig. 48.14A). Next, that lower extremity is returned to

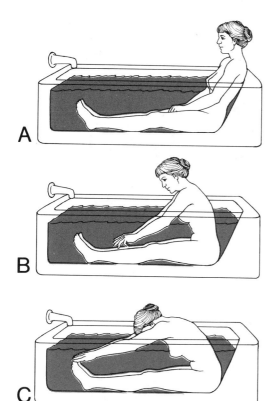

Figure 48.13. The In-bathtub Stretch Exercise. *A*, relaxed position in the bathtub with hot water covering the lower extremities and the lumbosacral area. *B*, partial stretch. A just tolerable stretch is maintained until the erector spinae and/or hamstring tightness releases enough to allow another step of the fingertips forward on the shins, ankles or feet. *C*, maximum stretch by reaching forward, while keeping the neck and back completely limp and relaxed. This long-sitting position puts a full stretch on both the hamstring and paraspinal muscles; tightness of either group of muscles limits this reach.

the straight-leg starting position, and the other thigh is flexed to the chest and returned. Finally, both legs are pulled to the chest (Fig. 48.14*B*), as also illustrated by Cailliet[15] and by Williams.[114]

Supplemental References, Case Reports

The senior author has presented the total management of patients with myofascial TPs of the paraspinal muscles.[110, 113]

References

1. Andersson BGJ, Murphy RW, Örtengren R, *et al.*: The influence of backrest inclination and lumbar support on lumbar lordosis. *Spine* 4:52–58, 1979.
2. Andersson BJ, Jonsson B, Örtengren R: Myoelectric activity in individual lumbar erector spinae muscles in sitting. A study with surface and wire electrodes. *Scand J Rehabil Med Suppl* 3:91–108, 1974.
3. Andersson BJG, Örtengren R: Myoelectric back muscle activity during sitting. *Scand J Rehab Med Suppl* 3:73–90, 1974.
4. Andersson GBJ, Örtengren R, Herberts P: Quantitative electromyographic studies of back muscle activity related to posture and loading. *Orthop Clin North Am* 8:85–96, 1977.
5. Andersson GBJ, Örtengren R, Nachemson A: Intradiskal pressure, intra-abdominal pressure and myoelectric back muscle activity related to posture and loading. *Clin Orthop* 129:156–164, 1977.
6. Baker DM: Changes in the corium and subcutaneous tissues as a cause of rheumatic pain. *Ann Rheum Dis* 14:385–391, 1955.
7. Basmajian JV: *Muscles Alive*, Ed. 4. Williams & Wilkins, Baltimore, 1978 (pp. 184, 282–285, 288).
8. Bates T, Grunwaldt E: Myofascial pain in childhood. *J Pediatr* 53:198–209, 1958.
9. Berges PU: Myofascial pain syndromes. *Postgrad Med* 53:161–168, 1973.
10. Blank VK: Bort bei Lumbalgien, Ischialgien, vertebragenen Syndromen und Muskulaeren Ver-

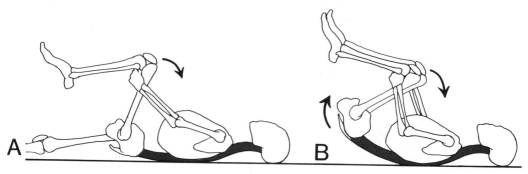

Figure 48.14. Low-back Stretching Exercise. *A*, first phase: flexion of *one* leg at a time by rhythmically and gently bringing the knee toward the corresponding armpit. *B*, second phase: flexion of *both* legs together onto the chest. The thighs, rather than the knees, are grasped to avoid forced knee flexion.

spannungszustaenden. *Hippokrates 38*:528–530, 1967.

11. Bourdillon JF: *Spinal Manipulation*, Ed. 2. Appleton-Century-Crofts, New York, 1973.

12. Broer MR, Houtz SJ: *Patterns of Muscular Activity in Selected Sport Skills, an Electromyographic Study.* Charles C Thomas, Springfield, Ill., 1967.

13. Brown BR: Diagnosis and therapy of common myofascial syndromes. *JAMA 239*:646–648, 1978.

14. Cailliet, R: *Soft Tissue Pain and Disability*, F.A. Davis, Philadelphia, 1977.

15. Cailliet R: *Low Back Pain Syndrome*. Ed. 3. F.A. Davis, Philadelphia, 1981 (pp. 109–115 Figs. 76, 77, 98).

16. Campbell EJM: Accessory muscles, Chapter 9. In *The Respiratory Muscles*, edited by E.J.M. Campbell, E. Agostoni, J.N. Davis, Ed. 2. W.B. Saunders, Philadelphia, 1970 (p. 188).

17. Carter BL, Morehead J, Wolpert SM, *et al.*: *Cross-Sectional Anatomy.* Appleton-Century-Crofts, New York, 1977 (Sects. 20–35).

18. *Ibid.* (Sects. 23–26, 28, 29).

19. Copeman WSC, Ackerman WL: Edema or herniations of fat lobules as a cause of lumbar and gluteal "fibrositis." *Arch Intern Med 79*:22–35, 1947.

20. Crow NE, Brogdon BG: The "normal" lumbosacral spine. *Radiology 72*:97, 1959.

21. Cyriax J: *Textbook of Orthopaedic Medicine*, Ed. 8, Vol. 2 *Treatment by Manipulation, Massage and Injection.* Williams & Wilkins, Baltimore, 1971.

22. Dittrich RJ: Coccygodynia as referred pain. *J Bone Joint Surg 33-A*:715–718, 1951.

23. Dittrich RJ: Low back pain—referred pain from deep somatic structure of the back. *J Lancet 73*:63–68, 1953.

24. Dittrich RJ: Somatic pain and autonomic concomitants. *Am J Surg 87*:66–73, 1954.

25. Dittrich RJ: Soft tissue lesions as cause of low back pain: anatomic study. *Am J Surg 91*:80–85, 1956.

26. Donisch EW, Basmajian JV: Electromyography of deep back muscles in man. *Am J Anat 133*:25–36, 1972.

27. Duchenne GB: *Physiology of Motion*, translated by E.B. Kaplan. J.B. Lippincott, Philadelphia, 1949 (pp. 505, 506).

28. Dyck P: The stoop-test in lumbar entrapment radiculopathy. *Spine 4*:89–92, 1979.

29. Edeiken J, Pitt MJ: The radiologic diagnosis of disc disease. *Orthop Clin North Am 2*:405–417, 1971.

30. Eisler P: *Die Muskeln des Stammes*. Gustav Fischer, Jena, 1912 (Fig. 56).

31. *Ibid.* (Fig. 59).

32. *Ibid.* (Fig. 62).

33. Finneson BE: *Low Back Pain*. J.B. Lippincott, Philadelphia, 1973 (pp. 31–33, 99, 100).

34. Good MG: The role of skeletal muscles in the pathogenesis of diseases. *Acta Med Scand 138*:285–292, 1950 (p. 286).

35. Goodgold J, Eberstein A: *Electrodiagnosis of Neuromuscular Diseases*, Ed. 2. Williams & Wilkins, Baltimore, 1977 (pp. 194–244).

36. Gough JG, Koepke GH: Electromyographic determination of motor root levels in erector spinae muscles. *Arch Phys Med Rehabil 47*:9–11, 1966.

37. Gould N: Back-pocket sciatica. *N Engl J Med 290*:633, 1974.

38. Grant JCB: *An Atlas of Human Anatomy*, Ed. 7. Williams & Wilkins, Baltimore, 1978 (Fig. 5–27).

39. *Ibid.* (Fig. 5–28).

40. *Ibid.* (Fig. 5–31).

41. Gray H: *Anatomy of the Human Body*, edited by C.M. Goss, American Ed. 29. Lea & Febiger, Philadelphia, 1973 (pp. 405–407, 953, Fig. 12-32).

42. Gunn CC, Milbrandt WE: Tenderness at motor points. *J Bone Joint Surg 58-A*:815–825, 1976.

43. Gunn CC, Milbrandt WE: Early and subtle signs in low-back sprain. *Spine 3*:267–281, 1978.

44. Gutstein M: Diagnosis and treatment of muscular rheumatism. *Br J Phys Med 1*:302–321, 1938.

45. Harman JB, Young RH: Muscle lesions simulating visceral disease. *Lancet 1*:1111–1113, 1940.

46. Hench PK: Nonarticular rheumatism. In *Rheumatic Diseases: Diagnosis and Management*, edited by W.A. Katz. J.B. Lippincott, Philadelphia, 1977 (p. 624).

47. Hirschberg GG, Froetscher L, Naeim F: Iliolumbar syndrome as a common cause of low back pain: Diagnosis and prognosis. *Arch Phys Med Rehabil 60*:415–419, 1979.

48. Hollinshead WH: *Anatomy for Surgeons*, Ed. 2, Vol. 3. *The Back and Limbs*, Harper & Row, New York, 1969 (p. 81, Fig. 2.2).

49. Hollinshead WH: *Functional Anatomy of the Limbs and Back*, Ed. 4. W.B. Saunders, Philadelphia, 1976 (pp. 229, 230).

50. Jayasinghe WJ, Harding RH, Anderson JAD, *et al.*: An electromyographic investigation of postural fatigue in low back pain—a preliminary study. *Electromyogr Clin Neurophysiol 18*:191–198, 1978.

51. Jonsson B: Morphology, innervation, and electromyographic study of the erector spinae. *Arch Phys Med Rehabil 50*:638–641, 1969.

52. Jonsson B: Topography of the lumbar part of the erector spinae muscle. *Z Anat Entwickl Gesch 130*:177–191, 1970.

53. Jonsson B: Electromyography of the erector spinae muscle. In *Medicine and Sport*, Vol. 8: *Biomechanics III*, edited by E. Jokl. Karger, Basel, 1973.

54. Kellgren JH: Observations on referred pain arising from muscle. *Clin Sci 3*:175–190, 1938 (pp. 180, 181, 185, 186; Figs. 3, 5, 9).

55. Kellgren JH: The anatomical source of back pain. *Rheumatol Rehabil 16*:3–12, 1977 (p. 7, Fig. 3; and p. 9, Fig. 4).

56. Kelly M: Pain in the chest: observations on the use of local anaesthesia in its investigation and treatment. *Med J Aust 1*:4–7, 1944 (pp. 5, 6, Case 4).

57. Korr IM, Wright HM, Chace JA: Cutaneous patterns of sympathetic activity in clinical abnormalities of the musculoskeletal system. *Acta Neurovegetativa 25*:489–606, 1964.

58. Korr IM, Wright HM, Thomas PE: Effects of experimental myofascial insults on cutaneous patterns of sympathetic activity in man. *Acta Neurovegetativa 23*:329–355, 1962.

PART 4

59. Kraus H: *Clinical Treatment of Back and Neck Pain.* McGraw-Hill, New York, 1970 (pp. 83, 98, 105, 106).

60. Lange M: *Die Muskelhaerten (Myogelosen); Ihre Entstehung und Heilung.* J.F. Lehmanns, Muenchen, 1931 (pp. 30, 91, 137, 138, 152, 158).

61. Lewis T, Kellgren JH: Observations relating to referred pain, viscero-motor reflexes and other associated phenomena. *Clin Sci* 1:47–71, 1939.

62. Lindstedt F: Zur Kenntnis der Aetiologie und Pathogenese der Lumbago und ähnlicher Rückenschmerzen. *Acta Med Scand* 55:248–280, 1921.

63. Lindstedt F: Ueber die Nature der muskelrheumatischen (myalgischen) Schmerzsymptome. *Acta Med Scand Suppl* 30:1–180, 1929.

64. Livingston WK: *Pain Mechanisms, A Physiologic Interpretation of Causalgia and Its Related States.* Macmillan, New York, 1943, reprinted by Plenum Press, New York, 1976 (pp. 134, 135).

65. Llewellyn LJ, Jones AB: *Fibrositis.* Rebman, New York, 1915 (Fig. 39).

66. Lundervold A: Electromyographic investigations during sedentary work, especially typing. *Br J Phys Med* 14:32–36, 1951.

67. Maigne R: *Orthopedic Medicine, A New Approach to Vertebral Manipulations,* translated and edited by W.T. Liberson. Charles C Thomas, Springfield, Ill., 1972 (pp. 282–310).

68. McMinn RMH, Hutchings RT: *Color Atlas of Human Anatomy.* Year Book Medical Publishers, Chicago, 1977 (p. 157).

69. *Ibid.* (p. 88).

70. Mennell J McM: *Back Pain.* Little, Brown & Company, Boston, 1960.

71. Morris JM, Banner G, Lucas DB: An electromyographic study of the intrinsic muscles of the back in man. *J Anat (Lond)* 96:509–520, 1962.

72. Morris JM, Lucas DB, Bresler B: Role of the trunk in stability of the spine. *J Bone Joint Surg* 43A:327–351, 1961.

73. Nachemson A: The effect of forward leaning on lumbar intradiscal pressure. *Acta Orthop Scand* 35:314–328, 1965.

74. Nachemson A, Lindh M: Measurement of abdominal and back muscle strength with and without low back pain. *Scan J Rehabil Med* 1:60–65, 1969.

75. Nichols PJR: Short-leg syndrome. *Br Med J* 1:1863–1865, 1960.

76. Orr LM, Mathers F, Butt T: Somatic pain due to fibrolipomatous nodules, simulating ureterorenal disease: a preliminary report. *J Urol* 59:1061–1069, 1948.

77. Osler W: *The Principles and Practice of Medicine.* D. Appleton and Co., New York, 1912 (p. 1131).

78. Patton IJ, Williamson JA: Fibrositis as a factor in the differential diagnosis of visceral pain. *Can Med Assoc J* 58:162–166, 1948 (Cases 2 and 3).

79. Pauly JE: An electromyographic analysis of certain movements and exercises, I—some deep muscles of the back. *Anat Rec* 155:223–234, 1966.

80. Pernkopf E: *Atlas of Topographical and Applied Human Anatomy,* Vol. 2. W.B. Saunders, Philadelphia, 1964 (Fig. 30).

81. *Ibid.* (p. 35).

82. Price JP, Clare MN, Ewerhardt FH: Studies in low backache with persistent muscle spasm. *Arch Phys Med* 29:703–709, 1948.

83. Rask MR: Thermography of the human spine: study of 150 cases with back pain and sciatica. *Orthop Rev* 8:73–82, 1979.

84. Reynolds MD: Myofascial trigger point syndromes in the practice of rheumatology. *Arch Phys Med Rehabil* 62:111–114, 1981.

85. Richter HR: Fettgewebe "Hernien". In *Der Weichteilrheumatismus,* Vol. 1, Fortbildungskunde Rheumatol. Karger, Basel, 1971 (pp. 49–59).

86. Richter HR: Einklemmungsneuropathien der Rami Dorsales als Ursache von akuten und chronischen Rueckenschmerzen. *Ther Umsch* 34:435–438, 1977.

87. Rubin D: An approach to the management of myofascial trigger point syndromes. *Arch Phys Med Rehabil* 62:107–110, 1981 (p. 110).

88. Samberg HH: The trigger point syndromes. *GP* 35:115–117, 1967.

89. Sicuranza BJ, Richards J, Tisdall L: The short leg syndrome in obstetrics & gynecology. *Am J Obstet Gynecol* 107:217–219, 1970.

90. Simmons EE: Referred low back pain. *J Omaha Mid-West Clin Soc* 1:3–6, 1954.

91. Simons DG, Travell J: Common myofascial origins of low back pain. *Postgrad Med,* early 1983. (In Press).

92. Sobotta J, Figge FHJ: *Atlas of Human Anatomy,* Ed. 9, Vol. 1. Hafner Divison of Macmillan, New York, 1974 (pp. 144, 146).

93. *Ibid.* (pp. 148, 152).

94. *Ibid.* (p. 152).

95. Sobotta J, Figge J: *Atlas of Human Anatomy,* Ed. 9, Vol. 3. Hafner Division of Macmillan, New York, 1974 (p. 253).

96. Spalteholz W: *Handatlas der Anatomie des Menschen,* Ed. 11, Vol. 2. S. Hirzel, Leipzig, 1922 (p. 309).

97. *Ibid.* (p. 311).

98. *Ibid.* (p. 312).

99. *Ibid.* (p. 313).

100. Stimson BB: The low back problem. *Psychosom Med* 9:210–212, 1947.

101. Terry AF, DeYoung R: Hip disease mimicking low back disorders. *Orthop Rev* 8:95–104, 1979.

102. Tichauer ER: Ergonomics: the state of the art. *Am Ind Hyg Assoc J* 28:105–116, 1967.

103. Tichauer ER: Industrial engineering in the rehabilitation of the handicapped. *J Ind Eng* 19:96–104, 1968.

104. Tichauer ER: A pilot study of the biomechanics of lifting in simulated industrial work situations. *J Safety Res* 3:98–115, 1971.

105. Toldt C: *An Atlas of Human Anatomy,* translated by M.E. Paul, Ed. 2, Vol. 1. Macmillan, New York, 1919 (pp. 268, 269).

106. *Ibid.* (p. 270).

107. *Ibid.* (p. 271).

108. *Ibid.* (p. 272).

109. *Ibid.* (p. 343).

110. Travell J: Basis for the multiple uses of local block of somatic trigger areas (procaine infiltration and ethyl chloride spray). *Miss Valley Med J* 71:13–22, 1949 (pp. 19, 20; Case 4).

111. Travell J: Symposium on mechanism and management of pain syndromes. *Proc Rudolf Virchow Med Soc* 16:128–136, (p. 135) 1957.

112. Travell J, Rinzler SH: The myofascial genesis of

pain. *Postgrad Med* 11:425–434, 1952.
113. Travell J, Travell W: Therapy of low back pain by manipulation and of referred pain in the lower extremity by procaine infiltration. *Arch Phys Med* 27:537–547, 1946 (pp. 544, 545; Case 3).
114. Williams PC: *Low Back and Neck Pain, Causes and Conservative Treatment.* Charles C

Thomas, Springfield, Ill., 1974 (Fig. 19, Panel 3).
115. Young D: The effects of novocain injections on simulated visceral pain. *Ann Intern Med* 19:749–756, 1943.
116. Zohn DA, Mennell JMcM: *Musculoskeletal pain.* Little, Brown & Company, Boston, 1976 (p. 193, Fig. 9–14).

CHAPTER 49

Abdominal Muscles
"Pseudo-visceral Pain"

HIGHLIGHTS: Myofascial phenomena of the abdominal musculature show strong reciprocal somatovisceral and viscerosomatic interactions. **REFERRED PAIN** from myofascial trigger points (TPs) in the abdominal musculature is likely to appear in the same quadrant and, occasionally, in any other quadrant of the abdomen, as well as in the back. These TPs are capable of initiating somatovisceral responses, including projectile vomiting, anorexia and nausea, intestinal colic, diarrhea, urinary bladder and sphincter spasm, and dysmenorrhea. When such visceral symptoms occur with abdominal pain and tenderness, the combination can strongly mimic acute visceral disease, especially appendicitis and cholelithiasis. **ANATOMICAL ATTACHMENTS** of the three lateral abdominal wall muscles, the internal and external obliques, and the transversus abdominis, produce a criss-cross fiber arrangement like plies in a tire. The fibers of the two medial muscles, the rectus abdominis and its pubic appendage, the pyramidalis muscle, are aligned vertically. **ACTIONS** of the abdominal musculature are chiefly to increase intra-abdominal pressure, and to flex and rotate the spine. **ACTIVATION OF TRIGGER POINTS** in the abdominal wall musculature secondary to visceral disease represents a viscerosomatic response. Examples of TP-initiating visceral diseases include peptic ulcer, intestinal parasites, dysentery, ulcerative colitis, diverticulosis, diverticulitis, and cholelithiasis. Once activated, TPs may then be perpetuated by emotional stress, occupational strain, faulty posture, and over-enthusiasm for "fitness" exercises. **ASSOCIATED TRIGGER POINTS** may occur in the iliopsoas and thoracic paraspinal muscles. **STRETCH AND SPRAY** of the involved abdominal muscles call for hyperextension of the spine, protrusion of the abdomen and a down-sweep spray pattern. **INJECTION AND STRETCH** begin with a pincer grasp, when possible, and injection proceeds with careful attention to the depth of needle penetration. **CORRECTIVE ACTIONS** include self-administration of ischemic compression, learning how to breathe with the abdomen, and doing the Pelvic-tilt and the Sit-back Exercises. Laughter is good medicine.

---

1. REFERRED PAIN
(Figs. 49.1 and 49.2)

Abdominal trigger points (TPs) may cause as much distress from induced visceral dysfunction as from referred pain. Symptoms referred from these myofascial TPs commonly confuse the diagnosis by mimicking visceral pathology. Pain patterns of TPs in the abdominal muscles, especially the obliques, are less consistent from patient to patient than are the patterns for most other muscles. Abdominal pain referred from TPs has little respect for the midline; abdominal TPs on one side frequently cause bilateral pain. Gutstein[36] observed that the patient is likely to describe the distress caused by abdominal TPs as "burning," "fullness," "bloating," "swelling," or "gas," although objective evidence of the symptom is frequently missing. Patterns repeatedly observed by the authors are presented, in addition to those reported by other authors. Each of the abdominal muscles will be considered separately.

PART 4

Abdominal Obliques
(Fig 49.1)

The abdominal oblique TPs have multiple referred pain patterns that may reach up into the chest, may travel straight or diagonally across the abdomen, and may extend downward. Whether this variability represents different characteristics of the successively deeper layers of muscle, or less consistency in the patterns of pain referred from TPs in this musculature, is not clear. One must palpate the abdomen carefully and thoroughly to identify all of the TPs potentially responsible for abdominal symptoms.

Active TPs in the upper portion of the abdominal external oblique muscle, which overlies the rib cage anteriorly, are likely to produce "heartburn" (Fig. 49.1A) and other symptoms commonly associated with hiatal hernia.[61] These "costal" and "subcostal" TPs in abdominal muscles also may produce deep epigastric pain that occasionally extends to other parts of the abdomen.[62]

Active TPs located in the musculature of the lower lateral abdominal wall, possibly in any one of the three layers of muscle, refer pain into the groin and testicle, and may project fingers of pain to other parts of the abdomen (Fig. 49.1C). The experimental injection of hypertonic saline into the external obliques near the anterior superior iliac spine induced referred pain over the lower portion of that quadrant of the abdomen, along the inguinal ligament and into the testicle.[44]

Active TPs along the upper rim of the pubis and the lateral half of the inguinal ligament may lie in the lower internal oblique muscle, and possibly in the lower rectus abdominis. These TPs can cause increased irritability and spasm of the detrusor and urinary sphincter muscles, producing urinary frequency, retention of urine and groin pain;[24, 59, 81] they have been associated with enuresis in older children. When needled, such TPs often refer pain to the region of the urinary bladder.

Melnick[61, 62] identified TPs in the muscles of the lower abdomen as sources of chronic diarrhea (Fig 49.1D). In our experience, when TPs that produce this symptom are identified and injected in a fold of the abdominal wall between the fingers,

they seem to be in the superficial layer of the lateral abdominal wall musculature.

Transversus Abdominis

Active TPs in the transversus abdominis near its costal attachments refer pain as a band across the upper abdomen between the anterior costal margins.

"Belch Button"

The "belch button" is a TP that is uncommon, but may be of critical importance to the patient who has one. It has not been accurately localized to a specific muscle. It is a dorsal TP that may lie in the posterior fringe of a lateral abdominal wall muscle, such as the external oblique, or it may be a fascial TP in the lumbodorsal fascia. The patient is likely to complain of a "stomach problem" with much belching of gas. In our experience, this TP is found on the left or right side usually at, or just below, the angle of the twelfth rib. When one locates it by palpation, a rib is beneath the finger (Fig. 49.1B), and the patient belches as pressure is applied to the TP. When sufficiently active, this TP causes spontaneous belching and in severe cases, projectile vomiting, which can be deeply embarrassing and a serious postoperative complication. Alvarez[2] reported that some patients belched every time the physician touched a trigger area in the back. Gutstein[36] reported that seven patients responded with belching following injection of fibrositic spots (interpreted by us as TPs) in the abdominal musculature, and that a few patients belched in response to pressure applied to tender abdominal spots.

Rectus Abdominis
(Fig 49.2)

The symptoms caused by TPs in this muscle are varied, but largely dependent on the location of the TPs. Symptoms will be considered in three groups, those due to TPs in the upper half of the muscle (above the umbilicus), those caused by periumbilical TPs, and those from TPs in the lower rectus abdominis.

Upper Rectus Abdominis. An active TP high in the rectus abdominis muscle on either side can refer pain to the mid-back bilaterally, which is described by the pa-

PART 4

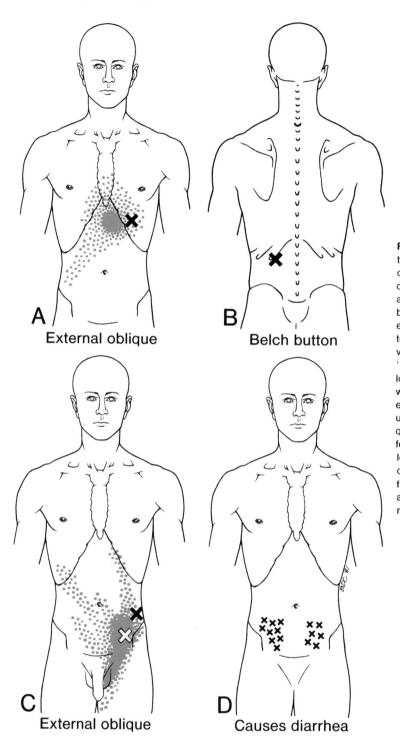

A External oblique

B Belch button

C External oblique

D Causes diarrhea

Figure 49.1. Referred pain patterns (*red*) and visceral symptoms of trigger points (×s) in the oblique (and possibly transverse abdominal muscles. *A*, "heartburn" from a trigger point in the external oblique overlying the anterior chest wall. *B*, projectile vomiting and belching from the "belch button", which is usually located in the posterior abdominal wall musculature and may be on either side. *C*, groin and/or testicular pain, as well as chiefly lower quadrant abdominal pain, referred from trigger points in the lower lateral abdominal wall musculature of either side. *D*, diarrhea from trigger points in the lower abdominal quadrants (after Melnick[61]).

tient as running horizontally *across* the back on both sides at the thoracolumbar level (Fig. 49.2A). Gutstein[36] also noted that treatment that relieved tender spots in abdominal wall muscles relieved pain in the back. Unilateral backache at this level, however, more frequently originates in TPs of the latissimus dorsi muscle.

Several authors have described symptoms of abdominal fullness, "heartburn," indigestion and sometimes nausea and vomiting due to paraxiphoid TPs located in the upper rectus abdominis.[24, 59, 61, 62] In our experience, nausea and epigastric distress occur more often when these uppermost rectus abdominis TPs are on the left, rather than on the right side. These TPs also may refer pain across the upper abdomen between the costal margins.

Injection of hypertonic saline into the rectus abdominis at about 2.5 cm (1 in) above the umbilicus caused brief referred pain throughout the same quadrant of the abdomen and on the same side in the back.[44] A TP in the upper rectus abdominis, when located on the left side, also may produce precordial pain.[24, 48, 59] When it has been established that the chest pain is myofascial and not cardiac in origin, it is usually due to TPs in the pectoralis or sternalis muscles; a rectus abdominis source of the pain is easily overlooked.

TPs in the upper rectus abdominis and focal tender points characteristic of TPs were observed to refer pain to the same abdominal quadrant,[23, 49] and to simulate the symptoms of cholecystitis, gynecological disease[59] and peptic ulcer.[59, 62]

Periumbilical Rectus Abdominis. Lateral border, periumbilical TPs are likely to produce sensations of abdominal cramping or colic.[61, 62] The patient often bends forward for relief. Infants, especially neonates who burp and cry persistently with colic, are likely to suffer from these periumbilical TPs, which may be relieved by the application of vapocoolant spray to the abdomen.[5] Lateral TPs in the rectus abdominis near the umbilicus may evoke diffuse abdominal pain,[24, 49-51] which is accentuated by movement.[47, 87]

Lewis and Kellgren[54] demonstrated experimentally that this muscle can generate the pain of intestinal colic. Injection of hypertonic saline into normal rectus abdominis muscle induced a familiar colic-like pain, which was much stronger anteriorly than toward the back, and which extended diffusely over several segments in front.[44]

Lower Rectus Abdominis. Inactivation of TPs in the lower rectus abdominis, about half-way between the umbilicus and the symphysis pubis (or in the overlying skin), may relieve dysmenorrhea[81] (Fig. 49.2C). (See Section 6 for a relevant experiment by Theobald.)

In the lowest part of the rectus abdominis, TPs may refer pain bilaterally to the sacroiliac and low back regions, which the patient portrays with a crosswise motion of the hand (Fig. 49.2A), rather than the up-and-down pain pattern characteristic of the iliocostalis thoracis and other paraspinal muscles.

Several authors have noted that a TP in the lateral border of the right rectus abdominis in the region of McBurney's point, which is halfway between the anterior superior iliac spine and the umbilicus (Fig. 49.2B), is likely to produce symptoms closely simulating those of acute appendicitis.[24, 25, 56, 59] This pain pattern was reported as often occurring when the patient was tired, worried or premenstrual.[24] In one case, the myalgic spot for this "pseudo-appendicitis" pain was reported in the rectus abdominis just above the level of the umbilicus.[25]

Other authors also have observed that TPs in the region of McBurney's point may refer pain to the same lower quadrant,[23, 56] throughout the abdomen,[18] and to the right upper quadrant.[49] These TPs also may refer sharp pain to the iliac fossa, the iliacus muscle and to the penis[24]; the pain may simulate renal colic.[59] An active TP in the right lower rectus abdominis also may cause diarrhea,[24, 62] and symptoms mimicking diverticulosis and gynecological disease.[59] A TP just above the pubis may cause spasm of the detrusor and urinary sphincter muscles.

Pyramidalis

The pyramidalis refers pain close to the midline between the symphysis pubis and the umbilicus (Fig. 49.2D).

2. ANATOMICAL ATTACHMENTS
(Figs. 49.3–49.5)

External Oblique
(Fig. 49.3A)

The fibers of the external oblique muscle travel diagonally downward and forward to join the abdominal aponeurosis which attaches **anteriorly** to the linea alba in the midline and to the anterior half of the iliac crest (Fig. 49.3A). **Laterally** and **cephalad** the fibers attach to the external surfaces and inferior borders of the lower eight ribs. The lower three of these rib attachments interdigitate with the latissi-

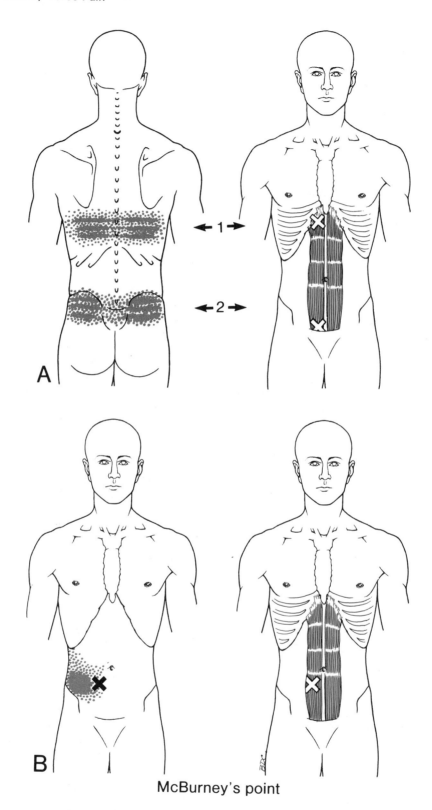

McBurney's point

Figure 49.2 A and B.

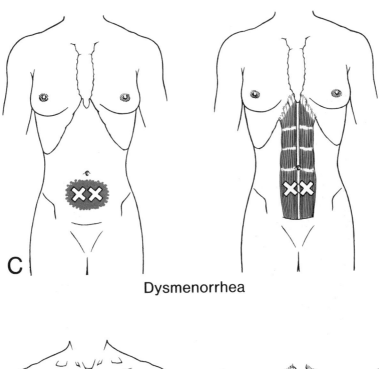

Dysmenorrhea

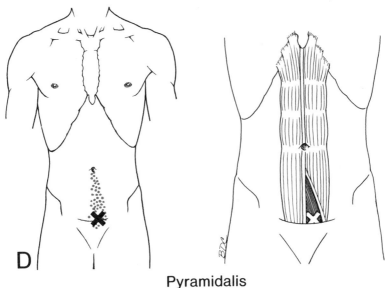

Pyramidalis

Figure 49.2A–D.   Referred pain patterns (*dark red*) and visceral symptoms of trigger points (×s) in the rectus abdominis and pyramidalis muscles (*medium red*). *A,* bilateral pain across the back, precordial pain, and/or a feeling of abdominal fullness, nausea and vomiting can be caused by a trigger point (*1*) in the left (or right) upper rectus abdominis. A similar pattern of bilateral low back pain is referred from a trigger point (*2*) in the caudal end of the rectus muscle on either side. *B,* lower right quadrant pain and tenderness may occur in the region of McBurney's point due to a nearby trigger point in the lateral border of the rectus abdominis. *C,* dysmenorrhea may be greatly intensified by trigger points in the lower rectus. *D,* referred pain pattern of the pyramidalis muscle.

mus dorsi, and the upper five, with the serratus anterior muscle. Although these three muscles appear in anatomy books to be quite separate, in dissection the external oblique may seem to form with the other two an unbroken sheet of muscle.

PART 4

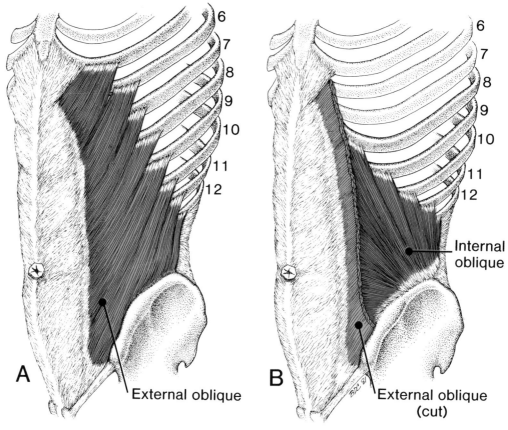

Figure 49.3. Attachments of two lateral abdominal wall muscles. *A*, external oblique (*light red*). *B*, internal oblique (*dark red*); external oblique (*light red*) is cut.

The fasciculi from the lowest two ribs lie nearly vertically, and thus are parallel and adjacent to those fibers of the quadratus lumborum that also connect the iliac crest and the twelfth rib.[31]

Internal Oblique
(Fig. 49.3*B*)

The direction of fibers in the fan-shaped internal oblique abdominal muscle in the upright body ranges from nearly vertical, *posteriorly*, through a diagonally upward and medial direction among its intermediate fibers, to horizontal for the most caudal fibers (Fig. 49.3*B*). *Laterally* all fibers converge onto the lateral half of the inguinal ligament, the anterior two-thirds of the iliac crest, and the lower portion of the lumbar aponeurosis. *Above* the nearly vertical fibers attach to the cartilages of the last three or four ribs. *Above* and *medially* diagonal fibers attach to the linea alba through the anterior and posterior rectus sheath. *Medially* the horizontal fibers from the inguinal ligament attach to the arch of the pubis through the conjoined tendon, which this muscle forms with the transversus abdominis.

Transversus Abdominis
(Fig. 49.4)

These fibers travel nearly horizontally across the abdomen and attach *anteriorly* to the midline linea alba *via* the rectus sheath (Fig. 49.4), which surrounds the rectus abdominis muscle above the arcuate line, and to the pubis through the conjoined tendon. Below that line, the sheath occurs only anterior to the rectus. *Laterally* the transversus muscle attaches to the lateral one-third of the inguinal ligament, to the anterior three-quarters of the crest of the ilium, to the thoracolumbar fascia, and to the inner surface of the cartilages of the last six ribs, where it interdigitates with fibers of the diaphragm.[33]

Rectus Abdominis
(Fig. 49.5)

The rectus abdominis attaches **below** along the crest of the pubic bone (Fig. 49.5). The fibers of the bilateral muscles interlace across the symphysis. **Above** the muscle attaches to the cartilages of the fifth, sixth, and seventh ribs.

The fibers of the rectus abdominis are usually interrupted by three or four, more or less complete, transverse tendinous inscriptions. The three most constant inscriptions are found near the tip of the xiphoid process, close to the level of the umbilicus, and one midway between them. Sometimes, there are also one or two partial inscriptions below the umbilicus.[34] In 115 cadavers, the total number of inscriptions per muscle ranged from one to four.[64]

The abdominal section of the pectoralis major muscle (see Fig. 42.5) may overlap the upper rectus abdominis, and thus may account for the occasional reference of pain to the anterior chest from TPs in this region.

Pyramidalis
(Fig. 49.5)

The pyramidalis is a variable muscle that attaches **below** to the symphysis pubis, and **above** to the linea alba approximately mid-way between the symphysis and the umbilicus. It lies within the anterior rectus sheath.[15, 34]

In several studies of 100 or more bodies,[15] the pyramidalis was absent bilaterally in 3.3% of Japanese, in 25% of Scottish, and generally in 15%–20% of bodies. Also, unilateral absence was somewhat more common than bilateral absence.[15] A subsequent study of 430 sides reported the pyramidalis absent in 17.7%.[6]

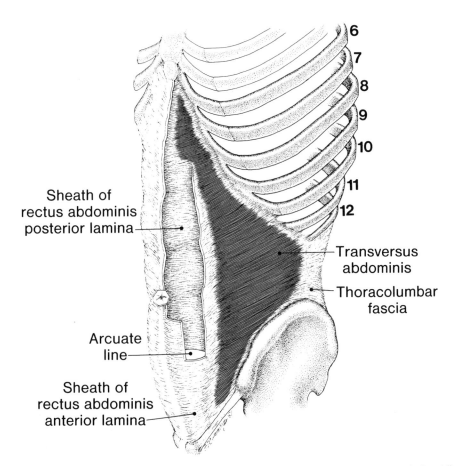

Figure 49.4.   Attachments of the transversus abdominis muscle (*red*), which lies beneath the obliques.

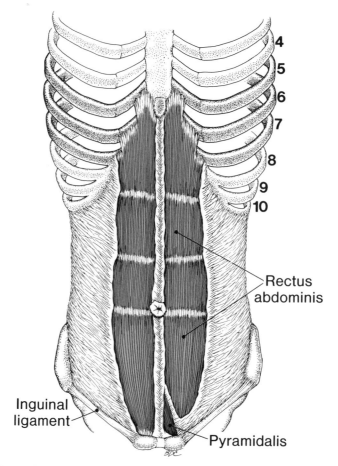

Figure 49.5. Attachments of the rectus abdominis muscle (*light red*), which connects the anterior rib cage to the pubic bone close to the symphysis, and of the variable pyramidalis muscle (*dark red*), which lies just above the symphysis pubis within the anterior rectus sheath.

Supplemental References

Other authors have presented clear drawings of the external oblique,[27, 29, 31, 58, 75] internal oblique,[28, 32, 58, 76] transversus abdominis,[33, 58, 77] rectus abdominis,[66, 77, 79, 85] and pyramidalis muscles.[15, 66, 76, 79] The anterior abdominal muscles are shown in cross section.[30, 66, 78]

3. INNERVATION

The three lateral abdominal wall muscles, the external and internal obliques and the transversus abdominis, are innervated by branches of the eighth through the twelfth intercostal nerves, and by branches of the iliohypogastric and the ilioinguinal nerves. Segmental innervation is from T_8–T_{12}. The transversus is supplied,

in addition, by the seventh intercostal nerve.[31–33]

The rectus abdominis is innervated by the seventh through the twelfth intercostal nerves derived from the corresponding spinal nerves; usually different segmental nerves innervate fibers between different tendinous inscriptions, especially in the upper half of the muscle.[34]

The pyramidalis is supplied by a branch of the twelfth thoracic nerve.[34]

4. ACTIONS

Lateral Abdominal Wall Muscles

The internal and external abdominal oblique muscles function: (1) bilaterally, to increase intra-abdominal pressure, e.g. for micturition, defecation, emesis, parturition

PART 4

and forced expiration; (2) bilaterally, to flex the spine; (3) unilaterally, to bend the spine toward the same side; and (4) unilaterally, to assist spinal rotation. The external oblique muscle rotates the homolateral shoulder forward; most of the internal oblique fibers rotate it backward.[31, 32]

The transversus abdominis increases intra-abdominal pressure.[33]

Stimulation experiments on these lateral abdominal wall muscles produced a powerful expiration which seriously compromised normal respiration.[12] The abdominal wall muscles as a group help to *complete* expiration quickly during rapid breathing.[4]

Electromyographically,[4] the external and internal obliques showed some activity during walking, modulated by the gait cycle. All three lateral wall muscles showed marked increase in activity with a sudden or sustained increase in intra-abdominal pressure. During lateral bending, the internal obliques were more strongly activated than the external obliques. The fibers of both the transversus and internal oblique muscles in the region of the inguinal canal were activated continuously during standing, with further increase in motor unit discharges during activities that would increase intra-abdominal pressure.

Activity of the abdominal muscles helps to pump venous blood out of the abdomen. Relaxation of the abdominal wall during inhalation increases blood flow into the abdominal veins from the lower extremities. As the abdominal wall muscles contract for exhalation, the blood is forced upward toward the heart if the valves of the lower extremity veins are competent.

Surface electrodes placed obliquely over each upper quadrant consistently disclosed more "external oblique" activity on the left than on the right side during most right-handed throwing activities in sports.[8] Since the left internal oblique, not the external oblique, brings the right shoulder forward, and since this type of electrode in this position should respond to both internal and external oblique activity, these results are compatible with kinesiology and the findings of other authors, provided the recorded potentials are interpreted as coming from the internal, rather than the external, oblique. Surface electrodes in this location would not distin-

guish between the motor unit activity of these two muscles. In none of these 13 sport activities was the rectus abdominis muscle as active as the oblique muscles. Usually the rectus abdominis showed little, if any, activity; it was most active during the tennis serve.[8]

Discus throwers develop greatly hypertrophied abdominal oblique musculature.

Rectus Abdominis

This muscle serves as the prime mover for spinal flexion, especially of the lumbar spine, and it tenses the anterior abdominal wall to increase intra-abdominal pressure.[34] Experimental stimulation of all portions of the rectus abdominis produced strong forward flexion of the trunk.[12]

Electromyographically, the rectus abdominis is active when a weight is carried on the back, but not when the weight is carried anterior to the thighs. The muscle responds consistently and clearly to the gait cycle during walking, but is not generally activated by efforts that increase intra-abdominal pressure, except by vigorous maneuvers, such as coughing.[4, 67] This muscle is consistently active as the feet leave the ground when jumping, and inconsistently active during landing from the jump.[43]

Electromyographically, sit-ups generated much more electrical activity in the rectus abdominis than did let-backs (sit-backs).[4, 18, 22, 89] The muscular activity was greatest during the initial phase of the sit-up: between 15°–45°,[18] or between scapular lift and hip lift from the floor.[22] Little difference was seen in this muscle's electrical activity whether the knees were bent to 65°, or were straight.[18] Flexing the knees and holding the feet down during a sit-up increased the activity of the abdominal muscles as compared to the rectus femoris, the fibers of which were said to become too short to pull effectively.[22]

The abdominal muscles are more active when walking uphill than on level ground.

Pyramidalis

The pyramidalis muscle tenses the linea alba.[34]

5. MYOTATIC UNIT

To increase intra-abdominal pressure, the four muscles of the belly wall are synergistic with the quadratus lumborum, and with the diaphragm when the increased pressure is for other than expiration.

For gross spinal rotation and extension, anatomically, the external abdominal oblique appears synergistic with the lower serratus anterior and vertical costal fibers of the latissimus dorsi, with which it interdigitates and forms a continuous line of pull.[31]

For side bending, the lateral, most vertical, fibers of the external and internal oblique muscles are synergistic with the vertical fibers of the quadratus lumborum, and with the most lateral of the paraspinal muscles, the iliocostalis.

During flexion/extension, the rectus abdominis is antagonistic to the paraspinal group, especially the longissimus thoracis muscle, and synergistic with the psoas muscle if the lumbosacral spine is flexed.

For rotation, the external oblique muscle on one side is synergistic with the deepest (most diagonal) paraspinal muscles on the same side, and with the contralateral serratus posterior inferior and internal abdominal oblique muscles.

6. SYMPTOMS

Abdominal symptoms are a common source of diagnostic confusion. Understanding the reciprocal somatovisceral and viscerosomatic effects helps greatly to unravel this confusion. Myofascial TPs in an abdominal muscle may produce referred abdominal pain and visceral disorders (somatovisceral effects) that, together, closely mimic visceral disease. Conversely, visceral disease can profoundly influence somatic sensory perception and can activate TPs in somatic structures that then may perpetuate pain and other symptoms long after the patient has recovered from the initiating visceral disease.

Symptoms Due to Myofascial Trigger Points in Abdominal Muscles

Melnick[60] reported the relative frequency of serious symptoms arising from trigger areas in the abdominal musculature among 56 patients (Table 49.1).

Long[56] distinguished the "anterior abdominal wall syndrome" from visceral disease. The syndrome was attributed to TPs in the musculature of the abdominal wall.

Table 49.1
Frequency of Serious Complaints among 56 Patients with Abdominal Trigger Points.[a]

Symptoms	Number of Patients	Prevalence[b]
		%
Pain	40	71
Pressure and bloating	14	25
Heartburn	6	11
Vomiting	6	11
Diarrhea	2	4

[a] Adapted from Melnick.[60]
[b] Percentage and numbers total more than 100% because some patients had more than one symptom.

Its distinguishing feature was nearly continuous pain that might relate to movement, but not to the ingestion of food or to evacuation. On careful inquiry, some of his patients localized the pain to the abdominal wall.

Good[23] observed that abdominal pain referred from TPs in the lateral border of the rectus abdominis muscle near mid-abdomen was typically aggravated by bending over when lifting (an activity which shortens and often causes contraction of the rectus abdominis). In the experience of the authors of this manual, prolonged vigorous activity that requires forceful abdominal breathing also may increase the pain referred from abdominal wall TPs.

Kelly[47] noted that patients with myalgic lesions (described like TPs) of the abdominal wall musculature were likely to complain of abdominal discomfort or distress, rather than of pain per se. In the authors' experience, active TPs of the abdominal muscles, especially in the rectus abdominis, may cause a lax, distended abdomen with excessive flatus. Contraction of the abdominal muscles is inhibited by the TPs so that the patient cannot "pull the stomach in." This distension is readily distinguished from that due to ascites.

Right upper quadrant pain due to TPs in either the oblique abdominal muscles, or in the lateral border of the rectus abdominis of the same quadrant, is easily confused with the pain of gallbladder disease. Pain simulating appendicitis was projected from "fibrositic nodules" (described like palpable bands and TPs) in the region covered by the costal portion of the external oblique,[93] and from TPs in the lateral border of the rectus abdominis in the right lower quadrant.[25, 41, 59]

Weiss and Davis[90] eloquently demonstrated that local anesthetic injection of a visceral pain reference zone can relieve the pain just as does infiltrating the area of pain referred from a TP in a muscle.[39, 45] Relief of pain in this way does not identify the source of the pain.

Symptoms Due to Trigger Points NOT in Abdominal Muscles

Although one first thinks of TPs in the abdominal musculature to explain non-visceral abdominal pain, there are numerous other TP sites to be considered. Epigastric pain suggestive of a duodenal ulcer may arise from "fibrositic nodules" (TPs) in the region of the serratus anterior muscle, and has been effectively treated by digital pressure on the nodules.[93]

Occasionally, abdominal pain in an upper quadrant may be due to Tietze's syndrome of the costal cartilages,[84] reported also as affecting the xiphisternal joint,[42] or to abnormal mobility of the lower intercostal joints, which has been variously referred to as the "slipping rib syndrome,"[37] or the "rib-tip syndrome."[57] This may be diagnosed by the "hooking maneuver," in which the fingers are hooked under the costal margin to pull the ribs forward, demonstrating their abnormal mobility and reproducing the pain.[57] Temporary, sometimes permanent, relief was obtained from this symptom by the local injection of an anesthetic agent.[57] Some patients required surgical removal of the hypermobile rib segment to obtain permanent relief.[37]

Abdominal pain, particularly in the lower quadrant of the abdomen, may be referred from TPs in the paravertebral muscles,[36, 60, 62, 95] (Chapter 48). Gastrointestinal pain and cramping has been reported from TPs specifically in the erector spinae bilaterally.[19] Also, nausea and belching may result from TP activity in the paraspinal muscles at the upper thoracic level.[2, 10] Three examples of abdominal pain were attributed to remote TPs in the skin itself.[72] Lower abdominal pain, tenderness and muscle spasm may be referred from TPs located in the vaginal wall

about 2.5–3.8 cm (1 to 1½ in) inside the introitus, in a region that is normally insensitive to digital pressure.[61]

Urinary frequency, urinary urgency and "kidney" pain may be referred from TPs in the skin of the lower abdomen, as well as from TPs in lower abdominal muscles. Injection of a TP in an old appendectomy scar in the right lower quadrant has relieved frequency and urgency, and increased the bladder capacity from 240 ml to 420 ml. Similar symptoms from a TP in the skin close to McBurney's point were relieved for at least 8 months by its injection with a local anesthetic.[40]

A TP high in the adductor muscles of the thigh may refer pain upward into the groin and to the lower lateral abdominal wall.[86]

Feinstein, et al.[17] injected hypertonic saline into paraspinal musculotendinous tissues, 1.3–2.5 cm (½ to 1 in) from the midline at each segmental level. The abdominal pain patterns referred from paraspinal muscles at the T_7 to T_{12} levels were similar, but without the precise degree of segmental correspondence suggested by Melnick.[61] Clinically, these authors found only an approximate anterior segmental correspondence.

Lewis and Kellgren,[54] and later Kellgren,[45] described pain referred to the abdomen from interspinous ligaments when they were injected with hypertonic saline; Hockaday and Whitty[39] subsequently found that pain was referred from these ligaments only to dorsal areas. The more extensive pain patterns observed by Kellgren[46] may have been due to his injection of paraspinal (non-midline) structures, which Hockaday and Whitty scrupulously avoided.

Differential Diagnosis

Non-abdominal diseases that may cause abdominal symptoms include coronary artery insufficiency,[52] which may present as acute "indigestion"[83]; pneumonia of the lower lobe with pleurisy; herpes zoster; a ruptured upper lumbar vertebral disc with nerve root compression; diabetic acidosis; and abdominal migraine.

The abdominal distress[52] and referred pain patterns[74] caused by a number of abdominal diseases is mimicked by the abdominal symptoms produced by myofascial TPs. These diseases include diaphragmatic hernia, peptic ulcer,[36, 62] gastric carcinoma, chronic cholecystitis or gallstone colic,[36] ureteral colic, inguinal hernia, hepatitis, pancreatitis, appendicitis,[25, 36] diverticulitis, colitis,[36] and cystitis.[52] Relatively common medical problems that also may cause abdominal pain include esophagitis, hiatus hernia with reflux, and spastic colon. Less frequent are aortic aneurysm, pancreatic carcinoma, bowel obstruction, ovarian cyst, endometriosis, and psychogenic pain.[52] Acute abdominal pain also may be due to epilepsy (diagnosed by EEG),[71] hydronephrosis, and ascariasis infestation with bowel obstruction (diagnosed by radiography and stool culture).[1]

Active TPs in the lateral border of the rectus abdominis may induce recurrent pain in the area of McBurney's point,[41] or pain in the iliac fossa.[25] These TPs simulate the symptoms of appendicitis,[36, 80] with marked local tenderness and rigidity. Surgeons who are unaware of the common myofascial sources of lower right quadrant pain are understandably frustrated by the poor correlation between the patient's symptoms and the pathological state of the excised appendix.[26] Nearly 40% of the appendices removed in one large series were normal.[91] One would suspect that many of the 22.4% of these operated patients who obtained only partial relief, and most of the 8.2% who had no relief from their "appendicular" pain by surgery,[91] had active TPs which contributed to their symptoms. A recent study found normal appendices in 12.4% of "appendicitis" patients.[94]

When the abdomianl pain suggestive of appendicitis is due to TPs in the rectus abdominis, that muscle shows palpable ropiness, which differs from the more generalized, board-like rigidity of all layers of the abdominal musculature found in acute appendicitis. Pain relief by the Abdominal Tension Test (Section 8, Patient Examination) and positive laboratory findings indicative of infection favor appendicitis. Rovsing's sign (pain from pressure on the left side of the abdomen due to colonic gas being pushed to the right),[83] and rebound tenderness are usually present only in visceral disease.

Abnormal sensitivity of the iliopsoas or obturator internus muscles to passive stretch due to an inflamed retrocaecal appendix[83] must be distinguished from a similarly reduced range of motion due to active TPs in these two pelvic muscles. In the latter case, it is specifically the muscles that are tender to palpation.

The leucocyte count and erythrocyte sedimentation rate are normal in the uncomplicated myofascial pain syndromes, but elevated in acute appendicitis and other acute inflammatory visceral disease.

An unusual source of continuous severe lower abdominal pain is hematoma of the rectus abdominis muscle;[14, 67, 68, 73] Murray[65] reported three such cases in 55,900 pregnancies, and all three had been coughing heavily when the pain began.

Somatovisceral Effects

Good[24] reported that a myalgic condition of the abdominal musculature (description compatible with TPs) often caused functional disturbance of an abdominal viscus.[24] Abdominal TPs may induce diarrhea, vomiting, food intolerance,[36] colic in an adult or excessive burping in an infant, and dysmenorrhea. Diarrhea may be a concomitant of TP activity in the rectus abdominis, but is more likely to depend on TPs in the lower-quadrant oblique muscles (Fig. 49.1D). These abdominal-TP-dependent symptoms could occur secondary to an autonomically controlled change in the activity of smooth muscle and secretory activity. Myofascial TPs also can induce pain in the urinary bladder,[40] with associated sphincter spasm and residual urine; some of these patients have received urethral dilation and urethrotomy without relief.

Three other somatic TPs produce reflex phenomena that are at least partly abdominal-visceral. One is the "cough" TP in the lower end of the sternal division of the sternocleidomastoid muscle (see Chapter 7). Another is the "belch button" (Fig. 49.1B). The third is a TP in the tip of the uvula that causes hiccup. Lifting the uvula with the handle of a spoon or fork, during and followed by small breaths with the chest held in a collapsed position for a period of time, consistently terminates an attack of hiccup; this stimulation of the uvula is still effective under general anesthesia.[87] It is not known whether the focus of irritation (possibly a TP) responsible for the hiccup is located in the muscular or mucosal tissue of the uvula.

A less specific somatic stimulus, caused by a massive hematoma of the rectus abdominis muscle, induced nausea, vomiting and brown watery diarrhea.[73]

Lewis and Kellgren[54] established experimentally that the clinical symptom of intestinal colic can be referred from normal rectus abdominis muscle by injecting 0.3 ml of 6% sodium chloride solution just *below*, and 2.5 cm (1 in) *outside*, the navel. This irritant solution produced continuous pain for 3–5 min; the pain was referred deeply in the front of the body, and was indistinguishable from the pain of colic.

Weiss and Davis[90] demonstrated another somatovisceral relationship by modulating the somatic limb of primarily visceral pain. They relieved the pain referred to the abdominal wall from a diseased viscus by infiltrating the pain reference zone subcutaneously (not intramuscularly) with a local anesthetic. This effectively anesthetized the skin of the painful area, and probably the underlying superficial layers of muscle. Three patients were tested who suffered from acute gallbladder disease; one felt pain over the epigastrium, the other two in the right upper quadrant. Subcutaneous infiltration of from 12–30 ml of 2% procaine solution into the area of referred pain provided relief lasting from 30 min to several hours. In one case, following the infiltration, pain appeared in an adjacent area, and this pain also was relieved by local anesthetic infiltration. One patient with acute, and another with chronic, appendicitis had pain and tenderness in the right lower quadrant. Subcutaneous infiltration of the painful zone with 8 and 15 ml of 2% procaine, respectively, completely relieved pain temporarily in both patients. Similar results were reported for pain due to nephrolithiasis, salpingitis and carcinoma of the esophagus.

Relief of this somatic abdominal expression of viscerally induced pain by local anesthesia of the painful area indicates that the pain was produced primarily by convergence facilitation.[69] This mechanism of referred pain may be based on the theory that visceral noxious stimuli modulate central nervous system transmission, producing referred pain by facilitating (or disinhibiting) the normal somatic sensory input from the pain reference zone. Local anesthesia would have reduced this latter afferent input, thereby eliminating the exaggerated perception of it as pain.

Experimentally, Trinca[88] irritated the skin of the abdomen with a rubefacient and produced a fluoroscopically demonstrable increase in peristalsis of the barium-filled stomach. Ruhmann[70] demonstrated marked radiological changes in gastric motility in response to hot or cold stimuli applied to the skin of the upper abdomen. This substantiated the importance of somatic influences on ulcer pain, which is as dependent on gastric motility as it is on gastric acidity.[7]

Theobald[82] electrically stimulated the endometrium to simulate dysmenorrhea by producing abdominal wall pain centrally over the rectus abdominis muscles midway between the umbilicus and the pubis. The visceral-referred uterine pain was eliminated somatically by procaine infiltration of the painful skin and subcutaneous tissues in the reference zone, again indicating a convergence-facilitation mechanism of referred pain.[69] However, referred abdominal pain produced by sufficiently strong electrical stimulation of the uterus was not blocked by local anesthetic infiltration of the abdominal reference zone. This observation is typical of the convergence-projection mechanism of referred pain,[69] which is not a viscerosomatic phenomenon because the soma is bypassed. Clinically, complete relief was usually, but not always, obtained when dysmenorrhea was treated by procaine infiltration of this painful area over the rectus abdominis muscles.[82]

Viscerosomatic Effects

The reciprocal influence of visceral structures on the somatic musculature is equally impressive. Well known is the reflex spasm (rigidity) of the abdominal muscles in response to the inflammation of acute appendicitis.[63] Pain, which previously had responded to medical therapy for a duodenal ulcer, became unresponsive and persisted until TPs in the abdominal musculature were found and inactivated.[62] The ulcer apparently had activated these abdominal TPs before it was healed by medical treatment. Then the TPs continued to refer pain that was similar to that previously caused by the ulcer.

In normal subjects, stimulation of the splenic flexure of the small intestine by acute distention induced pain referred to the upper abdomen.[13] In patients with an irritable colon, this stimulus projected pain also to the precordium, left shoulder, neck and arm.[13]

Reversal of the above somatovisceral rubefacient experiment by Trinca,[88] described above, demonstrated a viscerosomatic reflex. When the gastric mucosa was stimulated by drinking a cup of hot tea, it caused a reddening of the epigastric skin previously irritated by a rubefacient.

Specific viscero-rectus abdominis and viscero-pannicular reflexes were reported in the cat. Pinching the pancreas, or the mesentery, or a loop of the duodenum consistently produced a marked contraction of the rectus abdominis muscle.[54] Dilatation of the gallbladder by a balloon caused contraction of the subcutaneous panniculus carnosus muscle over the lateral and dorsal thorax of the cat.[3]

7. ACTIVATION OF TRIGGER POINTS

Abdominal TPs are likely to develop in a muscle that is subject to acute or chronic overload, or in muscles that lie within the zone of pain referred from a viscus. In general, these TPs may develop in response to visceral disease, direct trauma, and mechanical, toxic or emotional stress.

Visceral Disease

As indicated above, visceral diseases in general,[36] and specifically peptic ulcer,[60, 62] have been identified as often responsible for abdominal myofascial TPs. Abdominal TPs are especially likely to develop during an infestation with such intestinal parasites as *Entamoeba histolytica*, and beef or fish tapeworm. Such an infestation is a potent factor for the perpetuation of myofascial TPs, and also may activate TPs, in the abdominal musculature.

Trauma

Acute trauma[62] and chronic occupational strain[36] are important activating factors. In the authors' experience, TPs are likely to occur close to an abdominal scar, as after an appendectomy or hysterectomy; the initiating stresses during surgery may be the combination of excessive stretch on the muscles by retractors and associated ischemia. Cutaneous TPs within the scar tissue itself also are seen.[35] The skin and muscles around an incision have been infiltrated effectively with procaine at the time of suturing the wound to prevent the development of active TPs following surgery and to reduce postoperative incisional discomfort.

Rectus abdominis TPs may be initiated in conjunction with an abdominal operation and perpetuated by paradoxical breathing learned as a result of post-operative abdominal soreness.

Stress

Several commonly encountered stress factors may activate abdominal TPs: total body fatigue,[62] over-exercise (too many sit-ups), emotional tension,[36, 62] cold exposure, viral infections, straining at stool due to constipation, and poor posture[36] (such as sitting and leaning forward for hours on a bed or at a desk with the abdominal muscles shortened and tense, with the back not supported). Structural inadequacies, such as a short leg or small hemipelvis, may add unnecessary overload. These stresses are additive.

The external oblique is vulnerable to a sustained twisted position (sitting at a desk, turned sideways because of lighting). This muscle also is vulnerable in sports activities that require a vigorous twisting body motion (throwing the discus).

8. PATIENT EXAMINATION

Several authors have noted the value of *increasing* the abdominal muscle tension during examination to help distinguish the pain that is due to muscular TPs from that due to underlying visceral disease. To do the Abdominal Tension Test according to Long,[56] the sensitive area is compressed with sufficient pressure to cause steady pain. When the supine patient then raises the legs high enough to bring *both* heels a few inches above the examining surface, the tensed abdominal muscles lift the palpating finger away from the viscera, while the digital pressure on the muscle itself is increased. If the pain increases, that indicates that it originates in the abdominal wall; if it decreases, that shows that it arises inside the abdomen. To achieve increased abdominal tension, Llewellyn and Jones[55] recommended that the patient hold a partial sit-up. Wilson,[93] like Long,[56] asked the supine patient to lift both heels off the bed, while de Valera and Raftery[96] had the patient elevate both the feet and the head. Hunter[41] and Kelsey[52] merely requested the patient to tense the abdominal muscles.

Abdominal Obliques

To insure contraction of the lateral wall abdominal muscles when performing the Abdominal Tension Test, the supine patient must elevate the heels, or elevate the head and shoulders high enough to lift both scapulae off any support. When the patient elevates only the head, usually only the rectus abdominis muscles contract, and not the obliques.

Rectus Abdominis

When the patient with active TPs in the rectus abdominis muscle stands, the abdomen is likely to sag and become pendulous. Clinically, TPs in this muscle inhibit its supportive function. The tense palpable band associated with an active TP would extend through and shorten only the segment of muscle (between inscriptions) in which it lies. However, the TP activity apparently inhibits contraction of adjacent segments to reduce tension on the involved fibers, thereby causing lengthening, rather than shortening, of the muscle as a whole. The rectus abdominis has no parallel muscle, except its mate, that contracts, unloads it, and provides protective splinting.

If asked to take a deep breath, these patients are likely to exhibit paradoxical breathing (see Chapter 20). Apparently, the threat of pain due to stretching of the involved rectus abdominis subconciously inhibits the normal diaphragmatic contraction on inspiration. When the patient inhales deeply with the diaphragm, thus protruding the abdomen, referred pain due to rectus abdominis TPs may be exacerbated.

The bilateral, transverse, mid-back pain referred from TPs high in the rectus abdominis muscle is usually aggravated by taking a deep breath, especially when the back is arched in marked lumbar lordosis, which further stretches the rectus abdominis. Back pain from paraspinal TPs is not usually influenced by respiration.

Herniation through the abdominal musculature is more easily detected in some cases with the patient standing rather than recumbent.

9. TRIGGER POINT EXAMINATION

When the abdomen is examined for myofascial TPs, the supine patient should hold a deep abdominal breath to passively stretch these muscles and increase their sensitivity to palpation. To optimize palpation of lateral abdominal TPs, the patient lies on the opposite side and holds a similar deep breath.[55] Gutstein[36] warned that a few TPs are more easily found when the *relaxed* abdomen is palpated, and repeated palpation may be required before TP tenderness is definitely established.

External Oblique

Active TPs in the external oblique are found along the lower border of the rib cage[36] and along the line where this muscle attaches to the iliac crest.[36, 53] The authors of this manual frequently find TPs in superficial palpable bands that extend between the tip of the twelfth rib and the crest of the ilium.

In addition to examining the abdomen of the supine patient by flat palpation, the patient's hips may be flexed to slacken the abdominal muscles, so that the abdominal wall in the flank area (external, internal obliques and transversus muscles) can be grasped between the fingers and thumb, as shown later in Figure 49.7A. When the most tender part of a palpable band is briskly rolled within the pincer grasp, the band usually responds with a vigorous local twitch response. Some thin patients with lax abdominal musculature may be examined in this way with their hips extended.

Internal Oblique

"Fibrositic nodules" (most likely TPs) in this muscle were described along the inferior margins of the tips of the six lower ribs, and also close to the pubic bone.[55] In our experience, to find them, the examiner must press down against the *upper edge* of the pubic arch, not on the flat anterior surface of the pubis. These TPs feel like small buttons, or short bands.

Rectus Abdominis

Active TPs in this muscle are commonly found in the angle between the costal arch and the xiphoid process,[36, 55] or between the xiphoid process and the umbilicus. In addition, they may be found in the middle or lower portions of the rectus abdominis, especially along its lateral border and at its attachment to the pubic bone.

10. ENTRAPMENTS

An anterior branch of a spinal nerve may become entrapped in the rectus abdominis muscle or sheath, and thus produce lower abdominal and pelvic pain that can simulate gynecological disease in female patients. This was diagnosed by a test injection of procaine to block the nerve; if the test injection afforded relief, the entrapped nerve was cauterized by injection of 0.5 ml of 6% aqueous phenol solution.[96] Others injected 5% and 7% phenol into the lateral border of the rectus sheath.[11, 59]

When the entrapment is due to tension from TP activity in fibers of the rectus abdominis, inactivation of the TPs by injecting them with 0.5% procaine solution relieves the symptoms.

11. ASSOCIATED TRIGGER POINTS

Abdominal pain referred from TPs in muscles not in the abdominal wall is re-viewed above in Section 6. The TPs in the lower lateral abdominal wall are often associated with active TPs high in the adductor muscles of the thigh, which may refer pain upward inside the abdomen.

Gutstein[36] emphasized, and we agree, that it is important to look for additional tender points above and below the inguinal ligament on the same side as the pain and, if found, for corresponding points on the opposite side.

12. STRETCH AND SPRAY
(Fig. 49.6)

Active TPs in the abdominal muscles of infants and young children are particularly responsive to stretch and spray. In adults, one should first look for and inactivate any TPs in the back muscles that refer pain to the abdomen, before injecting the abdominal TPs, since the latter may be satellites of the dorsal TPs.

To stretch and spray the rectus abdominis muscle, (Fig. 49.6), the patient lies supine on a plinth or firm support with the legs hanging over the end, with the hands over the head, and with the feet supported approximately 60 cm (2 feet) below the level of the hips. The patient arches the back and protrudes the abdomen by strongly contracting the diaphragm, which is facilitated by first taking a deep breath. At the same time, the jet of vapocoolant spray is swept in parallel lines from above

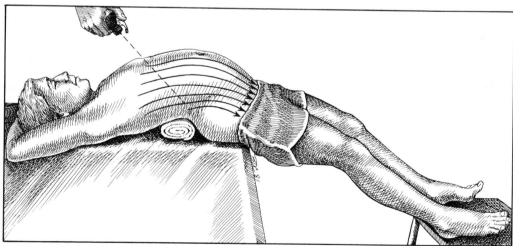

Figure 49.6.   Stretch position and spray pattern (*arrows*) for the abdominal musculature. In the supine position with the arms raised, the back fully arched, the legs extended over the edge of the table, and the feet supported at a lower level on a chair seat, the patient first takes a deep breath and then strongly contracts the diaphragm to protrude the abdomen and stretch the abdominal muscles. The vapocoolant spray is applied in a caudal direction, in parallel sweeps over the involved muscles.

downward across the involved muscles and over the pain reference zones. In the authors' clinical experience, an up-pattern of vapocooling, which was recommended by others,[60] is not as effective as the down-pattern (Fig. 49.6). Both right and left rectus abdominis muscles should always be treated, since they function as a team and usually are both involved. The operator should lift the patient's legs to return them to a more comfortable recumbent position.

To stretch the more lateral external oblique muscle, the patient lies on the opposite side and the upper shoulder is lowered backward toward the table. This rotates the thoracolumbar spine, as when stretching the serratus anterior muscle (see Fig. 46.4B). The spray pattern follows the line of the muscle fibers in an anterocaudal direction.

A moist hot pack or pad is applied promptly over the treated muscles.

Dysmenorrhea may be relieved by directing parallel sweeps of vapocoolant spray downward over the painful region of the abdomen[20] for 15 or 20 sec.[16] The authors of this volume are careful to avoid frosting the skin, by continuously moving the stream of spray in parallel lines. The patient may be taught to apply the Fluori-Methane spray herself, if repeated applications are necessary.

Effective ischemic compression applied to individual TPs in the abdominal muscles requires that the muscle be placed on sufficient tension. Compression is most successful for the TPs close to the arch of the pubic bones, and less successful in patients with excess adipose tissue.

13. INJECTION AND STRETCH
(Figs. 49.7–49.9)

Melnick[62] reported that in a series of 36 patients whose epigastric pain had become refractory to ulcer treatment, 32 responded successfully to myofascial TP inactivation and were returned to a normal diet without symptoms or need for medication. He injected their abdominal TPs once or twice weekly until no further muscular hypersensitivity was present.

Most TPs in abdominal muscles can be reached with a 3.8-cm (1½-in) needle unless the patient is obese. Better control is obtained by inserting it at a shallow angle, than by inserting it nearly perpendicular to the skin. The shallower angle makes it easier to align the shaft of the needle with the muscle fibers and to feel the changes in consistency of fat, fascia, and muscle as the needle penetrates successive layers. One should be careful to avoid penetrating the peritoneal cavity and its intestinal contents.

Stretching, together with repetition of vapocooling, should be done at once after the TP injection and then followed by a hot pack.

Lateral Abdominal Muscles
(Figs. 49.7 and 49.8)

Injection of TPs in that part of the external oblique muscle overlying the ribs employs a technique similar to the injection of the serratus anterior or serratus posterior muscles, with precautions to avoid penetrating an intercostal space and the pleura.

Injection of the lateral wall obliques is preferably done by pinching the abdominal wall between the fingers and thumb, so that no abdominal contents remain within the pincer grasp (Fig. 49.7 A and C). The TP is located by rolling the musculature between the digits to identify a palpable band and the spot tenderness of the TP, and to test for a local twitch response. The needle is then directed precisely into the TP, which is fixed within the operator's grasp.

Suprapubic TPs are felt as little buttons or bands where the musculature attaches to the upper border of the pubic bone (Fig. 49.7B). These are injected from above, directing the needle toward the pubis. These TPs may be responsive also to ischemic compression.

Injection of the transversus abdominis TPs along the costal margin (Fig. 49.8) requires special care. The muscle attaches to the underside of the costal margin where the fibers interdigitate with the diaphragm, beyond which lies the pleura. The exact position of the needle tip can be established by gently contacting the costal cartilage.

Rectus Abdominis
(Fig. 49.9)

Several authors have noted the effectiveness of injecting TPs in the rectus abdominis muscle for relief of abdominal pain.[49, 56, 81] Gutstein[36] warned of postinjection soreness and stiffness for 6–12 hr fol-

PART 4

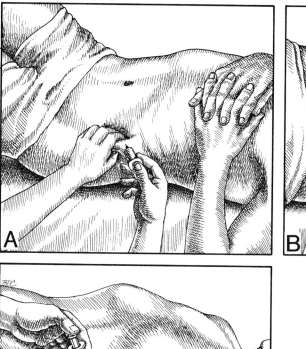
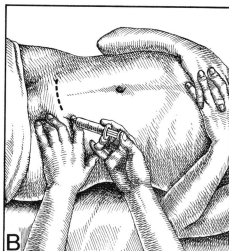
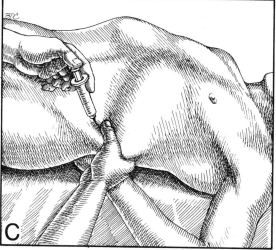

Figure 49.7. Injection of the external abdominal oblique muscle. *A*, pinching the abdominal wall permits grasping the muscle and its trigger points between the digits without any abdominal contents, *B*, suprapubic trigger points are injected against the upper border of the pubic arch. *Dashed line* marks upper border of the pubic bones. *C*, alternate manner of grasping the abdominal wall to eliminate abdominal contents while injecting myofascial trigger points in the oblique or transverse abdominal muscles.

lowing injection of the upper rectus abdominis. Kelly[50] estimated that only one-third of these injections relieved the patient's pain as compared with Melnick's 91% success rate[62]; the patients were selected very differently. Hunter[41] emphasized to his patients the importance of their emancipation from the fear of pain. Among 21 cases, he reported that 12 (57%) were fully relieved, and 5 (24%) were partly relieved of pain. We find that close attention to perpetuating factors is essential to a high success rate.

Injection of upper rectus abdominis TPs

in the costal arch beside the xiphoid process (Fig. 49.9A) again requires careful technique with attention to the depth of needle penetration. Experience gained by injecting TPs in other muscles teaches one to recognize the difference in the feel of the tissue as the needle penetrates skin, subcutaneous fat, epimysium, and then muscle, in the rectus abdominis. Penetration beyond the second layer of epimysium (the posterior rectus sheath) is avoided; it must be remembered that there is no posterior sheath below the arcuate line, which lies below the navel.

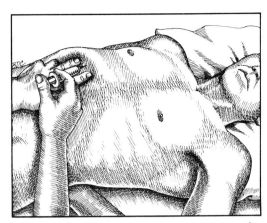

Figure 49.8.   Injection of the right transversus abdominis muscle for trigger points along the costal margin. The needle is directed at the caudal edge of the rib, not beneath it.

In supine subjects who are relatively thin, the needle can be inserted horizontally into the lateral border of the rectus abdominis by depressing the abdominal wall lateral to the rectus sheath (Fig. 49.9C). This muscle is likely to respond with marked local twitch responses. In one case, with the patient's hips and knees flexed, when the needle penetrated a rectus abdominis TP, the feet were lifted 10 cm (4 in) off the table by the vigor of the local twitch response,.

Injection of the fibers close to the pubic attachment of the rectus abdominis is accomplished by directing the needle toward the pubic bone (Fig. 49.9B).

Injection of TPs in the pyramidalis muscle is accomplished by directing the needle

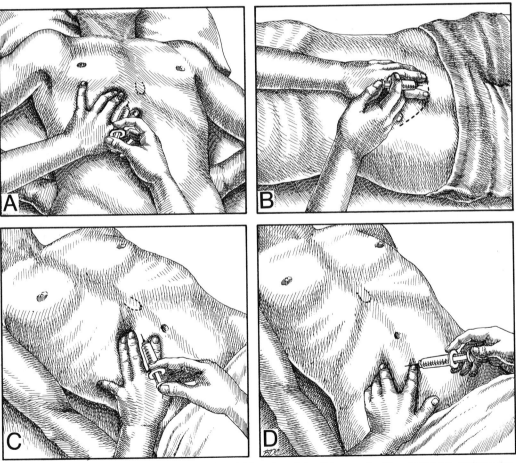

Figure 49.9.   Injection of trigger points in the right rectus abdominis muscle. The *dotted line* outlines the xiphoid process in *Parts A, C* and *D*, and in *B the dotted line* outlines the upper border of the inguinal ligament and pubis. *A*, in the para-xiphoid space, with close attention to the depth of needle penetration. *B*, in the suprapubic region. The pyramidalis muscle lies in this region, but the needle is directed cephalad to inject it. *C*, along the lateral border of the muscle, just above the umbilicus. *D*, in the lower rectus abdominis adjacent to McBurney's point.

PART 4

cephalad close to the midline, away from the pubis, rather than toward the bone.

14. CORRECTIVE ACTIONS
(Figs. 49.10 and 49.11)

Visceral Disease and Other Causal Factors

Myofascial TP activity may persist long after the initiating acute visceral disease has terminated. However, if the initiating visceral lesion persists (*e.g.* peptic ulcer, neoplasm, or intestinal parasites), treatment directed only to the TPs provides merely transient or partial relief. Causative factors must be resolved for lasting relief.[62, 81]

Likewise, perpetuating stresses on the muscles must be reduced or eliminated to obtain prolonged relief. Included are emotional stress, viral infections, and mechanical distortions to compensate for an awkward or stooped sitting posture. The patient should use a small pillow for lumbar support and should lean against the backrest of the chair. This increases lumbar lordosis and raises the thoracic cage anteriorly, which places the more longitudinal abdominal muscles on gentle stretch. A very tight elastic belt or girdle may compress the abdominal muscles, interfering with their circulation.

Exercises

Helpful exercises for the abdominal musculature include abdominal breathing, the Pelvic-tilt and the Sit-back/Sit-up Exercises, and laughter.

Abdominal Breathing. The most effective active stretch-exercise for these muscles is abdominal breathing[21] (see Chapter 20). Abdominal breathing, with the patient *prone*, particularly stretches the lateral abdominal wall muscles.

Pelvic Tilt. The Pelvic-tilt Exercise is a gentle and effective strengthening movement for the rectus abdominis. It is illustrated as a flexion exercise, by Williams,[92] and as "pelvic tilting" by Cailliet.[9] The exercise is done in three steps. The supine patient initially places one hand over the pubis and the other over the xiphoid, with the knees bent (Fig. 49.10A). For the second step, the lumbar spine is pressed to the floor, which tilts the pelvis so as to bring the hands closer together (Fig.

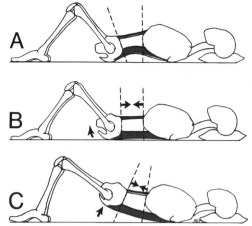

Figure 49.10.   The Pelvic-tilt Exercise stretches the lumbar spinal muscles and strengthens the abdominal muscles. *A*, normal relaxed starting position, with hands (not shown) separated, and resting on the pelvis and epigastrium (indicated by *dashed lines*). *B*, first step: abdominal muscular contraction flattens the spine and brings the symphysis pubis toward the xiphoid process, approximating the hands. *C*, second step: raising the hips and pelvis. The thoracolumbar junction remains firmly supported while the back remains flattened, not arched. This brings the hands closer together. The patient returns to position in *Part A* by rolling the back down, then relaxes and breathes deeply with the diaphragm.

49.10*B*). The third step of lifting the buttocks must be properly done with lumbar *flexion*, not extension (Fig. 49.10*C*). The patient returns to the initial position by rolling the back down, relaxing, and inhaling deeply with the abdomen. Standing with the back flat against a wall gives the patient practice in applying the pelvic tilt while upright. However, ordinarily when standing and walking, the lumbar spine should be held in mid-position with a moderately lordotic lumbar curve, not in a forced, completely flat position.

Sit-back/Sit-up. The Sit-back/Sit-up Exercise is the smooth combination of three exercises (Fig. 49.11). The combination exercise should always *begin with the* Sit-back Exercise (Fig. 49.11*A*), which is presented by Cailliet[9] as a progressive "uncurl." It results in a *lengthening*, not shortening contraction of the abdominal musculature. The lengthening contraction of the Sit-back places relatively less load on the involved abdominal muscles because of the greater strength and efficiency of a lengthening, as compared with a

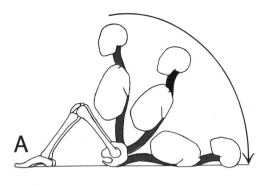

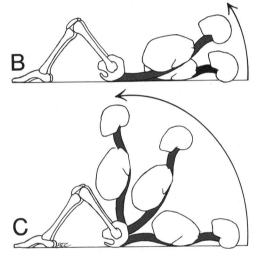

Figure 49.11. *A*, The Sit-back Exercise starts in the sitting position and ends supine. The initial sitting position is attained with the help of the arms (not shown). Knees and hips should be bent and the feet fixed. *B*, The Abdominal-curl Exercise starts with the patient supine. Progressively, the head is raised free of support, then the shoulders, and finally the scapulae, while the lumbar spine remains firmly supported. *C*, the Sit-up Exercise rolls up through an abdominal curl to the full sitting position. The strength required to do this exercise increases as the hands (not shown) are held, first at the level of the hips, next at the abdomen, then at the chest and, finally, at the back of the head. The Sit-up should not be done unless it is pain-free.

shortening contraction.[38] First, the patient pushes himself up into the sit-up position, and then does a slow Sit-back (Fig. 49.11*A*). The curl-down movement of the Sit-back should be made smoothly and slowly, without jerks.

The pause between each cycle of the exercise is as important as the movement, and should be equally long. During the pause, the muscle has time to recharge with blood and to wash out waste products. A full inspiration/expiration at the end of each Sit-back helps to reestablish complete relaxation of the muscles and to pace the exercise.

The patient starts by doing the exercise on alternate days or, if the abdominal musculature is still sore, skips two days; then the number of Sit-backs is gradually increased to a goal of 10 per daily session.

Abdominal-curl. Only when this goal is reached does the patient proceed to the Abdominal-curl (Fig. 49.11*B*), which is a partial Sit-up, described by Williams[92] as a flexion exercise. This is done as a "peel-up" with the spine flexed, so that each successive vertebra leaves the floor in turn.

Sit-up. When the Sit-back and Abdominal-curl Exercises can be done comfortably 10 times, the patient may start the Sit-up Exercise (Fig. 49.11*C*), as illustrated by Williams[92] and by Cailliet[9] as an abdominal flexion exercise.

Laughter. Laughter is a vigorous isometric exercise for all of the abdominal muscles and "pleasant medicine."

Other Actions

The patient should learn how to apply ischemic compression to individual TPs. While lying in a tub of hot bath water, the patient locates a tender spot, protrudes the abdomen and then applies steady and increasing pressure directly on the sore spot until it is no longer sensitive to the sustained pressure. Subsequently, that spot should still be non-tender, but others that remain can be similarly inactivated, TP by TP. This self-treatment is especially valuable, between menstrual periods, to relieve dysmenorrhea.

Skin-rolling (see *Panniculosis* in Chapter 3) over the affected abdominal muscles also may be effectively performed by the patient, while relaxing in a hot bath.

Patients with paradoxical breathing (asynchrony of the chest *versus* the diaphragm and abdominal muscles) must learn proper respiratory mechanics (see Fig. 20.13).

References

1. Aiken DW, Dickman FN: Surgery in obstruction of small intestine due to ascariasis. *JAMA 164(12)*:1317–1323, 1957.

2. Alvarez WC: *An Introduction to Gastro-enterology*, Ed. 3. Paul B. Hoeber, New York, 1940 (p. 144).

3. Ashkenaz DM, Spiegel EA: The viscero-pannicular reflex. *Am J Physiol* 112:573–576, 1935.

4. Basmajian JV: *Muscles Alive*, Ed. 4., Williams & Wilkins, Baltimore, 1978 (pp. 185, 314–315, 321–327).

5. Bates T, Grunwaldt E: Myofascial pain in childhood. *J Pediatr* 53:198–209, 1958.

6. Beaton LE, Anson BJ: The pyramidalis muscle: its occurrence and size in American white and negroes. *Am J Phys Anthropol* 25:261–269, 1939.

7. Bloomfield AL: Mechanism of pain with peptic ulcer. *Am J Med* 17:165–167, 1954.

8. Broer MR, Houtz SJ: *Patterns of Muscular Activity in Selected Sport Skills*. Charles C Thomas, Springfield, Ill., 1967.

9. Cailliet R: *Low Back Pain Syndrome*, Ed. 3. F.A. Davis, Philadelphia, 1981 (pp. 115–121; Figs. 81, 85, 86).

10. DonTigny RL: Inhibition of nausea and headaches. *Phys Ther* 54:864–865, 1974.

11. Doouss TW, Boas RA: The abdominal cutaneous nerve entrapment syndrome. *NZ Med J* 81:473–475, 1975.

12. Duchenne GB: *Physiology of Motion*, translated by E.B. Kaplan. J.B. Lippincott, Philadelphia, 1949 (pp. 488–490).

13. Dworken HJ, Biel FJ, Machella TE: Subdiaphragmatic reference of pain from the colon. *Gastroenterology* 22: 222–228, 1952.

14. Egan TF: Zenker's degeneration of rectus abdominis complicated by spontaneous rupture. *J Ir Med Assoc* 41:127–128, 1957.

15. Eisler P: *Die Muskeln des Stammes*. Gustav Fischer, Jena, 1912 (pp. 571–575, Fig. 93).

16. Ellis M: The relief of pain by cooling of the skin. *Br Med J* 1:250–252, 1961.

17. Feinstein B, Langton JNK, Jameson RM, Schiller F: Experiments on pain referred from deep somatic tissues. *J Bone Joint Surg* 36A:981–997, 1954.

18. Flint MM: An electromyographic comparison of the function of the iliacus and the rectus abdominis muscles. *J Am Phys Ther Assoc* 45:248–253, 1965.

19. Gardner DA: The use of ethyl chloride spray to relieve somatic pain. *J Am Osteopath Assoc* 49:525–528, 1950.

20. Gardner DA: Dysmenorrhea: a case report. *J Osteopath* 58:19–22, 1951.

21. Gelb H: *Killing Pain Without Prescription*. Harper & Row, 1980 (pp. 138, 139).

22. Godfrey KE, Kindig LE, Windell J: Electromyographic study of duration of muscle activity in sit-up variation. *Arch Phys Med Rehabil* 58:132–135, 1977.

23. Good MG: What is "fibrositis"? *Rheumatism* 5:117–123, 1949 (pp. 120, 121; Fig. 8).

24. Good MG: The role of skeletal muscles in the pathogenesis of diseases. *Acta Med Scand* 138:285–292, 1950.

25. Good MG: Pseudo-appendicitis. *Acta Med Scand* 138:348–353, 1950.

26. Gorrell RL: Appendicitis: failure to correlate clinical and pathologic diagnoses. *Minn Med* 34:137–138, 151, 1951.

27. Grant JCB: *An Atlas of Human Anatomy*, Ed. 7. Williams & Wilkins, Baltimore, 1978 (Fig. 2-6).

28. *Ibid.* (Figs. 2-8, 2-11).

29. *Ibid.* (Fig. 2-9).

30. *Ibid.* (Fig. 2-125).

31. Gray H: *Anatomy of the Human Body*, edited by C.M. Goss, American Ed. 29. Lea & Febiger, Philadelphia, 1973 (pp. 417–419, Fig. 6-18).

32. *Ibid.* (pp. 421–423, Fig. 6-21).

33. *Ibid.* (pp. 423–425, Fig. 6-23).

34. *Ibid.* (pp. 424–427).

35. Gross D: *Therapeutische Lokalanästhesie.* Hippokrates, Stuttgart, 1972.

36. Gutstein RR: The role of abdominal fibrositis in functional indigestion. *Mississippi Valley Med J* 66:114–24, 1944.

37. Heinz GJ III, Zavala DC: Slipping rib syndrome. *JAMA* 237:794–795, 1977.

38. Hill AV: The mechanics of voluntary muscle. *Lancet* 2:947–951, 1951.

39. Hockaday JM, Whitty CWM: Patterns of referred pain in the normal subject. *Brain* 90:481–496, 1967.

40. Hoyt HS: Segmental nerve lesions as a cause of the trigonitis syndrome. *Stanford Med Bulletin* 11:61–64, 1953.

41. Hunter C: Myalgia of the abdominal wall. *Can Med Assoc J* 28:157–161, 1933.

42. Jelenko C III: Tietze's disease predates "chest wall syndrome". *JAMA* 242: 2556, 1979.

43. Kamon E: Electromyographic kinesiology of jumping. *Arch Phys Med Rehabil* 52:152–157, 1971.

44. Kellgren JH: Observations on referred pain arising from muscle. *Clin Sci* 3:175–190, 1938 (pp. 180, 181, 185).

45. Kellgren JH: On the distribution of pain arising from deep somatic structures with charts of segmental pain areas. *Clin Sci* 4:35–46, 1939.

46. Kellgren JH: The anatomical source of back pain. *Rheumatol Rehabil* 16:3–12, (Plates facing p. 16) 1977.

47. Kelly M: Lumbago and abdominal pain. *Med J Aust* 1:311–317, 1942.

48. Kelly M: Pain in the Chest: Observations on the use of local anaesthesia in its investigation and treatment. *Med J Aust* 1:4–7, 1944 (p. 6, Case V, Fig. 3).

49. Kelly M: The nature of fibrositis. II. A study of the causation of the myalgic lesion (rheumatic, traumatic, infective). *Ann Rheum Dis* 5:69–77, 1946.

50. Kelly M: Some rules for the employment of local analgesia in the treatment of somatic pain. *Med J Aust* 1:235–239, 1947.

51. Kelly M: The relief of facial pain by procaine (novocaine) injections. *J Am Geriatr Soc* 11:586–596, 1963.

52. Kelsey MP: Diagnosis of upper abdominal pain. *Tex State J Med* 47:82–86, 1951.

53. Lange M: *Die Muskelhärten (Myogelosen)*. J.F. Lehmanns, München, 1931.

54. Lewis T, Kellgren JH: Observations relating to referred pain, visceromotor reflexes and other associated phenomena. *Clin Sci* 4:47–71, 1939 (pp. 50, 51, 58, 61).

55. Llewellyn LJ, Jones AB: *Fibrositis*. Rebman, New York, 1915 (pp. 266–268, Fig. 47).

56. Long C II: Myofascial pain syndromes, part III—some syndromes of the trunk and thigh. *Henry Ford Hosp Med Bull* 4:102–106, 1956 (pp. 103, 104).

57. McBeath AA, Keene JS: The rib-tip syndrome. *J*

Bone Joint Surg 57A:795–797, 1975.

58. McMinn RMH, Hutchings RT: *Color Atlas of Human Anatomy.* Year Book Medical Publishers, Chicago, 1977 (pp. 208, 210).

59. Mehta M, Ranger I: Persistent abdominal pain: treatment by nerve block. *Anaesthesia* 26:330–333, 1971.

60. Melnick J: Treatment of trigger mechanisms in gastrointestinal disease. *NY State J Med* 54:1324–1330, 1954.

61. Melnick J: Symposium on mechanism and management of pain syndromes. *Proc Rudolf Virchow Med Soc City NY* 16:135–142, 160, 1957.

62. Melnick J: Trigger areas and refractory pain in duodenal ulcer. *NY State J Med* 57:1073–1076, 1957.

63. Mendeloff AI, Seligman AM: Acute appendicitis, Chapt. 287. In *Harrison's Principles of Internal Medicine*, edited by M. W. Wintrobe, G.W. Thorn, R.D. Adams, et al., Ed. 7. McGraw-Hill, New York, 1974 (p. 1486).

64. Milloy FJ, Anson BJ: The rectus abdominis muscle and the epigastric arteries, *Surg Gynecol Obstet* 110:293–302, 1960.

65. Murray J: Rectus abdominis haematoma in pregnancy. *Aust NZ J Obstet Gynaecol* 15:173–176, 1975.

66. Pernkopf E: *Atlas of Topographical and Applied Human Anatomy*, Vol. 2, W.B. Saunders, Philadelphia, 1964 (Figs. 177, 181, 186–188).

67. Reid JD, Kommareddi S, Lankerani M, et al.: Chronic expanding hematomas. *JAMA* 244:2441–2442, 1980.

68. Rogatz P and Rubin IL: Hematoma of the rectus abdominis muscle. *NY State J Med* 54:675–679, 1954.

69. Ruch TC, Patton HD: *Physiology and Biophysics*, Ed. 19. W.B. Saunders, 1965 (pp. 357–359).

70. Ruhmann W: Über viscerale Reflexe auf lokale thermische Hautreize. *Z. Gesamte Exp Med* 52:338–376, 1926.

71. Sheehy BN, Little SC, Stone JJ: Abdominal epilepsy. *J Pediatr* 56:355–363, 1960.

72. Sinclair DC: The remote reference of pain aroused in the skin. *Brain* 72:364–372, 1949.

73. Slipyan A, Batongbacal VI: Massive right rectus muscle hematoma simulating signs and symptoms of coarctation of the aorta. *NY State J Med* 58:3851–3852, 1958.

74. Smith LA: The pattern of pain in the diagnosis of upper abdominal disorders. *JAMA* 156:1566–1573, 1954.

75. Sobotta J, Figge FHJ: *Atlas of Human Anatomy*, Ed. 9, Vol. 1. Hafner Division of Macmillan, New York, 1974 (p. 154).

76. *Ibid.* (pp. 156, 159).

77. *Ibid.* (pp. 158, 160).

78. *Ibid.* (p. 161).

79. Spalteholz W: *Handatlas der Anatomie des Menschen*, Ed. 11, Vol. 2. S. Hirzel, Leipzig, 1922 (pp. 291, 294).

80. Telling WH: The clinical importance of fibrositis in general practice. *Br Med J* 1:689–692, 1935.

81. Theobald GW: The relief and prevention of referred pain. *J Obstet Gynaecol Br Commonw* 56:447–460, 1949 (pp. 451, 452; Case 3; Fig. 3).

82. Theobald GW: The role of the cerebral cortex in the apperception of pain. *Lancet* 2:41–47, 94–97, 1949 (p. 41, Fig. 3).

83. Thorek P: The acute abdomen. *Can Med Assoc J* 62:550–556, 1950.

84. Tietze A: Ueber eine eigenartige Häufung von Fällen mit Dystrophie der Rippen Knorpel. *Berl Klin Wochenschr* 58:829–831, 1921.

85. Toldt C: *An Atlas of Human Anatomy*, translated by M.E.Paul, Ed. 2, Vol. 1. Macmillan, New York, 1919 (pp. 274, 276).

86. Travell J: The adductor longus syndrome: A cause of groin pain; Its treatment by local block of trigger areas (procaine infiltration and ethyl chloride spray). *Bull NY Acad Med* 26:284–285, 1950.

87. Travell JG: A trigger point for hiccup. *J Am Osteopath Assoc* 77:308–312, 1977.

88. Trinca F: New diagnostic method: manipulation of the hypersensitive visceral reflex as a clue to more exact diagnosis. *Med J Aust* 2:493–495, 1940.

89. Walters CE, Partridge MJ: Electromyographic study of the differential action of the abdominal muscles during exercise. *Am J Phys Med* 36:259–268, 1957.

90. Weiss S, Davis D: The significance of the afferent impulses from the skin in the mechanism of visceral pain. Skin infiltration as a useful therapeutic measure. *Am J Med Sci* 176:517–536, 1928.

91. Willauer GJ, O'Neill JF: Late postoperative follow-up studies on patients with recurrent appendicitis. *Am J Med Sci* 205:334–342, 1943.

92. Williams PC: *Low Back and Neck Pain, Causes and Conservative Treatment.* Charles C Thomas, Springfield, Ill., 1974 (Panels 1A, 1B, and 2, Fig. 19).

93. Wilson TS: Manipulative treatment of subacute and chronic fibrositis. *Br Med J* 1:298–302, 1936.

94. Wittman A, Bigler FC: Preoperative diagnosis. *J Kans Med Soc* 78:411–414, 1977.

95. Young D: The effects of novocaine injections on simulated visceral pain. *Ann Intern Med* 19:749–756, 1943.

96. deValera E, Raftery H: Lower abdominal and pelvic pain in women. In *Advances in Pain Research and Therapy*, edited by J.J. Bonica and D. Albe-Fessard, Vol. 1. Raven Press, New York, 1976 (pp. 933–937).

Index

With a few exceptions, individual anatomical structures are listed individually according to the descriptive adjective that identifies it, rather than collectively according to the noun category.

Thus, for instance, the subscapularis muscle will be found under **S**, subscapularis, not under **M**, muscle.

The page numbers of the definitive presentation on a topic are set in **bold face** type. The page number of a topic that refers to an illustration or table is *italicized*.

Muscles and Triggers